COLLINS-BRIDE & SAXE'S
Clinical Guidelines for Advanced Practice Nursing

Yoonmee Joo
PhD, RN, ANP-C

J. V. Gatewood
PhD, RN, MSN, AGPCNP-BC

Mary Anne M. Israel
RN, MS, CPNP-PC

Kelly Wong McGrath
CNM, AGPCNP-BC, RN, IBCLC

Becca Neuwirth
RN, MS, WHNP-BC, ANP-C

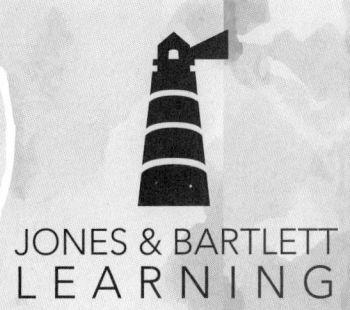

JONES & BARTLETT
LEARNING

World Headquarters
Jones & Bartlett Learning
25 Mall Road
Burlington, MA 01803
978-443-5000
info@jblearning.com
www.jblearning.com

Jones & Bartlett Learning books and products are available through most bookstores and online booksellers. To contact Jones & Bartlett Learning directly, call 800-832-0034, fax 978-443-8000, or visit our website, www.jblearning.com.

Substantial discounts on bulk quantities of Jones & Bartlett Learning publications are available to corporations, professional associations, and other qualified organizations. For details and specific discount information, contact the special sales department at Jones & Bartlett Learning via the above contact information or send an email to specialsales@jblearning.com.

Copyright © 2024 by Jones & Bartlett Learning, LLC, an Ascend Learning Company

All rights reserved. No part of the material protected by this copyright may be reproduced or utilized in any form, electronic or mechanical, including photocopying, recording, or by any information storage and retrieval system, without written permission from the copyright owner.

The content, statements, views, and opinions herein are the sole expression of the respective authors and not that of Jones & Bartlett Learning, LLC. Reference herein to any specific commercial product, process, or service by trade name, trademark, manufacturer, or otherwise does not constitute or imply its endorsement or recommendation by Jones & Bartlett Learning, LLC and such reference shall not be used for advertising or product endorsement purposes. All trademarks displayed are the trademarks of the parties noted herein. *Collins-Bride & Saxe's Clinical Guidelines for Advanced Practice Nursing, Fourth Edition* is an independent publication and has not been authorized, sponsored, or otherwise approved by the owners of the trademarks or service marks referenced in this product.

There may be images in this book that feature models; these models do not necessarily endorse, represent, or participate in the activities represented in the images. Any screenshots in this product are for educational and instructive purposes only. Any individuals and scenarios featured in the case studies throughout this product may be real or fictitious but are used for instructional purposes only.

The authors, editor, and publisher have made every effort to provide accurate information. However, they are not responsible for errors, omissions, or for any outcomes related to the use of the contents of this book and take no responsibility for the use of the products and procedures described. Treatments and side effects described in this book may not be applicable to all people; likewise, some people may require a dose or experience a side effect that is not described herein. Drugs and medical devices are discussed that may have limited availability controlled by the Food and Drug Administration (FDA) for use only in a research study or clinical trial. Research, clinical practice, and government regulations often change the accepted standard in this field. When consideration is being given to use of any drug in the clinical setting, the healthcare provider or reader is responsible for determining FDA status of the drug, reading the package insert, and reviewing prescribing information for the most up-to-date recommendations on dose, precautions, and contraindications, and determining the appropriate usage for the product. This is especially important in the case of drugs that are new or seldom used.

27218-5

Production Credits
Vice President, Product Management: Marisa R. Urbano
Vice President, Content Strategy and Implementation: Christine Emerton
Director, Product Management: Matthew Kane
Product Manager: Tina Chen
Director, Content Management: Donna Gridley
Manager, Content Strategy: Orsolya Gall
Content Coordinator: Samantha Gillespie
Director, Project Management and Content Services: Karen Scott
Manager, Program Management: Kristen Rogers
Project Manager: Belinda Thresher
Senior Product Marketing Manager: Lindsay White
Procurement Manager: Wendy Kilborn
Composition: S4Carlisle Publishing Services
Project Management: S4Carlisle Publishing Services
Cover Design: Michael O'Donnell
Text Design: Michael O'Donnell
Senior Media Development Editor: Troy Liston
Rights & Permissions Manager: John Rusk
Rights Specialist: Maria Leon Maimone
Cover Image (Title Page, Section Opener, Chapter Opener):
 © DrAfter123/DigitalVision Vectors/Getty Images
Printing and Binding: Sheridan Michigan

Library of Congress Cataloging-in-Publication Data
Library in Congress Cataloging-in-Publication unavailable at the time of printing.
LCCN: 2023035570

6048

Printed in the United States of America
28 27 26 25 24   10 9 8 7 6 5 4 3 2 1

To my husband, Jihwi, and my sons, Jooahn and Joohyung, who always support and respect my work. Thank you for the love and for making me laugh! To my patients and students, I appreciate the many lessons and the trust from you over the years.
—YJ

To my two favorite nurses, Patricia V. Gatewood and June S. Gatewood. Patty, thank you for inspiring me to be a better person every day. Mum, thank you for always being such a great role model.
—JVG

To my family and friends, who have supported and honored my dedication to my patients and my work. To Karen Duderstadt for her steadfast mentorship for the past 20 years. And to the children and families I have been privileged to work with and for all they have taught me over the years!
—MI

To my mom, Carol, for inspiring my love of learning, and my dad, Don, for inspiring my love of teaching.
—BN

To my partner, Benny, who always pushes me to achieve more than I think I can, and to my girls, Mícara, Sabrina, and Maisy, who keep life exciting. To my parents and siblings for their love and support. And to all the community birth workers and birthing families, who have been my greatest teachers of all.
—KWM

A Special Dedication

We dedicate this text to our beloved colleague and friend **Rebekah Kaplan, RN, MS, CNM**. Rebekah was an exceptional midwife, educator, and mentor. As reported by Karen Breslau (2021) and acknowledged by many, Rebekah was "dedicated to advancing equity and anti-racism in maternal and reproductive health." Her husband David Burk noted that Rebekah valued "teaching, learning, listening, and understanding the truths that we all communicate beyond the surface of our words" (Breslau, 2021). Rebekah brought this commitment and her clinical expertise to the second through fourth editions of this book as a contributing author and an associate editor to the third edition. Thank you, Rebekah, for all that you have given to patients, students, colleagues, and the community. You are always in our hearts.

Breslau, K. (2021). Remembering Rebekah Kaplan, midwife to midwives and dispenser of wisdom. Obituaries. https://www.berkeleyside.org/2021/11/24/rebekah-kaplan-berkeley-obituary

Brief Contents

Contributors xviii
Reviewers xxi
Introduction.. xxv

SECTION I — Pediatric Health Maintenance and Promotion 1

CHAPTER 1 First Well-Baby Visit 3

CHAPTER 2 Care of the Postneonatal Intensive Care Unit Graduate 9

CHAPTER 3 0 to 3 Years of Age Interval Visit 17

CHAPTER 4 3 to 6 Years of Age Interval Visit 25

CHAPTER 5 6 to 11 Years of Age Interval Visit 29

CHAPTER 6 The Adolescent and Young Adult (12–26 Years of Age) Interval Visit 35

CHAPTER 7 Care of Transgender and Gender Diverse Youth 41

CHAPTER 8 Developmental Assessment: Screening for Developmental Delay and Autism 53

SECTION II — Common Complex Pediatric Presentations 75

CHAPTER 9 Childhood Asthma 77

CHAPTER 10 Atopic Dermatitis in Children 89

CHAPTER 11 Attention-Deficit/Hyperactivity Disorder in Children and Adolescents 101

CHAPTER 12	**Pediatric Depression**	115
CHAPTER 13	**Child Maltreatment**	129
CHAPTER 14	**Childhood Overweight and Obesity**	145
CHAPTER 15	**Urinary Incontinence in Children**	155

SECTION III — Common Sexual and Reproductive Health Presentations ... 171

CHAPTER 16	**Abnormal Uterine Bleeding**	173
CHAPTER 17	**Abortion Care in the Primary Care Setting**	187
CHAPTER 18	**Amenorrhea and Polycystic Ovary Syndrome**	211
CHAPTER 19	**Benign Prostatic Hyperplasia**	223
CHAPTER 20	**Early Pregnancy Loss**	231
CHAPTER 21	**Contraception**	243
CHAPTER 22	**Menopause Transition**	275
CHAPTER 23	**Chronic Pelvic Pain in Persons Assigned Female at Birth**	289
CHAPTER 24	**Sexual Dysfunction**	301
CHAPTER 25	**Urinary Incontinence in Persons Assigned Female at Birth**	309

SECTION IV — Obstetric Health Maintenance and Promotion ... 319

CHAPTER 26	**The Initial Prenatal Visit**	321
CHAPTER 27	**Prenatal Genetic Screening and Diagnosis**	329
CHAPTER 28	**The Return Prenatal Visit**	337
CHAPTER 29	**The Postpartum Visit**	345
CHAPTER 30	**Guidelines for Medical Consultation, Interprofessional Collaboration, and Transfer of Care During Pregnancy and Childbirth**	355

SECTION V: Common Obstetric Presentations 361

- **CHAPTER 31** Birth Choices for Pregnant People With a Previous Cesarean Delivery 363
- **CHAPTER 32** Common Discomforts of Pregnancy 371
- **CHAPTER 33** Gestational Diabetes Mellitus: Early Detection and Management in Pregnancy 389
- **CHAPTER 34** Hypertension Disorders in Pregnancy: Gestational Hypertension and Preeclampsia 397
- **CHAPTER 35** Preterm Labor Management 405
- **CHAPTER 36** Perinatal Mood and Anxiety Disorders (PMADs) 413
- **CHAPTER 37** Human Lactation 423

SECTION VI: Adult Gerontology Health Maintenance and Promotion 441

- **CHAPTER 38** Adult Health Maintenance and Promotion 443
- **CHAPTER 39** Healthcare Maintenance for Adults With Developmental Disabilities 479
- **CHAPTER 40** Healthcare Maintenance for Transgender and Gender Expansive (TGE) Adults 495

SECTION VII: Common Complex Adult Gerontology Presentations 503

- **CHAPTER 41** Anemia 505
- **CHAPTER 42** Anxiety 521
- **CHAPTER 43** Asthma in Adolescents and Adults 529
- **CHAPTER 44** Cancer Survivorship 545
- **CHAPTER 45** Chronic Obstructive Pulmonary Disease 553
- **CHAPTER 46** Chronic Nonmalignant Pain Management 569

CHAPTER 47	**Chronic Wound Care**	579
CHAPTER 48	**Dementia**	587
CHAPTER 49	**Depression**	599
CHAPTER 50	**Diabetes Mellitus**	615
CHAPTER 51	**Epilepsy**	627
CHAPTER 52	**Gastroesophageal Reflux Disease**	637
CHAPTER 53	**Geriatric Syndromes**	645
CHAPTER 54	**Heart Failure**	655
CHAPTER 55	**Herpes Simplex Virus**	665
CHAPTER 56	**HIV Infection in Adolescents and Adults**	675
CHAPTER 57	**Hypertension**	701
CHAPTER 58	**Intimate Partner Violence (Domestic Violence)**	711
CHAPTER 59	**Irritable Bowel Syndrome**	721
CHAPTER 60	**Lipid Disorders**	729
CHAPTER 61	**Low Back Pain**	743
CHAPTER 62	**Nonalcoholic Fatty Liver Disease (NAFLD)**	757
CHAPTER 63	**Weight**	765
CHAPTER 64	**Substance Use and Substance Use Disorders**	775
CHAPTER 65	**Thyroid Disorders**	805
CHAPTER 66	**Upper Back and Neck Pain Syndromes**	817
CHAPTER 67	**Upper Extremity Tendinopathy: Shoulder (Bicipital and Rotator Cuff), Elbow, and De Quervain Tendinopathy**	833

Index **847**

Contents

Contributors xviii
Reviewers xxi
Introduction xxv

SECTION I Pediatric Health Maintenance and Promotion 1

CHAPTER 1 First Well-Baby Visit 3
Annette Carley

I. Introduction and general background 3
II. Database 4
III. Assessment 5
IV. Goals of first well-baby visit 5
V. Plan 5
VI. Resources and tools 6

CHAPTER 2 Care of the Postneonatal Intensive Care Unit Graduate 9
Annette Carley

I. Introduction and general background 9
II. Database 12
III. Assessment 13
IV. Goals of clinical management 13
V. Plan 13
VI. Resources and tools 14

CHAPTER 3 0 to 3 Years of Age Interval Visit 17
Pallavi Parthasarathy Sheth

I. Introduction and general background 17
II. Database 18
III. Assessment 21
IV. Plan 21

CHAPTER 4 3 to 6 Years of Age Interval Visit 25
Mary Anne M. Israel

I. Introduction and general background 25
II. Database 25
III. Assessment 27
IV. Plan 27

CHAPTER 5 6 to 11 Years of Age Interval Visit 29
Bridget Ward Gramkowski

I. Introduction and general background 29
II. Database 29
III. Assessment 31
IV. Plan 31

CHAPTER 6 The Adolescent and Young Adult (12–26 Years of Age) Interval Visit 35
Lisa Mihaly and Erica Monasterio

I. Introduction and general background 35
II. Database 36
III. Assessment 38
IV. Plan 38
V. Resources 39

CHAPTER 7 Care of Transgender and Gender Diverse Youth 41
Meredith Russell

I. Introduction and general background 41
II. Database 41
III. Assessment 43

IV. Plan 43
　　V. Treatment 44
　　VI. Self-management resources
　　　 and tools 50

CHAPTER 8　Developmental Assessment: Screening for Developmental Delay and Autism 53
Janis Mandac-Dy and Abbey Alkon

　　I. Introduction 53
　　II. Developmental surveillance and
　　　 screening algorithm 55
　　III. Developmental Screening Tests 70
　　IV. Psychometrics 70
　　V. Conclusion 71
　　VI. Clinician resources 71

SECTION II　Common Complex Pediatric Presentations 75

CHAPTER 9　Childhood Asthma 77
Christine Mayor

　　I. Introduction and general background 77
　　II. Database 77
　　III. Assessment 78
　　IV. Goals of clinical management 81
　　V. Plan 82
　　VI. Resources 86

CHAPTER 10　Atopic Dermatitis in Children 89
Nanette Madden and Karen G. Duderstadt

　　I. Introduction and general background 89
　　II. Database 90
　　III. Assessment 91
　　IV. Goals of clinical management 91
　　V. Plan 92
　　VI. Self-management 98
　　VII. Psychosocial and emotional support 98

CHAPTER 11　Attention-Deficit/Hyperactivity Disorder in Children and Adolescents 101
Naomi A. Schapiro

　　I. Introduction and general background 101
　　II. Overview 101
　　III. Database: History 104
　　IV. Physical examination 106
　　V. Assessment 106
　　VI. Plan 107

CHAPTER 12　Pediatric Depression ... 115
Monifa C. Willis

　　I. Introduction and general background 115
　　II. Gathering data 116
　　III. Assessment 119
　　IV. Plan and treatment 122
　　V. Referral 125
　　VI. Self-management tools 125

CHAPTER 13　Child Maltreatment 129
Naomi Schapiro and Tiffany Lambright

　　I. Introduction and general background 129
　　II. Database 133
　　III. Assessment 138
　　IV. Plan 139
　　V. Resources 141

CHAPTER 14　Childhood Overweight and Obesity 145
Mary Anne M. Israel and Amy Beck

　　I. Introduction and general background 145
　　II. Database 147
　　III. Assessment 149
　　IV. Plan 149
　　V. Helpful online resources 151

CHAPTER 15　Urinary Incontinence in Children 155
Angel C. Kuo

　　I. Introduction and general background 155
　　II. Database 158
　　III. Assessment 160

IV. Goals of clinical management 160
V. Plan 162
VI. Resources 169

SECTION III Common Sexual and Reproductive Health Presentations 171

CHAPTER 16 Abnormal Uterine Bleeding 173
Pilar Bernal de Pheils, Lisa Mihaly, and Sarah Nathan

I. Introduction and general background 173
II. Database 176

CHAPTER 17 Abortion Care in the Primary Care Setting 187
Gwendolyn Riddell

I. Introduction and general background 187
II. Database 193
III. Assessment 199
IV. Goals of clinical management 200
V. Plan 200
VI. Resources and further learning 205

CHAPTER 18 Amenorrhea and Polycystic Ovary Syndrome 211
Pilar Bernal de Pheils, Sarah Nathan, and Lisa Mihaly

I. Introduction and general background 211
II. Database 213
III. Assessment 215
IV. Goals of clinical management 216
V. Plan 216
VI. Self-management resources and tools ... 221

CHAPTER 19 Benign Prostatic Hyperplasia 223
Jean N. Taylor-Woodbury and Catherine D. Tanner

I. Introduction and general background 223
II. Database 224
III. Assessment 227
IV. Goals of clinical management 227

V. Plan 227
VI. Self-management resources and tools ... 228

CHAPTER 20 Early Pregnancy Loss 231
Gwendolyn Riddell

I. Introduction and general background 231
II. Database 233
III. Assessment 235
IV. Goals of clinical management 236
V. Review of systems 236
VI. Plan 236

CHAPTER 21 Contraception 243
Simran Tagore

I. Introduction and general background 243
II. Database 264
III. Assessment 265
IV. Goals of clinical management 265
V. Plan 265
VI. Patient and provider education resources 269

CHAPTER 22 Menopause Transition 275
Zaineh Khalil and Joleen D. Bishop

I. Introduction 275
II. Assessment 278
III. Goals of clinical management 279
IV. Plan 279
V. Patient education 285
VI. Resources 285

CHAPTER 23 Chronic Pelvic Pain in Persons Assigned Female at Birth 289
Becca Neuwirth

I. Introduction and general background 289
II. Database 292
III. Assessment 293
IV. Goals of clinical management 293
V. Plan 293
VI. Resources 297

CHAPTER 24 Sexual Dysfunction ...301
Milan Chavarkar

 I. Introduction and general background 301
 II. Database 303
 III. Assessment 303
 IV. Goals of clinical management 303
 V. Plan 303
 VI. Self-management resources and tools............................307

CHAPTER 25 Urinary Incontinence in Persons Assigned Female at Birth 309
Janis Luft

 I. Introduction and general background 309
 II. Initial evaluation 310
 III. Assessment 311
 IV. Goals of clinical management 312
 V. Plan 312
 VI. Self-management resources and tools...316

SECTION IV Obstetric Health Maintenance and Promotion........ 319

CHAPTER 26 The Initial Prenatal Visit 321
Rebekah Kaplan

 I. Definition and background 321
 II. Database 322
 III. Assessment 323
 IV. Goals of clinical management 323
 V. Plan 323
 VI. Internet resources..................327

CHAPTER 27 Prenatal Genetic Screening and Diagnosis 329
Kelly Wong McGrath and Deborah Anderson

 I. Introduction and general background 329
 II. Database 332
 III. Assessment 333
 IV. Goals for clinical management 333
 V. Plan 333
 VI. Prenatal genetic diagnosis: Introduction and general background 334
 VII. Database 335
 VIII. Assessment 335
 IX. Goals for clinical management 335
 X. Plan 335

CHAPTER 28 The Return Prenatal Visit 337
Rebekah Kaplan and Margaret Hutchison

 I. Definition and background 337
 II. Database 338
 III. Assessment 341
 IV. Goals of clinical management 341
 V. Plan 342

CHAPTER 29 The Postpartum Visit 345
Jenna Shaw-Battista and Holly Cost

 I. Introduction and general background 345
 II. Database 346
 III. Assessment 349
 IV. Goals for clinical management 349
 V. Plan 349

CHAPTER 30 Guidelines for Medical Consultation, Interprofessional Collaboration, and Transfer of Care During Pregnancy and Childbirth 355
Jenna Shaw-Battista and Annette Fineberg

 I. Introduction and general background 355

SECTION V Common Obstetric Presentations..... 361

CHAPTER 31 Birth Choices for Pregnant People With a Previous Cesarean Delivery................... 363
Rebekah Kaplan

 I. Introduction and general background 363
 II. Risks and benefits of TOLAC versus repeat cesarean birth 365

III. Data collection..................367
IV. Goals for clinical
management/assessment............367
V. Plan.........................368
VI. Internet resources for providers,
patients, and families.............368

CHAPTER 32 Common Discomforts of Pregnancy...........371
Jamie Meyerhoff and Cynthia Belew

I. Introduction to common
discomforts of pregnancy..........371
II. Poor quality of sleep..............372
III. Musculoskeletal..................373
IV. Gastrointestinal tract.............376
V. Heartburn......................380
VI. Constipation....................381

CHAPTER 33 Gestational Diabetes Mellitus: Early Detection and Management in Pregnancy.......................389
Kelly Wong McGrath, Maribeth Inturrisi, Julio Diaz-Abarca, and JoAnne M. Saxe

I. Introduction and general background....389
II. Database........................390
III. Goals of clinical management.........391
IV. Plan...........................392

CHAPTER 34 Hypertension Disorders in Pregnancy: Gestational Hypertension and Preeclampsia......................397
Colleen Moreno and Jenna Shaw-Battista

I. Introduction and general background....397
II. Database........................400
III. Assessment......................401
IV. Goals of clinical management.........401
V. Plan...........................401

CHAPTER 35 Preterm Labor Management......................405
Lisa Jensen

I. Introduction and general background....405
II. Database........................406

III. Assessment......................407
IV. Goals of clinical management.........408
V. Plan...........................408

CHAPTER 36 Perinatal Mood and Anxiety Disorders (PMADs).....413
Laura Todaro

I. Introduction and general background....413
II. Prevalence......................413
III. Screening recommendations..........413
IV. Diagnosis.......................414
V. Types of disorders.................414
VI. Health disparities and special
populations....................418
VII. Summary.......................419
VIII. Resources......................419

CHAPTER 37 Human Lactation.....423
Serena Saeed-Winn

I. Introduction and background..........423
II. Stages of lactation.................423
III. Common issues with lactation........425
IV. Contraindications to nursing..........435
V. Medications and nursing.............436
VI. Resources......................437

SECTION VI Adult Gerontology Health Maintenance and Promotion...441

CHAPTER 38 Adult Health Maintenance and Promotion.......443
Helen R. Horvath

I. Introduction and general background....443
II. Individualizing screening decisions
in the geriatric population..........468
III. Database........................470
IV. Assessment......................470
V. Plan...........................470
VI. Goals of clinical management.........470
VII. Resources for health professionals
and consumers..................474

CHAPTER 39 Healthcare Maintenance for Adults With Developmental Disabilities 479
Geraldine Collins-Bride and Clarissa Kripke

- I. Introduction and general background 479
- II. Database 483
- III. Assessment 485
- IV. Plan 486
- V. Self-management resources and tools.........493

CHAPTER 40 Healthcare Maintenance for Transgender and Gender Expansive (TGE) Adults 495
Bennett Lareau-Meredith and Isabella Ventura

- I. Introduction and general background 495
- II. Database 497
- III. Assessment 498
- IV. Plan 498

SECTION VII Common Complex Adult Gerontology Presentations ...503

CHAPTER 41 Anemia................ 505
Michelle M. Marin

- I. Introduction and general background 505
- II. Database 510
- III. Assessment 512
- IV. Goals of clinical management 515
- V. Plan 515
- VI. Self-management resources and tools.........517

CHAPTER 42 Anxiety 521
Amanda Ling and Esker-D Ligon

- I. Introduction and general background 521
- II. Database 522
- III. Assessment 522
- IV. Plan 524
- V. Special populations.........527
- VI. Self-management resources and tools...527

CHAPTER 43 Asthma in Adolescents and Adults 529
Susan L. Janson and Shaadi Settecase

- I. Introduction and general background 529
- II. Database 530
- III. Assessment 531
- IV. Goals of clinical management to control asthma 534
- V. Plan 534
- VI. Future update topics in asthma 541

CHAPTER 44 Cancer Survivorship... 545
Tara D. Lacey and Sheila N. Lindsay

- I. Introduction and background 545
- II. Database 547
- III. Assessment 549
- IV. Goals of clinical management 549
- V. Plan 550
- VI. Self-management resources 551

CHAPTER 45 Chronic Obstructive Pulmonary Disease 553
Emily Casabar

- I. Introduction and background 553
- II. Confirming COPD diagnosis.........554
- III. Management 558
- IV. Specific population considerations 564

CHAPTER 46 Chronic Nonmalignant Pain Management... 569
Caitlin Garvey and JoAnne M. Saxe

- I. Introduction 569
- II. Database 570
- III. Assessment 571
- IV. Goals of clinical management 571
- V. Plan 571
- VI. Patient education and care plan implementation 576
- VII. CP support resources and tools.........576

CHAPTER 47 Chronic Wound Care 579
Diana Roberts Mitchell and Eleanor Pascual

- I. Introduction and general background 579
- II. Database 581

III. Assessment 583
IV. Plan 584

CHAPTER 48 Dementia 587
Nhat Bui and Jennifer Merrilees

I. Introduction and general background 587
II. Database 589
III. Assessment 593
IV. Goals of clinical management 593
V. Plan 593
VI. Assessment and management of concomitant conditions 595
VII. Assessment of the status of the family caregiver 596
VIII. Resources and tools 596

CHAPTER 49 Depression 599
Beth Phoenix and Kathleen McDermott

I. Introduction and general background 599
II. Database 601
III. Assessment 602
IV. Goals of clinical management 603
V. Plan 604
VI. Self-management resources and tools 611

CHAPTER 50 Diabetes Mellitus 615
Anjali Asrani

I. Introduction and general background 615
II. Database 615
III. Assessment 617
IV. Goals of clinical management 617
V. Plan 618
VI. Diabetes and Language 625
VII. Self-management resources and tools 626

CHAPTER 51 Epilepsy 627
Maritza López and Paul Garcia

I. Introduction and general background 627
II. Database 627
III. Assessment 628
IV. Goals of clinical management 628
V. Plan 629
VI. Self-management resources 634

CHAPTER 52 Gastroesophageal Reflux Disease 637
Elizabeth Gatewood

I. Definition and overview 637
II. Database 638
III. Assessment 639
IV. Goals of clinical management 640
V. Plan 640
VI. Self-management resources 643

CHAPTER 53 Geriatric Syndromes 645
Courtney Gordon

I. Introduction and general background 645
II. Database 647
III. Assessment 650
IV. Goals of clinical management 651
V. Plan 651
VI. Online resources for clinicians, patients, and caregivers 654

CHAPTER 54 Heart Failure 655
Lisa Guertin

I. Introduction and general background 655
II. Database 656
III. Assessment 657
IV. Goals of clinical management 657
V. Plan 657
VI. Self-management resources and tools...663

CHAPTER 55 Herpes Simplex Virus 665
Natalie L. Wilson and Geraldine Collins-Bride

I. Introduction and general background 665
II. Database 667
III. Assessment 668
IV. Goals of clinical management 668
V. Plan 668
VI. Self-management resources and tools...672

CHAPTER 56 HIV Infection in Adolescents and Adults.......... 675
Christopher Berryhill Fox

I. Introduction and general background 675
II. HIV testing 688

III. Database 689
IV. Assessment 691
V. Goals of clinical management 691
VI. Plan 691
VII. Resources 697

CHAPTER 57 Hypertension..........701
Sarah Goodman

I. Introduction and definition 701
II. Database 702
III. Assessment 703
IV. Goals of clinical management 705
V. Plan and management 705

CHAPTER 58 Intimate Partner Violence (Domestic Violence) 711
Jessica Draughon Moret and JoAnne Saxe

I. Introduction and general background 711
II. The focused IPV assessment and database 715
III. Treatment 715
IV. Goals of clinical management 715
V. Plan 716
VI. Self-management resources and tools 716

CHAPTER 59 Irritable Bowel Syndrome 721
Elizabeth Gatewood

I. Introduction and general background 721
II. Database 723
III. Assessment 723
IV. Goals of clinical management 723
V. Plan 723
VI. Self-management e-resources 727

CHAPTER 60 Lipid Disorders....... 729
Lewis Fannon and J.V. Gatewood

I. Introduction and general background 729
II. Database 731
III. Assessment 732
IV. Goals of clinical management 732
V. Plan 732
VI. Resources and self-management tools ...740

CHAPTER 61 Low Back Pain 743
H. Kate Lawlor and Brandon Sessler

I. Introduction and general background 743
II. Database 743
III. Assessment 749
IV. Plan 749

CHAPTER 62 Nonalcoholic Fatty Liver Disease (NAFLD).................757
Miranda Surjadi

I. Introduction and general background 757
II. Database 758
III. Assessment 759
IV. Goals of clinical management 761
V. Plan 762
VI. Self-management resources and tools 762

CHAPTER 63 Weight................ 765
Morgan Weinert

I. Introduction and general background 765
II. Database 766
III. Assessment 768
IV. Plan 769
V. Management 769
VI. Resources 772

CHAPTER 64 Substance Use and Substance Use Disorders........775
Pierre-Cedric Crouch and Pauli Grey

I. Introduction and general background 775
II. Impact of stigmatizing language, language, and health disparities 775
III. Assessment 777
IV. Database 780
V. Goals of clinical management 786
VI. Assessment 786
VII. Plan 787
VIII. Harm reduction 789
IX. Follow-up 800
X. Resources for patients who use substances 800
XI. Resources for clinicians 800

CHAPTER 65 Thyroid Disorders 805
JoAnne M. Saxe

    I. Introduction and general background 805
    II. Database 807
    III. Assessment........................808
    IV. Goals of clinical management 808
    V. Plan 811
    VI. Self-management resources and tools...814

CHAPTER 66 Upper Back and Neck Pain Syndromes 817
Sandra Jo Domeracki and Rossana Segovia

    I. Introduction and general background 817
    II. Database 822
    III. Assessment........................825
    IV. Goals of clinical management 825
    V. Plan 826
    VI. Self-management resources and tools...826

    VII. Clinical evaluation of patients in medically underserved areas and low- and middle-income communities with spine-related complaints 829

CHAPTER 67 Upper Extremity Tendinopathy: Shoulder (Bicipital and Rotator Cuff), Elbow, and De Quervain Tendinopathy 833
Nicole L. Collman

    I. Introduction and general background 833
    II. Database 835
    III. Assessment........................838
    IV. Goals of clinical management 840
    V. Plan 841
    VI. Self-management resources and tools...843

Acknowledgments.....................843

Index 847

Contributors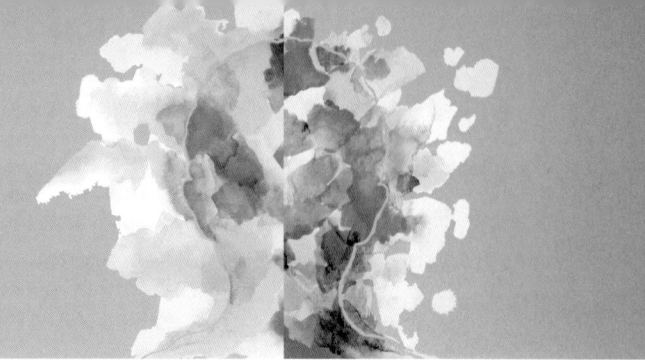

Anjali Asrani, RN, MSN, AGNP-BC
Endocrinology, Diabetes & Osteoporosis Division
Sutter Pacific Medical Foundation
San Francisco, CA

Joleen D. Bishop, MSN, WHNP-AC, MSCP
Marin Community Clinics
Novato, California

Annette Carley, DNP, RN, NNP-BC, PPCNP-BC
University of California San Francisco (UCSF)
   School of Nursing
San Francisco, CA

Emily Casabar, MSN, NP-C, AE-C
Stanford Health Care
Palo Alto, CA

Milan Chavarkar, DNP, RN, FNP-BC, CNM, IFMCP
Lotus Integrative Health and Nursing
Campbell, CA

Gerri Collins-Bride, RN, MS, ANP-BC, FAAN
Clinical Professor
Department of Community Health Systems
UCSF School of Nursing
San Francisco, CA

Nicole L. Collman, RN, MS, ANP-BC, CNS
University of California San Francisco (UCSF)
San Francisco, CA

Sandra Jo Domeracki, MSN, RN, FNP-BC, COHN-S, FAAOHN
University of California San Francisco (UCSF) School of
   Nursing; VA Health Care System, San Francisco, CA

Lewis Fannon, PhD, DDS, RN, ANP-BC
University of California San Francisco (UCSF)
   School of Nursing
San Francisco, CA

Christopher Berryhill Fox, MSN, RN, ANP-BC, AAHIVS
Oregon Health & Science University
Portland, OR

Elizabeth Gatewood, DNP, FNP-C, CNE, FAANP, FAAN
University of California San Francisco (UCSF)
San Francisco, CA

Jim V. Gatewood, PhD, MSN, AGPNCP-BC, RN
University of California San Francisco (UCSF)
   School of Nursing
San Francisco, CA

Courtney Gordon, DNP, MSN, GNP-BC, ACHPN
University of California San Francisco (UCSF)
San Francisco, CA

Pauli Grey
San Francisco, CA

Lisa Guertin, DNP, MS, ACNP-BC
University of California San Francisco (UCSF)
   School of Nursing
San Francisco, CA

Helen R. Horvath, RN, MS, ANP-BC
University of California San Francisco (UCSF)
   School of Nursing
San Francisco, CA

Lisa Jensen, CNM
San Francisco Birth Center
San Francisco, CA

Zaineh Khalil, MSN, FNP-BC
University of California San Francisco (UCSF)
San Francisco, CA

Clarissa Kripke, MD, FAAFP
University of California San Francisco (UCSF)
San Francisco, CA

Angel C. Kuo, EdD, MSN, RN, CPNP-PC
University of California San Francisco (UCSF)
   School of Nursing
San Francisco, CA

Bennett Lareau-Meredith, MSN, NP
University of California San Francisco (UCSF)
San Francisco, CA

Amanda Ling, MS, RN, PMHNP
University of California San Francisco (UCSF)
San Francisco, CA

Janis Luft, RN, NP, MSN
Retired
University of San Francisco (UCSF) Medical Center,
    UCSF School of Nursing, Adjunct Associate Professor
San Francisco, CA

Janis Mandac-Dy, MSN, RN, CPNP-PC, PMHS
Department of Public Health, City & County
    of San Francisco, University of California (UCSF)
    San Francisco
San Francisco, CA

Christine Mayor, MSN, RN, CPNP
Pediatric Asthma & Allergy Clinic,
Zuckerberg San Francisco General Hospital and Trauma
    Center
UCSF School of Nursing
San Francisco, CA

Jamie Meyerhoff, CNM, RN, WHNP, MSN
Natividad Medical Center
Salinas, California

Diana Roberts Mitchell, MSN, FNP, WCS
Kaiser Permanente, South San Francisco
South San Francisco, CA

Colleen Moreno, CNM/DNP
Stanford University School of Medicine
Palo Alto, CA

Jessica Draughon Moret, PhD, RN
Betty Irene Moore School of Nursing at UC Davis
Sacramento, CA

Karen G. Duderstadt, PhD, RN, CPNP-PC, PCNS, FAAN
University of California San Francisco (UCSF) School of
    Nursing
San Francisco, CA

Paul Garcia, MD
University of California San Francisco (UCSF)
San Francisco, CA

Margaret Hutchison, MSN, CNM
Professor, UCSF Department of Obstetrics, Gynecology
    and Reproductive Sciences
Midwifery Service Lead, San Francisco General Hospital
San Francisco, CA

Mary Anne M. Israel, RN, MS, CPNP-PC
Assistant Adjunct Professor
University of California San Francisco (UCSF) School of
    Nursing, Department of Family Health Care Nursing
San Francisco, CA

Susan L. Janson, PhD, ANP, RN, FAAN
University of California San Francisco (UCSF)
San Francisco, CA

Tara D. Lacey, RN, GNP-BC, AOCNP
Geriatric Nurse Practitioner
University of California San Francisco (UCSF) Medical
    Center
San Francisco, CA

Sheila N. Lindsay, MS, RN, ANP-BC, AOCNP
University of California San Francisco (UCSF)
    Medical Center
San Francisco, CA

Maritza López, RN, MS, NP
University of California San Francisco (UCSF)
San Francisco, CA

Nanette Madden, RN, MS, PNP
Associate Clinical Professor, Department of Family
    Health Care Nursing, University of California
San Francisco, CA

Michelle M. Marin, ANP, MS

Kathleen McDermott, DNP, PMHNP-BC
University of California San Francisco (UCSF)
San Francisco, CA

Kelly Wong McGrath, CNM, NP, RN, IBCLC
Clinical Director, San Francisco Birth Center

Lisa Mihaly, MS, RN, FNP
University of California San Francisco (UCSF)
San Francisco, CA

Sarah Nathan, MS, RN, FNP-C
University of California San Francisco (UCSF) School of
    Nursing
San Francisco, CA

Becca Neuwirth, MS, ANP-C, WHNP-BC
Kaiser Permanente, San Francisco
University of California (UCSF) San Francisco

Eleanor Pascual, BSN, RN, CWCN
The Permanente Group
South San Francisco, CA

Beth Phoenix, PhD, RN, CNS, FAAN
Professor, Dept. of Community Health Systems,
    UCSF School of Nursing
San Francisco, CA

Gwendolyn Riddell, CNM, MSN
Santa Rosa, CA

Nhat Bui, RN, MSN, AGNP-C
University of California San Francisco (UCSF)
San Francisco, CA

Meredith Russell, DNP, MSN, AC-CPNP
University of California San Francsisco (UCSF)
    Benioff Children's Hospital
San Francisco, CA

Serena Saeed-Winn, Mom, IBCLC, CNM, WHNP, RN
San Francisco, CA

JoAnne M. Saxe, RN, ANP-BC, MS, DNP, FAAN
Senior Editor, Professor Emerita, Department of Community Health Systems, UCSF School of Nursing
San Francisco, CA

Naomi A. Schapiro, PhD, RN, CPNP-PC
Professor Emerita, University of California San Francisco (UCSF)
San Francisco, CA

Shaadi Settecase, MSN, ANP-BC
University of California San Francisco (UCSF) Medical Center
San Francisco, CA

Jenna Shaw-Battista, PhD, NP, CNM, FACNM
Sutter Medical Group
Davis, CA

Pallavi Parthasarathy Sheth, BA, BSN, MSN
Zuckerberg San Francisco General Hospital,
San Francisco, CA
University of California San Francisco School of Nursing,
San Francisco, CA

Simranjeet K. Tagore, RN, BA, MSN, FNP
Kaiser Permanente, San Leandro, CA
Department of Obstetrics and Gynecology

Catherine D. Tanner, DNP, APRN, FNPC
Samuel Merritt University
Oakland, CA

Laura Todaro, MS, CNM, IBCLC, PMH-C
Kaiser Permanente, Walnut Creek
Walnut Creek, CA

Monifa C. Willis, PMHNP-BC
University of California San Francisco (UCSF)
San Francisco, CA

Natalie L. Wilson, PhD, DNP, MPH, APRN-BC
University of California San Francisco (UCSF)
San Francisco, CA

Esker-D Ligon, ANP-BC, PMHNP-BC
Kaiser Permanente
Oakland, CA

Sarah Goodman, RN, MS, AGPCNP-BC
San Francisco VA Medical Center
San Francisco, CA

H. Kate Lawlor, RN, MS, ANP
University of California San Francisco School of Nursing
San Francisco, CA

Brandon Sessler, MMS, PA-C
University of California
San Francisco, CA

Morgan Weinert, RN, AGPCNP-BC, PMHNP-BC, AAHIVS-BC
University of Minnesota CUHCC

Pierre-Cedric Crouch, PhD, ANP-BC, PMHNP-BC, ACRN, CARN-AP
University of California San Francisco
San Francisco, CA

Rossana Segovia, RN, MS, ANP-BC, COHN-S
University of California, San Francisco
San Francisco, CA

Jennifer Merrilees, RN, PhD
University of California, San Francisco
San Francisco, CA

Miranda Sujardi, RN, MS, ANP-BC
University of California, San Francisco
San Francisco, CA

Reviewers

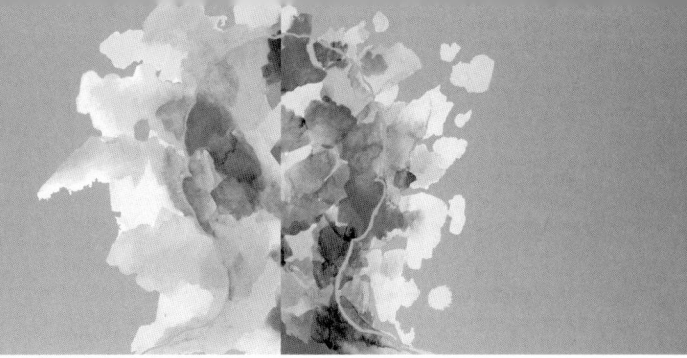

Pediatric Section

Mary Anne M. Israel, RN, MS, CPNP-PC
Assistant Adjunct Professor
Specialty Coordinator, Pediatric Primary Care Nurse
  Practitioner Program
Pediatric Nurse Practitioner, Healthy Lifestyles Clinic
Zuckerberg San Francisco General Hospital
San Francisco, CA

Courtney Giraudo, RN, MS, CNS, CPNP
Pediatric Nurse Practitioner
Whitney Newborn Follow-up Clinic
California Pacific Medical Center
San Francisco, CA

Carol A. Miller, MD
Professor, Pediatrics
University of California San Francisco School of Medicine
San Francisco, CA

Vera Goldberg, MD, FAAP
International Pediatrics
Kensington, MD

Jessica Axelrod, RN, MS, CPNP-PC
Children's Health Center
Zuckerberg San Francisco General Hospital
San Francisco, CA

Kaitlyn Basnett, MSN, RN, CPNP-PC
Stanford Medicine Children's Health
Palo Alto, CA

Layla Welborn, RN, MS, FNP-C
Gender Health SF, San Francisco Department of
  Public Health
Dimensions Clinic for Trans and Queer Youth, Castro
  Mission Health Center
San Francisco, CA

Neal Rojas, MD, MPH
Health Sciences Clinical Professor
Department of Pediatrics, Division of Developmental
  Medicine
University of California San Francisco (UCSF) School
  of Medicine
(Benioff Children's Hospital)
San Francisco, CA

Andrea Shah, RN, MS, FNP-C
Children's Health Center
Zuckerberg San Francisco General Hospital
San Francisco, CA

Grace J. Ko, MPH, MS, RN, CPNP-PC
Newborn Medicine
UC San Diego Health
San Francisco, CA

Michell Nakaishi, RN, MS, CPNP
Pediatric Primary Care Mental Health Specialist
University of California San Francisco (UCSF) Benioff
  Children's Hospital, Psychiatry
Oakland, CA

Eleanor Chung, MD
Associate Clinical Professor of Pediatrics
University of California San Francisco (UCSF) School
  of Medicine
Zuckerberg San Francisco General Hospital
Associate Medical Director for Children's Health Center
  (CHC) Specialty Care
Co-Medical Director for CHC Bridges Clinic for
  Newcomer Children
Children's Health Center
San Francisco, CA

Victoria F. Keeton, PhD, RN, CPNP-PC
Assistant professor
University of California Davis
Davis, CA
University of California San Francisco (UCSF)
  (Benioff Center for Microbiome Medicine)
San Francisco, CA

Wendy Gwirtzman Lane, MD, MPH
Medical Director
Center for Hope, Lifebridge Health
Child Abuse Pediatrician
Howard County Child Advocacy Center
Associate Professor
Department of Epidemiology & Public Health
Department of Pediatrics
University of Maryland School of Medicine
Baltimore, MD

Kelly Wong McGrath
Midwife and Lactation Consultant Hatch Midwifery
  San Francisco, CA

Sexual and Reproductive Section

Michalle Ramirez-McLaughlin, MS, FNP-C
Department of General Internal Medicine
University of California San Francisco
San Francisco, CA

Panna Lossy, MD
Clinical Professor
University of California San Francisco
San Francisco, CA
Santa Rosa Family Medicine Residency
Cotati, CA

JoAnne M. Saxe, RN, ANP-BC, MS, DNP, FAAN
Senior Editor
Professor Emerita
Former Director, Adult Gerontology Primary Nurse
  Practitioner Program
Department of Community Health Systems
University of California San Francisco School of Nursing
San Francisco, CA

Ann Griego, MS, MD
West County Health Centers
Oakland, CA
Director of Women's Health, Santa Rosa Family
  Medicine Residency
Santa Rosa, CA
TEACH (Training in Early Abortion for
  Comprehensive Healthcare)
San Francisco, CA

Kristen Sligar, MN, FNP
Nurse Practitioner
Zuckerberg San Francisco General, Obstetrics,
  Midwifery, and Gynecology Clinic (5M)
Clinical Professor
Department of Family Healthcare Nursing
University of San Francisco School of Nursing
San Francisco, CA

Susannah Ewing, MSN, NP
Department of Gynecology
University of California, San Francisco Medical Center
  San Francisco, CA

Jessica Opoku-Anane, MD, MS, FACOG
Director, Columbia University Comprehensive
  Endometriosis Center
Co-Director, OBGYN Office of Diversity,
  Equity, & Inclusion
Minimally Invasive Gynecologic Surgery
Columbia University Medical Center/New York
  Presbyterian
New York, NY

Lynn West, MSN, FNP
Nurse Practitioner
Department of OB/GYN
Kaiser Permanente Northern California
Redwood City, CA

Arielle Bivas
Nurse Practitioner
Penn Medicine Internal Medicine
Philadelphia, PA

Anne Linderman
Nurse Practitioner
Department of OB/GYN
Kaiser Permanente Northern California
Redwood City, CA

Obstetric Section

Cassandra Blot Simmons, MD
Division Director, General OB/GYN
Assistant Professor
Department of Obstetrics, Gynecology and
  Women's Health
Einstein Montefiore Medical Center
Bronx, NY

Kayon Donaldson, DNP, APRN, FNP-C
Nurse Practitioner (NP)
NP Team Lead and Educator
Department of Obstetrics, Gynecology and
  Women's Health
Einstein Montefiore Medical Center
Bronx NY

Allyson Scott, MS, CGC
Genetic Counselor
Associate Director, Graduate Program in Genetic
  Counseling
Health Sciences Clinical Instructor
Department of Pediatrics, Prenatal Diagnostic Center
University of California San Francisco
San Francisco, CA

Becca Neuwirth, RN, MS, WHNP-BC, ANP-C
Nurse Practitioner
Department of Obstetrics and Gynecology
Kaiser Permanente
San Francisco, CA
Assistant Adjunct Clinical Professor
Department of Family Health Care Nursing
University of California San Francisco School of Nursing
San Francsisco, CA

Mari-Paule Thiet, MD
Professor
Department of Obstetrics, Gynecology and Reproductive Sciences
Division of Maternal-Fetal Medicine
University of California San Francisco
San Francisco, CA

Sharon Quayle, MD
Director of Obstetrical Services
Weiler Hospital, Montefiore Medical Center
Assistant Professor of Obstetrics and Gynecology and Women's Health
Albert Einstein College of Medicine
Bronx, NY

Kelly Wong McGrath, CNM, AGPCNP-BC, RN, IBCLC
Midwife and Lactation Consultant
Hatch Midwifery
San Francisco, CA

Mason Wilson-Tanev, MA, LM
PhD Student, Anthropology and Social Change
California Institute of Integral Studies
San Francisco, CA
Psychedelic Journey Guide
Nova Health Services
Oakland, CA

Ami Burnham, LDM, RN, IBCLC
San Fransisco, CA

Adult Section

Lucy S. Crain, MD, MPH, FAAP
Clinical Professor of Pediatrics, Emerita
University of California San Francisco
San Francisco, CA

Layla Welborn, FNP
Gender Health SF, San Francisco Department of Public Health
Dimensions Clinic for Trans and Queer, Castro Mission Health Center (CMHC)
San Francisco, CA

Loree Skidmore, FNP-C
Nurse Practitioner
Canyon Manor
Novato, CA

Beth Phoenix, PhD, RN, FAAN
Clinical Professor, Health Sciences
Vice-Chair, Department of Community Health Systems
University of California San Francisco School of Nursing
San Francisco, CA

Stephanie Tsao, MSN, ANP-BC
Adult Nurse Practitioner
Zuckerberg San Francisco General Hospital
San Francisco, CA

Carol S. Viele, RN, MS, OCN
Associate Clinical Professor
Department of Physiological Nursing
University of California San Francisco School of Nursing
San Francisco, CA

Stephany Rodriguez, MSN, ANP-BC
Adult Nurse Practitioner
University of California San Francisco Medical Center
San Francisco, CA

Elika Rad, MS, RN, NP-C
Nurse Practitioner IV
Adult Cystic Fibrosis
Center for Advanced Lung Disease
Stanford Health Care
Palo Alto, CA

Jasmine Silva, DO, FAOAAM
Director, Chronic Pain Course
Touro University College of Osteopathic Medicine
New York, NY

Charleen Singh, PhD, FNP-BC, CWOCN, RN
Assistant Clinical Professor
Betty Irene Moore School of Nursing
University of California, Davis
Davis, CA

Lisa Kritikos, RN, MSN, AGNP-C
Nurse Practitioner
University of California San Francisco Memory and Aging Center
San Francisco, CA

Aaron Miller, RN, MS, NP
Associate Clinical Professor
Department of Community Health Systems
University of California San Francisco School of Nursing
San Francisco, CA

Bessa Malkoni, RN, MS, NP
San Francisco Department of Public Health
San Francisco, CA

Sara Benson, AGPCNP-BC, ACHPN
Nurse Practitioner
Center for Elders' Independence
Berkeley, CA

Fran Dreier, RN, MHS, FNP
University of California San Francisco School of Nursing
San Francisco, CA

Laura Wagner, PhD, RN, GNP, FAAN
Associate Professor
Department of Community Health Systems
University of California San Francisco School of Nursing
San Francisco, CA

Mary Wong, RN, MSN, ANP-BC
Adult Nurse Practitioner
Division of Cardiology
University of California San Francisco Medical Center
San Francisco, CA

Deepika Goyal, PhD, MS, FNPD, MS, FNP
Professor, Family Nurse Practitioner Program
Valley Foundation School of Nursing
San Jose State University
San Jose, CA

Kevin Miles, NP
UCSF 360 Wellness Clinic
University of California San Francisco Health
San Francisco, CA

Kristen Peek, MSN, FNP, RN
Assistant Professor, Family Health Care Nursing
University of California San Francisco School of Nursing
Nurse Practitioner
Zuckerburg San Francisco General Hospital
San Francisco, CA

Diana Teng, RN, MS, AGNP-BC
Assistant Clinical Professor of Nursing (Volunteer)
University of California San Francisco School of Nursing
San Francisco, CA
Adult-Gerontology Primary Care Nurse Practitioner
Palo Alto Medical Foundation, Internal Medicine
Burlingame, CA

Dana Drew-Nord, PhD, ANP-BC
Associate Clinical Professor (Retired)
School of Nursing, Community Health Systems
Occupational and Environmental Health Nursing
University of California San Francisco
San Francisco, CA

Lisa Catalli, MSN, NP-C
Hepatology and Liver Transplant Clinics
University of California San Francisco Medical Center
San Francisco, CA

Carissa Perkins, MSN, AGPCNP-BC, RN
Nurse Practitioner
East Bay Advanced Care–Alta Bates Summit Outpatient
Oakland, CA

Lou Fannon, DDS, PhD, MSN, ANP-BC, RN
Associate Clinical Professor
Nurse Practitioner
Interprofessional Primary Care Outreach for Persons with Mental Illness (IPCOM)
University of California San Francisco School of Nursing
San Francisco, CA

Jessica (Jesse) Ristau, MD
Assistant Professor
Division of General Internal Medicine
Consultant
National Clinician Consultation Center (NCCC) Substance Use Warmline
University of California San Francisco Health
San Francisco, CA

Hiu Yan (Joan) Chow, MSN
Nurse Practitioner
Division of General Medicine
University of California San Francisco Health
San Fransisco, CA

Sarah Balys Pawlowsky, PT, DPT, MS
Board Certified Orthopedic Clinical Specialist
Core Faculty for UCSF/SFSU Graduate Program in Physical Therapy
Per Diem Physical Therapist and WOS Associate Clinical Professor at UCSF
Associate Clinical Professor at SFSU
Assistant DCE for the UCSF/SFSU Graduate Program in Physical Therapy
San Francisco State University
San Francisco, CA

Michael Fischman, MD, MPH
Clinical Professor
Occupational & Environmental Medicine
University of California San Francisco School of Medicine
San Francisco, CA
Fellow, American College of Occupational and Environmental Medicine (ACOEM)
Elk Grove Village, IL

Introduction

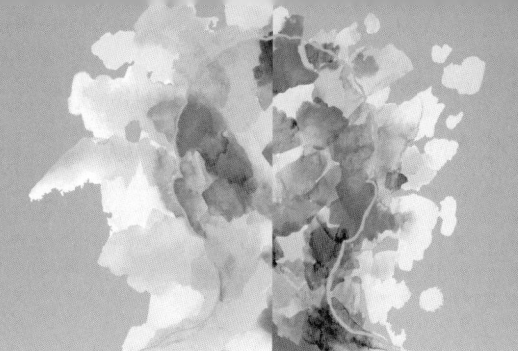

In 1998, Gerri Collins-Bride and Joanne Saxe, both pioneers in the field of advanced practice nursing and professors in the School of Nursing at the University of California San Francisco (UCSF), published the first edition of the book you are now holding, the forerunner to *Clinical Guidelines for Advanced Practice Nursing*. The title of that first edition, along with much of its content, was different from its successors, but its guiding principles have remained constant: to provide timely, relevant, evidence-based information that meets the day-to-day needs of clinicians working in primary care settings across the lifespan. Each iteration of *Clinical Guidelines* has furthered our understanding of important but often overlooked topics not adequately addressed in the training of primary care clinicians, including healthcare maintenance for adults with developmental disabilities, cancer survivorship in primary care, intimate partner violence, and care for transgender patients, among many other important topics. The widespread adoption of *Clinical Guidelines* by educators and advanced practice nurses both in the United States and abroad speaks both to the value of the book's content and to the integral role that advanced practice nurses play in the global healthcare system today.

The *First Edition* appeared at a time when online resources were few and far between, in many cases prohibitively expensive, and not altogether useful for community-based clinicians. Working in 2023, when we have nearly instant access to such resources as UpToDate®, Epocrates®, and PubMed® from our mobile devices, one might assume that this has always been the case, but in the years leading up to these incredible innovations, it was books like *Clinical Guidelines* that set the standard for practice. An advanced practice registered nurse (APRN) working in a busy clinic didn't necessarily have time between—or even during—patient visits to search through multiple textbooks for answers about differential diagnoses, diagnostic testing, or treatment plans. They relied on books like *Clinical Guidelines* as a one-stop source for information that guided their practice and furthered their education as primary care clinicians. Books like these are still of incredible value to many clinicians who work in communities without significant resources.

The fourth edition of *Clinical Guidelines*—now edited by Yoonmee Joo and J. V. Gatewood—continues to advance the important work that Collins-Bride and Saxe started over 40 years ago when they were affiliated with the Ambulatory Care Center at UCSF. In collaboration with Collins-Bride and Saxe, who remain as senior editors on this project, we have gone through the chapters that appeared in the previous edition of *Clinical Guidelines*, evaluated each in terms of its timeliness and clinical relevance, and made a collective decision about what topics would appear in the new edition of this text. The major emphasis of this text continues to be on chronic health problems—their prevention, pathophysiology, diagnosis, and treatment—with chapters dedicated to specific patient populations. Several new chapters appear in this new edition that speak to some of the challenges and chronic health conditions prevalent in health care today: care of transgender/gender-diverse youth, abortion, early pregnancy loss, pelvic pain, postpartum depression/anxiety, breastfeeding/chestfeeding concerns, nonalcoholic fatty liver disease (NAFLD), and substance use disorders.

For this new edition, we have asked our authors to incorporate diversity, equity, and inclusion (DEI) into their approach to writing the chapters and to include information that speaks to the ways in which structural racism, sexism, ageism, transphobia, biphobia, homophobia, ableism, and religious discrimination affect the lives and health of our patients. Healthcare organizations and the clinicians who work in them have a responsibility to understand the needs of our diverse patient populations and promote equity in practice to ensure the best long-term health outcomes for our patients.

This new edition retains the structure of its predecessors and will look familiar to those readers who have used this textbook in the past. For those who are new to this book, the current edition of *Clinical Guidelines* includes several outstanding features:

- An emphasis on clinical practice across the life span
- An interdisciplinary and team-based approach to clinical practice that includes chapters written by certified nurse midwives, clinical nurse specialists, nurse practitioners, physician assistants, and physicians
- A subjective–objective–assessment–plan (SOAP) format that is easily accessible to clinicians
- Timely and relevant information carefully selected by the editorial team to be practical for both advanced practice clinicians and students alike
- Test bank questions that reinforce student learning for each of the chapters
- Close affiliation with clinicians who teach, work, or have studied at UCSF, 1 of 10 campuses in the University of California system and the only one dedicated

to health sciences. UCSF has an outstanding international reputation for research, teaching, and clinical care. The School of Nursing is ranked within the top 10 of all nursing schools in the United States by *U.S. News & World Report*.

Welcome to the fourth edition of *Clinical Guidelines for Advanced Practice Nursing*. We hope that this text will be the one resource that students and APRNs will rely on to answer questions on common clinical presentations and chronic health conditions.

SECTION I

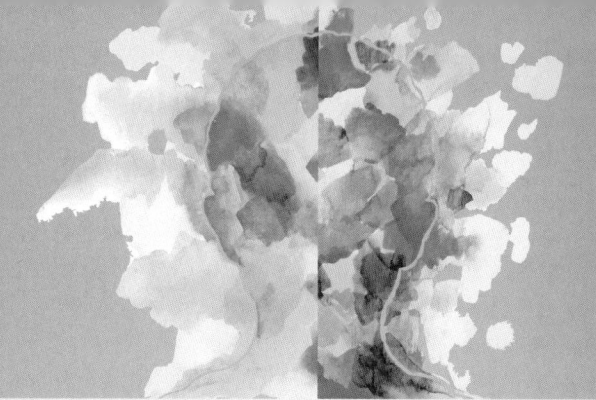

Pediatric Health Maintenance and Promotion

CHAPTER 1	First Well-Baby Visit	3
CHAPTER 2	Care of the Postneonatal Intensive Care Unit Graduate	9
CHAPTER 3	0 to 3 Years of Age Interval Visit	17
CHAPTER 4	3 to 6 Years of Age Interval Visit	25
CHAPTER 5	6 to 11 Years of Age Interval Visit	29
CHAPTER 6	The Adolescent and Young Adult (12-26 Years of Age) Interval Visit	35
CHAPTER 7	Care of Transgender and Gender Diverse Youth	41
CHAPTER 8	Developmental Assessment: Screening for Developmental Delay and Autism	53

CHAPTER 1

First Well-Baby Visit

Annette Carley

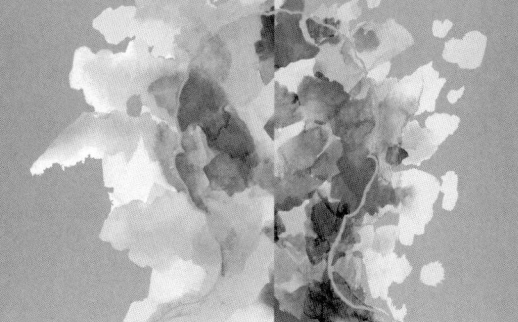

I. Introduction and general background

The birth of a child creates new challenges for a family. The initial outpatient visit affords the provider an opportunity to establish an ongoing relationship with the infant and family, follow up on residual issues from birth, and individualize and prioritize healthcare needs. For healthy infants, this initial visit should occur within the first week following discharge (March of Dimes, 2021b).

A. Follow-up of healthy infant after vaginal or cesarean delivery
   1. For vaginal delivery, where discharge is typically at 48 hours, follow-up should occur within 48 hours of discharge (Benitz & Committee on Fetus and Newborn, 2015).
   2. For cesarean delivery, where discharge typically occurs at 96 hours, follow-up should occur within 1 week of discharge (Hagan et al., 2008).
B. Follow-up of infant after early discharge
   1. Early discharge (i.e., hospital discharge between 24 and 48 hours) may be offered to healthy singleton infants, born at 37–41 weeks' gestation, who are appropriately grown for gestational age, have no abnormal physical findings, and were born vaginally after an uncomplicated prenatal course. Family, environmental, and social risks should be identified and addressed. Before discharge, the infant must have completed a minimum of two successful feedings, had such issues as jaundice (if present) adequately addressed, and demonstrated adequate voiding and stooling (Benitz & Committee on Fetus and Newborn, 2015; Committee on Fetus and Newborn, 2010). However, healthy newborns may not void or stool within the first day of life. If discharge of the otherwise healthy infant who has not voided or stooled is being considered, a documented plan for follow-up must be ensured, and parents must be instructed about findings that warrant immediate follow-up (e.g., vomiting, inconsolability, or abdominal distention).
   2. The plan for follow-up care should be confirmed and documented before discharge (Benitz & Committee on Fetus and Newborn, 2015).
C. Follow-up of premature and late premature infant after discharge
   1. Premature infants less than 37 weeks' gestational age are commonly discharged at or near their due date. At discharge, they should demonstrate cardiorespiratory, hemodynamic, and thermal stability and adequate weight gain. Exact standards for discharge are lacking, but most centers consider discharge after completion of the 35th to 37th postconceptual week and stabilization of weight at 1,800–2,000 g.
      a. Those with a complicated clinical course or birth weight less than 1,500 g are typically also followed by a specialty clinic versed in premature infant care and outcome.
   2. Late preterm (i.e., 34–37 weeks' gestation), also known as "near-term" infants, are frequently discharged using the same guidelines as term infants; however, this may underestimate some ongoing needs because of their immaturity or small size. To support a successful transition, it is recommended that the infant be seen within 48 hours of discharge (Quinn et al., 2017).
      a. Enhanced risks in this population that may complicate the early neonatal period or result in rehospitalization after discharge include hyperbilirubinemia, poor feeding, dehydration, sepsis, and respiratory and thermal instability (Huff et al., 2019; Phillips et al., 2013; Quinn et al., 2017). Up to 4% of late preterm infants may be readmitted, most within 2 weeks after discharge, most commonly due to jaundice and/or feeding difficulty (Hannan et al., 2020).

II. Database (may include but is not limited to)
A. *Subjective*
   1. History and review of systems
      a. Parental concerns, including feelings of readiness, stress, adequacy, and support
      b. Birth and health history to date
         i. Gestational parent age, gravida, and parity
         ii. Pregnancy complications, including substance exposure, infections, hypertensive disorders, gestational diabetes, and inadequate prenatal care
         iii. Duration of labor, delivery method, complications, use of anesthesia, timing of umbilical cord clamping
         iv. Birth complications, including premature rupture of membranes, meconium, need for resuscitation, and low Apgar scores at birth
         v. Birth date
         vi. Gestational age
         vii. Birth weight
         viii. Review of pertinent gestational parent and newborn lab work, including blood type and Coombs testing and bilirubin (if indicated)
         ix. Discharge weight and age at discharge
         x. Nursery complications, including jaundice
      c. Family, social, and environmental history
         i. Parent/co-parent/caretaker's age, health, occupation, level of education, and literacy
         ii. Siblings' age and health
         iii. Family history, including such conditions as asthma, allergies, atopic dermatitis, chronic lung disease, diabetes, renal dysfunction, mental health disorders, heart disease, hematologic disorders, and tuberculosis
         iv. Social or environmental concerns, such as unemployment, relationship stressors, physical abuse, substance exposure, and adjustment to newborn in home. Unmet social needs may affect immediate health and access to preventive care. Assess for needs such as housing, transportation, and food security (Hardy et al., 2021). The perinatal period is a vulnerable time for many families. Attending to cultural humility, maintaining awareness of biases, and applying a trauma-informed approach to care are paramount (Roosevelt et al., 2021).
         v. Family source of support and religious affiliation
      d. Nutrition history (American Academy of Pediatrics [AAP], 2018)
         i. For infants feeding from bottles: type, frequency, and volume of feedings; proper preparation of formula; strength of suck; burping
         ii. For infants feeding at the breast or chest: frequency; duration; perceived satiety; strength of suck; one versus two breasts used for feeding; breast fullness before and after feeding; use of breast pump; use of other devices, such as breast shields or supplemental nursing systems; care of milk, including labeling, storing (refrigerator vs. freezer), and rewarming; use of donor milk
         iii. The Academy of Breastfeeding Medicine recommends gender-inclusive/de-sexed language, such as "birthing people," "lactating person," and "human milk feeding," based on the individual family's preferences for terms used when describing human milk feeding (Bartick et al., 2021).
      e. Review of systems and clinical findings
B. *Objective*
   1. Physical examination findings (Tappero & Honeyfield, 2018)
      a. Skin: turgor, color, perfusion; presence of rashes, birthmarks, dermal breaks, skin tags or pits, or jaundice
      b. Head–eyes–ears–nose–throat–mouth
         i. Assess size, shape, symmetry of head and fontanels; note presence of cephalohematoma, caput, or cranial molding.
         ii. Assess red reflex, ocular mobility; note scleral color and presence of ocular opacification, drainage, and dacryostenosis.
         iii. Assess nares: patency, drainage, and symmetry of septum.
         iv. Assess placement of ears, external shape/contour, and patency of canals. Note that the natural accumulation of vernix may obscure assessment of tympanic membranes in the early neonatal period.
         v. Assess intactness of palate, strength of suck, presence of natal teeth, and presence of inclusion cysts.
      c. Chest and thorax
         i. Assess character of respirations, respiratory rate (normal, 30–60 breaths per minute), shape and contour of thorax, and breast size and shape; note presence of chest asymmetry, nipple discharge, or tenderness. Assess for increased work of breathing, including retractions and abnormal lung sounds on auscultation.
      d. Cardiovascular
         i. Assess heart rate (normal, 100–180 beats per minute), rhythm, perfusion, and quality of pulses; note presence of arrhythmias or murmurs.
      e. Abdomen and rectum
         i. Assess symmetry, tone, presence of bowel sounds, anal patency, timing of first stool, and stage of umbilical healing; note presence of distension and tenderness.
         ii. Assess liver size and note presence of hepatomegaly.

f. Genitourinary
      i. Assess appearance of external genitalia, timing of first void, voiding pattern, and kidney size by palpation (normally 4–5 cm in size); note presence of ambiguous genitalia or abnormal kidney size.
   g. Musculoskeletal
      i. Assess extremities, presence of digits, intactness of spine, and movement and stability of hips; note presence of deviation of gluteal cleft, hair tufts, or sacral dimple; note presence of click or clunk with hip exam.
   h. Neurobehavioral
      i. Assess activity, tone, state regulation, and symmetry of movements; note presence of clonus, irritability, inconsolability, or excess sleepiness or difficulty awakening.
2. Establish a growth trend, including comparative measurements of head circumference, weight, and length from birth, and adjust for gestational age as indicated. The Centers for Disease Control and Prevention (CDC) recommends the use of World Health Organization (WHO) growth records for infants up to 2 years of age (CDC, 2010).
3. Observe parent–child interactions, including holding, comforting, responsiveness, confidence, and mutual support. Postpartum depression occurs in approximately 12% of families and can affect the infant's development. Assess for evidence of parental depression, including use of the Edinburgh Postnatal Depression Scale (EPDS), at multiple intervals during the first 4–6 months (Turner, 2018).
4. Review supportive data from relevant diagnostic tests, including:
   a. Results of neonatal screening. All states require newborn screening, although there is variation in the conditions that are included in screening. Most states include those recommended in the federal Recommended Uniform Screening Panel (RUSP), which currently includes 34 core and 26 secondary conditions (CDC, 2020a; March of Dimes, 2021a; National Conference of State Legislatures, 2021).
      i. Phenylketonuria (PKU) screening is mandated in all states. Screening should occur prior to discharge; if screened within the first 24 hours, the test should be repeated by a postnatal age of 2 weeks to eliminate erroneous results. Preterm and ill infants are best screened near the 7th postnatal day but must be screened prior to discharge (Agency for Healthcare Research and Quality [AHRQ], 2014).
      ii. Sickle cell screening is mandatory in all states and should occur before discharge, with confirmation of positive results prior to 2 months of age (AAP, 2021c; AHRQ, 2014).
      iii. Congenital hypothyroid screening is required in all infants and is done at the 2nd to 4th postnatal day or immediately before discharge if discharge occurs before 48 hours of age. Positive screens require confirmatory testing and initiation of treatment by 2 weeks of age (AAP, 2006; AHRQ, 2014).
   b. Hearing screening is recommended for all infants at no later than 1 month of age, ideally prior to hospital discharge (CDC, 2020b).
   c. Screening for the presence of a critical congenital heart defect (CCHD) using pulse oximetry is recommended (AAP, 2021b).
   d. Ongoing monitoring for the development of jaundice is recommended. Approximately 60% of term and up to 80% of preterm infants develop some clinical jaundice in postnatal week 1. Infants who develop jaundice within 24 hours of birth should have direct serologic or transcutaneous bilirubin assessment and a management plan established (Muniyappa & Kelley, 2020). The National Perinatal Association further recommends that preterm/late preterm infants have direct bilirubin assessment (serum or transcutaneous testing) at 24 hours of age and prior to discharge (Phillips et al., 2013).
   e. Immunizations are deferred until 2 months postnatal age (AAP, 2021a). Hepatitis B vaccine is recommended for all infants at birth, with a second dose at 1–2 months (AAP, 2021a).

III. Assessment
A. *Determine the diagnosis*
   Determine patient's current health status, and identify general health risks based on gender, age, ethnicity, or other socioeconomic factors and the effects of structural racism.
B. *Motivation and ability*
   Determine caregiver and family willingness and ability to follow through with treatment plans and overcome barriers.

IV. Goals of first well-baby visit
A. *Screening or diagnosing*
   Choose a practical, cost-effective approach to screening and diagnosis while abiding by mandated screening protocols.
B. *Treatment*
   Select a treatment plan that achieves appropriate growth and development, is individualized for the caregiver and child, and maximizes caregiver success.

V. Plan
A. *Screening*
   Elicit a thorough history and perform a thorough physical examination, with growth and development assessments at the initial and all well-child visits.

B. Diagnostic tests
1. Newborn screening is performed as required by individual states, but it must include assessment for congenital hypothyroidism, PKU, and sickle cell (AHRQ, 2014).
2. Hearing screening is recommended for all infants.

C. Patient education and anticipatory guidance
1. Nutrition
   a. Support the gestational parent's nutritional needs for calories, liquids, adequate rest, and emotional and social support.
   b. Encourage breast-/chestfeeding or support bottle feeding as indicated.
   c. Milk intake is considered adequate if baby has five to eight wet diapers and three to four stools per day and is gaining weight appropriately (15 g/kg/day). Initial stools with human milk intake may be loose and occur after each feeding.
   d. Healthy infants should need no extra water because both human milk and formula provide adequate fluid for the newborn.
   e. Exclusive human milk feeding is considered the ideal source of nutrition for the first 4–6 months; for formula feeders, always use iron-fortified formula, and provide 2–3 oz every 2–3 hours; increase if infant seems hungry.
   f. Counsel about safety with milk preparation and storage.
2. Growth and development
3. Safety, including use of car seats; exposures, such as tobacco; back-to-sleep positioning; cardiopulmonary resuscitation; when to call the provider; and illness prevention
4. Referrals as indicated, including encouraging birthing parent and partner to seek appropriate postpartum follow-up if needed
5. Special Supplemental Nutrition Program for Women, Infants, and Children (WIC) referral should be initiated for eligible families (see https://www.fns.usda.gov/wic).
6. Family transition to parenthood and well-being, including obtaining adequate rest and developing routines

VI. Resources and tools

A. Patient education
1. The AAP website contains a variety of links of interest to parents, including the Healthy Children resources. https://www.healthychildren.org/English/Pages/default.aspx
2. The American Academy of Family Physicians sponsors a website called Family Doctor.org, which provides resources and links about infants of interest to parents. https://www.familydoctor.org
3. The National Institutes of Health sponsors a website, MedlinePlus, that contains infant and newborn care resources for parents. https://medlineplus.gov/infantandnewborncare.html

References

Agency for Healthcare Research and Quality. (2014). *The guide to clinical preventive services 2014. Recommendations of the U.S. Preventive Services Task Force.* https://www.ahrq.gov/sites/default/files/wysiwyg/professionals/clinicians-providers/guidelines-recommendations/guide/cpsguide.pdf

American Academy of Pediatrics. (2006). Update of newborn screening and therapy for congenital hypothyroidism. *Pediatrics, 117*(6), 2290–2303. Reaffirmed December 2011. https://pediatrics.aappublications.org/content/117/6/2290

American Academy of Pediatrics. (2018). *Amount and schedule of formula feedings.* https://www.healthychildren.org/English/ages-stages/baby/formula-feeding/Pages/Amount-and-Schedule-of-Formula-Feedings.aspx

American Academy of Pediatrics. (2021a). *Immunization schedule for 2021.* https://redbook.solutions.aap.org/selfserve/ssPage.aspx?SelfServeContentId=Immunization_Schedules

American Academy of Pediatrics. (2021b). *Newborn pulse oximetry screening to detect critical congenital heart disease.* https://www.healthychildren.org/English/ages-stages/baby/Pages/Newborn-Pulse-Oximetry-Screening-to-Detect-Critical-Congenital-Heart-Disease.aspx

American Academy of Pediatrics. (2021c). *Sickle cell disease: Information for parents.* https://www.healthychildren.org/English/health-issues/conditions/chronic/Pages/Sickle-Cell-Disease-in-Children.aspx

Bartick, M., Stehel, E. K., Calhoun, S. L., Feldman-Winter, L., Zimmerman, D., Noble, L., Rosen-Carole, C., Kair, L. R., & Academy of Breastfeeding Medicine. (2021). Academy of Breastfeeding Medicine position statement and guideline: Infant feeding and lactation-related language and gender. *Breastfeeding Medicine, 16*(8), 587–590. doi:10.1089/bfm.2021.29188.abm

Benitz, W., & Committee on Fetus and Newborn. (2015). Hospital stay for healthy term newborn infants. *Pediatrics, 135*(5), 948–953. doi:1-.1542/peds.2015-0699

Centers for Disease Control and Prevention. (2010). *Growth charts.* https://www.cdc.gov/growthcharts/

Centers for Disease Control and Prevention. (2020a). *Newborn screening portal.* https://www.cdc.gov/newbornscreening/index.html

Centers for Disease Control and Prevention. (2020b). *Screening and diagnosis of hearing loss.* https://www.cdc.gov/ncbddd/hearingloss/screening.html

Committee on Fetus and Newborn. (2010). Policy statement: Hospital stay for healthy term newborns. *Pediatrics, 125*(2), 405–409. http://pediatrics.aappublications.org/content/113/5/1434.full.pdf

Hagan, J. F., Shaw, J. S., & Duncan, P. M. (2008). Supervision: First week visit. In J. F. Hagan, J. S. Shaw, & P. M. Duncan (Eds.), *Bright futures: Guidelines for health supervision of infants, children, and adolescents* (3rd ed., pp. 289–302). American Academy of Pediatrics.

Hannan, K. E., Hwang, S. S., & Bourque, S. L. (2020). Readmissions among NICU graduates: Who, when and why? *Seminars in Perinatology, 44*(4), 1–7. doi:10.1016/j.semperi.2020.151245

Hardy, R., Boch, S., Keedy, H., & Chisolm, D. (2021). Social determinants of health needs and pediatric health care use. *Journal of Pediatrics, 238*, 275-281.e1. doi:10.1016/j.jpeds.2021.07.056

Huff, K., Rose, R., & Engle, W. A. (2019). Late preterm infants: Morbidities, mortality, and management. *Pediatric Clinics of North America, 66*(2), 387–402. doi:10.1016/j.pcl.2018.12.008

March of Dimes. (2021a). *Newborn screening tests for your baby.* https://www.marchofdimes.org/baby/newborn-screening-tests-for-your-baby.aspx

March of Dimes. (2021b). *Your baby's checkups.* https://www.marchofdimes.org/baby/your-babys-checkups.aspx

Muniyappa, P., & Kelley, D. (2020). Hyperbilirubinemia in pediatrics: Evaluation and care. *Current Problems in Pediatric & Adolescent Health Care, 50*(8), 1–9. doi:10.1016/j.cppeds.2020.100842

National Conference of State Legislatures. (2021). *State newborn health screening policies.* https://www.ncsl.org/research/health/state-newborn-health-screening-policies.aspx

Phillips, R. M., Goldstein, M., Houghland, K., Nandyal, R., Pizzica, A., Santa-Donato, A., Staebler, S., Stark, A. R., Treiger, T. M., & Yost, E. (2013). Multidisciplinary guidelines for the care of late preterm infants. *Journal of Perinatology, 33*(Suppl. 2), S5–82. doi:10.1038/jp.2013.53

Quinn, J. M., Sparks, M., & Gephart, S. M. (2017). Discharge criteria for the late preterm infant: A review of the literature. *Advances in Neonatal Care, 17*(5), 362–371. doi:10.1038/jp.2013.53

Roosevelt, L. K., Pietzmeier, S., & Reed, R. (2021). Clinically and culturally competent care for transgender and nonbinary people: A challenge to providers of perinatal care. *Journal of Perinatal & Neonatal Nursing, 35*(2), 142–149. doi:10.1097/JPN.0000000000000560

Tappero, E. P., & Honeyfield, M. E. (Eds.). (2018). *Physical assessment of the newborn: A comprehensive approach to the art of physical examination* (6th ed.). Springer.

Turner, K. (2018). Well-child visits for infants and young children. *American Family Physician, 98*(6), 347–354.

CHAPTER 2

Care of the Postneonatal Intensive Care Unit Graduate

Annette Carley

I. Introduction and general background

The need for expert, comprehensive postneonatal intensive care unit (post-NICU) care is never more apparent. Although survival to discharge has improved across gestational ages, survivors may have residual disabilities that will need expert follow-up care by providers well prepared to address the needs of these fragile infants and intervene early and effectively (Carley, 2008; Goldstein & Malcolm, 2019; Kelly, 2006a). The American Academy of Pediatrics (AAP) has identified four categories of post-NICU infants who are considered high risk at discharge: (1) premature infants, (2) those with special health needs or who are dependent on technology, (3) those at risk because of social or family issues, and (4) those for whom early death is anticipated. Benchmarks recommended by the AAP that support readiness for NICU discharge include physiologic stability, caretaker involvement and readiness to assume care, and an integrated plan for follow-up care and management of the infant (AAP, Committee on Fetus and Newborn, 2008; McInerny et al., 2017).

A. Common issues for the post-NICU population

1. The infant who is premature at discharge
   Premature births (i.e., less than 37 weeks' gestational age) account for 10% of births in the United States annually (Centers for Disease Control and Prevention [CDC], 2020), of whom late preterm infants (those born between gestational age 34 0/7 and 36 6/7 weeks) account for nearly three-quarters (March of Dimes Foundation, 2021). As gestational age decreases, the rate of neonatal complications increases; however, even late preterm infants are at risk for complications such as impaired thermoregulation, poor feeding and nutrition, gastroesophageal reflux and other gastrointestinal issues, late-onset sepsis, jaundice, or neurodevelopment impairment. Late preterm infants are at risk for rehospitalization in the early postnatal period (Darcy, 2009; Loftin et al., 2010; Quinn et al., 2017) and have up to a four-times-higher rate of infant mortality than their full-term peers, based on worldwide data (Delnord & Zeitlin, 2019). For successful transition, the post-NICU premature infant must be physiologically stable, feeding sufficiently well to support appropriate growth, able to maintain thermal neutrality in the post-NICU environment, and capable of sustaining mature respiratory system behavior (AAP, Committee on Fetus and Newborn, 2008; Barkemeyer, 2015; CDC, 2020; Goldstein & Malcolm, 2019; Smith & Stewart, 2021; Whyte, 2012).

2. Chronic lung disease (CLD)
   CLD is the leading cause of pediatric lung disease, and bronchopulmonary dysplasia (BPD) as a complication in NICU infants is the most common adverse pulmonary outcome in the preterm population. BPD results from pulmonary system immaturity or dysfunction and the additive effects of therapies, such as oxygen or mechanical ventilation support (Tracy & Berkelhamer, 2019). BPD commonly affects the premature infant, and despite overall improved survival and advances, such as gentler postnatal ventilation strategies and exogenous surfactant therapy, it affects approximately 10,000 neonates annually in the United States, based on its being defined as the need for oxygen support at 36 weeks' postmenstrual

age (Thekkeveedu et al., 2017). The incidence of CLD/BPD increases with decreasing gestational age at birth, and rates as high as 68% in infants born less than 28 weeks' gestational age have been reported (Thekkeveedu et al., 2017).

Infants with CLD/BPD are at increased risk for adverse health outcomes, including chronic pulmonary morbidity, pulmonary infections, long-term growth failure, sensory deficits, developmental delay, and mortality (Jensen & Schmidt, 2014).

   a. Postdischarge therapies that may be used to optimize pulmonary function and growth include supplemental oxygen or ventilation, cardiorespiratory monitors, diuretics, and bronchodilators, as well as enhanced nutritional strategies (Kelly, 2006b; Tracy & Berkelhamer, 2019).
   b. Supplemental oxygen aims to optimize growth and stamina and prevent the development of cor pulmonale. For those discharged on supplemental oxygen, adequate caretaker training and team planning for weaning should be assured (Andrews et al., 2014; Barkemeyer, 2015).
   c. Home mechanical ventilation, although rarely needed, may be used for those infants unable to wean from mechanical ventilation before hospital discharge. Careful caretaker training and establishment of outpatient support is essential (AAP, Committee on Fetus and Newborn, 2008; Andrews et al., 2014; Goldstein & Malcolm, 2019).

3. Apnea
   Apnea is a serious condition for the neonate and may result from pulmonary disorders; infection; brain injury; or metabolic derangements, such as hypoglycemia. Apnea is also a common complication in the preterm population, caused by immature central regulation of respiratory effort, and may be managed with oxygen or ventilator support, respiratory stimulants (e.g., methylxanthines), and cardiopulmonary monitoring. Although typically resolved by 36–40 weeks' postconceptual age, apnea caused by immaturity in some infants, or "apnea of prematurity," may persist until the time of discharge. It is recommended that infants be free of significant apnea for 3–8 days prior to discharge (Andrews et al., 2014; McInerny et al., 2017).

4. Gastroesophageal reflux disease (GERD)
   Infants born prematurely, those whose early course included structural or functional disorders of the gastrointestinal tract, those with pulmonary conditions requiring surgical intervention, and those with neurologic compromise are at risk for GERD. GERD may lead to erosive esophageal injury and may be associated with serious conditions, such as apnea, bronchospasm, aspiration, or long-term growth failure.
   a. Physiologic reflux is common in infants; up to half of all infants less than 3 months of age exhibit regurgitation.
   b. Pathologic reflux, also known as *GERD*, is associated with complications including apnea, bronchospasm, esophagitis, esophageal strictures, and failure to thrive. It may be managed conservatively with small, frequent feedings; upright positioning; and medications to optimize gastric emptying, or it may necessitate surgical management for intractable cases. The use of thickened feedings has shown variable results, and this practice may carry risks for the immature gastrointestinal tract. In otherwise healthy infants beyond their due date, it may be cautiously considered (Andrews et al., 2014; Martin & Hibbs, 2020).

5. Postnatal growth restriction
   Premature infants are at increased risk for poor feeding and growth failure, and at discharge, they are typically below their healthy term counterparts in weight. Growth risks are compounded by the effects of chronic illness and genetic potential. Premature infants frequently need higher calories and nutrients than their healthy term counterparts. Diligently applied nutritional support plays a key role in supporting adequate long-term growth and optimal neurologic development.
   a. Human milk is the ideal food for all infants regardless of gestational age. However, a diet of exclusively human milk may contribute to nutritional deficiencies in the recuperating post-NICU infant who has not attained adequate prenatal stores and has robust growth and recuperative needs. It is often necessary to supplement calories, protein, sodium, and calcium in these infants (Barkemeyer, 2015).
   b. If human milk is not available or appropriate, premature, transitional, or postdischarge formula may be indicated to optimize catch-up growth (McInerny et al., 2017).
   c. Premature infants may require additional supplementation to support nutrient requirements for protein; calcium; phosphorus; sodium; vitamins, such as B_{12}, B_6, D, E, and K; and trace minerals, such as zinc, copper, magnesium, selenium, and carnitine (Voller, 2018).
   d. Recuperating infants, especially preterm infants, need up to 130 kcal/kg/d to achieve adequate growth (Billimoria, 2014). Those born small for gestational age or those attempting to achieve adequate catch-up growth may require up to 165 kcal/kg/d. Chronic health issues creating increased nutritional demands, such as CLD or growth failure, may warrant increased caloric goals. Early and ongoing nutritional assessment and follow-up are important to optimize growth gains (Zhang et al., 2020).
   e. Structural or functional comorbidities, such as orofacial anomalies or altered tone, may complicate the nutritional plan (Kelly, 2006b).

6. Neurobehavioral and sensory deficits
Infants recovering from the effects of initial illness or prematurity and the NICU environment may have residual neurobehavioral challenges. This risk increases with decreasing gestational age (Billimoria, 2014) and may include developmental delays, learning disabilities, hyperactivity, and cerebral palsy. Additionally, sensory deficits may include hearing or vision loss, auditory processing disorders, or language delay.
   a. Hearing screening is recommended universally for all infants and indicated for the NICU infant before discharge. Hearing loss occurs in as many as 1.5% of all post-NICU infants (Andrews et al., 2014), and up to 50% of abnormal infant hearing screening occurs in NICU graduates (Kelly, 2006b). Special risks for the NICU population include a history of assisted ventilation, use of ototoxic pharmaceuticals, hyperbilirubinemia, infection, and craniofacial disorders (Andrews et al., 2014; Billimoria, 2014). Early intervention (i.e., at age <6 months) enhances language development (Kelly, 2006b). Those with risks should have ongoing assessment, including formal audiology evaluation by 8–12 months of age, even in cases with a normal initial hearing screen (McInerny et al., 2017).
7. Vision screening is recommended for preterm infants of less than 1,500 g birth weight (or <30 weeks' gestation), those with a complicated medical course, and those exposed to supplemental oxygen. Severe retinopathy occurs in approximately 7% of infants born between 24 and 28 weeks' gestation. Even without established retinopathy of prematurity, NICU infants are at risk for impaired visual acuity, refractive errors, and strabismus (Andrews et al., 2014). The first examination typically occurs at 31–34 weeks' postconceptual age, with regular follow-up until vascular maturity is ensured at 3–6 months (Billimoria, 2014; Kelly, 2006b). As part of health surveillance, infants at corrected age 3–4 months should be screened for strabismus and referred for ophthalmologic follow-up even if predischarge screening is normal (McInerny et al., 2017)
8. Formal developmental assessment is indicated for all at-risk infants, including those born preterm or with a complicated clinical course.
   a. Goals of developmental follow-up include optimizing growth and development to maximize long-term potential; integrating the infant into the family and community; and providing early intervention to reduce medical, social, and emotional burden (Kuppala et al., 2012)
   b. Due to their enhanced risk for adverse developmental sequelae, infants born at <1,000 g birth weight or <28 weeks' gestation and those whose history has included neurologic complications or congenital malformations of the CNS require close neurobehavioral follow-up. Infants who experienced extreme cases of hypoglycemia or hyperbilirubinemia or whose histories include prenatal substance exposure are also at risk and will need screening/follow-up until 30–36 months of age (McInerny et al., 2017)
9. Dependence on technology
Infants with unresolved cardiopulmonary issues, such as apnea, chronic hypoxia, or growth failure, may require technologic support in the home after discharge.
   a. Pulmonary support may be achieved with supplemental oxygen, cardiopulmonary monitoring, or the use of mechanical ventilation.
   b. Weaning from ventilatory support is dictated by the infant demonstrating normal oxygen saturation, resolution of apnea or bradycardia, and appropriate growth (Goldstein & Malcolm, 2019).
   c. The use of in-home technology requires vigilant attention to safety and hygiene, consistent education, and support of caretakers. Mechanical ventilation requires dedicated personnel and ongoing caregiver support, including respite care (McInerny et al., 2017)
   d. Nutritional support may be achieved with complementary enteral feedings or parenteral nutrition. In-home use of intermittent orogastric gavage or gastrostomy feedings requires vigilant attention to safety, hygiene, and education and support of caregivers. Efforts should concentrate on encouraging oral feeding skills.
   e. Weaning from supplemental nutritional support can be considered when the infant demonstrates consistent appropriate growth, under the supervision of a nutrition specialist (Barkemeyer, 2015; Kelly, 2006b).
   f. A plan for emergency management in the case of equipment malfunction must be in place (AAP, Committee on Fetus and Newborn, 2008).
10. Postnatal infection
Convalescing post-NICU patients, especially preterm infants, are at risk for complications related to infections, including respiratory syncytial virus (RSV) and influenza virus. Their increased vulnerability to infections may result in acute decompensation and the need for rehospitalization. At-risk infants discharged during peak RSV transmission seasons (i.e., October through March in the United States) should receive routine immunizations given at recommended intervals and RSV prophylaxis if indicated based on the most current recommendations (AAP, 2021).

B. *Additional issues for the post-NICU population*
1. Social and environmental risks
The AAP identifies premature birth, need for hospitalization, presence of birth defects, and infant disability as risks for family dysfunction and child abuse. These risks are compounded by family and

environmental risks, such as low socioeconomic status, lack of social support, substance exposure, and lack of family involvement during the infant's hospitalization. Identifying strategies to enhance infant safety and family functioning before discharge is encouraged (AAP, Committee on Fetus and Newborn, 2008; McInerny et al., 2017).
- a. The ongoing stress of hospitalization and uncertainty of neonatal outcome may have a negative impact on the quality of interactions with the infant as well as between the birth partners and between the family and providers. It is especially important to identify stress and depression in all birth partners. For example, stress and depression in partners may be overlooked because of a primary focus on the birthing parent (Hynan et al., 2013; Hoge et al., 2020; Purdy et al., 2015; Shaw et al., 2009). Evolving evidence suggests that both birthing parents and partners may be at high risk for traumatic stress and/or major depression (Cole et al., 2018). Although it is recognized that other co-parents and birth partners may experience stress, depression, and stigma during the perinatal period, there is limited research focusing on their mental health needs or appropriate strategies for assessment and support (Darwin et al., 2021).
- b. A relationship exists between parental mental health and infant developmental outcomes such as emotional adjustment, IQ, and growth (Bernardo et al., 2021)
- c. Vulnerable child syndrome has been described in the literature since the 1960s and is now recognized as a potential outcome caused by the effects of protracted neonatal hospitalization, parental anxiety or depression, impact of the illness on the family, or lack of social support. It has been associated with the risk of adverse health and neurobehavioral outcomes in infants (Hoge et al., 2020; Kokotos, 2009).
- d. A growing body of literature is focusing on the impact of stress as an environmental influence on fetal programming. Both chronic and acute stress can have a detrimental impact on pregnancy and result in suppression of normal immune responses with heightened risk for infection, as well as increased risk for preterm birth; low birth weight; and later impairment of physiologic, cognitive and behavioral development in the child. Mindfulness-based interventions have been advocated for birthing people as a strategy for perinatal stress management (Isgut et al., 2017).
- e. Infant with anticipated early death
  A family-centered and culturally sensitive approach to family support should be offered, with the goal of providing the family and the infant as much comfort as possible. To enhance the quality of remaining life, infants with terminal disorders may be discharged to the home for hospice care. Discharge planning and follow-up care attend to family needs and concerns and occur with the involvement of home nursing. Necessary elements include creating a plan for management of infant pain and discomfort; securing arrangements for equipment or supplies; and providing ongoing support to parents, siblings, or extended family members (AAP, Committee on Fetus and Newborn, 2008; Kenner et al., 2015).

II. Database (may include but is not limited to)
A. *Subjective database*
   1. History and review of systems
      a. Parental concerns, including feelings of readiness, stress, adequacy, and support, or parent-specific concerns about development or medical issues
      b. Birth and health history to date
         i. Birth history, including gravida and parity, pregnancy complications, delivery method and birth complications, Apgar scores
         ii. Infant birth date, weight, and gestational age (average for gestational age [AGA], large for gestational age [LGA], or small for gestational age [SGA]/intrauterine growth restriction [IUGR])
         iii. Neonatal course, including complications
      c. Family, social, and environmental history
         i. Biological parents' individual and family health history, including chronic conditions or any familial neurodevelopmental disorders or mental health concerns
         ii. Parental ages, health, occupation, and level of education
         iii. Sibling ages, health, and history of prematurity
         iv. Genetic parental head circumference and stature to compare with infant measurements
         v. Social or environmental concerns, such as unemployment, abuse, marital problems, and lack of support
      d. Nutrition history
         i. Date feedings initiated, formula versus human milk, nipple versus gavage, feeding tolerance, complications
         ii. Parenteral nutrition support, use of hyperalimentation, peripheral versus central vascular access
      e. Review of systems and clinical findings
         i. Dysmorphic features, which may suggest a genetic syndrome
         ii. Skin, including rashes, birthmarks, scars, or jaundice
         iii. Head, ears, eyes, nose, and throat, including:
            a. High arched palate caused by oral intubation
            b. Nostril distortion caused by feeding tube

c. Head circumference—appropriate head growth (as well as weight gain and linear growth) is associated with neurodevelopmental outcome (Skinner & Narchi, 2021).
d. Head shape may be transiently distorted as a consequence of NICU care practices that create positional deformities such as dolichocephaly (Billimoria, 2014).

iv. Chest and thorax, including character of respirations, respiratory rate, and shape and contour of the thorax; findings may include:
   a. Hyperexpansion caused by air trapping
   b. Tachypnea caused by chronic hypoxia
   c. Hypercarbia
v. Cardiovascular, including presence of murmurs; perfusion; and quality of pulses
vi. Abdomen and rectum, including stool pattern, distention, and inguinal or umbilical hernias
vii. Genitourinary, including voiding pattern
viii. Musculoskeletal, including symmetry of movements, strength, and tone
ix. Neurobehavioral, including activity, tone, state regulation, and tremulousness
x. Immune, including immunizations received before discharge
   a. Follow AAP and CDC recommendations for dosing by chronologic age.
xi. Supportive data from relevant diagnostic tests, including:
   a. Results of neonatal screen (phenylketonuria, sickle cell, and congenital hypothyroidism screening mandated in all states)
   b. Hearing screening
   c. Vision screening
   d. Developmental screening
   e. Laboratory studies, including baseline blood gas, oxygen saturation, electrolytes
   f. Imaging studies, including most recent chest radiograph, cranial ultrasound, or other cranial imaging study

B. Objective
1. Physical examination findings
   a. Establish a growth trend, including comparative measurements of head circumference, weight, and length, from birth. Plot and adjust for gestational age until 2 years of age.
   b. Thorough physical examination, including vital signs.
   c. For accurate assessment of postnatal growth, it is essential to take into account size at birth (**Table 2-1**) and use growth charts corrected for gestational age.
   d. The Fenton growth chart available at http://peditools.org/fenton2013/ is most commonly used in the NICU and remains appropriate until the infant reaches 50 weeks' postmenstrual age. Beyond that age, the World Health Organization chart is recommended for all infants (Billimoria, 2014).
2. Observation of parent–child interactions, including holding, comforting, responsiveness, confidence, and mutual support
3. Laboratory studies as clinically indicated, such as blood gas, electrolytes, or complete blood count
4. Chest radiograph as clinically indicated

Table 2-1 Birth-Weight Classifications

Extremely Low Birth Weight (ELBW)	Very Low Birth Weight (VLBW)	Low Birth Weight (LBW)
<1,000 g at birth	<1,500 g at birth	<2,500 g at birth

Data from Cutland, C. L., Lackritz, E. M., Mallett-Moore, T., Bardaji, A., Chandrasekaran, R., Lahariya, C., Nisar, M. I., Tapia, M. D., Pathirana, J., Kochhar, S., Munoz, F. M., & The Brighton Collaboration Low Birth Weight Working Group. (2017). Low birth weight: Case definitions & guidelines for data collection, analysis, and presentation of maternal immunization safety data. Vaccine, 35(48-A), 6492-6500.

III. Assessment
A. *Determine the diagnosis.*
Determine patient's current health status and identify general health risks based on gender, age, and other factors based on unconscious bias or systemic racism.
B. *Severity*
Assess the severity of illness, as indicated.
C. *Motivation and ability*
Determine family willingness to understand and comply with the treatment plan.

IV. Goals of clinical management
A. *Screening or diagnosing*
Choose a practical, cost-effective approach to screening and diagnosis while abiding by mandated screening protocols. Post-NICU infants need careful, ongoing assessment related to neurobehavioral and growth risks, and individualized screening based on clinical findings.
B. *Treatment*
Select a treatment plan that optimizes growth and development, is individualized for the caregiver and child, and maximizes caregiver acceptance.

V. Plan
A. *Screening*
Elicit a thorough history and perform a thorough physical examination, including growth and developmental assessment, at all visits.
B. *Diagnostic tests*
If not already performed before discharge, these should include:
1. Newborn screen as required by individual state
2. Hearing screen
3. Vision screen
4. Developmental assessment, often done by referral to a specified neonatal follow-up clinic facility. Premature

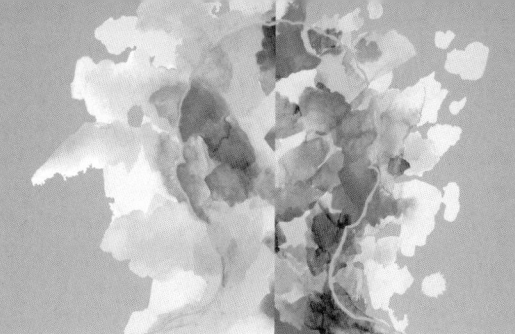

CHAPTER 3

0 to 3 Years of Age Interval Visit

Pallavi Parthasarathy Sheth

I. Introduction and general background

The pediatric health visit at 0–3 years of age involves assessing a wide range of physical and developmental growth. Infants go through dramatic physical growth while constantly developing gross and fine-motor, language, and social skills that allow them to respond to their environment. As infants reach early childhood, their physical growth slows as they begin an intense exploration of their environment (Hockenberry et al., 2016). This patient population requires additional consideration at each visit due to their developmental and physical diversity.

Health maintenance is a mutual goal for the patient and healthcare provider at each well-child visit and is aimed at potentiating the patient's state of well-being. During periodic well-child visits, growth and development are assessed, an update on changes to the caregiver's health and psychosocial stressors is performed and documented, relevant medical and family histories are updated, a complete history and review of systems is obtained, a thorough and age-appropriate physical examination is performed, potential physical and mental health risks are identified, and social determinants of health such as food and housing insecurities are assessed.

Infants and children may adjust optimally to a healthcare provider if they are first given the opportunity to observe the interaction between the examiner and their parent or caregiver during the parent interview (Duderstadt, 2019). During this time, respecting the child's personal space and avoiding eye contact may help them become comfortable before the physical examination. The physical examination of infants and children aged 0–3 years requires a different approach than for other age groups because they do not consistently respond to verbal instruction and developmentally may have stranger anxiety. Indirect examination can be a useful strategy in this age group. Breathing patterns; skin characteristics; symmetry of movement; musculoskeletal integrity; and gross-motor, fine-motor, and communication skills are examples of assessments that can be performed noninvasively. Encouraging the parent to actively participate by undressing the child, moving or gently holding body parts to aid in the provider's examination, or placing the stethoscope on the chest can also help to reduce a younger child's anxiety. Infants up to 6 months of age can usually be examined on the examining table, whereas infants older than 6 months and in early childhood may feel more comfortable being examined in their parent's lap (Duderstadt, 2019). Instead of a head-to-toe examination, a more system-focused approach may be necessary with some patients. For example, auscultation and palpation for pulses can be completed first in infants before they become more active or upset and uncomfortable as the examination proceeds.

In addition to assessing the child, it is also important to observe the parent–child interaction (Duderstadt, 2019). This interaction can give the provider clues to the parent–child dynamic, which is an important element of the health assessment. Once the physical examination is completed, counseling and anticipatory guidance are provided in the areas of physical, behavioral, and emotional development.

The healthcare provider should make every effort to address health disparities related to race or ethnicity during the pediatric health visit. It is important to consider the family's language and literacy barriers, cultural identity, beliefs and values, use of alternative or integrative health practices, and social history when conducting the pediatric health visit (Duderstadt, 2019). Providers should also be cognizant of stressors that a caregiver may be experiencing when caring for a child with special needs. For children with special needs, promoting self-empowerment and self-esteem and maximizing development and function are also important considerations (Duderstadt, 2019).

Given the increasing need for and frequent barriers to accessing behavioral and mental health services, the pediatric health visit can provide an important opportunity to integrate behavioral health into the care of vulnerable children and families. Routine screening for trauma and other behavioral and developmental challenges may be an effective early intervention strategy to identify and support families before they require more complex care (Sala-Hamrick et al., 2021). If a provider chooses to use one of the standard adverse childhood experience (ACE) screeners, they should exercise extreme care, caution, and discretion to avoid triggering retraumatization of the child and/or caregiver.

In addition to screening for risks, it is imperative that the healthcare provider simultaneously screen for positive family experiences and relationships that build resilience and protect children from the effects of trauma. The pediatric provider should build an understanding of a family's strengths, resources, and experiences during the health visit and subsequently encourage the family to identify and build on these protective factors. (California Early Start, 2014). Uplifting families' strengths can also allow caregivers to actively participate in creating and prioritizing solutions (Boynton-Jarrett & Flacks, 2018). Active listening, recognition of the effects of trauma, and strategies that families can use in the home should be implemented and discussed, in partnership with the primary care provider and available behavioral health providers.

The pediatric health visit can certainly be a venue to refer and connect children and families exposed to trauma to essential behavioral health services in the community. However, the thought of identifying family needs without having the ability to connect families to appropriate support or resources can be daunting for a pediatric provider. A clinical environment where all staff members have the appropriate training, knowledge, and skills to support families with trauma would allow providers to develop a safe and trusting relationship with their patients and families and provide optimal trauma-informed care (Sala-Hamrick et al., 2021)

II. Database (may include, but is not limited to)
A. *Subjective*
   1. Parental concerns
   2. Screening and risk assessment: A periodicity schedule for preventive pediatric health care and screening is available through the American Academy of Pediatrics (AAP) at https://downloads.aap.org/AAP/PDF/periodicity_schedule.pdf.
      a. COVID-19 screening
      b. Tuberculosis (TB)
         i. Administer validated questions to determine risk of latent TB. Consult local public health department screening guidelines.
      c. Tobacco/smoke exposure (Hagan et al., 2017)
         i. Assess use of cigarettes or e-cigarettes of household members.
         ii. Assess motivation of identified smokers to stop smoking.
      d. Travel screening can help assess risk for communicable diseases.
      e. Blood pressure (Hagan et al., 2017)
         i. Selective screening for children younger than 3 years with risk factors
            1. History of prematurity, very low birth weight, or other complication requiring intensive care
            2. Congenital heart disease (repaired or nonrepaired)
            3. Renal or urinary tract infection, renal disease, or urological malformations
            4. Solid-organ or bone marrow transplant
            5. Malignancy
            6. Treatment with medications known to elevate blood pressure
            7. Signs of increased intracranial pressure
         ii. Routine measurement of blood pressure at the 3-year visit
      f. Hearing (Hagan et al., 2017)
         i. Assessment of parental concern regarding hearing, speech, language, or developmental delay
         ii. Assessment of risk factors for hearing impairment
            At each health visit, children should be monitored for auditory skills, middle ear status, and developmental milestones.
            1. Failed newborn hearing screen
            2. Family history of permanent childhood hearing loss
            3. Maternal history of in utero infections
            4. Neonatal intensive care unit (NICU) stay of >5 days or postnatal course significant for history of requirement of extracorporeal membrane oxygenation (ECMO), assisted ventilation, exposure to ototoxic medications or loop diuretics, hyperbilirubinemia requiring exchange transfusion, or postnatal culture-positive infections associated with sensorineural hearing loss
            5. Child with craniofacial anomalies, including those that involve external and internal structures of the ear, physical findings associated with a syndrome known to include hearing loss, neurodegenerative disorders, head trauma, or current or past history of chemotherapy treatment
      g. Vision (Hagan et al., 2017)
         i. Assess ocular history and/or parental concern for:
            1. External appearance of eyes
            2. Difficulty with near or distance vision
            3. Crossed eyes

4. Eyelid drooping or asymmetrical eyelid closure
5. Eye injury
ii. Consider family history of eye disorders, history of genetic disorders, syndromes or complex medical problems, or early childhood use of glasses in parents or siblings of child.
iii. Direct assessment of visual acuity in early childhood to comply with vision screening test (AAP, 2021)

h. Anemia (Hagan et al., 2017)
 i. Risk assessment screening at 4, 15, 18, 24, 30, and 36 months of age
  1. At 4 months, risk assessment includes history of prematurity, low birth weight, use of formula not adequately fortified with iron, and early introduction of cow's milk.
  2. After 1 year, risk assessment includes special health needs, food insecurity, and a diet low in iron.

i. Oral health (American Academy of Pediatric Dentistry [AAPD], 2016)
 i. Review of parental oral health
 ii. Assessment of social/biological caries risk factors; protective factors against caries, including application of fluoride varnish in the primary care setting; and other common oral conditions in newborns and infants
 iii. Caries risk assessment tool available at http://www.aapd.org/media/Policies_Guidelines/G_CariesRiskAssessment.pdf

j. Lead (Hagan et al., 2017)
 i. Review state and local recommendations for lead risk assessment (e.g., https://www.cdc.gov/nceh/lead/programs/default.htm)
 ii. Inhabitation or visitation of a home or childcare facility with an identified lead hazard or a home built before 1960 that is in poor repair or was renovated in the past 6 months
 iii. Immigrant and refugee children 6 months of age and older

k. Dyslipidemia (Hagan et al., 2017)
 i. Selective screening for risk factors at age 2
  1. Parent, grandparent, aunt or uncle, or sibling with myocardial infarction, angina, stroke, or coronary artery bypass graft/stent/angioplasty at <55 years in males and <65 years in females
  2. Parent with total cholesterol >240 mg/dL or known dyslipidemia
  3. Child has diabetes, hypertension, or total body weight >95%.
  4. Child has moderate- or high-risk medical condition (organ transplant, systemic lupus erythematosus, nephrotic syndrome, protease inhibitor treatment).

3. Interval history (if new patient, include birth, patient and family medical history, and review of symptoms)
 a. Type, duration, and frequency of illness since last visit
 b. Trauma, surgery, emergency department visits or hospitalizations since last visit
 c. Medications, alternative (nonpharmacological) treatments, complementary therapies
 d. Status of chronic illness management or specialty care

4. Immunizations
 a. Review childhood immunization status (see http://www.cdc.gov/vaccines/schedules/).
 b. Influenza and COVID-19 immunization status

5. Family and social history
 a. Changes from previous visit, including new stressors
 b. Family planning
 c. Emotional support
 d. Means of financial support
  i. Food and housing stability
 e. Childcare arrangements
 f. Peer or social interactions, including siblings, other children, adults, and parents
 g. Home safety (presence of firearms, storage of medications/cleaning products, infant safety locks, working fire alarm, carbon monoxide monitor)

6. Review of systems
Birthing parent's obstetric and prenatal history (medical and social), birth history, neonatal history (including congenital anomalies, chronic health conditions, and hospitalizations), and family medical history are important elements of the review of symptoms for this age group (Duderstadt, 2019).
 a. Skin: birth skin trauma, skin tags, dimples, cysts, extra digits, birthmarks, hair, nails, diapering habits, clothing habits, behavioral history related to potential skin trauma, rashes, eczema, skin allergies
 b. Head: head growth, head trauma
 c. Eyes: focusing, eye discharge or swelling, infant history of being shaken, visual alignment and tracking, vision concerns, abnormal head positioning
 d. Ears: newborn hearing screening results, infant response to sound, infant vocalization, and history of recurrent otitis media or middle ear effusion
 e. Nose, mouth, and throat: frequent nasal congestion, runny nose, nasal allergy, difficulty sucking, feeding or swallowing, mouth sores or lesions, tooth eruption, breastfeeding, bottle use,

sucking on finger or pacifier, mouthing habits, language acquisition, childcare attendance, oral health and dental care
  f. Respiratory: frequent coughs or colds, respiratory distress, nasal flaring, retractions, tachypnea, wheezing, history of reactive airway disease or asthma, secondhand smoke exposure, childcare attendance
  g. Cardiovascular: heart murmur, cyanosis, failure to thrive, tachycardia
  h. Gastrointestinal: stooling and voiding patterns, vomiting or reflux, weight gain, linear growth pattern, constipation, toilet-training status, rectal bleeding
  i. Genitourinary: urinary stream, urinary tract infections, voiding pattern, dysuria, hematuria, testes descended, vaginal discharge
  j. Skeletal: gross and fine motor milestones, toe-walking, deformities, gait, bowing of legs, in-toeing, injuries or trauma
  k. Neurologic: difficulty feeding, tongue thrust, developmental milestones, toe-walking, hand dominance, feeds self, poor coordination, seizures, staring spells, loss of consciousness, speech development, muscle tone
  l. Lymph and endocrine: newborn screening results, weight gain, linear growth pattern, lymphadenopathy
7. Activities of daily living
  a. Nutrition
    i. Milk
      1. Type: human milk, donor human milk, iron-fortified formula, cow's milk, alternative formula/milk product
      2. Amount in 24 hours
      3. Method: breast/chest feeding, bottle (held or propped), cup
    ii. Type, amount, and frequency of solid foods
    iii. Self-feeding: use of fingers or utensils
    iv. Meal routine: number of meals per day, where eaten and with whom
    v. Vitamins, iron, dietary supplements
  b. Oral health (AAPD, 2016)
    i. Brushing and flossing (frequency, consistency, with or without assistance of parent)
    ii. Use of fluoridated toothpaste
    iii. Established and routine care at a pediatric dental home
  c. Sleep patterns
    i. Daytime and nighttime sleeping: hours and routine
    ii. Sleep training, bedtime resistance
    iii. Sleep location, co-sleeping, crib, separate bed, own room
    iv. Sleep positioning
    v. Nightmares and night terrors
  d. Elimination pattern and, if age appropriate, toilet-training history
  e. Developmental and behavioral surveillance and screening (Lipkin et al., 2020)
    i. Surveillance
      1. Parental concerns
      2. History of developmental milestones
      3. Observation of parent–child interaction
      4. Identification of risk and protective factors
    ii. Behavioral health screening
      a. Standardized screening tests
        1. 9 months: vision, hearing, motor skills, communication skills, Ages and Stages Questionnaire (ASQ; https://agesandstages.com/free-resources/)
        2. 18 months: motor skills, communication and language skills, autism spectrum disorder screen with M-CHAT (https://www.m-chat.org/), ASQ
        3. 24 months: motor, language, and cognitive skills; repeat autism screening with M-CHAT
        4. 30 months: motor, language, and cognitive skills; ASQ
        5. Consider an ASQ Social–Emotional, 2nd edition (ASQ:SE-2) screening once annually to screen for self-regulation, compliance, adaptive functioning, autonomy, affect, social communication, and interaction with people in the first 6 years of life.
    iii. Standardized developmental screening tools (see Chapter 8, Developmental Assessment: Screening for Developmental Delay and Autism)
  f. Age-related behavioral/developmental issues
    i. Crying
    ii. Temper tantrums
    iii. Head banging/body rocking
    iv. Pacifier use
    v. Thumb sucking, mouthing habits
    vi. Stranger anxiety
    vii. Approach to discipline/limit setting
    viii. Play, screen time
B. Objective
  1. Physical examination (Duderstadt, 2019)
    a. Obtain height, weight, and head circumference through 36 months of age.
    b. The Centers for Disease Control and Prevention (CDC) recommends that healthcare providers:
      i. Use the World Health Organization (WHO) growth charts (https://www.cdc.gov/growthcharts/who_charts.htm#The%20WHO%20Growth%20Charts) to monitor

growth for infants and children ages 0 to 2 years of age in the United States.
ii. Use the CDC growth charts (https://www.cdc.gov/growthcharts/clinical_charts.htm) to monitor growth for children age 2 years and older in the United States
c. Vital signs and pain assessment: heart rate, respirations, temperature, blood pressure (in children who are at risk or have chronic conditions), pain score, and O_2 saturation when indicated
d. General appearance: state of alertness, nutrition
e. Skin: hydration, rashes, birthmarks, dimpling, pits, nevi, scars, bruises, signs of trauma
f. Head: head shape, anterior fontanel size (palpate for swelling), sutures, condition of hair and scalp
g. Eyes: eyelids, discharge, subconjunctival hemorrhage, reactivity of pupils, corneal light reflex, red reflex, focus and follow, cover–uncover test (perform with infant sitting in parent's lap beginning at 9 months to 1 year of age), strabismus, nystagmus (Biousse & Newman, 2012)
h. Ears: external ear, external canal, tympanic membranes, pneumatic otoscopy, cerumen, presence of foreign body
i. Nose: patency, discharge, turbinates, deviated septum, presence of foreign body
j. Mouth and throat: presence and number of teeth, caries, occlusion status, tonsillar development
k. Neck: supple, rigid, palpation for lymph nodes
l. Chest: work of breathing, quality of lung sounds, chest wall shape, symmetry, breast swelling in infants
m. Heart: rhythm, quality of heart sounds, presence of murmur, gallop or click, pulses, precordium, perfusion, color
n. Abdomen: presence and quality of bowel sounds in all four quadrants, umbilicus, palpation for liver and spleen edge, palpation for abdominal mass, tenderness, or fecal impaction
o. Genitalia
i. Assigned sex at birth
1. Assigned male: general appearance of penis, presence and location of urethral meatus, circumcision healing in newborn, foreskin retraction if uncircumcised, palpation for testes in scrotum, inguinal canal, anus
2. Assigned female: appearance of perineum, clitoris, vaginal introitus, hymen, labial adhesion, vulvitis, discharge, anus
p. Musculoskeletal: muscle strength, range of motion of joints, inspection of extremities, spine, Ortolani and Barlow maneuvers for infants
q. Neurologic: motor function, symmetry, muscle tone, primitive reflexes, postural reflexes, gait, language, social development

III. Assessment
A. *Identify the child's general health risks based on age, gender, ethnicity, family history, medical history, and social determinants of health.*
B. *Determine the child's current health status.*
C. *Determine parent's or caregiver's motivation to promote and maintain positive health behaviors.*
D. *Assess the child's developmental milestones and ability to accomplish and master skills.*
E. *Assess the parent's and child's need for behavioral health support and socioeconomic support.*

IV. Plan
A. *Diagnostics (Hagan et al., 2017)*
A periodicity schedule for preventive pediatric secondary prevention tests is available through the AAP at https://downloads.aap.org/AAP/PDF/periodicity_schedule.pdf.
1. Tuberculosis
a. Tuberculin skin test (TST) for children infected with human immunodeficiency virus (HIV) or any children with risk factors
2. Anemia (AAP, 2021)
a. Hemoglobin or hematocrit at 12 and 24 months of age and at interim visits from 0 to 3 years of age for any child with risk factors
3. Lead
a. The Committee on Practice and Ambulatory Medicine, Bright Futures Periodicity Schedule Workgroup (2021) recommends universal blood lead screening at 12 months of age.
i. Routine screening is mandated in many states at 12 months and 2 years of age; interval lead screening is recommended for areas with a high prevalence of elevated blood lead levels or history of environmental risks.
b. Universal screening is also recommended for recent immigrants, refugees, foster children, or adopted children.
4. Dyslipidemia
a. Routine measurement of full fasting lipid profile twice with results averaged for any child with risk factors
B. *Treatment and referrals*
1. Immunizations appropriate for age are available at http://www.cdc.gov/vaccines/schedules/ or the CDC Vaccine Schedules mobile app available for download at https://www.cdc.gov/vaccines/schedules/hcp/schedule-app.html
2. Vitamin D supplementation for breastfed infants and any child who is taking less than 32 oz of vitamin D–fortified formula or milk per day (Simon & Ahrens, 2020)
3. Hearing
a. If an infant fails their newborn hearing screen, they should be referred for an audiological evaluation before 3 months of age (Yoeli & Nicklas, 2021).

b. If the child does not pass the speech–language portion of the global screening, or there is a physician or parental concern, the child should be referred to an audiologist and a speech and language pathologist for further evaluation.
c. All children with a risk factor for hearing loss should be referred for an audiological assessment at least once by 24 to 30 months of age (Hagan et. al., 2017).
4. Vision
a. All children with a risk factor for visual impairment or physical exam finding concerning for an ocular anomaly should be referred for an ophthalmological assessment (Hagan et al., 2017).
5. Oral health (AAPD, 2016)
a. Fluoride varnish application to the teeth of all infants and children at least once every 6 months and every 3 months for children at elevated risk of caries
b. Fluoride supplementation (if not consuming optimally fluoridated water)
c. Referral to dental home for routine dental visits by 12 months of age
6. Other specialty referral based on history of present illness, physical exam findings, and/or diagnostic test results
7. Referral for resources for food, housing, items for infants, childcare/preschool enrollment, school issues, transportation, employment, utilities, legal services, parenting resources

C. *Counseling, education, and anticipatory guidance*
1. Counseling and education regarding presenting concerns
2. Review of growth chart and physical exam findings in discussing age-appropriate growth and physiologic development
3. Age-appropriate nutritional counseling
4. Diapering, genital hygiene, and toilet training
5. Oral health (AAPD, 2016)
a. Caries prevention education
6. Anticipatory guidance on developmental milestones
a. Counseling on discipline and limit setting
7. Safety and injury prevention appropriate to age and developmental stage. Caregivers can access a comprehensive "Home Safety Checklist" can be found at https://kidshealth.org/en/parents/household-checklist.html.
8. Tobacco/smoke exposure (Hagan et al., 2017)
a. Counsel on keeping places where the child spends time free of tobacco, smoke, and vapor from e-cigarettes.
b. Advise that smokers change clothes and wash hands prior to contact with child.
c. Offer smoking cessation resources.
9. Dyslipidemia (Stewart et al., 2020)
a. Discuss lifestyle modification of diet and exercise as first-line therapies for preventing and treating hyperlipidemia in this age group.
10. Immunizations
a. Review vaccines being administered, risks/benefits, and possible reactions to obtain informed consent.
b. Review options for pharmacological treatment of fever or pain after immunization.

D. *Optimal parent outcomes*
At the end of a pediatric health visit, a parent should feel confident that all concerns about their child(ren) have been addressed. They should be well informed about any screening tests, treatments, or immunizations being administered to their child. Parents should leave the health visit with adequate knowledge of providing age-appropriate nutrition, sleep, oral and physical hygiene, developmental stimulation, and safety for their child. They should also be supported in meeting their family's social–emotional needs through community resources and referrals.

References

American Academy of Pediatric Dentistry. (2016). *Guideline on perinatal and infant oral health care*. http://www.aapd.org/media/Policies_Guidelines/G_InfantOralHealthCare.pdf

American Academy of Pediatrics. (2021). *Recommendations for pediatric preventive health care*. https://downloads.aap.org/AAP/PDF/periodicity_schedule.pdf

Biousse, V., & Newman, N. J. (2012). Cover-uncover test. [Illustration]. In *Neuro-ophthalmology illustrated* (2nd ed.). Thieme Medical Publishers. https://neuro-ophthalmology.stanford.edu/2018/03/noi13-diplopia-2-assessment/

Boynton-Jarrett, R., & Flacks, J. (2018). *Strengths-based approaches to screening families for health-related social needs in the healthcare setting*. https://cssp.org/resource/strengths-based-approaches-screening-families-final/

California Early Start. (2014). *Assessment of family Strengths and needs*. https://www.ceitan-earlystart.org/wp-content/uploads/es_family-assessment_standalone_v14.pdf

Centers for Disease Control and Prevention. (2021). *CDC's childhood lead poisoning prevention program*. http://www.cdc.gov/nceh/lead/about/program.htm

Committee on Practice and Ambulatory Medicine, Bright Futures Periodicity Schedule Workgroup. (2021). 2021 Recommendations for preventive pediatric health care. *Pediatrics*, 147(3):e2020049776. doi:10.1542/peds.2020-049776

Duderstadt, K. G. (Ed.). (2019). *Pediatric physical examination: An illustrated handbook* (3rd ed.). Elsevier.

Hagan, J. F., Shaw, J. S., & Duncan, P. M. (Eds.). (2017). *Bright futures: Guidelines for health supervision of infants, children, and adolescents* (4th ed.). American Academy of Pediatrics.

Hockenberry, M. J., Wilson, D. W., & Rogers, C. (2016). Communication and physical assessment of the child. *Wong's nursing care of infants and children* (10th ed.). Mosby.

Lipkin, P. H., Macias, M. M., Council on Children with Disabilities Section on Developmental and Behavioral Pediatrics. (2020). Promoting optimal development: Identifying infants and young children with developmental disorders through developmental surveillance and screening. *Pediatrics, 145*(1), 1–19. doi:10.1542/peds.2019-3449

Sala-Hamrick, K. J., Isakson, B., De Gonzalez, S. D. C., Cooper, A., Buchan J., Aceves, J., Van Orton, E., Holtz, J., & Waggoner, D. M. (2021). Trauma-informed pediatric primary care: Facilitators and challenges to the implementation process. *Journal of Behavioral Health Services and Research, 48*(3), 363–381. doi:10.1007/s11414-020-09741-1

Simon, A. E., & Ahrens, K. A. (2020). Adherence to vitamin D intake guidelines in the United States. *Pediatrics, 145*(6), e20193574. doi:10.1542/peds.2019-3574

Stewart, J., McCallin, T., Martinez, J., Chacko, S., & Yusuf, S. (2020). Hyperlipidemia. *Pediatrics in Review, 41*(8), 393–402. doi:10.1542/pir.2019-0053

Yoeli, J. K., & Nicklas, D. (2021). Hearing screening in pediatric primary care. *Pediatrics in Review, 42*(5), 275–277. doi:10.1542/pir.2020-000901

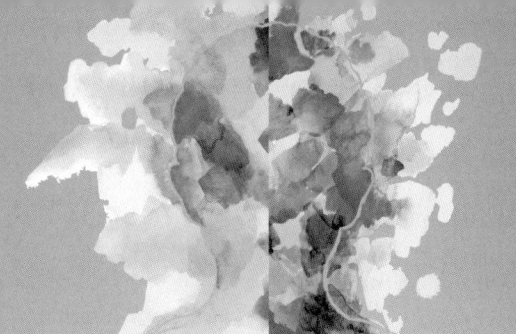

CHAPTER 4

3 to 6 Years of Age Interval Visit

Mary Anne M. Israel

I. Introduction and general background

Health supervision and well-child visits are opportunities for the healthcare provider to assess a child's foundation for optimal physical and emotional well-being, including nutrition, sleep, social–emotional and intellectual development, and secure emotional attachments. It also offers an opportunity to address risks and barriers to the child's individual thriving and to evaluate for and support positive parenting strategies and skills that promote wellness in the child and family system. Furthermore, the provider needs to address disease detection and prevention and offer proper anticipatory guidance during the visit (Turner, 2018).

The approach to early childhood during the well-child visit is twofold: although most of the history may still be provided by the parent or caretaker, children at this age may now participate in some of the interview and actively engage with the provider. Careful observation of their behavior in the examination room is also useful, including their interaction with the parent or caretaker, the environment, and the provider (Duderstadt, 2014). Healthcare maintenance visits in this age range include comprehensive history, physical examination, screening tests (as appropriate), immunizations, anticipatory guidance, counseling on a yearly basis, and follow-up as needed.

II. Database (may include but is not limited to)

A. *Subjective*
  1. Parental and child concerns (chief complaint)
     a. History of present illness
  2. Interval history
     a. Changes in health status
     b. Consultations with specialists since last well-check visit, including treatments
     c. Visits to urgent care or the emergency department
  3. Past medical history
     a. Birth history
     b. Trauma, surgeries, or hospitalizations
     c. Dental home: date of last examination (if any); caries or dental work
     d. History of COVID-19
  4. Medication (include homeopathic or herbal supplements and vitamins)
  5. Allergies (medication, environmental, and food)
     a. Type of reaction (anaphylactic, urticaria, gastrointestinal [GI])
  6. Immunization status
  7. Family history
  8. Social history (American Academy of Family Physicians [AAFP], 2018)
     a. Language spoken at home
     b. Family and household members
     c. Daycare, preschool, or school attendance
     d. Means of financial support, food insecurity
     e. Adverse childhood events
  9. Environmental health history (National Environmental Education Foundation, 2015)
     a. Indoor exposures: smoke, mold, cockroaches, rodents, damp walls, strong odors, broken windows, lead exposure, and parental occupation
     b. Outdoor exposures: sun, industrial smokestack, and housing proximity to heavy traffic
  10. Nutrition/Higher body weight prevention (American Academy of Pediatrics [AAP], 2021
      a. Foods—intake of fruits, vegetables, lean meat/beans and other protein sources, iron-rich foods, whole grains; calcium sources: milk, cheese, and yogurt; and juice and water intake (source of water and fluoride)
      b. Eating habits, mealtime behavior, and family meals

c. Amount of time spent in physical play each day
d. Amount of screen time per day
e. Supplements such as vitamin D, probiotics, fish oil, multivitamin
11. Elimination
    a. Potty training process and status; voiding habits
    b. Stooling patterns and consistency
12. Sleep (quality and quantity): bedtime routine
13. Developmental (see Chapter 8: Developmental Assessment: Screening for Developmental Delay and Autism); evaluate overall school readiness
    a. Social–emotional: self-care skills, typical play, emotional regulation and description of self, sharing
    b. Language (expressive and receptive)
        i. 3-year-old: speech is approximately 75% clear, three-word sentences, intelligible by strangers, tells stories, uses comparisons
        ii. 4-year-old: four-word sentences, 100% intelligible to strangers, tells story from a book (Hagan et al., 2017)
        iii. 5- to 6-year-old: communicates easily to adults and children, long and imaginative stories, enjoys listening to stories, and has full comprehension of age-appropriate language
    c. Cognitive
        i. 3- to 4-year-old: repeats two numbers, imaginative play, eats independently (Duderstadt, 2019)
        ii. 5- to 6-year-old: increases memory capacity, follows directions, able to listen and attend, advances pretend play
    d. Physical (gross motor and fine motor)
        i. 3-year-old: builds tower of cubes, throws ball overhand, rides tricycle, walks upstairs, draws, toilet-training progress
        ii. 4-year-old: hops on one foot; balances for 2 seconds; climbs stairs alternating feet without support; copies cross; dresses and undresses with minimal assistance; pours, cuts, and mashes own food
        iii. 5- to 6-year-old: balances on one foot, hops and skips, ties a knot, grasps a pencil, draws a person with at least six body parts, recognizes letters and numbers, copies squares and triangles, dresses and undresses without assistance
14. Review of systems
    a. General
    b. Skin, hair, and nails: birthmarks, rashes
    c. Head–eyes–ears–nose–throat: headaches; ocular history (vision, eyes straight, eyelid droop, eye injury, allergies); hearing and history of otitis media; nasal congestion, allergies, snoring, and nosebleeds; oral health, dental hygiene; sore throats and difficulty swallowing
    d. Chest and lungs: history of asthma or reactive airway disease, croup, bronchitis, or persistent cough
    e. Cardiac and heart: history of heart murmur, cyanosis, shortness of breath, and energy level
    f. Abdomen and gastrointestinal: appetite, diet, abdominal pain, constipation, vomiting, and diarrhea
    g. Genitourinary: incontinence if potty trained, urinary tract infections, dysuria, frequency, hematuria, vaginal discharge, and phimosis or balanitis
    h. Musculoskeletal: deformities, limb pains, injuries, and orthopedic appliances
    i. Neurologic: seizures, fainting spells, loss of consciousness, concussion, inattention, learning difficulties, headache, and gait
    j. Endocrine: recent weight gain or loss and linear growth patterns

B. Objective
1. Physical examination
    a. Weight, height, and BMI
    b. Pulse, respiratory rate, and blood pressure
    c. General: state of alertness and quality of interaction with parent and staff
    d. Skin, hair, and nails: hydration, rashes, birthmarks, scars, nail and hair health, and infestations (lice and scabies)
    e. Head–eyes–ears–nose–throat: symmetry of head; external inspection of eyes and lids, extraocular movement assessment, pupil examination, red light reflex examination, corneal light reflex, cover–uncover examination, ophthalmoscopic examination of optic nerve and retinal vessels (in 5- and 6-year-olds); tympanic membrane description and mobility; nasal septal deviation, nasal discharge, and turbinate status; dental condition, dental caries, gingival inflammation, and malocclusion; throat and tonsils
    f. Neck: supple, presence of palpable lymph nodes
    g. Chest and lungs: symmetry of chest, auscultation of lungs
    h. Cardiac and heart: rhythm, rate, murmur, gallop, click, pulses, and capillary refill time
    i. Abdomen: liver, spleen, masses, palpable stool, and bowel sounds
    j. Genitalia
        i. Assigned male at birth: circumcision or retractable foreskin, meatus midline, testes descended bilaterally
        ii. Assigned female at birth: inspect urethra, vaginal introitus, labial condition
    k. Musculoskeletal: muscle strength; range of motion; inspection of spine, back, and gait
    l. Neurologic: cranial nerves II–XII; deep tendon reflexes; symmetry, tone, gait, strength; observation of fine- and gross-motor skills
    m. Developmental: assessment of language acquisition, speech fluency, and clarity; thought content and ability to understand abstract thinking

III. Assessment
A. *Summary of health, growth, and development*
   1. Identify general health risks related to age, past medical history, systemic racism, and social determinants of health (SDOH).
   2. Determine caregiver's personal strengths and motivation, as well as structural barriers to promoting and maintaining positive health behaviors.
   3. Identify patient ability and needs to achieve optimal well-being for age.

IV. Plan
A. *Screening (AAP screening recommendations can be found at https://www.aap.org/en-us/documents/periodicity_schedule.pdf)*
   1. Vision screening
   2. Audiometric screening
   3. Lead screening and risk assessment
   4. Anemia screening and risk assessment: Those at high risk and children with diet low in iron, with limited access to food, and/or with special needs should have screening labs.
   5. Tuberculosis screening and risk assessment
   6. Dyslipidemia screening and risk assessment
   7. Hypertension
   8. Blood pressure based on age and height
   9. Developmental screening and surveillance
   10. Psychosocial assessment
B. *Treatment*
   1. Immunizations appropriate for ages 3–6 years old are available at http://www.cdc.gov/vaccines/schedules/hcp/imz/child-adolescent.html (CDC, 2022).
   2. COVID-19 vaccination as recommended for 3–6 years old
   3. Influenza vaccination annually as recommended
   4. Oral fluoride (if primary water source is deficient in fluoride)
   5. Iron supplementation: Consider for children not meeting dietary iron requirements through foods (American Family Physician, 2016).
   6. Vitamin D supplementation (National Institutes of Health, Office of Dietary Supplements, 2021)
C. *Anticipatory guidance and family education*
   1. Address child and parental or caregiver concerns
   2. Family support and routine
      a. Parent-led decisions and guidance related to sleep, nutrition, screen time and safety, sibling rivalry, work balance, and discipline methods
      b. Temperament
   3. Reading literacy and comprehension, speech and language skills
   4. Peers
      a. Interactive games, play opportunities, social interactions, and taking turns
   5. School readiness
      a. Preschool: structured learning experiences; friends; socialization; and able to express feelings of joy, anger, sadness, fear, and frustration
      b. Kindergarten and elementary school: establishment of routine, after-school care and activities, parent–teacher communication, friends, bullying, maturity, management of disappointments, and fears
   6. Physical activity
      a. Limit screen time (television, computer, mobile device) to no more than 2 hours per day of appropriate programming; no television in child's room; no electronics during mealtime.
      b. Encourage physical activity throughout the day; for 3- to 5-year-olds, 60 minutes of physical activity per day is recommended (Centers for Disease Control and Prevention [CDC], 2019).
   7. Personal health habits
      a. Daily routines, including bedtime routine
      b. Oral health: daily brushing and flossing, adequate fluoride intake
      c. Discuss proper nutrition for age: well-balanced diet, breakfast every day, five servings of fruits and vegetables per day, increased whole-grain consumption, 2 cups of milk or equivalent calcium intake per day, 3–4 oz protein daily—lean meat/beans/soy; limited high-fat and low-nutrient foods and drinks
   8. Safety
      a. Car safety: seat or booster. Toddlers and preschoolers: forward-facing convertibles or forward facing with harness (up to highest weight or height allowed by car seat manufacturer). School-age-children: belt-positioning booster seats from the time they outgrow forward-facing seats for most children through at least 8 years of age (Durbin et al., 2018).
      b. Street safety, falls from windows, outdoor safety, swimming safety, smoke detectors and carbon monoxide detectors, and guns and other weapons in the home
      c. Stranger safety: Reinforce rules about talking with and going with strangers if approached.
      d. Sexual abuse prevention: establishing healthy boundaries, reviewing inappropriate touch, and fostering healthy sexual development (National Sexual Violence Resource Center, 2020)
D. *Expected outcomes*
   1. Reassure and educate parents and child about health concerns.
   2. Promote optimal health for children and their families.
   3. Promote family support and acceptable discipline approach.
   4. Promote social development.
   5. Encourage literacy activities.
   6. Empower parents to provide healthy eating habits and encourage physical activity; limit amount of screen time.
   7. Promote safety parameters.
   8. Support school readiness.

E. Consultation and referral
   1. Dental home if not already established
   2. Further developmental testing if indicated
   3. Subspecialty referral if indicated
F. Resources for families
   1. Healthy Children (AAP): http://www.healthychildren.org (includes special section on preschoolers in "Ages and Stages"; in English and Spanish)
   2. Kids Health (Nemours Center for Child Health Media): http://www.kidshealth.org
   3. Bright Futures for Families: http://www.brightfuturesforfamilies.org
G. Resources for providers
   1. National Association of Pediatric Nurse Practitioners: https://www.napnap.org
   2. AAP: https://www.aap.org
   3. Bright Futures: http://www.brightfutures.org

References

American Academy of Pediatrics. (2021). *Bright Futures: Recommendations for preventive pediatric health care.* http://www.publications.aap.org

Centers for Disease Control and Prevention. (2019). *Physical activity recommendations for different age groups.* http://www.cdc.gov/physicalactivity

Centers for Disease Control and Prevention. (2022). *Child & adolescent immunization schedule: Recommendations for Ages 18 years or younger, United States, 2022.* https://www.cdc.gov/vaccines/schedules/hcp/imz/child-adolescent.html

Duderstadt, K. (2014). Approach to care and assessment of children & adolescents. In K. Duderstadt (Ed.), *Pediatric physical examination: An illustrated handbook* (2nd ed., pp. 1–8). Elsevier.

Durbin, D. R., Hoffman, B. D., Council on Injury, Violence, and Poison Prevention, Argan, P. F., Denny, S. A. Hirssh, M., Johnston, B., Lee, J. K., Monroe, K., Schaechter, J., Tenebein, M., Zonfrillo, M. R., & Quinlan, K. (2018). Child passenger safety. *Pediatrics,* 142(5), e20182460. doi:10.1542/peds.2018-2460

Hagan, J. F. Jr., Shaw, J. S., & Duncan, P. M. (Eds.). (2017). *Bright Futures pocket guide* (4th ed.). American Academy of Pediatrics.

National Environmental Education Foundation. (2015). *Pediatric environmental history form.* http://neefusa.org

National Institutes of Health, Office of Dietary Supplements. (2021). *Vitamin D: Fact sheet for health professionals.* http://ods.od.nih.gov

National Sexual Violence Resource Center. (2020). *Preventing child sexual abuse: Resources.* https://nsvrc.org

Turner, K. (2018). *Well-child visits for infants and young children.* American Academy of Family Physicians. http://aafp.org/afp/2018/0915/p.347.html

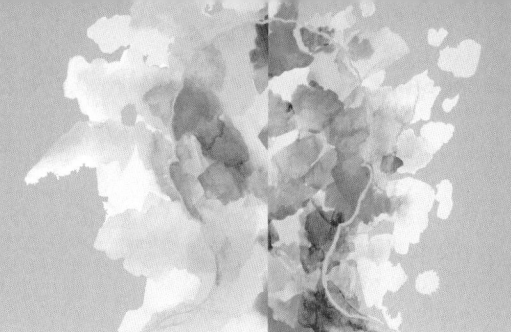

CHAPTER 5

6 to 11 Years of Age Interval Visit

Bridget Ward Gramkowski

I. Introduction and general background

Children in middle childhood spend less than half as much time with their parents as they did in early childhood. Although parents are still the most important influence in their child's emotional and physical development, teachers and peers become increasingly important as the child approaches adolescence. Children in middle childhood have their own identities and sense of self; for example, their gender identity is established by the age of 4 years (Mayo Clinic, 2022). Using inclusive language throughout the visit both supports parental communication and increases the participation of the child in the visit. These early patterns of openness promote opportunities for questions and shared decision making in their health.

During annual well-child visits, clinical data are collected from both a detailed history and a complete "head-to-toe" physical examination. Throughout the pediatric lifespan, clinicians will continue to use appropriate evidence-based screening tools. "School performance remains a functional marker of a child's development and accomplishments" (Hagan et al., 2017, p. 677). Opportunities for mastery and early identification of learning issues are critical to promoting self-esteem and academic success; student work habits at the age of 6 have been correlated to career and academic attainment at age 26 (Simpkins et al., 2020). Screening at well-child visits should include assessing for adverse childhood experiences (ACEs) and social determinats of health (SDOH). Children with greater ACE exposure before the age of 5 are more likely to have both externalizing and internalizing behaviors and have an increased likelihood of attention-deficit/hyperactivity disorder (ADHD) diagnosis in middle childhood (Hunt et al., 2017). The influence of media in middle childhood continues to increase, with "screen time" for children ages 6–8 years averaging roughly 3 hours a day. Additionally, we see different exposures to screen time within populations, with children living in families with higher incomes or higher parental education levels having less overall screen time (Common Sense Media, 2017).

In terms of physical growth, children in middle childhood have very steady growth that should continue to track on appropriate growth curves. Roughly, children grow 2.5 inches and increase weight by 4–7 pounds a year (Hagan et al., 2017). The timing of puberty varies widely and is known to be influenced by gender, health, genetics, hormones, and nutrition. Children with certain conditions or genetic syndromes should use a growth chart specific to their diagnosis; for example, there are growth charts for children with trisomy 21, Turner syndrome, Marfan syndrome, and Achondroplasia (Duran et al., 2019).

Promoting health equity comes hand in hand with the well-child exam. Middle childhood continues to be influenced by all the SDOH that affect the child's family, including healthcare access and quality, school access and quality, neighborhoods and social communities, and economic stability (Centers for Disease Control and Prevention [CDC], 2021). These powerful forces that affect health should be assessed at least annually at every well-child visit. Combining our goals for health maintenance with a partnership within our communities to address health disparities is essential to reducing health disparities across the life span. Finally, as the global pandemic continues to have a unique and disproportionate impact on children, we as clinicians will need to continuously monitor and support their needs as they evolve.

II. Database (may include but is not limited to the following elements) (Hagan et al., 2017)

A. *Subjective*
  1. Parent and child concerns
  2. Interval history
     a. Frequency and type of illness since last visit

b. Chronic illnesses: current status, treatment plan, any pending referrals or barriers to care
c. Medications, including supplements such as melatonin
d. Trauma, hospitalizations, or emergency room visits
e. Dental care status
f. History of COVID-19
3. Immunization status: View the American Academy of Pediatrics (AAP) periodicity schedule online for vaccination completion and catch-up scheduling.
4. Family and social history
   a. Changes from previous visit: SDOH, emotional support, means of financial support/parental employment status, childcare arrangements, changes to family medical history, and impact of the pandemic
   b. Sibling rivalry, parental stress, living arrangements, and childcare
   c. Safety: Screen for domestic violence, sexual abuse, substance abuse, neighborhood safety, school bullying, and internet use, as well as access to medicines, drugs, or weapons.
   d. Environmental risk factors: cigarette smoke, sun exposure, pollution, lead, and allergens
5. Developmental and behavioral history
   a. Problems or concerns
   b. Appraisal of coping styles: anxiety, anger, frustration, fear, and happiness
   c. Interaction with peers, teachers, adults, and family
   d. Amount and type of screen time per day and per week, supervised versus alone, academic versus entertainment purposes
   e. Child's strengths and self-esteem
   f. Child's socialization skills and peer activities
   g. Parent's approach to gender identity, sexuality, and pubertal development
   h. Exposure to ACEs
6. Activities of daily living
   a. Nutrition
      i. Calcium: type and amount in 24 hours
      ii. Meal routine: 24- to 48-hour dietary recall; number of meals per day, at home and at school; frequency and type of snacks, family meals, eating or snacking while watching TV
      iii. Attitude toward body image and food
      iv. Intake of sugar-sweetened beverages, intake of caffeinated beverages
      v. Fast-food or snack-food frequency and type
   b. Physical activity: frequency, type, duration, and safety
   c. Sleep patterns
      i. Amount of sleep, scheduled bedtime, sleep hygiene (routines and sleep-promoting habits), sleep environment (co-sleeping, devices in room)
      ii. Sleepwalking
      iii. Teeth grinding, snoring, apnea, and daytime sleepiness
      iv. Nocturnal enuresis
      v. Nightmares
   d. School
      i. Name of school, teacher, and grade; new or continuing at previous year's school
      ii. Scholastic achievement or grades, other areas of achievement, changes in performance, attention concerns
      iii. Attitude toward school and teachers, favorite subject, and future goals
      iv. Peer relationships
      v. School attendance and participation in activities
      vi. Reading, writing skills (have child demonstrate)
      vii. Additional school support: learning differences, disabilities, and delays; individual educational plan (IEP) or special education classes
7. Review of systems
   a. Constitutional: fatigue, unusual weight loss or gain, temperature sensitivity, pattern of growth, and pubescence (time and pattern)
   b. Skin: birthmarks, rashes, texture, problems with hair, and acne
   c. Head–eyes–ears–nose–throat (HEENT): headaches, head injuries, vision, corrective lenses or glasses, hearing, history of otitis media or effusion, nasal allergies, frequent colds, snoring, nosebleeds, loss or change of smell, dental hygiene, dentist visit, orthodontics, difficulty swallowing, hoarseness, and sore throats
   d. Respiratory: reactive airway disease or asthma, bronchitis, persistent cough, and cough at night or with exercise
   e. Cardiovascular: heart murmur, cyanosis, shortness of breath, syncope, chest pain, and change in energy level
   f. Gastrointestinal: appetite, food restriction, weight gain or loss, abdominal pain, vomiting, and diarrhea or constipation
   g. Genitourinary: polydipsia or polyuria, enuresis, urinary tract infection, dysuria, frequency, hematuria, penile discharge, vaginal discharge, and menstrual history
   h. Musculoskeletal: deformities, scoliosis, limb pains, injuries, orthopedic appliances, and linear growth
   i. Endocrine: heat or cold intolerance, disturbance in growth, polyphagia, and thyroid disease
   j. Hematologic: easy bruising, difficulty stopping bleeds, and fevers
   k. Neurologic: involuntary abnormal movements, concussion, loss of consciousness, headaches, changes in gait, and cognitive disorders

l. Lymph: lymphadenopathy, enlarged tonsils or adenoids, or enlarged spleen
m. Psychiatric/Behavioral: changes in mood, behavior, or learning (loss, regression, or arrest of milestones)

B. *Objective*
1. Physical examination
   a. Height, weight, and BMI—using appropriate chart from CDC growth charts (http://www.cdc.gov/growthcharts/charts.htm)
   b. Vital signs and pain assessment: blood pressure, heart rate, pulse, and respirations; pain score
   c. Vision/Hearing: AAP periodicity screening guidelines
   d. General appearance: state of health and alertness, mood
   e. Skin: hydration, lesions or rashes, acne, scars, nevi, and birthmarks. Assess for bruising and/or signs of nonaccidental trauma (NAD).
   f. Head: hair growth and distribution, asymmetry
   g. Eyes: reactivity of pupils, red reflexes, fundus, extraocular movements, and cover–uncover test
   h. Ears: tympanic membrane description and mobility, cerumen, and external canal
   i. Nose: presence or absence of discharge, color of turbinates, and swelling
   j. Mouth: number of teeth, caries, occlusion, orthodontics, and lesions
   k. Neck: palpable nodes and presence of nuchal rigidity
   l. Chest: presence of rhonchi, coarseness, wheeze, or diminished breath sounds in lung fields; breast development (females) with Tanner stage
   m. Cardiac: rate, rhythm, pulses; presence of murmur, gallop, or click
   n. Abdomen: palpable organs, masses, tenderness, and guarding
   o. Genitalia: Tanner stage; circumcision, foreskin retractability, and testes (designated male at birth); general description of vaginal introitus, clitoris, labia (designated female at birth), again with Tanner stage
   p. Musculoskeletal: muscle strength, range of motion, and scoliosis
   q. Neurologic: mental status examination; cerebellar testing; sensory, motor (fine and gross) status; deep tendon reflexes; and cranial nerves II–XII, may include CN I (olfactory) if concerns in history

III. Assessment
A. *Determine the child's current health status.*
B. *Identify the child's general health risks.*
C. *Determine child and caregiver's motivation and access to resources to promote and maintain positive health behaviors.*
D. *Delineate the child's ability to accomplish and master milestones of middle childhood.*

IV. Plan
A. *Diagnostics (screening and secondary prevention tests)*
The periodicity schedule for preventive pediatric health care is updated annually by the AAP and is available online via the AAP website.
1. Hearing risk assessment: auditory skills monitoring annually or if indicated by parental or teacher concerns
2. Vision screen: Assess for defects in visual acuity annually or if indicated by parental or teacher concerns.
3. Oral health screening
   a. Assessment for caries, gingival health, and orthodontic needs.
   b. Recommend routine dental visit every 6 months.
4. Lead poisoning: for known communities at risk, including individuals who have recently immigrated, adoptees from other countries, and children between ages 6 months and 16 years who are refugees
5. Tuberculosis (TB) risk assessment annually
6. Dyslipidemia risk assessment at ages 2, 4, 6, and annually after 8 years
   a. Screen once between ages 9 and 11, regardless of risk factors (AAP, 2021).
7. Depression screening as indicated based on history

B. *Therapeutics and treatments*
1. Immunizations appropriate for age are available at http://www.cdc.gov/vaccines/schedules/.
2. Oral fluoride supplementation (if primary water source is deficient in fluoride)
3. Vitamin D supplementation: Consider for all children 6 to 11 years of age

C. *Patient and family education (Box 5-1)*
1. Discussion of parent and child concerns
2. Discussion of nutritional requirements, sleep, physical activities appropriate for age, and both supervision and limitation of entertainment screen time
3. Child–parent discussion of safety: personal safety, helmet use, car (booster seats, seatbelts), protective sports and recreational equipment, water safety, and pedestrian safety; exposure to bullying through school, texting, or social media
4. Discussion of approaches to discipline within the family
5. Discussion of middle childhood needs for peer interaction and socialization
6. Discussion of child adjustment to classroom and school setting
7. Discussion of opportunities for skill mastery and self-esteem building
8. Ages 8–11 years: discussions of child's pubertal development, diversity of gender identity, hygiene, and body image
9. Discussion of child's relationship with peers, school, and family

D. *Expected child–parent outcomes*
1. Anticipatory guidance and reassurance when indicted in relation to parent and child's concerns

Box 5-1 Safety, Nutrition, and Activity Guidelines for Your School-Aged Child

- ***Teach*** your child to think carefully about his or her surroundings, particularly around new animals or people. Review the use of 911 and what to do if a child gets lost or separated. Model safe habits, such as seat-belt use, and instruct your child to use a booster or seat belt as recommended by the AAP for age and weight.
- ***Prepare and practice*** for emergency situations in the home, such as a fire or natural disaster. Make sure you have a planned reunification point (a school, firehouse, and so forth) in the event of a catastrophe. Have emergency supplies for at least 3 days. Have an emergency "go bag" with essential items in case you are forced to leave home quickly. Include in the bag any medical needs, emergency instructions, and contact information. Instruct all your caregivers regarding the emergency plan and location of the go bag.
- ***Media access and use*** should be closely monitored. Use should be supervised, and parents should review clear limits and enact parental controls on media as indicated.
- ***Nutrition*** (U.S. Department of Agriculture, 2021):
  - ***Try whole grains:*** whole-wheat bread, oatmeal, brown rice
  - ***Eat more fruit and veggies:*** Make half of your plate fruits and vegetables every day.
  - ***Think about your drink:*** Choose water or fat-free milk.
  - ***Mix up your protein foods:*** Include different foods like seafood, beans, lentils, nuts, eggs, meats, or poultry.
  - ***Get involved:*** Help out by putting away groceries, stirring ingredients, peeling fruits, assembling salads, or setting the table.
- ***Activity*** (CDC, 2021):
  - ***Get 60 minutes or more EVERY day!***
  - ***Get vigorous exercise*** at least 3 days a week. Examples of this include outdoor activities, such as running, bicycle riding, jumping rope, or swimming, and organized sports, including soccer, basketball, baseball, tennis, martial arts, and gymnastics.
  - ***Strengthen muscles*** at least 3 days a week. Strength training examples include throwing, hitting or kicking a ball, and using outdoor recreational equipment.
  - ***Strengthen bones*** at least 3 days a week. Some examples of bone-strengthening activities include hopscotch, hopping, skipping, jumping, and jumping rope.
  - ***Recreational activities*** should always be supervised, and full protective sports gear should be used. Helmets should be used with any wheeled devices.
    - ***Review setting and device-specific safety:***
      - *Traffic and pedestrian safety*
      - Vehicle safety: bicycle, scooter, skateboard, and motorized devices
      - Water safety: swim lessons; pool, river, ice, and ocean safety
  - ***Chronic conditions:*** These may influence or require additional support for certain activities; the child's interests should be encouraged and accommodations made following the Americans With Disabilities Act.
  - ***Sleep for children ages 6–12 years*** (AAP, 2016): minimum of 9 hours and maximum of 12 hours

2. Nutrition and physical activity: Understands nutritional and physical activity recommendations appropriate for age
3. Safety measures understood
4. Discipline and behavior: Parents agree on an approach to discipline and implement it with consistency; address any behavioral problems in home and school settings.
5. Developmental needs: Parental understanding of child's need for peer interaction, socialization, and opportunities for skill mastery
6. Education: Parents assess child's performance in school and adjustment to current teacher/class; address parental concerns and provide anticipatory guidance.
7. Sexuality: Developmentally appropriate discussion and anticipatory guidance on pubertal developmental stages, body image, and diversity of gender identity
8. Ages 8–11 years: Encourage child able to verbalize "body concerns" and understanding of puberty in the presence of a trusted adult.

References

American Academy of Pediatrics. (2016). *AAP endorses new recommendations on sleep times.* https://publications.aap.org/aapnews/news/6630

American Academy of Pediatrics. (2021). 2021 recommendations for pediatric preventive healthcare. *Pediatrics, 147*(3), e2020049776. doi:10.1542/peds.2020-049776

Centers for Disease Control and Prevention. (2021). *How much physical activity do children need?* http://www.cdc.gov/physical-activity/everyone/guidelines/children.html

Common Sense Media. (2017). *Common Sense Media Census: Media use by kids age zero to eight.* https://www.commonsensemedia.org/sites/default/files/uploads/research/csm_zerotoeight_fullreport_release_2.pdf

Duran, I., Martakis, K., Stark, C., Ballmann, M., Hamacher, S., Schoenau, E., Semler, O., & Hellmich, M. (2019). Suitability of growth standards for growth monitoring in children with genetic diseases. *Anthropologischer Anzeiger; Bericht uber die biologisch-anthropologische Literatur, 76*(1), 15–28. doi:10.1127/anthranz/2019/0932

Hagan, J. F., Shaw, J. S., & Duncan, P. M. (Eds.). (2017). *Bright Futures: Guidelines for health supervision of infants, children, and adolescents* (4th ed.). American Academy of Pediatrics.

Hunt, T., Slack, K. S., & Berger, L. M. (2017). Adverse childhood experiences and behavioral problems in middle childhood. *Child Abuse & Neglect, 67*, 391–402. doi:10.1016/j.chiabu.2016.11.005

Mayo Clinic. (2022). *Children and gender identity.* https://www.mayoclinic.org/healthy-lifestyle/childrens-health/in-depth/children-and-gender-identity/art-20266811

Simpkins, S. D., Tulagan, N., Lee, G., Ma, T. L., Zarrett, N., & Vandell, D. L. (2020). Children's developing work habits from middle childhood to early adolescence: Cascading effects for academic outcomes in adolescence and adulthood. *Developmental Psychology, 56*(12), 2281–2292. doi:10.1037/dev0001113

U.S. Department of Agriculture, Food and Nutrition Service. (2021). *MyPlate: Life stages: Kids.* https://www.myplate.gov/life-stages/kids

CHAPTER 6

The Adolescent and Young Adult (12–26 Years of Age) Interval Visit

Lisa Mihaly and Erica Monasterio

I. Introduction and general background
A. *Developmental considerations*
   Adolescence, generally considered to encompass ages 12–21, is a time of enormous development and change in all domains of a young person's and a family's life. Bridging and overlapping childhood and young adulthood, adolescents experience the physical changes of growth and sexual maturation; continued developmental changes in both the structure and function of their brains (a process not completed until the mid- to late 20s); and cognitive, psychological, and social changes related to both their physical changes and the roles and expectations of the culture and society in which they live.
B. *Adolescent consent and confidentiality*
   1. For the healthcare provider, the care of the adolescent may also be a time of transition because the relationship between the youth and the provider becomes central (Neinstein et al., 2016). The provider must develop an alliance with the youth, and addressing issues of confidentiality is the cornerstone of this alliance. Without assurances of confidentiality, many youth will not disclose important concerns to their providers or may avoid care altogether. This is especially true for the most vulnerable youth in need of attention and intervention—those who engage in behaviors that present a risk to their health; those who are depressed, anxious, or suicidal; and those who report poor communication and lack of perceived support from their parents or caregivers (Neinstein et al., 2016). For these reasons, providers seeing adolescents should be prepared to spend time in the visit with both the adolescent and adult together and with the adolescent alone to get a full picture of the youth's strengths, risks, and overall physical and psychological health status (Neinstein et al., 2016).
   2. Although the involvement and participation of a caring adult in the provision of adolescent services are desirable, there are situations in which a young person may not feel able to involve an adult or in which adult involvement could impair the youth's ability to seek or receive services. All states give adolescents some rights to both consent to care and maintain privacy related to care for confidential issues (Pathak & Chou, 2019). Laws vary significantly from state to state, as do the services to which youth can independently consent; therefore, healthcare providers should familiarize themselves with consent and confidentiality laws for minors in their state.
   3. Effective communication with youth and their caregivers about adolescent consent and confidentiality rights (and limitations) is essential to establishing rapport, eliciting pertinent information, and providing appropriate care. At the beginning of healthcare encounters (whether in person or telehealth), a brief discussion of adolescent consent and confidentiality with youths and adults, emphasizing the benefit of developing self-reliance and skills to manage their own health care, helps to set the stage. Assuring the parent or caregiver that youth are always encouraged to communicate with adults and that their presence and participation are valued helps reassure them that they are not being "shut out" of their child's care. Additionally, it is important for youths to become more familiar with their own past

health history and their family history as they transition into becoming the main source of their own health information. Both adults and youths should be informed of the conditional nature of adolescent confidentiality rights, given provider obligations to break confidentiality in the event that youth pose a danger to themselves or others or have been subjected to any reportable abuse. Once alone with the adolescent, it is helpful for the provider to confirm the youth's understanding of conditional confidentiality and explain the personal nature of the questions that will be asked.

C. *Rationale for the psychosocial assessment*
  1. The leading causes of morbidity and mortality in adolescents (accidents, homicides, and suicides) are rooted in behavioral risk that the astute provider can identify and in which they can attempt to intervene (Centers for Disease Control and Prevention [CDC], 2020). For this reason, the major consensus guidelines focused on the care of adolescents (*Guidelines for Adolescent Preventative Services* from the American Medical Association and *Bright Futures* from the American Academy of Pediatrics [AAP]) concur that a psychosocial assessment, focused to determine the strengths and risks of the youth and guide the physical and psychological assessment and intervention process, is recommended (Alderman & Breuner, 2019; Hagan et al., 2017).

D. *Periodicity and focus of well-adolescent care*
  1. Yearly well-adolescent visits are recommended, with an emphasis on prevention, education, and counseling for both youth and their adults, screening for risk behaviors and their consequences, and counseling on healthy lifestyles. *Healthy People 2030* identified critical objectives for youth, focusing on the social determinants of adolescent health, including reproductive health care; increased safety of lesbian, gay, bisexual, and transgender (LGBT) youth; healthy development; school completion; injury and violence prevention; mental health; substance abuse; sexual health; and prevention of chronic diseases of adulthood (Office of Disease Prevention and Health Promotion, 2020).
  2. According to *Bright Futures*, priority areas to address in the well-adolescent visit include the following (Hagen et al., 2017):
     a. Physical growth and development (physical and oral health, body image, healthy eating, and physical activity)
     b. Social and academic competence (connectedness with family, peers, and community; interpersonal relationships; and school performance)
     c. Emotional well-being (coping, mood regulation, and mental health)
     d. Sexuality and sexual health
     e. Risk reduction (tobacco, alcohol, or other drugs; pregnancy; and sexually transmitted infections [STIs])
     f. Violence and injury prevention (safety belt and helmet use, driving and substance abuse, guns, interpersonal violence [dating violence], and bullying)

II. **Database** (may include but is not limited to)
A. *Subjective (to be obtained with both the youth and parent or caregiver present)*
  1. Patient and parent or caregiver concerns
  2. Past medical history
     a. Congenital or chronic conditions, including mental health diagnoses
     b. Surgery or hospitalizations
     c. Accidents or injuries, including injuries in sports that have required exclusion from play and head injuries resulting in loss of consciousness and/or concussions
  3. Medications inclusive of over-the-counter and complementary and alternative medications
     a. Drug, dose, prescriber, and medication adherence
     b. Revisit topic of medications once alone with the youth to determine if they are using any medications to treat or suppress STIs or to prevent pregnancy
  4. Dental
     a. Last dental visit
  5. Communicable diseases
     a. Varicella (documented disease or vaccination)
     b. Hepatitis (travel to or recent emigrant from endemic areas, perinatal acquisition)
     c. Exposure to tuberculosis
     d. STIs (discussed confidentially)
  6. Immunizations
     a. Completion of childhood immunizations if necessary
     b. Initiation or completion of adolescent immunizations—current schedule available at http://www.cdc.gov/vaccines/schedules/
  7. Allergies
     a. Food allergies or intolerances
     b. Drug reactions
  8. Family history
     a. First-degree relatives with a history of
        i. Hypertension
        ii. Hyperlipidemia
        iii. Cardiovascular disease
        iv. Sudden cardiac or unexplained death
        v. Cerebrovascular accidents
        vi. Seizure disorder
        vii. Diabetes
        viii. Cancer
        ix. Mental health diagnoses
        x. Substance abuse
        xi. Other medical or mental health problems

B. *Subjective history (to be obtained only with the youth)*
The psychosocial history, obtained after the adult has left the exam room, must be adapted to the age, developmental stage, and interactive style of the adolescent.

The mnemonic HEEADDSSS (for Home, Education/employment, Eating, Activities, Drugs, Diet, Sexuality, Suicide/depression/Self-image, and Safety) provides a flexible tool for guiding a discussion with an adolescent about the protective and risk factors in their lives (Klein et al., 2014). A slight variation of that approach, SSHADESS (for Strengths, School, Home, Activities, Drugs/substance use, Emotions/depression, Sexuality, and Safety) ensures that the provider starts with a focus on strengths that can then be built on in the context of the assessment and counseling (Ginsburg, 2007).

1. Home
    a. Where do you live?
    b. Whom do you live with?
    c. How is the stress level where you live?
    d. Connectedness and engagement with and monitoring by parents or caregiver
2. Education and employment
    a. School attendance
    b. School achievement (grades)
    c. School experience and connectedness to school (including direct queries about bullying)
    d. Concerns about school
    e. Attitude toward school
    f. Work: type of work and how many hours
    g. Goals: academic and beyond
3. Eating
    a. Body image
    b. Recent changes in weight
    c. Nutritional intake
    d. Eating patterns
    e. Family meals
    f. Dieting and weight control
4. Activities
    a. Peers: relationship quality (friends and/or romantic and sexual partners)
    b. Peer relationships
    c. Outside interests
    d. Amount of daily screen time, especially social media
5. Drugs and alcohol
    a. Tobacco, alcohol, and drug use (quantify frequency, intensity, patterns, and context of use)
    b. Family and friends' substance use patterns
6. Sexuality
    a. Information appropriate for age
    b. Attracted to same, opposite, or all genders
    c. Romantic/sexual relationships
    d. Sexual behavior
        i. Age of sexual debut
        ii. Number of partners (if relevant)
        iii. Genders of partners
        iv. Contraception type and frequency of use
        v. Partner support or resistance to pregnancy and STI prevention efforts
        vi. Protected or unprotected sex
        vii. Comfort and satisfaction with sexual activity
        viii. History of/risk for STIs
7. Suicide and depression
    a. Mood or energy level
    b. Stress and coping
    c. Depression and/or anxiety
    d. Self-harm
    e. Suicidal thoughts or suicide attempts
    f. History of mental health services or experience with counseling
8. Safety
    a. Use of seat belts; riding in or driving a car under the influence
    b. Use of protective equipment for sports activities
    c. Sense of safety, experienced bullying or violence, or history of abuse in the following:
        i. Home
        ii. School and/or work (including being a target of or witnessing bullying)
        iii. Relationships (peer and romantic)
        iv. Community

C. Review of systems
1. General health: fatigue, fever, weight change, appetite change, mood change, and sleep problems
2. Skin: lesions, rashes, and acne
3. Hematology: excessive bleeding, bruising, and lymphadenopathy
4. Head–ears–eyes–noes–throat (HEENT): headaches, head injuries, vision problems, need for or current glasses, ear pain, decreased hearing, allergies, frequent colds, snoring, dental hygiene, last dentist visit, difficulty swallowing, hoarseness, or sore throats
5. Respiratory: asthma, frequent colds or cough, wheezing, shortness of breath, and exercise-induced cough or wheezing
6. Cardiovascular: chest pain, palpitations, syncope or near syncope, and shortness of breath on exertion
7. Gastrointestinal: abdominal pain, nausea, vomiting, diarrhea, constipation, and bloody stool
8. Genitourinary: enuresis, dysuria, frequency, hematuria, unusual vaginal discharge, urethral discharge, testicular pain, vulvar lesions, and genital lesions
9. Skeletal: joint pain, joint swelling, injuries, and back pain
10. Neurologic: headache, seizures, syncope, dizziness, and numbness
11. Endocrine: polyuria and polydipsia
12. Designated female at birth: menarche, last menstrual period, regularity and frequency, duration, dysmenorrhea, and premenstrual symptoms
13. Designated male at birth: body hair, genital changes, and voice change
14. Psychological and emotional: mood, stress, and emotional or mental health problems or diagnoses

D. Objective
1. Physical examination
    a. Height and weight (measure and plot on growth chart if under 18)—refer to the following link for CDC growth charts: http://www.cdc.gov/growthcharts/data/set1clinical/set1color.pdf.

b. BMI (calculate and plot on graph if under 18): https://www.cdc.gov/growthcharts/index.htm
  c. Blood pressure, pulse, and respiration
  d. Vision (Snellen once in early, middle, and late adolescence—12, 15, and 18 years old; more frequently based on risk assessment)
  e. Hearing screen
  f. Mental status
  g. State of nutrition
  h. Skin: scars, tattoos, piercings, signs of self-injurious behavior, acne, and acanthosis nigricans
  i. Ears
  j. Eyes: include fundoscopic examination
  k. Nose: patency, nasal mucosa, turbinates, septum, piercings
  l. Mouth: teeth (gums, caries, and occlusion), piercings
  m. Pharynx: tonsillar size
  n. Thyroid
  o. Lymph nodes
     i. Cervical
     ii. Axillary
     iii. Inguinal
  p. Breasts: inspect for sexual maturity rating (SMR) or Tanner stage; gynecomastia in patients designated male at birth
  q. Lungs: wheezing and adventitious sounds
  r. Heart: murmurs (upright and supine), rate, rhythm, lower extremity pulses, and radial/femoral pulse delay
  s. Abdomen: masses and hepatosplenomegaly
  t. Genitalia
     i. Assigned male at birth: inspect for SMR, signs of STIs, palpation of scrotum and testes for masses, presence of hernia
     ii. Assigned female at birth: inspect for SMR, signs of STIs and dermatologic conditions of the vulva; use of screening tests for gonorrhea and chlamydia when possible (urine-based test or high vaginal swab)
     iii. Pelvic examination indicated at 21 years of age to obtain first Pap smear, earlier if signs and symptoms of STI, pregnancy, or pelvic infection or to evaluate abnormal pubertal development or abnormal vaginal bleeding
  u. Musculoskeletal
     i. Back: range of motion and presence of scoliosis
     ii. Extremities: strength, joint pain, swelling, and stability; range of motion
     iii. Neurologic: strength, deep tendon reflexes, coordination and gait, cranial nerves II–XII

III. Assessment
A. *Identify the strengths and protective factors that will support the youth and family in successfully negotiating challenges in adolescence.*
B. *Identify the youth's specific health risks, based on structural racism, family history, past medical history, and behavioral choices and activities.*
C. *Determine the youth's current health status.*
D. *Determine the youth's motivation to modify health-damaging behaviors and promote and maintain health-promoting behaviors.*
E. *Determine the parent or caregiver's motivation to support the youth's behavior change as appropriate.*

IV. Plan
A. *Screening* (Hagan et al., 2017)
   1. Psychosocial assessment (annually)
   2. Major depressive disorder screening when systems for diagnosis, treatment, and follow-up are in place, using such tools as the Patient Health Questionnaire for Adolescents or the Beck Depression Inventory–Primary Care Version
   3. Alcohol and drug use risk assessment (annually), with follow-up in-depth assessment based on findings using a youth-specific alcohol and drug screening assessment tool, such as CRAFFT
   4. Hematocrit or hemoglobin as indicated based on risk
   5. Dyslipidemia screening (fasting total cholesterol, low-density lipoprotein [LDL], high-density lipoprotein [HDL], and triglycerides)
      a. 9–11 years: old one screen
      b. 17–21 years old: universal screening once during this time period, more frequently if patient or family elevated risk
   6. Tuberculosis testing based on risk assessment
   7. Chlamydia screening annually for all sexually active females ≤24 years old, men who have sex with men, and other men as clinically indicated (CDC, 2021)
   8. Gonorrhea screening annually for all sexually active females ≤24 years old, young men who have sex with men, and other men as clinically indicated (CDC, 2021)
   9. Syphilis screening for all pregnant women, young men who have sex with men and engage in high-risk sexual behaviors, commercial sex workers, youth who exchange sex for drugs, and youth in adult correctional facilities (CDC, 2021)
   10. HIV screening once for all individuals between 13 and 64 years of age regardless of recognized risk factors (CDC, 2021). Repeat HIV screening should be offered with any new risk.
   11. Cervical cancer screening (Pap smear) for all women at age 21 regardless of sexual history, then every 3 years if normal Pap smear (Melnikow et al., 2018)
B. *Immunization update*
   1. Immunizations for adolescents—current schedule available at https://www.cdc.gov/vaccines/schedules/hcp/imz/child-adolescent.html

C. Anticipatory guidance
 1. Normative development and developmental progression (discuss with youth and parent or caregiver as appropriate)
    a. Adapt to youth's developmental stage, developmental delays, and any concerns of youth or parent or caregiver.
    b. Include counseling regarding physical and psychosocial development.
    c. Address levels of stress in youth and family and discuss healthy coping strategies.
    d. Use an approach that is dynamic, interactive, and inclusive of the youth, prioritizing behaviors that the young person is interested in modifying and developing a plan *with* the youth rather than *for* the youth (Neinstein et al., 2016).
    e. Address parenting issues; emphasize continued importance of parental support as developmentally appropriate.
 2. Nutrition and activity counseling (discuss with youth and parent as appropriate):
    a. Support regular meals and snacks.
    b. Drink adequate fluids; emphasize hydration and limit juice, sports drinks, and caffeinated drinks.
    c. Encourage intake of fruits and vegetables.
    d. Limit high-calorie and low-nutritional-value snacks
    e. Build physical activity into everyday routine and limit screen time.
 3. Safety, injury, and violence prevention counseling as appropriate to age and developmental stage and individual risk
    a. Use of protective gear for sports and leisure activities
    b. Automobile safety
       i. Seat-belt use
       ii. Counseling regarding alcohol and drug use and driving or riding with an impaired driver
    c. Nonviolent conflict resolution
    d. Relationship safety and healthy interactions with romantic and sexual partners
 4. Tobacco, alcohol, and other drug counseling as appropriate to age and developmental stage and individual risk (with youth alone, using a motivational counseling approach)
 5. Sexual health and risk reduction as appropriate to age and developmental stage and individual risk (with youth alone, using a motivational counseling approach)
    a. Relationship quality and sexual decision making
    b. Contraception and pregnancy prevention
       i. Discuss access to emergency contraception with all youth regardless of current sexual activity.
       ii. Counsel regarding contraceptive choice as appropriate to current and anticipated sexual activity, using a patient-centered approach (Dehlendorf et al., 2016).
    c. STI and HIV risk reduction
       i. Discuss risk-reduction approaches with all youth regardless of current sexual activity.

V. Resources
A. *For adolescents*
 1. The Adolescent Health Working Group has resources for youth, providers and parents available at https://ahwg.org/.
 2. The Society for Adolescent Health and Medicine (SAHM) has resources for adolescents and parents available at https://www.adolescenthealth.org/Resources/Resources-for-Adolescents-and-Parents.aspx. Clinical resources are also available for members of SAHM.
B. *For healthcare providers*
 1. *Bright Futures: Guidelines for Health Supervision of Adolescents* (4th ed.), developed by the American Academy of Pediatrics, is available at https://web.p.ebscohost.com/ehost/ebookviewer/ebook/bmxlYmtfXzE0NzE3NzVfX0FO0?sid=e11845ae-a1a3-4a2e-b196-c2656bdbbf77@redis&vid=0&format=EB&rid=1.

References

Alderman, E. M., & Breuner, C. C. (2019). Unique needs of the adolescent. *Pediatrics*, *144*(6), e20193150. doi:10.1542/peds.2019-3150

Centers for Disease Control and Prevention. (2020). *About underlying cause of death*. https://wonder.cdc.gov/controller/saved/D76/D266F033

Centers for Disease Control and Prevention. (2021). *Screening recommendations and considerations referenced in treatment guidelines and original sources*. https://www.cdc.gov/std/treatment-guidelines/screening-recommendations.htm

Dehlendorf, C., Fox, E., Sobel, L., & Borerro, S. (2016). Patient-centered contraceptive counseling: Evidence to inform practice. *Current Obstetrics and Gynecology Reports*, *5*, 55–63. doi:10.1007/s13669-016-0139-1

Ginsburg, K. R. (2007). Viewing our adolescent patients through a positive lens. *Contemporary Pediatrics*, *24*(1), 6–76.

Hagan, J. F., Shaw, J. S., & Duncan, P. M. (Eds.). (2017). *Bright futures*. American Academy of Pediatrics.

Klein, D. A., Goldenring, J. M., & Adelman, W. P. (2014, January 1). HEEADSSS 3.0: The psychosocial interview for adolescents *updated for a new century fueled by media.* Contemporary Pediatrics. http://contemporarypediatrics.modernmedicine.com/contemporary-pediatrics/content/tags/adolescent-medicine/heeadsss-30-psychosocial-interview-adolesce?page=0,2

Melnikow, J., Henderson, J. T., Burda, B. U., Senger, C. A., Durbin, S., & Soulsby, M. A. (2018). *Screening for cervical cancer with high-risk human papillomavirus testing: A systematic evidence review for the U.S. Preventive Services Task Force* [Internet]. Agency for Healthcare Research and Quality. https://www.ncbi.nlm.nih.gov/books/NBK526306/

Neinstein, L. S., Katzman, D., & Callahan, T. (2016). *Neinstein's adolescent and young adult health care: A practical guide* (6th ed.). Lippincott Williams & Wilkins.

Office of Disease Prevention and Health Promotion. (2020). *Healthy people 2030: Adolescent health*. U.S. Department of Health and Human Services. https://health.gov/healthypeople/objectives-and-data/browse-objectives/adolescents

Pathak, P. R., & Chou, A. (2019). Confidential care for adolescents in the U.S. health care system. *Journal of Patient-Centered Research and Reviews*, 6(1), 46–50. doi:10.17294/2330-0698.1656

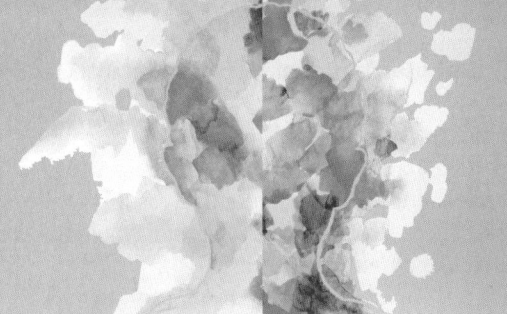

CHAPTER 7

Care of Transgender and Gender Diverse Youth

Meredith Russell

I. Introduction and general background

Compared to cisgender peers, transgender and gender diverse (TGD) youth experience health disparities, with higher rates of affective disorders, suicidal ideation, substance abuse, risky sexual behaviors, sexually transmitted infections, and violence victimization (Becerra-Culqui et al., 2018; Clark et al., 2017; Johns et al., 2019; Perez-Brumer et al., 2017; Reisner et al., 2015; Travers et al., 2012; Vance et al., 2021; Wilson et al., 2017). These health disparities are theorized to result from a combination of social stigmatization and gender dysphoria, which can be ameliorated by access to quality social, psychological, and medical care (Turban et al., 2020; Vance et al., 2014). Strengthening resilience against environmental factors that increase the risk for health disparities includes promoting parental support of gender identity, facilitating social transition to the affirmed gender when desired, and removing the barriers to gender-affirming health care (de Vries et al., 2014; Durwood et al., 2017; Travers et al., 2012; Vance et al., 2021).

Access to gender-affirming medications such as puberty blockers (gonadotropin-releasing hormone agonists) and sex hormones (estradiol or testosterone) is critically important for TGD youth who seek medical transition because delaying medication treatment is associated with increased poor mental health outcomes, whereas facilitating access improves mental health, well-being, and function (de Vries et al., 2011, 2014; T'Sjoen et al., 2019; Turban et al., 2020). However, TGD youth face significant barriers to care due to fear of discrimination and a lack of providers trained to deliver gender-affirming health care within a feasible geographic location (Gridley et al., 2016; Hamnvik et al., 2020; Klein et al., 2018). Therefore, both primary care providers (PCPs) and interdisciplinary clinics with mental health, medical, social, and nursing gender specialists can form a network and use clinical practice guidelines to improve access to care (Coleman et al., 2012; Deutsch, 2016; Hembree et al., 2017; Rafferty et al., 2018).

A. Definition and overview

Approximately 0.6% of adults and 0.7%–1.8% of adolescents in the United States identify as TGD, a term used to describe individuals whose gender identity and/or gender expression differs from their sex designated at birth (Hembree et al., 2017; Johns et al., 2019; Wilson et al., 2017). *Cisgender* is an alternative term for nontransgender persons, and *gender nonbinary* (GNB) encompasses a broad spectrum of gender identities and expressions (Deutsch, 2016). *Gender dysphoria* is a mental health diagnostic label that describes the distress or functional problems experienced by some TGD individuals due to the mismatch between their gender identity and sex designated at birth (American Psychiatric Association, 2013; Hembree et al., 2017). *Gender incongruence* is a sexual health diagnostic label that describes the discrepancy between an individual's gender identity and their designated sex at birth and does not imply pathology or preference for treatment (Klein et al., 2018). Although diagnostic labels are necessary for medical care, including insurance approval of gender-affirming medications, they can be pathologizing and may not reflect an individual's gender experience. Therefore, clinicians should explain the rationale regarding the use of diagnostic labels and use the TGD youth's preferred terminology for gender concepts and sexual characteristics when providing health care.

II. Database (may include but is not limited to)
A. *Subjective*
Ask, record, and use the patient's provided name and pronouns. This helps build trust, improving the therapeutic alliance and likelihood that TGD youth will

seek healthcare services. In addition, consistent use of provided names and pronouns across social contexts (home, school, work, friends) results in decreased depression, suicidal ideation, and suicidal behaviors (Russell et al., 2018; Vance, 2018).

1. Sexual orientation/gender identity (SOGI)
   Ask about and record sexual orientation, gender identity, and primary and secondary sexual characteristics.
2. Gender history
   Determine onset and development of gender identity, age of social transition to affirmed gender, and gender dysphoria symptoms such as discomfort with primary and secondary sexual characteristics or functions such as menses.
   Determine gender expression goals and past experiences with gender expression.
3. Puberty history
   Assess thelarche and menarche in TGD youth with ovaries and gonadarche (testicular volume ≥ 4 mL) in TGD youth with testes, along with any associated increase in gender dysphoria.
4. Pertinent past medical history
   Evaluate pertinent past medical history as outlined in Chapter 6: The Adolescent and Young Adult (12–26 Years of Age) Interval Visit, with a focus on the following additional data:
   a. Medications: emphasis on hormone use (prescribed and nonprescribed); birth control; human immunodeficiency virus (HIV) treatment; or medications that reduce bone mineral density (BMD), such as chronic systemic corticosteroids
   b. Immunization status: emphasis on human papillomavirus (HPV) and hepatitis A and B vaccination
   c. Sexually transmitted infection (STI) history, with emphasis on hepatitis C and HIV risk factors and serology status
   d. Previous medical disorders, with emphasis on a history of low BMD for age or risk of BMD accrual, cardiovascular disease, thromboembolism, metabolic syndrome (higher body weight, diabetes, dyslipidemia, hypertension), or estrogen-sensitive cancer
   e. Nonpharmacologic body modification: breast binders, breast binding or taping, genitalia tucking and/or taping, use of genitalia compression garments such as gaff, and breast or penile prosthesis
   f. Surgeries: emphasis on gender-affirming surgeries, such as masculinizing chest reconstruction, breast augmentation, facial feminization, chondrolaryngoplasty (tracheal shave), or vaginoplasty/phalloplasty surgeries
   g. Other gender-affirming procedures: emphasis on permanent hair removal/reduction and procedures by nonlicensed individuals, such as silicone/filler injections
   h. Psychiatric history: emphasis on history of affective disorders, suicidal ideation or attempts, psychiatric hospitalizations, residential treatment, or intensive outpatient program treatment
   i. Adverse childhood experiences (ACEs): abuse, neglect, and/or household challenges
5. Family history
   Emphasis on cardiovascular disease, thromboembolism, metabolic syndrome (higher body weight, diabetes, dyslipidemia, hypertension), osteoporosis, sex-steroid–sensitive cancer, psychiatric conditions
6. Psychosocial history: HEEADDSSS (for Home, Education/employment, Eating, Activities, Drugs, Diet, Sexuality, Suicide/depression/Self-image, and Safety) assessment, with emphasis on:
   a. Home: housing status, legal guardian status, caregiver and family support for gender
   b. Education/Employment: school attendance, social transition status, school gender support plan, bullying, violence victimization, employment status
   c. Activities: peer support groups, sports participation
   d. Drugs: illicit, nonprescribed hormones; supplements; filler injectables; tobacco or vaporized nicotine
   e. Sexuality: sexual behaviors, family planning, STI prevention and testing, HIV preexposure prophylaxis (HIV PrEP)
   f. Suicide/Depression/Self-Image: depression and suicidal ideation screen
   g. Safety: ACEs
7. Disordered eating screen
   There is a higher incidence of disordered eating in TGD youth compared to the general population, which has been theorized to result from stigma, gender dysphoria, or intentional weight manipulation to affirm gender, including weight loss to achieve menses cessation and breast reduction in transmasculine people or weight gain to achieve breast development in transfeminine people (Avila et al., 2019; Coelho et al., 2019; Watson et al., 2017).
   Screen using a validated tool, such as SCOFF or Eating Disorders Examination Questionnaire (EDE-Q) (Avila et al., 2019; Hautala et al., 2009).

B. Objective
1. Physical examination: Due to a history of gender dysphoria or trauma, TGD youth may experience significant stress from a physical examination. First, establish a trusting provider–patient relationship unless a review of systems indicates the need for an urgent physical exam. Ask permission to do an exam, explain what you would like to examine and why, and allow the patient to express feelings or preferences about the exam. Screening and healthcare maintenance exams are based on current anatomy, regardless of the patient's gender identity (Deutsch, 2016).

a. Ask, record, and use the patient's preferred terms for primary and secondary sexual characteristics.
   b. Vital signs, height, and weight
2. Pubertal examination: With the patient's consent, conduct a pubertal exam to stage endogenous puberty or effects of hormone replacement therapy. For TGD youth designated female at birth, the first physical sign of puberty is breast buds, or sexual maturity rating (SMR) stage 2. The first sign of puberty for youth designated male at birth is testicular growth to 4 mL, or SMR stage 2. Pubic hair, axillary hair, and body odor alone do not reflect gonadarche/puberty and may instead result from adrenarche.
3. Surgery: For patients who have had gender-affirming surgery such as masculinizing chest reconstruction, evaluate pain, wound healing, infection, and edema.
4. Nonsurgical body modification: For assigned male at birth and transgender females who are tucking, screen for skin irritation/infection from taping, inguinal hernia, or urinary tract infection. For individuals assigned female at birth and transgender males who use breast binders, screen for skin irritation/infection and costochondritis.
5. Acne: Examine the skin for acne, which can be caused or exacerbated by testosterone hormone replacement.

III. Assessment

A. *Health status and risk status*

The current risk factors and health status of the patient should be identified, the patient's motivation to change unhealthy habits should be assessed, and the patient's ability to successfully accomplish pediatric developmental milestones should be determined as outlined in Chapter 06.

B. *Pubertal status*

Determine the pubertal stage based on SMR staging of the patient, as well as the impact of the pubertal development on the patient's gender identity (Hembree et al., 2017).

C. *Diagnosis*

The *Diagnostic and Statistical Manual of Mental Disorders* (*DSM*) has diagnostic criteria for gender dysphoria, and the World Health Organization (WHO) *International Classification of Diseases* (*ICD*) has diagnostic codes for gender dysphoria (10th ed. [*ICD-10*]) under the mental and behavioral disorders classification and gender incongruence (11th ed. [*ICD-11*]) under the chapter on conditions relating to sexual health (American Psychiatric Association, 2013; WHO, 2021). Since the DSM classification of gender dysphoria as a mental health disorder can be pathologizing, the reclassification to gender incongruence under by ICD-11 in the conditions related to sexual health chapter better reflects current understanding of gender identity and sexual health.

Gender dysphoria refers to the psychological distress experienced from the incongruence between an individual's sex designated at birth and their gender identity or affirmed gender.

For TGD youth, a mental health provider (MHP) who has training/experience in child and adolescent gender development should make the diagnosis of gender dysphoria/gender incongruence. Providers prescribing hormones and who are involved in the diagnosis and psychosocial assessment should be competent in using the *DSM* and/or *ICD* for diagnosing gender dysphoria/gender incongruence and psychiatric conditions, be able to undertake or refer for appropriate treatment, be able to evaluate the patient's ability to consent to treatment, and regularly attend relevant continuing education (Hembree et al., 2017).

D. *Gender affirmation*
1. Identify the patient's gender expression goals and barriers.
2. Identify the potential benefits and risks of gender-affirming care across the (1) medical domain (hormone therapy, surgery, voice therapy), (2) psychological domain (psychological or psychiatric needs), (3) social domain (social transition), and (4) legal domain (legal name or gender change, school activity participation).

IV. Plan

A. *Diagnostics (screening and secondary prevention tests)*
1. Screening for disease: Screen for diseases and conditions based on the patient's risk profile. When evaluating laboratory values, use the normal reference interval that corresponds to the patient's biologic sex before sex-steroid treatment and reference interval for their gender identity when administering sex-steroid treatment (Hembree et al., 2017). The CDC 2021 publication *STD Treatment Guidelines* includes guidance on how to take a sexual history and the recommended frequency of STIs by gender and risk group; it also include risk assessment of transgender individuals based on current anatomy and sexual behaviors (Workowski et al., 2021). In the United States, transgender individuals are disproportionately affected by HIV infection, and transgender females have a higher HIV prevalence compared to their cisgender peers (Clark et al., 2017). In line with the CDC and U.S. Preventative Services Taskforce (USPSTF) guidelines for all adults, all transgender individuals should be screened at least once for HIV and then as needed based on HIV risk assessment (Deutsch, 2016; Workowski et al., 2021).
2. Healthcare maintenance: similar healthcare maintenance and screening needs as general populations, with emphasis on screening for depression, suicidal ideation, violence victimization, substance abuse, and risky sexual behaviors

V. Treatment

Immunization recommendations are not sex specific. Follow general guidelines for the primary prevention of STIs (vaccination and counseling) in children and adolescents (CDC, 2015).

Gender-affirming health care is the process of affirming gender identity across the social, psychological, legal, and medical domains. An interdisciplinary team of medical and mental healthcare providers should collaborate to meet the needs of TGD youth.

A. *Social gender affirmation*
Social transition and use of the provided name and pronouns

B. *Psychological gender affirmation*
Ensure access to mental health gender specialists, reflect gender identity, mitigate risk, and promote resilience.

C. *Legal gender affirmation*
Legal name and gender change identity documents

D. *Medical gender affirmation*
Pubertal suppression with gonadotropin-releasing hormone agonists (GnRHas)/puberty blockers, amenorrhea induction of TGD youth, sex-steroid treatment, androgen receptor blockade, gender-affirming surgery, and voice therapy

E. *Fertility and family planning*
Discuss fertility preservation (oocyte or sperm cryopreservation) and family planning with TGD youth seeking gender-affirming medical treatment and their guardians prior to initiating puberty suppression or hormone replacement therapy (Bonnington et al., 2020; Hembree et al., 2017). Although GnRHas are reversible, TGD youth who take GnRHa and then sex hormone treatment may experience reduced fertility. Standard fertility preservation options exist for SMR 3 or greater, and experimental fertility preservation for SMR 1 or 2 exists (Rosenthal, 2021).

F. *Gender-affirming medications*
For medication guidelines for hormonal therapy, see **Tables 7-1 to 7-7**. Use the appropriate drug interaction database when prescribing hormone therapy to avoid adverse drug interactions, especially for patients taking HIV treatment medications, antidepressants, and anticonvulsant medications. Gender-affirming hormone medications are used off-label for the diagnosis of gender dysphoria/gender incongruence, and there are brands approved for the pediatric and adult populations.

G. *Prepubertal TGD youth*
Create safe environments at home, school, and in the community to promote healthy growth and development of prepubertal TGD youth. Social transition has been shown to result in positive mental health and self-worth in TGD youth (Durwood et al., 2017). Gender-affirming medications are not indicated in prepubertal children.

H. *Eligibility criteria*
TGD youth are eligible for pubertal suppression with GnRHa if (1) a qualified MHP has diagnosed gender dysphoria/gender incongruence and confirmed that there are no mental health conditions that interfere with the diagnosis or treatment; (2) the prescribing provider has confirmed the onset of puberty ($\geq$SMR 2); the treatment is indicated, and there are no contraindications; and (3) the adolescent and legal guardians have provided informed assent/consent, respectively (including fertility and family planning). TGD youth are eligible for sex-steroid treatment if these criteria are met and the adolescent has reached the age of legal medical consent, which most have by age 16 years. However, guidelines suggest that there may be compelling reasons to begin sex steroids prior to the age of 16 years, such as an increased risk of low bone density for age, inappropriate height, or poor psychosocial function if the development of secondary sexual characteristics is delayed until 16 years of age (Hembree et al., 2017).

I. *Pubertal suppression*
Pubertal suppression with GnRHa can provide more time for gender identity development and the exploration of gender expression options, prevent the development of irreversible secondary sexual characteristics, improve mental health and function, and allow for the use of physiologic doses of sex steroids, which may reduce side effects. Pediatric GnRHas are available in depot formulations of leuprolide acetate (1, 3, or 6 month IM and 6 month SQ), triptorelin (6-month IM) and histrelin acetate subcutaneous (SQ) implant (1-year SQ). Evidence suggests that the SQ implant effectively suppresses puberty for up to 36 months (Deutsch, 2016; Olson-Kennedy et al., 2020). There are also GnRHa forms approved for adults by the U.S. Food and Drug Administration (FDA), including depot leuprolide acetate. The main risks of GnRHa use include reduced bone mineralization, delayed brain maturation, more complex vaginoplasty if started at SMR 2 or 3 in individuals designated male at birth, and reduced fertility if the TGD youth is subsequently treated with sex steroids (Rosenthal, 2021; van de Grift et al., 2020). Evidence demonstrates a reduction in BMD z-scores with GnRHa treatment and an increase with sex-steroid treatment, but peak BMD may be decreased in individuals treated with GnRHas, particularly for TGD youth assigned male at birth (Klink et al., 2015; Lee et al., 2020; Rosenthal, 2021; Stoffers et al., 2019; Vlot et al., 2016). GnRHa decreases linear velocity to the prepubertal rate and delays epiphyseal fusion, prolonging the growth period before final height is achieved in TGD youth with open epiphyses. See **Table 7-1** for forms and adverse reactions and **Table 7-2** for monitoring parameters. If SMR or laboratory monitoring indicates that puberty is inadequately suppressed, the dose of GnRHa can be increased, or the interval between administration can be decreased. GnRHas may be continued until the TGD youth reaches adulthood and has gonadectomy. However, TGD youth assigned male at birth may choose to discontinue them earlier and start an androgen receptor blocker, and TGD youth assigned

female at birth may discontinue GnRHa treatment after reaching adult doses of testosterone therapy because testosterone alone can suppress gonadotropins, estradiol, and menses.

Table 7-1 Gonadotropin-Releasing Hormone Agonists (Puberty Blockers)

GnRHa Form	Potential Adverse Reactions
Pediatric Histrelin acetate (Supprelin LA) 50 mg SQ implant 1 year Leuprolide acetate (Lupron Depot Ped): 7.5 mg, 11.25 mg, 15 mg 1 month and 11.25, 30 mg 3 month IM and SQ 6 month Triptorelin (Triptodur): 22.5 mg IM 6 month	Pain at injection/insertion site Reduced bone mineralization Reduced fertility if followed by sex steroid Increased fat mass/reduced lean body mass Arterial hypertension Mood changes/depression Hot flashes Fatigue Reduced libido/sexual function Decreased growth rate to prepubertal rate Unknown effects on brain development Sterile abscess (leuprolide acetate) Vaginoplasty challenges due to decreased tissue if GnRHa started at SMR 2 or 3 in designated males at birth

Data from Hembree, W. C., Cohen-Kettenis, P. T., Gooren, L., Hannema, S. E., Meyer, W. J., Murad, H. M., Rosenthal, S. M., Safer, J. D., Tangpricha, V., & T'Sjoen, G. G. (2017). Endocrine Treatment of Gender-Dysphoric/Gender-Incongruent Persons: An Endocrine Society Clinical Practice Guideline. The Journal of Clinical Endocrinology & Metabolism, 102(11), 3869-3903. https://doi.org/10.1210/jc.2017-01658

J. Feminizing protocol

After initiating GnRHa and confirming eligibility criteria for estradiol are met, obtain baseline labs, and initiate 17-beta estradiol (transdermal/oral/sublingual) using a gradually increasing dose regimen. See **Table 7-3** for dosing and **Table 7-4** for adverse reactions. The initial dose and frequency of dose escalations depend on age and the stage of endogenous puberty prior to sex-steroid initiation. For TGD youth assigned male at birth in which GnRHa therapy was initiated at SMR stage 2 or 3, the dose regimen is similar to that cisgender females with hypogonadism, starting at a low dose of estradiol and increasing every 6 months. Higher initial

Table 7-2 Pubertal Suppression Baseline and Follow-Up Monitoring

Physical Exam: Every 3–6 Months	Laboratory: Every 6–12 Months	Imaging: Every 1–2 Years
Vital signs, height, weight, sexual maturity rating	Ultrasensitive LH, FSH, E2/T, 25OHD	Pediatric bone density using DXA Bone age X-ray (if clinically indicated, such as short stature or deficient linear velocity)

DXA, dual-energy X-ray absorptiometry; E2, estradiol; FSH, follicle-stimulating hormone; LH, luteinizing hormone; T, total testosterone.

Data from Hembree, W. C., Cohen-Kettenis, P. T., Gooren, L., Hannema, S. E., Meyer, W. J., Murad, H. M., Rosenthal, S. M., Safer, J. D., Tangpricha, V., & T'Sjoen, G. G. (2017). Endocrine Treatment of Gender-Dysphoric/Gender-Incongruent Persons: An Endocrine Society Clinical Practice Guideline. The Journal of Clinical Endocrinology & Metabolism, 102(11), 3869-3903. https://doi.org/10.1210/jc.2017-01658

Table 7-3 Induction of Puberty: Suggested Feminization Regimens*

Estrogen Form	Estrogen Start at SMR 2 or 3: Increase Every 6 Months Over 2–3 Years Until Reaching Adult Dose	Estrogen Start at SMR 4 or 5 and <16 Years of Age: Increase Every 3 Months Over 1 Year Until Reaching Adult Dose	Estrogen Start at SMR 5 in Adolescents ≥16 Years: Increase Every 3–6 Months Until Reaching Adult Dose
17-beta estradiol transdermal	6.25–12.5 mcg/24 h 25 mcg/24 h 37.5 mcg/24 h 50 mcg/24 h 75 mcg/24 h 100 mcg/24 h Adult dose: 50–200 mcg/24 h	25 mcg/24 h 37.5 mcg/24 h 50 mcg/24 h 100 mcg/24 h Adult dose: 50–200 mcg/24 h	50 mcg/24 h 100 mcg/24 h Adult dose: 50–200 mg/24 h
Micronized 17-beta estradiol oral/sublingual	0.25 mg/d 0.5 mg/d 0.75 mg/d 1 mg/d Adult dose: 2–6 mg/d or divided BID	0.5 mg/d 1 mg/d 2 mg/d or divided BID Adult dose: 2–6 mg/d or divided BID	1 mg/d 2 mg/d or divided BID Adult dose: 2–6 mg/d or divided BID

(continues)

Table 7-3 Induction of Puberty: Suggested Feminization Regimens* (continued)

Estrogen Form	Estrogen Start at SMR 2 or 3: Increase Every 6 Months Over 2–3 Years Until Reaching Adult Dose	Estrogen Start at SMR 4 or 5 and <16 Years of Age: Increase Every 3 Months Over 1 Year Until Reaching Adult Dose	Estrogen Start at SMR 5 in Adolescents ≥16 Years: Increase Every 3–6 Months Until Reaching Adult Dose
Estradiol valerate or cypionate (synthetic esters of 17B-esetradiol) parenteral SQ	Insufficient evidence for pubertal induction in this population	Estradiol cypionate: 0.25 mg/week 0.5 mg/week 1 mg/week Adult: max 2.5 mg/week Estradiol valerate: 2.5 mg/week 5 mg/week 10 mg/week Adult: max 20 mg/week Or double dose and administer q 2 weeks IM	Estradiol cypionate: 0.5 mg/week 1 mg/week Adult: max 2.5 mg/week Estradiol valerate: 5 mg/week 10 mg/week Adult: max 20 mg/week Or double dose and administer q 2 weeks IM
Androgen receptor blockers, oral	N/A: GnRHa recommended	Without GnRHa: Spironolactone: increase every 2–4 weeks 25 mg/day 25 mg BID 50 mg BID 100 mg BID Max dose: 200 mg BID (400 mg/day) Monitor electrolytes, creatinine, and blood pressure for orthostasis	Without GnRHa: Spironolactone: increase every 2–4 weeks 25 mg BID 50 mg BID 100 mg BID Max dose: 200 mg BID Monitor electrolytes, creatinine, and blood pressure for orthostasis

* Continuation of GnRHa treatment is recommended during gradually increasing estradiol doses until gonadectomy to suppress endogenous sex steroids. Alternatively, an androgen receptor blocker can be administered if GnRHa treatment is unavailable.

Data from Hembree, W. C., Cohen-Kettenis, P. T., Gooren, L., Hannema, S. E., Meyer, W. J., Murad, H. M., Rosenthal, S. M., Safer, J. D., Tangpricha, V., & T'Sjoen, G. G. (2017). Endocrine Treatment of Gender-Dysphoric/Gender-Incongruent Persons: An Endocrine Society Clinical Practice Guideline. The Journal of Clinical Endocrinology & Metabolism, 102(11), 3869-3903. https://doi.org/10.1210/jc.2017-01658 and Deutsch, M. (2016). Guidelines for the Primary and Gender-Affirming Care of Transgender and Gender Nonbinary People. UCSF Transgender Care, Department of Family and Community Medicine, University of California San Francisco. https://transcare.ucsf.edu/guidelines

Table 7-4 Estrogen Effects and Potential Adverse Reactions

Irreversible	Partially Reversible	Reversible	Adverse Reactions
Breasts > SMR 2	Reduced fertility	Improved psychosocial function Reduced gender dysphoria Body fat redistribution Skin softening Decreased libido Testicular atrophy	Thromboembolic disease Coronary artery disease Cerebrovascular disease Hypertriglyceridemia Cholelithiasis Breast cancer Macroprolactinoma Mood changes Migraine exacerbation Premature epiphyseal fusion

Data from Hembree, W. C., Cohen-Kettenis, P. T., Gooren, L., Hannema, S. E., Meyer, W. J., Murad, H. M., Rosenthal, S. M., Safer, J. D., Tangpricha, V., & T'Sjoen, G. G. (2017). Endocrine Treatment of Gender-Dysphoric/Gender-Incongruent Persons: An Endocrine Society Clinical Practice Guideline. The Journal of Clinical Endocrinology & Metabolism, 102(11), 3869-3903. https://doi.org/10.1210/jc.2017-01658

Table 7-5 Induction of Puberty: Suggested Masculinizing Regimens*

Testosterone Form	Testosterone Start at SMR 2 or 3: Increase Every 6 Months Over 2–3 Years Until Reaching Adult Dose	Testosterone Start at SMR 4 or 5 and <16 Years of Age: Increase Every 3 Months Over 1 Year Until Reaching Adult Dose	Testosterone SMR 5 in Adolescents ≥16 Years: Increase Every 3–6 Months Until Reaching Adult Dose
Parenteral	Testosterone cypionate/enanthate 200 mg/mL SQ: 10 mg/week 20 mg/week 30 mg/week 40 mg/week 50 mg/week Adult dose: 50–100 mg/week IM: double the dose and administer q 2 weeks	Testosterone cypionate/enanthate 200 mg/mL SQ: 20 mg/week 30 mg/week 40 mg/week 50 mg/week Adult dose: 50–100 mg/week Max dose: 100 mg/week	Testosterone cypionate/enanthate 200 mg/mL SQ: 30 mg/week 40 mg/week 50 mg/week Adult dose: 50–100 mg/week Max dose: 100 mg/week
Transdermal	1% Gel or compounded cream: 10 mg/d 20 mg/d 30 mg/d 40 mg/d 50 mg/d Adult: max 100 mg/d May use 1% or 1.62% gel to gradually escalate doses according to regimen	1% Gel: 25 mg/d 50 mg/d 75 mg/d Adult: max 100 mg/week 1.62% Gel: 20.25 mg/d 40.5 mg/d 60.75 mg/d Adult: max 81 mg/d	1% Gel: 50 mg/d 75 mg/d Adult: max 100 mg/week 1.62% Gel: 40.5 mg/d 60.75 mg/d Adult: max 81 mg/d

SQ: 1 mL syringe and 27 G ½" or 25 G 5/8" needle with 18G 1" needle for draw-up.

* Continuation of GnRHa treatment is recommended during gradually increasing testosterone doses until reaching an adult dose of testosterone to suppress endogenous sex steroids. If uterine bleeding occurs without GnRHa, menstrual suppression with progestin can be initiated.

Data from Hembree, W. C., Cohen-Kettenis, P. T., Gooren, L., Hannema, S. E., Meyer, W. J., Murad, H. M., Rosenthal, S. M., Safer, J. D., Tangpricha, V., & T'Sjoen, G. G. (2017). Endocrine Treatment of Gender-Dysphoric/Gender-Incongruent Persons: An Endocrine Society Clinical Practice Guideline. The Journal of Clinical Endocrinology & Metabolism, 102(11), 3869-3903. https://doi.org/10.1210/jc.2017-01658

doses of estradiol with more frequent dose increases can be used for older adolescents without GnRHa therapy, and an androgen receptor blocker can be used. In addition, older adolescents who are at SMR 4 or 5 prior to gender-affirming treatment can be offered the more rapid dose-increase regimens with GnRHa or an androgen receptor blocker because there is insufficient evidence to support the very slow dose-escalation schedule, and this may increase distress from slow feminization. During hormone replacement, continue to monitor with physical exams, vital signs, growth, laboratory, and imaging as indicated. Serum sex-steroid levels should be in the normal reference range for age, and gender- and age-based reference ranges for females should be used when interpreting lab results. See **Table 7-7** for monitoring of sex steroids.

K. *Masculinizing protocol*

After initiating GnRHa and confirming eligibility criteria for estradiol are met, obtain baseline labs and initiate testosterone using a gradually increasing dose regimen. See **Table 7-5** for dosing and **Table 7-6** for adverse reactions. Weekly SQ injections of testosterone cypionate/enanthate are effective, safe, and less painful compared to IM injections (McFarland et al., 2017). TGD youth with a needle phobia may benefit from daily transdermal testosterone gel or patch. The initial dose and frequency of dose escalations depend on age and stage of puberty prior to sex-steroid initiation. For TGD youth assigned female at birth in which GnRHa therapy was initiated at SMR stage 2 or 3, the dose regimen is similar to that for cisgender males with hypogonadism, starting at a low dose of testosterone and increasing every 6 months. GnRHa may be discontinued after reaching adult doses of testosterone because testosterone alone can then suppress gonadotropins. Higher initial doses of testosterone with more frequent dose increases can be used for adolescents presenting at SMR 3–5 without GnRHa therapy because testosterone at adult doses can suppress gonadotropins. Menstrual suppression with testosterone can take 3–6 months, and a progestin can be utilized for amenorrhea induction. Continue pubertal induction monitoring throughout treatment. Serum sex-steroid levels should be in the normal range for age, and gender- and age-based reference ranges for

Table 7-6 Testosterone Effects and Potential Adverse Reactions

Irreversible	Partially Reversible	Reversible	Adverse Reactions
Voice change Increased terminal hair Laryngeal prominence Facial structure changes	Clitoral hypertrophy Male-pattern hair loss Reduced fertility	Improved psychosocial function Decreased gender dysphoria Increased muscle mass Decreased lean tissue mass Body fat redistribution Increased libido Increased energy Menses cessation	Erythrocytosis/polycythemia Coronary artery disease Cerebrovascular disease Hypertension Metabolic syndrome: higher body weight, glucose intolerance, dyslipidemia (hypertriglyceridemia and low high-density lipoprotein [HDL]) Severe liver dysfunction (transaminases > 3× upper limit of normal) Breast or uterine cancer Mood problems Male-pattern hair loss Acne

Data from Hembree, W. C., Cohen-Kettenis, P. T., Gooren, L., Hannema, S. E., Meyer, W. J., Murad, H. M., Rosenthal, S. M., Safer, J. D., Tangpricha, V., & T'Sjoen, G. G. (2017). Endocrine Treatment of Gender-Dysphoric/Gender-Incongruent Persons: An Endocrine Society Clinical Practice Guideline. The Journal of Clinical Endocrinology & Metabolism, 102(11), 3869-3903. https://doi.org/10.1210/jc.2017-01658

Table 7-7 Puberty Induction Baseline and Follow-Up Monitoring

Physical Exam: Every 3–6 Months	Laboratory: Every 6–12 Months	Imaging: Every 1–2 Years
Vital signs, height, weight, sexual maturity rating	TGD assigned male at birth E2, prolactin, 25OHD TGD assigned female at birth T, HGB/HCT, 25OHD	Pediatric bone density using DXA (if history of GnRHa treatment) Bone age on X-ray (if clinically indicated)

BMD should be monitored into adulthood (until age 25-30 years or until peak bone density).

DXA, dual-energy X-ray absorptiometry; *E2*, estradiol; *FSH*, follicle-stimulating hormone; *HGB*, hemoglobin; *HCT*, hematocrit; *LH*, luteinizing hormone; *T*, total testosterone.

Data from Hembree, W. C., Cohen-Kettenis, P. T., Gooren, L., Hannema, S. E., Meyer, W. J., Murad, H. M., Rosenthal, S. M., Safer, J. D., Tangpricha, V., & T'Sjoen, G. G. (2017). Endocrine Treatment of Gender-Dysphoric/Gender-Incongruent Persons: An Endocrine Society Clinical Practice Guideline. The Journal of Clinical Endocrinology & Metabolism, 102(11), 3869-3903. https://doi.org/10.1210/jc.2017-01658

males should be used when interpreting lab results, including hemoglobin/hematocrit.

L. *Amenorrhea induction*

Induction of amenorrhea can be used for TGD youth (masculine and nonbinary) who desire menses cessation and are not eligible for or interested in testosterone therapy. This can be accomplished with GnRHa, continuous administration of oral contraceptive pills (OCPs), and progestogen-only long-acting reversible contraceptives (LARCs). TGD youth with breast dysphoria who prefer oral progestin for amenorrhea induction can be successfully treated with drospirenone 4 mg daily or Aygestin (norethindrone acetate) 2.5–20 mg divided daily, BID, or TID (Apter et al., 2020; Kaunitz et al., 2021; Palacios et al., 2019). However, low-dose combined OCPs and oral progestins have been shown to result in reduced BMD accrual, and there is insufficient evidence for BMD safety for use longer than 1–2 years in pediatrics (Agostino & Di Meglio, 2010; Tack et al., 2018).

M. *Gender nonbinary youth*

There is no consensus on the management of pubertal gender nonbinary (GNB) youth, and treatment approaches depend on the symptoms of gender dysphoria and goals for gender expression. For GNB youth with increased gender dysphoria with the onset or progression of puberty, GnRHa monotherapy can be considered until age 14–16 years, when sex steroids are critical for bone density accrual. GNB youth dysphoric about menses may benefit from amenorrhea induction with a progestin. Low-dose (micro-dose) estradiol with GnRHa or androgen receptor blocker therapy can provide gradual feminization, and low-dose testosterone with GnRHa or progestin can provide gradual masculinization. However, there is insufficient evidence to evaluate the safety in TGD youth, permanent secondary sexual characteristics from the sex steroids can develop, and there are concerns about compromised bone density accrual.

N. *Tobacco cessation*
   Screen for and treat tobacco use using a harm-reduction approach.
O. *HIV prevention*
   Condoms are first-line HIV prevention. PrEP is effective in preventing HIV when the medication is taken as prescribed, and there are no known contraindications with concomitant use of gender-affirming hormone therapy and PrEP (Deutsch, 2016). Nonoccupational postexposure prophylaxis (nPEP) should follow existing guidelines for the general population.
P. *HIV-positive youth*
   HIV-positive status or HIV treatment are not contraindications for gender-affirming hormone treatment. There are potential drug–drug interactions between 17-beta estradiol and antiretroviral therapy or non-nucleoside reverse transcriptase inhibitors (NNRTIs), although these do not change treatment recommendations for either HIV or gender dysphoria; there is no evidence to date of interactions with testosterone or testosterone receptor blockers (Deutsch, 2016).
Q. *Thrombosis screening and risk reduction*
   Prior to initiating gender-affirming sex steroids, screen for medical and family history of thrombosis, cardiovascular disease, metabolic disease, and genetic diagnoses of coagulation disorders, and assess for personal factors that increase thrombosis, such as immobility; injury; and lifestyle factors such as smoking, inactivity, and higher body weight. There is mixed evidence in adults that estradiol therapy increases the risk of venous thromboembolism (VTE) compared to no use, but there is no evidence that physiologic transdermal 17-beta estradiol increases the risk of VTE (Canonico et al., 2008; Connors & Middeldorp, 2019; Getahun et al., 2018; Iwamoto et al., 2019; Vinogradova et al., 2019). Therefore, this is the preferred route for patients with a history of VTE or risk factors for VTE. Testosterone increases the risk for erythrocytosis/polycythemia, and this may contribute to an increased risk of VTE. However, evidence from a large cohort study demonstrated that testosterone hormone replacement therapy (HRT) in transmasculine adults resulted in a similar risk for VTE, ischemic stroke, and myocardial infarction compared to cisgender women (Getahun et al., 2018). A large retrospective cohort study of transgender youth ($N = 611$) receiving either bioidentical estradiol or testosterone HRT for <2 years resulted in no thrombosis events (Mullins et al., 2021). However, long-term longitudinal research is needed in TGD youth to determine whether testosterone HRT increases the risk for acute and chronic cardiovascular disease.
R. *Surgical treatment*
   Gender-affirming genital surgery with gonadectomy and/or hysterectomy can be considered at the age of legal majority, which is 18 years or older in the United States. There is insufficient evidence to recommend a specific age requirement for other gender-affirming surgeries, such as masculinizing chest reconstruction, breast augmentation, facial feminization, or surgery/thyroid chondroplasty (chondrolaryngoplasty). The timing of these surgeries should be based on the TGD youth's gender expression goals and the physical and mental health evaluation by an interdisciplinary team of medical and mental health gender specialists.
   If the TGD youth is interested in gender-affirming surgery, evaluate the potential benefits and risks, discuss surgical options and preparation, and initiate the process of referral to plastic surgery.
   Eligibility criteria typically include a medical clearance letter from the primary care provider or endocrine provider responsible for gender-affirming medication therapy, as well as a letter of support from a mental health gender specialist.
   Although there is not a minimum length of time on testosterone required for masculinizing chest reconstruction, TGD youth assigned male at birth taking estradiol should delay breast augmentation until stage SMR 5 breast development occurs.
   Educate TGD youth and caregivers on preoperative thrombosis risk reduction, such as smoking cessation and body mass index normalization. There is no evidence to support withholding physiologic sex-steroid therapy in the perioperative period, but the prescribing clinician should ensure that serum estradiol or testosterone levels are within normal reference intervals for age to minimize the risk of adverse events. In addition, TGD youth assigned male at birth with thrombosis risk factors may consider transdermal estradiol because there is no evidence of increased thrombosis with this form compared to endogenous estradiol. Clinicians should screen hemoglobin/hematocrit prior to surgery for TGD youth assigned female at birth taking testosterone, and the dose of testosterone should be decreased if erythrocytosis is present.
S. *Patient education*
   1. Establish a trusting relationship with the TGD youth and their legal guardians. This can help overcome the past stigma and minority stress experienced by some TGD individuals in healthcare settings and builds the foundation for successful gender-affirming outcomes.
   2. Provide education to legal guardians on the importance of parental, school, and community support for the youth's gender identity in terms of psychosocial well-being and health outcomes.
   3. Provide health counseling, with an emphasis on STI prevention and mental health support.
   4. Harm reduction as indicated by subjective and objective assessments.
   5. Education on community resources, including gender-affirming psychological, social, medical, and legal resources.
   6. Periodic health counseling, as outlined in Chapter 06.

VI. **Self-management resources and tools**
A. *University of California, San Francisco's Center of Excellence for Transgender Health*
Provides education, advocacy, and current research around transgender health needs for both TGD youth, caregivers, and providers (https://transcare.ucsf.edu)
B. *Endocrine Society*
Provides academic education, advocacy, current research, and clinical practice guidelines regarding transgender health (https://www.endocrine.org)
C. *World Professional Association for Transgender Health*
Provides academic education, advocacy, current research, and clinical practice guidelines regarding transgender health (https://www.wpath.org)
D. *Gender Spectrum*
Provides professional and community education, school and youth-serving organization training, support groups, and advocacy for creating gender-sensitive and inclusive environments for all youth (https://genderspectrum.org)
E. *Transgender Law Center*
Provides advocacy for equity and justice for transgender individuals through legal work, programs, and education, such as name and/or gender marker changes on identity documents (https://transgenderlawcenter.org)
F. *National Center for Lesbian Rights*
A national legal organization committed to advancing the civil and human rights of lesbian, gay, bisexual, and transgender (LGBT) individuals through litigation, legislation, policy, and public education (https://www.nclrights.org)
G. *National Center for Transgender Equality*
An advocacy organization working to advance equality of transgender individuals (https://transequality.org)

References

Agostino, H., & Di Meglio, G. (2010). Low-dose oral contraceptives in adolescents: how low can you go? *Journal of Pediatric and Adolescent Gynecology*, 23(4), 195–201. doi:10.1016/j.jpag.2009.11.001

American Psychiatric Association. (2013). *Diagnostic and statistical manual of mental disorders* (5th ed.).

Apter, D., Colli, E., Gemzell-Danielsson, K., & Peters, K. (2020). Multicenter, open-label trial to assess the safety and tolerability of drospirenone 4.0 mg over 6 cycles in female adolescents, with a 7-cycle extension phase. *Contraception*, 101(6), 412–419. doi:10.1016/j.contraception.2020.02.004

Avila, J. T., Golden, N. H., & Aye, T. (2019). Eating disorder screening in transgender youth. *Journal of Adolescent Health*, 65(6), 815–817. doi:10.1016/j.jadohealth.2019.06.011

Becerra-Culqui, T. A., Liu, Y., Nash, R., Cromwell, L., Flanders, W. D., Getahun, D., Giammattei, S. V., Hunkeler, E. M., Lash, T. L., Millman, A., Quinn, V. P., Robinson, B., Roblin, D., Sandberg, D. E., Silverberg, M. J., Tangpricha, V., & Goodman, M. (2018). Mental health of transgender and gender nonconforming youth compared with their peers. *Pediatrics*, 141(5), e20173845. doi:10.1542/peds.2017-3845

Bonnington, A., Dianat, S., Kerns, J., Hastings, J., Hawkins, M., De Haan, G., & Obedin-Maliver, J. (2020). Society of Family Planning clinical recommendations: Contraceptive counseling for transgender and gender diverse people who were female sex assigned at birth. *Contraception*, 102(2), 70–82. doi:10.1016/j.contraception.2020.04.001

Canonico, M., Plu-Bureau, G., Lowe, G. D. O., & Scarabin, P.-Y. (2008). Hormone replacement therapy and risk of venous thromboembolism in postmenopausal women: systematic review and meta-analysis. *BMJ*, 336(7655), 1227–1231. doi:10.1136/bmj.39555.441944.BE

Centers for Disease Control and Prevention. (2015). Sexually transmitted diseases: Summary of 2015 CDC treatment guidelines. *Journal of the Mississippi State Medical Association*, 56(12), 372–375.

Clark, H., Babu, A. S., Wiewel, E., Opoku, J., & Crepaz, N. (2017). Diagnosed HIV infection in transgender adults and adolescents: Results from the National HIV Surveillance System, 2009–2014. *AIDS and Behavior*, 21(9), 2774–2783. doi:10.1007/s10461-016-1656-7

Coelho, J. S., Suen, J., Clark, B. A., Marshall, S. K., Geller, J., & Lam, P.-Y. (2019). Eating disorder diagnoses and symptom presentation in transgender youth: A scoping review. *Current Psychiatry Reports*, 21(11), 107. doi:10.1007/s11920-019-1097-x

Coleman, E., Bockting, W., Botzer, M., Cohen-Kettenis, P., DeCuypere, G., Feldman, J., Fraser, L., Green, J., Knudson, G., Meyer, W. J., Monstrey, S., Adler, R. K., Brown, G. R., Devor, A. H., Ehrbar, R., Ettner, R., Eyler, E., Garofalo, R., Karasic, D. H., . . . Zucker, K. (2012). Standards of care for the health of transsexual, transgender, and gender-nonconforming people, version 7. *International Journal of Transgenderism*, 13(4), 165–232. doi:10.1080/15532739.2011.700873

Connors, J. M., & Middeldorp, S. (2019). Transgender patients and the role of the coagulation clinician. *Journal of Thrombosis and Haemostasis*, 17(11), 1790–1797. doi:10.1111/jth.14626

de Vries, A. L. C., Doreleijers, T. A. H., Steensma, T. D., & Cohen-Kettenis, P. T. (2011). Psychiatric comorbidity in gender dysphoric adolescents. *Journal of Child Psychology and Psychiatry*, 52(11), 1195–1202. doi:10.1111/j.1469-7610.2011.02426.x

de Vries, A. L. C., McGuire, J. K., Steensma, T. D., Wagenaar, E. C. F., Doreleijers, T. A. H., & Cohen-Kettenis, P. T. (2014). Young adult psychological outcome after puberty suppression and gender reassignment. *Pediatrics*, 134(4), 696–704. doi:10.1542/peds.2013-2958

Deutsch, M. (2016). *Guidelines for the primary and gender-affirming care of transgender and gender nonbinary people*. UCSF Transgender Care, Department of Family and Community Medicine, University of California San Francisco. https://transcare.ucsf.edu/guidelines

Durwood, L. B. A., McLaughlin, K. A. P., & Olson, K. R. P. (2017). Mental health and self-worth in socially-transitioned transgender youth. *Journal of the American Academy of Child & Adolescent Psychiatry*, 56(2), 116–123.e112. doi:10.1016/j.jaac.2016.10.016

Getahun, D., Nash, R., Flanders, W. D., Baird, T. C., Becerra-Culqui, T. A., Cromwell, L., Hunkeler, E., Lash, T. L., Millman, A., Quinn, V. P., Robinson, B., Roblin, D., Silverberg, M. J., Safer, J.,

Slovis, J., Tangpricha, V., & Goodman, M. (2018). Cross-sex hormones and acute cardiovascular events in transgender persons: A cohort study. *Annals of Internal Medicine, 169*(4), 205–213. doi:10.7326/M17-2785

Gridley, S. J., Crouch, J. M., Evans, Y., Eng, W., Antoon, E., Lyapustina, M., Schimmel-Bristow, A., Woodward, J., Dundon, K., Schaff, R., McCarty, C., Ahrens, K., & Breland, D. J. (2016). Youth and caregiver perspectives on barriers to gender-affirming health care for transgender youth. *Journal of Adolescent Health, 59*(3), 254–261. doi:10.1016/j.jadohealth.2016.03.017

Hamnvik, O.-P. R., Agarwal, S., AhnAllen, C. G., Goldman, A. L., & Reisner, S. L. (2020). Telemedicine and inequities in health care access: The example of transgender health. *Transgender Health, 7*(2), 113–116. doi:10.1089/trgh.2020.0122

Hautala, L., Junnila, J., Alin, J., Grönroos, M., Maunula, A.-M., Karukivi, M., Liuksila, P.-R., Räihä, H., Välimäki, M., & Saarijärvi, S. (2009). Uncovering hidden eating disorders using the SCOFF questionnaire: Cross-sectional survey of adolescents and comparison with nurse assessments. *International Journal of Nursing Studies, 46*(11), 1439–1447. doi:10.1016/j.ijnurstu.2009.04.007

Hembree, W. C., Cohen-Kettenis, P. T., Gooren, L., Hannema, S. E., Meyer, W. J., Murad, H. M., Rosenthal, S. M., Safer, J. D., Tangpricha, V., & T'Sjoen, G. G. (2017). Endocrine treatment of gender-dysphoric/gender-incongruent persons: An endocrine society clinical practice guideline. *Journal of Clinical Endocrinology & Metabolism, 102*(11), 3869–3903. doi:10.1210/jc.2017-01658

Iwamoto, S. J., Defreyne, J., Rothman, M. S., Van Schuylenbergh, J., Van de Bruaene, L., Motmans, J., & T'Sjoen, G. (2019). Health considerations for transgender women and remaining unknowns: a narrative review. *Therapeutic Advances in Endocrinology and Metabolism, 10*, 204201881987116. doi:10.1177/2042018819871166

Johns, M. M., Lowry, R., Andrzejewski, J., Barrios, L. C., Demissie, Z., McManus, T., Rasberry, C. N., Robin, L., & Underwood, J. M. (2019). Transgender identity and experiences of violence victimization, substance use, suicide risk, and sexual risk behaviors among high school students—19 states and large urban school districts, 2017. *Morbidity and Mortality Weekly Report, 68*(3), 67–71. doi:10.15585/mmwr.mm6803a3

Kaunitz, A. M., Barbieri, R. L., & Eckler, K. (2021). *Hormonal contraception for suppression of menstruation.* UpToDate. http://uptodate.com

Klein, D. A., Paradise, S. L., & Goodwin, E. T. (2018). Caring for transgender and gender-diverse persons: What clinicians should know. *American Family Physician, 98*(11), 645. https://www.aafp.org/afp/2018/1201/p645.pdf

Klink, D., Caris, M., Heijboer, A., van Trotsenburg, M., & Rotteveel, J. (2015). Bone mass in young adulthood following gonadotropin-releasing hormone analog treatment and cross-sex hormone treatment in adolescents with gender dysphoria. *Journal of Clinical Endocrinology & Metabolism, 100*(2), E270–E275. doi:10.1210/jc.2014-2439

Lee, J. Y., Finlayson, C., Olson-Kennedy, J., Garofalo, R., Chan, Y.-M., Glidden, D. V., & Rosenthal, S. M. (2020). Low bone mineral density in early pubertal transgender/gender diverse youth: Findings from the Trans Youth Care Study. *Journal of the Endocrine Society, 4*(9), bvaa065-bvaa065. doi:10.1210/jendso/bvaa065

McFarland, J., Craig, W., Clarke, N. J., & Spratt, D. I. (2017). Serum testosterone concentrations remain stable between injections in patients receiving subcutaneous testosterone. *Journal of the Endocrine Society, 1*(8), 1095–1103. doi:10.1210/js.2017-00148

Mullins, E. S., Geer, R., Metcalf, M., Piccola, J., Lane, A., Conard, L. A. E., & Mullins, T. L. K. (2021). Thrombosis risk in transgender adolescents receiving gender-affirming hormone therapy. *Pediatrics, 147*(4), e2020023549. doi:10.1542/peds.2020-023549

Olson-Kennedy, J., Streeter, L. H., Garofalo, R., Chan, Y.-M., & Rosenthal, S. M. (2020). Histrelin implants for suppression of puberty in youth with gender dysphoria: A comparison of 50 mcg/day (Vantas) and 65 mcg/day (SupprelinLA). *Transgender Health, 6*(1), 36–42. doi:10.1089/trgh.2020.0055

Palacios, S., Colli, E., & Regidor, P.-A. (2019). Multicenter, phase III trials on the contraceptive efficacy, tolerability and safety of a new drospirenone-only pill *Acta Obstetricia et Gynecologica Scandinavica, 98*(12), 1549–1557. doi:10.1111/aogs.13688

Perez-Brumer, A., Day, J. K., Russell, S. T., & Hatzenbueler, M. L. (2017). Prevalence and correlates of suicidal ideation among transgender youth in California: Findings from a representative, population-based sample of high school students. *Journal of the American Academy of Child and Adolescent Psychiatry, 56*(9), 739–746. doi:10.1016/j.jaac.2017.06.010

Rafferty, J., Committee on Psychosocial Aspects of Child and Family Health, Committee on Adolescence, & Section on Lesbian, Gay, Bisexual, and Transgender Health and Wellness. (2018). Ensuring comprehensive care and support for transgender and gender-diverse children and adolescents. *Pediatrics, 142*(4), e20182162. doi:10.1542/peds.2018-2162

Reisner, S. L., Greytak, E. A., Parsons, J. T., & Ybarra, M. L. (2015). Gender minority social stress in adolescence: Disparities in adolescent bullying and substance use by gender identity. *Journal of Sex Research, 52*(3), 243–256. doi:10.1080/00224499.2014.886321

Rosenthal, S. M. (2021). Challenges in the care of transgender and gender-diverse youth: An endocrinologist's view. *Nature Reviews Endocrinology, 17*(10), 581–591. doi:10.1038/s41574-021-00535-9

Russell, S. T., Pollitt, A. M., Li, G., & Grossman, A. H. (2018). Chosen name use is linked to reduced depressive symptoms, suicidal ideation, and suicidal behavior among transgender youth. *Journal of Adolescent Health, 63*(4), 503–505. doi:10.1016/j.jadohealth.2018.02.003

Stoffers, I. E., de Vries, M. C., & Hannema, S. E. (2019). Physical changes, laboratory parameters, and bone mineral density during testosterone treatment in adolescents with gender dysphoria. *Journal of Sexual Medicine, 16*(9), 1459–1468. doi:10.1016/j.jsxm.2019.06.014

Tack, L. J. W., Craen, M., Lapauw, B., Goemaere, S., Toye, K., Kaufman, J. M., Vandewalle, S., T'Sjoen, G., Zmierczak, H. G., & Cools, M. (2018). Proandrogenic and antiandrogenic progestins in transgender youth: Differential effects on body composition and bone metabolism. *Journal of Clinical Endocrinology and Metabolism, 103*(6), 2147–2156. doi:10.1210/jc.2017-02316

Travers, R., Bauer, G., Pyne, J., & Bradley, L. (2012). *Impacts of strong parental support for trans youth.* Trans PULSE Project. http://transpulseproject.ca/wp-content/uploads/2012/10/Impacts-of-Strong-Parental-Support-for-Trans-Youth-vFINAL.pdf

T'Sjoen, G., Arcelus, J., Gooren, L., Klink, D. T., & Tangpricha, V. (2019). Endocrinology of transgender medicine. *Endocrine Reviews, 40*(1), 97–117. doi:10.1210/er.2018-00011

Turban, J. L., King, D., Carswell, J. M., & Keuroghlian, A. S. (2020). Pubertal suppression for transgender youth and risk of suicidal ideation. *Pediatrics, 145*(2), e20191725. doi:10.1542/peds.2019-1725

van de Grift, T. C., van Gelder, Z. J., Mullender, M. G., Steensma, T. D., de Vries, A. L. C., & Bouman, M. B. (2020). Timing of puberty suppression and surgical options for transgender youth. *Pediatrics, 146*(5), e20193653. doi:10.1542/peds.2019-3653

Vance, S. R., Jr. (2018). The importance of getting the name right for transgender and other gender expansive youth. *Journal of Adolescent Health, 63*(4), 379–380. doi:10.1016/j.jadohealth.2018.07.022

Vance, S. R., Jr., Boyer, C. B., Glidden, D. V., & Sevelius, J. (2021). Mental health and psychosocial risk and protective factors among black and Latinx transgender youth compared with peers. *JAMA Network Open*, *4*(3), e213256. doi:10.1001/jamanetworkopen.2021.3256

Vance, S. R., Jr., Ehrensaft, D., & Rosenthal, S. M. (2014). Psychological and medical care of gender nonconforming youth. *Pediatrics*, *134*(6), 1184–1192. doi:10.1542/peds.2014-0772

Vinogradova, Y., Coupland, C., & Hippisley-Cox, J. (2019). Use of hormone replacement therapy and risk of venous thromboembolism: Nested case-control studies using the QResearch and CPRD databases. *BMJ*, *364*, k4810-k4810. doi:10.1136/bmj.k4810

Vlot, M. C., Klink, D. T., den Heijer, M., Blankenstein, M. A., Rotteveel, J., & Heijboer, A. C. (2016). Effect of pubertal suppression and cross-sex hormone therapy on bone turnover markers and bone mineral apparent density (BMAD) in transgender adolescents. *Bone*, *95*, 11–19. doi:10.1016/j.bone.2016.11.008

Watson, R. J., Veale, J. F., & Saewyc, E. M. (2017). Disordered eating behaviors among transgender youth: Probability profiles from risk and protective factors. *International Journal of Eating Disorders*, *50*(5), 515–522. doi:10.1002/eat.22627

Wilson, B., Choi, S., Herman, J., Becker, T., & Conron, K. (2017). *Characteristics and mental health of gender nonconforming adolescents in California: Findings from the 2015n2016 California Health Interview Survey*. https://williamsinstitute.law.ucla.edu/wp-content/uploads/CHIS-Transgender-Teens-FINAL.pdf

Workowski, K. A., Bachmann, L. H., Chan, P. A., Johnston, C. M., Muzny, C. A., Park, I., Reno, H., Zenilman, J. M., & Bolan, G. A. (2021). Sexually transmitted infections treatment guidelines, 2021. *MMWR Recommendations and Reports*, *70*(4), 1–187. doi:10.15585/mmwr.rr7004a1

World Health Organization. (2021). *International statistical classification of diseases and related health problems (ICD)*. https://www.who.int/standards/classifications/classification-of-diseases

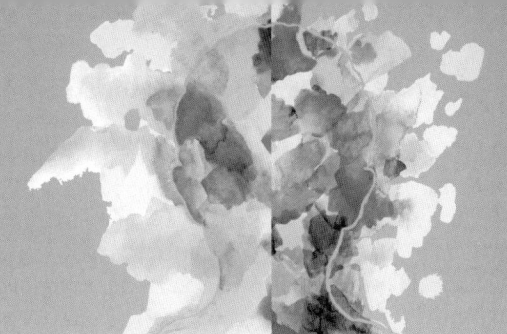

CHAPTER 8

Developmental Assessment: Screening for Developmental Delay and Autism

Janis Mandac-Dy and Abbey Alkon

I. Introduction

A. *General background*

The prevalence of children with developmental and behavioral problems is estimated to be 17% in the United States (Zablotsky et al., 2019). In the 2019–2020 National Survey of Children's Health, nearly 20% of children younger than 5 years of age were at risk for developmental and behavioral problems or social delays, but fewer than one in four received the recommended screening (U.S. Department of Health and Human Services et al., 2020). Screening instruments help identify children with possible developmental delays or disorders who may require follow-up or referrals to complete diagnostic evaluations.

There has been an increase in awareness of developmental and behavioral health in children, with more programs available at the national and state levels. In 2003, the President's New Freedom Commission on Mental Health included the goal for early mental health screening, assessment, and referral to services to be common practice and recommended that screening for mental disorders be included in primary health care and connected to treatment and support services. Title V of the Social Security Act and the Individuals With Disabilities Education Improvement Act (IDEA) of 2004 reaffirm the mandate for child health professionals to provide early identification of and intervention for children with developmental disabilities through community-based collaborative systems. The Early and Periodic Screening, Diagnostic, and Treatment (EPSDT) guidelines require that states provide regular health screenings and all medically necessary services to children and adolescents, including assessments of mental health development. The American Academy of Pediatrics (AAP) provides guidelines for screening for developmental and behavioral problems as part of the recommended primary care schedule (Lipkin et al., 2020). The *Birth to 5: Watch Me Thrive!* initiative by the U.S. Department of Health and Human Services and U.S. Department of Education provides a user guide on how to select and use developmental and behavioral screening tools for parents and providers (Administration for Children and Families, U.S. Department of Health and Human Services, 2020).

Under the Affordable Care Act (ACA), screening for children less than 3 years of age and surveillance throughout childhood are covered under preventive services. Current Procedural Terminology (CPT) code 96127 is used for billing for an emotional and behavioral assessment, and CPT code 96110 is used for a developmental assessment in primary care.

The Centers for Disease Control and Prevention (CDC) program *Learn the Signs. Act Early* is a resource for caregivers and parents that includes free milestone checklists and other online tools to help track children's development. The program also has printed materials as well as a mobile app to track developmental milestones. In 2021, the CDC funded a group of subject-matter experts in the AAP to help revise the developmental surveillance checklists (Zubler et al., 2022). The experts conducted a broad literature search and identified resources and commonly used screening tools. They categorized milestones into four developmental domains: social–emotional, language/communication, cognitive, and motor. They applied the criteria that a milestone represented those that most children (≥75%) would be expected to achieve by a certain age. This work resulted in the addition of well-child checklists for ages 15 and 30 months, identification of additional social and emotional milestones, removal of vague language and duplicate milestones, revision of tips and developmental activities, and addition of open-ended questions for pediatric primary care providers to use when discussing development with families. The new milestone criteria are based on 75% of children being able to achieve a developmental milestone, discouraging a wait-and-see approach and minimizing potential delays to diagnosis. Parents and providers are encouraged to learn and monitor the signs of healthy development and take action when there is a concern.

Pediatric nurse practitioners (PNPs) providing primary care via telehealth can continue to conduct surveillance and screening. The widespread utilization of telehealth due to the COVID-19 pandemic was facilitated through its emergency authorization by governmental agencies and by allowing providers to get reimbursed for such visits. PNPs in primary care should continue to use validated, caregiver-completed questionnaires, along with review of any concerning surveillance findings, to properly assess a child's developmental status. Observation alone through video telehealth is not sufficient due to limitations in screen and sound clarity and variations in how children interact via screens. Any positive surveillance and caregiver-completed screening findings may require an in-person visit to assess the child before making any referrals. Because parent-completed screening instruments have been validated, the primary care PNP can use these screening tests either in person or via telehealth. By contrast, diagnostic instruments have not been validated for use over telehealth, so they should only be administered in person at this time.

B. *Primary care and screening*

In 2004, Halfon et al. found that primary care practices failed to identify and refer 60%–80% of children with developmental delays in a timely manner (Halfon et al., 2004). Primary care practices continue to fall short, failing to screen more than 60% of children at primary care visits (U.S. Department of Health and Human Services et al., 2020). Although pediatric primary care practices are busy and primary care providers have a limited amount of time with children, children who are at risk for developing developmental and behavioral problems need to be identified early in life and referred for intervention services which can have significant impact on their ability to learn new skills and increase success in school and life (CDC, 2023). The AAP developed a policy statement, "Identifying Infants and Young Children with Developmental Disorders: An Algorithm for Developmental Surveillance and Screening," that provides a strategy to incorporate ongoing developmental surveillance and screening of all children into primary care visits (AAP Council on Children with Disabilities et al., 2006). In 2020, the AAP provided an update: "Promoting Optimal Development: Identifying Infants and Young Children With Developmental Disorders Through Developmental Surveillance and Screening" (Lipkin et al., 2020), which aimed to reduce confusion about when to be concerned by identifying the milestones most children (≥75%) would be expected to achieve by specific ages at health supervision visits. More in-depth surveillance and consideration for developmental screening are warranted for those children not meeting these revised criteria.

C. *Why screen?*

Standardized screening tests are more accurate than clinical impressions and thus are recommended at targeted ages to augment developmental surveillance. Screening programs are provided to all children or those at risk for behavioral, developmental, and emotional problems. Children with positive screening tests may need to be referred for diagnostic testing because screening is not a diagnostic tool.

The goal of screening is to identify children who will benefit from early intervention services. Early intervention services for children with developmental problems have been shown to be extremely effective if children enter these programs at an early age (Glascoe, 2005). Intervention programs can help children with behavior problems, autism, or developmental delays to reduce the likelihood of needing special education placement and increase the likelihood of future school success (Johnson & Myers, 2007).

D. *Where?*

Screening is most effective when embedded in a preventive services system in primary care, where screening is part of a preventive services schedule coordinated with other guidance and screening activities, and where concerns and observations always lead to a within-office guidance process even if a referral to an outside agency or service is made.

The AAP recommends that all children have a "medical home," which is defined as care that is accessible, continuous, comprehensive, family centered, coordinated, compassionate, and culturally effective (AAP, 2021). The 2019–2020 National Survey of Children's Health found that more than half of all children did not have a medical home, including nearly 6 of 10 children with special healthcare needs (U.S. Department of Health and Human Services et al., 2020). With only half of all children receiving the recommended screening in their primary care practices, new, innovative screening programs need to be developed in primary care or community settings, such as public health departments or childcare programs, to ensure that developmental disorders are identified, referrals to necessary diagnostic testing are made, and children can receive early intervention.

E. *Prevalence of disorders*

At least one in six children has a developmental concern at some point during their childhood (CDC, 2021). Of all children, 12%–17% have:
- Speech or language delay
- Intellectual disability
- Learning disability
- Hearing loss
- Emotional or behavioral concern
- Delay in growth or development

The prevalence of autism spectrum disorders in children aged 8 years is estimated at about 1 in 36 (Maenner et al., 2023). The prevalence differs for boys (1 in 23) compared to girls (1 in 88).

II. Developmental surveillance and screening algorithm

Figure 8-1 provides an overview of screening of all children in the primary care setting. **Figure 8-2** provides a flowchart algorithm with steps for screening a patient without identified risks for developmental problems at a health supervision visit (Lipkin et al., 2020).

A. *Patient without identified risks or developmental problems arrives for health supervision visit. (Step 1)*

The AAP recommends surveillance to be included in every well-child visit as outlined in the AAP's *Bright Futures*, 4th edition (Hagan et al., 2017). This includes developmental impressions and concerns raised by a parent or professional.

To enhance the accuracy of developmental surveillance, standardized screening should be included in well-child visits at 9, 18, and 30 months of age. Developmental surveillance alone, without screening, captures only 30% of children with delays and disabilities before the age of 5 years (Rice et al., 2014).

Although developmental surveillance and screening are recommended throughout childhood, it is important to conduct these assessments at the 4- or 5-year visit as the child prepares to enter elementary school.

B. *Is this a 9-, 18-, 24-, or 30-month visit? (Step 2)*

Any concerns raised by the parent or primary care provider during surveillance should be followed by the administration of a standardized screening tool. A standardized test should be used to perform developmental screening at the 9-, 18-, and 30-month visits. At a minimum, screening for behavioral and emotional problems is also recommended. In addition, visits at 18 and 24 months should include screening for autism spectrum disorders (ASDs). A general developmental screen is recommended at the 9-, 18-, 30-month, and prekindergarten visits according to the current well-child guidelines in *Bright Futures: Guidelines for Health Supervision for Infants, Children and Adolescents* (AAP, 2007). The AAP recommendations are based on recent research that credits standardized screening tools with capturing up to 80% of children with early developmental delays. Autism screening is recommended for all children before they are 24 months of age (Johnson & Myers, 2007; Robins, 2014).

C. *Administer screening test. (Step 3)*
1. Definition
   a. Screening is the use of standardized tools to identify and refine a recognized risk (AAP Council on Children With Disabilities et al., 2006).
   b. Assessments include gathering and synthesizing information across multiple domains, settings, and informants.
   c. A list of selected screening tools is provided in **Table 8-1**.

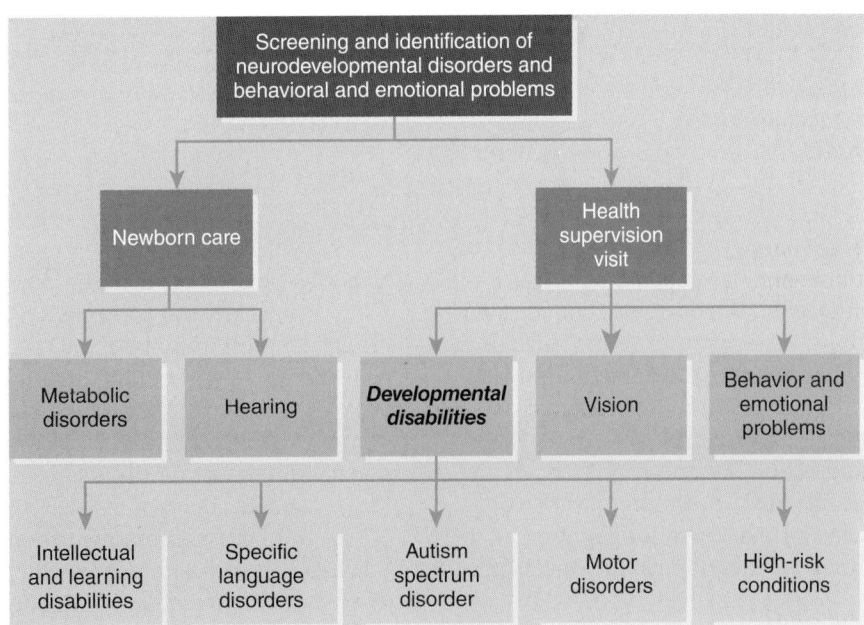

Figure 8-1 Early childhood screening for the identification of neurodevelopmental disorders and behavioral and emotional problems.

Data from Pediatrics, Vol. 145, number 1, January 2020:e20193449, Copyright © by the AAP.

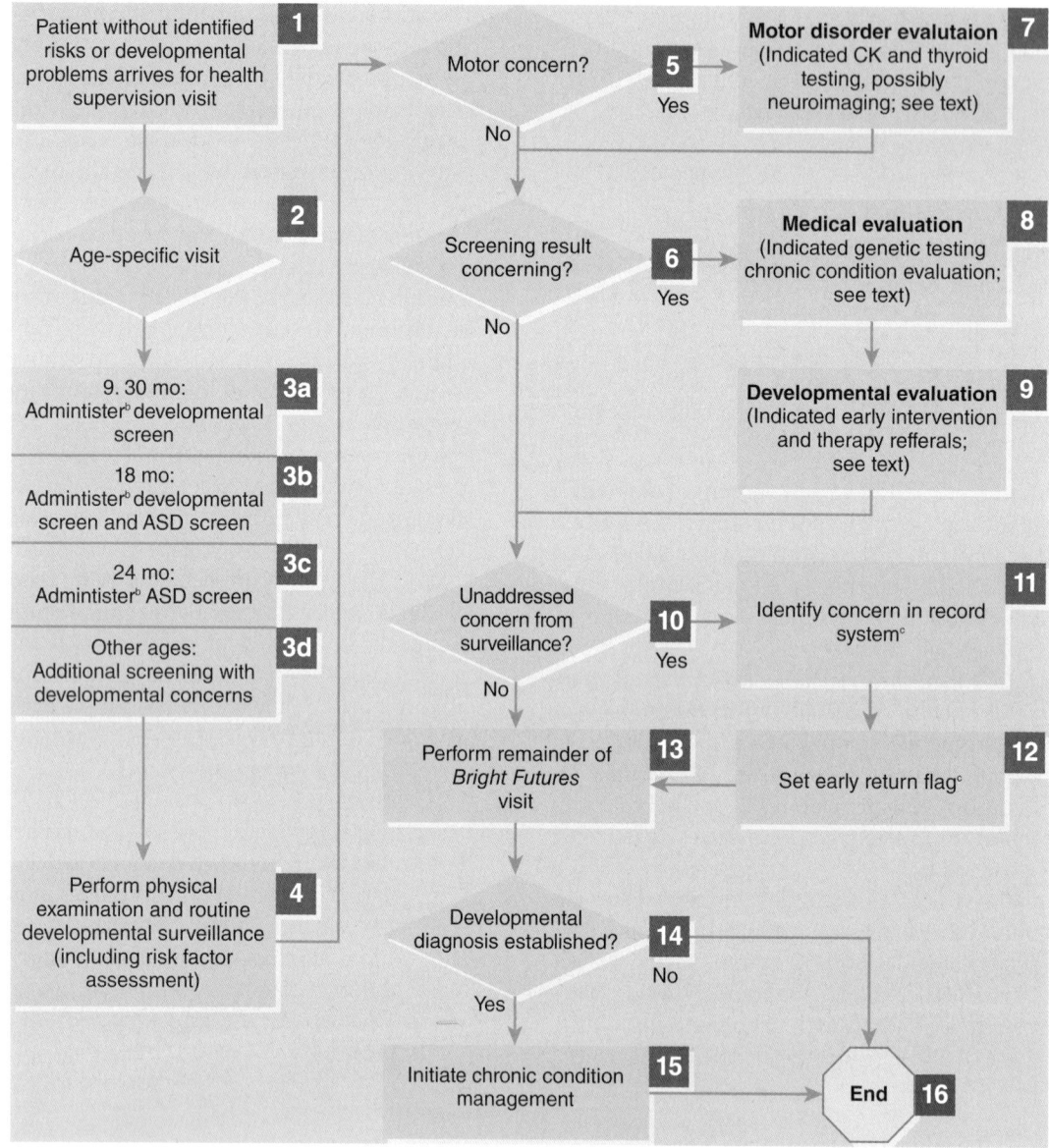

Figure 8-2 Algorithm for screening a patient without identified risks for developmental problems at a health supervision visit.
Data from Pediatrics, Vol. 145, number 1, January 2020:e20193449, Copyright © by the AAP.

2. Age-specific visits
   a. 9, 30 mo: Administer developmental screen.
      i. Screening at the 9-month visit provides an opportunity not only to monitor emerging motor and communication skills but also educate parents about developmental milestones and screening.
      ii. Screening at the 30-month visit allows for the identification of children who would qualify for early intervention services.
   b. 18 mo: Administer developmental screen and ASD screen.
      i. Delays in communication and fine motor skills are often evident by 18 months of age.
      ii. If surveillance and screening in earlier visits identified ASD symptomatology, accurate screening for ASD is possible at 18 months and provides the opportunity for effective early intervention.
   c. 24 mo: Administer ASD screen.
      i. A repeat of the ASD screen at the 24-month visit further ensures identification of children with ASD.
   d. Other ages: Additional screening with developmental concerns.
      i. It is appropriate to conduct screening using validated tests at other intervals, especially if parents or others involved in the child's care raise development concerns.
      ii. If any routine health supervision visit was missed, developmental screening should be administered at the next opportunity.

D. *Perform physical examination and routine surveillance (including risk factor assessment). (Step 4)*
Surveillance is the process of recognizing children who may be at risk of developmental delays. It is the process of gathering information about the family's well-being through report or observation, observing children's behavior, eliciting parents' concerns, and gathering data from the medical history and current physical examination (Glascoe, 2005). The components of surveillance are:
1. Eliciting and attending to the parents' concerns about their child's development
2. Obtaining, documenting, and maintaining the child's developmental history
3. Making informed and accurate observations of the child
4. Identifying risks, strengths, and protective factors
5. Maintaining an accurate record of the process and findings
6. Obtaining and sharing opinions and findings with other professionals with parental/guardian consent, such as childcare providers, home visitors, preschool teachers, and developmental therapists, especially when concerns arise.

E. *Does the screening suggest a motor concern? (Step 5)*
A motor disorder evaluation should be conducted if the screening results suggest a motor concern (see Step 7).

F. *Is the screening result concerning? (Step 6)*
If the screening results are negative or do not reveal a concern for developmental delay, the pediatric healthcare professional may proceed to Step 10: Unaddressed Concern From Surveillance? of the algorithm and proceed as directed with the remainder of the health supervision visit. Normal screening results provide an opportunity to focus on promoting health development.

If the results of the screening test are positive, review the child's strengths and then review the child's areas of difficulty. Explain the results to the parents and refer the child for further evaluation. A focused history and physical examination are also warranted (see Step 8: Perform Complete Medical Evaluation).

G. *Perform motor disorder evaluation. (Step 7)*
When motor concerns are identified on surveillance or screening, a comprehensive neurologic examination should be performed. Brain imaging should be considered for increase tone. Laboratory testing of creatine kinase and thyroid-stimulating hormone should be ordered for child with normal or decreased tone whose screening identifies a motor concern.

H. *Perform complete medical evaluation. (Step 8)*
When there is a concern for developmental delay in a child, a medical diagnostic evaluation should be completed to identify any underlying etiology. Consideration should be given to biological, environmental, and established risk factors for delayed development. Vision screening and an audiologic evaluation should be performed, as well as a thorough review of prenatal and birth history, metabolic screening, and growth measurements. Additional risk factors, such as environmental and family medical and social histories, must also be considered. Consider laboratory testing, such as chromosomal microarray and fragile X testing for children with suspected global developmental delay. If further evaluation is warranted, additional referrals should be made to specialties, such as neurology or genetics.

Identification of an etiology may provide parents and caregivers with a better understanding of their child's disability and can affect treatment planning. Once referrals are made to outside providers for further developmental or medical evaluation, it is crucial for the pediatric healthcare professional within the medical home to develop an explicit co-management plan with those subspecialists and coordinate care with the family.

I. *Perform or refer for developmental evaluation and refer to early intervention or early childhood education. (Step 9)*
Once a child has been identified as at risk for a developmental disorder with proper surveillance and screening, a comprehensive developmental evaluation should be performed as quickly as possible. A diagnostic evaluation helps to identify a specific developmental disorder or disorders and allows for prognostic information and specific recommendations for early therapeutic interventions.

Diagnostic evaluations can be performed by pediatric medical or developmental subspecialists, such as developmental–behavioral pediatricians, pediatric psychiatrists or neurologists, advanced practice nurses, psychologists, speech–language pathologists, occupational and physical therapists, and other trained early childhood professionals. Ideally, an interdisciplinary assessment, along with communication and coordination with the medical home, can provide the child and family with the most comprehensive care.

Referral to early intervention programs can and should be made as soon as developmental concerns are identified. Early intervention and early childhood education programs include federally funded programs and preschool and parent education programs.

J. *Unaddressed concern from surveillance? (Steps 10–12)*
If developmental concerns were raised during surveillance but screening did not identify a disorder or condition, the concern should be documented in the patient's record (Step 11). The child's developmental progress should be closely monitored, which would include a return visit earlier than the recommended interval for healthcare supervision (Step 12).

K. *Perform remainder of health supervision visit. (Step 13)*
When formal screening indicates that the child is within the range of normal development, pediatric healthcare providers can discuss the negative screening results and the low risk for a developmental disorder (Hagan et al., 2017). This is also an opportunity to provide

Table 8-1 Supplemental Information

	Description	Age Range	No. Items	Administration Time	Forms Available EHR Compatible	Psychometric Properties[a]
General Developmental Screening Tests						
Ages and Stages Questionnaires – 3	Parent-completed questionnaire. Series of 21 questions screening communication, gross motor, fine motor, problem-solving, and personal adaptive skills. Results in pass, monitor, or fail score for domains	2–60 mo	30	10–15 min	Electronic format that can be adapted for an EH	Standardized on 2008 children from diverse ethnic and socioeconomic backgrounds, including Spanish-speaking Sensitivity: 0.70–0.90 (moderate to high) Specificity: 0.76–0.91 (moderate to high) Across ages: Sensitivity: 86% Specificity: 85% By domain: Sensitivity: 83% Specificity: 91%
PEDS	Parent interview form. Designed to screen for developmental and behavioral problems needing further evaluation. Single response form used for all ages. May be useful as a surveillance tool	0–8 y	10	2–5 min	Electronic format that can be adapted for an EHR	2013 restandardization (n = 47 531 families from diverse ethnic and socioeconomic backgrounds) Sensitivity: 96% Specificity: 83%
PEDS: Developmental Milestones Screening Version	Parent interview form. Designed to screen for developmental and social-emotional problems	0–8 y	6–8 items at each age level	4–6 min	Electronic format that can be adapted for an EHR	Standardized with 1600 children from diverse ethnic and socioeconomic backgrounds. Sensitivity: 0.70–0.94 Specificity: 0.77–0.93 across ages

Utility as Autism Screener	Scoring Method	Cultural Considerations	Purchase and Obtainment Information	Key References
General screen: Sensitivity: 0.86 Specificity: 0.85 Using the monitor cutoff in communication domain: identified 95% of children positive on ASD-specific screen	Risk categorization. Provides a cutoff score in 5 domains of development that indicates possible need for further evaluation and a monitoring zone that identifies children who should be monitored and rescreened	Available in multiple languages; see test information for details	Paul H. Brookes Publishing Co, Inc: 800-638-3775 or www.brookespublishing.com	Squires J, Potter L, Bricker D. *The ASQ User's Guide: Third Edition*. Baltimore, MD: Paul H. Brookes Publishing Co; 2009
At 12 mo, PEDS is 83% sensitive to an ASD diagnosis at 36 mo but 60% specific. Utility as a component of ongoing surveillance	Risk categorization. Provides algorithm to guide need for referral, additional screening, or continued surveillance	Available in multiple languages; see test information for details	Ellsworth and Vandermeer Press, LLC: 888-729-1697 or www.pedstest.com	Glascoe FP. *Collaborating with Parents: Using Parents' Evaluation of Developmental Status (PEDS) to Detect and Address Developmental and Behavioral Problems*. Second ed. Nolansville, TN: PEDSTest.com, LLC; 2013
—	Risk categorization. Tied to performance above and below the 16th percentile for each item and domain. Provides algorithm to guide need for referral, additional screening, or continued surveillance	Available in multiple languages; see test information for details	Ellsworth and Vandermeer Press, LLC: 888-729-1697 or www.pedstest.com	Brothers KB, Glascoe FP, Robertshaw NS. PEDS: developmental milestones—an accurate brief tool for surveillance and screening. *Clin Pediatr (Phila)*. 2008;47(3):271-279

(continues)

Table 8-1 Supplemental Information

	Description	Age Range	No. Items	Administration Time	Forms Available EHR Compatible	Psychometric Properties[a]
SWYC: milestones	12 age-specific forms, keyed to pediatric periodicity schedule. Includes cognitive, language, and motor skills	1–65 mo	10	~5 min	Available through Patient Tools, Epic, and CHADIS Available for free download as PDFs from www.theswyc.org	Sensitivity: Average across ages: 75.8% Specificity: Average across ages: 78.3%
Behavioral Screening Tests						
Ages and Stages Questionnaire: Social-Emotional-2 (2015)	Screening and surveillance of milestones in social-emotional and mental health. Items focus on self-regulation, compliance, communication, adaptive functioning, autonomy, affect, and interaction with people	1–72 mo	9 age-specific forms (each 4–6 pages long) with 19–33 items	10–15 min	Electronic format that can be adapted for an EHR	By age and disability (i.e., social-emotional problems) Sensitivity: 78% Specificity: 95%
PSC PSC-17b (17 items)	General psychosocial screening and functional assessment in the domains of attention, externalizing, and internalizing symptoms	4–16 y	17 items	<5 min	Yes	Subscales have obtained reasonable agreement with validated and accepted parent-report instruments. Cronbach a was high for each subscale.
PSC-35b (35 items)	Pictorial version available with English, Spanish, Filipino subtitles	Youth self-report: ≥11 y	35 items	<5 min	Yes Online form available	General psychosocial screen: Sensitivity: 80%–95% Specificity: 68%–100%

Utility as Autism Screener	Scoring Method	Cultural Considerations	Purchase and Obtainment Information	Key References
Not evaluated; see SWYC: POSI	Risk categorization. Provides a cutoff score that varies by age that indicates possible need for further evaluation	Available in multiple languages; see test information for details	Available for free download from www.theswyc.org	Sheldrick RC, Perrin EC. Evidence-based milestones for surveillance of cognitive, language, and motor development. *Acad Pediatr.* 2013; 13(6):577–586 Publications and User's Manual available at www.theswyc.org
Need Ages and Stages Questionnaire: Social-Emotional studies in ASD	Cutoff score indicating when further evaluation is needed; monitoring zone that identifies children who should be monitored and rescreened	Available in multiple languages; see test information for details	Paul H. Brookes Publishing Co, Inc: 800-638-3775 or www.agesandstages.com	Squires J, Bricker DD, Twombly E. *Ages & Stages Questionnaires: Social-Emotional -2(ASQ:SE-2). A Parent- Completed, Child-Monitoring System for Social-Emotional Behaviors.* Baltimore, MD: Paul H. Brookes Publishing Co, Inc; 2016 Briggs RD, Stettler EM, Johnson Silver, E, Schrag RDA, Nayak M, Chinitz S, Racine AD. Social-emotional screening for infants and toddlers in primary care. *Pediatrics.* 2012;129(2):1–8
Not examined	Cut points for overall screen and subscales	Available in multiple languages; see test information for details.	http://www.massgeneral.org/psychiatry/services/psc_about.aspx	Gardner W, Lucas A, Kolko DJ, Campo JV. Comparison of the PSC-17 and alternative mental health screens in an at-risk primary care sample. *J Am Acad Child Adolesc Psychiatry.* 2007;46:611–618
Not examined	Cut points for overall screen and subscales	Available in multiple languages; see test information for details.	http://www.massgeneral.org/psychiatry/services/psc_about.aspx	Jellinek MS, Bishop SJ, Murphy JM, Biederman J, Rosenbaum JF. Screening for dysfunction in the children of outpatients at a psychopharmacology clinic. *Am J Psychiatry.* 1991;148:1031–1036 Jellinek MS, Murphy JM, Little M, Pagano ME, Comer DM, Kelleher KJ. Use of the Pediatric Symptom Checklist to screen for psychosocial problems in pediatric primary care: a national feasibility study. *Arch Pediatr Adolesc Med.* 1999;153: 254–260

Table 8-1 Supplemental Information

	Description	Age Range	No. Items	Administration Time	Forms Available EHR Compatible	Psychometric Properties[a]
SDQ	Resilience and psychosocial risk for mental health and social-emotional, behavioral skills. Generates indicators for conduct problems, hyperactivity, emotional symptoms, peer problems, and prosocial behavior. Youth self-report and parent and teacher report	4–17; 3- to 4-y-old version available. Youth self-report: 11–16 y	25; 22 items for 3- to 4-y-olds	5–10 min	Yes, but must first contact youthinmind@gmail.com	Reliable and valid in various populations and for a No. general mental health conditions Sensitivity: 63–94% Specificity: 88%–98% Cross-cultural research and translations
SWYC: Baby PSC	Screening of social-emotional health and behavior	1–18 mo	12	~5 min	Available through Patient Tools, Epic, and CHADIS. Available for free download as PDFs from www.theswyc.org	Correlation 0.61–0.70 with ASQ-SE
SWYC: Preschool PSC	Screening of social-emotional health and behavior	18–65 mo	18	~5 min	Available through Patient Tools, Epic, and CHADIS. Available for free download as PDFs from www.theswyc.org	Correlation 0.88–0.89 with ASQ-SE
Promising Tests: Behavioral Screening						
Brief Early Childhood Screening Assessment	Screening tool developed to facilitate primary care pediatrician's identification of young children who need further assessment of their emotional and social development	1.5–5 y	22 items. 4 items on maternal distress	5 min	No	Fifth-grade reading level. Normative studies conducted in New Orleans, Louisiana; Providence, Rhode Island; and Florida. Sensitivity: 89% Specificity: 85%

Utility as Autism Screener	Scoring Method	Cultural Considerations	Purchase and Obtainment Information	Key References
Not examined	Produces a total strengths versus total difficulties score	Available in multiple languages; see test information for details	Not in the public domain. Downloadable in multiple languages. For permission to use the SDQ, contact Robert Goodman at www.sdqinfo.org	Stone LL, Otten R, Engels RC, Vermulst AA, Janssens JM. Psychometric properties of the parent and teacher versions of the strengths and difficulties questionnaire for 4- to 12-y-olds: a review. *Clin Child Fam Psychol Rev.* 2010;13(3): 254–274
Not evaluated, see SWYC: POSI	Cutoff score of 3 for each of 3 subscales	Available in multiple languages; see test information for details	Available for free download from www.theswyc.org	Publications and User's Manual available at www.theswyc.org Sheldrick RC, Henson BS, Neger EN, Merchant S, Murphy JM, Perrin EC. The Baby Pediatric Symptom Checklist: development and initial validation of a new social/emotional screening instrument for very young children. *Acad Pediatr.* 2013;13(1):72–80
Not evaluated, see SWYC: POSI	Single cutoff score of 9	Available in multiple languages; see test information for details	Available for free download from www.theswyc.org	Publications and User's Manual available at www.theswyc.org Sheldrick RC, Henson BS, Merchant S, Neger EN, Murphy JM, Perrin EC. The Preschool Pediatric Symptom Checklist (PPSC): development and initial validation of a new social/emotional screening instrument. *Acad Pediatr.* 2012; 12(5):456–467
No	Single cutoff score of 9	English	https://medicine.tulane.edu/centers-institutes/tecc/provider-resources/general-screens	Fallucco EM, Wysocki T, James L, Kozikowski C, Williams A, Gleason MM. Brief Early Childhood Screening Assessment: preliminary validity in pediatric primary care. *J Dev Behav Pediatr.* 2017; 38(2):89–98

Table 8-1 Supplemental Information

	Description	Age Range	No. Items	Administration Time	Forms Available EHR Compatible	Psychometric Properties[a]
Language Screening Test						
Communication and Symbolic Behavior Scales Developmental Profile: Infant Toddler Checklist	Standardized tool for screening of communication and symbolic abilities up to the 24-mo level. The Infant Toddler Checklist is a 1-page parent-completed screening tool	6–24 mo	24	5–10 min	No	Standardized on 2188 North American children 6–24 mo of age. Correlations 0.39–0.75 with Mullen Scales at 2 y of age. Sensitivity: 0.76–0.88 in low- and at-risk children at 2 y of age (moderate). Specificity: 0.82–0.87 in low- and at-risk children at 2 y of age (moderate)
Autism Screening Tests						
Modified Checklist for Autism in Toddlers, Revised with Follow-up	Parent-completed questionnaire designed to identify children at risk for autism from the general population. Follow-up clinician administered questions and repeat questionnaire required for specificity	16–30 mo	20 (averaged)	5–10 min	Yes	Standardization sample included 16,071 children screened, 115 had a positive result, 348 needed evaluation, 221 evaluated, and 105 diagnosed with ASD. Validated using ADI-R, ADOS-G, CARS, DSM-IV-TR. Sensitivity: 0.91 Specificity: 0.95 for low-risk 18- and 24-mo-olds with follow-up questionnaire and interview. 45% of children with score ≥3 on initial screen and ≥2 on follow-up have ASD; 95% have clinically significant developmental delay

Utility as Autism Screener	Scoring Method	Cultural Considerations	Purchase and Obtainment Information	Key References
Identifies language delays, discriminates language delay alone from ASD risk for ASD by 12 mo. Risk status for social, speech, symbolic composites and total score	Risk categorization (concern or no concern) in 3 categories (social, speech, and symbolic) and overall total score	Available in multiple languages; see test information for details	Paul H. Brookes Publishing Co, Inc: 800-638-3775 or www.brookes publishing.com	Wetherby AM, Prizant BM. *Communication and Symbolic Behavior Scales: Developmental Profile*. Baltimore, MD: Paul H. Brookes Publishing Co, Inc; 2002
Yes	Risk categorization for questionnaire (pass, need interview, fail). After interview (pass, fail)	Available in multiple languages; see test information for details	http://mchatscreen.com/	Robins DL, Casagrande K, Barton M, Chen CM, Dumont-Mathieu T, Fein D. Validation of the modified checklist for autism in toddlers, revised with follow-up (M-CHAT-R/F). *Pediatrics*. 2014;133(1):37–45

(continued)

(continues)

Table 8-1 Supplemental Information

	Description	Age Range	No. Items	Administration Time	Forms Available EHR Compatible	Psychometric Properties[a]
Social Communication Questionnaire	Parent-completed questionnaire. Designed to identify children at risk for ASD from the general population. Based on items in the ADI-R.	41 y	40 (averaged)	5–10 min	No	Validated using the ADI-R and DSMIV on 200 subjects (160 with pervasive developmental disorder, 40 without pervasive developmental disorder). For use in children with mental age of at least 2 y and chronologic age 41 y. Available in 2 forms: lifetime and current. Overall test sensitivity: 0.85 (moderate). Specificity: 0.75 (moderate). Varies by age. Sensitivity can be improved with lowering cutoff for children 5 y and 5–7 y, specifically poor for younger children
Screening Tool for Autism in Toddlers and Young Children, 24–35 mo	Clinician-directed, interactive and observation measure. Requires training of clinician for standardized administration. Not for population screening	24–35 mo, <24 mo (exploratory)	12 (averaged)	20–30 min	No	Validated by comparison with ADOSG results in 52 children 24–35 mo (26 autism, 26 developmental delay). Sensitivity: 0.83 Specificity: 0.86 PPV: 0.77 NPV: 0.90. For <24 mo: Sensitivity: 0.95 Specificity: 0.73 PPV: 0.56 NPV: 0.97. Screening properties improved for 14-mo-old

Utility as Autism Screener	Scoring Method	Cultural Considerations	Purchase and Obtainment Information	Key References
Yes	Risk categorization (pass, fail).	Available in multiple languages; see test information for details	Western Psychological Corporation: www.wpspublish.com	Rutter M, Bailey A, Lord C. *The Social Communication Questionnaire (SCQ) Manual.* Los Angeles, CA: Western Psychological Services; 2003 Corsello C, Hus V, Pickles A, Risi S, Cook EH Jr, Leventhal BL, Lord C. Between a ROC and a hard place: decision making and making decisions about using the SCQ. *J Child Psychol Psychiatry.* 2007; 48(9):932–940
Yes	12 activities to observe early social-communicative behavior; risk categorization (high risk, low risk)	English	http://stat.vueinnovations.com	Stone WL, Coonrod EE, Ousley O. Brief report: screening tool for autism in 2-year-olds (STAT): development and preliminary data. *J Autism Dev Disord.* 2000; 30:607–612 Stone WL, Coonrod EE, Turner LM, Pozdol SL. Psychometric properties of the STAT for early autism screening. *J Autism Dev Disord* 2004;34:691–701

Table 8-1 Supplemental Information

	Description	Age Range	No. Items	Administration Time	Forms Available EHR Compatible	Psychometric Properties[a]
Autism Screening: Promising Tests						
The Infant and Toddler Checklist (Communication and Symbolic Behavior Scales Developmental Profile) usefulness for autism screening	Parent questionnaire: screens for language delay	6–24 mo	24 (averaged)	15 min	Yes	PPV DD: 0.43 (6–8 mo) PPV DD: 0.79 (21–24 mo)
Early Screening for Autism and Communication Disorders	Parent questionnaire: research edition, 47 items	12–36 mo	47 (averaged)	10–15 min	No	Sensitivity: 0.85–0.91 Specificity: 0.82–0.84 PPV: 0.55–0.81 NPV: 0.88–0.98
First Year Inventory	Parent questionnaire: population screening tool to identify 12-mo-old infants	12 mo	63 (averaged)	10 min	No	Sensitivity, specificity, PPV not reported
SWYC: POSI	7 questions; assesses autism risk	16–35 mo	7 (averaged)	~5 min	Available through Patient Tools, Epic, and CHADIS. Available for free download as PDFs from www.theswyc.org	Sensitivity: 83%–93% (average: 88.5%) Specificity: 42%–75% (average: 56.9%)
Rapid Interactive Screening Test for Autism in Toddlers 1	Clinician observation: administered by trained examiner	12–36 mo	9 interactive items (averaged)	20–30 min	No	Cutoff .15: Sensitivity: 1 Specificity: 0.84 PPV: 0.88 NPV: 0.94. Needs further study in larger samples

The AAP does not approve or endorse any specific tool for screening purposes. This table is not exhaustive, and other tests may be available. ADI-R, Autism Diagnostic Interview, Revised; ADOS-G, Autism Diagnostic Observation Schedule, Generic; CARS, Childhood Autism Rating Scale; DD, developmental disorder; DSM-IV, *Diagnostic and Statistical Manual of Mental Disorders, Fourth Edition*; DSM-IV-TR, *Diagnostic and Statistical Manual of Mental Disorders, Fourth Edition*, Text Revision; EHR, electronic health record; IMFAR, International Meeting for Autism Research (now International Society for Autism Research [INSAR]); PEDS, Parents' Evaluation of Developmental Status; POSI, Parent's Observations of Social Interactions; PSC, Pediatric Symptom Checklist; SDQ, Strengths and Difficulties Questionnaire; SWYC, The Survey of Wellbeing of Young Children; —, not evaluated.

[a] Sensitivity and specificity were categorized as follows: low, ≤69; moderate, 70–89; high, ≥90.

Data from Lipkin, P.H., Macias, M. M. (2020). Council on Children with Disabilities, Section on Developmental and Behavioral Pediatrics. Promoting optimal development: Identifying infants and young children with developmental disorders through developmental surveillance and screening. Pediatrics, 145(1): e20193449. https://publications.aap.org/pediatrics/article/145/1/e20193449/36971/Promoting-Optimal-Development-Identifying-Infants?autologincheck=redirected

(continued)

Utility as Autism Screener	Scoring Method	Cultural Considerations	Purchase and Obtainment Information	Key References
Yes	Identifies language delays (alone, with ASD), risk for ASD; risk status for social, speech, symbolic composites and total score	Available in multiple languages; see test information for details	Paul H. Brookes Publishing Co, Inc: 800-638-3775 or www.brookespublishing.com	Wetherby AM, Brosnan-Maddox S, Peace V, Newton L. Validation of the Infant-Toddler Checklist as a broadband screener for autism spectrum disorders from 9–24 mo of age. *Autism*. 2008 Sep;12(5):487-511
Yes	Investigation ongoing of subset (24 items)	English	https://firstwordsproject.com/screen-my-child/	Not in peer-reviewed literature; presented at IMFAR 2009, 2015. First Words Project (http://med.fsu.edu/index.cfm?page=autismInstitute.firstwords)
Yes	Scores at risk. Promising in high-risk (infant sibling) cohort (Rowberry et al).	English	https://www.med.unc.edu/ahs/pearls/research/first-year-inventory-fyidevelopment/	Rowberry JJ. Screening for autism spectrum disorders in 12-mo-old high-risk siblings by parental report. *J Autism Dev Disord*. 2015;45:221-229
Included on 18-, 24-, and 30-mo SWYC forms	3 of 7 symptoms in at-risk range	Available in multiple languages; see test information for details	Available for free download from www.theswyc.org	Publications and User's Manual available at www.theswyc.org. Smith N, Sheldrick R, Perrin E. An Abbreviated Screening Instrument for Autism Spectrum Disorders. *Infant Mental Health J*. 2013;34(2):149–155 Salisbury LA, Nyce JD, Hannum CD, Sheldrick RC, Perrin EC. Sensitivity and specificity of 2 autism screeners among referred children between 16 and 48 mo of age. *J Dev Behav Pediatr*. 2018;39(3):254–258
Yes	9 interactive activities. Total score summed, cutoff score of 15 (for that sample)	English	https://umassmed.edu/AutismRITA-T/about-thetest/	Choueiri R, Wagner S. A new interactive screening test for autism spectrum disorders in toddlers. *J Pediatr*. 2015;167:460–466

anticipatory guidance on promoting development and behavior using a strength-based approach. If developmental surveillance did not reveal a concern, the next healthcare supervision visit should be scheduled after completion of the current visit.

L. *Developmental diagnosis established? Also, initiate chronic condition management. (Steps 14 and 15)*
A child meets the criteria for a child with special healthcare needs (CSHCN) when a developmental disorder has been diagnosed (McPherson et al., 1998). Once the child has been identified as CSHCN by the medical home, proper care management includes regular monitoring, referral to appropriate subspecialties, and practice or community resources to help ensure that all needed services can be accessed.

   In addition to close monitoring of the CSHCN, the pediatric healthcare provider should be an active participant in the coordination of care services. Consultation between the child's parents, involved healthcare providers, therapists, and educators should take place regularly and as needed to ensure that the child receives evidence-based treatments that are both timely and appropriate for the specific needs of the child.

   Referrals to community-based family support services, such as parent training or support groups, advocacy groups, and respite care, should also be made to provide parents with information they may find helpful. The pediatric healthcare provider should be familiar with local, state, and national programs that may provide additional benefits for CSHCNs.

III. Developmental Screening Tests

Table 8-1 lists a selected group of screening instruments that can be administered in a primary care office by the type of screening instrument, description of who completes the tool and why it is administered, age range, number of items, time for administration, psychometrics, utility as an autism screener, scoring method, languages available, how to purchase or obtain the tool, and primary references if available (Lipkin et al., 2020).

The list is not exhaustive, with numerous developmental tools available and others under development. Providers should familiarize themselves with a variety of screening tests, taking into consideration their patient population, practice needs and resources, and skill level.

A. *General Developmental Screening Tools*
   1. Ages and Stages Questionnaires, 3rd edition (Squires et al., 2009)
   2. Parents' Evaluation of Developmental Status (PEDS) (Glascoe, 2013)
   3. PEDS: Developmental Milestones Screening Version (Brothers et al., 2008)
   4. Survey of Well-Being of Young Children (SWYC): Milestones (Sheldrick & Perrin, 2013)

B. *Behavioral Screening Tests*
   1. Ages and Stages Questionnaire: Social-Emotional, 2nd edition (Squires et al., 2016)
   2. Pediatric Symptom Checklist (PSC): PSC-17b (17 items) (Gardner et al., 2007)
   3. PSC: PSC-35b (35 items) (Jellinek et al., 1999)
   4. Strengths and Difficulties Questionnaire (SDQ) (Stone et al., 2010)
   5. SWYC: Baby PSC (Sheldrick et al., 2013)
   6. SWYC: Preschool PSC (Sheldrick et al., 2012)

C. *Promising Tests: Behavioral Screening*
   1. Brief Early Childhood Screening Assessment (Fallucco et al., 2017)

D. *Language Screening Test*
   1. Communication and Symbolic Behavior Scales Developmental Profile: Infant Toddler Checklist (Wetherby & Prizant, 2002)

E. *Autism Screening Tests*
   1. Modified Checklist for Autism in Toddlers, Revised With Follow-Up (Robins et al., 2014)
   2. Social Communication Questionnaire (Rutter et al., 2003)
   3. Screening Tool for Autism in Toddlers and Young Children, 24–35 mo (Stone et al., 2000)

F. *Autism Screening: Promising Tests*
   1. The Infant and Toddler Checklist (Communication and Symbolic Behavior Scales Developmental Profile) (Wetherby et al., 2008)
   2. Early Screening for Autism and Communication Disorders (Wetherby et al., 2021)
   3. First Year Inventory (Rowberry, 2015)
   4. SWYC: Parent's Observations of Social Interactions (POSI) (Smith et al., 2013)

IV. Psychometrics (Lipkin et al., 2020)

A. *Characteristics of accurate screening tests*
Developmental screening tests should be both reliable and valid, with good sensitivity and specificity. Properties of screening tests that should be considered are:
1. Reliability
   Definition: the ability of a measure to produce consistent results. There are different types of reliability:
   a. Test–retest reliability: the stability or consistency of results across different administrations.
   b. Interrater reliability: the stability or consistency of results across different raters.
   c. Internal consistency: the correlation across items on an instrument to show consistency or responses. Usually shown as the Cronbach's alpha coefficient.
2. Validity
   Definition: the ability of a measure to discriminate between a child at a determined level of risk for delay and the rest of the population. There are many types of validity:
   a. Concurrent validity: high correlation between the screening tool and a diagnostic measure with similar domains.
   b. Discriminant validity: how well the screening tool distinguishes children with the problem or

condition compared to those without the problem or condition.
   c. Predictive validity: screening test results are compared to performance on diagnostic measures administered at a later time.
3. Sensitivity
   Definition: the accuracy of the test in identifying delayed development. Sensitivity is also seen as the percentage of children with true problems correctly identified on a screening tool.
   a. Example: if the screening tool has 70% sensitivity, it means that 70% of the children who receive a positive screening result truly have a developmental problem.
   b. Standards: 70%–80% sensitivity is considered moderate, and 90% or higher is strong.
4. Specificity
   Definition: the accuracy of a test in identifying children who are not delayed. Specificity is also seen as the percentage of children without true difficulties correctly identified by a negative result on a screening tool.
   a. Example: if the test has 80% specificity, it means that 80% of the children screened who have a negative result have no developmental problem.
   b. Standards: 80% or higher specificity is considered moderate to strong. This minimizes referrals for diagnostic tests for children with no developmental delays or problems.
5. Positive predictive value (PPV)
   Definition: the proportion of children with a positive test result who are truly delayed. The PPV tells the primary care provider what a positive test result means for the individual child. PPV is frequently used by primary care providers.
   a. Example: if four out of five children have positive screening test results and are found to have a developmental problem, then the PPV is 80%. Therefore, for the screening test, there is an 80% chance that the child actually has a developmental problem.
   b. Standards: there is no agreed-on standard for PPV for screening tests. In reality, PPVs are rarely very high and can range between 30% and 50%.
6. Negative predictive value (NPV)
   Definition: the proportion of children with negative test results who do not have a developmental disorder. The NPV informs the primary care provider of the chance that a child truly does not have a developmental disorder when the screening result is negative.
7. Prevalence rate: number of children in the population with a disorder, measured at a given time
8. Base rate: rate of a given disorder
9. General screening test: a test that evaluates multiple areas of development
10. Domain-specific screening test: a test that evaluates one area of development, such as gross motor or language
11. Disorder-specific screening test: a test aimed at identifying a specific developmental disorder, such as ASD

V. Conclusion

Regular surveillance and routine screening at recommended intervals help identify children at risk for behavioral, developmental, and emotional problems and facilitate referral for diagnostic tests and early intervention services. Children develop at different paces, and surveillance and screening tests can help differentiate normal, intermittent changes in behavior from persistent challenging behaviors. In addition, valid and reliable screening tests can help identify children whose development has changed or shows a loss of developmental milestones. Early identification of developmental, behavioral, and emotional problems during childhood may help children succeed in school, develop social relationships, and contribute to society.

In addition to performing regular developmental surveillance and screening, the pediatric healthcare provider should become versed in early intervention services and programs at the local, state, and national levels. Awareness of these programs, as well as the challenges in accessing early intervention services, will help the pediatric healthcare provider facilitate the coordination of care for children with special healthcare needs.

VI. Clinician resources

A. *AAP National Center of Medical Home Initiatives for Children With Special Needs*
   Resources developed by the AAP and pilot projects implementing the AAP algorithm for developmental screening, including policies and protocols, screening algorithms, resources and tips on Medicaid billing, and parent resources; available at www.medicalhomeinfo.org

B. *AAP, Caring for Children With Autism Spectrum Disorders: A Resource Toolkit for Clinicians*
   Includes identification, surveillance, and screening tools, as well as referrals, fact sheets, and family handouts; available at https://publications.aap.org/toolkits/pages/Autism-Toolkit

C. *AAP's Bright Futures*
   Provides health supervision guidelines and developmental, behavioral, and psychosocial screening and assessment tools for use in primary care, including questions to ask parents during the interview; available at https://brightfutures.aap.org/Pages/default.aspx

D. *Assuring Better Child Health and Development (ABCD Initiative)*
   Research and resources promoting child health and development; includes tools for clinicians and state resources; available at http://www.nashp.org/abcd-map/

E. Center on the Social and Emotional Foundations for Early Learning
Available at http://csefel.vanderbilt.edu

F. Developmental Monitoring and Screening for Health Professionals, CDC
Includes guidance on child health developmental monitoring with links to AAP and *Bright Futures*; available at https://www.cdc.gov/ncbddd/childdevelopment/screening-hcp.html

G. Early Childhood Technical Assistance Center "Early Identification: Screening"
Available at https://ectacenter.org/topics/earlyid/screeneval.asp

H. The Commonwealth Fund
Research on innovations in child health and development, including the work of the ABCD initiative and screening in primary care settings; available at http://www.commonwealthfund.org

References

Administration for Children and Families, U.S. Department of Health and Human Services. (2020). *Birth to 5: Watch Me Thrive!* https://www.acf.hhs.gov/archive/ecd/child-health-development/watch-me-thrive

American Academy of Pediatrics. (2007). *Bright Futures: Guidelines for health supervision of infants, children, and adolescents* (3rd ed.).

American Academy of Pediatrics. (2021). *The medical home definition.* https://medicalhomeinfo.aap.org/overview/Pages/Whatisthemedicalhome.aspx

American Academy of Pediatrics Council on Children With Disabilities, AAP Section on Developmental Behavioral Pediatrics, Bright Futures Steering Committee, & AAP Medical Home Initiatives for Children With Special Needs Project Advisory Committee. (2006). Identifying infants and young children with developmental disorders in the medical home: An algorithm for developmental surveillance and screening. *Pediatrics, 118*(1), 405–420. doi:10.1542/peds.2006-1231

Brothers, K. B., Glascoe, F. P., & Robertshaw, N. S. (2008). PEDS: Developmental milestones—an accurate brief tool for surveillance and screening. *Clinical Pediatrics, 47*(3), 271–279. doi:10.1177/0009922807309419

Centers for Disease Control and Prevention. (2021). *Developmental disabilities.* https://www.cdc.gov/ncbddd/developmentaldisabilities/index.html

Centers for Disease Control and Prevention. (2023). *Learn the signs. Act early.* https://www.cdc.gov/ncbddd/actearly/index.html

Fallucco, E. M., Wysocki, T., James, L., Kozikowski, C., Williams, A., & Gleason, M. M. (2017). Brief Early Childhood Screening Assessment: Preliminary validity in pediatric primary care. *Journal of Developmental & Behavioral Pediatrics, 38*(2), 89–98. doi:10.1097/DBP.0000000000000384

Gardner, W., Lucas, A., Kolko, D. J., & Campo, J. V. (2007). Comparison of the PSC-17 and alternative mental health screens in an at-risk primary care sample. *Journal of the American Academy of Child & Adolescent Psychiatry, 46*(5), 611–618. doi:10.1097/chi.0b013e318032384b

Glascoe, F. P. (2005). Screening for developmental and behavioral problems. *Mental Retardation and Developmental Disabilities Research Reviews, 11*(3), 173–179. doi:10.1002/mrdd.20068

Glascoe, F. P. (2013). *Collaborating with parents: Using Parents' Evaluation of Developmental Status (PEDS) to detect and address developmental and behavioral problems* (2nd ed.). PEDSTest.com.

Hagan, J. F., Shaw, J. S., & Duncan, P. M. (Eds.). (2017). *Bright Futures: Guidelines for health supervision of infants, children, and adolescents* (4th ed.). American Academy of Pediatrics.

Halfon, N., Regalado, M., Sareen, H., Inkelas, M., Reuland, C. P., Glascoe, F. P., & Olson, L. M. (2004). Assessing development in the pediatric office. *Pediatrics, 113*(6), 1926–1933.

Jellinek, M., Murphy, J. M., Little, M., Pagano, M. E., Comer, D. M., & Kelleher, K. J. (1999). Use of the Pediatric Symptom Checklist (PSC) to screen for psychosocial problems in pediatric primary care: A national feasibility study. *Archives of Pediatric and Adolescent Medicine, 153*(3), 254–260. doi:10.1001/archpedi.153.3.254

Johnson, C., & Myers, S. (2007). Identification and evaluation of children with autism spectrum disorders. *Pediatrics, 120*, 1183–1215. doi:10.1542/peds.2007-2361

Lipkin, P. H., Macias, M. M., & Council on Children with Disabilities, Section on Developmental and Behavioral Pediatrics. (2020). Promoting optimal development: Identifying infants and young children with developmental disorders through developmental surveillance and screening. *Pediatrics, 145*(1), e20193449. doi:10.1542/peds.2019-3449

Maenner, M. J., Warren, Z., Williams, A. R., Amoakohene, E., Bakian, A. V., Bilder, D. A., Durkin., M. S., Fitzgerald, R. T., Furnier, S. M., Hughes, M. M., Ladd-Acosta, C. M., McArthur, D., Pas, E. T., Salinas, A., Vehorn, A., Williams, S., Esler, A., Grzybowski, A.,...Shaw., K., A. (2023). Prevalence and characteristics of autism spectrum disorder among children aged 8 years—Autism and Developmental Disabilities Monitoring Network, 11 Sites, United States, 2020. *MMWR Surveillance Summaries, 72*(2), 1–14. DOI: doi:10.15585/mmwr.ss7202a1

McPherson, M., Arango, P., Fox, H., Lauver, C., McManus, C., Newacheck, P. W., Perrin, J. M., Shonkoff, J. P., & Strickland, B. (1998). A new definition of children with special health care needs. *Pediatrics, 101*(1), 137–140. doi:10.1542/peds.102.1.137

Rice, C. E., Van Naarden Braun, K., Kogan, M. D., Smith, C., Kavanaugh, L., Strickland, B., & Blumberg, S. J. (2014). Screening for developmental delays among young children—National Survey of Children's Health, United States, 2007. *MMWR Supplement, 63*(02), 27–35.

Robins, D., Casagrande, K., Barton, M. L., Chen, C. A., Dumont-Mathieu, T. M., & Fein, D. (2014). Validation of the Modified Checklist for Autism in Toddlers, Revised With Follow-Up (M-CHAT-R/F). *Pediatrics, 133*(1), 37–45. doi:10.1542/peds.2013-1813

Rowberry, J. J. (2015). Screening for autism spectrum disorders in 12-mo-old high-risk siblings by parental report. *Journal of Autism and Developmental Disorders, 45*(1), 221–229. doi:10.1007/s10803-014-2211-x

Rutter, M., Bailey, A., & Lord, C. (2003). *The Social Communication Questionnaire (SCQ) manual.* Western Psychological Services.

Sheldrick, R., & Perrin, E. C. (2013). Evidence-based milestones for surveillance of cognitive, language, and motor development. *Academic Pediatrics*, *13*(6), 577–586. doi:10.1016/j.acap.2013.07.001

Sheldrick, R. C., Henson, B. S., Merchant, S., Neger, E. N., Murphy, J., & Perrin, E. C. (2012). The Preschool Pediatric Symptom Checklist (PPSC): Development and initial validation of a new social/emotional screening instrument. *Academic Pediatrics*, *12*(5), 456–467. doi:10.1016/j.acap.2012.06.008

Sheldrick, R. C., Henson, B. S., Neger, E. N., Merchant, S., Murphy, J. M., & Perrin, E. C. (2013). The Baby Pediatric Symptom Checklist: Development and initial validation of a new social/emotional screening instrument for very young children. *Academic Pediatrics*, *12*(1), 72–80. doi:10.1016/j.acap.2012.08.003

Smith, N., Sheldrick, R., & Perrin, E. (2013). An abbreviated screening instrument for autism spectrum disorders. *Infant Mental Health Journal*, *34*(2), 149–155. doi:10.1002/imhj.21356

Squires, J., Bricker, D., & Twombly, E. (2016). *Ages and Stages Questionnaires: Social-Emotional-2 (ASQ SE-2). A parent-completed, child-monitoring system for social-emotional behaviors*. Paul H. Brookes.

Squires, J., Potter, L., & Bricker, D. (2009). *The ASQ user's guide: Third edition*. Paul H. Brookes.

Stone, L. L., Otten, R., Engels, R. C., Vermulst, A. A., & Janssens, J. M. (2010). Psychometric properties of the parent and teacher versions of the Strengths and Difficulties Questionnaire for 4- to 12-y-olds: A review. *Clinical Child and Family Psychology Review*, *13*(3), 254–274. doi:10.1007/s10567-010-0071-2

Stone, W. L., Coonrod, E. E., & Ousley, O. (2000). Brief report: Screening Tool for Autism in 2-Year-Olds (STAT): Development and preliminary data. *Journal of Autism and Developmental Disorders*, *30*(6), 607–612. doi:10.1023/a:1005647629002

U.S. Department of Health and Human Services, Health Resources and Services Administration, & Maternal and Child Health Bureau. (2020). *The National Survey of Children's Health*. https://www.childhealthdata.org/learn-about-the-nsch/NSCH

Wetherby, A. M., Brosnan-Maddox, S., Peace, V., & Newton, L. (2008). Validation of the Infant-Toddler Checklist as a broadband screener for autism spectrum disorders from 9–24 mo of age. *Autism*, *12*(5), 487–511. doi:10.1177/1362361308094501

Wetherby, A. M., Guthrie, W., Hooker, J. L., Delehanty, A., Day, T. N., Woods, J., Pierce, K., Manwaring, S. S., Thurm, A., Ozonoff, S., Petkova, E., & Lord, C. (2021). The Early Screening for Autism and Communication Disorders: Field-testing an autism-specific screening tool for children 12 to 36 months of age. *Autism*, *25*(7), 2112–2123. doi:10.1177/13623613211012526

Wetherby, A. M., & Prizant, B. M. (2002). *Communication and Symbolic Behavior Scales: Developmental profile*. Paul H. Brookes.

Zablotsky, B., Black, L., Maenner, M., Schieve, L., Danielson, M., Bitsko, R., Blumberg, S., Kogan, M., & Boyle, C. (2019). Prevalence and trends of developmental disabilities among children in the United States: 2009–2017. *Pediatrics*, *144*(4), e20190811. doi:10.1542/peds.2019-0811

Zubler, J. M., Wiggins, L. D., Macias, M. M., Whitaker, T. M., Shaw, J. S., Squires, J. K., Pajek, J. A., Wolf, R. B., Slaughter, K. S., Broughton, A. S., Gerndt, K. L., Mlodoch, B. J., & Lipkin, P. H. (2022). Evidence-informed milestones for developmental surveillance tools. *Pediatrics*, *149*(3), e2021052138. doi:10.1542/peds.2021-052138

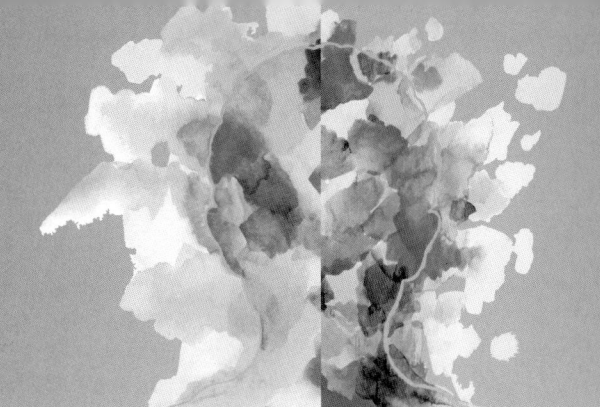

SECTION II

Common Complex Pediatric Presentations

CHAPTER 9	Childhood Asthma	77
CHAPTER 10	Atopic Dermatitis in Children	89
CHAPTER 11	Attention-Deficit/Hyperactivity Disorder in Children and Adolescents	101
CHAPTER 12	Pediatric Depression	115
CHAPTER 13	Child Maltreatment	129
CHAPTER 14	Childhood Overweight and Obesity	145
CHAPTER 15	Urinary Incontinence in Children	155

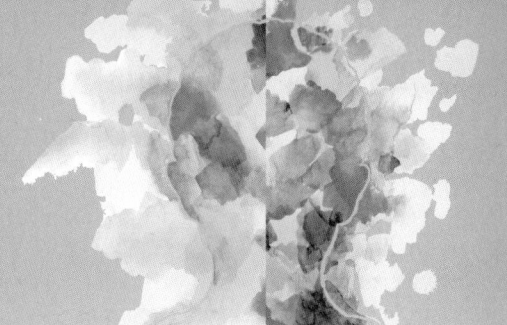

CHAPTER 9

Childhood Asthma

Christine Mayor

I. Introduction and general background

A. *Definition and overview*

Asthma is a chronic lung disease causing narrowing of the airways and airway obstruction. It is characterized by underlying inflammation that can be acute or chronic, bronchial hyperresponsiveness and constriction, and excess mucus production (National Asthma Education and Prevention Program [NAEPP], 2007). Symptoms are variable and episodic and include coughing, wheezing, shortness of breath, and chest tightness. Airway obstruction is generally reversible; however, chronic inflammation may lead to permanent airway remodeling that is only partially responsive to treatment (NAEPP, 2007). There is no cure for asthma, although asthma symptoms can be absent for quite some time, even years.

B. *Prevalence and incidence*

The onset of asthma often occurs during childhood (NAEPP, 2007). In the United States, 6.5% of individuals younger than 18 years old have asthma (Centers for Disease Control and Prevention [CDC], 2021a). Subgroups with higher rates of asthma include boys (7.3%), teenagers (15-17 years, 9.5%), and children living below the poverty threshold (10.4%) (CDC, 2021a). In addition, non-Hispanic Black, American Indian/Alaska Native, non-Mexican Hispanic, and non-Hispanic multiracial children are more likely to be diagnosed with asthma, whereas non-Hispanic Asian and Mexican children have the lowest rates of asthma (CDC, 2021b). The rates of asthma in children are also higher in urban environments (Gern, 2010).

C. *Health outcomes*

In general, the health outcomes for individuals with asthma have improved over time; however, disparities do exist for certain racial and ethnic groups. For all ages, Black individuals are five times more likely to be seen in the emergency department for asthma, twice as likely to be hospitalized for asthma, and three times more likely to die from asthma compared to non-Hispanic White individuals (Asthma and Allergy Foundation of America [AAFA], 2020). Higher morbidity also exists for Puerto Ricans and Indigenous populations in the United States (AAFA, 2020). The causal factors are complex but can be categorized into four groups: (1) structural determinants, such as systemic racism; (2) social determinants, such as socioeconomic status, education, and neighborhood; (3) biological determinants, such as genetics and ancestry; and (4) behavioral determinants, such as tobacco use and medication adherence (AAFA, 2020).

II. Database (may include but is not limited to)

A. *Subjective*
1. Past health history
   a. Prematurity (particularly with known lung disease)
   b. Birth via cesarean section
   c. Breastfed
   d. Respiratory syncytial virus infection in infancy or toddlerhood
   e. Rhinovirus infection in childhood
   f. Hospitalization for respiratory issues
   g. Wheezing in first years of life
   h. Gastroesophageal reflux
   i. Progression of atopic disease ("atopic march"): atopic dermatitis (eczema), food allergy, allergic rhinitis, asthma (Hill & Spergel, 2018)
   j. Frequency of emergency room (ER)/urgent care visits for asthma, particularly a history of needing oral steroids
   k. Known allergies to medications, food, or environmental factors
2. Family history
   a. Asthma
   b. Allergic rhinitis
   c. Atopic dermatitis

3. Occupational and environmental history
   a. Maternal smoking during pregnancy
   b. Maternal stress and experience of trauma during pregnancy
   c. Exposure to tobacco smoke
   d. Exposure to environmental toxins and pollution (through parental occupation, neighborhood of residence, etc.)
   e. Exposure to environmental allergens (dust, animals with dander, mold, cockroaches, etc.) at home, school, or daycare
   f. Exposure to different microbes during the development of the immune system
   g. Stress and adverse childhood experiences (ACEs)
4. Review of systems
   a. Constitutional: poor sleep patterns; other problems related to poor sleep, sedentary lifestyle, and avoidance of physical activity
   b. Ocular: itchy, irritated, red, and/or watery eyes; swollen eyelids
   c. Ear, nose, and throat: runny nose, nasal congestion, sneezing, snoring, mouth-breathing, itchy nose, itchy throat, throat-clearing
   d. Pulmonary: chronic cough, wheezing, shortness of breath, chest pain, nocturnal dry cough, exercise intolerance, cough with exertion
   e. Skin: pruritis, rash
5. Medications
   a. Past and current medications, including over-the-counter medications, medications obtained abroad, alternative therapies, and home remedies
   b. Actual use, as opposed to prescribed use, of medications (medication strength, amount, timing of use, adherence)
   c. Response of symptoms to past and current medications
   d. Side effects, especially for medications with a black-box warning
   e. Device technique

B. Objective
1. Physical examination findings
   a. General: general appearance, body habitus, level of distress, and interaction with caregiver and provider
   b. Vital signs: heart rate, respiratory rate, and oxygen saturation
   c. Eyes: "allergic shiners" (dark circles under eyes), Dennie-Morgan lines, boggy conjunctivae, discharge, and eyelid edema
   d. Ear, nose, and throat: rhinorrhea, boggy nasal turbinates, ear effusion, cobblestoning of posterior oropharynx (from chronic postnasal drip), and "allergic crease" (a crease across the nose caused by habitual upward wiping or rubbing of nose a.k.a. "allergic salute")
   e. Pulmonary exam findings are largely normal when not in an acute flare.
   f. Skin: hydration, presence of scarring or rashes
   g. In severe acute flare:
      i. Overall appearance: general state of distress and anxiety because of "air hunger," posturing (leaning forward to increase air entry), grunting, nasal flaring, inability to speak in full sentences, pallor
      ii. Pulmonary examination findings: cough, tachypnea, wheezing (expiratory more common than inspiratory), decreased air movement (may result in minimal to no wheezing, which is a warning sign), prolonged expiratory phase, intercostal and/or supraclavicular retractions
      iii. Abdomen: increased use of accessory muscles to improve air entry
2. Supporting data from relevant diagnostic tests (not required for diagnosis and further detailed under the Plan section)
   a. Spirometry (pre- and post-bronchodilator)
   b. Allergy testing for response to environmental allergens
   c. Radiology: chest radiograph
   d. Laboratory measures: complete blood count and arterial blood gas

III. Assessment
A. *Differential diagnosis* (NAEPP, 2007)
1. Asthma
2. Allergic rhinitis
3. Sinusitis
4. Gastroesophageal reflux
5. Viral upper respiratory infection
6. Other causes of large airway obstruction
   a. Foreign body in trachea or bronchus
   b. Viral infection (e.g., croup)
   c. Vocal cord dysfunction
   d. Vascular rings or laryngeal webs
   e. Laryngotracheomalacia, tracheal stenosis, or bronchostenosis
   f. Enlarged lymph nodes or tumor
7. Other causes of small airway obstruction
   a. Bronchiolitis
   b. Cystic fibrosis
   c. Bronchopulmonary dysplasia
   d. Pulmonary edema (e.g., from congenital heart disease)
8. Habit cough or psychogenic cough
9. Anxiety/stress (in the case of chest pain as the primary symptom)

B. Classify severity or control (**Tables 9-1** and **9-2**)
1. Classify **severity** if child *is not* currently on any controller medications, considering domains of both impairment and risk. *Impairment* refers to how the patient feels presently or in a typical week; *risk* refers to the likelihood that exacerbations will occur over time. A patient's severity level is defined by the most severe category for any

Table 9-1 Classifying Asthma Severity in Children 0–11 Years of Age

	Components of Severity	Intermittent Asthma	Mild Persistent Asthma	Moderate Persistent Asthma	Severe Persistent Asthma
Impairment	Symptom Frequency (not with exercise)	≤2 d/wk	>2 d/wk but not daily	Daily	Throughout the day
	Nighttime Awakenings	Children 0–4 years: 0 Children 5–11 years: ≤2x/mo	Children 0–4 years: 1–2x/mo Children 5–11 years: 3–4x/mo	Children 0–4 years: 3–4x/mo Children 5–11 years: >1x/wk but not nightly	Children 0–4 years: >1x/wk Children 5–11 years: 7x/wk
	Short-acting β_2-agonist for symptom control (not prevention of EIB)	≤2 d/wk	>2 d/wk but not daily	Daily	Several times per day
	Inference with normal activity	None	Minor limitation	Some limitation	Extremely limited
	Lung function (ages 5–11 years)	Normal FEV_1 between exacerbations FEV_1 > 80% predicted FEV_1/FVC > 85%	FEV_1 > 80% predicted FEV_1/FVC > 80%	FEV_1 = 60%–80% predicted FEV_1/FVC = 75–80%	FEV_1 < 60% predicted FEV_1/FVC < 75%
Risk	Exacerbations requiring oral systemic corticosteroids	0–1/year	Children 0–4 years: ≥2 exacerbations in 6 mo requiring oral systemic corticosteroids, or ≥4 wheezing episodes/yr lasting >1 d AND risk factors for persistent asthma. Children 5–11 years: ≥2/year More frequent and intense exacerbations indicate greater severity.		
		Consider severity and interval since last exacerbation. Frequency and severity may fluctuate over time. Relative annual risk may be related to FEV_1. Exacerbations of any severity may occur in patients in any severity category.			
Recommended Step for Initiating Therapy (see Table 9-3 for recommended treatment steps)		Step 1	Step 2	Step 3 and consider short course of oral systemic corticosteroids	
		In 2–6 wk, depending on severity, evaluate level of asthma control that is achieved. If no clear benefit is observed in 4–6 wk, consider adjusting therapy or alternative diagnosis.			

EIB, exercise-induced bronchospasm; FEV_1, forced expiratory volume in the first second of expiration; FVC, forced vital capacity. U.S. Department of Health and Human Services, National Institutes of Health, National Heart, Lung, and Blood Institute. (2008). National Asthma Education and Prevention Program Expert Panel Report 3: Guidelines for the diagnosis and management of asthma—Summary Report 2007 (NIH Publication Number 08-5846, pp. 40–42). Bethesda, MD: Author.

Table 9-2 Classifying Asthma Control and Adjusting Therapy in Children 0–11 Years of Age

	Components of Control	Well Controlled Asthma	Not Well Controlled Asthma	Very Poorly Controlled Asthma
Impairment	Symptom Frequency (not with exercise)	≤2 d/wk and not more than once a day for children age 5–11 years	>2 d/wk or multiple times on ≤2 d/wk for children age 5–11 years	Throughout the day
	Nighttime Awakenings	≤1x/mo	Children 0–4 years: >1x/mo Children 5–11 years: ≥2x/month	Children 0–4 years: >1x/wk Children 5–11 years: ≥2x/wk
	Short-acting β_2-agonist for symptom control (not prevention of EIB)	≤2 d/wk	>2 d/wk	Several times per day
	Lung function (ages 5–11 years)	FEV_1 > 80% predicted FEV_1/FVC > 80%	FEV_1 60–80% predicted FEV_1/FVC 75–80%	FEV_1 < 60% predicted FEV_1/FVC < 75%
Risk	Exacerbations requiring oral systemic corticosteroids	0–1/year	Children 0–4 years: 2–3/year Children 5–11 years: ≥2/year	Children 0–4 years: >3/year Children 5–11 years: ≥2/year
		Consider severity and interval since last exacerbation.		
	Reduction in lung growth (ages 5–11)	Evaluation requires long-term follow-up care.		
	Treatment-related adverse effects	Medication side effects may vary in intensity from none to very troublesome and worrisome. The level of intensity does not correlate to specific levels of control but should be considered in the overall assessment of risk.		
	Recommended Action for Treatment (see Table 9-3 for treatment steps) The stepwise approach is meant to assist, not replace, clinical decision making required to meet individual patient needs.	Maintain current step Regular follow-up every 1–6 mo. Consider step-down if well controlled for at least 3 mo.	Children 0–4 years: Step up 1 step Children 5–11 years: Step up at least 1 step Reevalute in 2–4 wks to achieve control. For children 0–4 years, if no clear benefit observed in 4–6 wks, consider adjusting therapy or alternative diagnosis.	Step up 1–2 steps and consider short course of oral systemic corticosteroids. Reevaluate in 2 wks to achieve control.
			Before step-up: Review adherence to medication, device technique, and environmental control. If alternative treatment was used, discontinue it and use preferred treatment for that step. For side effects, consider alternative treatment options.	

EIB, exercise-induced bronchospasm; FEV_1, forced expiratory volume in the first second of expiration; FVC, forced vital capacity.

U.S. Department of Health and Human Services, National Institutes of Health, National Heart, Lung, and Blood Institute. (2008). National Asthma Education and Prevention Program Expert Panel Report 3: Guidelines for the diagnosis and management of asthma–Summary Report 2007 (NIH Publication Number 08-5846, pp. 40–42). Bethesda, MD: Author.

particular component of severity. For example, if a patient has no symptoms during the day but wheezes every night, the severity level would be defined as severe persistent. The severity level is used to determine if a patient should be started on a daily controller medicine. Once the severity level is determined, pharmacotherapy may be initiated based on a stepwise approach. The higher steps correspond to more potent medications (**Table 9-3**). Asthma severity classifications are as follows:
   a. Intermittent
   b. Mild persistent
   c. Moderate persistent
   d. Severe persistent
2. Classify **control** if the child is currently on a controller medication, again considering domains of both impairment and risk. As with the severity domain, the control level is defined by the most severe category for any particular component of control. Identifying a child's level of control helps determine if the patient's asthma medications should be stepped up or stepped down. For example, if a child has been symptom-free for at least 3 months with no more than one exacerbation requiring oral steroids on the current controller therapy in the last 12 months, a step-down of the controller medication could be considered. On the other hand, if the child's asthma is not well controlled, due to either impairment or risk, the child's controller medication should be stepped up at least one step, and asthma control should be reevaluated in 2 to 6 weeks. Asthma control levels are defined as follows:
   a. Well controlled
   b. Not well controlled
   c. Very poorly controlled

IV. Goals of clinical management

A. Infrequent or no daytime asthma symptoms
B. No nighttime awakenings caused by asthma symptoms
C. Normal spirometry
D. Ability to do normal physical activity and sports
E. Child should not miss school, and caregiver should not need to miss work.
F. Not more than one exacerbation requiring oral corticosteroids per rolling 6-month period in children 0–4 years and per rolling 12-month period in children >4 years
G. Child is on the safest form and lowest dose of controller medication needed to achieve these goals.

Table 9-3 Stepwise Approach for Managing Asthma Long Term in Children 0–11 Years of Age: Preferred Medications*

Intermittent Asthma	Persistent Asthma				
Step 1	Step 2	Step 3	Step 4	Step 5	Step 6
Children age 0–4 years: PRN SABA and add 7–10 day course of daily ICS at the start of RTI Children age 5–11 years: PRN SABA	Children age 0–11 years: Daily low-dose ICS and PRN SABA	Children age 0–3 years: Daily medium-dose ICS and PRN SABA Children age 4–11 years: Daily and PRN combination low-dose ICS-formoterol.	Children age 0–3 years: Daily medium-dose ICS-LABA and PRN SABA Children age 4–11 years: Daily and PRN combination medium-dose ICS-formoterol.	Children age 0–11 years: Daily high-dose ICS-LABA and PRN SABA	Children age 0–11 years: Daily high-dose ICS-LABA + oral systemic corticosteroid and PRN SABA

Check adherence, inhaler technique, environmental factors, and comorbid conditions.

Consider step down if asthma is well controlled for at least 3 consecutive months.

Children age 0–4 years: Reasess in 4–6 wks after step up. Consider consultation with asthma specialist at Step 2. Consult with asthma specialist if Step 3 or higher is required.

Children age 5–11 years: Reasess in 2–6 wks after step up. Consider consultation with asthma specialist at Step 3. Consult with asthma specialist if Step 4 or higher is required.

ICS, inhaled corticosteroid; LABA, inhaled long-acting beta2-agonist; PRN, as needed; RTI, respiratory tract infection; SABA, inhaled short-acting beta2-agonist.
* See U.S. Department of Health and Human Services et al. (2020a, 2020b) focused updates for full details of stepwise treatment, including alternative therapies.
Data from U.S. Department of Health and Human Services, National Institutes of Health, National Heart, Lung, and Blood Institute. (2020b). 2020 Focused updates to the asthma management guidelines: At-a-glance guide (NIH Publication No. 20-HL-8142). Retrieved from https://www.nhlbi.nih.gov/health-topics/all-publications-and-resources/at-glance-2020-focused-updates-asthma-management-guidelines

V. Plan

A. *Diagnostic tests*
  1. Spirometry
     a. Obtain a baseline in children ages 5 years and older, and repeat with changes in clinical status and/or major changes in medication regimen. Developmental delays and anatomical abnormalities of the face and/or trunk may affect performance and results.
     b. Forced expiratory volume in the first second of expiration (FEV_1), forced vital capacity (FVC), and forced expiratory flow in the mid-expiratory phase (FEF 25%–75%) are most useful in children.
     c. It may be difficult to obtain accurate results in children, but trends over time may be helpful even if values remain in normal range.
     d. Most often normal in children between asthma flares
     e. May be abnormal in children during a respiratory illness or flares of allergic rhinitis without abnormal physical exam lung findings
     f. May be falsely normal due to inhaled short-acting beta$_2$-agonist (SABA) use in the preceding 4 hours or inhaled long-acting beta$_2$-agonist (LABA) use in the preceding 12 hours
     g. The comparison of the results of spirometry performed before and after the administration of a bronchodilator demonstrates obstruction and assesses reversibility. An increase of greater than or equal to 12% in the FEV_1 and/or in the FEF 25%–75% shows significant reversibility and is diagnostic for asthma.
     h. Aerosol-generating procedure that requires appropriate precautions if the patient may have a communicable airborne respiratory disease (e.g., COVID-19, tuberculosis)
  2. Chest radiograph
     a. May be needed to exclude differential diagnoses, such as anatomical abnormalities
     b. May show hyperinflation, infiltrates, and bronchiolar cuffing
  3. Allergy testing
     a. Indicated in children with persistent or uncontrolled asthma, allergy symptoms, or severe eczema
     b. Tests for common environmental allergens and known or possible triggers
     c. Testing to detect specific immunoglobulin E (IgE) sensitization can be done on children of any age.
     d. Referral to a subspecialty clinic may be necessary for testing.
     e. When access to specialists or testing is limited, clinicians should interview patients for allergy symptoms and known exposures.
     f. Skin testing
        i. Results are immediate and generally considered more sensitive than in vitro testing.
        ii. Results will not be accurate if an antihistamine was taken recently or if the child has dermatographism.
        iii. Will yield more meaningful results after the age of 2 years when sensitization is more likely to have occurred
     g. Specific IgE immunoassay (in vitro)
        i. Not affected by recent doses of antihistamines or a history of dermatographism
        ii. Indicated if severe atopic dermatitis or an episode of urticaria makes it difficult to find clear skin on which to perform the prick tests
        iii. More expensive and less sensitive than skin testing
        iv. Requires a blood draw but allows for more comprehensive testing without additional discomfort to the child
        v. May be a more feasible testing option in under-resourced areas and healthcare settings
  4. Laboratory measures
     a. Laboratory tests should not be routinely performed in the diagnosis or management of pediatric asthma patients. Consider only if results will help with differential diagnosis or meaningfully change management.
     b. Complete blood count: Eosinophilia may be supportive of allergic component to child's asthma.
     c. Blood gas: In acute asthma flare, can show retention of carbon dioxide, suggestive of impending respiratory failure. Should not be used alone to determine need for intubation

B. *Management*
  1. Environmental controls
     a. Allergens: Identify and minimize exposure to common allergens (animal dander and saliva, cockroaches, dust mites, molds, rodents, and pollens).
        i. Animal dander and saliva (from pets with hair or fur and rodents)
           a. Found on all surfaces of the home, but especially in carpet and cloth furniture
           b. Animal saliva can be a contact irritant to skin but also can dry on surfaces and then become airborne (Polovic et al., 2013)
        ii. Cockroaches (allergen is the feces): found in air and on flooring
        iii. Dust mite (allergen is the feces): found in air and on all surfaces of the home, but especially in carpet and rugs, cloth furniture, cloth window coverings, mattresses, pillows, stuffed animals
        iv. Molds: found in air, walls and ceilings, and in more severe instances, furniture and clothing
        v. Pollens: found outdoors and in indoor areas of the home adjacent to windows and doors
        vi. General mitigation strategies for all environmental aeroallergens
           a. Replace carpet with hard, nonporous flooring; otherwise, vacuum carpet one to two

times a week with vacuum with a high-efficiency particulate air (HEPA) filter.
- b. Replace cloth window coverings with nonporous window coverings or wash them regularly in hot water.
- c. Use allergen-proof encasements for mattress and pillow, and wash all other bedding weekly in hot water and dry in a dryer.
- d. Limit stuffed animals to one or two and wash them every 2 weeks in hot water or place them in a freezer and then dry in a dryer.
- e. Vacuum flooring, furniture, and window coverings regularly with a vacuum with a HEPA filter.
- f. Regularly wipe hard surfaces with a damp cloth.
- g. Limit clutter and avoid decorations that cannot be easily cleaned (e.g., dried flowers).
- h. Use an air purifier with a HEPA filter. The child's sleeping area is the priority, and the best effects are achieved when it is constantly on.

vii. Additional allergen-specific mitigation strategies
- a. Pets: If a child with asthma exhibits allergy symptoms around a pet, the pet should be kept out of sleeping areas or outdoors. The emotional and psychological benefits of a pet should be considered before recommending removal.
- b. Cockroaches and rodents: pest control strategies that do not compromise air quality
- c. Mold: Increase airflow through home, especially in areas of humidity (bathroom, kitchen), use a dehumidifier, and discard furniture and clothing with mold. Mold removal from walls and ceilings should be performed by professionals.
- d. Pollen: Use air-conditioning in warm weather, avoid opening windows and doors for long periods of time on windy or high-pollen-count days, and avoid placing sleeping area next to the window. If a child with asthma exhibits allergy symptoms with exposure to pollen, the child should wear a hat and sunglasses on windy or high-pollen-count days when outdoors, wash hands and face upon returning home, and shower in the evening. Due to the physical, emotional, and psychological benefits of being outdoors, especially in nature, it is not typically recommended to limit time spent outside due to asthma or allergies.

viii. Allergen mitigation should not be recommended universally for those with asthma. Providers should first consider a child's exposures, symptoms, and likelihood of sensitization or allergy testing results (U.S. Department of Health and Human Services et al., 2020a).

b. Irritants (smoke, scented products, fumes from cleaning solutions, air pollution)
- i. Tobacco smoke particles: Children are exposed through second- and third-hand smoke, even if the child is not present at the time of smoking. Family and friends who choose to smoke should smoke outside and wear a smoking jacket that is never brought into the house, as well as brush their teeth and wash their hands after smoking. There should be absolutely no smoking in the home or in a vehicle. Refer smokers to smoking cessation programs and/or provide nicotine-replacement therapy.
- ii. Wildfire smoke: Monitor air quality regularly during wildfire season, keep windows and doors closed during times there are smoke particles in the air, use an air-conditioner during warm weather, and run air purifiers with HEPA filters; time spent exercising outside may need to be limited.
- iii. Scents: Do not use items that infuse the air or clothing with scent, such as air fresheners, oil diffusers, or scented dryer sheets.
- iv. Cleaning products: Bleach, powders, and sprays are particularly harmful. Use environmentally safe, nonscented products that are applied directly to the cleaning surface, and clean when the child is out of the home.
- v. Air pollution: In areas adjacent to heavy construction or freeways, avoid opening windows and doors for extensive periods of time during active construction or heavy traffic. Use an air-conditioner during warm weather and run air purifiers with HEPA filters.

c. Structuralized racism and other factors that result in social inequities create circumstances that expose certain groups to more allergens, irritants, and toxins. The cost and inaccessibility of some mitigation strategies, as well as a lack of home ownership, exacerbate disparities in asthma management and outcomes. Recommendations should be personalized, considering cost, feasibility, and the potential benefit to the individual.

2. Medication (Table 9-3)
  a. Rescue medication
    i. Steps 1, 2, 3 (for age 0–3 years), 4 (for age 0–3 years), 5, and 6 rescue medications are

inhaled SABAs (albuterol or levalbuterol, available in hydrofluoroalkaline [HFA] or nebules).
  a. Typical use is every 4 hours as needed for any signs of asthma, including cough.
  b. The frequency and intensity of treatment may be altered depending on severity of symptoms, up to three treatments every 20 minutes as needed.
 ii. Steps 3 and 4 for ages 4-11 yrs rescue medications are inhaled corticosteroid-formoterol (ICS-formoterol) (budesonide-formoterol HFA or mometasone-formoterol HFA).
  a. ICS dosing is low dose for Step 3 and medium dose for Step 4.
  b. Use is 1–2 puffs as needed.
  c. Number of puffs should not exceed 8 puffs/day, including controller doses, in children <12 years and should not exceed 12 puffs/day, including controller doses, in children >11 years.
  d. Off-label use, so there may be issues in insurance coverage and supply
b. Controller medication
 i. Prescribe controller medications for children with persistent asthma.
  a. ICSs are the first-line treatment because they offer the best and safest long-term control therapy (NAEPP, 2007).
  b. Start with a low to medium dose, depending on the child's risk and severity of symptoms.
  c. Assess control after 2–6 weeks, and if well controlled, continue treatment for at least 3 months. Step down to a lower dose if asthma remains under control. Goal is for the child to use the minimum dose at which asthma is well controlled.
  d. If asthma is not well controlled after 2–6 weeks, assess medication adherence and device technique. If both are appropriate, step up therapy and/or consider an alternative diagnosis.
  e. The use of a leukotriene receptor antagonist is less desirable due to an increased risk of adverse consequences and the need for monitoring. The U.S. Food and Drug Administration (FDA) issued a black-box warning for montelukast in March 2020. Evaluate for side effects at each visit for children using this medication (U.S. Department of Health and Human Services et al., 2020b).
  f. In December 2017, the FDA removed the black-box warning for ICS-LABA medications after multiple large clinical safety trials found that ICS-LABA medications do not result in a higher risk of asthma-related hospitalizations or death compared to ICS alone. Single-ingredient LABA medications (e.g., salmeterol, formoterol, olodaterol), which are not appropriate for managing pediatric asthma, are associated with an increased risk of asthma-related death and continue to have a black-box warning.
c. Antihistamines
 i. Medication to decrease allergy symptoms, such as runny nose, itchy eyes, frequent sneezing, itchy nose or throat, and itchy skin without rashes, should also be considered. Besides negatively affecting a child's quality of life and academic performance, allergies can trigger bronchoconstriction (Mahr & Sneth, 2005; NAEPP, 2007).
d. Oral systemic corticosteroids
 i. A short course is used to decrease airway inflammation during moderate or severe exacerbations or for patients who fail to respond promptly and completely to a rescue medication.
 ii. Oral prednisone and dexamethasone are equally effective. Usually requires 2–10 days of therapy. No evidence that tapering "pulse" dose prevents relapse (NAEPP, 2007).
 iii. Daily long-term use of oral steroids is a treatment of last resort and is reserved for children with severe asthma who do not respond adequately to other controller medications.
e. Omalizumab (Xolair)
 i. A monoclonal IgE antibody, administered in subcutaneous injections.
 ii. Recommended for consideration for children older than 4 years of age who require Step 5 or 6 controller therapy (U.S. Department of Health and Human Services et al., 2020b).
 iii. Dosing and frequency of injections are based on age, weight, and pretreatment serum IgE level.
 iv. Omalizumab's major potential side effect is anaphylaxis, and it is therefore administered in a specialist's office.
3. Treat comorbid conditions and protect against communicable respiratory infections.
 a. Treatment of the following conditions that are frequently seen with asthma may improve asthma control: allergic rhinitis, sinusitis, obstructive sleep apnea, gastroesophageal reflux, higher body weight, depression, and allergic bronchopulmonary aspergillosis. Additionally, stressors, such as food insecurity, housing instability, and stressful family circumstances, affect asthma severity and outcomes. Clinicians should make appropriate referrals to social support services as needed.

b. Vaccinations
   i. Vaccinate all children over the age of 6 months with the influenza vaccine. Children younger than 2 years or those with asthma or wheezing in the preceding 12 months should receive the inactivated influenza vaccine (CDC, 2021). Children with an egg allergy of any severity should also receive the influenza vaccine. Observation following vaccination is no longer recommended, but those with a severe egg allergy should be vaccinated in a medical setting under the supervision of a healthcare provider who is able to recognize and manage severe allergic reactions (CDC, National Center for Immunization and Respiratory Diseases, 2021).
   ii. All eligible children, including those with asthma, should complete the full series of the COVID-19 vaccine, including any boosters recommended by the CDC. This includes children using daily inhaled corticosteroids to control their asthma. Children who are receiving omalizumab injections should wait 1–7 days after their injection before getting the COVID-19 vaccine. The only contraindication to the COVID-19 vaccine is an allergy to the vaccine or any of its ingredients (Allergy & Asthma Network, 2021).
c. When possible, young children should avoid contact with people who have viral respiratory infections, a common trigger and a major factor in the development, persistence, and possibly severity of asthma (NAEPP, 2007).
4. Encourage physical activity.
   a. If necessary, treat exercise-induced bronchospasm by use of a rescue medication 15–20 minutes before exercise. Increase or start a daily controller medication if exercise-induced symptoms persist or if symptoms occur during daily activities.
   b. Cost and inaccessibility of sports and exercise programs may be challenging to families with lower income and communities with fewer resources. Additionally, neighborhood safety concerns may be prohibitive to outdoor physical activity. Clinicians should partner with families to think creatively about feasible options and refer to community agencies as needed.
5. Consider allergy immunotherapy.
   a. Referral may be appropriate if there is a correlation between the child's asthma symptoms and their exposure to allergens, and allergy symptom relief is inadequate despite the use of antihistamines.
6. Involve the family and child (if old enough) in all treatment decision making to encourage a partnership in the care and control of the child's asthma.
7. Follow-up
   a. Patients with well-controlled asthma should be seen every 3–6 months by a specialist or primary care provider, depending on the patient's past asthma history, the family's need for reinforcement and education, and social factors that might put the child at high risk.
   b. At each follow-up visit, reassess asthma severity or control, adjust medications as needed, evaluate for environmental triggers, review medication regimen, and review device technique.
   c. Telehealth has been shown to be an effective alternative to in-person visits for children with intermittent or well-controlled asthma (Portnoy, 2016) and may increase adherence to follow-up visits, especially in areas with limited health care.
8. Referral to subspecialist
   a. Primary provider is uncertain about the diagnosis of asthma in a child.
   b. Child has severe asthma (multiple hospitalizations, history of intubation, requires step 3 controller therapy or higher for ages 0–4 years, requires step 4 controller therapy or higher for ages 5–11 years).
   c. Symptoms are not responding to appropriate treatment.
   d. Allergy testing or spirometry is desired and cannot be performed by primary provider.
   e. Child is candidate for allergy immunotherapy or omalizumab therapy.

C. *Patient and family education*
1. Basic asthma education
   a. Determine family's knowledge about asthma and the diagnosis.
   b. Show diagrams of the lungs and where they are located in the body to both the caregiver and child. Explain that asthma is a chronic, inflammatory disease of the lungs. Although the child's asthma can be controlled and the child can lead a normal life, the asthma itself will not be cured. This is an important and difficult concept for some families and children to understand and accept.
2. Environmental controls
   Allergy and trigger reduction or avoidance (see the Management section)
3. Medications
   a. Explain the difference between rescue medication and controller medication. Lung diagrams showing normal lungs versus lungs affected by asthma and other diagrams showing the muscle-relaxing effect of bronchodilators and the anti-inflammatory effects of ICS medications can be very useful.
   b. Review the use of the asthma action plan, the identification of symptoms, and when to seek emergency care (see the Self-Management Resources and Tools section).

c. Demonstrate the proper device technique and have the family or older child perform a "teach-back" demonstration.
   d. Address, if necessary, the family's concerns about asthma medications. Long-term studies have shown that children reach predicted adult height despite ongoing use of inhaled steroids (Guill, 2004). If needed, point out that the risks of inadequately treated asthma include death.
   e. Teach methods of obtaining refills from a pharmacy.
   f. Discuss the importance of always having rescue medication at home, daycare or school, and after-school programs. Rescue medication should be taken along with the child to all other settings (e.g., park, sports, errands, visits to other homes, etc.).
   g. If the child lives in multiple homes, each home should have a set of all medications for ease and to optimize adherence. Each caregiver should be given education about medications and device technique.
4. Emergency care
   a. Recognition of severe asthma symptoms
   b. Use of medications for severe symptoms
   c. When to call the medical provider
   d. When to bring the child to the emergency room or call 911
   e. Due to social and/or economic reasons (e.g. immigration status, lack of insurance, cost, lost work time, or fear of receiving poor care due to social status, race, or language discordance) families may delay seeking emergency care. Clinicians should have frank discussions about these concerns and reinforce the importance of seeking emergency care to prevent a life-threatening situation.
5. Follow-up telephone calls or emails
   a. Answer questions.
   b. Identify any issues obtaining medications.
   c. Review the asthma action plan.
   d. Review knowledge of emergency care of the child.
   e. Remind the family of follow-up appointments.
6. Educational tools
   a. Education on device technique should be given in person or via synchronous video with the child's own device or a sample device.
   b. Written material should be available to those who are interested, with consideration of the family's preferred language and literacy level.
   c. Videos and patient-centered webinars can be used instead of or in addition to written materials, especially if the family has a low literacy level.
   d. Computer programs, peer education, and other school-based programs can be effective educational tools for school-aged children and adolescents.
7. Barriers to learning
   a. Family: Caregivers may have difficulty accepting that a child has a chronic disease. Denial of the chronic nature of asthma is very common and frequently leads to nonadherence to medication routines, laxity in environmental controls, and delay in seeking care. Fear of addiction to, or side effects from, medications is another common barrier.
   b. Patient: The child or teenager may also have difficulty accepting the diagnosis of asthma. After acknowledging this difficulty, naming famous athletes or celebrities who have controlled asthma might be reassuring.
   c. Language, culture, and/or race discordance between a clinician and family may be a barrier to creating a trusting relationship. The use of community health workers ("promotoras") to provide education and nonclinical follow-up has been shown to create a stronger, more positive relationship between families and the healthcare system and optimizes asthma outcomes.
8. Adherence
   a. Provide calendars with boxes for the parent or child to check when medicine has been given. Cellphone alarms and alerts can also be effective.
   b. Help the family or child coordinate the timing of medication use with another well-established habit, such as brushing the teeth.
   c. Remind the family and child that adherence helps them achieve their desired outcomes, improves general quality of life, and minimizes visits to the emergency department, as well as the use of stronger medications.
9. Goal setting: It might help for a child or teenager to set a goal for improvement. An example of a very concrete goal is being able to blow out all the candles during the next pulmonary function test or being able to sleep all night without symptoms by the next office or clinic visit.

VI. Resources
A. *Self-management resources and tools*
   1. At home
      a. Asthma action plan (See sample Action Plan, Figure 43-2, in Chapter 43, Asthma in Adolescents and Adults.)
         i. Complete a written asthma action plan, with a copy for any secondary home and for school or daycare.
            a. To avoid confusion, keep the medication regimen as uncomplicated as the child's condition allows.
            b. Provide a new plan at every visit, even if the plan does not change.
            c. The plan should be given in the family's preferred language. If the caregiver and an older child have different

preferred languages, give one plan in each language.
   d. Some electronic health records can create an electronic version of the asthma action plan that the family can access using a smartphone or computer.
  b. Peak flow meter
    i. May be helpful in identifying airway obstruction before overt symptoms appear in children over 5 years. Usefulness of peak flow meter depends on correct technique and interpretation and adherence to using the device at least once a day.
 2. At child's school
   i. It is imperative that a school knows if a child has asthma, no matter how intermittent or well controlled, and has rescue medication and an emergency care plan in place. Most schools require written permission from the health provider and from the parent for the child to be able to use or receive rescue medication in school. Ensuring that the school has this permission should be part of the routine care of all children with asthma. This is also true of after-school programs, camps, and athletics.
B. Asthma education resources
 1. Allergy & Asthma Network: http://www.allergyasthmanetwork.org
 2. American Academy of Allergy, Asthma, and Immunology: http://www.aaaai.org
 3. American Lung Association: http://www.lungusa.org
 4. CDC: http://www.cdc.gov/asthma
 5. NHLBI Information Center: http://www.nhlbi.nih.gov
 6. National Jewish Medical and Research Center (Lung Line): http://www.nationaljewish.org

References

Asthma and Allergy Foundation of America. (2020). *Asthma disparities in America: A roadmap to reducing burden on racial and ethnic minorities.* http://aaafa.org/asthmadisparities

Allergy & Asthma Network. (2021). *COVID-19 vaccine and asthma: What you need to know.* https://allergyasthmanetwork.org/news/covid-vaccine-and-asthma/

Centers for Disease Control and Prevention. (2021). *2021 National Health Interview Survey (NHIS) data.* https://www.cdc.gov/asthma/most_recent_national_asthma_data.htm

Centers for Disease Control and Prevention. (2021). *2019-2021 National Health Interview Survey (NHIS) data.* https://www.cdc.gov/asthma/most_recent_national_asthma_data.htm

Centers for Disease Control and Prevention. (2021). *Live, intranasal influenza vaccine information statement.* https://www.cdc.gov/vaccines/hcp/vis/vis-statements/flulive.html

Centers for Disease Control and Prevention, National Center for Immunization and Respiratory Diseases. (2021). *Flu vaccine and people with egg allergies.* https://www.cdc.gov/flu/prevent/egg-allergies.htm

Gern, J. (2010). The Urban Environment and Childhood Asthma Study. *Journal of Allergy and Clinical Immunology, 125*(3), 545–549. doi:10.1016/j.jaci.2010.01.037

Guill, M. F. (2004). Asthma update: Clinical aspects and management. *Pediatrics in Review, 25*(10), 338–342. doi:10.1542/pir.25-10-335

Hill, D. A., & Spergel, J. M. (2018). The atopic march: Critical evidence and clinical relevance. *Annals of Allergy, Asthma & Immunology 120*(2018): 131–137. doi:10.1016/j.anai.2017.10.037

Mahr, T. A., & Sneth, K. (2005). Update on allergic rhinitis. *Pediatrics in Review, 25*(8), 284–289. doi:10.1542/pir.26-8-284

National Asthma Education and Prevention Program. (2007). *Expert Panel Report 3: Guidelines for the diagnosis and management of asthma* (NIH Publication No. 08-4051). http://www.nhlbi.nih.gov/healthpro/resources/lung/naci/asthma-info/asthma-guidelines.htm

Polovic, N., Wadén, K., Binnmyr, J., Hamsten, C., Grönneberg, R., Palmberg, C., Milcic-Matic, N., Bergman, T., Grönlund, H., & van Hage, M. (2013). Dog saliva—an important source of dog allergens. *Allergy 68*(5): 585–592. doi:10.1111/all.12130

Portnoy, J. M., Waller, M., De Lurgio, S., & Dinakar, C. (2016). Telemedicine is as effective as in-person visits for patients with asthma. *Annals of Allergy, Asthma & Immunology, 117*(3), 241-245. doi:10.1016/j.anai.2016.07.012

U.S. Department of Health and Human Services, National Institutes of Health, & National Heart, Lung, and Blood Institute. (2020a). *2020 Focused updates to the asthma management guidelines: A report from the National Asthma Education and Prevention Program Coordinating Committee Expert Panel Working Group.* https://www.nhlbi.nih.gov/health-topics/all-publications-and-resources/2020-focused-updates-asthma-management-guidelines

U.S. Department of Health and Human Services, National Institutes of Health, & National Heart, Lung, and Blood Institute. (2020b). *2020 Focused updates to the asthma management guidelines: At-a-glance guide* (NIH Publication No. 20-HL-8142). https://www.nhlbi.nih.gov/health-topics/all-publications-and-resources/at-glance-2020-focused-updates-asthma-management-guidelines

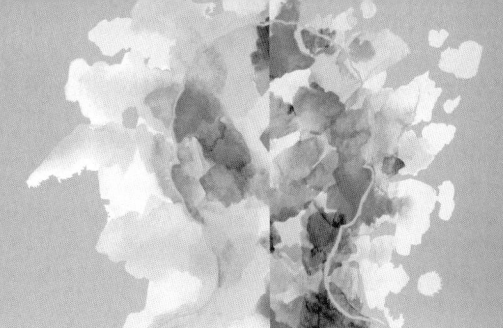

CHAPTER 10

Atopic Dermatitis in Children

Nanette Madden and Karen G. Duderstadt

I. Introduction and general background

A. Definition and overview

Atopic dermatitis (AD) is a chronic, relapsing inflammatory skin disorder that usually begins in infants and children (Grey & Maguiness, 2016). The term *eczema* is often used interchangeably with *AD*. However, AD is a more specific term to describe this type of dermatitis. The word *eczema* comes from the Greek word meaning "to boil," which describes the acute symptoms of AD, including erythema, scaling, crusting, oozing, and sometimes bleeding due to scratching (National Eczema Society, 2017). When the protective barrier of the skin is impaired, it has an increased susceptibility to bacterial, viral, and fungal infections, as well as to aeroallergens. Aeroallergens are airborne substances or inhalants and cutaneous contacts that cause allergic disorders. The most common aeroallergens are pollens and house dust mites.

AD is often the initial manifestation of atopic disease in children and is thought to trigger the "atopic march" that predisposes children to other atopic disorders, such as asthma and allergic rhinitis, later in life (Yang et al., 2018). This is particularly true for children who have severe AD during infancy and if they have elevated total and specific immunoglobulin E (IgE) antibodies to common environmental allergens at a young age (Bantz et al., 2014). Quality of life is often diminished for children with AD due to the chronicity of the condition, constant pruritus, and difficulty in identifying and avoiding triggers.

B. Prevalence and incidence

AD is the most common skin disorder in young children and affects approximately 5% to 20% of the pediatric population globally. It is increasing in prevalence in economically developed countries and in developing countries as well, such as Chile, Kenya, and Algeria (Urban et al., 2021). In the United States, the overall prevalence is 16%, with the highest incidence reported in African American children (19%) (Fu et al., 2014; McKenzie & Silverberg, 2019). AD develops in 60% of affected children in the first year of life and 90% by 5 years of age, with a slight prevalence in females. Onset in the first 6 months of life is often associated with more severe disease. AD occurs more commonly in urban populations and those with a family history of atopic disease. Most children with AD have resolution of their disease by adulthood. However, recent research has shown a prevalence of 7.3% in U.S. adults, ranging from mild to severe (Chiesa Fuxench et al., 2019).

Several air pollutants have been found to be related to the prevalence and development of AD. These air pollutant chemicals include nitrogen oxide compounds, benzene, formaldehyde, sulfur dioxide, and tobacco smoke (Kim, 2015).

C. Etiology

The exact etiology or immune mechanism of AD remains unknown. Epidermal barrier dysfunction is now recognized as having a key role in the development of AD. Defects in the outer layer of the skin, the stratum corneum, reduce the ability of keratinocytes to maintain hydration and restrict transepidermal water loss. This leads to extreme dryness of the skin, which produces itching and, subsequently, AD (Tollefson & Bruckner, 2014). About 75% of children with AD have a positive family history of the atopic disease, indicating a genetic predisposition for the dysfunction of the skin barrier (Eichenfield et al., 2014). Filaggrin is a structural protein found in cells that make up the epidermis and maintains the epidermal barrier. Defects in the filaggrin gene are strong predisposing factors in the development of atopic disease (Grey & Maguiness, 2016).

Skin barrier dysfunction may also allow for the entry of environmental aeroallergens. When aeroallergens enter the skin, they activate local immune cells. Activation of cytokines, such as interleukins, leads to increased production of IgE and eosinophilia. This triggers the itch–scratch cycle: itching leads to scratching or rubbing of the skin, and scratching causes the release of cytokines from the epidermal cells, which perpetuates the inflammation and causes more rash. Exposure to endotoxins, farm animals, and dogs as an infant may protect against AD due to the early microbial contact that activates the critical postnatal period of immune response, often called the *hygiene hypothesis* (Flohr & Yeo., 2011). Other probable protective factors include living in an environment with higher ultraviolet (UV) irradiation, maternal intake of fish and probiotics during pregnancy, and vitamin D supplementation (Kantor & Silverberg, 2017).

II. Database (may include but is not limited to)

A. *Subjective*

1. History of the presenting illness and relevant past health history
   a. Feeding history: Breastfed or formula fed? When were solids started? Any foods avoided?
   b. When did rash or lesions first appear and on what areas of the body?
   c. Has infant or child had periods without lesions or rash?
   d. Bathing routine and how often? Soaps or shampoos used?
   e. Moisturizers used and on what part of body? How often?
   f. Sleep history? Quality of sleep and nighttime symptoms?
   g. Any known food or drug allergies?
   h. Any history of exposure to known allergens? Pets in household?
   i. What does the parent, caregiver, or child think makes the rash or lesions better or worse?
   j. History of other atopic skin disease or urticaria (hives)?
   k. History of allergic rhinitis or asthma?
   l. History of bacterial skin infections, herpes, or fungal infections?
   m. History of other chronic conditions or developmental delay?
2. Medication history
   a. Over-the-counter medications used, topical and/or oral?
   b. Prescription medications used, topical and/or oral?
   c. Frequency of medication use, daily or with flares?
   d. Complementary or alternative medications or therapies used?
   e. Has child been on antibiotics in the past year?
   f. Has child been on oral steroids in the past year?
   g. Taking vitamins? How often?
3. Family history
   a. Any family history of allergies, AD, eczema, allergic rhinitis, hay fever, or asthma?
   b. Siblings with atopic skin disease or asthma?
   c. Known food allergies in parent or sibling?
4. Environmental history
   a. Known environmental allergy triggers? (**Figure 10-1**)

TRIGGER	ASSOCIATED FINDINGS (may or may not include)
Food:	Food items include eggs, peanuts, cow's milk, fish, shellfish, soy, and wheat. Food preservatives and food color may trigger allergies but no testing mechanism exists for these substances.
Decreased humidity:	Cold seasons with reduced humidity often herald a flare-up for children with AD. Skin holds less moisture, dry skin becomes irritated, pruritus develops, and scratching begins.
Emotional stress:	Physical and emotional stress can precipitate flares of AD. It is not causative but worsens the condition.
Aeroallergens:	Most common trigger of aeroallergens: • Dust mites in household • Grass pollens • Animal dander • Molds
Temperature change and sweating:	Increased scratching and rubbing caused by sudden change in temperature are common in infants and children with AD. Sweating particularly causes scratching and flares of AD.

Figure 10-1 Common triggering factors

Data from Habif, T. P. (2010). Atopic dermatitis. In T. P. Habif (Ed.), Clinical dermatology: A color guide to diagnosis and therapy (5th ed.). Philadelphia, PA: Elsevier.

b. Exposure to known household chemicals or pollutants?
c. Pests or insects noted in home?
d. Exposure to aerosols or fumigants in home or workplace?
5. Social history
   a. Sleep disturbances for child or caregiver?
   b. Missed school days for child?
   c. Missed work or school days for parent?
   d. Interference with sports, social activities, friendships
   e. Any behavioral changes or problems?
6. Current family stressors
   a. Any concerns about food insecurity in home?
   b. Any concerns about housing security?
7. Symptom history
   a. Common constitutional signs and symptoms of AD: pruritus, age-specific patterns or distribution of skin involvement, sparing of diaper area in infants, and sparing of groin and axillae in older children and adolescents; occasionally irritability in infants with moderate to severe disease.
   b. Skin, hair, and nails
      i. Dry skin (xerosis), erythema, occasional papules, vesicles, weeping lesions, crusting
      ii. Chronic skin changes include hyperpigmentation on lighter skin; hypopigmentation on darker skin; lichenification or leathery, thickened skin; scarring from scratching.
      iii. Patchy alopecia (hair loss) is common in children with severe AD affecting the scalp. The hair regrows when the inflammation is effectively treated.
   c. Lymphadenopathy
      i. Enlarged lymph glands can be a common associated finding of children with AD, particularly in areas localized to exacerbations of AD or in children with associated bacterial, viral, or fungal infections.
   d. Respiratory
      i. Pulmonary findings of wheezing are common in children with atopic disease, and asthma is a common associated condition.

B. Objective
1. Physical examination findings
   a. General physical examination findings of AD:
      i. General appearance: pallor, allergic shiners, allergic salute, Dennie-Morgan folds, and xerosis
      ii. Head, eye, ear, nose, and throat: periorbital puffiness; tympanic membranes with effusion unilaterally or bilaterally; boggy nasal mucosa or erythematous turbinates with enlarged adenoids; and tonsillar hypertrophy, nonerythematous, nonexudative
      iii. Neck: enlarged lymph nodes (cervical, occipital, postauricular)
      iv. Chest: adventitious sounds such as wheezing
2. AD presents differently at different ages. There are three distinct phases of clinical features: (1) infantile phase, (2) childhood phase, and (3) adult phase (**Figure 10-2**).
3. Conditions and features often associated with AD in children and adolescents (**Figure 10-3**).
4. Opportunistic infections are common in infants and children with AD (**Figure 10-4**).
5. Supporting data from relevant diagnostic tests
   a. Diagnosis of AD is most often a clinical diagnosis, and immunologic testing is reserved for moderate to severe disease (**Table 10-1**).
      i. IgE-mediated food allergy testing may not be necessary when only one food is suspected.
      ii. Diagnostic testing for skin allergies should be reserved for children who are nonresponsive to traditional food elimination challenges or who may have gastrointestinal symptoms of AD, such as diarrhea, vomiting, and reflux.
      iii. IgE immunoassay values in children have been established for egg, milk, peanut, tree nuts, and fish, and a negative skin-prick test (SPT) corresponds to a 90% to 95% accuracy for excluding IgE-mediated food allergy in infants and young children (Sicherer & Sampson, 2018).

III. Assessment
A. Determine the diagnosis
   1. Common differential diagnoses (**Figure 10-5**)
B. Assess the severity of the disease.
   Scoring Atopic Dermatitis (SCORAD) and Eczema Area and Severity Index (EASI) are two scoring systems tools used by dermatologists to assess the extent and severity of AD in children and determine the effectiveness of the treatment regimen; these are available at http://scorad.corti.li/ and http://dermnetnz.org/topics/easi-score/.
C. *Assess the significance of the problem to the child and family.*
D. *Assess the family functioning and ability to follow the treatment regimen.*

IV. Goals of clinical management
A. Improve quality of life for children with AD and their families.
   1. No nighttime awakening because of itching
   2. No daytime discomfort or itching
   3. No missed school because of AD
   4. Normalization of child's appearance
   5. No missed workdays for the parents because of their child's symptoms

PHASES	CLINICAL FEATURES (may or may not include)
Infantile phase	Begins from birth to 6 months of age: • May begin on cheeks and progress to scalp, arms, trunk, and legs; generalized dry skin (xerosis) including scalp • Progresses to lateral extensor surfaces of arms and legs • Pruritus and itch-scratch-itch cycle develops • Acute phase with intense itching causing irritability in infant; vesicle formation, oozing, and crusting with excoriated areas on the skin • Hallmark sign is diaper area and groin are usually spared of lesions • May resolve by 2 years of age but can continue into childhood; symptoms may become milder as the child ages and disappear at adolescence or may continue throughout life
Childhood phase	Begins around 2 years of age: • Involves wrists, hands, neck, ankles, popliteal and antecubital spaces, commonly on flexural surfaces • Lesions tend to be dry, papular, circumscribed, scaly patches • Pruritus is often severe Chronic manifestations include: • Lichenification, thickening of skin causing leathery appearance • Hyperpigmentation • Scratch marks Often worse during winter dryness or summer heat.
Adult phase	Begins at puberty or ~12 years of age: • Most commonly involves flexural skin folds; bends of elbows and knees; face; neck; upper arms; back; and dorsa of the hands, feet, fingers, and toes • May be a new occurrence or reoccurrence of chronic condition Often postinflammatory hyperpigmentation and hypopigmentation disappear in adolescence or young adulthood.

Figure 10-2 Phases of atopic dermatitis in children

Data from Habif, T. P. (2010). Atopic dermatitis. In T. P. Habif (Ed.), Clinical dermatology: A color guide to diagnosis and therapy (5th ed.). Philadelphia, PA: Elsevier.

B. Prescribe medications that allow the minimum effective dose to prevent adverse reactions.
C. Educate families so that they understand and adhere to optimum skin-care and medication regimens.
D. Control environmental factors that may adversely affect the child's skin. (Note: Food avoidance is no longer the first-line management or mainstay of treatment for AD.)
E. Provide ongoing emotional and medical support for children and their families.

V. Plan
A. *Develop an optimum skin-care routine with the family.* AD results from primary abnormalities of the skin barrier and the inability to maintain skin hydration. Therefore, gentle skin care with moisturization is a key component of managing AD (Tollefson & Bruckner, 2014). Developing an optimum skin-care routine with the family or caregiver is an important first step to symptom control. The following "soak and seal" technique is recommended:
1. Daily bath with lukewarm water for about 10 to 15 minutes or short lukewarm shower. Use a minimal amount of fragrance-free and dye-free gentle soap or cleanser that is formulated for sensitive skin, such as Cetaphil Cleanser™, at the end of the bath. If the child is not too dirty, use soap or cleanser only on hands, feet, armpits, and genital area, not all over the body.
2. If the child complains of burning sensation of the skin when sitting in a bathtub, the addition of 1 cup of table salt may make the bath more soothing (Paller & Mancini, 2015).

ASSOCIATED CONDITIONS (may or may not include)	CLINICAL FEATURES
Dennie line or Dennie-Morgan fold	Extra grooves or accentuated lines seen below lower eyelids bilaterally; may result from chronic edema of the eyelids and skin thickening
Allergic shiners	Dark discoloration below lower eyelids in lighter skin; slate-gray discoloration in individuals with darker skin; a result of vascular stasis
Allergic salute	Crease over the nasal bridge or exaggerated linear nasal crease caused by frequent rubbing of nose or nasal tip; most often associated with allergic rhinitis but common in atopic children
Pityriasis alba	Hypopigmented, slightly elevated plaques; occasionally with fine scaling, irregular borders; nonpruritic; occurring most often on the face of young children; also may appear on the upper arms and thighs; ~2–4 cm in diameter round-to-oval, often occur in summer or fall
Keratosis pilaris	Most predominant on the lateral aspects of the upper arms, buttocks, and thighs; appears in early childhood and persists into adulthood; papular with plugged hair follicles and surrounding inflammation; characterized by redness on lighter skin
Nummular eczema	Coin-shaped lesions or plaques ~1 cm or greater in diameter; erythematous and formed by confluent papules or occasionally vesicles
Ichthyosis vulgaris	Transmitted as an autosomal-dominant trait; can be associated with AD but a separate disease; may occur as early as 3 months of age, but most common onset in later childhood; characterized by large scales on extensor surfaces of extremities, particularly on lateral aspect of the lower legs in plate-like scales; flexural surfaces are spared

Figure 10-3 Conditions and features associated with atopic dermatitis

Data from Habif, T. P. (2010). Atopic dermatitis. In T. P. Habif (Ed.), Clinical dermatology: A color guide to diagnosis and therapy (5th ed.). Philadelphia, PA: Elsevier.

OPPORTUNISTIC INFECTIONS	ASSOCIATED FINDINGS (may or may not include)
Staphylococcus aureus	Erythematous with pustular, exudative lesions and crusting; the most common opportunistic infection in AD and recovered in 93% of patients with AD lesions, 79% from nares of atopic children
Streptococcus pyogenes	A less common opportunistic infection in children with AD than *S. aureus*; skin findings as above
Herpes simplex	Vesicles often become umbilicated; eczema herpeticum, rapid development of vesiculopustular lesions over the sites of dermatitis, can occur in individuals with AD
Viral molluscum contagiosum	Small, dome-shaped papules often with central umbilication; commonly affect trunk, axillae, and antecubital and popliteal fossae in 25% of children with AD

Figure 10-4 Secondary opportunistic skin infections

Data from Habif, T. P. (2015). Atopic dermatitis. In T. P. Habif (Ed.), Clinical dermatology: A color guide to diagnosis and therapy (6th ed.). Philadelphia, PA: Elsevier.

Table 10-1 Common Laboratory Tests

Test	Definition	Clinical Implications	Comments
Skin-prick test	Wheal response after skin prick with antigen	IgE-mediated food hypersensitivity	Often does not correlate with clinical manifestations in children with AD
Radioallergosorbent test	Circulating specific IgE	IgE-mediated food hypersensitivity	False-positive findings are common, particularly in older children

Data from Paller, A. S., & Mancini, A. J. (2011). Eczematous eruptions in childhood. In A. S. Paller & A. J. Mancini (Eds.), *Hurwitz clinical pediatric dermatology: A textbook of skin disorders of childhood and adolescence* (4th ed., pp. 49–64). Elsevier.

CONDITION	ASSOCIATED FINDINGS (may or may not include)
Contact dermatitis	Irritant or allergic contact dermatitis is generally milder than AD; occurs on the cheeks and chin, extensor surfaces or diaper area of infants and young children; caused by harsh soaps, vigorous bathing, or saliva on cheek and chin area.
Seborrheic dermatitis	Greasy, yellow scales that involve the scalp, eyebrows, behind the ears, cheeks, and can spread to neck and chest area; generally nonpruritic. Often AD appears as seborrheic dermatitis subsides.
Psoriasis	Round, erythematous, well-marginated plaques; covered by grayish or silvery-white scales; ~1 cm or greater in diameter; commonly found on the scalp, elbows, knees, and lumbosacral area.
Scabies	Pruritic papules, nodules, vesiculopustules, and burrowing lesions; commonly occur on infants and young children; seen on trunk, between the fingers, wrists, ankles, axillae, waist, groin, palms of hands, and soles of feet; occasionally seen on the head of infants.

Figure 10-5 Common differential diagnoses for atopic dermatitis

Data from Paller A. S., & Mancini, A. J. (2011). Eczematous eruptions in childhood. In A. S. Paller & A. J. Mancini (Eds.), *Hurwitz clinical pediatric dermatology: A textbook of skin disorders of childhood and adolescence* (4th ed.). Philadelphia, PA: Elsevier.

3. Gently pat away excess water after bathing, leaving skin slightly damp.
4. If AD skin lesions are present, apply topical anti-inflammatory medications or prescription medications to areas of the skin that are red, rough, or itchy or where there is a rash when the skin is slightly damp. Apply in a thin layer and rub in well.
5. While skin is still slightly moist, apply a generous amount of an AD therapeutic moisturizing cream or emollient to the entire body and face. This seals in the water from bathing and makes the skin less dry and itchy. Eucerin Eczema Body Cream™ and Cetaphil Restoraderm Moisturizer and Wash™ cream are examples of effective products (Hebert et al., 2020). There are many good over-the-counter products to control skin hydration for AD on the market. Lotions are not recommended for adequate moisturizing in children with AD because their content has a high percentage of water. Petroleum jelly can be used as a sealer, and it is a good occlusive preparation, although it is not a moisturizer. Several new "barrier repair" formulations are also now available for use as moisturizers, including some over-the-counter products (e.g., Cerave™ cream). The application of moisturizing creams should be done within 3 minutes of exiting the bath before water loss in the skin occurs from evaporation. Ideally, the moisturizer should be applied twice daily. It can also be repeated as needed on dry, itchy skin (Paller & Mancini, 2015). This bathing routine should be

continued even after the skin has improved and prescription medication is no longer necessary.
   6. Applying moisturizer to the skin of a young infant with a family history of AD reduces the risk of future development of both AD and asthma, possibly due to skin barrier properties. This should be considered for newborns at high risk of developing AD (Bantz et al., 2014; de la O-Escamilia & Sidbury, 2020; Horimukai et al., 2014).
B. *Avoid known factors or allergic triggers that lead to flares.*
   1. Some irritants in the home or school environment may cause the skin to be red or itchy or to burn:
      a. Wash all new clothes before wearing to remove chemicals. Double-rinse the child's laundry so that the skin is not in contact with residual detergent in clothing.
      b. Do not use fabric softeners.
      c. Avoid clothes made of wool and artificial fibers. Dress the child in loose-fitting clothing and lighter cotton-blend clothing that allows air to pass freely to the skin.
      d. Avoid contact with harsh household cleaners. Use natural, environmentally safe products.
      e. Wear long pants and long sleeves when playing around irritating substances, such as sand, dirt, and plants.
      f. Eliminate the child's exposure to secondhand smoke because it can increase irritation and pruritus and may also increase the tendency for the development of asthma (Paller & Mancini, 2015).
      g. Keep the child's fingernails short, smooth, and clean to help prevent skin irritation, infection, and damage caused by scratching. Explain to the family or caregiver that when the child scratches, the rash becomes worse, and the skin becomes thicker. AD is a condition that is sometimes referred to as "the itch that rashes."
   2. Prevent or delay the onset of specific food allergies with early dietary interventions.
   In 2019, the American Academy of Pediatric published an updated clinical report on dietary recommendations for infants and children (Greer et al., 2019).
      a. There is evidence that exclusive breastfeeding for the first 3 to 4 months of life decreases the evidence of AD in the first 2 years of life.
      b. There is no evidence that commercial hydrolyzed formulas prevent AD in infants and children, even in those who are at high risk for AD.
      c. There is a lack of evidence that delaying the introduction of allergenic foods beyond 4 to 6 months, including peanuts, fish, and eggs, prevents AD.
      d. There is evidence that the early introduction of infant-safe forms of peanuts for infants at high risk for peanut allergy reduces the risk for peanut allergies. This should be done as early as 4 to 6 months of age in the healthcare provider's office after the appropriate tests have been done (specific IgE, SPTs, and/or oral food challenges). For infants who have already developed mild to moderate AD, peanut-containing food can be introduced at around 6 months of age (Greer et al., 2019). See the guidelines from the National Institute of Allergy and Infectious Diseases (NIAID) for the amount and frequency of these feedings (Togias et al., 2017).
   3. Proved or suspected food allergens
      a. Consider food allergy only in children who have reacted immediately to a certain food and in infants and young children with moderate or severe uncontrolled AD, particularly with gastrointestinal symptoms or failure to thrive (Walsh & O'Flinn, 2011). Indiscriminate allergy testing without a history that suggests allergy triggers is not recommended because radioallergosorbent tests (RASTs) have a low positive predictive value (Sidbury et al., 2014). NIAID guidelines state that allergy evaluation, specifically for milk, eggs, peanuts, wheat, and soy, should be considered in children less than 5 years of age with severe AD if the child has persistent AD despite optimal management. The guidelines state that food allergies can induce hives and itching, which may aggravate AD but do not cause AD. Egg allergy may be one exception. Up to half of infants with egg-specific IgE may have an improvement in their AD when following an egg-free diet (Tollefson & Bruckner, 2014).
      b. Consider inhalant allergy in children with seasonal flares, associated asthma, and allergic rhinitis and in children older than 3 years of age with AD on the face. After 3 years of age, many children outgrow food allergies but become sensitive to airborne allergens, such as dust mites (Yang et al., 2018). Some children have shown improvement in symptoms when dust mites are controlled in their environment, especially in their bedroom:
         i. Eliminate floor coverings and curtains.
            a. Eliminate all upholstered furniture except the bed.
            b. Cover box springs, mattress, and pillows in plastic zippered covers or allergy-proof covers.
            c. Eliminate clutter and limit toys, especially stuffed animals.
            d. Wash all bedcovers and stuffed animals at least once a week in hot water.
            e. Keep pets with fur or feathers out of the room because they attract dust.
      c. Avoid only substances that are documented to cause an increase in symptoms. It is important

not to deny children things unnecessarily, such as foods or outdoor activities.
   d. Most children with AD do not need diagnostic testing for allergies independent of clinical assessment (Eichenfield et al., 2017).
   e. Dust mite avoidance strategies do not decrease the risk of developing AD and should not be recommended for this purpose (Bremmer & Simpson, 2015).
C. *Treat symptoms when they occur.*
   1. Topical corticosteroids are the therapeutic mainstay for AD and have been proven to be effective for children for several decades (Yang et al., 2018). They not only suppress the inflammation and pruritus associated with AD, but they may also prevent bacterial colonization. Choosing which corticosteroid to prescribe depends on the severity and distribution of the lesions and the age of the child. Preparations are divided into seven groups based on relative potency, from very low preparations, such as hydrocortisone acetate, to very high preparations, such as clobetasol propionate. Ointment-based preparations are more potent, more occlusive, and less drying than chemically equivalent cream-based agents. The most effective, but least potent, medication should be used to minimize the risk of adverse side effects, such as thinning of the skin. For children with mild to moderate disease, a group VII drug, such as hydrocortisone ointment 1% or 2.5%, is usually sufficient. When corticosteroids are prescribed, consider the following:
      a. Prescribe in adequate amounts to optimize control. Prescriptions that require frequent refills may lead to undertreatment or nonadherence.
      b. Prescribe for application only once or twice a day.
      c. Corticosteroids should be applied to areas of active lesions, not to clear skin for prophylaxis.
      d. Consider the possibility of secondary bacterial or viral infection if the regular application of corticosteroids by parent or caregiver has not controlled the AD within 2 weeks.
      e. Consider changing to a different topical corticosteroid of the same potency as an alternative to stepping up treatment if a diminishing response or tachyphylaxis is suspected.
      f. Do not use potent topical corticosteroids on the face, neck, or groin. When inflammation is widespread, avoid high-potency corticosteroids because of the risk of systemic adverse effects.
      g. Refer to dermatology if potent corticosteroids are needed for children younger than 12 months of age or infants and children with moderate to severe disease unresponsive to treatment.
      h. Explain to families that the benefits of topical corticosteroids outweigh the risks if applied correctly.
   2. Topical calcineurin inhibitors are an option for treatment if the child's AD has not shown a satisfactory clinical response to adequate use of topical corticosteroids or if the parent/caregiver or the provider has concerns about long-term effects of topical steroid use, such as skin atrophy, striae development, or systemic effects (Yang et al., 2018). Pimecrolimus cream 1% (Elidel) and tacrolimus ointment 0.03% (Protopic) are approved for treating AD in children 2 years of age and older. Tacrolimus ointment 0.1% (Protopic) is approved for adolescents 16 years of age and older.
      a. Pimecrolimus is efficacious in children with mild to moderate AD. It is comparable to low-potency steroids.
      b. Tacrolimus is appropriate for children with moderate to severe disease. The efficacy of the 0.03% ointment is comparable to that of low-potency steroids, and the efficacy of the 0.1% ointment is comparable to that of medium- to high-potency topical steroids (Ohtsuki et al., 2018).
      c. Both medications are safe for use in the periorbital areas and on the head, neck, and intertriginous area because they do not thin the skin or cause adverse effects to the eyes (Luger et al., 2020; Paller & Mancini, 2015).
      d. A burning sensation may occur during the first few days of application in children with either medication, especially in children with more severe dermatitis.
      e. Use sun protection regularly when using these medications.
   3. Crisaborole is a topical phosphodiesterase-4 (PDE-4) inhibitor approved in 2016 for the treatment of mild to moderate AD in children 2 years of age and older. PDE-4 inhibition decreases pro-inflammatory cytokine release. In general, it is well tolerated. A small percentage of patients (4.4%) experience burning or stinging in the first 4 weeks of use, with decreased symptoms over time (Yang et al., 2018).
   4. Dupilumab (injection) is a human monoclonal antibody approved for the treatment of moderate to severe AD in children 6 years of age and older. Studies have documented several ways in which the use of dupilumab can potentially lead to skin normalization, including downregulation of inflammatory mediators, downregulation of markers of epidermal proliferation, and upgrading of genes involved in skin barrier function. (Fishbein et al., 2020). The most common adverse reactions are conjunctivitis (4%–5%) and injection site reactions (8%–14%). Topical therapies can be combined with dupilumab for additional benefit for those patients with recalcitrant disease (Yang et al., 2018).
   5. Wet-wrap dressings reduce itching and inflammation by cooling the skin and improving the

penetration of topical corticosteroids for acute exacerbations. They also prevent excoriation from scratching. In the hospital, gauze is usually used for this procedure. At home, a method used for years at the National Jewish Medical and Research Center in Denver, Colorado, is a simpler approach. It uses clothing, such as long underwear and cotton socks, moistened in warm water until slightly damp. It is applied to the skin after bathing, moisturizing, and applying medication, with a dry layer of clothing on top. This is to be left on for several hours or overnight.
    a. Use blankets to prevent chilling.
    b. This treatment should not be used for more than 7–14 consecutive nights. Prolonged therapy could lead to folliculitis, secondary infection, or skin maceration (Eichenfield et al., 2017).
6. Antihistamines are thought to have little direct effect on pruritus. However, the tranquilizing and sedating effects of sedating antihistamines, such as hydroxyzine, diphenhydramine, and doxepin, may provide symptomatic relief if given at bedtime when a child is having a flare (Eichenfield et al., 2017). Cetirizine may have limited value, but it is also somewhat sedating. Nonsedating antihistamines are not effective in alleviating pruritus (Paller & Mancini, 2015).
    a. Ensure that the medication does not interfere with the child's functioning during the daytime. Sedating therapies should only be used short term because of their negative effect on school performance (Yang et al., 2018).
    b. Topical antihistamines should be avoided because of possible local allergic reactions.
7. Phototherapy could be considered for severe AD or when other management options have failed. This therapy requires frequent treatments in a clinical setting, often two to three times a week. Refer to a pediatric specialty clinic where staff is experienced in dealing with children.
8. Systemic corticosteroids should be avoided except in rare instances. Although effective for most patients with AD, the rapid rebound after discontinuation and high risk of potential side effects make their use impractical in children (Fishbein et al., 2020; Yu et al., 2018).
9. Give written instructions, such as an eczema action plan, on how to manage the child's AD by stepping up or decreasing medications according to the child's symptoms. The treatment plan and medication are often quite confusing to parents or caregivers, especially when several medications have been prescribed. Knowing when to start a medication and for how long to apply the medication is an important part of the eczema action plan. An action plan can help parents or caregivers feel more confident in managing their child's AD over time, especially when there is a flare in symptoms. (Gilliam et al., 2016). It can also be helpful for the parent or caregiver to bring the patient's moisturizers and medications for AD to follow-up appointments. This will enable the provider to know what products and medications are being used and to clarify any confusion about the medication regimen.
10. Treating flares of symptoms is an important area of patient education. Flares can occur at any time, and the family should be prepared to step up treatment when needed. Treatment of flares should be started as soon as symptoms appear and should be continued for 48 hours after acute symptoms subside.
D. Treat complications
    1. Bacterial superinfection with *Staphylococcus aureus* is common in children with AD and should be suspected if a rash is excoriated. First-generation cephalosporins, such as cephalexin, 25–50 mg/kg divided two or three times daily for 10 days, are commonly used, although in some communities it may be advisable to culture for methicillin-resistant *S. aureus* and then treat accordingly. Bleach baths are recommended for children with moderate to severe AD with signs of a secondary bacterial infection and for maintenance treatment of those suffering from recurrent infections. These children should bathe twice a week in a tub filled with 40 gallons of water mixed with 0.5 cups of household bleach. Bleach baths can be used daily if the child has severe disease (Yang et al., 2018). Control of pruritus and prevention of excoriation with proper skin care and medications also decreases the recurrence of secondary bacterial infections.
    2. Herpes simplex virus infection (*eczema herpeticum*) is a potentially life-threatening complication of AD.
        a. Observe for the following symptoms:
            i. Areas of rapidly worsening and painful dermatitis
            ii. Systemic symptoms, such as fever, lethargy, or distress
            iii. Clustered blisters with the appearance of early-stage cold sores
            iv. Punched-out erosions that are uniform in appearance and that may coalesce
            v. Child's infected dermatitis fails to respond to antibiotic treatment and appropriate corticosteroids.
        b. If eczema herpeticum is suspected, treat immediately with systemic acyclovir, and refer for urgent dermatologic consultation.
        c. If there are facial lesions around the eyes, refer for a same-day consultation with an ophthalmologist.

VI. Self-management

A. Patient and family education and home management of bathing and medication regimens are the key factors in determining successful outcomes for children with AD. It is important to:
   1. Involve the family or caregiver in all treatment decisions. The child and the family or caregiver are likely to be more adherent to the treatment plan if they have been part of the decision-making process. Consider the family's cultural skin-care and bathing practices when discussing options.
   2. Explain that AD often improves with time, but not all children grow out of the condition; at times, it becomes worse as the child gets older.
   3. Educate families regarding the avoidance of environmental, behavioral, or emotional factors that may trigger symptoms. Consider referral to a public health nurse or community health worker, if available, for an environmental assessment in the home.
   4. Clearly explain the quantity of moisturizer to use on the child's skin. Applying an insufficient amount of moisturizer is a common problem.
B. Families need comprehensive written and verbal information in their native language regarding maintenance therapy, when and how to step treatment up and down, how to treat flares, and how to recognize complications. All procedures, even the application of ointments, should be demonstrated.
C. Discuss complementary therapies with the family and explain that often, their effectiveness and safety for AD have not been adequately studied.

VII. Psychosocial and emotional support

A. Considering the effect of AD on the quality of life of patients and their families, it is important to address possible psychosocial issues and offer support:
   1. Parents may feel guilty about the child's condition, and they may be exhausted from sleep deprivation and caring for the child's needs.
   2. School-age children may be bullied by their peers about the appearance of their skin and may also fall behind in their schoolwork because of school absences.
   3. Adolescents may be particularly self-conscious about their appearance and may self-isolate.
B. Refer the family and child or adolescent for counseling when indicated.

References

Bantz, S. K., Zhu, Z., & Zheng, T. (2014). The atopic march: Progression from atopic dermatitis to allergic rhinitis and asthma. *Journal of Clinical Cell Immunology, 5*(2), 202. doi:10.4172/2155-9899.1000202

Bremmer, S. F., & Simpson, E. L. (2015). Dust mite avoidance for the primary prevention of atopic dermatitis: A systematic review and meta-analysis. *Pediatric Allergy and Immunology, 26*(7), 646–654. doi:10.1111/pai.12452

Chiesa Fuxench, Z. C., Block, J. K., Boguniewicz, M., Boyle, J., Fonacier, L., Gelfand, J. M., Grayson, M. H., Margolis, D. J., Mitchell, L., Silverberg, J. I., Schwartz, L., Simpson, E. L., Ong, P. Y. (2019). Atopic Dermatitis in America Study: A cross-sectional study examining the prevalence and disease burden of atopic dermatitis in the US adult population. *Journal of Investigative Dermatology, 139*(3), 583–590. doi:10.1016/j.jid.2018.08.028

de la O-Escamilla, N. O., & Sidbury, R. (2020). Atopic dermatitis: Update on pathogenesis and therapy. *Pediatric Annals, 49*(3), 140–146. doi:10.39.28/10382359-20200217-01

Eichenfield, L. F., Ahluwalia, J., Waldman, A., Borok, J., Udkoff, J., & Boguniewicz, M. (2017). Current guidelines for the evaluation and management of atopic dermatitis: A comparison of the Joint Task Force Practice Parameter and American Academy of Dermatology guidelines. *Journal of American Clinical Immunology, 139*(4), 49–57. doi:10.1016/j.jaci.2017.01.009

Eichenfield, L. F., Tom, W. L., Chamlin, S. L., Feldman, S. R., Hanifin, J. M., Simpson, E. L., Berger, T. G., Berman, J. N., Cohen, D. E., Cooper, K. D., Cordoro, K., Davis, D. M., Krol, A., Margolis, D. J., Paller, A. S., Schwarzenberger, K., Silverman, R. A., Williams, H. C., Elmets, C. A., . . . Sidbury, R. (2014). Guidelines of care for the management of atopic dermatitis. *Journal of the American Academy of Dermatology, 70*, 338–351. doi:101016/j.jaad.2013.10.010

Fishbein, A. B., Silverberg, J. I., Wilson, E. J., & Ong, P. Y. (2020). Update on atopic dermatitis: Diagnosis, severity assessment, and treatment selection. *Journal of Allergy and Clinical Immunology: In Practice, 8*(1), 91–101. doi:10.1016/j.jaip.2019.06.044

Flohr, C., & Yeo, L. (2011). Atopic dermatitis and the hygiene hypothesis revisited. *Current Problems in Dermatology, 41*, 1–34. doi:10.1159/000323290

Fu, T., Keiser, E., Linos, E., Rotatori, R. M., Sainani, K., Lingala, B., Lane, A. T., Schneider, L., & Tang, J. Y. (2014). Eczema and sensitization to common allergens in the United States: A multiethnic, population-based study. *Pediatric Dermatology, 31*(1), 21–26. doi:10.1111/pde.12237

Gilliam, A. E., Madden, N., Sendowski, M., Mioduszewski, M., & Duderstadt, K. G. (2016). Use of eczema action plans (EAPs) to improve parental understanding of treatment regimens in pediatric atopic dermatitis (AD): A randomized controlled trial. *Journal of American Academic Dermatology, 74*(2), 375–377. doi:10.1016/j.jaad.2015.08.067

Greer, F. R., Sicherer, S. H., & Burks, A. W. (2019). The effects of early nutritional interventions on the development of atopic disease in infants and children: The role of maternal dietary restriction, breastfeeding, hydrolyzed formulas, and timing of the introduction of allergenic complementary foods. *Pediatrics, 143*(4), 1–11. doi:10.1542/peds.2019-0281

Grey, K., & Maguiness, S. (2016). Atopic dermatitis: Update for pediatricians. *Pediatric Annals, 45*(8), 280–286. doi:10.3928/19382359-20160720-05

Hebert, A. A., Rippke, F., Weber, T. M., & Nicol, N. H. (2020). Efficacy of nonprescription moisturizers for atopic dermatitis: An updated review of clinical evidence. *American Journal of Clinical Dermatology, 21*, 641–655. doi:10.1007/S40275-020-00529-9

Horimukai, K., Morita, J., Narita, M., Kondo, M., Kitazawa, H., Nozaki, M., Shigematsu, Y., Yoshida, J., Niizeki, H., Motomura, K., Sago, H., Takimoto, T., Eisukelnoue, Kamemura, N., Kido, H., Hisatsune, J., Sugai, M., Murota, H., & Ohya, Y. (2014). Application of moisturizer to neonates prevents development of topic dermatitis. *Journal of Allergy and Clinical Immunology, 134*(4), 824–830. doi:101016/jaci.2014.07.060

Kantor, R., & Silverberg, J. I. (2017). Environmental risk factors and their role in the management of atopic dermatitis. *Expert Review of Clinical Immunology, 13*(1), 15–26. doi:10.10.18/1744666X.2016.1212660

Kim, K. (2015). Influences of environmental chemicals on atopic dermatitis. *Toxicology Research, 31*(2), 89–96. doi:10.5487/tr.2015.31.2.089

Luger, T., Augustin, M., Lambert, J., Paul, C., Pincelli, C., Torrelo, A., Vestergaard, C., Wahn, U., & Werfel, T. (2021). Unmet medical needs in the treatment of atopic dermatitis in infants: An expert consensus on safety and efficacy of pimecrolimus. *Pediatric Allergy and Immunology, 32*, 414–424. doi:10.1111/pai.13422

McKenzie, C., & Silverberg, J. I. (2019). The prevalence and persistence of atopic dermatitis in urban United States children. *Annals of Allergy, Asthma, & Immunology, 123*(2), 173. doi:10.1016/j.anai.2019.05.014

National Eczema Society. (n.d.) Our skin and eczema. https://eczema.org/information-and-advice/our-skin-and-eczema/2017

Ohtsuki, M., Morimoto, H., & Nakagawa, H. (2018). Tacrolimus ointment for the treatment of adult and pediatric atopic dermatitis: Review on safety and benefits. *Journal of Dermatology, 45*, 936–942. doi:10.1111/1346-8138.14501

Paller, A. S., & Mancini, A. J. (2015). Eczematous eruptions in childhood. In A. S. Paller & A. J. Mancini (Eds.), *Hurwitz clinical pediatric dermatology: A textbook of skin disorders of childhood and adolescence* (5th ed., pp. 38–72) Elsevier.

Sicherer, S. H., & Sampson, H. A. (2018). Food allergy: A review and update on epidemiology, pathogenesis, diagnosis, prevention, and management. *Journal of Allergy and Clinical Immunology, 141*(1), 41–58. doi:10.1016/j.jaci.2017.11.003

Sidbury, R., Tom, W. L., Bergman, J. N., Cooper, K. D., Silverman, R. A., Berger, T. G., Chamlin, S. L., Cohen, D. E., Cordoro, K. M., Davis, D. M., Feldman, S. R., Hanifin, J. M., Krol, A., Margolis, D. J., Paller, A. S., Schwarzenberger, K., Simpson, E. L., Williams, H. C., & Eichenfield, L. F. (2014). Guidelines of care for the management of atopic dermatitis: section 4: Prevention of disease flares and the use of adjunctive therapies and approaches. *Journal of the American Academy of Dermatology, 7*(16), 1218–1233. https://doi.org/101016/j.jaad.2014.08.038

Togias, A., Cooper, S. F., Acebal, M. L., Assa'ad, A., Baker, J. R., Beck, L. A., Block, J., Byrd-Bredbenner, C., Chan, E., Eichenfield, L. F., Fleischer, D. M., Fuchs, G. J., Fureta, G. T., Greenhawt, M. J., Gupta, R. S., Habich, M., Jones, S. M., Keaton, K., Muraro, A., . . . Boyce, J. A. (2017). Addendum guidelines for the prevention of peanut allergy in the United States: Report of the National Institute of Allergy and Infectious Disease—sponsored expert panel. *Annals of Allergy, Asthma, & Immunology, 118*(2), 166–173.e7. doi:10.1016/j.anai.2016.10.004

Tollefson, M. M., & Bruckner, A. L. (2014). Atopic dermatitis: Skin-directed management. *Pediatrics, 135*(6), 1735–1744. doi:10.1542/peds.2014-2812

Urban, K., Chu, S., Giesey, R., Mehrmal, S., Uppal, P., Nedley, N., & Delost, G. R. (2021). The global, regional, and national burden of atopic dermatitis in 195 countries and territories: An ecological study from global burden of disease study. *Journal of the American Academy of Dermatology International, 2*, 12–18. doi:10.1016/j.jdin.2020.10.002

Walsh, J., & O'Flinn, N. (2011). Diagnosis and assessment of food allergy in children and young people in primary and community settings: NICE clinical guideline. *British Journal of General Practice, 61*(588), 473–475. doi:10.3399/bjgp11X583498

Yang, E. J., Sekhon, S., Sanchez, I. M., Beck, K. M., & Bhutani, T. (2018). Recent developments in atopic dermatitis. *Pediatrics, 142*(4), e20181102. doi:10.1542/peds.2018-1102

Yu, S. H., Drucker, A. M., Lebwohl, M., & Silverberg, J. I. (2018). A systematic review of the safety and efficacy of systemic corticosteroids in atopic dermatitis. *Journal of the American Academy of Dermatology, 78*(4), 733–740. doi:10.1016/j.jaad.2017.09.074

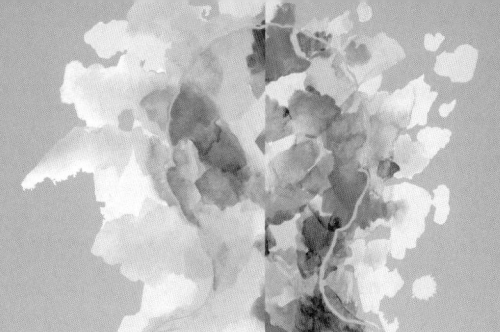

CHAPTER 11

Attention-Deficit/Hyperactivity Disorder in Children and Adolescents

Naomi A. Schapiro

I. Introduction and general background

Attention-deficit/hyperactivity disorder (ADHD) is one of the most common chronic conditions in childhood and the most common of the chronic neuropsychiatric conditions (Perou et al., 2013), with an estimated parent-reported prevalence rate of 9.6% (Zablotsky & Black, 2020). The major pediatric and child psychiatric organizations recognize the benefits and role of primary care providers in diagnosing and treating ADHD in childhood and adolescence (Barbaresi et al., 2020; Pliszka & AACAP Work Group on Quality Issues, 2007; Wolraich, Hagan, et al., 2019). Advanced practice nurses (APNs) are well suited to provide holistic and multifaceted care of children and adolescents with chronic conditions and can detect, follow, refer, and manage children with ADHD (McCoy et al., 2019; Vierhile et al., 2017).

II. Overview

A. Definitions

ADHD is defined by its features as a syndrome involving inattentiveness, hyperactivity, impulsivity, or a combination (Cabral et al., 2020). The most recent practice guidelines for ADHD from the American Academy of Pediatrics (AAP) define ADHD as a chronic condition, recommending that providers manage children and adolescents with ADHD as they would other children with special healthcare needs (Wolraich, Hagan, et al., 2019).

Diagnostic criteria for ADHD have been set historically by the *Diagnostic and Statistical Manual for Mental Disorders* (*DSM*). The current edition, *DSM-5* (American Psychiatric Association [APA], 2013, p. 61), describes the "essential feature" of ADHD as "a persistent pattern of inattention and/or hyperactivity-impulsivity that interferes with functioning or development." Under the current diagnostic criteria, the individual must have displayed some of these behaviors before 12 years of age, and they must be present in at least two areas of the child's life, such as home and school. Changes from the *DSM-IV-TR* (APA, 2000) include a move in the upper limit for the appearance of first symptoms from age 7 to age 12, a lowering of the number of required symptoms in the categories described next for older adolescents and young adults, and the addition of examples of core behaviors that are more applicable to adolescents and adults (APA, 2013). These changes were made in recognition of the developmental changes in behaviors across the life span and the difficulties adults might have in recalling childhood symptoms when presenting for diagnosis. The core behaviors of ADHD remain the same across *DSM* versions (Dalsgaard, 2013), and current practice guidelines are consistent with the *DSM-5* criteria (Barbaresi et al., 2020; Wolraich, Hagan, et al., 2019).

To be diagnosed with ADHD under *DSM-5* criteria, the child or adolescent (under 17) must display at least six inattentive behaviors and/or at least six impulsive or hyperactive behaviors, and these core symptoms must impair function in academic, social, or occupational activities (APA, 2013). Adolescents and adults 17 and older must display at least five behaviors in either or both categories. Examples of inattentive behaviors include difficulty in performing tasks that require sustained attention, distractibility, difficulty in organizing sequential tasks, poor time management, forgetfulness, and appearing not to listen when spoken to directly. Examples of hyperactive or impulsive behaviors include fidgeting, leaving one's seat or running around in inappropriate settings or difficulty staying still in restaurants or meetings, difficulty taking turns, blurting out answers, taking over what others are doing, and acting as if "driven by a motor" (APA, 2013, p. 60). In adolescents and young adults, inattentive behaviors are more prominent; hyperactive behaviors may be more subtle; and impulsivity may manifest as impaired concentration, decision making, or impulsive driving errors (Aduen et al., 2019; Asherson & Agnew-Blais, 2019; Niina et al., 2022). In addition to specifying whether the symptoms are predominantly inattentive, predominantly hyperactive/impulsive, or combined, the diagnosing clinician should specify whether the severity is mild, moderate, or severe, depending on the number of symptoms and degree of impairment in social, educational, or occupational functioning (APA, 2013).

Many of the symptoms and behaviors diagnostic of ADHD can be considered developmentally normal in younger children. Nevertheless, the current AAP guidelines state that primary care clinicians can diagnose ADHD in children as young as 4 years of age, as long as the child is showing behavior that is out of range for developmentally appropriate peers and functional impairment in two domains (Wolraich, Hagan, et al., 2019).

B. *Incidence and prevalence*

According to the 2015–2018 National Health Interview Survey (NHIS), 9.6% of U.S. children were reported by their parents to have ever been diagnosed with ADHD (Zablotsky & Black, 2020). Using data from the 2016 National Survey of Children's Health, an estimated 5.4 million children had a current ADHD diagnosis, or 8.4% of children ages 2–17 (Danielson et al., 2018). Less than two-thirds of these children (62%) were taking medication, 46.7% were receiving behavioral treatment, and 23% had not received either treatment. Fairman and colleagues (2017) used pediatric and adult data from a national survey of physician offices between 2008 and 2013 to track changes in ADHD diagnosis with the transition to *DSM-5* criteria. Rates of diagnosis and drug treatment trended upward for all ages and both assigned males and females, with a more rapid increase in rates for youth assigned female at birth compared with those assigned MALE. The authors attribute this difference to an increased focus on inattention, rather than just hyperactivity, in ADHD diagnosis (Fairman et al., 2017)

A review of 2014–2018 NHIS data for racial and ethnic differences in ADHD diagnosis found that Latinx (6%) and Asian (2.2%) children had lower rates of ADHD diagnosis when compared with non-Latinx Native American (11.9%), White (11.3%), and Black (10.7%) children (Wong & Landes, 2022). A national birth cohort analysis of over 200,000 commercially insured children found that the cumulative incidence of ADHD at 12 years was over 14% for White children, almost 12% for Black children, over 10% for Latinx children, and 6% for Asian children (Shi et al., 2021). In this sample, children living in lower-income families and children living in the South were more likely to be diagnosed with ADHD, and children living in the Midwest and West were least likely (Shi et al., 2021). The underlying mechanisms for these inequities are unclear and may include socioeconomic and cultural factors, including a lack of access to health care, variations in the interpretation of children's behavior, and variations in the application of the diagnostic criteria (DuPaul et al., 2020; Haack et al., 2018; Rowland et al., 2018).

There are no biomarkers for ADHD, and diagnosis is affected by access to care, as well as the potential implicit biases of teachers, caregivers, and clinicians. Wexler and colleagues (2022) compared parent and teacher ratings of ADHD symptoms on diagnostic scales and found that teachers were more likely to rate Black children higher on inattentive and impulsive symptoms and conduct problems, regardless of ADHD diagnosis or insurance status (Wexler et al., 2022). In another study, female-identified parenting adults were asked to view videotapes of a Black or white children displaying behaviors consistent with an ADHD diagnosis (Barrett & DuPaul, 2018). Black participants rated the behavior of both Black and White children higher for ADHD symptoms than White participants (Barrett & DuPaul, 2018). Other studies have shown that parents and teachers respond differently to standard questions in ADHD rating scales, depending on the age, assumed gender, and race of the child (DuPaul et al., 2020). Pediatric and adult practices are more likely to diagnose and treat patients with ADHD if they have a coexisting mood, anxiety, or conduct disorder (Fairman et al., 2017), yet Black children, assumed girls, and children of parents with lower educational levels have been less likely to receive a comprehensive neurodevelopmental evaluation for coexisting conditions (Gipson et al., 2015; Shi et al., 2021). Implicit bias affects differential assessments of similar behaviors, provider-patient communication, and provider decisions about whether or not to comprehensively evaluate a child with behavioral and educational problems for a full range of neuro-psychiatric conditions (Schnierle et al., 2019).

The majority of children with ADHD have at least one coexisting behavioral or psychiatric condition, commonly learning or sleep problems, oppositional defiant disorder (ODD), anxiety, or a mood disorder (Reale et al., 2017; Wolraich, Hagan, et al., 2019). Up to 50% of children with ADHD have a coexisting anxiety diagnosis. A systematic review found that both the level and types of ADHD and anxiety symptoms had more to do with social impairment than their mere coexistence (Bishop et al., 2019). Children with Tourette syndrome (TS), characterized by chronic motor and vocal tics, have high rates of coexisting ADHD, ranging from 17% to 68% of children with TS, depending on the study (Cravedi et al., 2017). Of note is that ADHD symptoms appear on average 2 years before diagnosis with TS. Children with seizure disorders, autism, and other neurodevelopmental conditions also have a greater prevalence of ADHD than the general pediatric population (Bélanger et al., 2018). Given the highlighted inequities in the comprehensive evaluation of coexisting conditions in children diagnosed with ADHD (Gipson et al., 2015), it's possible that current data are underestimates of true prevalence.

C. *Developmental trajectory and outcomes of ADHD*
Longitudinal studies suggest that there may be four different developmental variants of ADHD: early childhood (3–5 years) onset, middle childhood (6–14 years) onset with either a persistent course or a resolution of symptoms in adolescence, and adolescent or adult onset (Posner et al., 2020). One 6-year follow-up study of adolescents with ADHD found that 79% of adolescents with ADHD still met diagnostic criteria for ADHD into adulthood, with hyperactivity and parent ratings in childhood predicting adult persistence and low income and lower cognitive function in childhood predicting higher adult functional impairment (Cheung et al., 2015). A recent nationwide survey found that almost 70% of adolescents with ADHD had at least one coexisting behavioral health condition (Sultan et al., 2021). They were also more likely than adolescents without ADHD to have been expelled from school or fired from a job, have problems with alcohol use, and have attempted suicide.

In an earlier 10-year longitudinal study, boys with ADHD who were treated with stimulants had lower rates of psychiatric problems and academic failure than boys with ADHD who were not treated (Biederman et al., 2009). A more recent follow-up of young adults who were treated in the Multi-Modal Treatment Study of Children with ADHD (MTA) found that initial symptom severity, mental health of caregivers, and coexisting childhood mental health conditions were most predictive of persisting ADHD symptoms in young adults (Roy et al., 2016). However, socioeconomic status, childhood scores on intelligence tests, caregiver education levels, and parent–child relationships did not predict persistence into adulthood. These findings reinforce the importance of early diagnosis, evaluation of all children for coexisting conditions, and effective treatment.

D. *Theories of pathophysiology*
Studies of heritability have found that 70%–80% of the variance in ADHD can be explained by genetic factors, although only 22% of possible genome-wide risk locations have been identified (Posner et al., 2020). Genome-wide association studies have shown that heritability is polygenic, with a mixture of common and rare DNA variants (Faraone, 2014). Researchers are exploring the possibility that there are genetic differences between early and childhood-onset ADHD and adolescent- or adult-onset ADHD (Palladino et al., 2019; Posner et al., 2020). Although more assigned males than females are diagnosed in childhood, genetic studies show no differences, leading to speculations about differing symptom expression and underdiagnosis, as well as later emergence of symptoms in females (Palladino et al., 2019). Gene–environment interactions, including epigenetic changes, may explain the gap between identified genes and heritability; however, inconsistency between studies and potential observer bias in retrospective research have limited the usefulness of emerging data so far (Palladino et al., 2019).

Prematurity and low birth weight have been consistently associated with ADHD diagnosis (Posner et al., 2020). Children with fetal alcohol spectrum disorder (FASD) and those exposed to other toxic agents in utero, such as pesticides, also have a higher incidence of ADHD and other neurological disorders, due to direct toxicity to neurons or disruption of neuroendocrine pathways (Arab & Mostafalou, 2021; Kingdon et al., 2016).

Adverse childhood experiences (ACEs), including child maltreatment and other household dysfunctions, can have long-lasting effects on pediatric and adult health outcomes (Rariden et al., 2020). A regression analysis of the National Survey of Children's Health showed that children with no ACEs had an ADHD prevalence of 5.6%, and those with three or more ACEs had an ADHD prevalence of 19.4% (Walker et al., 2021). The adverse experiences most associated with an ADHD diagnosis were parental mental illness and parental incarceration. A meta-analysis of 28 studies examining the relationship between posttraumatic stress disorder (PTSD) and ADHD showed a bidirectional association between the two conditions (Spencer et al., 2016); however, more research is needed to elucidate the mechanisms underlying this association.

Dopamine and adrenergic systems have been implicated in the core symptoms of ADHD, with alpha-2-adrenergic receptors responsible for inhibitory control of motor activity (Cortese, 2012). There may be involvement of serotonin and cholinergic systems, although animal studies are less consistent, and there is no animal model that completely replicates the core symptoms of ADHD. Earlier research suggested the implication of structural abnormalities and delays in maturation in the prefrontal cortex, caudate, and cerebellum (Sharma & Couture, 2014), and the current focus is on abnormalities in neural networks, including the default mode network, and frontostriatal and mesocorticolimbic circuits (Posner et al., 2020). These circuits affect attention, distractibility, motivation and reward behaviors. To date, neuroimaging studies are small and cross-sectional, and they show poor reproducibility (Posner et al., 2020). Up to 45% of children with ADHD exhibit emotional dysregulation, with less sensitivity to positive stimuli than children without ADHD, problems regulating attention to emotional stimuli, and misperception of the emotions of others (Shaw et al., 2014). Some researchers consider emotional impulsivity and deficient emotional self-regulation to be core symptoms of ADHD, but at this point, there is no consensus on how to define and measure these constructs for diagnostic purposes (Faraone et al., 2019).

III. Database: History

A. *Chief complaint: referrals from parents, teachers, and family members*

Parents may initiate care if they have noticed disruptive behaviors or attention problems at home or at school and are also frequently encouraged by school personnel to have their child evaluated for ADHD. The initiating symptoms and motivation for seeking a diagnosis or treatment are an important part of the history. Because specific behaviors are both part of the diagnostic criteria and help guide the treatment plan, it is important to have parents and children be as specific as possible about the core behavioral symptoms and how they manifest in all the areas or domains of the child's life, particularly at home, at school, and with friends. Just as with a purely physical chief complaint, the APN can be guided in diagnosis by asking for the duration of the behaviors, specifically when they manifest (during which activities at home or which parts of the school day), any environmental characteristics or interventions that have made the behaviors better or worse, any associated problems, and any previous efforts by parents or teachers to manage the behaviors. Eliciting information about social determinants of health is an important part of this history (Barbaresi et al., 2020; McCoy et al., 2019), and some experts also recommend formal screening for ACEs (Walker et al., 2021). For older adolescents and young adults, the functional impairment in school- and work-related settings may be the most salient part of the presenting complaint, and it may take skillful questioning to elicit the core behavioral symptoms that fit the diagnostic criteria for ADHD and the age at which they began to manifest (Niina et al., 2022). Because ADHD is highly heritable, it is useful to take a detailed family history of ADHD or other behavioral or mental health conditions and to a detailed history of any cardiac conditions in the child or family, including histories of arrhythmias, to determine if any cardiac workup might be needed before starting medication (Wolraich, Hagan, et al., 2019). Supplement 1 of the AAP 2019 guidelines also provides detailed guidance on evaluation for ADHD, available at https://www.ncbi.nlm.nih.gov/pmc/articles/PMC7067282/.

Sleep problems, including sleep apnea, may result in daytime fatigue and inattention. Seizure disorders, especially absence seizures, may masquerade as inattention. Allergy symptoms, and the medications used to treat them, can also be related to inattention. The APN's documentation of patient history should include questions about sleep, snoring, and nighttime awakening and specific descriptions of inattentive behavior (Wolraich, Hagan, et al., 2019).

Children with hearing impairments or learning disabilities, such as reading disorders and receptive language delays, and other psychiatric and neurodevelopmental conditions, such as autism spectrum disorder, anxiety, or depression, may also seem distractible and inattentive (Barbaresi et al., 2020). History should include questions about any unusual movements or habits, such as tics or obsessive–compulsive behaviors, which may coexist with ADHD.

B. *Screening for ADHD*

The AAP states that primary care clinicians may use ADHD-specific screening scales to aid in the diagnosis of ADHD (Wolraich, Hagan, et al., 2019). Screening questionnaires such as the Vanderbilt questionnaire in the AAP ADHD Toolkit (Bard et al., 2013; Wolraich et al., 2003) and the Swanson, Nolan and Pelham Teacher and Parent Rating Scale (SNAP-IV) questionnaire (Hall et al., 2020) are available without cost on several websites in English and Spanish (**Table 11-1**). Broader questionnaires, such as the Achenbach Child Behavior Checklist, have not been found to be specific or sensitive enough for the diagnosis of ADHD in primary care settings but can be used to identify possible coexisting conditions to guide treatment and co-management with a behavioral health clinician (Biederman et al., 2021). Most clinical questionnaires for identifying ADHD include parent forms and teacher forms, and it is crucial to collect information directly from the child's teacher(s). Asking the parent to deliver and retrieve screening forms from the teacher saves the APN time and ensures parent consent to the collection of this information. The AAP Toolkit is designed for use with children from 4 to 18 years and does not include a child or adolescent self-report form. However, many pediatric and adolescent practices see emerging adults up to their mid-20s and will need to use other questionnaires. See Table 11-1 for the American Academy of Family Practice guide to adult screeners.

Because ADHD symptoms in adolescents shift to inattentive manifestations and difficulties with organization, which are more internal and may be reported more accurately by the adolescent than by adult caregivers (Niina et al., 2022; Posner et al., 2020), some research has validated adult self-report scales for ADHD in middle and high school students (Green et al., 2019).

C. *Screening for coexisting psychiatric and behavioral issues*

Screening questionnaires, such as the Vanderbilt, SNAP-IV, and Conners forms, include questions whose positive answers raise the clinician's suspicion of coexisting oppositional, anxiety, or mood disorders. Children who are suffering the sequelae of family disruption, child maltreatment, or other traumas may exhibit distractibility, inattention, disruptive behavior,

Table 11-1 Screening Tools for ADHD (Partial List)

Name and Contact Info	Cost	Individuals Screened	Languages	Additional Information
Vanderbilt Forms in *Caring for Children With ADHD: A Practical Resource Toolkit for Clinicians*, 3rd ed. American Academy of Pediatrics (2019) https://toolkits.solutions.aap.org/adhd/home	$150.00	Parents Teachers	English Spanish	Screening forms Educational handouts Behavioral treatment guidelines
Vanderbilt Forms, 2nd edition National Institute for Children's Health Quality (NICHQ) https://www.nichq.org/resource/caring-children-adhd-resource-toolkit-clinicians	No cost	Parents Teachers	English	Screening forms (2nd ed. of AAP) Educational handouts
Swanson, Nolan and Pelham Teacher and Parent Rating Scale (SNAP-IV) ADHD Screening Questions http://www.shared-care.ca/files/Scoring_for_SNAP_IV_Guide_26-item.pdf	No cost	Parents Teachers	English	26-item questionnaire
Columbia Community Pediatrics http://www.columbia.edu/itc/hs/medical/residency/peds/new_compeds_site/genpeds_menthealthres_dxandscreening-tools.html	No cost	Parents Teachers Children	Spanish English	Various screening forms (ADHD/anxiety/depression)
Conners forms https://www.pearsonassessments.com/store/usassessments/en/Store/Professional-Assessments/Behavior/Comprehensive/Conners-3rd-Edition/p/100000523.html	Up to $497.40, paper, online, software	Parents Teachers Youth (8–18)	English Spanish	Screening—long and short forms, including Abbreviated Symptoms Questionnaire (ASQ)
Barkley scales, resources for children and adults http://www.guilford.com/search-products/ADHD	Variable	Parents Teachers Adults	English	
American Academy of Family Practice ADHD and Quality of Life Screeners (2021) https://www.aafp.org/dam/AAFP/documents/patient_care/adhd_toolkit/adhd19-assessment-screeners.pdf	Free comprehensive diagnosis/treatment resources for families	Adults	English Some Spanish	
Children and Adults with AD/HD (CHADD) toolkit https://chadd.org/nrc-toolkit/	Information packets for families and health professionals		English Spanish Chinese	

and fatigue from sleep problems related to posttraumatic stress symptoms, anxiety, or mood changes (Klein et al., 2015; Song et al., 2021; Walker et al., 2021). Careful history taking, including the use of additional screening questionnaires for depression, anxiety, and substance use (Levy et al., 2016; Mossman et al., 2017; Trafalis et al., 2021; Zuckerbrot et al., 2018), will aid in the assessment of children with more complex behavioral and emotional symptoms. Some APNs and collaborating clinicians are experienced in diagnosing and managing mental health conditions in the primary care setting or work in integrated primary care and behavioral health settings. Others should consult with developmental/behavioral or mental health clinicians and refer children who may have coexisting conditions for diagnosis and co-management (Barbaresi et al., 2020).

D. *Screening for learning disabilities*
If the child's functioning at school indicates the possibility of both learning disabilities and ADHD, both evaluations should proceed (Barbaresi et al., 2020).

Most health insurance plans, private or public, do not cover learning evaluations, which must be requested by the parent from an overburdened public school system. Although these evaluations are legally required for children who may need special education services, parents may need assistance from the APN and guidance from family support organizations in advocating for them (Wolraich, Chan, et al., 2019). (See Table 11-1 for parent resources.) For children who seem to have ADHD without learning disabilities but whose academic performance does not improve on pharmacologic and appropriate behavioral interventions, an evaluation by the school for learning disabilities, such as dyslexia or processing difficulties, should be requested (Barbaresi et al., 2020; Wolraich, Hagan, et al., 2019).

IV. Physical examination

A. *Overview*

The physical examination in ADHD should help the APN eliminate potential physical causes of inattention, hyperactivity, and disruptive behavior and any contraindications to medication that might be used to treat ADHD. Observing the child–caregiver interaction and the child at play in the waiting area or exam room may provide the APN with additional information, although shy or fearful children may not display impulsive behaviors in a clinic setting. There are no specific physical findings that confirm or rule out a diagnosis of ADHD.

B. *Important to eliminate other potential physical causes of attention issues and disruptive behavior*

The physical examination should include a thorough head, eye, ear, nose, and throat examination, including documentation of any dysmorphic facial features; a thorough cardiovascular evaluation; a thorough neurologic examination, including a mental status exam; documentation of any tics; and hearing and vision screening. If the history or other findings on physical examination suggest hyperthyroidism, hypothyroidism, anemia, or lead poisoning, then appropriate laboratory and other tests are indicated (Wolraich, Hagan, et al., 2019). Children with sleep apnea may have fatigue and inattention during the day (Honaker & Meltzer, 2016). Most children with ADHD have a normal physical examination, although some children may have "soft neurologic signs" (Barbaresi et al., 2020), demonstrating more clumsiness on tasks requiring cerebellar integration, such as rapid-finger or alternating-hand tests, than most children of their age. A history of traumatic brain injury or tumors or a frankly abnormal neurologic or mental status examination should prompt a search for other diagnoses; additional testing, including imaging; and referral for any positive results (Wolraich, Hagan, et al., 2019).

Children with normal examinations do not need laboratory or other imaging tests (Wolraich, Hagan, et al., 2019). If the child also has symptoms of anxiety, mood disturbances, or sleep disturbances (e.g., restless leg syndrome), complete blood count, ferritin, thyroid, lead, and metabolic panels may be indicated.

C. *Monitor for possible cautions or contraindications to treatments.*

Concerns about possible cases of sudden death in children treated with stimulants for ADHD prompted concerns about screening all children with ADHD for cardiovascular disease before initiating treatment with medications (AAP & American Heart Association, 2008). Children with congenital heart disease have a higher incidence of ADHD than the general population, and many of these children have been managed successfully on stimulants in consultation with their cardiologists (Batra et al., 2012). A longitudinal case-control study of adolescents with long-QT syndrome who were taking ADHD medications indicated that episodes of syncope and risk for sudden death were higher in this group (Zhang et al., 2015). The current recommendations from the AAP Section on Cardiology and Cardiac Surgery (2020) are that providers should take a thorough history of child and family incidence of cardiac disease, especially connective tissue disorders, cardiomyopathies, arrhythmias, any need for pacemaker or implanted defibrillator, storage diseases, sudden unexplained death, and any premature cardiovascular disease before age 50. For asymptomatic children with a normal exam and without this family history, no prescreening electrocardiogram (ECG) is needed (AAP Section on Cardiology and Cardiac Surgery, 2020)

When a range of medications is being considered, consulting mental health professionals may ask for chemistry panels that could reassure prescribers about kidney function (creatinine and blood urea nitrogen) and a lack of liver inflammation (aspartate aminotransferase and alanine aminotransferase).

D. *Neuropsychiatric conditions and ADHD: tic disorders, autism spectrum*

Between 3% and 6% of all school-age children exhibit chronic vocal or motor tics, lasting over 1 year, and fewer than 1% have TS. However, among children with TS, ADHD is the most common coexisting condition, with a prevalence of up to 68%, and children with tics or TS should be evaluated for ADHD (Cravedi et al., 2017). Although most children with tics can suppress them for a time in public settings, they may show up on examination. An estimated 2.5% of U.S. children from ages 3 to 17 have been diagnosed with autism spectrum disorder (ASD) (Zablotsky & Black, 2020). Children with ASD, genetic syndromes such as fragile X, or FASD may have additional functional impairment from ADHD; the evaluation and management of these coexisting conditions should involve consultation with or referral to behavioral and developmental specialists (Barbaresi et al., 2020; Wolraich, Hagan, et al., 2019).

V. Assessment

A. *History and examination that support a diagnosis of ADHD*

No coexisting mental or behavioral health conditions are present. The child may be treated in a primary care setting or co-managed with mental health and learning professionals.

B. *History and examination that support a diagnosis of ADHD and coexisting conditions*

If additional coexisting conditions are suspected, consultation or referral to behavioral–developmental or mental health and learning professionals for more definitive diagnosis is recommended, with co-management by the APN (Barbaresi et al., 2020). Coexistence of anxiety, mood disorders, or tic disorders may complicate treatment, and children with a family history of bipolar disorder may react poorly to stimulant medications, even if they themselves do not have coexisting conditions. Conversely, oppositional and anxious symptoms may be related to worries or frustration with academic performance and may diminish with effective treatment for ADHD (Wolraich, Hagan, et al., 2019).

C. *History and examination that do not support a diagnosis of ADHD*

Refer to behavioral–developmental or mental health professionals or a neurologist, as indicated by the findings. Consider workup for sleep apnea.

VI. Plan

Current practice guidelines recommend treating the child or youth with ADHD as a child or youth with special healthcare needs (CYSHCN); centering management in the healthcare home; and collaborating with the child, family, and school to determine the best treatment plans (Wolraich, Hagan, et al., 2019). These plans may start with medication, psychosocial treatment, or both, depending on the age of the child (Barbaresi et al., 2020; Wolraich, Hagan, et al., 2019). As evidence emerges from long-term follow-up of individuals with ADHD across the lifespan (Posner et al., 2020), recommendations increasingly emphasize the importance of teaching self-management skills, with a focus on training parents and teachers in positive behavioral management rather than relying on medication alone (Barbaresi et al., 2020; Schoenfelder & Sasser, 2016; Wolraich, Chan, et al., 2019; Wolraich, Hagan, et al., 2019). The AAP recommends encouraging the family and child to choose three of the most concerning target behaviors affecting the child's function at home and school to address initially (Wolraich, Hagan, et al., 2019). One study comparing parent and teacher Vanderbilt scale ratings of symptoms of children with ADHD found that "avoiding tasks" and "making careless mistakes" predicted writing difficulties in elementary school grades and overall academic performance in higher grades (Zoromski et al., 2021), and the authors suggested school-based interventions to address these functional impairments.

For school-age children and adolescents, the AAP and the Society for Developmental and Behavioral Pediatrics (SDBP) have found that multimodal treatment, including behavioral management and medication, is the most effective treatment option for core symptoms of ADHD and that child and family collaboration is essential in deciding on medication (Barbaresi et al., 2020; Wolraich, Hagan, et al., 2019). For children from 4 to 6 years of age, the AAP and SDBP recommend coordinated family and school behavioral interventions as first-line treatment, with medication considered if behavioral treatments are insufficient (APA, 2000; Barbaresi et al., 2020). Barbaresi and colleagues note that medications may be less effective and adverse effects more common in this age group.

A. *Behavioral approaches (AAP and SDBP recommendations)*
  1. Psychoeducation (for child/adolescent and all family members)
     a. Long-term developmental implications of ADHD
     b. Effects on self-esteem and strategies for positive parenting
     c. Goals of treatment
     d. Bringing in school personnel as part of the team
  2. Behavioral parent training to help parents work more effectively with their children, specifically using the following techniques:
     a. Positive reinforcement (including point systems, token economy)
     b. Methods of negative reinforcement (e.g., cost response)
     c. Giving commands, shaping behavior effectively
     d. Setting up schedules, helping to organize backpack, homework
  3. School-based interventions
     a. Classroom-wide interventions (posted rules, positive reinforcement for appropriate behavior and accurate work completion, appropriate consequences for misbehavior, reading out loud)
     b. Individual interventions, such as a daily report card with clear goals and feedback
     c. More intensive treatment as outlined in an individual educational plan (IEP) or a plan developed under Section 504 of the Americans With Disabilities Act.

B. *Medication*
  1. Stimulant medications
     Methylphenidate and amphetamine both block presynaptic transporters of dopamine and norepinephrine, increasing the supply of both; amphetamine additionally increases the presynaptic release of dopamine (Posner et al., 2020). Although the exact mechanism of action is unclear, stimulant medications improve the core symptoms of ADHD in up to 90% of children if dosed appropriately (Pliszka, 2016) and are considered first-line treatment by most clinicians (see **Table 11-2**). All stimulant medications have potential side effects of appetite suppression, sleep disturbance (although this is also a core ADHD symptom), headaches, constipation, and irritability during the day as the medication wears off. Although stimulants can increase symptoms of anxiety, many children with diagnosed ADHD and anxiety can have fewer anxious symptoms if their attention and academic performance improve on stimulants (Pliszka, 2019; Wolraich, Hagan, et al., 2019). Stimulants can increase mania in children with bipolar disorder (Lexicomp Online, 2021). If

Table 11-2 ADHD Medications: U.S. Food and Drug Administration (FDA) Approved

Class of Medication	Duration	Examples	Advantages	Disadvantages	Dosing
Stimulants	Short acting (3–6 h)	Methylphenidate (chewable, liquid available) Dextroamphetamine Dexmethylphenidate	Quick onset Ease of making dosage adjustments without changing prescription	Must be dosed midday to last through school or workday Higher abuse potential	Individualized, not mg/kg dosing, but starting dose adjusted to weight
	Medium acting (4–8 h)	Mixed amphetamine salts (sometimes listed as short acting; however effects may last through school day)	May last during school day, lower abuse potential	Steady release during day, less effective for some children than bursts of medication	Individualized, not mg/kg dosing, but starting dose adjusted to weight
	Long acting, variable forms of absorption/ release (8–12 h)	OROS methylphenidate Methylphenidate ER, SR Methylphenidate–LA* Methylphenidate CD* Methylphenidate patch Methylphenidate XR solution Dextroamphetamine XR Dexmethylphenidate XR* Mixed amphetamine salts XR* Lisdexamfetamine**	Last during entire school day, better coverage for driving, lower abuse potential	Cannot be crushed or altered, may effect sleep more	Dosing less flexible, conversion charts available from short-acting medications
Norepinephrine reuptake inhibitor	Long acting, 24-h effect, half-life 5–21 h	Atomoxetine Viloxazine	24-h coverage, low abuse potential, may be effective for depression	Extensive drug interactions, black-box warnings for suicidality	Weight-based dosing for children <70 kg
Alpha-2-agonist	Short or long acting (only extended release FDA approved 2009), half-life 17 h	Guanfacine Guanfacine ER Clonidine Kapvay	More effective for impulsivity and hyperactivity than for inattention	Rebound hypertension if withdrawn too quickly, some children have headache, somnolence; drug interactions	Guanfacine/ER: Start with 1 mg oral daily, may increase in increments of 1 mg/wk, weight-based suggested upper limits Clonidine/Kapvay: start with 0.1, ½ tab at qhs; max is 0.3 mg qhs and 0.4 mg/day

* Capsule may be opened and sprinkled on applesauce.
** Capsule may be opened and dissolved in water.

Data from Lexicomp Online, Pediatric and Neonatal Lexi-Drugs Online, Hudson, Ohio: UpToDate, Inc.; 2013; August 2, 2021; Posner, J., Polanczyk, G. V., & Sonuga-Barke, E. (2020). Attention-deficit hyperactivity disorder. Lancet, 395(10222), 450-462. https://doi.org/10.1016/s0140-6736(19)33004-1 ; Wolraich, M. L., Hagan, J. F., Allan, C., Chan, E., Davison, D., Earls, M., Evans, S. W., Flinn, S. K., Froehlich, T., Frost, J., Holbrook, J. R., Lehmann, C. U., Lessin, H. R., Okechukwu, K., Pierce, K. L., Winner, J. D., & Zurhellen, W. (2019). Clinical Practice Guideline for the Diagnosis, Evaluation, and Treatment of Attention-Deficit/Hyperactivity Disorder in Children and Adolescents. Pediatrics, 144(4), e20192528. https://doi.org/10.1542/peds.2019-2528

there is a family history of bipolar disorder or any concerns about mania from the child's mental status exam, the APN should consider co-management with a mental health clinician before prescribing medications.

Although dextroamphetamine and mixed amphetamine salts are approved for children as young as 3, stimulants are not generally recommended for preschool-age children because they seem to have increased adverse effects and may not be as effective as behavioral treatment in this age group (Barbaresi et al., 2020; Wolraich, Hagan, et al., 2019). Methylphenidate is the first-line treatment for preschool-age youth after behavior management interventions. Extended-release medications can last anywhere from 6 to 12 hours, depending on the medication and absorption formulation. These medications obviate the need for midday dosing, may decrease irritability because the medication wears off more slowly, and may have less potential for abuse. Adolescents and emerging adults benefit from dosing that is directly related to their school and work schedules, including late-night driving (Aduen et al., 2019; Barbaresi et al., 2020; Lexicomp Online, 2021; Wolraich, Hagan, et al., 2019).

  a. Short-acting medication: rapid onset, duration of action 3–4 hours
      i. Advantages: dose clears system rapidly, effect rapid
      ii. Disadvantages: given two or three times a day, including midday; issues of convenience (parent, school personnel), training, safety, and child's embarrassment; and more reports of irritability as medication wears off
  b. Intermediate- and long-acting medication
      i. Longer acting: 6–12 hours, no need for midday dose
      ii. May start long acting directly, no need to start with short acting first, except in very young children
      iii. May have slower onset, depending on formulation
      iv. May have decreased abuse potential relative to short-acting medication
      v. If slower, steady release, the child may not "feel" that the medication is working as much as the short-acting medication or medication released in several bursts, but the literature shows an equivalent effect.
  c. Absorption mechanisms available in long-acting medications (current available medications in parentheses accurate at time of publication)
      i. Osmotically released oral therapy: shorter release and nonabsorbable plastic shell contains some medication for later release; later onset; longer effect than spheroidal oral drug absorption system (methylphenidate)
      ii. Spheroidal oral drug absorption system: Combination of immediate-release and longer-release beads; capsules may be opened up and sprinkled on food (methylphenidate, dexmethylphenidate). One version can be taken at night, with peak effect in the daytime.
      iii. Transdermal patch: releases medication over 9 hours; onset within 2 hours; duration 12 hours; applied on hip; site and patch changed daily (methylphenidate); lower abuse potential
      iv. Prodrug, converted slowly to active drug in intestines and liver; slower onset and 10 hours of active effect; lower abuse potential (lisdexamfetamine to dexamphetamine)
2. Nonstimulant medication
  a. Norepinephrine reuptake inhibitors
      i. Atomoxetine: slow onset, effects may not be felt for several weeks, 24-hour coverage, cannot be chewed or crushed
      ii. Viloxazine: approved in 2021; ages 6–17 only; capsule may be opened, sprinkled on applesauce; reputed to take effect more quickly than atomoxetine
      iii. More acceptable to child and adolescent if first medication, rather than switching from stimulant (patient may not "feel" that medication is taking effect)
      iv. Rare reports of liver toxicity (atomoxetine), cleared through CYP2D6 pathway, half-life up to 21 hours (atomoxetine) in individuals with less active CYP2D6; half-life of viloxazine up to 11 hours; recommend monitoring liver enzymes with viloxazine
      v. May increase effects of albuterol, sympathomimetic drugs in general
      vi. Black-box warnings for suicidality
  b. α_2-Adrenergic agonists
      i. More effective for impulsivity than for inattention
      ii. Guanfacine and clonidine approved for children 6 years and older, extended-release form available
      iii. Clonidine patch available when steady dose reached; medication must be tapered off slowly
      iv. Sometimes used for children with impulsive ADHD and tics
      v. Clonidine approved for sleep in children with neurodevelopmental disorders
      vi. Side effects: depression, headache, dizziness, fatigue, constipation, decreased appetite; rebound hypertension if discontinued suddenly; drug interactions

c. Bupropion
   i. Not recommended as first-line treatment for ADHD, dosing available for 6–18 years and for adults
   ii. May be used in refractory depression (8–18 years), not considered a first-line treatment, may be more effective children/adolescents with depression and ADHD
   iii. Side effects: insomnia, fatigue, agitation, dry mouth, headaches, rash, and lower seizure threshold
   iv. Contraindicated if history of seizures, traumatic head injury, eating disorders, or undergoing abrupt discontinuation of ethanol or other sedatives

C. *General considerations about medication*
   1. Contraindications for stimulants
      a. Symptomatic cardiovascular disease (adults and children)
      b. Glaucoma
      c. The U.S. Food and Drug Administration lists tics as a contraindication to some stimulant medication and a caution for others; however, several studies of children with TS randomized to various treatment arms for ADHD showed no increase in tics with stimulant medicine.
   2. Strategies for starting medication, tracking, and managing short-term effects
      a. Start medications on the weekend, so caregivers can monitor for side effects, before administering on a school day.
      b. Discuss potential impact on mood; ask parents to call immediately if any changes, agitation, or suicidal ideation.
      c. Initial dose should be increased every 4 to 7 days until core symptoms show improvement or side effects increase.
         i. Clinician and family should expect some loss of appetite during the dosing period for stimulants, with normal appetite before dose and after wearing off; lack of this effect may indicate subtherapeutic dose; weight should be monitored and addressed if changes in growth curve.
         ii. Carefully monitor side effects if child is on nonstimulant medication or if taking additional medications.
         iii. Check in weekly with parent and child by telephone or in the office when starting medication and increasing dose. Stimulants are Schedule II medications: no refills by telephone, and new prescriptions must be written and picked up when continuing these medications. The Drug Enforcement Agency does allow electronic prescribing of stimulants; check with your institutional and state guidelines for electronic prescriptions.
         iv. Follow blood pressure, heart rate, and weight for stimulants and norepinephrine reuptake inhibitors (Hennissen et al., 2017).
         v. Follow side effects of other medications as indicated (e.g., possible liver inflammation for atomoxetine, viloxazine).
      d. Sleep issues are common with ADHD, with or without medication.
         i. Take detailed sleep history before starting medications.
         ii. Counsel patient and family on sleep hygiene and sleep environment.
         iii. Adjust dose or duration of medication, if indicated.
         iv. Consider melatonin or clonidine.
      e. Track adherence and diversion: especially an issue for adolescent and young adult patients taking shorter-acting stimulant medication and those with a history of substance abuse in the family or the patient.
      f. Stimulant medication holidays
         i. Medication holidays are sometimes used or recommended on weekends and summer if core symptoms are manageable outside of school and there are weight-loss concerns; however, medication holidays are controversial.
         ii. May increase side effects on restarting
         iii. May not be beneficial for adolescents, especially if they drive or work in evening
   3. Tracking medication long-term effects
      a. Effects on academic and job performance and home and peer relationships
         i. Most documented benefits early in treatment (first 3 years) may be partly caused by more intensive management.
         ii. May be more effective if started earlier in the course of ADHD
         iii. The interaction of ADHD and substance abuse is complex; in general, adolescents and adults with ADHD have higher rates of substance abuse compared to non-ADHD peers, but effective treatment with stimulants seems to lower this risk while treatment is maintained.
      b. Emergence or persistence of any mood-related symptoms
      c. Growth (height, weight) and blood pressure
         i. Some decreased height velocity and possible shorter adult height by up to 2 cm
         ii. Possible long-term increase in blood pressure
      d. Diversion or substance use issues: in-depth psychosocial screen for adolescents, screening for substance use recommended from age 9 on, awareness of parental substance abuse

Box 11-1 Resources

National Institute for Children's Health Quality (NICHQ)
Caring for Children with ADHD: A Resource Toolkit for Clinicians (3rd ed., 2019, open access)
https://www.nichq.org/resource/caring-children-adhd-resource-toolkit-clinicians
American Academy of Pediatrics, healthy children.org—parent handouts about ADHD and related issues (in English and Spanish)
https://www.healthychildren.org/English/health-issues/conditions/adhd/Pages/default.aspx
https://www.healthychildren.org/spanish/health-issues/conditions/adhd/paginas/default.aspx
American Academy of Child and Adolescent Psychiatry ADHD Resource Center
https://www.aacap.org/AACAP/Families_and_Youth/Resource_Centers/ADHD_Resource_Center/Home.aspx
https://www.aacap.org/App_Themes/AACAP/docs/resource_centers/resources/med_guides/adhd_parents_medication_guide_english.pdf
ADDitude Magazine: Inside the ADHD Mind
https://www.additudemag.com/
Children and Adults with Attention-Deficit/Hyperactivity Disorder (CHADD) (resources in English and Spanish)
http://www.chadd.org/
Support for Families of Children with Disabilities—information packets in English, Spanish, Chinese
https://www.supportforfamilies.org/adhd-info-packet

D. *Follow-up and indications for referral*
   1. Lack of expected improvement
      a. Most children respond to stimulants, but some may require a switch in the specific type, adjustments in dose, or addition or switch to a nonstimulant medication.
      b. Response to behavioral approaches
   2. Coexisting learning, mood, or behavioral problems not improving or worsening
E. *Parental/patient education/school interventions*
   Encourage parental connection with other parents, peer support for children and youth, and use of community resources (**Box 11-1**).
F. *Long-term issues and transition to adulthood* (Aduen et al., 2019; Niina et al., 2022; Posner et al., 2020; Schoenfelder & Sasser, 2016; Sultan et al., 2021; Swanson et al., 2017)
   1. Condition trajectory
      a. Initial presenting behavioral symptoms may change or diminish; functional impairments may improve or worsen.
      b. Behavioral, academic, and self-regulatory skills and supports are crucial for optimal adult functioning.
      c. Adolescents with ADHD have significantly increased risks of driving accidents, tickets, and impulsive errors, especially if not properly medicated; additional driving strategies may help.
      d. Increasing appearance of coexisting conditions (anxiety, mood, conduct, substance abuse); may be mitigated by appropriate medication and behavioral treatment in childhood and adolescence
   2. Long-term planning should begin with early adolescent and parent
      a. Skill building to increase confidence, offer alternatives to risky behavior, and aid in career planning
         i. Reframing ADHD to highlight positive aspects of behavioral characteristics for appropriate careers
         ii. Jobs and/or chores to give youth a sense of accomplishment and instill work ethic
         iii. Focusing on strengths and interests
      b. Advocating for educational accommodations as needed throughout academic career, involving the adolescent as a self-advocate, and preparing for job skills and higher education
      c. Shift to long-acting medication with decreased abuse potential and greater coverage for evening behaviors, especially driving
   3. Transition to adult systems of care
      a. Adult providers are often unfamiliar with ADHD relative to pediatric providers
      b. Loss of insurance coverage and difficulty continuing stimulant medications through publicly funded or indigent mental health care
         i. Issues have been mitigated through the Affordable Care Act.
         ii. Decreased access to care affects educational and job trajectories.
         iii. Severities of coexisting conditions may increase the risk of substance abuse increases without access to effective care.

References

Aduen, P. A., Cox, D. J., Fabiano, G. A., Garner, A. A., & Kofler, M. J. (2019). Expert recommendations for improving driving safety for teens and adult drivers with ADHD. *ADHD Reports*, 27(4), 8–14. doi:10.1521/adhd.2019.27.4.8

American Academy of Pediatrics & American Heart Association. (2008). American Academy of Pediatrics/American Heart Association clarification of statement on cardiovascular evaluation and monitoring of children and adolescents with heart disease receiving medications for ADHD: May 16, 2008. *Journal of Developmental and Behavioral Pediatrics*, 29(4), 335. doi:10.1097/DBP.0b013e31318185dc14

American Academy of Pediatrics Section on Cardiology and Cardiac Surgery. (2020). *Five things physicians and patients should question*. ABIM Foundation. https://www.choosingwisely.org/wp-content/uploads/2020/11/AAP_Cardio-5things-List_Draft-3.pdf

American Psychiatric Association. (2000). *Diagnostic and statistical manual of mental disorders* (4th ed., Text rev.).

American Psychiatric Association. (2013). *Diagnostic and statistical manual of mental disorders* (5fth ed.).

Arab, A., & Mostafalou, S. (2021). Neurotoxicity of pesticides in the context of CNS chronic diseases. *International Journal of Environmental Health Research*, 32(12), 2718–2755. doi:10.1080/09603123.2021.1987396

Asherson, P., & Agnew-Blais, J. (2019). Annual research review: Does late-onset attention-deficit/hyperactivity disorder exist? *Journal of Child Psychology and Psychiatry*, 60(4), 333–352. doi:10.1111/jcpp.13020

Barbaresi, W. J., Campbell, L., Diekroger, E. A., Froehlich, T. E., Liu, Y. H., O'Malley, E., Pelham, W. E., Jr., Power, T. J., Zinner, S. H., & Chan, E. (2020). Society for Developmental and Behavioral Pediatrics clinical practice guideline for the assessment and treatment of children and adolescents with complex attention-deficit/hyperactivity disorder. *Journal of Developmental & Behavioral Pediatrics*, 41(Suppl. 2S), S35-s57. doi:10.1097/dbp.0000000000000770

Bard, D. E., Wolraich, M. L., Neas, B., Doffing, M., & Beck, L. (2013). The psychometric properties of the Vanderbilt attention-deficit hyperactivity disorder diagnostic parent rating scale in a community population. *Journal of Developmental & Behavioral Pediatrics*, 34(2), 72–82. doi:10.1097/DBP.0b013e31827a3a22

Barrett, C., & DuPaul, G. J. (2018). Impact of maternal and child race on maternal ratings of ADHD symptoms in Black and White boys. *Journal of Attention Disorders*, 22(13), 1246–1254. doi:10.1177/1087054715616489

Batra, A. S., Alexander, M. E., & Silka, M. J. (2012). Attention-deficit/hyperactivity disorder, stimulant therapy, and the patient with congenital heart disease: Evidence and reason. *Pediatric Cardiology*, 33(3), 394–401. doi:10.1007/s00246-012-0162-6

Bélanger, S. A., Andrews, D., Gray, C., & Korczak, D. (2018). ADHD in children and youth: Part 1—Etiology, diagnosis, and comorbidity. *Paediatrics & Child Health*, 23(7), 447–453. doi:10.1093/pch/pxy109

Biederman, J., DiSalvo, M., Vaudreuil, C., Wozniak, J., Uchida, M., Woodworth, K. Y., Green, A., Farrell, A., & Faraone, S. V. (2021). The Child Behavior Checklist can aid in characterizing suspected comorbid psychopathology in clinically referred youth with ADHD. *Journal of Psychiatric Research*, 138, 477–484. doi:10.1016/j.jpsychires.2021.04.028

Biederman, J., Monuteaux, M. C., Spencer, T., Wilens, T. E., & Faraone, S. V. (2009). Do stimulants protect against psychiatric disorders in youth with ADHD? A 10-year follow-up study. *Pediatrics*, 124(1), 71–78. doi:10.1542/peds.2008-3347

Bishop, C., Mulraney, M., Rinehart, N., & Sciberras, E. (2019). An examination of the association between anxiety and social functioning in youth with ADHD: A systematic review. *Psychiatry Research*, 273, 402–421. doi:10.1016/j.psychres.2019.01.039

Cabral, M. D. I., Liu, S., & Soares, N. (2020). Attention-deficit/hyperactivity disorder: diagnostic criteria, epidemiology, risk factors and evaluation in youth. *Translational Pediatrics*, 9(Suppl. 1), S104-s113. doi:10.21037/tp.2019.09.08

Cheung, C. H., Rijdijk, F., McLoughlin, G., Faraone, S. V., Asherson, P., & Kuntsi, J. (2015). Childhood predictors of adolescent and young adult outcome in ADHD. *Journal of Psychiatric Research*, 62, 92–100. https://doi.org/10.1016/j.jpsychires.2015.01.011

Cortese, S. (2012). The neurobiology and genetics of attention-deficit/hyperactivity disorder (ADHD): what every clinician should know. *European Journal of Paediatric Neurology*, 16(5), 422–433. doi:10.1016/j.ejpn.2012.01.009

Cravedi, E., Deniau, E., Giannitelli, M., Xavier, J., Hartmann, A., & Cohen, D. (2017). Tourette syndrome and other neurodevelopmental disorders: a comprehensive review. *Child and Adolescent Psychiatry and Mental Health*, 11, 59. doi:10.1186/s13034-017-0196-x

Dalsgaard, S. (2013). Attention-deficit/hyperactivity disorder (ADHD). *European Child and Adolescent Psychiatry*, 22(Suppl. 1), S43–48. doi:10.1007/s00787-012-0360-z

Danielson, M. L., Bitsko, R. H., Ghandour, R. M., Holbrook, J. R., Kogan, M. D., & Blumberg, S. J. (2018). Prevalence of parent-reported ADHD diagnosis and associated treatment among U.S. Children and adolescents, 2016. *Journal of Clinical Child & Adolescent Psychology*, 47(2), 199–212. doi:10.1080/15374416.2017.1417860

DuPaul, G. J., Fu, Q., Anastopoulos, A. D., Reid, R., & Power, T. J. (2020). ADHD parent and teacher symptom ratings: Differential item functioning across gender, age, race, and ethnicity. *Journal of Abnormal Child Psychology*, 48(5), 679–691. doi:10.1007/s10802-020-00618-7

Fairman, K. A., Peckham, A. M., & Sclar, D. A. (2017). Diagnosis and treatment of ADHD in the United States: Update by gender and race. *Journal of Attention Disorders*, 24(1), 10–19. doi:10.1177/1087054716688534

Faraone, S. V. (2014). Advances in the genetics of attention-deficit/hyperactivity disorder. *Biological Psychiatry*, 76(8), 599–600. doi:10.1016/j.biopsych.2014.07.016

Faraone, S. V., Rostain, A. L., Blader, J., Busch, B., Childress, A. C., Connor, D. F., & Newcorn, J. H. (2019). Practitioner review: Emotional dysregulation in attention-deficit/hyperactivity disorder—implications for clinical recognition and intervention. *Journal of Child Psychology and Psychiatry*, 60(2), 133–150. doi:10.1111/jcpp.12899

Gipson, T. T., Lance, E. I., Albury, R. A., Gentner, M. B., & Leppert, M. L. (2015). Disparities in identification of comorbid diagnoses in children with ADHD. *Clinical Pediatrics*, 54(4), 376–381. doi:10.1177/0009922814553434

Green, J. G., DeYoung, G., Wogan, M. E., Wolf, E. J., Lane, K. L., & Adler, L. A. (2019). Evidence for the reliability and preliminary validity of the Adult ADHD Self-Report Scale v1.1 (ASRS v1.1) screener in an adolescent community sample. *International Journal of Methods in Psychiatric Research*, 28(1), e1751. doi:10.1002/mpr.1751

Haack, L. M., Meza, J., Jiang, Y., Araujo, E. J., & Pfiffner, L. (2018). Influences to ADHD problem recognition: Mixed-method investigation and recommendations to reduce disparities for Latino youth. *Administration and Policy in Mental Health and Mental Health Services, 45*(6), 958–977. doi:10.1007/s10488-018-0877-7

Hall, C. L., Guo, B., Valentine, A. Z., Groom, M. J., Daley, D., Sayal, K., & Hollis, C. (2020). The validity of the SNAP-IV in children displaying ADHD symptoms. *Assessment, 27*(6), 1258–1271. doi:10.1177/1073191119842255

Hennissen, L., Bakker, M. J., Banaschewski, T., Carucci, S., Coghill, D., Danckaerts, M., Dittmann, R. W., Hollis, C., Kovshoff, H., McCarthy, S., Nagy, P., Sonuga-Barke, E., Wong, I. C., Zuddas, A., Rosenthal, E., & Buitelaar, J. K. (2017). Cardiovascular effects of stimulant and non-stimulant medication for children and adolescents with ADHD: A systematic review and meta-analysis of trials of methylphenidate, amphetamines and atomoxetine. *CNS Drugs, 31*(3), 199–215. doi:10.1007/s40263-017-0410-7

Honaker, S. M., & Meltzer, L. J. (2016). Sleep in pediatric primary care: A review of the literature. *Sleep Medicine Reviews, 25*, 31–39. doi:10.1016/j.smrv.2015.01.004

Kingdon, D., Cardoso, C., & McGrath, J. J. (2016). Research review: Executive function deficits in fetal alcohol spectrum disorders and attention-deficit/hyperactivity disorder—a meta-analysis. *Journal of Child Psychology and Psychiatry, 57*(2), 116–131. doi:10.1111/jcpp.12451

Klein, B., Damiani-Taraba, G., Koster, A., Campbell, J., & Scholz, C. (2015). Diagnosing attention-deficit hyperactivity disorder (ADHD) in children involved with child protection services: Are current diagnostic guidelines acceptable for vulnerable populations? *Child: Care, Health and Development, 41*(2), 178–185. doi:10.1111/cch.12168

Lexicomp Online, Pediatric and Neonatal Lexi-Drugs Online. UpToDate, Inc. Accessed August 2, 2021.

Levy, S. J., Williams, J. F., & Committee on Substance Abuse and Prevention. (2016). Substance use screening, brief intervention, and referral to treatment. *Pediatrics, 138*(1), e20161210. doi:10.1542/peds.2016-1210

McCoy, K. T., Pancione, K., Hammonds, L. S., & Costa, C. B. (2019). Management of attention-deficit/hyperactivity disorder in primary care. *Nursing Clinics of North America, 54*(4), 517–532. doi:10.1016/j.cnur.2019.08.001

Mossman, S. A., Luft, M. J., Schroeder, H. K., Varney, S. T., Fleck, D. E., Barzman, D. H., Gilman, R., DelBello, M. P., & Strawn, J. R. (2017). The Generalized Anxiety Disorder 7-item scale in adolescents with generalized anxiety disorder: Signal detection and validation. *Annals of Clinical Psychiatry, 29*(4), 227–234a.

Niina, A., Eyre, O., Wootton, R., Stergiakouli, E., Thapar, A., & Riglin, L. (2022). Exploring ADHD symptoms and associated impairment across development. *Journal of Attention Disorders, 26*(6), 822–830. doi:10.1177/10870547211025612

Palladino, V. S., McNeill, R., Reif, A., & Kittel-Schneider, S. (2019). Genetic risk factors and gene-environment interactions in adult and childhood attention-deficit/hyperactivity disorder. *Psychiatric Genetics, 29*(3), 63–78. doi:10.1097/ypg.0000000000000220

Perou, R., Bitsko, R. H., Blumberg, S. J., Pastor, P., Ghandour, R. M., Gfroerer, J. C., Hedden, S. L., Crosby, A. E., Visser, S. N., Schieve, L. A., Parks, S. E., Hall, J. E., Brody, D., Simile, C. M., Thompson, W. W., Baio, J., Avenevoli, S., Kogan, M. D., Huang, L. N., . . . Centers for Disease Control and Prevention. (2013). Mental health surveillance among children—United States, 2005–2011. *MMWR Surveillance Summaries, 62*(2), 1–35. http://www.ncbi.nlm.nih.gov/pubmed/23677130

Pliszka, S., & AACAP Work Group on Quality Issues. (2007). Practice parameter for the assessment and treatment of children and adolescents with attention-deficit/hyperactivity disorder. *Journal of the American Academy of Child and Adolescent Psychiatry, 46*(7), 894–921. doi:10.1097/chi.0b013e318054e724

Pliszka, S. R. (2016). Attention-deficit hyperactivity disorder across the lifespan. *Focus: The Journal of Lifelong Learning in Psychiatry, 14*(1), 46–53. doi:10.1176/appi.focus.20150022

Pliszka, S. R. (2019). ADHD and anxiety: Clinical implications. *Journal of Attention Disorders, 23*(3), 203–205. doi:10.1177/1087054718817365

Posner, J., Polanczyk, G. V., & Sonuga-Barke, E. (2020). Attention-deficit hyperactivity disorder. *Lancet, 395*(10222), 450–462. doi:10.1016/s0140-6736(19)33004-1

Rariden, C., SmithBattle, L., Yoo, J. H., Cibulka, N., & Loman, D. (2020). Screening for adverse childhood experiences: Literature review and practice implications. *Journal for Nurse Practitioners, 17*(1), 98–104. doi:10.1016/j.nurpra.2020.08.002

Reale, L., Bartoli, B., Cartabia, M., Zanetti, M., Costantino, M. A., Canevini, M. P., Termine, C., Bonati, M., Conte, S., Renzetti, V., Salvoni, L., Molteni, M., Salandi, A., Trabattoni, S., Effedri, P., Filippini, E., Pedercini, E., Zanetti, E., Fteita, N., . . . Lombardy, A. G. (2017). Comorbidity prevalence and treatment outcome in children and adolescents with ADHD. *European Child & Adolescent Psychiatry, 26*(12), 1443–1457. doi:10.1007/s00787-017-1005-z

Rowland, A. S., Skipper, B. J., Rabiner, D. L., Qeadan, F., Campbell, R. A., Naftel, A. J., & Umbach, D. M. (2018). Attention-deficit/hyperactivity disorder (ADHD): Interaction between socioeconomic status and parental history of ADHD determines prevalence. *Journal of Child Psychology and Psychiatry, 59*(3), 213–222. doi:10.1111/jcpp.12775

Roy, A., Hechtman, L., Arnold, L. E., Sibley, M. H., Molina, B. S. G., Swanson, J. M., Howard, A. L., Vitiello, B., Severe, J. B., Jensen, P. S., Arnold, L. E., Hoagwood, K., Richters, J., Vereen, D., Hinshaw, S. P., Elliott, G. R., Wells, K. C., Epstein, J. N., Murray, D. W., . . . Stern, K. (2016). Childhood factors affecting persistence and desistence of attention-deficit/hyperactivity disorder symptoms in adulthood: Results from the MTA. *Journal of the American Academy of Child & Adolescent Psychiatry, 55*(11), 937–944.e934. doi:10.1016/j.jaac.2016.05.027

Schnierle, J., Christian-Brathwaite, N., & Louisias, M. (2019). Implicit Bias: What Every Pediatrician Should Know About the Effect of Bias on Health and Future Directions. *Current Problems in Pediatric and Adolescent Health Care, 49*(2), 34-44. https://doi.org/10.1016/j.cppeds.2019.01.003

Schoenfelder, E. N., & Sasser, T. (2016). Skills versus pills: Psychosocial treatments for ADHD in childhood and adolescence. *Pediatric Annals, 45*(10), e367–e372. doi:10.3928/19382359-20160920-04

Sharma, A., & Couture, J. (2014). A review of the pathophysiology, etiology, and treatment of attention-deficit hyperactivity disorder (ADHD). *Annals of Pharmacotherapy, 48*(2), 209–225. doi:10.1177/1060028013510699

Shaw, P., Stringaris, A., Nigg, J., & Leibenluft, E. (2014). Emotion dysregulation in attention deficit hyperactivity disorder. *American Journal of Psychiatry, 171*(3), 276–293. doi:10.1176/appi.ajp.2013.13070966

Shi, Y., Hunter Guevara, L. R., Dykhoff, H. J., Sangaralingham, L. R., Phelan, S., Zaccariello, M. J., & Warner, D. O. (2021). Racial disparities in diagnosis of attention-deficit/hyperactivity disorder in a US national birth cohort. *JAMA Networks Open, 4*(3), e210321. doi:10.1001/jamanetworkopen.2021.0321

Song, J., Fogarty, K., Suk, R., & Gillen, M. (2021). Behavioral and mental health problems in adolescents with ADHD: Exploring the role of family resilience. *Journal of Affective Disorders, 294*, 450–458. doi:10.1016/j.jad.2021.07.073

Spencer, A. E., Faraone, S. V., Bogucki, O. E., Pope, A. L., Uchida, M., Milad, M. R., Spencer, T. J., Woodworth, K. Y., & Biederman, J. (2016). Examining the association between posttraumatic stress disorder and attention-deficit/hyperactivity disorder: A systematic review and meta-analysis. *Journal of Clinical Psychiatry*, 77(1), 72–83. doi:10.4088/JCP.14r09479

Sultan, R. S., Liu, S. M., Hacker, K. A., & Olfson, M. (2021). Adolescents with attention-deficit/hyperactivity disorder: Adverse behaviors and comorbidity. *Journal of Adolescent Health*, 68(2), 284–291. doi:10.1016/j.jadohealth.2020.09.036

Swanson, J. M., Arnold, L. E., Molina, B. S. G., Sibley, M. H., Hechtman, L. T., Hinshaw, S. P., Abikoff, H. B., Stehli, A., Owens, E. B., Mitchell, J. T., Nichols, Q., Howard, A., Greenhill, L. L., Hoza, B., Newcorn, J. H., Jensen, P. S., Vitiello, B., Wigal, T., Epstein, J. N., . . . Kraemer, H. C. (2017). Young adult outcomes in the follow-up of the multimodal treatment study of attention-deficit/hyperactivity disorder: Symptom persistence, source discrepancy, and height suppression. *Journal of Child Psychology and Psychiatry*, 58(6), 663–678. doi:10.1111/jcpp.12684

Trafalis, S., Giannini, C., Joves, J., Portera, S., Toyama, H., Mehta, A., Basile, K., & Friedberg, R. D. (2021). A pediatrician-friendly review of three common behavioral health screeners in pediatric practice: Findings and recommendations. *Pediatric Investigation*, 5(1), 58–64. doi:10.1002/ped4.12246

Vierhile, A. E., Palumbo, D., & Belden, H. (2017). Diagnosis and treatment of attention deficit hyperactivity disorder. *Nurse Practitioner*, 42(10), 48–54. doi:10.1097/01.NPR.0000521995.38311.e7

Walker, C. S., Walker, B. H., Brown, D. C., Buttross, S., & Sarver, D. E. (2021). Defining the role of exposure to ACEs in ADHD: Examination in a national sample of US children. *Child Abuse & Neglect*, 112, 104884. doi:10.1016/j.chiabu.2020.104884

Wexler, D., Salgado, R., Gornik, A., Peterson, R., & Pritchard, A. (2022). What's race got to do with it? Informant rating discrepancies in neuropsychological evaluations for children with ADHD. *Clinical Neuropsychology*, 36(2), 264–286. doi:10.1080/13854046.2021.1944671

Wolraich, M. L., Chan, E., Froehlich, T., Lynch, R. L., Bax, A., Redwine, S. T., Ihyembe, D., & Hagan, J. F., Jr. (2019). ADHD Diagnosis and treatment guidelines: A historical perspective. *Pediatrics*, 144(4), e20191682. doi:10.1542/peds.2019-1682

Wolraich, M. L., Hagan, J. F., Allan, C., Chan, E., Davison, D., Earls, M., Evans, S. W., Flinn, S. K., Froehlich, T., Frost, J., Holbrook, J. R., Lehmann, C. U., Lessin, H. R., Okechukwu, K., Pierce, K. L., Winner, J. D., & Zurhellen, W. (2019). Clinical practice guideline for the diagnosis, evaluation, and treatment of attention-deficit/hyperactivity disorder in children and adolescents. *Pediatrics*, 144(4), e20192528. doi:10.1542/peds.2019-2528

Wolraich, M. L., Lambert, W., Doffing, M. A., Bickman, L., Simmons, T., & Worley, K. (2003). Psychometric properties of the Vanderbilt ADHD diagnostic parent rating scale in a referred population. *Journal of Pediatric Psychology*, 28(8), 559–567. doi:10.1093/jpepsy/jsg046

Wong, A., & Landes, S. D. (2022). Expanding understanding of racial-ethnic differences in ADHD prevalence rates among children to include Asians and Alaskan Natives/American Indians. *Journal of Attention Disorders*, 26(5), 747–754. doi:10.1177/10870547211027932

Zablotsky, B., & Black, L. I. (2020). Prevalence of children aged 3–17 years with developmental disabilities, by urbanicity: United States, 2015–2018. *National Health Statistics Reports*, 139, 1–7.

Zhang, C., Kutyifa, V., Moss, A. J., McNitt, S., Zareba, W., & Kaufman, E. S. (2015). Long-QT syndrome and therapy for attention deficit/hyperactivity disorder. *Journal of Cardiovascular Electrophysiology*, 26(10), 1039–1044. doi:10.1111/jce.12739

Zoromski, A. K., Epstein, J. N., & Ciesielski, H. A. (2021). Unique associations between specific attention-deficit hyperactivity disorder symptoms and related functional impairments. *Journal of Developmental & Behavioral Pediatrics*, 42(5), 343–354. doi:10.1097/DBP.0000000000000904

Zuckerbrot, R. A., Cheung, A., Jensen, P. S., Stein, R. E. K., & Laraque, D. (2018). Guidelines for Adolescent Depression in Primary Care (GLAD-PC): Part I. Practice preparation, identification, assessment, and initial management. *Pediatrics*, 141(3), e20174081. doi:10.1542/peds.2017-4081

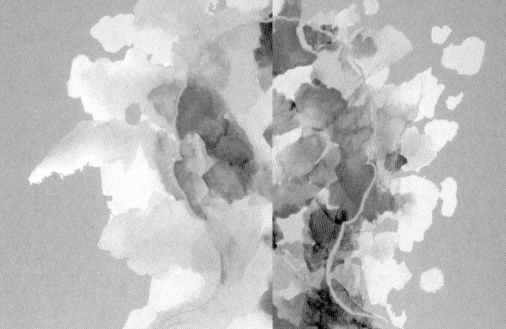

CHAPTER 12

Pediatric Depression

Monifa C. Willis

I. Introduction and general background

A. *Overview, clinical definition, and epidemiology*

Childhood and adolescence are a time when rapid growth and development take place in the brain, and therefore they are also crucial stages for mental health. Causes of depression can be linked to interactions between biological, psychological, social, and structural factors. For example, a history of depression or exposure to an adverse life event can be a contributing factor to the degree of severity of an individual's experience of and ability to cope with depression and other mental health conditions.

Depression is a mood state with distinct physical, emotional, and cognitive effects that impair psychosocial functioning and is often accompanied by comorbid psychopathology, such as anxiety disorders. It is characterized by a constellation of symptoms, including persistent low mood, loss of interest/pleasure (anhedonia), and disturbed sleep and appetite. Moreover, an individual with depression may experience excessive guilt or low self-worth, hopelessness about the future, tiredness, poor concentration, and/or thoughts about dying or suicide. Symptomology is typically subjectively reported and/or objectively observed. Importantly, the intensity and chronicity of depressive symptoms determine the degree of severity.

In young children, notable irritability, anger, and/or aggressive outbursts can characterize a depressive presentation. In general, one may expect adolescents to experience phases of depression or irritability (Arnett, 1999), largely as a result of hormonal changes during development. Although this may be true to a minor degree, the typically developing child or adolescent should not go through an extended period of depression, irritability, or rebelliousness as a part of normative development. More so, any prolonged period of irritability or oppositional behavior reported by the parent/caretaker or child should trigger suspicion of depressive a and/or other psychiatric illness, thus warranting further inquiry (Hines & Paulson, 2006).

Additionally, a presenting recurrent or acute somatic complaint (stomachache, headache, etc.), particularly in younger children, or feeling "blah," appetite loss, appetite increase, weight fluctuation, or anxiety complaints may indicate the presence of depressive illness (American Psychiatric Association [APA], 2013).

Lastly, when a child presents with any of the mood and/or physical changes previously mentioned, the safety of the child should be assessed to rule out the possibility of a traumatic event, such as bullying, sexual or physical abuse, exposure to violence (in home or community), and neglect.

The primary care provider is encouraged to appreciate the importance of their position as gatekeepers who can identify and assist depressed youth in their practice settings (Zuckerbrot et al., 2007). Additionally, it should be kept in mind that although reassurance and normalizing are useful practices, the primary care provider should not prioritize these activities above appropriate screening, assessment, and treatment when warranted, especially when considering safety.

According to the World Health Organization (WHO, n.d.), depression is a leading cause of disability worldwide. Per data gathered from the Substance Abuse Mental Health Services Administration (SAMHSA) in 2020, an estimated 4.1 million adolescents aged 12 to 17 in the United States had at least one major depressive episode. This number represented 17% of the U.S. population aged 12 to 17. The risk for developing depression increases for females during puberty. The SAMHSA data show that the prevalence of major depressive episodes was higher among adolescent females (25.2%) compared to males (9.2%). The prevalence of a major depressive episode was highest among adolescents reporting two or more races (29.9%). Increases in depression during pandemic, a meta-analysis of 53 longitudinal cohort studies with data on prepandemic to pandemic estimates of depression showed an increase in depressive symptoms during the pandemic, primarily among girls (Madigan et al., 2023)

Depression in younger children is not as prevalent, but it does occur. According to Cheung et al. (2013), it has been "reliably diagnosed in children as young as 3 years of age." Depression in children, particularly those under 5 years of age, rarely arises de novo as a result of purely internal biologic or psychologic factors because the young child's psyche is developmentally predicated upon the family environment, especially the relationship with the primary caregiver(s). Therefore, the onset of depressive symptoms in a young child warrants careful consideration for child abuse, neglect, and other forms of trauma. More broadly, atypical mood changes in young children warrant further consideration of family dynamics, including parental mental health, parenting and disciplinary approaches, parental/family conflict, and sibling interactions.

The U.S. Preventive Task Force strongly recommends primary care providers to continually perform screenings for depression among patients aged 12–18 years old in order to assess for and treat depression as early as possible (Cheung et al., 2013). A review of longitudinal studies by Birmaher et al. (2002) found that children experience a depressive episode for an average duration of 8–13 months. Moreover, those who are seen in clinical settings show a reduction in episode duration, and 50%–90% of children experience full recovery, defined as the absence of depressive symptoms. Relapse or recurrence occurs in 30%–70% of children after 24 to 70 months of recovery. Children and adolescents who experience two or more depressive episodes have more recurrences. Lastly, it is important to note that children and adolescents were found to have an increased risk of becoming depressed adults when not adequately treated for depression during their childhood years.

If depressive episodes are inadequately treated, the brain can become sensitized to being in a depressed state, which is then more likely to recur in the future. This phenomenon, called *kindling*, may lead to depressive episodes that are more frequent, more severe, and of longer duration, with incomplete recovery between episodes. Genetic, biologic, and environmental etiologic factors are suggested as contributing to depression (Rao & Chen, 2009). Despite clear evidence of familial transmission of depression in the case of children and adolescents, it is unclear to what degree childhood depression is influenced by genetics, environment, or some combination thereof (Rao & Chen, 2009). In any case, it is believed that the single greatest risk factor for developing major depressive disorder (MDD) in childhood or adolescence is a paternal or maternal history of the disorder (Birmaher & Brent, 2007). Thus, the subjective and family history should include any history of depression in the family, especially the child's parents or siblings and any parental or family history of bipolar disorder or alcohol or substance abuse.

Evidence suggests that depression is associated with altered brain structure and function. Ming et al. (2017) emphasize the structural dysfunction of the hypothalamic–pituitary–adrenal axis (HPA) as a neurobiological factor in depression. According to Ming et al. (2017), individuals with acute and remitted unipolar major depression display overproduction of corticotropin-releasing hormone, which leads to an overactive HPA. This finding drives the connection between depression and anxiety. Patients who had long-standing and/or untreated depression were found to have an increased ventricular–brain ratio, smaller frontal lobe volumes, and smaller hippocampal volumes (Lui et al., 2016), further supporting the notion that immediate treatment for depression is beneficial.

Historical theory proposed that depression was due to diminished neurotransmission of monoamines, namely, serotonin and norepinephrine. However, it has been determined that the dysfunction is far more complex and nuanced. Depression also involves abnormal functioning of several neurotransmitters, including monoamines, gamma-aminobutyric acid (GABA), and glutamate. Current theory proposes that serotonin and norepinephrine synthesis is of more concern versus depleted transmission. This explains the first-line pharmacologic treatment of selective serotonin reuptake inhibitors (SSRIs) and serotonin–norepinephrine reuptake inhibitors (SNRIs). Moreover, depletion of dopamine has been associated with treatment-resistant depression, which further explains adjunct treatments with antipsychotic agents.

Lastly, numerous studies (e.g., Lener et al., 2017) implicate elevated levels of glutamate and lowered levels of GABA in the etiology of depression. Increased glutamate has been found to be associated with symptoms of anhedonia and motor slowing, whereas the lowered levels of GABA present in depression emphasize the anxiety symptoms noted in depressive disorders.

Other researchers have theorized that depression, from a strictly behavioral perspective, is caused by a loss of environmental reward (positive reinforcement) leading to avoidance, withdrawal, and isolation via negative reinforcement (Dimidjian et al., 2011; Dobson et al., 2008).

The clinical evaluation of youth with a suspected depressive disorder includes a medical and psychiatric history, mental status and physical examination, and focused laboratory tests. Moreover, specific diagnostic screening tools can be useful for identifying symptomology and acuity. Evaluations should be responsive to the patient's age and cultural, ethnic, and religious or spiritual backgrounds.

II. Gathering data

The primary care provider (PCP) evaluating the child or adolescent is in an excellent position to assess for depression. The PCP can establish a trusting relationship with the child and family and gain insight into family dynamics and their potential impact on the child's developmental and other medical history, which are all essential components of a competent evaluation for pediatric depression.

However, even if this is the provider's first encounter with a completely new patient, the treating clinician should always consider information from the child and parents about the family situation and the child's emotional, physical, and cognitive development and history since birth, including intrauterine conditions.

Prior to an in-depth screening and assessment for depression with the child and family, it is important to clarify the parameters of confidentiality, what information will and will not be shared with caregivers, and how this will occur. Clarity around confidentiality is essential for maintaining rapport with the child and the caregivers throughout this process and may assist in greater disclosure during the data-gathering process. However, always frame the discussion of confidentiality with specific instances where the provider is obligated to breach confidentiality, such as when there is a significant risk to safety for self and/or others. Screening always opens the possibility of disclosure of suicidality or other self-endangerment behaviors, whether the initial screening of a new patient or a subsequent screening for a well-known patient who seems "stable," and if the youth is aware that there are certain situations in which confidentiality may be breached, the patient may feel less betrayed if information must be shared. Confidentiality also extends to third parties with significant involvement in a child's life, such as schools, counselors, and therapists.

Gathering data may take several visits, especially with adolescents, because the clinician may choose to meet first with the family together, then on separate occasions with the child/adolescent alone, and then the parents alone (or vice versa). Regardless of the number of visits, always prioritize the safety screening in each encounter. The safety screening can help determine the urgency of referral and the treatment course, if indicated.

Depending on the age and developmental stage, the patient database review should include the elements in the following section.

A. *Subjective data*
1. Current psychiatric: Assessing the current psychiatric symptom presentation is important to appreciate the impact of symptoms on the patient's current daily life. When assessing symptoms, it is important to gather information on when symptoms were first experienced, triggering events, duration, and alleviating and exacerbating factors. It's important to get this information from the young person and the parent when possible.
2. Psychiatric history: This includes any previous psychiatric diagnosis, symptoms, and outpatient mental health treatments and/or inpatient psychiatric hospitalizations. When interviewing the child or parent, it is important to distinguish between psychiatric evaluations versus inpatient hospitalizations. Some youth are evaluated for danger to self and/or others but not hospitalized because appropriate safety planning was achieved. It is also important to ask about previous exposure to psychiatric medication and the child's response if medication was administered in the past. It is also important to directly inquire about past behaviors or symptoms of self-injurious behaviors, such as "cutting," suicidal ideation or attempts (including type and lethality), anxiety, hallucinations, inattention, and hyperactivity.
3. Medical history: When assessing medical history, it is particularly important to perform a comprehensive review of health concerns, signs, and symptoms that could be contributing to the clinical presentation. Particularly, the patient should be screened for cardiovascular health, seizures and other neurological disorders, and endocrine and metabolic problems, in addition to chronic conditions such as diabetes, asthma, and sleep-related disorders. Moreover, appreciating chronic illnesses and/or chronic pain would be prudent in a holistic understanding of the young person's health. Lastly, the clinician will want to assess for any medications (prescribed and over the counter), including herbs, supplements, and herbal teas, because some of these may have psychotropic side effects.
4. Social and family history: The clinician assesses the young person's family dynamic ("How does your family get along?"; "Who lives with you?"; "Do you have siblings?"), community safety ("Where do you live?; "Do you feel safe in your community?"), the health of peer relationships (ability to name friends, assessing for peer bullying), romantic/intimate relationships ("Are you dating anybody?"; "Any break-ups recently?"), sexual debut and safety ("Have you ever had sex with anyone?"), traumatic events ("Has anything really bad ever happened to you?"; "Has anything happened that you think about a lot or can't stop thinking about?"), sexual or physical abuse ("Has anyone ever touched you when you didn't want them to?"; "Has anyone ever hit you?").
5. Education and/or occupational history: Typically, a clinician would want to know where the young person attends school, the highest grade completed, and the current grade. Moreover, the clinician should ask the child about favored and disliked subjects. A general sense of the child's appraisal of school can be useful as well ("How is school going for you?"; "What kind of grades are you getting?"). Asking the parents or child about specific learning disabilities and learning plans, such as an individual educational plan (IEP) or Section 504 plan, will allow the clinician to appreciate current school supports or lack thereof. In-depth school assessment is important for a full understanding of the accuracy of diagnosis, comorbid conditions, and consequently, the treatment plan. Assessing for desire to work or actual engagement in the workforce is useful for youth of working age (15 years or older) when seeking to understand the youth's goal orientation and social development.
6. Substance use: Youth may be hesitant to share this information for fear of disclosure to parents.

As mentioned, it is important to incorporate the confidentiality preface to the health visit. It is recommended to frame questions around substance use from a safety lens ("I'm going to ask questions about drugs for the sake of safety, not to tell your parents"). Teens are more forthcoming when the clinician educates them regarding confidentiality and the fact that, in most cases, there is not an obligation to report such use to parents or law enforcement (reference your local laws, policies, and other professional guidelines). Moreover, using terms like "recreational drugs" and "experimentation" can also be useful. During this screening, you want to include the use of caffeine, cigarettes, alcohol, and marijuana or any illicit or licit drug use.

7. Birth and developmental history: While asking routine questions regarding birth and development, it is also recommended to speak with the parent confidentially to encourage and support a safe space for the parent to disclose any concerns they may not have otherwise disclosed in front of the child. The birth history is helpful for understanding the prenatal course, whether there were any unique circumstantial factors resulting in pregnancy, adequate prenatal care, exposures to trauma or environmental hazards, domestic violence, usage of drugs (illicit or prescribed), and any actual or perceived complications during delivery. The clinician should then inquire about the young person's temperament as an infant (difficult, easy) and parental response (overwhelmed, attuned). This allows the clinician to appreciate the parent's ability to form a healthy attachment with the young person in the early years. Lastly, assessing for physical (crawling, walking, talking, toileting), emotional (cooing, smiling, ability to cope with feelings over time), and relational (ability to play with peers) development is important in assessing a young person's behavioral and mood history, patterns, and changes.

B. *Objective data*

The mental status examination (MSE) is the psychiatric equivalent to the physical examination, and it must be included in any evaluation of depressive conditions or other psychiatric illness. However, the MSE does not substitute for the physical examination to rule out organic factors in a depressive presentation or identify other comorbid medical illness.

The MSE begins with gross observations and progresses to description of the internal cognitive and emotional processes as observed by the clinician during the interview, visit, or interaction, however brief.

C. *Mental status examination*

The MSE typically includes the following observations, adapted from Saddock and Saddock (2007); common findings with depressed youth are exemplified.

1. Appearance: Appearance includes grooming (remarkable identifiers). Depressed teens may look disheveled or unkempt and/or have poor hygiene.
2. Behavior: Behavior includes general demeanor and response to the clinician. The youth may present as irritable and avoidant, with a lack of engagement. Younger children may present as fearful, reserved, and timid.
3. Motor function: Observe the physical motor function of the client. Depression may present with slowed motor function and/or agitation.
4. Mood: The patient's direct report of how they feel, noted in quotation marks (e.g., "sad," "tired," "bored," "none of your business," etc.).
5. Affect: Depressed youths can present with a flat or restricted affect. In some cases, they may present with anxious distress along with lowered mood.
6. Language: The clinician wants to assess flow and volume. In youth, this may present as lowered speech with few words and/or anxious pressure.
7. Thought process: Assess the youth's thought patterns—for example, organized, linear, cogent versus disorganized, circumstantial/tangential, loose. In depressed youth, the clinician may notice slowed responses.
8. Thought content: This includes suicidal and homicidal ideation, perceptual changes, paranoia, intrusive thoughts/memories/worries, and hallucinatory experiences. When young people report suicidal and homicidal ideation, it is important to assess for any established plans or means because this would warrant an emergency psychiatric evaluation if safety planning cannot be achieved. Depressed thoughts in youth are often perseverative, negative in nature, and hopeless, sometimes presenting with detachment. Psychotic depression may include auditory and visual hallucinations or delusions.
9. Cognition: For depressed individuals, the clinician will want to appreciate changes in orientation, concentration, and memory.
10. Insight: This is rated good, fair, or poor based on the youth's awareness of their depressive symptoms. Individuals who are unsure or unaware of their symptoms are typically rated fair or poor.
11. Judgment: This is rated good, fair, or poor based on the youth's ability to organize information and make plans toward improving function. In this category, impulsivity is also considered because some youth may not have fully developed executive functioning, thus increasing the risk for impulsive actions that could be harmful.

D. *Physical examination findings*

1. Vital signs, including weight—specifically, monitoring for no significant changes from prior trends in growth parameters, blood pressure, and heart rate
2. Thyroid examination
3. Any lymphadenopathy, pallor, jaundice, hepatosplenomegaly, bruising, neurocutaneous stigmata (e.g., neurofibromas, café au lait macules)
4. Neurologic exam. Assessment may uncover depressive symptoms caused by an organic brain illness (traumatic brain or spinal cord injuries).

E. *Data from diagnostic tests*

There is no definitive diagnostic test to assess depression. However, the following tests are recommended to rule out other possible reasons to explain depressive symptoms.
1. Complete blood count to rule out anemia
2. Comprehensive metabolic panel to rule out possible medical causes, such as diabetes, electrolyte abnormalities, and vitamin D deficiency
3. Thyroid-stimulating hormone and free T_4 to rule out a dysregulated thyroid
4. Drug abuse screen to rule out substance abuse disorders and/or substances that may be contributing to depressed presentation. However, it is important to note that adolescents require consent to test.
5. Hormone levels to rule out endocrine dysregulation

III. Assessment

A. *Determine the diagnosis*

A formal diagnosis of a depressive disorder follows clinical guidelines and criteria set forth by the *Diagnostic and Statistical Manual of Mental Disorders*, 5th edition (*DSM-5*; APA, 2013). This manual contains the classification of all mental health disorders and is the collective effort of hundreds of international experts. In March 2022, the *DSM-5-TR* (text revision) was released, with updates such as the inclusion of prolonged grief disorders, improved clarification of criteria, and a comprehensive review of the impact of racism and discrimination on the diagnosis and manifestation of mental disorders (APA, 2022).

Although *DSM-5* criteria are important to assess, it is equally important for the clinician to determine how the patient got to their current state using the biopsycho-social-structural model. The provider should consider predisposing, precipitating, perpetuating, and protective factors from biological, psychological, social, and structural perspectives. When applying this more holistic approach to the foundation of assessment, the provider can better inform their treatment and safety decisions.

The *DSM-5* includes the following depressive disorders:
- MDD
- Persistent depressive disorder
- Unspecified depressive disorder

Disorders that may have depressive features are as follows:
- Bipolar disorder I and II (variously abbreviated as BD)
- Cyclothymia
- Seasonal affective disorder
- Disruptive mood dysregulation disorder
- Adjustment disorder with depressed mood or mixed depression and anxiety
- Anxiety disorders
- Prodromal psychosis

Note: An in-depth review of the latter seven diagnoses is beyond the scope of this chapter, and the reader is referred to the 2022 *DSM-5-TR*.

B. *Major depressive disorder*

MDD is the prototypical disease usually referred to when depression is spoken of generically. It is diagnosed based on the occurrence of one or more major depressive episodes (APA, 2022). A major depressive episode consists of 2 (or more) weeks of depressed mood/irritability or anhedonia and a minimum of four additional depressive symptoms (APA, 2022).

C. *Persistent depressive disorder (formerly dysthymia)*

Persistent depressive disorder is similar in symptom profile to MDD but lacks its severity and demonstrates a course that is constant over a longer period (at least 2 years) without distinct episodes (APA, 2022). The *DSM-5* criteria for persistent depressive disorder are not significantly different from the *DSM-IV* (APA, 1994) criteria for dysthymia. The major difference is that chronic MDD, which had been a distinct and separate diagnosis, was integrated into the single diagnosis of persistent depressive disorder, along with dysthymia (APA, 2022).

The presence of MDD and comorbid dysthymia identified in a single individual is commonly known as *double depression*. The clinician should keep in mind that 5%–10% of children and adolescents have depressive symptoms that are not severe enough to warrant the diagnosis of a depressive syndrome, such as MDD or dysthymia, but that are debilitating nonetheless (Birmaher & Brent, 2007); in some cases, these depressive symptoms are attributable to an adjustment disorder caused by an acute stressor. Additionally, of those children and adolescents with diagnosable depressive syndromes, 40%–90% have other psychiatric disorders (Birmaher & Brent, 2007). Thus, the clinician should observe for any potential signs of other comorbid psychiatric illness, such as attention-deficit/hyperactivity disorder, anxiety disorders, eating disorders, substance abuse disorders, and autism spectrum disorder.

In terms of the diagnostic nomenclature used by the *DSM-5*, a child with depressive symptoms who does not have enough signs and symptoms to meet the criteria for MDD or dysthymia could be identified as having unspecified depressive disorder—formerly depressive disorder not otherwise specified (NOS) in the *DSM-IV-TR* (APA, 2000).

D. *Other conditions that may explain the patient's presentation*

1. Grief and adjustment disorders: It is important to assess for any recent loss, whether it be through death, loss of relationship (friend, intimate partner, pet) or change in environment. It is important to normalize feelings of grief during significant life events and refer the youth and family to the appropriate supportive resources.
2. Anxiety disorders: Clinically, clients often express symptoms of anxiety and depression. In community

samples, it is estimated that 25%–50% of youth with depression also meet the criteria for an anxiety disorder (Garber & Weersing, 2010). Symptoms that commonly overlap are sleep disturbances, fatigue, poor concentration, and suicidal thinking. From a clinical perspective, it can be postulated that depressed youth find themselves "falling behind" in life, which fuels feelings of anxiousness, and the constant worries exacerbate or deepen depressed symptomology, such as a sense of hopelessness for their future. From a pathophysiological perspective, anxiety and depression share dysfunction in many of the same key neurotransmitters.

3. Bipolar spectrum disorder: Clinical depression is also a significant component of the bipolar "spectrum" of illnesses, which includes bipolar disorder I, bipolar disorder II, and cyclothymia. As would be suggested by the idea of a "spectrum," these three illnesses are differentiated from one another by severity and duration, but all show similar cyclical episodic variations in mood reflecting elevated, expansive, energized mood symptoms (mania or hypomania) alternating or sometimes even intermixed with depressive symptoms. Patients experiencing a bipolar spectrum illness, like those with MDD, may also spend a period in a euthymic ("normal") mood state. Mania is differentiated from (less severe) hypomania by a greater duration (at least 1 week) and greater intensity of symptoms (more symptoms, need for hospitalization, or presence of psychotic symptoms) (APA, 2013). One might characterize the bipolar spectrum from most severe to least severe as follows: bipolar disorder I, bipolar disorder II, and cyclothymia. The *DSM-5*, to address the controversy over the upswing in pediatric patients with bipolar disorder, also now includes a diagnosis called *disruptive mood dysregulation disorder* (DMDD; APA, 2013). Distinguishing between bipolar and DMDD is best performed by pediatric mental health specialists. DMDD categorizes "children who present with chronic, persistent irritability relative to children who present with classic (i.e., episodic) bipolar disorder" (APA, 2013, p. 157). Children and adults with bipolar illness often present in a depressed, rather than elevated, state. In these cases, the clinician may mistakenly diagnose unipolar depression rather than bipolar depression if inquiry is not made about elevated mood and behavior over the lifetime of the patient rather than the limited course of the current episode alone. In cases of undiagnosed bipolar disorder, psychotropic medications (especially antidepressants) may precipitate hypomanic or manic mood or behavior when administered—this is known as *activation* or an *activated mania*. Thus, in the interest of "doing no harm," the clinician evaluating clinical depression in the child, adolescent, or adult must always entertain the possibility of a bipolar illness presenting in its depressed phase, especially if antidepressant medication is being considered. This evaluation can be assisted by asking about a family history of mood lability or bipolar disorder and substance abuse, although the absence of these in the family history does not rule out bipolar disorder. Finally, in many cases of MDD, bipolar spectrum illness remains a "rule out" diagnosis; one should advise the patient and family about the possibility of activation when reviewing the risks and benefits of antidepressant medication.

4. Prodromal psychosis: Youth experiencing early stages of psychotic disorders often present with *negative symptoms* that can last several weeks to years and are typically not diagnosed until after the initial psychotic break. Negative symptoms present as withdrawal, disengagement in usual activities, decline in hygiene, sleep disturbances, and cognitive decline—specifically, deficits in memory, information processing, and inattention.

5. Thought disorders: Youth with depression can also present with paranoia or feelings like "everyone is looking at me," usually driven by a decrease in self-confidence versus a true psychotic disorder. Asking clarification questions can assist with understanding the genesis of this paranoid thinking.

6. Substance use disorder: The clinician will want to assess if the symptom presentation is better accounted for by substance intoxication or withdrawal. A urine toxicology screen (UTOX) and thorough substance abuse history can assist in ruling this out.

7. Other medical conditions should be considered, such as endocrine disorders, thyroid dysfunction, and malnutrition. Gathering labs and medical history will assist with ruling other conditions out.

E. *Risk assessment*

No assessment of depressive illness in the child or adolescent is complete without an assessment of suicide risk and any self-injurious behaviors. Suicide risk increases with the interaction of mental disorders and other factors. Since 2020, suicide has been the leading cause of death among 10- to 14-year-olds and the second-leading cause among 15- to 24-year-olds in the United States (Centers for Disease Control and Prevention [CDC], 2020). According to CDC (2020), girls account for an increasingly large share of youth suicides. A study in 2018 first identified the alarming finding of Black youth suicide rates doubling those of their White counterparts, and this trend continues to rise (Caron, 2021). It is postulated that factors of the COVID-19 pandemic, structural racism, and underidentified depression in the Black community have been contributing factors to this trend, leading to the implementation of a policy by the American Academy of Child and Adolescent Psychiatry (AACAP) in March of 2022 encouraging providers to explore the impact of racism and unconscious bias, improve identification of risk and access, support resiliency programs, and advocate for increased investment in programs and funds that target Black youth (AACAP, 2022).

Risk of suicide and lethality must be assessed on an individual basis. Keeping this in mind, the clinician must be aware that the following factors (not listed in order of importance) increase the risk for suicide and may warrant emergent referral to a psychiatric provider or hospital emergency room (Bilsen, 2018):

- Existing mental or substance abuse disorders: Of youth who completed suicide, 90% had at least one preexisting mental disorder. Criteria for depression were met in 50% to 65% of suicide cases. Alcohol abuse is strongly associated with suicide among older adolescents and males.
- Previous suicide attempts: A history of self-harm and suicide attempts is strongly linked to subsequent suicide attempts.
- Personality characteristics: Impulsivity is associated with increased suicide attempts among adolescents. Additionally, the youth's neurobiological development, such as an underdeveloped frontal lobe and prefrontal cortex, coupled with hormonal and biological mood dysregulation, can contribute to emotional and/or suicidal crisis.
- Family factors: Youth with family members who have mental health disorders and/or a history of suicide have a higher risk of suicidal behavior, likely due to genetics and imitation behavior. Moreover, conflicts with parents and absent or unsupportive parents have also been found to be contributing factors.
- Special life events: Certain life events are more associated with suicide in youth, particularly events related to relationships, such as interpersonal losses, breakups, peer rejection, and death of friends. In addition, 14% of deaths by suicide are linked to youth who were exhibiting school troubles or youth who were neither attending school nor working. Lastly, events like bullying, physical/sexual abuse, and disciplinary troubles have also been triggering events to suicide among youth.
- Contagion–imitation: Youth are learning through modeling. Therefore, suicide risk increases when suicides are "modeled" by individuals with significant value to the youth, such as celebrities and social media influencers. In addition, social media perpetuates the extent to which the model's behavior is reinforced, condoned, and/or frequently headlined. Such imitation behavior has been found to have large impacts, known as *suicide clusters*.
- Availability of means: In most cases, youth are ambivalent about suicide. It is typically a stressor that triggers the urge, followed by an impulsive reaction to complete suicide. Therefore, limiting lethal means is crucial to suicide prevention.

A comprehensive review of the assessment, evaluation, and treatment of suicidal ideation in the child or adolescent is beyond the scope of this chapter. However, the reader is referred to the AACAP's Practice Parameter on the topic. This parameter includes a more thorough treatment of risk factors, safety planning, national resources on suicide for the family and clinician, and a comparative review of suicide-screening instruments for the child and adolescent. It is available for free from the AACAP website; a link is provided in the "Resources" section.

1. **Suicide risk screeners**

    Screeners can be a useful tool to assist with initial risk assessment and ongoing monitoring of symptom severity and safety. Although useful, it is recommended that the provider use subjectivity when assessing safety or decisions. Some screeners commonly used to support risk assessments are as follows:

    a. Patient Health Questionnaire (PHQ-9). The following two questions, sometimes referred to as the *Patient Health Questionnaire* (PHQ-2), are highly effective in identifying most cases of depression (Manea et al., 2016): "Over the past 2 weeks, have you felt down, depressed, or hopeless?" and "Over the past 2 weeks, have you felt little interest or pleasure in doing things?" A positive response to either of these questions warrants a more thorough screening for depression. The PHQ-9, a commonly used tool for depression screening and monitoring response to treatment, incorporates *DSM* diagnostic criteria for MDD. In addition to being a reliable tool for diagnosis, it measures depression severity, which can be useful for ongoing monitoring of symptom progression once treatment is administered (Kroenke et al., 2001).

    b. Ask Suicide-Screening Questions (ASQ). This validated tool is easily used in primary care and emergency room settings to identify individuals at risk for suicide. It has been validated for ages 8 years and above. It consists of four screening questions. A "yes" response to any of the four questions warrants further suicide risk assessment (Horowitz et al., 2014).

    c. Suicide Assessment Five-Step Evaluation and Triage (SAFE-T). This tool uses the APA practice guidelines for the assessment and treatment of patients with suicidal behavior (AACAP, 2001). The five-step guide provides prompting questions that help assign suicide risk levels of high, moderate, and low, followed by possible interventions based on assessed acuity. It is a free, downloadable pocket-sized card.

IV. Plan and treatment

A. *Health maintenance*

Exercise, adequate sleep, healthy diet and eating hygiene, and multivitamin supplementation are recommended.

B. *Client education and counseling*

Your counseling may help break down the stigma around mental health. Approaching these conversations in a nonjudgmental, inclusive way honors the family's cultural lens and is an effective approach in fostering acceptance of the situation.

C. *Diagnosis*

For many youth and families, this may be the first time they learn of a mental health diagnosis. It will be important to provide education on the signs and symptoms of depression and instill hope based on prognosis data. Provide anticipatory guidance that diagnoses can change with evolving circumstances and development of the youth.

D. *Approaches to treatment*

It is important to explore the many options for the treatment of depression aside from psychotropic intervention—namely, therapy (individual, group). The emphasis is on maintaining health, building on existing positive factors, and help youth/family identify resiliency factors. Importantly, in designing any treatment plan, the provider must use shared decision making with the individual (shared goals of treatment) to improve motivation and treatment adherence.

E. *Family inclusion*

Include family members in discussions when appropriate and possible. When engaging in safety planning, family/caregivers must be involved in the construction of the safety plan. If the conversation is not related to treatment approach or safety, it is not necessary to include the parental figures because confidentiality is important in gaining patient trust. However, consider preemptively counseling the patient that, as for all patients, you provide crisis resources (i.e., suicide hotlines) for caregivers, regardless of mental health status.

F. *Diagnostic tests*

As previously discussed, it will be important to educate families on the rationale for ruling out medical causes of depression. Sometimes, in this education, family members recall medical history that may better inform your assessment and treatment plan.

G. *Medication management*

The goal of psychotropic intervention is to find an option that can lead to sustained full remission of depressive symptoms. However, less than one-third of depressed patients achieve remission with the first medication trial, and another third fail to respond to two or more trials. Therefore, it is important to educate youth and families on the possibility of trialing more than one medication option.

1. Treatment phases: Treatment in pediatric depression is divided into the acute, maintenance, and continuation phases (Patra, 2019).

   a. The acute phase aims to reduce symptoms by 50%, which can be a period ranging from 2 weeks to 3 months. Visits should be weekly while monitoring for side effects. Once stable on a dose and without significant side effects, visits can be reduced to monthly.

   b. The maintenance phase focuses on stabilization and prevention of relapse. This is typically reached/achieved once a patient is symptom-free for 6 months. Visits are typically every 2–3 months.

   c. The continuation phase is also known as the *recovery phase*, where much of the focus is on preventing the recurrence of depression. Visits remain 2–3 months apart. This is a great time to begin discussion of discontinuation of medication and bolstering of therapeutic skills.

2. Discontinuation of medication is considered after the patient has been free of symptoms for greater than 12 months. Medication should be tapered off slowly, ranging 4 weeks apart, to mitigate withdrawal symptoms or return of symptomology. Coordinated discontinuation of medication with family and therapeutic support systems is advised. Patients may abruptly discontinue their medication independently of your advice for various reasons (e.g., feeling better, not allowing time for medication to take effect, mistaking symptoms for side effects, missing refills). Thus, frequent check-ins on medication are recommended. *Patient adherence:* It is important to ensure the patient and family agree with medication treatment because this directly affects adherence. In addition, giving proper education on what to expect and side effects can improve adherence outcomes. Moreover, think about the complexity of the medication regimen and what may work best for the patient and family. If you find that a patient is not taking their medication regularly, this should warrant an assessment of barriers.

3. Side effects and management: Read the medication guidelines that come with the antidepressant medicine because these include all risks and benefits. However, side effects like stomachache and headache typically remit after 1 week and can be mitigated through eating food before administration and taking ibuprofen for headache. If any side effects persist and/or worsen beyond 1 week, it is advised to stop the medication completely and reconsider alternative medication options. If the medication is at a high dose, consider a gradual taper to avoid withdrawal syndrome.

4. Black-box warning: The U.S. Food and Drug Administration (FDA) issued a ruling in 2007 directing antidepressant manufacturers to include black-box labeling identifying the possibility of increased suicidal ideation in children and adolescents up through age 24. The announcement of this black-box warning was widely reported in the

media. Since that time, there has been a marked drop in the prescription of first-line antidepressant treatment by PCPs (Gibbons et al., 2007) and a subsequent increase in deaths by suicide. The prudent clinician should continue vigilant monitoring for increased suicidal ideation or behavior in the child or adolescent (through age 24) during the initiation and continuation of an antidepressant medication. However, considerable data continue to accumulate regarding the benefit of antidepressant treatment in children and adolescents and the importance of early intervention and potential negative sequelae associated with failure to prescribe (Gibbons et al., 2007; Hammad et al., 2006a, 2006b; March et al., 2004). The PCP who has identified a child or adolescent with uncomplicated unipolar depression is encouraged to consider, with the family, the benefits and risks of cautiously initiating first-line antidepressant treatment. Otherwise, the provider should promptly consult and/or refer to a psychiatric provider for medication treatment plans, keeping in mind that these referrals often take months.

In addition to the very small but real potential risk of increased suicidal ideation and behavior, SSRIs, including escitalopram and fluoxetine, often have significant gastrointestinal, nervous system, and sexual side effects, predominantly because of the effect on nontargeted serotonin receptors. The risk of various potential side effects (additional to suicidal ideation) must be reviewed with the child and their parents or guardians as part of the process for obtaining informed consent (**Table 12-1**). The medication guide in Table 12-1 may be helpful in assisting families through this process. For the most current version and other prescriber-directed medication advisories, see http://www.fda.gov. The process of initiating first-line antidepressant treatment for the child or adolescent with uncomplicated unipolar depression may be done in tandem with referral to a pediatric psychiatric specialist.

5. FDA-approved antidepressant agents and consent
Only two agents have FDA approval for use as antidepressants in children and adolescents: the SSRIs fluoxetine (Prozac™) and escitalopram (Lexapro™). **Table 12-2** summarizes data on these agents. Note that sertraline (Zoloft™) and fluvoxamine (Luvox™)—also SSRIs—do not have FDA approval for use in the pediatric age group for depressive disorders. They do, however, have FDA approval for the treatment of obsessive–compulsive disorder (OCD) in children and adolescents, sertraline for ages 6–17 years and fluvoxamine for ages 8–17, and have been used off-label for the treatment of depressive disorders.

After gaining appropriate consent, the clinician choosing to initiate antidepressant treatment in an uncomplicated case of MDD should begin with the lowest dose possible (often one-quarter to one-half the recommended adult dose, depending on other factors) and titrate in very slow intervals, generally not sooner than every 3–4 weeks. However, face-to-face monitoring at more frequent intervals, even without dosing changes, is recommended for children and adolescents receiving antidepressant medication. Vigilance is especially warranted when initiating, increasing, reducing, or otherwise changing dosage. The FDA recommends "at least weekly face-to-face contact with the prescriber during the first 4 weeks of treatment, then visits every other week for the next 4 weeks, then at 12 weeks, and as clinically indicated beyond 12 weeks" (Hughes et al., 2007, pp. 667–686), and this is now generally accepted as the standard of care. The provider should enlist parents in monitoring for adverse effects and, with proper consent, could consider educating the child's psychotherapist(s) and teachers to assist in monitoring.

At a minimum, medication monitoring visits should include the following parameters:
a. Patient's subjective response to the medication
b. Objective evaluation of demeanor, energy, and affect
c. Report of any adverse effects, including any changes in weight, sleep, behavior (activation), and sexual problems (adolescents). The clinician is referred to the manufacturer's literature for a comprehensive listing of drug side effects with frequency of occurrence.
d. Dosing record and any difficulties with or obstacles to adherence, such as gastrointestinal complaints or sleep changes
e. Suicidal ideation and self-harming behaviors
f. Progress with psychiatric referral or response to psychotherapy or other nonpharmacologic treatments

H. *Therapy*

Psychotherapy, either alone or combined with pharmacotherapy, is effective in treating pediatric depression. Specifically, cognitive–behavioral therapy (CBT) shows the strongest evidence for improved outcome (March et al., 2004; Weisz et al., 2006). Developed by Aaron Beck (and since elaborated by many other clinician-researchers), CBT uses behavioral interventions, structured exercises, and talk therapy to change negative thinking. In a depressed child, CBT is thought to exert a therapeutic effect because it leads to restructuring of the negatively distorted cognitions that engender and accompany depressive symptoms.

The best data concerning CBT and depression in the pediatric population come from the Treatment for Adolescents with Depression Study (TADS). The TADS is a highly powered, 13-site, national study funded by the National Institute of Mental Health that tested three conditions in a randomized, controlled trial design from spring through summer 2003 (March et al., 2004): fluoxetine alone, CBT alone, and fluoxetine plus CBT. The study was conducted with the adolescent population,

Table 12-1 Revisions to Medication Guide

What is the most important information I should know about antidepressant medicines, depression and other serious mental illness, and suicidal thoughts or actions?

1. Antidepressant medicines may increase suicidal thoughts or actions in some children, teenagers, and young adults when the medicine is first started.
2. Depression and other serious mental illnesses are the most important causes of suicidal thoughts and actions. Some people may have a particularly high risk of having suicidal thoughts or actions. These include people who have (or have a family history of) bipolar illness (also called *manic-depressive illness*) or suicidal thoughts or actions.
3. How can I watch for and try to prevent suicidal thoughts and actions in a family member or myself?
   - Pay close attention to any changes, especially sudden changes, in mood, behaviors, thoughts, or feelings. This is very important when an antidepressant medicine is first started or when the dose is changed.
   - Call the healthcare provider right away to report new or sudden changes in mood, behavior, thoughts, or feelings.
   - Keep all follow-up visits with the healthcare provider as scheduled. Call the healthcare provider between visits as needed, especially if you have concerns about symptoms.

Call a healthcare provider right away if you or your family member has any of the following symptoms, especially if they are new, worse, or worry you:
- Thoughts about suicide or dying
- Attempts to commit suicide
- New or worse depression
- New or worse anxiety
- Feeling very agitated or restless
- Panic attacks
- Trouble sleeping (insomnia)
- New or worse irritability
- Acting aggressive, being angry or violent
- Acting on dangerous impulses
- An extreme increase in activity and talking (mania)
- Other unusual changes in behavior or mood

What else do I need to know about antidepressant medicines?
- **Never stop an antidepressant medicine without first talking to a healthcare provider.** Stopping an antidepressant medicine suddenly can cause other symptoms.
- **Antidepressants are medicines used to treat depression and other illnesses.** It is important to discuss all the risks of treating depression and also the risks of not treating it. Patients and their families or other caregivers should discuss all treatment choices with the healthcare provider, not just the use of antidepressants.
- **Antidepressant medicines have other side effects.** Talk to the healthcare provider about the side effects of the medicine prescribed for you or your family member.
- **Antidepressant medicines can interact with other medicines.** Know all of the medicines that you or your family member takes. Keep a list of all medicine to show the healthcare provider. Do not start new medicines without first checking with your healthcare provider.
- **Not all antidepressant medicines prescribed for children are approved by the U.S. Food and Drug Administration (FDA) for use in children.** Talk to your child's healthcare provider for more information.

The FDA has approved this Medication Guide for all antidepressants.

U.S. Food and Drug Administration. *Medication Guide: Antidepressant medicines, depression and other serious mental illnesses, and suicidal thoughts or actions.* Retrieved from http://www.fda.gov/downloads/drugs/drugsafety/informationbydrugclass/ucm100211.pdf

---

so conclusions should be applied only to that population. Among the conclusions reached by the TADS team are the following:

- "Despite calls to restrict access to medications, medical management of MDD with fluoxetine, including careful monitoring for adverse events, should be made widely available, not discouraged" (March et al., 2004, p. 819).

- "Given incremental improvement in outcome when CBT is combined with medication and, as importantly, increased protection from suicidality, CBT also should be readily available as part of comprehensive treatment for depressed adolescents" (March et al., 2004, p. 819).

In addition to CBT, family therapy and interpersonal therapy are often used in the treatment of

Table 12-2 Antidepressant Medications With U.S. Food and Drug Administration (FDA) Approval for Use in the Pediatric Population

Proprietary Name	Generic Name	Generic Available	FDA-Approved Pediatric Indication	Dosage
Prozac™	Fluoxetine hydrochloride	Yes	MDD, 8–18 years (also OCD, 7–17 years)	Initial: 10–20 mg/day, depending on weight (initial dose in OCD is 10 mg)
Lexapro™	Escitalopram	Yes	MDD, 12–17 years	Initial: 10 mg once daily Recommended: 10 mg once daily Maximum: 20 mg once daily

MDD, major depressive disorder; OCD, obsessive–compulsive disorder.
Data from U.S. Food and Drug Administration.

pediatric depression (Weisz et al., 2006). The clinician should keep in mind that all therapeutic interventions must be chosen based on the child's particular context, family situation, and unique presentation.

It should be noted that most of the research into psychotherapy treatment of pediatric depression has focused particularly on adolescents and only rarely on young school-age children. Although some CBT models have been adapted for use in younger children, for a chronologically preadolescent child (or developmentally young older child), play psychotherapies are both more accessible and developmentally appropriate, although they may seem like a waste of time or simply esoteric to the parent or caregiver. CBT requires a certain level of cognitive, verbal, and social development on the part of the child. Very young or developmentally impaired persons do not and cannot process thoughts and feelings like some adolescents and adults. For these young children, expressing themselves with and through play is the developmental equivalent of talking through something using spoken words and conversation for the adult or older adolescent. Typically, a play psychotherapist will use the play itself to help the child explore feelings and thoughts by acting them out in the therapy room using toys, puppets, paint, drawing, and the like. The primary provider can facilitate a successful referral for evaluation or psychotherapy of the young child by helping to frame the caretaker's expectations of psychotherapy in a developmentally appropriate way.

V. Referral

Children and adolescents with depression and other psychiatric illnesses are optimally treated in the context of their families, school, and community within a developmental framework. Often, the collateral contacts required for optimal assessment and treatment are not easily conducted within the confines of the 15-minute medical office visit. Thus, the primary care clinician should always feel free to consult with or refer to a pediatric psychiatric specialist. Referral or consultation should be sought depending on the severity, lethality, complexity, and comorbidity of the case. Cases in which emergent or urgent referral to a psychiatric colleague or hospital emergency room should be made include the following:

1. Suspected bipolar illness
2. Presence of suspected or identified suicidal ideation or suicide-related behavior or nonsuicidal self-harming behavior
3. Aggressive behavior
4. Comorbid or suspected psychiatric or medical illnesses
5. Comorbid or suspected substance abuse
6. Impaired parent–child functioning or other dysfunction in the family or support system
7. Significant family pathology or history of suicide in the family
8. Comorbid or suspected learning disability
9. Any case in which the treating clinician desires consultation or believes that the presenting problem exceeds their scope or knowledge base in providing competent care

VI. Self-management tools

A. *For providers*
  1. Information on antidepressant use in children, adolescents, and adults with advisories from the FDA is available at http://www.fda.gov/Drugs/DrugSafety/InformationbyDrugClass/ucm096273.htm.
  2. A toolkit for child and adolescent depression treatment in primary care, developed from consensus guidelines, is available at http://www.glad-pc.org.
  3. The general AACAP website also offers parameters for competent prescribing and evaluation in the child and adolescent population for licensed professionals, available at http://www.aacap.org/AACAP/Resources_for_Primary_Care/Practice_Parameters_and_Resource_Centers/Practice_Parameters.aspx.

B. *For patients and families*
   1. The general AACAP website offers excellent educational materials for families on a number of topics, including medications, and is available at http://www.aacap.org/AACAP/Families_and_Youth/Facts_for_Families/Facts_for_Families_Keyword.aspx.
   2. Also available from the AACAP is the depression resource center at http://www.aacap.org/AACAP/Families_and_Youth/Resource_Centers/Depression_Resource_Center/Home.aspx.
   3. American Academy of Pediatrics resources on child health topics, including depression and suicide, are available at https://healthychildren.org/English/health-issues/conditions/emotional-problems/Pages/default.aspx.
   4. Information on depression in children and adolescents is available at http://www.nami.org/Content/NavigationMenu/Mental_Illnesses/Depression/Depression_in_Children_and_Adolescents.htm.
   5. Child and adolescent mental health resources are available at http://www.nimh.nih.gov/health/topics/child-and-adolescent-mental-health/index.shtml.
   6. The National Center for Infants, Toddlers, and Families has excellent educational materials for parents and providers, available at http://www.zerotothree.org/child-development/temperament-behavior/.

References

American Academy of Child and Adolescent Psychiatry. (2001). Practice parameter for the assessment and treatment of children and adolescents with suicidal behavior. American Academy of Child and Adolescent Psychiatry. *Journal of the American Academy of Child and Adolescent Psychiatry*, 40(Suppl. 7), 24S–51S. doi:10.1097/00004583-200107001-00003

American Academy of Child and Adolescent Psychiatry. (2022, March). *AACAP policy statement on increased suicide among Black youth in the U.S.* https://www.aacap.org/AACAP/Policy_Statements/2022/AACAP_Policy_Statement_Increased_Suicide_Among_Black_Youth_US.aspx

American Psychiatric Association. (1994). *Diagnostic and statistical manual of mental disorders* (4th ed.).

American Psychiatric Association. (2000). *Diagnostic and statistical manual of mental disorders* (4th ed., text rev.).

American Psychiatric Association. (2013). *Diagnostic and statistical manual of mental disorders* (5th ed.).

American Psychiatric Association. (2022). *DSM-5-TR and diagnoses for children.* https://www.psychiatry.org/File%20Library/Psychiatrists/Practice/DSM/DSM-5-TR/APA-DSM5TR-DiagnosesforChildren.pdf

Arnett, J. J. (1999). Adolescent storm and stress, reconsidered. *American Psychologist*, 54(5), 317–326. doi:10.1037//0003-066x.54.5.317

Bilsen J. (2018). Suicide and youth: Risk factors. *Frontiers in Psychiatry*, 9, 540. doi:10.3389/fpsyt.2018.00540

Birmaher, B., Arbelaez, C., & Brent, D. (2002). Course and outcome of child and adolescent major depressive disorder. *Child and Adolescent Psychiatric Clinics of North America*, 11(3), 619–637. doi:10.1016/s1056-4993(02)00011-1

Birmaher, B., & Brent, D. (2007). Practice parameter for the assessment and treatment of children and adolescents with depressive disorders. *Journal of the American Academy of Child & Adolescent Psychiatry*, 46(11), 1503–1526. doi:10.1097/chi.0b013e318145ae1c

Caron, C. (2021, November 18). Why are more Black kids suicidal? A search for answers. *New York Times*. https://www.nytimes.com/2021/11/18/well/mind/suicide-black-kids.html

Centers for Disease Control and Prevention. (2020). *10 leading causes of death, United States.* https://www.cdc.gov/injury/wisqars/index.html

Cheung, A. H., Kozloff, N., & Sacks, D. (2013). Pediatric depression: An evidence-based update on treatment interventions. *Current Psychiatry Reports*, 15(8), 381. doi:10.1007/s11920-013-0381-4

Dimidjian, S., Barrera, M., Martell, C., Muñoz, R. F., & Lewinsohn, P. M. (2011). The origins and current status of behavioral activation treatments for depression. *Annual Review of Clinical Psychology*, 7, 1–38. doi:10.1146/annurev-clinpsy-032210-104535

Dobson, K. S., Hollon, S. D., Dimidjian, S., Schmaling, K. B., Kohlenberg, R. J., Gallop, R., Rizvi, S. L., Gollan, J. K., Dunner, D. L., & Jacobson, N. S. (2008). Randomized trial of behavioral activation, cognitive therapy, and antidepressant medication in the prevention of relapse and recurrence in major depression. *Journal of Consulting and Clinical Psychology*, 76(3), 468–477. doi:10.1037/0022-006X.76.3.468

Garber, J., & Weersing, V. R. (2010). Comorbidity of anxiety and depression in youth: Implications for treatment and prevention. *Clinical Psychology*, 17(4), 293–306. doi:10.1111/j.1468-2850.2010.01221.x

Gould, M. S., Greenberg, T., Velting, D. M., & Shaffer, D. (2003). Youth suicide risk and preventive interventions: A review of the past 10 years. *Journal of the American Academy of Child & Adolescent Psychiatry*, 42(4), 386–405. doi:10.1097/01.CHI.0000046821.95464.CF

Hines, A. R., & Paulson, S. E. (2006). Parents' and teachers' perceptions of adolescent storm and stress: Relations with parenting and teaching styles. *Adolescence*, 41(164), 597–614.

Horowitz, L. M., Bridge, J. A., Pao, M., & Boudreaux, E. D. (2014). Screening youth for suicide risk in medical settings: Time to ask questions. *American Journal of Preventive Medicine*, 47(3), S170–S175. doi:10.1016/j.amepre.2014.06.002

Kroenke, K., Spitzer, R. L., & Williams, J. B. (2001). The PHQ-9: Validity of a brief depression severity measure. *Journal of General Internal Medicine*, 16(9), 606–613. doi:10.1046/j.1525-1497.2001.016009606.x

Lener, M. S., Niciu, M. J., Ballard, E. D., Park, M., Park, L. T., Nugent, A. C., & Zarate, C. A., Jr. (2017). Glutamate and gamma-aminobutyric acid systems in the pathophysiology of major depression and antidepressant response to ketamine. *Biological Psychiatry*, 81(10), 886–897. doi:10.1016/j.biopsych.2016.05.005

Lui, S., Zhou, X. J., Sweeney, J. A., & Gong, Q. (2016). Psychoradiology: The frontier of neuroimaging in psychiatry. *Radiology, 281*(2), 357–372. doi:10.1148/radiol.2016152149

Madigan S, Racine N, Vaillancourt T, Korczak DJ, Hewitt JMA, Pador P, Park JL, McArthur BA, Holy C, Neville RD. Changes in Depression and Anxiety Among Children and Adolescents From Before to During the COVID-19 Pandemic: A Systematic Review and Meta-analysis. *JAMA Pediatr.* 2023 Jun 1;177(6):567-581. doi: 10.1001/jamapediatrics.2023.0846. PMID: 37126337; PMCID: PMC10152379.

Ming, Q., Zhong, X., Zhang, X., Pu, W., Dong, D., Jiang, Y., Gao, Y., Wang, X., Detre, J. A., Yao, S., & Rao, H. (2017). State-independent and dependent neural responses to psychosocial stress in current and remitted depression. *American Journal of Psychiatry, 174*(10), 971–979. doi:10.1176/appi.ajp.2017.16080974

Patra, S. (2019). Assessment and management of pediatric depression. *Indian Journal of Psychiatry, 61*(3), 300–306. doi:10.4103/psychiatry.IndianJPsychiatry_446_18

Perou, R., Bitsko, R. H., Blumberg, S. J., Pastor, P., Ghandour, R. M., Gfroerer, J. C., Hedden, S. L., Crosby, A. E., Visser, S. N., Schieve, L. A., Parks, S. E., Hall, J. E., Brody, D., Simile, C. M., Thompson, W. W., Baio, J., Avenevoli, S., Kogan, M. D., Huang, L. N., & Centers for Disease Control and Prevention. (2013). Mental health surveillance among children—United States, 2005–2011. *MMWR Supplements, 62*(2), 1–35.

Rao, U., & Chen, L. (2009). Characteristics, correlates, and outcomes of childhood and adolescent depressive disorders. *Dialogues in Clinical Neuroscience, 11*, 45–62. doi:10.31887/DCNS.2009.11.1/urao

Saddock, B. J., & Saddock, V. A. (2007). *Kaplan & Saddock's synopsis of psychiatry* (10th ed.). Lippincott, Williams & Wilkins.

World Health Organization. (n.d.). Depression. https://www.who.int/health-topics/depression#tab=tab_1

Zuckerbrot, R. A., Cheung, A. H., Jensen, P. S., Stein, R. E., Laraque, D., & GLAD-PC Steering Group. (2007). Guidelines for adolescent depression in primary care (GLAD-PC): I. Identification, assessment, and initial management. *Pediatrics, 120*(5), e1299–e1312. doi:10.1542/peds.2007-1144

CHAPTER 13

Child Maltreatment

Naomi Schapiro and Tiffany Lambright

I. Introduction and general background

Child maltreatment encompasses physical, sexual, and emotional abuse and child neglect, as well as trafficking of children. Healthcare providers have legal, professional, and ethical responsibilities to assess children for maltreatment and report suspected cases. In this chapter, "child" refers to any individual under the age of 18, related to the APN's legal responsibility to detect and report maltreatment. We refer to specific ages of children when discussing important physical, cognitive or emotional differences, we use the term "adolescent" as a subset of child, to refer to individuals aged 12 to 18, as their legal and reporting status changes at 18. (See Chapter 06, in which adolescents are defined as 12- to 21-year-olds for general health issues). Each of the 50 states, the District of Columbia, and the U.S. territories have their own definitions of child abuse and neglect, but all must conform to minimum federal standards set in the Child Abuse Prevention and Treatment Act (CAPTA): any recent act or failure to act on the part of a parent or caregiver that results in death, serious physical or emotional harm, sexual abuse, or exploitation or an act or failure to act that presents an imminent risk of serious harm (CAPTA, 1998; Child Welfare Information Gateway, 2019a). The Justice for Victims of Trafficking Act of 2015, which amended CAPTA, required all states receiving federal funding to include sex trafficking in their definitions and statutes that relate to child abuse and neglect and sexual abuse, making reporting of child abuse mandatory in cases of child sex trafficking (Child Welfare Information Gateway, 2019; Justice for Victims of Trafficking Act, 2015). Advanced practice nurses (APNs) can consult the website https://www.childwelfare.gov/topics/systemwide/laws-policies/state/ for the specific definitions and reporting responsibilities in their own states.

The professional and ethical responsibilities to assess for, detect, and report child maltreatment are reinforced by a steadily accumulating body of literature on the myriad and long-lasting effects of these adverse events, including greater rates of depression and substance abuse, early onset of sexual activity, greater likelihood of becoming a teenage parent, and higher rates of adult chronic health conditions (Merrick et al., 2017; Petrucelli et al., 2019; Rebbe et al., 2018; Shonkoff & Garner, 2012). Child maltreatment comprises 5 of the 10 adverse childhood experiences (ACE) that were part of a historic study by Kaiser and the Centers for Disease Control and Prevention (CDC) demonstrating strong epidemiological links to these long-lasting effects (Van Niel et al., 2014). Initiatives to ameliorate the impact of ACEs in many states have highlighted the importance of prevention, early recognition, and healing support for survivors of child maltreatment (Barnes et al., 2020; Bhushan et al., 2020).

In 2020, there were 3.9 million reports made to child protection, and an estimated 618,000 children were deemed to be victims of maltreatment (U.S. Department of Health and Human Services, 2022), in contrast to 4.4 million reports and an estimated 656,000 child victims in 2019 (U.S. Department of Health and Human Services, 2021). This decrease is believed to be a reflection of nationwide school closures during the COVID pandemic because educational staff are among the largest reporters of child abuse and neglect (Baron et al., 2020) and because of restrictions experienced by many child protection agencies in making in-person assessments (U.S. Department of Health and Human Services, 2022). An international review of 12 studies conducted during pandemic lockdowns found that hospital reports of child maltreatment increased, whereas reports from police and social service agencies decreased (Rapp et al., 2021). We have, therefore, opted to use reporting data from 2019 in this chapter (U.S. Department of Health and Human Services, 2021) because they are likely closer to the current incidence and prevalence than the 2020 data.

An estimated 1,840 children died as a result of abuse or neglect, with a rate of 2.50 deaths for 100,000 children. Children who were less than 1 year old comprised 45.4% of children who died from maltreatment, at a rate of 22.94 per 100,000 infants (U.S. Department of Health and Human Services, 2021). However, these annual reporting rates understate the prevalence of child abuse and neglect in the pediatric population. Cumulative estimates from the National Child Abuse and Neglect Data System (NCANDS) are that 11.7% of all children will be reported and confirmed as maltreated during their childhood (Yi et al., 2020). A 2014 household survey of 4,000 caregivers and older children found that 15% of children in the sample experienced some form of maltreatment in just the past year, and 38% of 14- to 17-year-olds reported a lifetime history of maltreatment (Finkelhor et al., 2015), indicating that many incidents of maltreatment are not reported. During the height of COVID-related social isolation, a survey of parents found increases in self-reported parental stress, neglect, and verbal aggression toward their children (Lee et al., 2022).

Increased risk for child maltreatment is associated in the literature with structural inequities, including family and community poverty, housing instability, lack of child health insurance, and low parental education levels (Hunter & Flores, 2021; Lane & Dubowitz, 2021). Rates of child abuse reporting are higher for children who are Black, Latinx, and Pacific Islander/Native Hawaiian, reflecting both the impact of structural racism on social determinants of health (SDOH) inequities and reporting and response bias in the medical and child welfare system (Luken et al., 2021). Research has shown that healthcare providers' reliance on intuition and social information about families influences their decisions to pursue evaluations for physical abuse or report neglect, leading to potential overreporting for poor and minoritized families and underdiagnosis for well-off and White families (Janson, 2021; Keenan et al., 2017). Just as it is important for the APN to explore the stresses, resources, and coping strategies of all families, including those who seem to have risk factors for maltreatment, it is also important to remember that child maltreatment can occur in families that do not have known risk factors.

Family and caregiver adversity, including intimate partner violence, substance abuse, and depression, are independently associated with child maltreatment and are in themselves classified as ACEs (Bhushan et al., 2020; Institute of Medicine [IOM] & National Research Council [NRC], 2014). Child maltreatment reports are greater for children with special healthcare needs and temperamental mismatch with a parent (Azzopardi et al., 2021; IOM & NRC, 2014). Protective factors may include extended family cohesiveness; personal, financial, and community resources; positive religious coping; and optimism on the part of the child and caregiver (IOM & NRC, 2014; Schaefer et al., 2018).

Assessing and responding to child maltreatment can be challenging for the APN because the abuse or neglect may not be readily apparent and may not be the specific reason that the child is presenting for care. The epidemiologic risk factors discussed previously for child maltreatment can be helpful in planning population-level interventions, but they can also reinforce implicit bias in the individual practitioner (Forkey et al., 2021; Schnierle et al., 2019). They should not be used to amplify or dismiss concerns in the clinical setting, where the APN should always keep maltreatment in mind as part of the differential diagnosis (Jordan & Steelman, 2015) and should follow established protocols for assessing potential maltreatment, regardless of their assumptions of which families are at lower or higher risk (Palusci & Botash, 2021). Child abuse and neglect involve injuries to children, failure to provide necessary care, and/or failure to protect them from harm. Maltreatment assessments and reports are made based on the impact on the child, including the risk of harm, not the provider's opinion of the caregivers (Keeshin & Dubowitz, 2013). Keeping the focus on the child can help the APN to sort through what is often a confusing and emotion-laden situation.

Trauma is defined as "a frightening, dangerous, or violent event that poses a threat to a child's life or bodily integrity" and can include physical, sexual, and psychological abuse and neglect (National Child Traumatic Stress Network, n.d., para. 1). Trauma-informed care (TIC) acknowledges the prevalence of trauma in patients and their caregivers and promotes the development of compassionate and collaborative relationships with families, in which the objective is to understand the family in social and relational contexts, determine their challenges and strengths, and support their own efforts to heal (Fleishman et al., 2019; Forkey et al., 2021). A complete discussion of TIC is beyond the scope of this chapter. However, because the assessment and mandatory reporting of suspected child abuse can be trauma inducing for a child and family, it is important to adhere to trauma-informed practices, including ensuring transparency about the purpose of history taking and diagnostic tests; discussing confidentiality and its limits; offering choices where possible, such as participating in the reporting process; and providing support for families, providers, and staff. For more information on TIC, see the Resources section at the end of this chapter.

A. *Physical abuse*
   1. Definition and overview
      Broadly, *physical abuse* is an inflicted (nonaccidental) injury to a child by a parent or caregiver that results in physical impairment. Mechanisms of injury may include biting, burning, kicking, striking, shaking, grabbing, stabbing, dragging, throwing, strangling, or poisoning. Legal definitions of reportable physical abuse vary widely from state to state (for details, use the State Statutes search at Child Welfare Information Gateway, 2019a).
   2. Incidence and prevalence
      During 2019, 17.5% of victims of child maltreatment were physically abused. Physical abuse accounted for 44.4% of child fatalities, either alone or in combination with another type of maltreatment (U.S. Department of Health and Human Services, 2021). A meta-analysis of global maltreatment

prevalence studies found that the lifetime prevalence of physical abuse in North America ranged from 14.1% to 33.3% (Moody et al., 2018). Widely differing definitions and overlap with nonabusive physical punishment make estimation of prevalence difficult.

B. *Sexual abuse*
1. Definition and overview
   Sexual abuse includes sexual contact between adults and children, including touching of breasts, genitals, and buttocks; penetration; exposure to sexual activity or involvement in pornography; and unwanted sexual contact between minors. This contact may be carried out through violence, coercion, emotional manipulation, or the child's developmental inability to understand or consent to the activity (Child Welfare Information Gateway, 2019b). Sexual abuse includes commercial sexual exploitation of children (see Section E). In many states, consensual sexual activity of a minor with either an older minor or an adult may be reportable under sexual abuse or statutory rape laws (Reproductive National Health Training Center, 2021), and APNs should consult their state laws for specific reporting requirements (see the State Statutes search at Child Welfare Information Gateway, 2019a).
2. Incidence and prevalence
   During 2019, 7.2% of child maltreatment victims were sexually abused (U.S. Department of Health and Human Services, 2021). Median lifetime prevalence rates in North America, calculated from a global meta-analysis of prevalence studies, were 20.4% for girls and 14.1% for boys (Moody et al., 2018).

C. *Psychologic or emotional abuse*
1. Definition and overview
   Under federal standards, emotional abuse involves "a pattern of behavior that impairs a child's emotional development or sense of self-worth. This may include constant criticism, threats, or rejection, as well as withholding love, support, or guidance" (Child Welfare Information Gateway, 2019b, p. 3). Emotional abuse is difficult to substantiate unless the child exhibits severe psychologic sequelae, including post-traumatic stress symptoms, depression and anxiety (Salloum at el., 2018, and see Chapter 12). Such abuse is also a component of other forms of child maltreatment, which impedes independent reporting and tracking of emotional abuse. In some states, committing intimate partner violence in the presence of a child may be considered a form of child abuse because of the potential emotional impact on the child (Child Welfare Information Gateway, 2021).
2. Incidence and prevalence
   In 2019, 6.1% of child maltreatment victims were psychologically abused (U.S. Department of Health and Human Services, 2021). Prevalence studies in North America range from 15.9% to 28.4% for girls and from 12.3% to 13.7% for boys (Moody et al., 2018).

D. *Neglect*
1. Definition and overview
   As the most commonly reported form of child maltreatment, neglect has been understudied, yet its long-term consequences may be just as devastating as other forms of maltreatment (Keeshin & Dubowitz, 2013; Vanderminden et al., 2019). Broadly, neglect occurs when a child's basic physical, emotional, and developmental needs are not being met (Keeshin & Dubowitz). These basic needs include food, clothing, shelter, educational needs, medical care, supervision, and emotional care (Child Welfare Information Gateway, 2019a). Although neglect may involve one instance of a dangerous failure of a parent or caretaker to supervise or provide care, it also may result from the accumulation of smaller lapses over time and have roots in poverty and lack of community resources, making assessment a challenge. States vary widely in their specific definitions of neglect, with some including or excluding drug use, homelessness, or parental refusal of health care for their child for personal or religious reasons. In some states, failure to educate is covered under truancy rather than child abuse law (Child Welfare Information Gateway, 2019a). The standard for reporting neglect also varies, with some states naming specific reportable parental behaviors or failure to provide care and others using suspicion of actual or imminent harm to a child as the reporting standard (Rebbe, 2018).
2. Incidence and prevalence
   In 2019, 74.9% of child maltreatment victims in the United States were neglected and 2.3% suffered from medical neglect , defined as a failure of the child's caregiver to provide "appropriate health care" for the child, despite having or being provided adequate financial resources (U.S. Department of Health and Human Services, 2021). North American prevalence studies, based on self-report, range from 40.5% of girls to 16.8% of boys (Moody et al., 2018). The authors theorized that there may have been gender differences in willingness to self-report instances of neglect, and different definitions of neglect compared with studies in other parts of the world.

E. *Medical child abuse*
1. Definition and overview
   Medical child abuse, also known as *fabricated* or *induced illness in a child* or *factitious disorder imposed on another*, may involve elements of physical abuse, psychological abuse, and child endangerment (a type of neglect). This rare and puzzling form of child maltreatment was initially known (and is still searchable) as *Munchausen syndrome by proxy*; however, most experts prefer to emphasize the harm to

the child and the role of pediatric providers who are induced to order and perform unnecessary and invasive diagnostic testing and treatment (Hornor, 2021; Schechter & Nurko, 2019). In this form of maltreatment, caregivers induce or falsify symptoms of illness in their children, presenting them as victims of rare and serious medical conditions (Hamilton et al., 2021; Hornor, 2021). The caregiver is typically a well-educated mother, often with training in a healthcare profession (Yates & Bass, 2017). Clinicians may not recognize medical child abuse, given the reliance on parent reports in pediatric histories and a reluctance to document any discrepancies between history and findings or finer details of interactions that would indicate a pattern of concern (Hamilton et al., 2021; Hornor, 2021). Although uncommon, this form of maltreatment should be in the differential when children have repeated visits or hospitalizations for serious symptoms with negative diagnostic tests and a lack of symptoms or abnormal exam findings within the clinical setting. It can be challenging to distinguish parental anxiety about a difficult-to-diagnose medical condition from symptom inducement or fabrication, and some children who are victims of medical child abuse also have complex medical conditions (Petska et al. 2017).

2. Incidence and prevalence

Prospective studies in the United Kingdom and Ireland found an incidence of 0.5 in 100,000 (McClure et al., 1996), and a more recent prospective study in Italy found an incidence of 0.53% (Ferrara et al., 2013). However, the true incidence and prevalence of medical child abuse are unknown because providers tend to report only the most egregious cases (Flaherty & MacMillan, 2013; Jenny & Metz, 2020), and the abuse may be classified as another type of maltreatment by child welfare agencies.

F. *Trafficking and exploitation of children*

1. Definition and overview

A United Nations Office on Drugs and Crime (2004) protocol defines human trafficking as follows:

"Trafficking in persons" shall mean the recruitment, transportation, transfer, harboring or receipt of persons, by means of the threat or use of force or other forms of coercion, of abduction, of fraud, of deception, of the abuse of power or of a position of vulnerability or of the giving or receiving of payments or benefits to achieve the consent of a person having control over another person, for the purpose of exploitation. (p. 42)

Human trafficking, including both labor and sex trafficking, may or may not involve the smuggling or movement of those being trafficked. Human trafficking in the United States includes both U.S.-born and foreign-born persons, and exploiters generally target vulnerable people, increasing the risk of trafficking for children and youth (Nazer & Greenbaum, 2020).

Labor trafficking is forced labor for little or no pay, and the definition under U.S. federal law requires an element of coercion, force, deception, or fraud, regardless of the age of the victim. Approximately 20 states include child labor trafficking in their definition of physical child abuse. Common examples of types of labor trafficking in which children may be exploited include the sale and transport of drugs, work in nail and hair salons and restaurants, agricultural and domestic labor, door-to-door sales, and begging (Child Welfare Information Gateway, 2018).

"Child sex trafficking" (CST), also commonly referred to as *commercial sexual exploitation of children* (CSEC), can be defined as the involvement of a minor in any sexual activity, including prostitution, child sexual exploitation materials (child pornography), or sexually explicit performance, in exchange for money or something of perceived value (Child Welfare Information Gateway, 2018, 2020; Greenbaum, 2018). Under federal law, if the victim of exploitation is a minor, the use of coercion, force, or fraud need not be present for the act to be considered sex trafficking (Child Welfare Information Gateway, 2020; Nazer & Greenbaum, 2020). According to the Justice for Victims of Trafficking Act, all states must consider any victim of CST to be a victim of "child abuse and neglect" as well as "sexual abuse" (Child Welfare Information Gateway, 2018; Justice for Victims of Trafficking Act, 2015).

2. Incidence and prevalence

Accurate data on the incidence and prevalence of human trafficking are nearly impossible to collect due to several factors: the covert nature of trafficking itself, the underidentification of victims, and the lack of standardized reporting and tracking systems. Children comprised 5.5 million of the 20.9 million persons, or 26%, estimated to be involved in forced labor globally at any point during the period from 2002 to 2011. This is equivalent to 3 in every 1,000 people in the global population at that time (International Labor Organization, 2012). Polaris, a national agency that operates the U.S. National Human Trafficking Hotline, estimates that minors were involved in approximately 26% of the 8,248 cases of sex trafficking and 14% of the 1,236 cases of labor trafficking reported to the hotline (National Human Trafficking Hotline, in 2019; Polaris, 2020).

States have the option to report sex trafficking in addition to their reports of child sexual abuse, which affects how cases are tracked, as well as the response of child protective services (CPS) and/or law enforcement. In 2020, 35 states reported a total of 953 unique victims of CST to the NCANDS, including partial-year data (U.S. Department of

Health and Human Services, 2022). The relatively low numbers, compared to other estimates, as well as a lack of uniformity in what and how states are reporting, highlight some of the challenges of capturing true numbers of trafficking victims. Additionally, the NCANDS reporting data do not capture the number of labor trafficking victims because labor trafficking is not considered a distinct form of child maltreatment in many states.

II. Database (may include but is not limited to)

Trusting family–provider relationships provide a basis for surveillance and screening for traumatic events, including maltreatment. Some practices are adopting universal questionnaires to uncover adverse events that include child maltreatment at preventive exams and asking about SDOH and coping mechanisms and supports (Barnes et al., 2020). Routinely asking families questions about physical punishment or fighting, forced or coerced sexual activity and inappropriate touching, and general safety can send a message to the child and parent that these subjects are open topics of discussion during the visit, even if they do not answer them at first. Whenever possible, talking to caregivers and children separately can be helpful in gathering history about potential maltreatment.

A. *Subjective*
1. Chief complaint
    a. Injuries
        Detailed history of any new or old injuries and context of injury: Is the history consistent with the injury and developmental capabilities of the child? Also include the following:
        History of similar injuries and general injury history
        Current or past history of delayed care for injuries
        History of seeking care for injuries at multiple facilities
    b. Injury sustained at work with no or inappropriate response from employer (suspicious for labor trafficking)
    c. Sudden changes in behavior
        Because children vary widely in temperament, and cultural influences may also affect their behavior in clinical settings, a sudden change, rather than the specific behavior, may be an important indicator of trauma (including but not limited to child maltreatment)—for example, the outgoing child who suddenly seems withdrawn, or the quiet child who suddenly seems driven by a motor.
    d. Sexual acting out
        Genital self-stimulation for pleasure, or masturbation, is a normal part of child development from toddlerhood through adolescence; children younger than school age may not have a well-developed sense of privacy and may masturbate in social settings considered inappropriate by adults. Sexual play between age mates, consisting of exploration of body parts and sexual jokes, is developmentally normal and not in itself a sign of sexual abuse (Chiesa & Goldson, 2017; Kellogg, 2010). In a media-saturated society in which sexual images are widely available, discerning age-appropriate from inappropriate sexual knowledge may be difficult, as may be distinguishing between a history of abuse and either accidental or neglectful exposure to sexually explicit material. However, some activities should raise a suspicion of sexual abuse:
        i. Sexual acts involving penetration or use of objects
        ii. Sexual play that closely mimics adult sexual activity
        iii. Sexual activity between children with age or developmental differences or suspicion of coercion
    e. Review of systems:
        Recurrent headache, abdominal pain, or genitourinary discomfort may be related to somatic symptoms of psychological distress or recurrent injury. A thorough review of systems from both caregiver and child, separately, may be helpful in cases in which the history is confusing or inconsistent.
    f. Social history
        i. How does the parent describe the child? Red flags include obvious lack of enjoyment of the child, labeling the child as bad, or inappropriate expectations for child's developmental stage.
        ii. Methods of discipline used and their perceived effectiveness
        iii. Expectations around chores and helping out with the household
        iv. For the minor that is employed, where and what hours are they working? What type of compensation is given?
2. Situations that may heighten family stress
    Children and families may need extra support and should be asked how they are coping if they are experiencing any of the following situations (Christian & Committee on Child Abuse, 2015; Forkey et al., 2021).
    a. Changes in family status and/or caregivers
        Job loss, loss of health insurance, death, divorce or other family separation, intimate partner violence, unstable housing, and caregiver or other family member illness, including mental health diagnoses and substance abuse, can all strain or overwhelm a parent's resources and ability to care for a child.
    b. History of foster care, of running away or being ejected from the home
        These situations may put children and youth at increased risk for maltreatment, both by legal guardians and by traffickers who look for vulnerability in their victims (Child Welfare

Information Gateway, 2018; Euser et al., 2014; Landers et al., 2021).
   c. Challenging stages in child development
      i. The inconsolable infant, the willful toddler, and normative developmental changes of adolescence can challenge all parents.
      ii. In some cases, these typical challenges of parenting can exacerbate a stressed family system.
   d. Children who are difficult to care for
      This category encompasses a wide variety of conditions, from children whose temperaments are not well matched with those of their parents and/or have difficulties with self-regulation to children with complex medical conditions, neuromuscular disabilities, and/or behavioral and learning difficulties, whose families may be struggling with limited time and financial capacity. Children who are less able to give the parent positive reinforcement for their care may also be at greater risk for maltreatment (Azzopardi et al., 2021; Turner et al., 2019).
   e. Sexual and gender minorities
      Children and youth who identify as lesbian, gay, bisexual, transgender/gender non-conforming, or questioning are at increased risk for victimization by family members, including ejection from the home, and by traffickers (Hornor et al., 2019; McGeough & Sterzing, 2018).
3. Special considerations for taking histories from children about suspected maltreatment
   The APN should approach history taking of injuries and physical complaints in a careful and systematic fashion. If children disclose abuse, the APN should avoid taking a comprehensive history of the disclosure, instead limiting questions to a brief review of who, what, and when, gathering just enough information to report to CPS or the police. The following are age-related considerations:
   a. Toddlers and preschool-aged children
      i. Children under the age of 6 have limited vocabularies and a relatively undeveloped sense of time and sequence and are best interviewed by a trained expert in child maltreatment (Adams et al., 2016).
      ii. Well-meaning parents and healthcare professionals can inadvertently feed the child information and unwittingly distort the story (Canning & Peterson, 2020).
   b. School-age children
      i. School-age children have a developed sense of time and sequence. The challenge for the healthcare provider is to speak briefly with the school-age child without the parent present.
      ii. If history taking is not possible, the APN with a reasonable suspicion of maltreatment should still file a CPS report.
   c. Adolescents
      i. Adolescents may come in alone for care, and many clinics have established policies for taking written questionnaires and verbal histories from children over 12 without a parent in the room (see Chapter 6).
      ii. Each state has its own parameters for confidential services (Guttmacher Institute, 2021), and it is important to let the adolescent know which parts of the history are truly confidential and what the APN must report related to sexual assault and consensual sexual activity between dissimilar-aged minors and between minors and adults, as well as disclosures regarding trafficking (Child Welfare Information Gateway, 2020, 2021; Hornor et al., 2019; Schapiro & Mejia, 2018).
      iii. Ask all adolescents a general question about trafficking, such as whether they have ever gone on dates or traded sex or sexual pictures for money, clothes, drugs, food, a place to stay, or other favors or have ever been asked or forced to do something sexual against their will (Hornor et al., 2019).
      iv. If your patient population warrants more detailed screening questions, or for follow-up to a positive answer, see the Resources section at the end of the chapter for links to additional questions.

B. *Objective*
   It is important to document any abnormal findings as thoroughly and accurately as possible, including measurement of injuries and drawings if appropriate. Photographic documentation may be useful if it conforms to local law enforcement standards for quality and chain of custody.
1. General overview of child's appearance and behavior
   The demeanor, appearance, clothing, accessories, and behavior of the child or adolescent in the clinic can provide the APN with valuable information. However, it is important to remember that the APN is seeing just a snapshot of the child in an artificial and sometimes stressful setting. Behavioral changes commonly seen in maltreated children may also occur after other adverse and traumatic events of childhood, including death, incarceration, or divorce of a parent; community violence; natural disasters; or sudden death of a close friend (Forkey et al., 2021; Oral et al., 2016). Children may also exhibit temporary behavioral changes and developmental regression after normative family changes, such as a move or new sibling. Children may be overly compliant for their developmental age, may be withdrawn or attach readily to adults they do not know well, may exhibit hypervigilance, or may fail to seek comfort in the clinical setting from parents or caregivers (Child Welfare Information Gateway, 2019b).

2. Physical examination findings consistent with physical abuse

   In some cases, an inflicted injury is obvious to the examiner. In other cases, it may be difficult to distinguish between inflicted and accidental injury or between injury and infection or a chronic medical condition. Yet timely identification of physical abuse can protect vulnerable children and may be able to prevent serious injury or fatalities, especially in infants and young children. Reviews of missed cases of physical abuse show that clinicians tend to miss "sentinel injuries" (Christian & Committee on Child Abuse, 2015, p. e1340), such as bruising; intraoral injuries, including lingual and labial frena tears; and fractures. Common errors include incomplete exams, failure to understand the significance of bruises in preambulatory children, failure to report discrepancies between the history and the physical findings, and failure to obtain imaging when recommended by protocols (Jackson et al., 2015; Keenan et al., 2017). It is important for the clinician to consult with a child abuse team when etiologies of injuries and next steps in evaluation are unclear. **Table 13-1** is a partial list of physical indicators of maltreatment and normal variants or medical conditions that may appear similar on exam and should be considered in a differential diagnosis.

   a. Bruises are the most common injuries in physically abused children. Dating of bruises by appearance has been found to be unreliable (Grossman et al., 2011), and studies evaluating the dating accuracy of bilirubinometers and artificial intelligence analysis of photos are underway (Mesli et al., 2019; Tirado & Mauricio, 2021). Bruising to the center of the face, ears, neck, back, buttocks, upper arms, and backs of the legs and any bruising in a premobile infant raise suspicions of inflicted injury. In one study, half of premobile infants with one or more bruises were found to have been abused, and the majority of these infants had additional occult injuries. Injuries in an additional 23% of cases could not be ruled out as nonaccidental (Feldman et al., 2020). These data support the need for maltreatment to be high on the list of differential diagnoses when premobile infants present with bruising. The mnemonic "TEN4" (bruising to torso, ears, or neck in a child under 4 or any bruising in an infant 4 months or less) is a reminder to order additional imaging and laboratory studies and refer to or consult with child maltreatment experts (Christian & Committee on Child Abuse and Neglect, 2015; Wallace et al., 2021). Bruises over bony prominences in ambulatory children are more consistent with accidental injury (Christian & Committee on Child Abuse and Neglect, 2015).

   b. Burns may be inflicted or accidental. Accidental burns from hot objects, such as heaters or irons, may be difficult to distinguish from inflicted burns because both have patterning. Splash burns, occurring, for example, when a toddler pulls a hot pot or cup off a surface, and burns from hot liquids and foods are more likely to be accidental (Loos et al., 2020). Immersion burns with a stocking or glove demarcation are nearly always inflicted. Hot tap water burns in general, burns with full or deep partial thickness, and burns located bilaterally or on the back of the torso are concerning for inflicted injury (Loos et al., 2020).

   c. Fractures are common in children, and distinguishing inflicted from accidental fractures can be difficult. Spiral fractures can be the result of inflicted or accidental trauma, and some preambulatory infants in walkers have sustained accidental fractures. The following findings on physical or radiologic examination should raise suspicions of physical abuse (Flaherty et al., 2014; Walker et al., 2016):
      i. Fractures in a preambulatory infant
      ii. Fractures in different stages of healing
      iii. Rib fractures, particularly in younger children and especially posteromedial and scapular, sternal, or spinous process fractures
      iv. Classic metaphyseal lesions (CMLs), including bucket-handle or corner fractures (from shaking or squeezing)

   d. Abusive head trauma (AHT) may be inflicted by shaking, striking, or throwing an infant and is implicated in most cases of fatal physical abuse. Presentations may be acute or subtle, with children often misdiagnosed in emergency settings as suffering from a viral illness because of lethargy, vomiting, and poor feeding (Narang et al., 2020). Even though an isolated skull fracture is consistent with a history of accidental fall, a recent review of infants with this history and injury indicates that they should be evaluated for AHT before discharge (Boruah et al., 2021). The following findings on exam or imaging can be associated with AHT and, when found together, are highly specific for abuse:
      i. Altered mental status
      ii. Apnea
      iii. Extensive retinal hemorrhages or retinal tears (retinoschisis)—seen on dilated examination by a pediatric ophthalmologist
      iv. Skull fractures, additional long-bone or rib fractures
      v. Intracranial hemorrhages—usually subdural (also may be present in coagulopathies and other medical conditions)

   e. Thoracoabdominal trauma: Squeezing or punching may result in rib fractures, trauma to underlying

Table 13-1 Physical Findings or Conditions That May Mimic Findings in Child Maltreatment

Findings	Inflicted Injury/Abuse	Normal Variant or Medical Condition
Circular crusted plaques with red margins	Burns from cigarettes or other hot circular-tipped objects	Impetigo Iatrogenic: wart removal
Bullae	Inflicted burns	Accidental burns Bullous impetigo
Marked erythema with or without vesicles or bullae	Immersion burns	Staphylococcal scalded skin syndrome Toxic epidermal necrolysis
Red or hyperpigmented handprint	Slapping	In sun-exposed areas: phytophotodermatitis
Ecchymoses	Inflicted injury from grabbing, pinching, punching, or slapping	Accidental injury Clotting or bleeding disorders, chronic or acute (e.g., hemophilia vs. idiopathic thrombocytopenic purpura) Infants: birthmarks (congenital dermal melanocytosis) Neonates: bruising from precipitous delivery Ambulatory children: accidental impact to forehead with movement of ecchymoses during healing Allergic "shiners"
Swollen red eyelid or orbital area	Fresh inflicted injury	Periorbital cellulitis
Scratches on wrists, popliteal spaces, back, genital area	Scratching, restraining child	Self-inflicted secondary to atopic dermatitis, lichen sclerosis, or neuropsychiatric conditions
Fractures inconsistent with history or child's developmental level; multiple fractures at different stages of healing	Grabbing, twisting, throwing, striking	Pathologic fractures related to osteogenesis imperfecta or other bone abnormalities
Skull fractures	Abusive head trauma from shaking, striking, or throwing an infant	Accidental fall or trauma
Prepubertal vulvovaginitis, including with mucopurulent vaginal discharge	*Neisseria gonorrhoeae* or *Chlamydia trachomatis* infection (Absence of discharge does not indicate lack of infection)	*Streptococcus pyogenes* or *Salmonella shigella* infection Intravaginal foreign body (e.g., toilet paper) Irritation from soaps/bath wash
Clear, gray, or whitish vaginal discharge in early puberty	Nonspecific or may indicate bacterial vaginosis, trichomoniasis	Physiologic leukorrhea common in sexual maturity rating stages 2 and 3
Vulvar/vaginal trauma	Penetration (penis, finger, or foreign object), nonpenetrative but forceful touching or groping	Straddle injuries, physiologic variations in the appearance of the hymen, variations in pigmentation of the tissues, labial adhesion, urethral prolapse
Anal fissure	Penetration (penis, finger, or foreign object)	Functional constipation/hard stools
Anal dilation	Penetration (penis, finger, or foreign object)	Stool in the vault, constipation, neuromuscular conditions
Weight loss or failure to thrive	Neglect	Metabolic, neuromuscular, or cardiac abnormalities, including malabsorption syndromes Depression Eating disorders

structures, or abdominal trauma. Children may not have surface bruising, and the examination can be confounded by other injuries or concurrent head injury. Laboratory testing, including blood counts, liver and pancreatic enzymes, and imaging studies, including skeletal survey and computed tomography with contrast, are indicated (Christian & Committee on Child Abuse and Neglect, 2015; Danaher et al., 2018). Nonspecific examination findings may include:
  i. Decreased or absent bowel sounds
  ii. Guarding or abdominal muscle rigidity
  iii. Shallow and painful breathing
3. Physical examination findings highly suggestive of sexual abuse
  a. In examinations of sexually abused children, physical findings are rare; over 95% of examinations of children who are evaluated for sexual abuse show no evidence of trauma or infection (Jenny & Crawford-Jakubiak, 2013; Smith et al., 2018). This lack of physical exam findings is due to a combination of factors. Many forms of child sexual abuse do not cause physical injury (e.g., touching or oral contact with genitalia or exposing a child to pornographic material). When present, minor irritation or superficial injury generally heal quickly, and even more involved injuries can heal completely before an exam occurs because delays in disclosure are common (Chiesa & Goldson, 2017).
  b. The APN who regularly examines the genital area of prepubertal children during well-child examinations will be more comfortable distinguishing normal from abnormal findings (Monasterio & Schapiro, 2019). However, abnormal findings are often difficult to determine without special magnification equipment. When sexual assault has been disclosed or is suspected, the examination should be performed by or in consultations with an expert in sexual abuse examinations. Similarly, in the event of incidental apparent abnormal exam findings, an expert should be consulted for confirmation and interpretation of findings. Please refer to Table 13-1, which includes a partial differential of certain physical exam findings that may be suspicious for sexual abuse.
  c. The following are findings that are highly suggestive of sexual abuse (Adams et al., 2018):
    i. Vulvar/vaginal trauma
      a. Vaginal laceration or acute laceration or bruising of the labia, posterior fourchette, or vestibule without a history of accidental injury
      b. Acute trauma to the hymen, including partial or complete transection, bruising, abrasions, or petechiae
      c. Healed hymenal transection—a cleft that extends to or beyond the base of the tissue, located between 3 o'clock and 9 o'clock
      d. Partial or complete removal of the clitoral hood, clitoris, labia minora, or labia majora can all be indicative of female genital mutilation.
    ii. Penile trauma: Although uncommon in sexual abuse, this may be associated with severe physical abuse. Acute lacerations or bruising of the penis, scrotum, or perineum are suggestive of abuse (Adams et al., 2018). Balanitis is not typically associated with sexual abuse and is most often caused by hygiene concerns.
    iii. Anorectal trauma: Acute perianal laceration that is deep enough to expose tissue below the dermis is concerning for abuse. On the other hand, although penetration may cause fissures, the most common cause of an anal fissure is a large, hard stool, so fissures in themselves are nonspecific. Although dilation of the anal sphincter may raise suspicion of abuse, there are a number of other potential etiologies, and there is no expert consensus on the significance of the finding in confirming abuse. In the nonacute period, perianal scarring is a rare finding and can be difficult to diagnose, especially in the absence of previous documentation of injury in the same location.
    iv. Sexually transmitted infections: When perinatal transmission, transmission by blood or contaminated needles, and transmission by consensual sexual activity in adolescents have all been ruled out, infection with gonorrhea, chlamydia, syphilis, *Trichomonas vaginalis*, or HIV in children is indicative of sexual contact. Infection in the genital or anal area with molluscum contagiosum, genital warts (caused by human papillomavirus), or herpes simplex virus (HSV) lesions can all result from either sexual or nonsexual transmission. Interpretation must consider the context, including the history, infection status of caregivers, and history of similar lesions in the child in the past (e.g., history of oral HSV lesions or molluscum on other parts of the body) (Adams et al., 2018). See Section A.2 under "Plan for further discussion of testing for sexually transmitted infections (STIs) in cases of suspected maltreatment."
    v. A positive pregnancy test and the presence of semen in a specimen taken directly from the child are confirmatory of sexual contact (Adams et al., 2018).
4. Physical examination findings consistent with neglect

a. Physical signs of neglect may include evidence of generally poor hygiene, inadequate clothing, and failure to grow and gain weight as expected during childhood. Failure to thrive has a variety of causes, including congenital heart disease, malabsorption syndromes, neuromuscular disorders, and relational dysfunctions between caregiver and child (Homan, 2016). These relational challenges may be related to neglect or to a caregiver's appropriate anxieties about a medically fragile child who does not respond easily to customary caretaking strategies.
b. A failure to gain weight may also be an outcome of medical child abuse, in which a child is not being fed or given laxatives or emetics to induce symptoms of a medical condition (Hornor, 2021).
5. Physical exam findings consistent with trafficking
Physical exam findings in trafficked children and youth are not always present and are nonspecific. The following findings may, however, raise concern about the minor's risk for being trafficked and warrant further assessment.
a. Physical injury—blunt-force trauma, cuts, burns, ligature marks, bruising to face/neck/upper arms, fractures, broken teeth
b. Poor diet or malnutrition—signs of dehydration, severe weight loss, dental decay
c. Sexual health concerns—frequent urinary tract infections (UTIs), recurrent STIs, a diagnosis of HIV/AIDS, pelvic pain, genital or anal/rectal trauma, pregnancy (especially multiple undesired pregnancies)
d. Tattoos of names, gang affiliation, sexually explicit content, or referencing property/sale (Greenbaum et al., 2017; Hornor et al., 2019; National Human Trafficking Resource Center, 2016)

III. Assessment

Child maltreatment does not always fit easily into a medical model or diagnostic algorithm in which one can "rule out" or "rule in" abuse or neglect. Many physical signs and behaviors associated with abuse are also associated with infections, serious chronic conditions, or variations of normal. Children and their caregivers may withhold elements of the history because of shame, fear, gaps in memory, or other reasons. This history, alone or considered together with physical findings, could aid in the determination or elimination of child maltreatment as a likely explanation for a given clinical picture.

However, the APN's legal responsibility usually hinges on a reasonable suspicion or concern rather than a firm or even likely diagnosis (Child Welfare Information Gateway, 2019a) (see **Table 13-2**). The elements listed in Table 13-2 should be carefully assessed when the APN suspects child maltreatment.

Table 13-2 Child Maltreatment: Associated Factors That May Trigger an Independent Report

Adverse Conditions	Specific Reportable Behaviors	Variations from State to State
Intimate partner violence	Intimate partner violence committed in front of a child Physical injury to a child reportable under child abuse laws	Reportable in some states but not others Adds to criminal charges or sentencing of offender in some states Offender may have to pay for child's counseling
Substance abuse	Exposure of a child to substance abuse Manufacturing or using methamphetamine in front of a child Substance abuse affecting parenting ability Prenatal use of substances affecting a fetus Newborn testing positive for drugs of abuse	Specifically reportable in some states but not others Providing substances to a child or failure to prevent access reportable in all states Some states have mandated follow-up for prenatally exposed newborns with evaluation by child protective services before discharge
Poverty	Homelessness Failure to provide adequate food, clothing, shelter, health care	Homelessness reportable in some states, specifically excluded in others Inability to provide stable, adequate housing may be related to reporting in some states Some states have exemptions for personal or religious beliefs
Truancy	Failure to send child to school or provide home schooling, failure to ensure child goes to school	Check individual state laws—in some states, a violation of truancy laws; not under child protection laws

Data from U.S. Department of Health and Human Services, Child Welfare Information Gateway. (n.d.). State statutes search. Retrieved from https://www.childwelfare.gov/topics/systemwide/laws-policies/state/

A. Determining need for further evaluation and safety
1. Is further testing or examination warranted by experts in child physical or sexual abuse?
   a. Sentinel injuries and/or serious physical injuries that need expert evaluation to determine whether inflicted, accidental, or a sign of physical illness
   b. Child is severely or critically ill (e.g., altered mental status, apnea or breathing difficulties, extensive bruising with concerns for myoglobinuria, significant burns).
   c. Equivocal examination, for example, an unusual finding on genital exam that needs further expertise for diagnosis and assessment of specificity for abuse
   d. Disclosure of sexual abuse or assault, especially involving penetration or exchange of body fluids. If the abuse or assault occurred recently, forensic evidence such as DNA, semen, or saliva may be present and can be collected in a forensic evidence kit. The post-assault time period defined as "acute" varies by jurisdiction, and clinicians should consult with their county's designated sexual abuse center or consultant to determine next steps because the child or adolescent may need to be transported to a specialized center for forensic examination, usually a designated emergency room or child advocacy center within or near the county where the abuse took place.
2. Is it safe for the child or adolescent to go home? Although CPS ultimately makes this decision, the APN's concerns will affect the urgency of reporting and referral.
   a. Do the suspected injuries or overall physical condition warrant hospitalization?
   b. Does the suspected abuser live with and/or provide care for the child, raising concern for imminent danger to the child?
   c. Is the caregiver with the child a possible suspect?
   d. Can the caregiver with the child keep the child safe?
      i. Willingness and ability to protect the child and prevent contact with the alleged offender.
      ii. Safe transport (e.g., Does the caregiver have access to transportation? Is the caregiver or anticipated driver sober?)
   e. Will the disclosure or reporting of maltreatment put the child or caregiver at increased risk?
      i. Family reactions to disclosure
      ii. Adolescents who experience harsh punishment after reporting nonfamilial sexual abuse or assault connected to behavior that breaks family rules (e.g., sneaking out to a party)
      iii. Risk for retaliation or further abuse by a trafficker who learns about the disclosure
      iv. Risk for loss of shelter
3. Are there potential safety issues for the APN in reporting?
   a. Suspected offending caregiver in the clinic
   b. Reactions of nonoffending caregiver of child or adolescent
   c. Retaliative action by a trafficker
B. Determining the need to report
   If a child maltreatment report is indicated, it is important to approach the family with transparency and compassion, balancing child safety with family support, and with the ultimate aim of maintaining child–caregiver relationships when possible.
   1. Does the situation warrant mandatory reporting in the state in which the APN is practicing?
      a. Consultation with other clinic providers
      b. Consultation with local child abuse reporting hotline
   2. How urgent is the report (related to safety issues described previously)?
      a. Immediate
         i. Immediate safety issues
         ii. Legal issues: evidence collection or documentation
      b. End of the day (disclosures of past abuse, child and caregiver currently safe, sexual abuse outside of home beyond acute period)
C. Are the child's and family's immediate needs being met?
   1. When suspected maltreatment is part of the family's chief complaint
      a. Determine their expectations for outcome regarding housing safety (e.g., shelter versus arrest of suspected offender, which is not always immediate, vs. a safety plan in which the alleged offender agrees to leave the home).
      b. Further testing desired by child and family
   2. If suspected maltreatment is not the chief complaint of the child or caregiver
      a. It is important for the APN not to lose sight of child and family priorities, which may be equally or more urgent than the investigation of maltreatment.
      b. If a report is necessary, a collaborative approach with the family and respect for their priorities can help preserve provider–family relationships.

IV. Plan
A. Diagnostic testing
   1. Imaging: Order in consultation with radiologist or child abuse specialist to determine occult, old, and healing fractures.
      a. If inflicted fractures are suspected in children younger than 2 years, a full skeletal survey should be ordered (Christian & Committee on Child Abuse and Neglect, 2015; Flaherty et al. 2014). A skeletal survey should be considered in children aged 2–5 with other severe injuries and/or a history that raises concern for possible fractures.

b. Rib fractures, especially posterior; oral injuries in children younger than 2; and bruising in premobile children should prompt a head computed tomography (CT) scan or ultrafast head magnetic resonance imaging (MRI) and ophthalmology consult to look for signs of AHT (Narang et al., 2020).
2. Laboratory testing
If there is a new disclosure of sexual assault or abuse within the time period for forensic evidence, examination and laboratory testing should be ordered by a specialized sexual abuse forensic testing center.
   a. Routine STI cultures are not recommended in the asymptomatic prepubertal child because both testing sensitivity and infection rates of prepubertal sexually abused children are low (Adams et al., 2016; Jenny & Crawford-Jakubiak, 2013). Screening of prepuberal children should be considered based on other risk factors: when there are STI signs or symptoms, when the child has already been diagnosed with an STI, when penetration has occurred, when the perpetrator was unknown to the child, when the perpetrator has a known STI or has high-risk behaviors, when a sibling or other household family member has an STI, when the incidence of STIs in the community is high, when the child is unable to verbalize details of the assault, or by parental request (CDC, 2021a; Jenny & Crawford-Jakubiak, 2013). Adolescents are at higher risk for STIs after sexual abuse or exploitation and should be screened for all STIs (Jenny & Crawford-Jakubiak, 2013).
   b. Many sites screen all children being evaluated for sexual abuse with nucleic acid amplification testing (NAAT) of urine samples for gonorrhea and chlamydia because collection is noninvasive and asymptomatic infection can be detected; positive NAAT tests are confirmed with additional testing (Adams et al., 2018; CDC, 2021a).
   c. NAAT is also available for *T. vaginalis* and can be used as a more sensitive alternative to wet mount. NAAT or viral culture for HSV should be used to test any genital or perianal vesicles, ulcers, or lesions. Wet mount can be used to detect bacterial vaginosis and candidiasis (CDC, 2021a).
   d. Serologic testing for antibodies should be as indicated for HIV, *Treponema pallidum*, and hepatitis B (CDC, 2021a).
   e. Due to the incubation period of infectious organisms, follow-up STI testing 2–6 weeks after the exam may be indicated when a single incident of sexual abuse occurred less than 2 weeks before the time of the examination (CDC, 2021a).

B. Management
1. Provide appropriate medical care, including treatment of injuries or infections as indicated.
   a. Prophylactic treatment of adolescents to prevent STIs in cases of sexual assault, including HIV prophylaxis if indicated (CDC, 2021b). Given the low incidence of STI infection after abuse in prepubertal children, prophylaxis of prepubertal children is not universally recommended, although there will be rare cases when it is indicated (CDC, 2021a).
   b. The decision to treat prepubertal children with postexposure prophylaxis (PEP) for HIV should be made with consideration for the local HIV epidemiology, and the circumstances of the assault, including the assailant's risk of HIV infection. Although PEP is safe and well tolerated in children, a provider specialized in treating children with HIV should be consulted regarding dosing, baseline lab tests, and follow-up (CDC, 2021a).
   c. When the assault involved vaginal contact, adolescents and postmenarchal children should be screened for pregnancy and offered emergency contraception if care is being provided within 120 hours of the time of the assault (CDC, 2021b).
2. As indicated previously, refer any child or adolescent with sexual abuse or assault of less than 72 hours (or up to 10 days in some localities) to police and specialized child sexual abuse forensic team. Beyond the acute exam cutoff time, the child can be referred to the local child advocacy center for medical evaluation.
3. Make a child abuse report if maltreatment is suspected, following state and local procedures for verbal (telephone) and written reporting; usually, both are required.
   a. Consider informing the parent about a report if it is safe for the provider, to maintain transparency and trust in the therapeutic relationship.
   b. Involve the adolescent in making a report.
      i. In most states, reporting of abuse is required by law, regardless of the adolescent's wishes; in some states, in the absence of confirmed or suspected trafficking, the provider has discretion, and the adolescent can decline to report extrafamilial sexual assault to law enforcement if the suspected offender is not a parent or caregiver (Child Welfare Information Gateway, 2019a).
      ii. Discuss APN legal responsibilities and adolescent decision making about disclosing versus withholding information.
4. Arrange follow-up care.
   a. Referral to counseling or local child advocacy center, if not arranged by law enforcement or CPS
   b. Follow-up supports for family
      i. Practical and material (food banks, shelter assistance, transportation vouchers, legal assistance)
      ii. Health supervision and support: public health nursing and health education
   c. Close clinic follow-up as indicated

V. Resources
A. Patient education and support

Many states have excellent websites with parent and child educational material in multiple languages. The Child Welfare and Information Gateway at https://www.childwelfare.gov/ is an excellent site for parent and provider education, with some materials available in Spanish. Following is a partial list of additional resources.

1. TIC resources
   a. Resources for child TIC (Substance Abuse and Mental Health Services Administration [SAMHSA]): https://www.samhsa.gov/childrens-awareness-day/past-events/2018/child-traumatic-stress-resources
   b. National Child Traumatic Stress Network: https://www.nctsn.org/trauma-informed-care
2. Screening for ACEs and other maltreatment risk factors
   a. Centers for Disease Control and Prevention: https://www.cdc.gov/violenceprevention/aces/index.html
   b. ACES Aware: https://www.acesaware.org
   c. Safe Environment for Every Kid (SEEK): https://seekwellbeing.org/seek-materials/
   d. Well Child Care, Evaluation, Community Resources, Advocacy, Referral, Education (WE CARE): https://sirenetwork.ucsf.edu/tools-resources/resources/we-care
3. Sexual abuse and assault: testing and treatment for STIs
   a. CDC 2021 guidelines: https://www.cdc.gov/std/treatment-guidelines/sexual-assault.htm
4. Trafficking resources
   a. VERA Institute: https://www.vera.org/downloads/publications/human-trafficking-identification-tool-and-user-guidelines.pdf
   b. West Coast Children's Center: https://www.westcoastcc.org/cse-it/
   c. Polaris Project: https://polarisproject.org/human-trafficking/
   d. Dignity PEARRS tool: https://www.dignityhealth.org/content/dam/dignity-health/pdfs/pearrtoolm15nofield2019.pdf

References

Adams, J. A., Farst, K. J., & Kellogg, N. D. (2018). Interpretation of medical findings in suspected child sexual abuse: An update for 2018. *Journal of Pediatric and Adolescent Gynecology, 31*(3), 225–231. doi:10.1016/j.jpag.2017.12.011

Adams, J. A., Kellogg, N. D., Farst, K. J., Harper, N. S., Palusci, V. J., Frasier, L. D., Levitt, C. J., Shapiro, R. A., Moles, R. L., & Starling, S. P. (2016). Updated guidelines for the medical assessment and care of children who may have been sexually abused. *Journal of Pediatric and Adolescent Gynecology, 29*(2), 81–87. doi:10.1016/j.jpag.2015.01.007

Azzopardi, C., Cohen, E., Pépin, K., Netten, K., Birken, C., & Madigan, S. (2021). Child welfare system involvement among children with medical complexity. *Child Maltreatment, 27*(2), 257–266. doi.org/10.1177/10775595211029713

Barnes, A. J., Anthony, B. J., Karatekin, C., Lingras, K. A., Mercado, R., & Thompson, L. A. (2020). Identifying adverse childhood experiences in pediatrics to prevent chronic health conditions. *Pediatric Research, 87*(2), 362–370. doi:10.1038/s41390-019-0613-3

Baron, E. J., Goldstein, E. G., & Wallace, C. T. (2020). Suffering in silence: How COVID-19 school closures inhibit the reporting of child maltreatment. *Journal of Public Economics, 190*, 104258. doi:10.1016/j.jpubeco.2020.104258

Bhushan, D., Kotz, K., McCall, J., Wirtz, S., Gilgoff, R., Dube, S., Powers, C., Olson-Morgan, J., Galeste, M., Patterson, K., Harris, L., Mills, A., Bethell, C., Burke Harris, N., & Office of the California Surgeon General. (2020). *Roadmap for resilience: The California Surgeon General's report on adverse childhood experiences, toxic stress and health*. Office of the California Surgeon General. https://osg.ca.gov/wp-content/uploads/sites/266/2020/12/Roadmap-For-Resilience_CA-Surgeon-Generals-Report-on-ACEs-Toxic-Stress-and-Health_12092020.pdf

Boruah, A. P., Potter, T. O., Shammassian, B. H., Hills, B. B., Dingeldein, M. W., & Tomei, K. L. (2021). Evaluation of nonaccidental trauma in infants presenting with skull fractures: A retrospective review. *Journal of Neurosurgery: Pediatrics, 28*(3), 268–277. doi:10.3171/2021.2.Peds20872

Canning, H. S., & Peterson, C. (2020). Encouraging more open-ended recall in child interviews. *Psychiatry Psychology and Law, 27*(1), 81–94. doi:10.1080/13218719.2019.1687045

Centers for Disease Control and Prevention. (2021a). *Sexual assault and abuse of children. Sexually transmitted infections treatment guidelines.* https://www.cdc.gov/std/treatment-guidelines/sexual-assault-children.htm

Centers for Disease Control and Prevention. (2021b). *Sexual assault and abuse and STIs—adolescents and adults. Sexually transmitted infections treatment guidelines.* https://www.cdc.gov/std/treatment-guidelines/sexual-assault-adults.htm

Chiesa, A., & Goldson, E. (2017). Child sexual abuse. *Pediatrics in Review, 38*(3), 105. doi:10.1542/pir.2016-0113

Child Abuse Prevention and Treatment Act (CAPTA). 42 USCA § 5106g(2) (West Supp. 1998).

Child Welfare Information Gateway. (2018). *Human trafficking: Protecting our youth.* U.S. Department of Health and Human Services, Children's Bureau. https://www.childwelfare.gov/pubPDFs/trafficking_ts_2018.pdf

Child Welfare Information Gateway. (2019a). *Definitions of child abuse and neglect: State statutes series.* U.S. Department of Health and Human Services, Children's Bureau. https://www.childwelfare.gov/pubPDFs/define.pdf

Child Welfare Information Gateway. (2019b). *What is child abuse and neglect? Recognizing the signs and symptoms.* U.S. Department of Health and Human Services, Children's Bureau. https://www.childwelfare.gov/pubs/factsheets/whatiscan/

Child Welfare Information Gateway. (2020). *Human trafficking.* U.S. Department of Health and Human Services, Children's Bureau. https://www.childwelfare.gov/topics/systemwide/trafficking/

Child Welfare Information Gateway. (2021). *Child witnesses to domestic violence: Summary of state laws.* U.S. Department of Health and Human Services, Children's Bureau. Rhttps://www.childwelfare.gov/pubPDFs/witnessdv.pdf

Christian, C. W., & Committee on Child Abuse and Neglect. (2015). The evaluation of suspected child physical abuse. *Pediatrics, 135,* e1337–1354. doi:10.1542/peds.2015-0356

Danaher, F., Vandeven, A., Blanchard, A., & Newton, A. W. (2018). Recognizing, diagnosing, and preventing child maltreatment: An update for pediatric clinicians. *Current Opinion in Pediatrics, 30*(4), 582–590. doi:10.1097/mop.0000000000000648

Euser, S., Alink, L. R., Tharner, A., van IJzendoorn, M. H., & Bakermans-Kranenburg, M. J. (2014). Out of home placement to promote safety? The prevalence of physical abuse in residential and foster care. *Children and Youth Services Review, 37,* 64–70. doi:10.1016/j.childyouth.2013.12.002

Feldman, K. W., Tayama, T. M., Strickler, L. E., Johnson, L. A., Kolhatkar, G., DeRidder, C. A., Matthews, D. C., Sidbury, R., & Taylor, J. A. (2020). A prospective study of the causes of bruises in premobile infants. *Pediatric Emergency Care, 36*(2), e43–e49. doi:10.1097/pec.0000000000001311

Ferrara, P., Vitelli, O., Bottaro, G., Gatto, A., Liberatore, P., Binetti, P., & Stabile, A. (2013). Factitious disorders and Munchausen syndrome: The tip of the iceberg. *Journal of Child Health Care, 17*(4), 366–374. doi:10.1177/1367493512462262

Finkelhor, D., Turner, H. A., Shattuck, A., & Hamby, S. L. (2015). Prevalence of childhood exposure to violence, crime, and abuse: Results from the National Survey of Children's Exposure to Violence. *JAMA Pediatrics, 169*(8), 746–754. doi:10.1001/jamapediatrics.2015.0676

Flaherty, E. G., & MacMillan, H. L. (2013). Caregiver-fabricated illness in a child: A manifestation of child maltreatment. *Pediatrics, 132,* 590–597. doi:10.1542/peds.2013-2045

Flaherty, E. G., Perez-Rossello, J. M., Levine, M. A., & Hennrikus, W. L. (2014). Evaluating children with fractures for child physical abuse. *Pediatrics, 133,* e477–e489. doi:10.1542/peds.2013-379

Fleishman, J., Kamsky, H., & Sundborg, S. (2019). Trauma-informed nursing practice. *OJIN: The Online Journal of Issues in Nursing, 24*(2), Manuscript 3. doi:10.3912/OJIN.Vol24No02Man03

Forkey, H., Szilagyi, M., Kelly, E. T., & Duffee, J. (2021). Trauma-informed care. *Pediatrics, 148*(2), e2021052580. doi:10.1542/peds.2021-052580

Greenbaum, J. (2018). Child sex trafficking and commercial sexual exploitation. *Advances in Pediatrics, 65*(1), 55–70. doi:10.1016/j.yapd.2018.04.003

Greenbaum, J., Bodrick, N., & Committee on Child Abuse and Neglect. (2017). Global human trafficking and child victimization. *Pediatrics, 140*(6), e20173138. doi:10.1542/peds.2017-3138

Grossman, S. E., Johnston, A., Vanezis, P., & Perrett, D. (2011). Can we assess the age of bruises? An attempt to develop an objective technique. *Medicine Science & Law, 51,* 170–176. doi:10.1258/msl.2011.010135

Guttmacher Institute. (2021, February 1). *An overview of consent to reproductive health services by young people.* Guttmacher Institute. https://www.guttmacher.org/state-policy/explore/overview-minors-consent-law

Hamilton, J. C., Leventhal, J. M., & Asnes, A. G. (2021). Origins and early management of medical child abuse in routine pediatric care. *JAMA Pediatrics, 175*(8), 771–772. doi:10.1001/jamapediatrics.2021.0919

Homan, G. J. (2016). Failure to thrive: A Practical guide. *American Family Physician, 94*(4), 295-299, https://www.aafp.org/pubs/afp/issues/2016/0815/p295.html

Hornor, G. (2021). Medical child abuse: Essentials for pediatric health care providers. *Journal of Pediatric Health Care.* doi:10.1016/j.pedhc.2021.01.006

Hornor, G., Quinones, S. G., Bretl, D., Courtney, A. B., Herendeen, P. A., Lewin, L., Loyke, J. A., Morris, K., Schapiro, N. A., & Williams, S. (2019). Commercial sexual exploitation of children: An update for the forensic nurse. *Journal of Forensic Nursing, 15*(2), 93–102. doi:10.1097/JFN.0000000000000243

Hunter, A. A., & Flores, G. (2021). Social determinants of health and child maltreatment: A systematic review. *Pediatric Research, 89*(2), 269–274. doi:10.1038/s41390-020-01175-x

Institute of Medicine & National Research Council. (2014). *New directions in child abuse and neglect research.* http://www.nap.edu/catalog/18331/new-directions-in-child-abuse-and-neglect-research.

International Labor Organization. (2012). *ILO global estimate of forced labour: Results and methodology.* http://www.ilo.org/wcmsp5/groups/public/—ed_norm/—declaration/documents/publication/wcms_182004.pdf

Jackson, A. M., Deye, K. P., Halley, T., Hinds, T., Rosenthal, E., Shalaby-Rana, E., & Goldman, E. F. (2015). Curiosity and critical thinking: Identifying child abuse before it is too late. *Clinical Pediatrics, 54,* 54–61. doi:10.1177/0009922814549314

Janson, S. (2021). Can we trust our gut feeling when we suspect child abuse? *Acta Paediatrica, 110*(6), 1713–1714. doi:10.1111/apa.15783

Jenny, C., & Crawford-Jakubiak, J. E. (2013). The evaluation of children in the primary care setting when sexual abuse is suspected. *Pediatrics, 132,* e558–e567. doi:10.1542/peds.2013-1741

Jenny, C., & Metz, J. B. (2020). Medical child abuse and medical neglect. *Pediatrics in Review, 41*(2), 49. doi:10.1542/pir.2017-0302

Jordan, K. S., & Steelman, S. H. (2015). Child maltreatment: Interventions to improve recognition and reporting. *Journal of Forensic Nursing, 11*(2), 107–113. doi:10.1097/jfn.0000000000000068

Justice for Victims of Trafficking Act, I U.S.C. § Section 104 (2015). https://www.congress.gov/bill/114th-congress/senate-bill/178

Keenan, H. T., Cook, L. J., Olson, L. M., Bardsley, T., & Campbell, K. A. (2017). Social intuition and social information in physical child abuse evaluation and diagnosis. *Pediatrics, 140*(5), e20171188. doi:10.1542/peds.2017-1188

Keeshin, B. R., & Dubowitz, H. (2013). Childhood neglect: The role of the paediatrician. *Paediatric Child Health, 18,* e39–e43.

Kellogg, N. D. (2010). Sexual behaviors in children: Evaluation and management. *American Family Physician, 82,* 1233–1238.

Landers, A. L., Danes, S. M., Campbell, A. R., & Hawk, S. W. (2021). Abuse after abuse: The recurrent maltreatment of American Indian children in foster care and adoption. *Child Abuse & Neglect, 111,* 104805. doi:10.1016/j.chiabu.2020.104805

Lane, W. G., & Dubowitz, H. (2021). Social determinants of health, personalized medicine, and child maltreatment. *Pediatric Research, 89*(2), 368–376. doi:10.1038/s41390-020-01290-9

Lee, S. J., Ward, K. P., Lee, J. Y., & Rodriguez, C. M. (2022). Parental social isolation and child maltreatment risk during the COVID-19 pandemic. *Journal of Family Violence, 37*(5), 813–824. doi:10.1007/s10896-020-00244-3

Loos, M. H. J., Almekinders, C. A. M., Heymans, M. W., de Vries, A., & Bakx, R. (2020). Incidence and characteristics of non-accidental burns in children: A systematic review. *Burns, 46*(6), 1243–1253. doi:10.1016/j.burns.2020.01.008

Luken, A., Nair, R., & Fix, R. L. (2021). On racial disparities in child abuse reports: Exploratory mapping the 2018 NCANDS. *Child Maltreatment, 26*(3), 267–281. doi:10.1177/10775595211001926

McClure, R. J., Davis, P. M., Meadow, S. R., & Sibert, J. R. (1996). Epidemiology of Munchausen syndrome by proxy, non-accidental poisoning, and non-accidental suffocation. *Archives of Disease in Childhood*, 75(1), 57–61. doi:10.1136/adc.75.1.57

McGeough, B. L., & Sterzing, P. R. (2018). A systematic review of family victimization experiences among sexual minority youth. *Journal of Primary Prevention*, 39(5), 491–528. doi:10.1007/s10935-018-0523-x

Merrick, M. T., Ports, K. A., Ford, D. C., Afifi, T. O., Gershoff, E. T., & Grogan-Kaylor, A. (2017). Unpacking the impact of adverse childhood experiences on adult mental health. *Child Abuse and Neglect*, 69, 10–19. doi:10.1016/j.chiabu.2017.03.016

Mesli, V., Le Garff, E., Marchand, E., Labreuche, J., Ramdane, N., Maynou, C., Delannoy, Y., & Hédouin, V. (2019). Determination of the age of bruises using a bilirubinometer. *Forensic Science International*, 302, 109831. doi:10.1016/j.forsciint.2019.05.047

Monasterio, E. B., & Schapiro, N. A. (2019). Female genitalia. In K. G. Duderstadt (Ed.), *Pediatric physical examination: An illustrated handbook* (3rd ed., pp. 284–301). Elsevier.

Moody, G., Cannings-John, R., Hood, K., Kemp, A., & Robling, M. (2018). Establishing the international prevalence of self-reported child maltreatment: a systematic review by maltreatment type and gender. *BMC Public Health*, 18(1), 1164. doi:10.1186/s12889-018-6044-y

Narang, S. K., Fingarson, A., Lukefahr, J., & Council on Child Abuse and Neglect. (2020). Abusive head trauma in infants and children. *Pediatrics*, 145(4), e20200203. doi:10.154/peds.2020-0203

National Child Traumatic Stress Network. (n.d.). *What is a traumatic event?* https://www.nctsn.org/what-is-child-trauma/about-child-trauma

National Human Trafficking Hotline. (2019, May 6). *What is human trafficking?* https://humantraffickinghotline.org/what-human-trafficking.

National Human Trafficking Resource Center. (2016, February 16). *Identifying victims of human trafficking: What to look for in a healthcare setting.* https://humantraffickinghotline.org/sites/default/files/What%20to%20Look%20for%20during%20a%20Medical%20Exam%20-%20FINAL%20-%202-16-16_0.pdf

Nazer, D., & Greenbaum, J. (2020). Human trafficking of children. *Pediatric Annals*, 49(5), e209–e214. doi:10.3928/19382359-20200417-01

Oral, R., Ramirez, M., Coohey, C., Nakada, S., Walz, A., Kuntz, A., Benoit, J., & Peek-Asa, C. (2016). Adverse childhood experiences and trauma informed care: The future of health care. *Pediatric Research*, 79(1–2), 227–233. doi:10.1038/pr.2015.197

Palusci, V. J., & Botash, A. S. (2021). Race and bias in child maltreatment diagnosis and reporting. *Pediatrics*, 148(1), e2020049625. doi:10.1542/peds.2020-049625

Petruccelli, K., Davis, J., & Berman, T. (2019). Adverse childhood experiences and associated health outcomes: A systematic review and meta-analysis. *Child Abuse & Neglect*, 97, 104127. doi:10.1016/j.chiabu.2019.104127

Petska, H. W., Gordon, J. B., Jablonski, D., & Sheets, L. K. (2017). The intersection of medical child abuse and medical complexity. *Pediatric Clinics of North America*, 64(1), 253–264. doi:10.1016/j.pcl.2016.08.016

Polaris. (2020, November 12). *2019 U.S. National Human Trafficking Hotline statistics.* https://polarisproject.org/2019-us-national-human-trafficking-hotline-statistics/.

Rapp, A., Fall, G., Radomsky, A. C., & Santarossa, S. (2021). Child maltreatment during the COVID-19 pandemic: A systematic rapid review. *Pediatric Clinics of North America*, 68(5), 991–1009. doi:10.1016/j.pcl.2021.05.006

Rebbe, R. (2018). What is neglect? State legal definitions in the United States. *Child Maltreatment*, 23(3), 303–315. doi:10.1177/1077559518767337

Rebbe, R., Nurius, P. S., Courtney, M. E., & Ahrens, K. R. (2018). Adverse childhood experiences and young adult health outcomes among youth aging out of foster care. *Academic Pediatrics*, 18(5), 502–509. doi:10.1016/j.acap.2018.04.011

Reproductive National Health Training Center. (2021). *Mandatory child abuse reporting state* Retrieved 9/27/2021 from https://rhntc.org/resources/mandatory-child-abuse-reporting-state-summaries

Salloum, A., Johnco, C., Smyth, K. M., Murphy, T. K., & Storch, E. A. (2018). Co-Occurring Posttraumatic Stress Disorder and Depression Among Young Children [Article]. *Child Psychiatry & Human Development*, 49(3), 452-459. https://doi.org/10.1007/s10578-017-0764-6

Schaefer, L. M., Howell, K. H., Schwartz, L. E., Bottomley, J. S., & Crossnine, C. B. (2018). A concurrent examination of protective factors associated with resilience and posttraumatic growth following childhood victimization. *Child Abuse & Neglect*, 85, 17–27. doi:10.1016/j.chiabu.2018.08.019

Schapiro, N. A., & Mejia, J. (2018). Adolescent confidentiality and women's health: History, rationale, and current threats. *Nursing Clinics*, 53(2), 145–156. doi:10.1016/j.cnur.2018.01

Schechter, N. L., & Nurko, S. (2019). Unintentional symptom intensification by doctors. *Pediatrics*, 144(5), e20183808. doi:10.1542/peds.2018-3808

Schnierle, J., Christian-Brathwaite, N., & Louisias, M. (2019). Implicit bias: What every pediatrician should know about the effect of bias on health and future directions. *Current Problems in Pediatric & Adolescent Health Care*, 49(2), 34–44. doi:10.1016/j.cppeds.2019.01.003

Shonkoff, J. P., & Garner, A. S. (2012). The lifelong effects of early childhood adversity and toxic stress. *Pediatrics*, 129, e232–e246. doi:10.1542/peds.2011-2663

Smith, T. D., Raman, S. R., Madigan, S., Waldman, J., & Shouldice, M. (2018). Anogenital findings in 3569 pediatric examinations for sexual abuse/assault. *Journal of Pediatric and Adolescent Gynecology*, 31(2), 79–83.

Tirado, J., & Mauricio, D. (2021). Bruise dating using deep learning. *Journal of Forensic Science*, 66(1), 336–346. doi:10.1111/1556-4029.14578

Turner, H. A., Vanderminden, J., Finkelhor, D., & Hamby, S. (2019). Child neglect and the broader context of child victimization. *Child Maltreatment*, 24(3), 265–274. doi:10.1177/1077559518825312

United Nations, Office on Drugs and Crime. (2004). *United Nations Convention Against Transnational Organized Crime and the Protocols Thereto.* https://www.unodc.org/documents/treaties/UNTOC/Publications/TOC%20Convention/TOCebook-e.pdf

U.S. Department of Health and Human Services. (2021). *Child maltreatment 2019.* https://www.acf.hhs.gov/cb/data-research/child-maltreatme

U.S. Department of Health and Human Services. (2022). *Child maltreatment 2020.* https://www.acf.hhs.gov/sites/default/files/documents/cb/cm2020.pdf

Van Niel, C., Pachter, L. M., Wade, R., Jr., Felitti, V. J., & Stein, M. T. (2014). Adverse events in children: Predictors of adult physical and mental conditions. *Journal of Developmental and Behavioral Pediatrics*, 35(8), 549–551. doi:10.1097/dbp.0000000000000102

Vanderminden, J., Hamby, S., David-Ferdon, C., Kacha-Ochana, A., Merrick, M., Simon, T. R., Finkelhor, D., & Turner, H. (2019). Rates of neglect in a national sample: Child and family characteristics and psychological impact. *Child Abuse & Neglect*, 88, 256–265. doi:10.1016/j.chiabu.2018.11.014

Walker, A., Kepron, C., & Milroy, C. M. (2016). Are there hallmarks of child abuse? I. Osseous injuries. *Academic Forensic Pathology*, 6(4), 568–590. doi:10.23907/2016.056

Wallace, F., Collins, J. A., Talawila Da Camara, N., Kemp, A. M., Prosser, I., & Mullen, S. (2021). Fifteen-minute consultation: Bruising in the premobile child. *Archives of Disease in Childhood—Education and Practice*. doi:10.1136/archdischild-2021-321661

Yates, G., & Bass, C. (2017). The perpetrators of medical child abuse (Munchausen syndrome by proxy)—a systematic review of 796 cases. *Child Abuse & Neglect*, 72, 45–53. doi:10.1016/j.chiabu.2017.07.008

Yi, Y., Edwards, F. R., & Wildeman, C. (2020). Cumulative prevalence of confirmed maltreatment and foster care placement for US children by race/ethnicity, 2011–2016. *American Journal of Public Health*, 110(5), 704–709. doi:10.2105/ajph.2019.305554

CHAPTER 14

Childhood Overweight and Obesity

Mary Anne M. Israel and Amy Beck

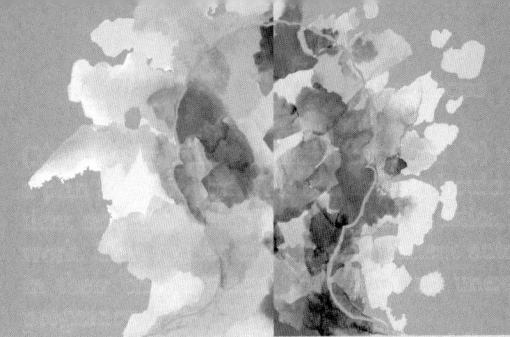

I. Introduction and general background

Pediatric overweight and obesity have been linked to numerous health consequences, including metabolic and cardiovascular disease, increased rates of mental health disorders and increased risk for obesity as an adult (de Onis et al., 2013; Harrington et al., 2013). Recent research indicates that children diagnosed with obesity at 3 years of age have a very high likelihood of having overweight or obesity in adolescence, making prevention and early detection critical (Evensen et al., 2016; Simmonds et al., 2016). *Overweight* is defined as a body mass index (BMI) equal to or greater than 85% and less than 95%, and *obesity* is defined as a BMI equal to or greater than 95%, using sex-specific BMI-for-age growth charts (Ogden et al., 2014). The use of BMI is recommended as the acceptable alternative method of approximating visceral adiposity, which is a predictor of comorbidities such as type II diabetes and metabolic dysfunction-associated steatotic liver disease.(MASLD The gold standard for measuring visceral adiposity is computed tomography (CT) imaging, which exposes patients to radiation and is costly. Given this, it is standard practice to use BMI as our guide in clinical decision making.

In the United States, 19.3% of children and adolescents between 2 and 19 years old have obesity (Centers for Disease Control and Prevention [CDC], 2022). Data from the National Health and Nutrition Examination Survey (NHANES) indicate racial/ethnic disparities in the prevalence of obesity. In 2017–2018, 16.1% of White children, 25.6% of Hispanic children, 24.2% of non-Hispanic Black children, and 8.7% of non-Hispanic Asian children had obesity. Obesity is a complex health condition, as it stems from the impacts of structural racism, biologic and genetic predisposition, health behaviors such as food environment, chronic toxic stress, the built environment, and the healthcare system (The National Institute of Minority Health and Health Disparities' Research Framework, 2021, Loos & Yeo, 2022). Of particular importance, there is increased awareness of the variability of genetic responses to obesogenic environments, where some people develop obesity and some do not, and genetic differences are the primary reason rather than individual choices.. Also critical, is that the impact of structural racism created an inequitable allocation of resources resulting in decreased access to healthy food and green space/recreation for communities of color. Targeted marketing of SSBs and high-calorie, low-nutrient foods to communities of color also contributes to disparities (Barnhill et al., 2022). Research indicates that the intake of sugar-sweetened beverages (SSBs) is strongly correlated to obesity (Acharya et al., 2011; Pan et al., 2014) as is high-calorie, low-nutrient foods and inadequate physical activity (Utesch et al., 2018) Although the prevalence of childhood overweight (BMI > 85%) has remained relatively stable in the United States over the last decade (CDC, 2022), there is still much work to be done to understand and address this epidemic, the underlying structural racism that contributes to disparities, and its effects on children and their families.

A. *Obesity in infancy*

According to NHANES data from 2017–2018, approximately 9.9% of U.S. infants younger than 2 years of age have a high weight for recumbent length (≥95% on the CDC growth chart). Although the diagnosis of overweight or obesity is not generally used in this age group, there is increasing research showing that infants with high weight for length or rapid weight gain are at greater risk of overweight and adverse metabolic and cardiovascular outcomes in both childhood and adulthood (Fryar et al., 2018; Roy et al., 2016). Contributing factors to overweight in infancy include maternal weight gain during pregnancy, maternal BMI at time of pregnancy, and presence of gestational diabetes (Larque et al., 2019; Michaliszyn et al., 2017).

B. Obesity in early childhood

Overweight and obesity in children between 2 and 5-years-old are particularly concerning, and much attention is being paid to prevention in this age group. During this time, BMI generally reaches its minimum point before beginning to increase again (known as the *adiposity rebound*) in early school age. This is a critical point for the prevention of obesity because there is evidence that an early adiposity rebound is predictive of obesity later in life (Brisbois et al., 2012; Hughes et al., 2014).

Key risk factors for the development of obesity in 2- to 5-year-olds include intake of SSBs, energy-dense dietary patterns, and excess screen time (Neshturuk et al., 2021; Pan et al., 2014; Utesch et al., 2018).

C. Obesity in school-age children

In addition to the risk factors in early childhood described previously, children in this group are also beginning to consume more food outside of the home, which can include high amounts of fast food or other "junk" foods. Disturbances in the social environment, such as family strain and insecurity, and other life changes that affect daily life can also be stressors leading to increased intake of junk foods (Hemmingsson, 2018). The COVID-19 pandemic affected children and adolescence in numerous ways, one of which was increased BMI related to increased stress, less access to nutritious foods, increased screen time, and decreased physical activity (Lange, 2021). Body awareness and teasing or bullying by peers may also surface during this period, which can negatively affect self-esteem and emotional health (Maggio et al., 2014; van Geel et al., 2014).

D. Obesity in adolescence

Some consider adolescence to be one of the most challenging periods with regard to overweight and obesity. Puberty brings physical and metabolic changes in the body that may exacerbate the risk for negative sequelae such as insulin resistance (Kelsey, 2016; Jeffrey, 2012). Developmentally, teens are increasingly more independent from their parents, which often includes unsupervised decision making related to food and beverage choices. Excessive sedentary behavior and screen time are also a significant problem when activities such as watching TV, using social media, texting, and playing video games become more common pastimes and sources of peer interaction (Li et al., 2013; Mitchell et al., 2013; Robinson et al., 2017; Tanaka et al., 2014). Studies have shown that physical activity levels decrease significantly in early adolescence, especially among girls (World Health Organization, 2022. Body image may be more of a concern in this age group, and negative mental health consequences associated with being overweight are more prevalent (Maggio et al., 2014; Marmorstein et al., 2014). Body positivity (Markula, 2022) is a movement that supports individuals having a positive body image regardless of how society and popular culture view ideal shape, size, and appearance. Body-positive content on social media (e.g., Instagram) attempts to challenge mainstream beauty ideas by encouraging acceptance of a variety of body types. Recent studies suggest that viewing body-positive content online is connected to increased positive mood and body satisfaction in young women, which might reduce the negative impact on mental health observed previously. More studies are necessary to investigate the impact of body-positive content because some studies suggest this content also increases self-objectification (Cohen et al., 2019). Body neutrality is a concept introduced by eating disorder specialist, Anne Poirier, that encourages a peaceful acceptance and appreciation for one's body and its abilities. For patients who have had years of a negative body image, body neutrality may be easier to achieve and also supports a healthy relationship with one's body.

E. Obesity in special populations

1. Children and adolescents with special health care needs (SHCNs)

There is increasing awareness of the high prevalence of overweight and obesity in children with SHCN or developmental disabilities. Although there are diverse conditions within this population, several factors may contribute to this issue (Abeysekara et al., 2014; CDC, 2019). Restrictive eating habits in some children with conditions such as sensory processing disorders and autism can provide challenges to caregivers' ability to consistently provide balanced and nutritious meals (Padmanabhan & Shroff, 2020). Some psychotropic medications, such as mood stabilizers or atypical antipsychotics, may lead to weight gain (Cockerill et al., 2013). Children with physical impairments or immobility may have decreased ability to participate in sufficient physical activity. Limited access to appropriate environments that can enable exercise or increased pain with activity are contributing factors (Abeysekara et al., 2014). The need for intense cognitive therapies, which are more often sedentary in nature, may also take precedence over physical activity.

2. Children and adolescents with mental health concerns

Proper prevention and management of childhood overweight must include the integration of physical and behavioral health considerations. Children with mental health conditions such as depression may have unique risk factors for overweight, as well as particular challenges in its prevention and management (Korczak et al., 2013). Especially when a mental health condition worsens, a child's or teen's motivation for and interest in physical activity may be negatively affected. The provider must also be aware of the potential for food and eating to be a significant source of coping for some patients and may become disordered as a result. Youth Risk Behavior Surveillance Survey responses indicated that 15% of teens practice some unhealthy eating behaviors, all teens should be evaluated for these symptoms. Providers should be especially concerned if weight loss is >2 lb/week in this age group and should evaluate patients for excessive energy restrictions by the parent or child or unhealthy forms of weight loss (meal skipping, purging, fasting, or excessive exercise; use of fixatives, diet pills, or weight loss supplements). Conversely, the presence of overweight in a child may also contribute to the emergence or worsening of mental health conditions, especially if negative self-esteem or bullying is present (Geoffroy et al., 2014; Rottenberg et al., 2014). Children report that this stigmatization can be experienced when interacting with the healthcare system as well (Pont et al., 2017). General mental health assessment of the parents or guardian should be considered as well because caregivers with impaired mental health may have a compromised ability to promote healthy behaviors in their children (Foster et al., 2020; Zarychta et al., 2020).

II. Database

Figure 14-1 shows the 2007 Expert Committee Recommendations for obesity risk assessment and recommended steps for prevention and treatment in all children (Barlow & Expert Committee, 2007). The following provides a comprehensive overview of pertinent assessment of the child with overweight or obesity. Of note, in January 2023, The American Academy of Pediatrics published, Clinical Practice Guideline for the Evaluation and Treatment of Children and Adolescents With Obesity. This guideline was made available after the chapter was sent for publication and has not been integrated into this chapter.

A. *Subjective*
  1. Past medical/developmental history
     a. Investigate for a history of any physical illnesses that may contribute to weight gain and/or limitations in physical activity, potential stressors such as changes in living situation or family, divorce, as well as any related comorbid conditions and their management plans.
     b. Review current medications and note whether significant changes in weight occurred with their initiation.
     c. If the child is 5 years old or younger or has a significant developmental delay, review the developmental history and note any impact of current or previous delays on nutrition or mobility status.
  2. Family history
     a. Take an accurate history of familial cardiovascular disease (including hypertension and/or hyperlipidemia) and diabetes in the immediate family, especially siblings and parents.
     b. Obtain a comprehensive family mental health history, including disordered eating.
  3. Diet
     Request a detailed history of intake that includes the type of food as well as serving size and overall quantity consumed per day or week. Consider having examples of cup sizes to help families accurately describe the quantity of intake.
     a. Beverages, including sodas, juices, lemonade, sports drinks, sweetened tea, and coffee drinks
     b. Breakfast consumption and what is consumed (e.g., sugar cereals, pastries, bagels)
     c. Nonnutritious snack foods (sweets, chips, etc.)
     d. Intake of fast food or other food prepared outside the home
     e. Fruit and vegetable consumption
     f. Starches low in fiber (made from white flour or white rice, etc.)
  4. Physical activity and sedentary behavior
     a. Minutes per day spent engaged in moderate to vigorous physical activity (breathing hard, sweating, etc.) and type of physical activity
     b. Minutes per day spent in screen-based activities (TV, computer, tablets, gaming, etc.)
     c. Quantity and quality of sleep
  5. Emotional and social history
     a. History of mental/behavioral health conditions and management
     b. Screen for the presence of active symptoms, for example, using a tool like the Pediatric Symptom Checklist (available at http://www.brightfutures.org).
     c. Discuss family eating and activity patterns.
     d. Screen for food and housing insecurity (Cutts & Cook, 2017).
  6. Body image and attitudes toward body
  7. Previous strategies for losing/maintaining weight, if any
  8. Level of readiness, confidence, and motivation for lifestyle changes
  9. Obesity-focused review of systems
     a. General/constitutional: fatigue, unexplained weight gain/loss
     b. Skin: presence of dark patches around neck, abdomen, or underarm area that can't be "scrubbed off"
     c. Head, eyes, ears, nose, and throat (HEENT): snoring and/or gasping for air during sleep
     d. Respiratory: shortness of breath, cough, or wheeze with exercise
     e. Cardiac: history of elevated blood pressure
     f. Gastrointestinal (GI): unexplained nausea or vomiting
     g. Endocrine: irregular/absent menses, polydipsia, polyuria, polyphagia
     h. Musculoskeletal: joint pain
     i. Psychiatric/behavioral: moods, self-harm, suicidal ideation, stress, coping

B. *Objective*
  1. Vital signs
     Measure blood pressure at every visit for children over 3 years of age. Be sure that the appropriate cuff size is used, and if using an electronic sphygmomanometer,

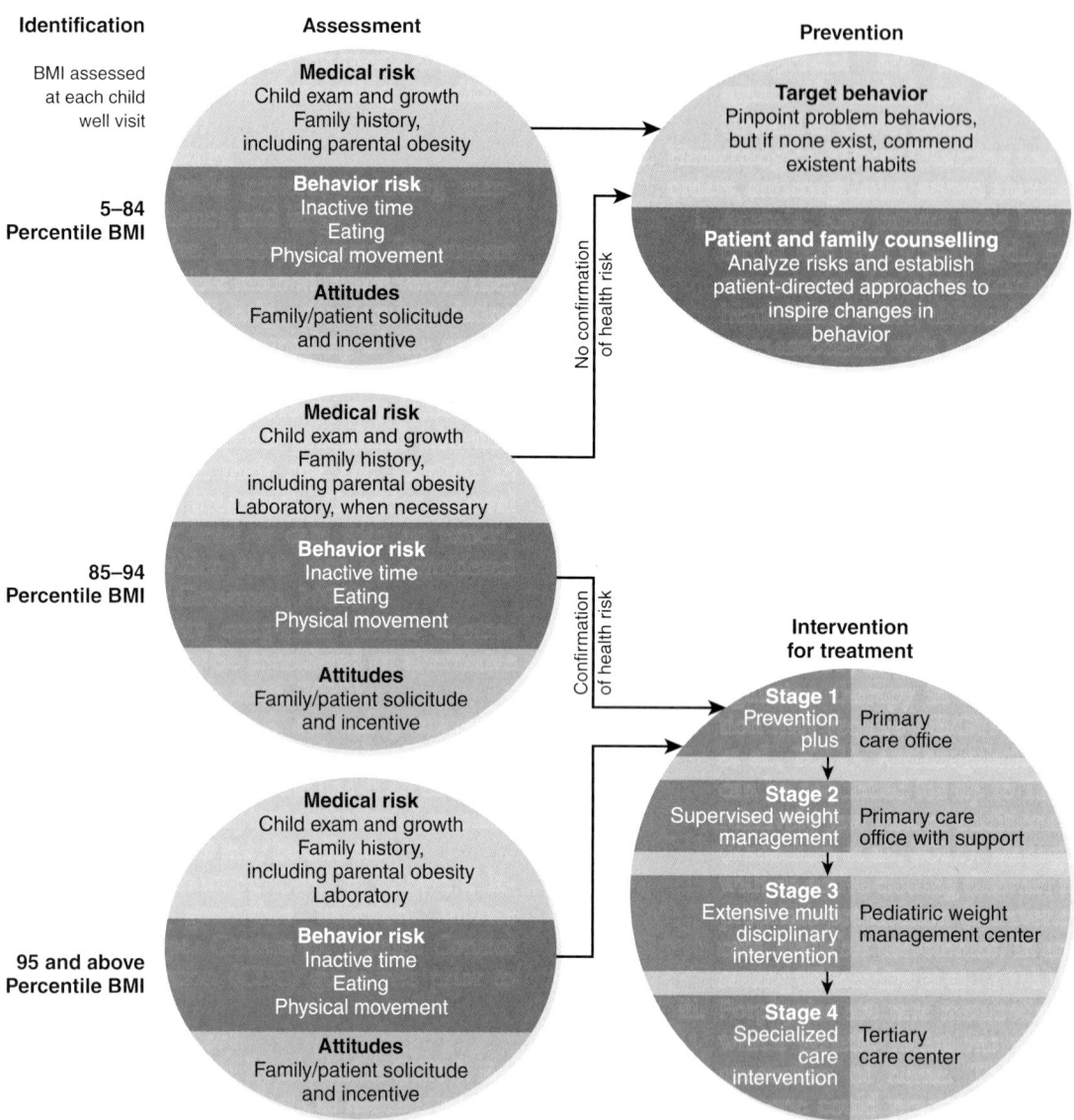

Figure 14-1 Assessment of obesity risk and steps to prevention and treatment.

Barlow, S. E., & Expert Committee. (2007). Expert committee recommendations regarding the prevention, assessment, and treatment of child and adolescent overweight and obesity: Summary report. *Pediatrics, 120*(Suppl. 4), S164–S192. doi:120/Supplement_4/S164

confirm elevated results with a manual cuff. Calculate blood pressure percentile for sex, age, and height percentile using a National Heart, Lung, and Blood Institute chart (Flynn et al., 2017).

2. Anthropometric measurements
   Accurate weight and height should be measured at each visit. Calculate BMI and BMI percentile whenever possible.
3. Physical exam
   a. General: Observe overall appearance of health.
   b. Skin: Inspect posterior neck, axilla, and lower abdomen for evidence of acanthosis nigricans.
   c. HEENT: Inspect tonsils for hypertrophy.
   d. Neck: Palpate thyroid in older children and adolescents.
   e. Chest: Auscultate breath and heart sounds.
   f. GI: Palpate for masses and hepatosplenomegaly.
   g. Musculoskeletal: Observe range of motion in all extremities.
   h. Psychiatric/behavioral: Note affect and mood.
4. Laboratory testing

The primary goal of laboratory analysis in the child with obesity is to evaluate for comorbid conditions, based on the presence of risk factors and/or any current symptoms (Barlow & Expert Committee, 2007). Elevated BMI, together with unhealthy lifestyle behaviors and/or a family history of obesity-related conditions, can be a strong predictor of metabolic and cardiovascular disease risk (de Onis et al., 2013; Friedemann et al., 2012; Harrington et al., 2013), and thus screening for these conditions should be considered.

When deciding whether to perform laboratory analysis, it is important to consider whether the results will in any way alter the treatment plan. If the answer is no, then the provider should consider whether there is true justification for the use of resources and subjecting the patient to the trauma of venipuncture. It is possible that abnormal lab results can be useful in patient/family education, regardless of whether they will affect the overall management plan. An example is a lab report that demonstrates mildly elevated lipids, which would most often be treated with lifestyle modifications but could still be a powerful visual indicator for the family that the child's condition has had a negative physical impact.

Although there are no clear guidelines for laboratory studies in the evaluation of pediatric obesity, consider risk-based screening for the following in children over 8–10 years of age and/or a child of any age with increased risk:

    a. Diabetes: HgbA1c, fasting glucose (or if strong concerns about presence of hyperglycemia in clinic, perform a random fingerstick glucose)
    b. Metabolic dysfunction-associated steatotic liver disease (MASLD): aspartate aminotransferase (AST), alanine aminotransferase (ALT)
    c. Hyperlipidemia: fasting lipid panel
    d. Hypertension: complete metabolic panel
    e. Hypovitaminosis D: 25-hydroxyvitamin D

5. Other diagnostics

Other diagnostic evaluations may be useful in the diagnosis of comorbid conditions, such as an ultrasound of the liver to confirm the diagnosis of NAFLD or a sleep study to confirm the diagnosis of obstructive sleep apnea or obesity hypoventilation syndrome. These conditions are generally co-managed with pediatric subspecialists, and thus it may be helpful to consult with such specialists prior to ordering additional studies to confirm what is needed.

III. Assessment

A. *Classification using BMI percentile*
B. *Although very uncommon, consider evaluating for an underlying cause of obesity (endocrine, genetic, cerebral, or medication induced), particularly if weight gain is sudden over a brief period and/or not well explained through patient and family history (Kleinendorst, 2020).*
C. *Identify co-occurring illnesses or conditions, including mental health concerns and social needs.*
D. *Motivation and confidence*
Use motivational interviewing methods to determine the patient's and family's perception of the child's weight and overall health, as well as the level of motivation and confidence in the ability to make lifestyle changes (Hooker et al., 2018). It is important to focus on current or potential future health outcomes rather than weight alone.

IV. Plan

The foundation for the prevention or management of childhood overweight is lifestyle modifications related to nutritional intake, physical activity, and adequate sleep, often by the entire family (CDC, 2022).

Figure 14-2 illustrates a staged approach to treatment according to the child's age and BMI percentile (Barlow & Expert Committee, 2007). The following presents a complete plan for managing the child or adolescent with overweight in primary care. It is important to note that it may not be possible to cover everything in one visit; rather, the plan should include frequent follow-up to provide continuing education, review goal setting, and monitor progress. It is also possible that the following would not be carried out by the PCP alone but in collaboration with other professionals. Ideally, holistic and comprehensive care for patients with overweight and obesity will involve an interdisciplinary team of clinicians that may include a registered dietician, behavioral health provider, and/or pediatric specialists as indicated.

A. *Although extremely rare, if secondary obesity is suspected, treat or refer for treatment of underlying cause.*
B. *Provide family-centered education.*
    1. Multifactorial etiology of obesity and associated health risks
    2. Importance of healthy nutrition, physical activity, and sleep routines for all members of the family
    3. All members involved in child/adolescent's daily life using supportive and body-positive approach
    4. Impact of weight and height changes on BMI for children who are still growing
    5. Realistic expectations for weight or BMI changes over time
C. *Encourage lifestyle modification where appropriate.*
    1. Nutrition counseling
        a. Use "My Plate" (**Figure 14-3**) to encourage a balanced distribution of nutrients and healthy portion sizes.
        b. Encourage reduction/elimination of all SSBs.
        c. Review healthy eating behaviors, such as eating meals at the table as a family and not eating in front of screens.
        d. Provide culturally tailored resources for grocery shopping and recipes for meals.
    2. Activity counseling and community referrals
        a. Review recommendations for at least 60 minutes (cumulative) of moderate to vigorous activity and less than 2 hours of nonacademic screen time daily.
        b. Discuss creative ways to find enjoyable physical activities for the family.
        c. Provide resources and referrals for low-cost, safe local activity options.

150 Chapter 14 Childhood Overweight and Obesity

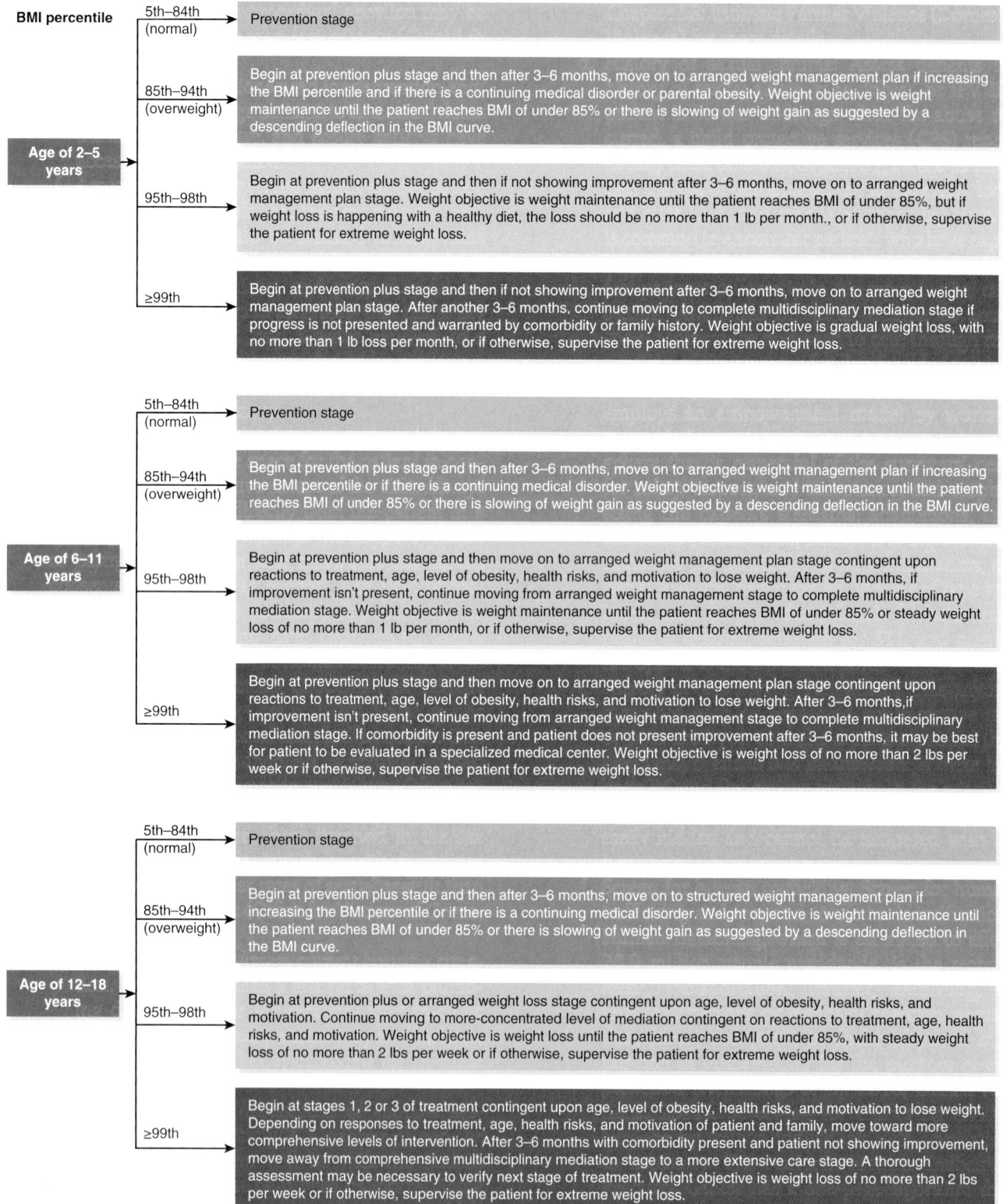

Figure 14-2 Staged Treatment of Obesity According to Age and BMI

Barlow, S. E., & Expert Committee. (2007). Expert committee recommendations regarding the prevention, assessment, and treatment of child and adolescent overweight and obesity: Summary report. *Pediatrics, 120*(Suppl. 4), S164–S192. doi:120/Supplement_4/S164

    d. For children with special needs, encourage participation in suitable physical activity whenever possible.

    e. Emphasize the importance of sleep hygiene to support adequate sleep for age.

3. Set SMART (Specific, Measurable, Achievable, Realistic, Timely) goals for nutrition and activity, to be followed up at next visit. Write them on a prescription pad for the family to take home and post in a visible location.

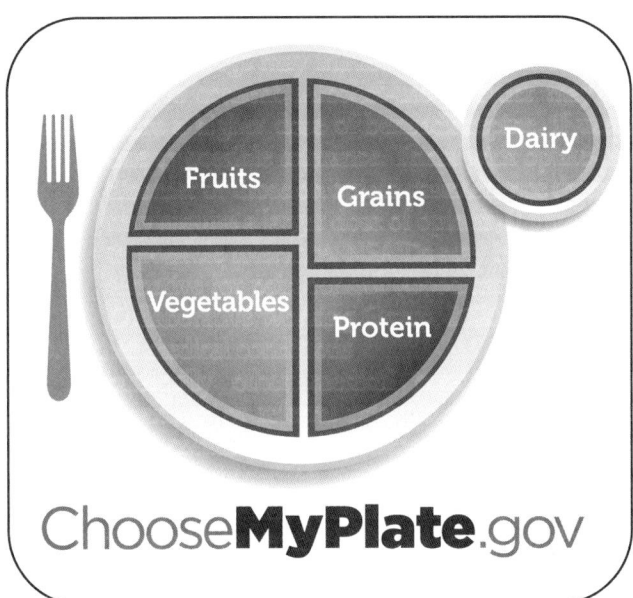

Figure 14-3 "My Plate" Guide for Making Healthy Eating Choices

U.S. Department of Agriculture. Retrieved from https://www.myplate.gov/

D. Refer to specialty care as needed for management of co-occurring conditions (otolaryngology, pulmonology, GI, endocrine, mental health, etc.).
E. Refer to tertiary obesity care if patient fails repeated attempts to lower BMI or if co-occurring conditions are not improving. Tertiary interventions may include the following:
  1. Medication management
    "In December 2022, the FDA approved the use of semaglutide for treatment of obesity among adolescents ages 12–17. In a randomized controlled trial, participants taking once weekly semaglutide had on average a 16% reduction in BMI, while participants who received placebo had a mean increase in BMI of 0.4%. There are challenges with access to the medication due to high cost and variable insurance coverage." (Weghuber et al., p. 2245, 2022).
  2. Bariatric surgery
    Adolescents who present with a BMI >120 percent of the 95% for age or BMI > 35kg/m^2, whichever is lower, with complications of obesity or a BMI > 140 percent of the 95th % of BMI or BMI >40kg/m^2 are candidates for bariatric surgery (Schmoke, 2021). Bariatric surgery is considered the most effective treatment for adolescents with severe obesity (Jaklevic, 2021). Between 2015–2018, 3.7% of the total bariatric surgery performed were on adolescents and young adults, despite the studies that establish its safety and efficacy (Schmoke, 2021).
F. The encouragement of weight maintenance versus weight loss depends on the age and BMI percentile of the child, as follows (Barlow & Expert Committee, 2007; Spear et al., 2007):
  1. Overweight (BMI 85%–94%)
    Children of any age should be encouraged to maintain weight and/or slow weight gain until a BMI of <85% is achieved.
  2. Obese (BMI 95%–98%)
    a. Children under 12 should be encouraged to maintain weight or lose weight at a rate of no greater than 1 lb per month.
    b. Adolescents 12 and older should be encouraged to lose weight at a rate of no greater than 2 lb per week.
  3. Severely obese (BMI >98%)
    a. Children under 6 years old should be encouraged to lose weight at a rate of no greater than 1 lb per month.
    b. Children 6 years and older should be encouraged to lose weight at a rate of no greater than 2 lb per week.
G. Follow up with the patient at least every 3–6 months for weight/BMI monitoring and further support in lifestyle modification.

V. Helpful online resources

A. http://www.aap.org
  Website for American Academy of Pediatrics, Clinical Practice Guideline for the Evaluation and Treatment of Children and Adolescents With Obesity
B. http://www.cdc.gov/obesity/childhood/
  CDC website that provides statistics and facts about obesity in the United States, tools for BMI measurement and tracking, and strategies for obesity prevention
C. http://ihcw.aap.org/
  Website for the American Academy of Pediatrics Institute for Healthy Childhood Weight; includes information about programs and practice resources aimed toward obesity prevention and treatment
D. http://www.choosemyplate.gov
  U.S. Department of Agriculture–sponsored website that offers resources and tools for dietary assessment and nutrition education
E. http://www.letsmove.gov
  Official website of the "Let's Move" campaign launched by former first lady Michelle Obama; provides information about nutrition, physical activity, and advocacy around obesity prevention initiatives in communities and schools
F. http://www.nchpad.org
  National Center on Health, Physical Activity and Disability website; provides information and resources to promote the health of people with disabilities through physical activity
G. http://www.chopchopmag.org
  Website and print magazine developed by the nonprofit organization ChopChopKids, whose mission is to promote nutrition by teaching children and families to cook and eat together; offers a wide selection of easy recipes from a variety of cultural cuisines

References

Abeysekara, P., Turchi, R., & O'Neil, M. (2014). Obesity and children with special needs: Special considerations for a special population. *Current Opinion Pediatrics*, 26(4), 508–515. doi:10.1097/MOP.000000000000012

Acharya, K., Feese, M., Franklin, F., & Kabagambe, E. (2011). Body mass index and dietary intake among Head Start children and caregivers. *Journal of American Dietetic Association*, 111(9), 1314–1321. doi:10.1016/j.jada.2011.06.013

Barlow, S. E., & Expert Committee. (2007). Expert Committee recommendations regarding the prevention, assessment, and treatment of child and adolescent overweight and obesity: Summary report. *Pediatrics*, 120(Suppl. 4), S164–S192. doi:120/Supplement_4/S164

Barnhill, A., Ramirez, A., Ashe, M., Berhaupt-Glickstein, A., Freudenberg, N., Grier, S.,Kumanyika, S. (2022). The racialized marketing of unhealthy foods and beverages: Perspectives and potential. *Journal of Law, Medicine & Ethics*, 50(1), 52–59. doi:10.1017/jme.2022.8

Brisbois, T. D., Farmer, A. P., & McCargar, L. J. (2012). Early markers of adult obesity: A review. *Obesity Reviews*, 13(4), 347–367. doi:10.1111/j.1467-789X.2011.00965.x

Center for Disease Control and Prevention. (2019). Disability and health promotion. *Disability & Obesity*. Https://www.cdc.gov/ncbddd/disabilityandhealth/obesity.html

Center for Disease Control and Prevention (2022). Overweight and Obesity. https://www.cdc.gov/obesity/index.html

Cockerill, R. G., Biggs, B. K., Oesterle, T. S., & Croarkin, P. E. (2014). Antidepressant use and body mass index change in overweight adolescents: A historical cohort study. *Innovations in Clinical Neuroscience*, 11(11–12), 14–21.

Cohen, R., Fardouly, J., Newton-John, T., & Slater, A. (2019). #BoPo on Instagram: An experimental investigation of the effects of viewing body positive content on young women's mood and body image. *New Media & Society*, 21(7), 1546–1564. doi:10.1177/1461444819826530

Cutts, D., & Cook, J. (2017). Screening for food insecurity: Short-term alleviation and long-term prevention. *American Journal of Public Health*, 107(11), 1699–1700. doi:10.2105.?AJPH.2017.304082

de Onis, M., Martinez-Costa, C., Nunez, F., Nguefack-Tsague, G., Montal, A., & Brines, J. (2013). Association between WHO cut-offs for childhood overweight and obesity and cardiometabolic risk. *Public Health Nutrition*, 16(4), 625–630. doi:10.1017/S1368980012004776

Evensen, E., Wilsgaard, T., Furberg, A., & Skeie, G. (2016). Tracking of overweight and obesity from early childhood to adolescence in a population-based cohort-the Tromso Study, Fit Futures. *BMC Pediatrics*, 16, 64. doi:10.1186/s12887-016-0599-5

Foster, B., Weinstein, K., & Davis, M. (2020). Parental mental health associated with child overweight and obesity, examined within rural and urban settings, stratified by income. *Journal of Rural Health*, 36(1), 27137. doi:10.1111/jrh.12395

Flynn, J. T., Kaelber, D. C., Baker-Smith, C. M., Blowey, D., Carroll, A. E., Daniels, S., de Ferranti, S. D., Dionne, J. M., Falkner, B., Flinn, S. K., Giding, S. S., Goodnwin, C., Leu, M. G., Powers, M. E., Rea, C., Samuels, J., Simasek, M., Thaker, V. V., & Urbina, E. (2017). Clinical practice guidelines for screening and management of high blood pressure in children and adolescents. *Pediatrics*, 140(3), e20171904. doi:10.1542/peds/2017-1904

Friedemann, C., Heneghan, C., Mahtani, K., Thompson, M., Perera, R., & Ward, A. M. (2012). Cardiovascular disease risk in healthy children and its association with body mass index: Systematic review and meta-analysis. *BMJ*, 345, e4759. doi:10.1136/bmj.e4759

Fryar, C., Carroll, M., & Afful, J. (2018). *Prevalence of high weight-for-recumbent length among infants and toddlers from birth to 24 months of age: United States, 1971–1974 through 2015–2016.* National Center for Health Statistics, Division of Health and Nutrition Examination Surveys.

Geoffroy, M. C., Li, L., & Power, C. (2014). Depressive symptoms and body mass index: Co-morbidity and direction of association in a British birth cohort followed over 50 years. *Psychological Medicine*, 44(12), 2641–2652. doi:10.1017/S0033291714000142

Harrington, D. M., Staiano, A. E., Broyles, S.T., Gupta, A. K., & Katzmarzyk, P. T. (2013). BMI percentiles for the identification of abdominal obesity and metabolic risk in children and adolescents: Evidence in support of the CDC 95th percentile. *European Journal of Clinical Nutrition*, 67(2), 218–222. doi:10.1038/ejcn.2012.203

Hemmingsson, E. (2018). Early childhood obesity risk factors: Socioeconomic adversity, family dysfunction, offspring distress, and junk food self-medication. *Current Obesity Reports*, 7, 204–209. doi:10.1007/s13679-018-0310-2

Hooker, S., Punjabi, A., Justesen, K., Boyle, L., & Sherman, M. (2018). Encouraging health behavior change: Eight evidence-based strategies. *American Academy of Family Practice*, 25(2), 31–36.

Hughes, A. R., Sherriff, A., Ness, A. R., & Reilly, J. J. (2014). Timing of adiposity rebound and adiposity in adolescence. *Pediatrics*, 134(5), e1354–e1361. doi:10.1542/peds.2014-1908

Jaklevic, M. C. (2021). The push for earlier bariatric surgery for adolescents with severe obesity. *Journal of American Medical Association*, 325(22), 2241–2242. doi:10.1001/jama.2021.7912

Jeffrey, A. N., Metcalf, B. S., Hosking, J., Streeter, A. J., Voss, L. D., Wilkin, T. J. (2012). Age before stage: Insulin resistance rises before the onset of puberty: A 9-year longitudinal study. *Diabetes Care*, 35(3), 536–541. doi:10.2337/dc11-1281

Kelly, A. S., Auerbach, P., Barrientos-Perez, M., Gies, I., Hale, P. M., Marcus, C., Mastrandrea, L. D., Prabhu, N., & Arslanian, S. (2020). A randomized, controlled trial of liraglutide for adolescents with obesity. *New England Journal of Medicine*, 382(22), 2117–2128. doi:10.1056/NEJMoa1916038

Kelsey, M. M., & Zeitler, P. S. (2016). Insulin resistance of puberty. *Current Diabetes Reports*, 16(7), 64. doi:10.1007/s11892-016-0751-5

Kleinendorst, L., Abawi, O., van der Voorn, B., Jongejan, H. T. M., Brandsma, A. E., Visser, J. A., van Rossum, E. F. C., van der Zwagg, B., Alders, M., Boon, E. M. J., van Haelst, M. M., & van den Akker, E. L. T. (2020). Identifying underlying medical causes of pediatric obesity: Results of a systemic diagnostic approach in a pediatric obesity center. *PLoS ONE*, 15(12), e0244508. doi:10.1371/journal.pone.0244508

Korczak, D. J., Lipman, E., Morrison, K., & Szatmari, P. (2013). Are children and adolescents with psychiatric illness at risk for increased future body weight? A systematic review. *Developmental Medicine and Child Neurology*, 55(11), 980–987. doi:10.1111/dmcn.12168

Lange, S. J., Kompaniyets, L., Freedman, D., Kraus, E., Porter, R., Blandk, H. M. & Goodman, A. (2021). Longitudinal trends in body mass index before and during COVID-19 pandemic among persons ages 2–19 years—United States, 2018—2020. *Morbidity and Mortality Weekly Report*, 70(37), 1278–1283. doi:10.15585/mmwr.mm7027a3

Larque, E., Labayen I., Flodmark, C., Lissau, I., Czernin., S., Moreno, L., Pietrobelli, A., & Widhalm, K. (2019). From conception to infancy-early risk factors for childhood obesity. *Nature Reviews Endocrinology*, 15, 456–478. doi:10.1038/s41574-019-0219-1

Lennerz, B. S., Wabitsch, M., Lippert, H., Wolff, S., Knoll, C., Weiner, R., Manger, T., Kiess, W., & Stroh, C. (2014). Bariatric surgery in adolescents and young adults—safety and effectiveness in a cohort of 345 patients. *International Journal of Obesity, 38*(3), 334–340. doi:10.1038/ijo.2013.182

Li, J. S., Barnett, T. A., Goodman, E., Wasserman, R. C., Kemper, A. R., & American Heart Association Atherosclerosis, Hypertension and Obesity in the Young Committee of the Council on Cardiovascular Disease in the Young, Council on Epidemiology and Prevention, and Council on Nutrition, Physical Activity and Metabolism. (2013). Approaches to the prevention and management of childhood obesity: The role of social networks and the use of social media and related electronic technologies: A scientific statement from the American Heart Association. *Circulation, 127*(2), 260–267. doi:10.1161/CIR.0b013e3182756d8e

Loos, R.J.F., Yeo, G.S.H. (2022). The genetics of obesity: from discovery to biology. *Nature Reviews Genetics (23),* 120-133. doi.org/10.1038?s41576-021-00414-z

Maggio, A. B., Martin, X. E., Saunders Gasser, C., Gal-Duding, C., Beghetti, M., Farpour-Lambert, N. J., & Chamay-Weber, C. (2014). Medical and non-medical complications among children and adolescents with excessive body weight. *BMC Pediatrics, 14,* 232. doi:10.1186/1471-2431-14-232

Markula, Pirko. (2022). Exploring the body positivity movement. *Psychology Today.* Https:www.psychologytoday.com

Marmorstein, N. R., Iacono, W. G., & Legrand, L. (2014). Obesity and depression in adolescence and beyond: Reciprocal risks. *International Journal of Obesity, 38*(7), 906–911. doi:10.1038/ijo.2014.19

Michaliszyn, SF., Sjaarda, LA, Scifres, C., Simhan, H., Arslanian, SA. (2017). Maternal excess gestational weight gain and infant waist circumference: a 2-y observational study. *Pediatric Research 81(1-1):* 63-67. doi:10.1038/pr.2016.174

Mitchell, J. A., Rodriguez, D., Schmitz, K. H., & Audrain-McGovern, J. (2013). Greater screentime is associated with adolescent obesity: A longitudinal study of the BMI distribution from ages 14 to 18. *Obesity, 21*(3), 572–575. doi:10.1002/oby.20157

National Association of Pediatric Nurse Associates and Practitioners. (2006). NAPNAP Healthy Eating and Activity Together (HEAT) initiative. *Journal of Pediatric Health Care, 20*(2Suppl. 2), S3–S63.

Neshteruk, C. D., Tripicchio, G., Lobaugh, S., Vaughn, A., Luecking, C., Mazzucca, S., & Ward, D. S. (2021). Screen time parenting practices and associations with preschool children's TV viewing and weight-related outcomes. *International Journal of Environmental Research and Public Health, 18*(14), 7359. doi:10.3390/ijerph18147359.

Ogden, C. L., Carroll, M. D., Kit, B. K., & Flegal, K. M. (2012). Prevalence of obesity and trends in body mass index among US children and adolescents, 1999–2010. *JAMA, 307*(5), 483–490. doi:10.1001/jama.2012.40

Ogden, C. L., Carroll, M. D., Kit, B. K., & Flegal, K. M. (2014). Prevalence of childhood and adult obesity in the United States, 2011–2012. *JAMA, 311*(8), 806–814. doi:10.1001/jama.2014.732

Padmanabhan, P., & Shroff, H. (2020). The relationship between sensory integration challenges and the dietary intake and nutritional status of children with autism spectrum disorders in Mumbai, India. *International Journal of Developmental Disabilities, 66*(2), 142–152. doi:10.1080/20473869.2018.1522816

Pan, L., Li, R., Park, S., Galuska, D. A., Sherry, B., & Freedman, D. S. (2014). A longitudinal analysis of sugar-sweetened beverages intake in infancy and obesity at 6 years. *Pediatrics, 134*(Suppl. 1), S29–S35. doi:10.1542/peds.2014-0646F

Pont, S.J., Puhl, R. Cook, S.R, Slusser, W.(2020). Stigma experienced by children and adolescents with obesity. *Pediatrics 140*(6). doi:10.1542/peds.2017-3034

Robinson, T. N., Banda, J. A., Hale, L., Lu, A. S., Fleming-Milici, F., Calvert, S. L., & Wartella, E. (2017). Screen media exposure and obesity in children and adolescents. *Pediatrics, 140*(Suppl. 2), S97S101. doi:10.1542/pes.2016-1758K

Rottenberg, J., Yaroslavsky, I., Carney, R. M., Freedland, K. E., George, C. J., Baji, I., Dochnal, R., Gádoros, J., Halas, K., Kapornai, K., Kiss, E., Osváth, V., Varga, H., Vetró, A., & Kovacs, M. (2014). The association between major depressive disorder in childhood and risk factors for cardiovascular disease in adolescence. *Psychosomatic Medicine, 76*(2), 122–127. doi:10.1097/PSY.0000000000000028

Roy, S. M., Spivack, J. G., Faith, M. S, Chesi, A., Mitchell, J. A., Kelly, A., Grant, S. F. A., Mccormack, S. E., & Zemel, B. S. (2016). Infant BMI or weight-for-length and obesity risk in early childhood. *Pediatrics, 137*(5), e20153492. doi:10.1542/peds.2015-3492

Schmoke, N, Ogle, S. Inge, T. (2021). Adolescent Bariatric Surgery. *Endotext.* Http://www.ncbi.nlm.nih.gov/books/NBK575728

Simmonds, M., Liewellyn, A., Owen, C. G., & Woolacott, N. (2016). Predicting adult obesity from childhood obesity: A systemic review and meta-analysis. *Obesity Reviews, 17*(2), 95–107. doi:10.1111/obr.12334

Tanaka, C., Reilly, J. J., & Huang, W. Y. (2014). Longitudinal changes in objectively measured sedentary behaviour and their relationship with adiposity in children and adolescents: Systematic review and evidence appraisal. *Obesity Reviews, 15*(10), 791–803. doi:10.1111/obr.12195

Utesch, T., Dreiskamper, D., Naul, R., & Geukes, K. (2018). Understanding physical (in)activity, overweight, and obesity in childhood: Effects of congruence between physical self-concept and motor competence. *Scientific Reports, 8,* 5908. doi:1038/s41598-028-24139-y

van Geel, M., Vedder, P., & Tanilon, J. (2014). Are overweight and obese youths more often bullied by their peers? A meta-analysis on the relation between weight status and bullying. *International Journal of Obesity, 38*(10), 1263–1267. doi:10.1038/ijo.2014.117

Weghuber, D, Barrett, T, Barrientos-Perez, M, Gies, I, Hesse, D, Jeppesen, O.K., Kelly, A. S., Mastrandrea, L.D., Sorrig, R., Arslanian, S. STEP TEENS Investigators. (2022). Once-Weekly Semaglutide in Adolescents with Obesity. *New England Journal of Medicine* (24).2245-2257. Doi:10.1056/NEJMoa2208601

World Health Organization (2022) Physical Activity. Https://www.who.int/news-room/fa...tivity%20per%20day

Zarychta, K., Banik, A., Kulis, E., Boberska, M., Radtke, T., Chan, C. K. Y., & Luszczynska, A. (2020). Parental depression predicts child body mass via parental support provision, child support receipt, and child physical activity: Findings from parent/caregiver-child dyads. *Frontiers in Psychology, 11,* 161. doi:10.3389//fpsyg2020.0061

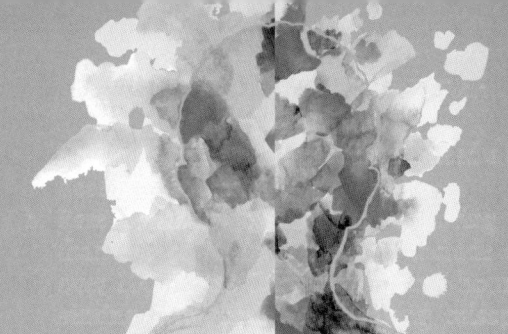

CHAPTER 15

Urinary Incontinence in Children

Angel C. Kuo

I. Introduction and general background

Urinary incontinence is the involuntary loss of urine (Austin et al., 2016). The bladder is responsible for the storage and emptying of urine. During infancy, this occurs as reflexive behavior by the complex pathway controlled by an "integration of sympathetic, parasympathetic, and somatic innervation that involves the lower urinary tract, the micturition center in the sacral spinal cord, the midbrain, and the higher cortical centers" (Champeau, 2018, p. 91). The infant also may not empty to completion (Feldman & Bauer, 2006). The cortical inhibitory pathway develops between 1 and 3 years of age, which inhibits bladder contraction and allows for voluntary control of the external sphincter (Feldman & Bauer, 2006). By age 4, a child has learned to control and coordinate the voiding process and can become dry between voids. The detrusor muscle (bladder wall muscle) is relaxed during the filling stage while the bladder neck remains closed to maintain continence. Once the bladder is full, the external sphincter relaxes while the detrusor muscle contracts during voiding to allow for complete emptying of the bladder. An estimated bladder capacity in milliliters for a child over 4 years of age is now defined by the International Children's Continence Society (ICCS) as **the child's age (in years) plus 1 $\times$ 30 mL** up until puberty (Austin et al., 2016); earlier literature has also defined estimated bladder capacity as the child's age (in years) plus 2 $\times$ 30 mL (Champeau, 2018; Dos Santos, 2014; Dos Santos et al., 2017; Greenfield & Cooper, 2019). The normal range of voiding is between three and seven times per day for children between the ages of 7 and 15 years (Austin et al., 2016). However, a wide range of conditions or dysfunctions may cause either continuous or intermittent urinary incontinence in children.

This chapter presents the latest standard terminology set forth by the ICCS to standardize the language and avoid confusion among clinicians and researchers (Austin et al., 2016). Urinary incontinence is categorized as either continuous (constant urinary leakage during day and night) or intermittent, which is further specified by daytime incontinence and enuresis (Austin et al., 2016). This chapter focuses on intermittent incontinence in children older than 5 years of age who are otherwise healthy and normal (who are otherwise healthy without anatomical nor neurological concerns), both anatomically and neurologically. The assessment and management of both daytime and nighttime urinary incontinence (nocturnal enuresis) are discussed. There is also a brief review of the assessment and management of the common comorbid conditions associated with urinary incontinence, including urinary tract infections (UTIs); stool retention; encopresis due to behavioral patterns; and the psychological, social, and cultural impact on children with incontinence.

As a child learns to contract the external sphincter muscle, the muscle inhibits both detrusor contraction and stool motility, which can affect both systems. It is referred to as *bladder and bowel dysfunction* (BBD) when both lower urinary tract (LUT) dysfunction and bowel dysfunction coexist (Austin et al., 2016). Chronic contraction of the sphincter muscle promotes further stool retention and distention and/or incomplete emptying of the bladder, potentially leading to recurrent UTIs. In addition, a full rectum may exert pressure on the bladder, inducing bladder symptoms, such as sudden urgency or decreased bladder capacity, described as the "cross-talk" mechanism (Bernal et al., 2018; Burgers et al., 2013; Dos Santos et al., 2017).

Possible early childhood risk factors, such as developmental delays in motor, communication, and social skills, or even difficult temperament, may contribute to a higher chance of daytime incontinence and soiling (Joinson et al., 2008). Children with urinary incontinence have also been found to have social and psychological distress that must be addressed at the same time (Dos Santos et al., 2017; Thibodeau et al., 2013). Although correction of incontinence may not alter internalizing problems, such as anxiety or obsessive–compulsive disorders, it does normalize the incidence of externalizing problems, such as conduct disorders (Glassberg & Combs, 2009). Additional considerations need to be taken regarding concurrent behavioral conditions that increase the risk of both urinary and bowel incontinence because these may interfere with the child's ability to get to the bathroom on time due to disorganized thinking, confusion, or inattention (Dos Santos et al., 2017). Children with attention-deficit/hyperactivity disorder (ADHD) may have more LUT symptoms and are more challenging to treat (Dos Santos et al., 2017). Medications used to treat the behavioral conditions (e.g., for anxiety or obsessive–compulsive disorders) may also interfere with the child's awareness of their need to void (Dos Santos et al., 2017). Our society has little tolerance for bladder and bowel incontinence; thus, children with such symptoms are at risk for further embarrassment and psychological and emotional distress, which can lead to issues with self-esteem, feelings of shame and isolation, or even poor school performance and aggressive behaviors (Dos Santos et al., 2017; Thibodeau et al., 2013) . Providers must handle both the initial workup and routine follow-up with much sensitivity and respect for the child's self-esteem, with a nonjudgmental attitude, language, and approach.

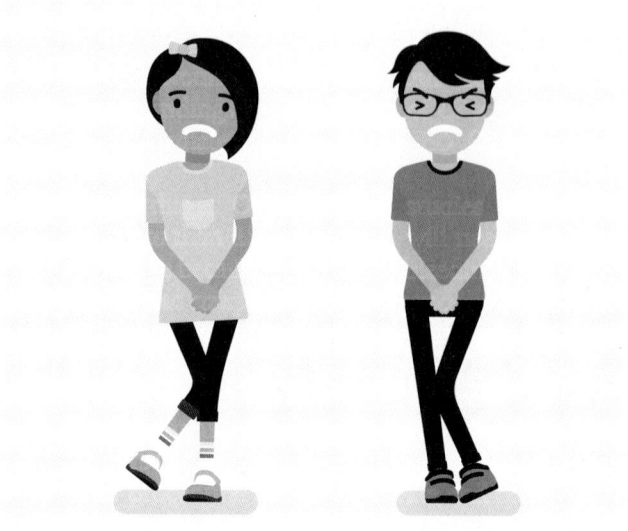

Figure 15-1 Holding maneuvers in females assigned at birth: Vincent Curtsy's sign.

© Andrew Rybalko/Shutterstock

A. *Daytime (intermittent) incontinence*
  1. Definition and overview
     Daytime urinary incontinence is the intermediate involuntary loss of urine while awake (Austin et al., 2016). It involves a wide array of clinical symptoms and causes, which differ in severity and reversibility. In addition, it may involve the maturation, functional, or behavioral process within the elimination cycle. Most commonly, children discover the power of controlling the external sphincter to postpone urination (by inhibiting the detrusor contraction) and thus eventually may reach a dyscoordination between the bladder and sphincter muscle control or have a delay in maturation of the bladder sphincter coordination (Dos Santos, 2014), both of which lead to daytime urinary leakage. Furthermore, after repeated dyscoordination, the child may also have a difficult time relaxing the external sphincter muscle enough to void to completion, thus increasing the risk of UTI and causing even more uninhibited contractions of the bladder (Dos Santos, 2014).
     Some of the major causes of daytime incontinence include the following:
     a. Vaginal reflux and postmicturition dribbling: involuntary leakage of urine immediately or within 10 minutes after voiding, which can be caused by urine trapped in the introitus during voiding or may occur with coughing, sneezing, or jumping; often due to voiding with adducted legs or presence of labial adhesions; may cause skin irritation. Generally, there is a lack of other LUT symptoms and nighttime wetting.
     b. Voiding postponement: typically with classic postponing maneuvers ("potty dance," crossing legs fully, squatting with heel pressed into perineum, or penile grabbing) (**Figure 15-1**) as strategies to externally contract the sphincter or compress urethra to temporarily suppress urgency, relax the detrusor, postpone urination, or prevent urinary leakage, but followed by a sudden urge to void. May experience psychological comorbidities or behavioral disturbances.
     c. Overactive bladder (OAB) and urge incontinence: increased detrusor contractions that lead to pelvic floor contraction; can be diagnosed by urodynamics or accurate voiding diary; may or may not involve urinary frequency; high association with UTIs; associated with strong desire to void with tendency to perform classic postponing maneuvers and leads to involuntary loss of urine (see item b). Approximately 60% of children who present with incontinence have OAB (Dos Santos, 2014).
     d. Dysfunctional voiding: incomplete relaxation of external sphincter during voiding in an otherwise neurologically intact patient; may be verified by urodynamics or uroflow evaluation with staccato urinary flow pattern and prolonged voiding time, potentially with incomplete emptying of the bladder (elevated postvoid residual [PVR]); associated with increased risk of UTI
     e. BBD: combination of both bladder and bowel dysfunction, without identifiable neurologic abnormality and potentially affecting the upper urinary tract system if severe
     f. Underactive bladder: decreased voiding frequency (three or less per day) with need for intra-abdominal pressure (Valsalva) or straining

to initiate, maintain, or complete voiding; caused by hypotonic detrusor muscle; large bladder volume with elevated PVR and increased risk for UTI
   g. Giggle incontinence (enuresis risoria): a rare condition with complete involuntary emptying of bladder that occurs during or after laughter; bladder function normal while not laughing; seen in females assigned at birth
   h. Stress incontinence: involuntary leakage of urine with physical exertion that increases intra-abdominal pressure; on urodynamics, leakage confirmed by lack of a detrusor muscle contraction
   i. Extraordinary daytime urinary frequency: frequent, small-volume voiding during the day only (>1 time per hour with voided volume of <50% estimated bladder capacity). More frequent in young males assigned at birth and generally self-limiting. Incontinence is rare, and comorbidities need to be ruled out.
2. Prevalence and incidence
Daytime urinary incontinence is generally considered a problem after 5 years of age (Austin et al., 2016). It may account for up to 40% of the visits in a pediatric urology clinic (Dos Santos et al., 2017). In addition, dysfunctional voiding is associated with an increased risk of UTIs, stool retention and encopresis, vesicoureteral reflux, and psychological distress (Bernal et al., 2018; Dos Santos et al., 2017; Thibodeau et al., 2013; Yang & Chua, 2018). Emotional stressors, such as sexual abuse, may sometimes trigger sudden dysfunctional voiding.

B. *Nighttime (intermittent) incontinence—nocturnal enuresis*
   1. Definition and overview
      a. Nighttime intermittent incontinence, also known as *nocturnal enuresis*, is the involuntary loss of urine in discrete episodes while asleep, beyond the age of anticipated control (~5 years of age) (Arnhym, 2018; Austin et al., 2016; Bogaert et al., 2020). Enuresis is thought to be caused by a lack of arousal during nighttime with resultant bladder contractions and wetting, reduced nighttime bladder capacity, nighttime polyuria, bladder overactivity, or an elevated threshold for nighttime arousal (Arnhym, 2018). To better understand nighttime incontinence, it is important to divide the children into subgroups based on symptoms or by onset of enuresis:
         i. Monosymptomatic enuresis: Enuresis is the sole symptom, without any bladder dysfunction or other LUT symptoms. The etiology is unclear, but possible cause is thought to be related to immaturity of the brainstem, with fluctuation or decreased production of serum arginine vasopressin, which leads to increased nocturnal urine production (Arnhym, 2018; Austin et al., 2016; Bogaert et al., 2020).
         ii. Non-monosymptomatic enuresis: enuresis along with additional daytime LUT symptoms (e.g., daytime incontinence, frequency, and urgency). The cause is thought to be overactive bladder or stool retention, or a combination of both (Austin et al., 2016; Dos Santos et al., 2017).
         iii. Primary enuresis: Child has never been dry at night—can be for either monosymptomatic or non-monosymptomatic enuresis.
         iv. Secondary enuresis: Child has had dry nights for at least 6 consecutive months but now presents with recurrence of enuresis; may have similar presentation as primary enuresis, with the difference in the degree of constipation or other behavioral comorbidities and age of toilet training.
      b. Risk factors such as difficult temperament or behavioral problems have been found to be associated with enuresis (Joinson et al., 2016). Additional causes of enuresis may include genetic factors, maturational delay, upper airway obstruction (rare), psychologic factors, UTI, or decreased nighttime bladder capacity. Severe stool retention may also lead to decreased bladder capacity. Secondary non-monosymptomatic enuresis requires further workup for neurologic involvement, especially if unresponsive to traditional treatments for enuresis or stool retention (Bernal et al., 2018).
   2. Prevalence and incidence
Approximately 15%–25% of 5-year-olds have nocturnal enuresis despite cultural differences (Arnhym, 2018; Bogaert et al., 2020). Children with non-monosymptomatic enuresis tend to have higher rates of comorbidity, including both bladder and bowel dysfunction (Butler et al., 2006). In addition, they tend to have more severe symptoms, including more wet episodes per night and more wet nights per week, than those with monosymptomatic enuresis because of persistent bladder overactivity throughout the night (Butler et al., 2006). The comorbid factors hinder the success of treatment for enuresis if left unresolved. The spontaneous cure rate in children is about 15% per year, depending on their culture. Approximately 2%–3% of older adolescents and 1%–2% of adults continue to experience nocturnal enuresis. This occurs more often in males assigned at birth than females assigned at birth (Bogaert et al., 2020). Although most children do outgrow enuresis, studies have shown reduced self-esteem in children with even just once-per-month enuresis. By providing treatment, self-esteem improves, regardless of the actual success of treatment (Bogaert et al., 2020). Another study by Butler and Heron (2008) reveals that 9-year-old children view enuresis as an extremely stressful life event, even more stressful than physical illnesses. Insurance companies may pay for bed alarm treatment for children over 7 years of age with monosymptomatic enuresis (Aetna, 2022), but daytime symptoms must be

ruled out initially. The decision about when to start treatment depends on the child's degree of concern and motivation rather than the family's concerns and motivation (Bogaert et al., 2020).

II. **Database (may include but is not limited to)**
A. *Subjective*
 1. Detailed voiding and elimination history: most useful and most important (**Table 15-1**). May also do a

Table 15-1 Detailed Voiding and Elimination History from Child and Parent

Daily Activities and Related Symptoms	Information Gathering
Voiding habits	Potty-training process (age, approach, and length of time) Number of voids throughout the day or at school (0–3 times) Postponing behavior ("potty dance") Urgency or frequency (number of times per hour; whether able to sit through a movie) Voiding volume Intermittent versus smooth urine stream Use of abdominal pressure to void (Valsalva) Nocturnal wetting or polyuria
Daytime incontinence	Frequency: number of times wet per day or per week Amount and severity: dampness versus soaking accidents <ul><li>Number of pads or liners used per day</li></ul>Pattern: morning versus afternoon<ul><li>Weekday versus weekend</li></ul>Sudden wetting versus wet along the way to the bathroom Amount of time between voiding and wetting (immediately, 10 min, or 2 h) Aware of wetting and changes clothes independently? Previous treatment and results
Nighttime incontinence	Frequency: number of nights per week Amount and frequency: wet before or after midnight<ul><li>Number of times per night (1 or >1)</li><li>Soak through pull-ups or diapers</li></ul>Previous treatment and results; compliance or appropriate use? Age when initial nighttime wetting resolved (if applicable) Family history of delayed resolution of nighttime wetting Responsible for changing wet sheets or clothing?
History of urinary tract infection	Bladder versus kidney infection Fever or other symptoms at presentation Symptoms after treatment Previous workup Total number of infections, dates, and treatment
Elimination habits	Frequency of stooling in toilet Size, shape, and consistency of stool; clog the toilet? Staining on underwear versus complete soiling Postponing of stooling (withholding behavior) Chronic abdominal pain Water, fruit, and fiber intake per day; evaluate timing of fluid intake Prior treatment and results Family history of constipation or infrequent stooling
Overall	Skin breakdown or rashes in perineum Awareness before or right after accident (urine or stool)? Which occurred first: urinary wetting or stool retention or soiling? Which is worse: daytime or nighttime wetting, or stool retention or soiling? Which is the child more motivated to correct? Which is the family more motivated to correct? Assess child's and family's readiness to address the issues

formal bladder diary to document 7-night incontinence episodes and nighttime voiding volume and a 48-hour daytime frequency and volume chart. For bowel diary, use the Bristol Stool Scale (**Figure 15-2**).
   a. The history provides critical information.
   b. Direct questions at both child and parent because the child knows best what occurs during the day; parents have been found to be unreliable in stating the voiding and elimination history alone.
2. Past health history
   a. Prenatal and birth history
   b. Medical illnesses: significant congenital conditions, especially of the genitourinary tract, heavy snoring. Concurrent behavioral/mental health

Date _____							
	Mon	Tues	Wed	Thurs	Fri	Sat	Sun
When you wake up	_____	_____	_____	_____	_____	_____	_____
Mid AM recess	_____	_____	_____	_____	_____	_____	_____
Lunch	_____	_____	_____	_____	_____	_____	_____
Mid PM (before leaving school)	_____	_____	_____	_____	_____	_____	_____
Dinner	_____	_____	_____	_____	_____	_____	_____
Bedtime	_____	_____	_____	_____	_____	_____	_____
Poop	_____	_____	_____	_____	_____	_____	_____
Dry Days	_____	_____	_____	_____	_____	_____	_____
Dry Nights	_____	_____	_____	_____	_____	_____	_____

Date _____							
	Mon	Tues	Wed	Thurs	Fri	Sat	Sun
When you wake up	_____	_____	_____	_____	_____	_____	_____
Mid AM recess	_____	_____	_____	_____	_____	_____	_____
Lunch	_____	_____	_____	_____	_____	_____	_____
Mid PM (before leaving school)	_____	_____	_____	_____	_____	_____	_____
Dinner	_____	_____	_____	_____	_____	_____	_____
Bedtime	_____	_____	_____	_____	_____	_____	_____
Poop	_____	_____	_____	_____	_____	_____	_____
Dry Days	_____	_____	_____	_____	_____	_____	_____
Dry Nights	_____	_____	_____	_____	_____	_____	_____

Date _____							
	Mon	Tues	Wed	Thurs	Fri	Sat	Sun
When you wake up	_____	_____	_____	_____	_____	_____	_____
Mid AM recess	_____	_____	_____	_____	_____	_____	_____
Lunch	_____	_____	_____	_____	_____	_____	_____
Mid PM (before leaving school)	_____	_____	_____	_____	_____	_____	_____
Dinner	_____	_____	_____	_____	_____	_____	_____
Bedtime	_____	_____	_____	_____	_____	_____	_____
Poop	_____	_____	_____	_____	_____	_____	_____
Dry Days	_____	_____	_____	_____	_____	_____	_____
Dry Nights	_____	_____	_____	_____	_____	_____	_____

Figure 15-2 Voiding and Elimination Diary

diagnosis such as ADHD, anxiety, autism spectrum disorder, obsessive–compulsive disorder, or others.
   c. Surgical history: urologic or neurologic surgery
   d. Obstetric and gynecological history: recent pregnancy
   e. Growth and development: developmental milestones and any challenges or delays, especially in neuromuscular area; ADHD; and school performance
   f. Family history: renal or urologic diseases and history of enuresis
   g. Diet: caffeine, soda, energy drinks, chocolate, or citrus intake (bladder irritants); fluid intake throughout the day and night; and fruit or fiber intake
   h. Personal–social–psychologic history: traumatic events or history of abuse, family and social support, reaction to accidents, recent major changes in the family; temperament in general
  3. Review of systems
   a. General: self-esteem, mood, attitude, patterns of behavior, fatigFue, weight loss
   b. Musculoskeletal and neurologic: gait and changes in lower extremity sensation or control
 B. Objective
  1. Physical examination findings (**Table 15-2**)
  2. Supporting data from relevant diagnostic tests gathered from workup and management plan (**Table 15-3**)

III. Assessment
 A. Determine the diagnosis
  1. Daytime (intermittent) urinary incontinence
  2. Nighttime (intermittent) urinary incontinence—nocturnal enuresis; monosymptomatic versus non-monosymptomatic; primary versus secondary
  3. Eliminate other conditions that may explain the patient's symptoms and presentation:
   a. UTIs
   b. Constipation or stool retention; bladder and bowel dysfunction
   c. Neurogenic bladder
   d. Diabetes insipidus or diabetes mellitus
   e. Ectopic ureter (typically continuous incontinence)
 B. Severity
   Assess the severity of the disease (mild, moderate, severe, or debilitating).
 C. Significance
   Assess the significance of the problem to the child and family.
 D. Motivation and ability
  1. Determine the child's motivation, willingness, and ability to follow an individualized treatment plan.
  2. Provide individualized program and set realistic goals.
  3. Provide frequent follow-up to monitor progress and sustain motivation.

Table 15-2 Physical Examination

System	Details
General	Assess self-esteem, attitude, and mood
Abdomen	Abdominal tenderness or distention Abdominal masses ■ Kidneys and bladder ■ Stool masses
Genitourinary	Overall hygiene Dampness or stool staining on underwear Tanner stage Anatomic abnormality Signs of skin breakdown, skin excoriation, or skin rash Signs of infection Male: urine pooled under foreskin, balanitis, or meatal stenosis Female: urine in introitus or perineum, discharge, or labial adhesion Active urine leakage at baseline versus with straining or coughing Rectum ■ Stool staining around rectum (or in underwear) ■ Rectal fissures ■ Sphincter tone and sensation; anal wink If positive stool symptoms, then consider digital rectal examination for assessment of rectal tone, presence of fecal or solid mass, or hemoccult testing
Spine	Sacral dimple, pit, or sinus tract Tuft of hair Hemangioma Subcutaneous lipoma Asymmetric gluteal crease
Neurologic	Gait Coordination Heel-and-toe walk Lower extremity muscle strength and tone Deep tendon reflexes Sensation in lower extremities

IV. Goals of clinical management
 A. Screening or diagnosing
  1. Choose a cost-effective approach for screening or diagnosing daytime and nighttime urinary incontinence in children.
  2. Eliminate other possible conditions causing urinary incontinence, which require referral to a specialty service.

Table 15-3 Common Urologic Tests

Test	Definition	Clinical Implications	Comments
Urinalysis (UA)	Analysis of the urine by urine dipstick and, when available, evaluation under the microscope with spun urine	Specific gravity ■ <1.000 may reveal concentrating defect ■ >1.020 may reveal dehydration and insufficient fluid intake Positive glucose on dipstick: rule out diabetes mellitus Positive protein on dipstick: repeat and rule out renal disease Positive leukocytes or nitrites on dipstick: proceed with microscopic evaluation and culture and sensitivity to rule out UTI	Urinary tract infections (UTIs) must be ruled out because they may be the cause of or the result of the incontinence. Can exacerbate bladder symptoms.
Urine culture and sensitivity (urine C&S)	Cultured urine specimen to evaluate organism causing UTI and sensitivity to panel of antibiotics	Positive urine culture indicates UTI and requires treatment with antibiotics May follow with prophylactic antibiotics to prevent further infections until voiding dysfunction resolved	Should not obtain for surveillance when child is asymptomatic. Method of obtaining specimen is important. Use a catheterized specimen if not fully toilet trained to avoid contamination.
Uroflowmetry (UF)	Noninvasive test measuring urinary flow rate, voiding pattern (degree of external sphincter relaxation), voiding volume, and time	Staccato flow (intermittent stream) indicates inability of sphincter to completely relax during voiding and may cause incomplete emptying in dysfunctional voiding Bell-shaped curve indicates proper sphincter relaxation during voiding Prolonged flow time with weak flow rate may indicate hypotonic bladder and detrusor contraction Best done with simultaneous pelvic floor electromyogram monitoring	Need to have at least half of estimated bladder capacity in the bladder to be effective. Can be evaluated by listening and observing the urine flow if machine is not available.
Bladder scan and postvoiding residual (PVR)	Ultrasound of the bladder after voiding to determine residual urine within the bladder; noninvasive	Ideal goal of <10% of expected bladder capacity Can detect bladder wall thickness (>5 mm; caused by voiding dysfunction) and any masses within the bladder Useful as prognostic indicator Prevoid bladder volume is also helpful	
Renal bladder ultrasound (RBUS)	Ultrasound of the kidneys and bladder; noninvasive	Assess renal size and parenchyma and any evidence of hydronephrosis Assess bladder volume, bladder wall thickness, and any masses within the bladder May assess rectal diameter and see rectal distention (indicate stool retention)	Normal renal bladder ultrasound can also be reassuring to both families and provider.

(continues)

Table 15-3 Common Urologic Tests (continued)

Test	Definition	Clinical Implications	Comments
Kidneys, ureter, bladder radiograph (KUB)	Plain film of kidneys, ureter, and bladder region	Assess degree of stool retention Assess for any spinal deformity	Complements clinical history and physical examination.
Urodynamics (UDS)	Invasive study involving urethral catheter and filling of bladder for evaluation of bladder pressure, compliance, detrusor and uninhibited contractions, and bladder capacity Also evaluates pelvic floor muscle coordination and condition of bladder at time of urinary leakage (if any) Fluoroscopic urodynamics also is able to reveal vesicoureteric reflux (VUR)	Reserved for those without improvement or concern for neurogenic cause	Results may vary depending on how fast the bladder is filled and how cooperative the patient is.
Spinal magnetic resonance imaging (MRI)	MRI of the spine to rule out tethered cord	Consider for those suspected of neurogenic bladder Should be MRI of entire spine	Children who require this workup should also receive a full neurologic examination.
Voiding cystourethrogram (VCUG)	Invasive fluoroscopic study with insertion of urinary catheter to fill the bladder and evaluate for signs of VUR; requires evaluation of voiding and PVR	Indicated if positive history of febrile UTI to rule out VUR Also reveals bladder volume, bladder trabeculation, sphincter relaxation during voiding, urethra, and PVR Includes scout film (kidneys, ureter, bladder radiograph); reveals spinal deformity and degree of stool retention Incomplete relaxation of external sphincter during urination is seen as "spinning top urethra" in females assigned at birth	Consider fluoroscopic urodynamics rather than VCUG only if the child has a history of incontinence and pyelonephritis.

B. Treatment
1. Improve the patient's bladder and bowel health, including skin integrity.
2. Properly treat conditions with minimal use of medication (both in dose and length of treatment).
3. Decrease the prevalence of UTIs.
4. Improve the quality of life for both patient and family.
5. Prevent psychological and emotional trauma caused by incontinence.
6. Foster a healthy and active lifestyle.
7. Empower the patient and family to manage bladder and bowel health.

C. Patient adherence
1. Select an approach that maximizes patient and family adherence, including positive reinforcement.
2. Provide close follow-up to maximize patient and family adherence.

V. Plan
A. Screening
1. Urinalysis or urine culture and sensitivities, if indicated, to rule out UTI and other abnormalities in the urine (Table 15-3)
2. Dysfunctional Voiding Scoring System (DVSS) Questionnaire—a 10-item questionnaire to quantify severity of symptoms (Dos Santos, 2014; Thibodeau et al., 2013)
3. Additional psychological questionnaires may be used to determine behavioral comorbidities.

B. Diagnostic tests (Table 15-3)
1. Bladder and bowel (voiding or elimination) diary as both a diagnostic tool and treatment via urotherapy—the timed voiding and elimination process (Figure 15-2).
2. Uroflowmetry: Consider after 3 months of behavioral modification. Alternatively, parents can watch

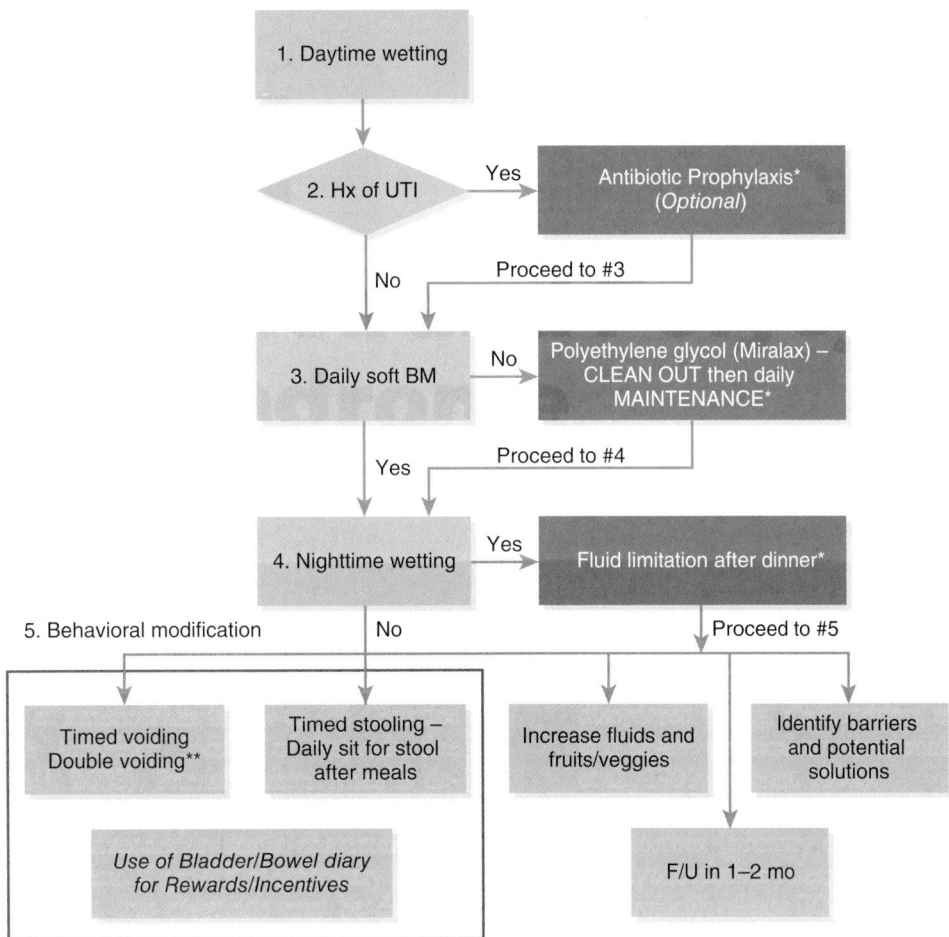

Figure 15-3 Algorithm for Diagnosis, Evaluation, and Treatment for Urinary Incontinence

child void and listen to urine flow for interruption or smooth flow. Review past history and bladder scan (if available); evaluate patient's voiding pattern and postvoiding residual (PVR).
3. Renal bladder ultrasound if positive for UTI or severe wetting (**Figures 15-3** and **15-4**).
4. Abdominal plain film if there is stool retention or unclear history of constipation
5. Voiding cystourethrogram (VCUG) if positive history of febrile UTI; or video urodynamics study, which includes fluoroscopic voiding cystourethrogram in addition to the urodynamics study of the bladder (Figures 15-3 and 15-4).
6. Urodynamics study and spinal magnetic resonance imaging if suspicion of neurogenic bladder for both day and nighttime incontinence or no improvement with initial treatment regimen (at least 3 months) of non-monosymptomatic enuresis

C. *Management, including treatment, consultation, referral, and follow-up care* (**Tables 15-4** *and* **15-5**; *Figures 15-3 and 15-4*) (Austin et al., 2016; Bernal et al., 2018; Burgers et al., 2013; Dos Santos et al., 2017; Maternik et al., 2015; Middleton & Ellsworth, 2019)

1. Daytime incontinence
   a. Bladder and bowel dysfunction: Adhere to strict urotherapy, including education on normal bladder function, regular voiding and elimination habits and posture, fluid intake, prevention of stool retention, and instruction on the use of voiding and elimination diaries. Of note, not enough data exist regarding benefits of fiber or probiotics for them to be recommended routinely.
   b. Vaginal reflux and postvoid dribbling: Sit on toilet with underwear all the way down by the ankles or sit backward on toilet to allow full abduction of legs during urination to prevent urine from backflowing into the vagina.
   c. Giggle incontinence and enuresis risoria: methylphenidate, 0.2–0.5 mg/kg orally daily for 2 months for trial
      i. Children less than 10 years of age: short-acting (4-h) form used midmorning
      ii. Children more than 10 years of age: intermediate-acting (8-h) form used before school (Middleton & Ellsworth, 2019)

164 Chapter 15 Urinary Incontinence in Children

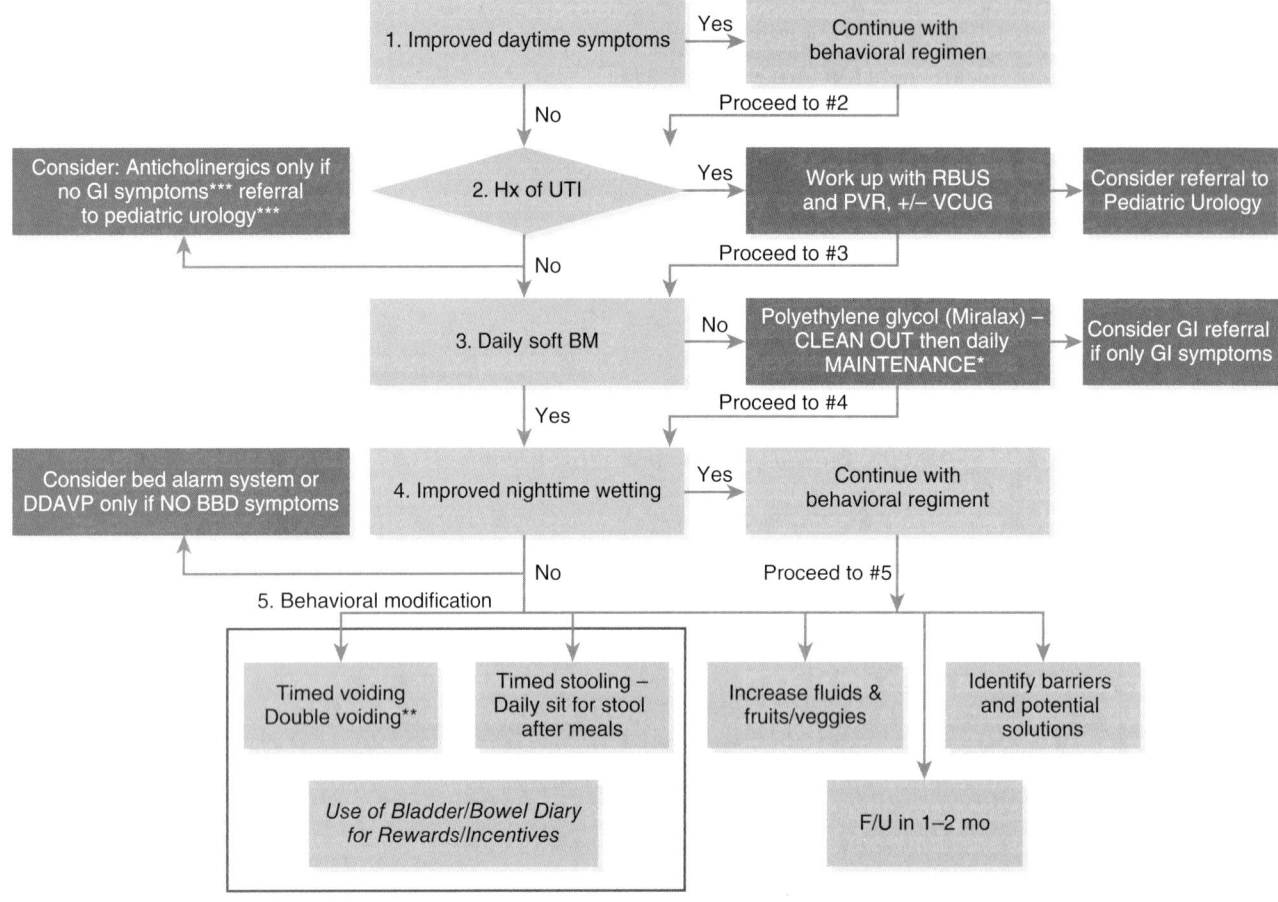

* Consider workup and management accordingly; see Tables 17-3, 17-4, and 17-5. Stool retention must be addressed/resolved.
** Void every 1–2 hr; double void if elevated postvoid residual.
***Consider anticholinergics only if (+) symptoms despite adherence to excellent behavioral modification.

Figure 15-4 Algorithm for Follow-Up of Urinary Incontinence

Table 15-4 Management of Daytime and Nighttime Urinary Incontinence*

Step	Recommendation	Comments
Step 1: Initial workup or treatment	Antibiotic prophylaxis if needed (Table 15-5)	If positive for recurrent urinary tract infection or incomplete emptying, consider daily low-dose prophylactic antibiotics at the same time as timed voiding and stooling May consider: ■ Trimethoprim-sulfamethoxazole ■ Nitrofurantoin
	Timed voiding and double voiding	Initiate voiding every 1–2 hours during the day whether or not the child "feels the need"; approximately 6 times per day: first thing in the morning, midmorning recess, lunch, midafternoon before coming home, dinner, and bedtime. May use an alarm but best to build into daily routine. Provide school note as needed. If elevated postvoid residual (>10% estimated bladder capacity), perform double voiding by returning to void a few minutes after initial voiding; may consider antibiotic prophylaxis and eventually potentially biofeedback AVOID POSTPONING BEHAVIOR!

Step	Recommendation	Comments
	Timed stooling	After a meal, typically dinner, sit on toilet for 10 minutes to attempt to have a bowel movement, and as needed. Avoid rushing through the attempt. Use of footstool to help with best posture in stooling.
	Voiding and elimination diary (Figure 15-2)	Document every voiding and elimination attempt each day, along with any dry days and nights. May do a frequency–volume chart of shorter duration (i.e., 2-day diary) that includes fluid intake and volume voided. Make note of size, shape, and consistency of stool.
	Rewards system	Use the results on voiding–elimination diary to provide positive reinforcement. Small treats, stickers, stamps, and privileges for voiding and elimination attempts rather than just for accident-free days and nights.
	Dietary adjustments	Encourage fluids throughout the day (water best); avoid sodas and caffeinated beverages. Aim for 1 cup of fluid after all voids. Increase fruit intake; natural best.
	Stool retention and encopresis management (Table 15-5)	If initial presentation with significant stool retention or encopresis, or on return with symptoms despite behavioral regimen, consider polyethylene glycol (Miralax) for cleanout and maintenance regimen. May consider footstool to achieve best posture to relax external sphincter for stooling and voiding. Refer to pediatric gastrointestinal service for further workup if no improvement or gastrointestinal symptoms more severe than genitourinary symptoms. Instruct families to expect 6–12 months of treatment, then wean therapy.
	Fluid restriction (for nocturnal enuresis)	Avoid large amounts of fluids ingested at dinner and beyond. Caution: children in afterschool sports activities require sufficient rehydration; thus, significant fluid restriction may cause further dehydration. Encourage fluid intake throughout the day.
	Follow-up	Return to clinic in 1 month for close follow-up; best to maintain frequent contact, especially if minor adjustments are necessary to behavior regimen.
Step 2: Follow-up evaluation or treatment	Reevaluate	On return, review voiding–elimination diary and symptoms since last visit. Repeat uroflowmetry and postvoid residual check (if available). If failed to comply with behavioral regimen, discuss barriers and possible ways to resolve barriers. Continue with timed voiding, timed stooling, use of diary, and reward system. Treatment outcome: ■ If <50% reduction in symptoms, considered as "No response" ■ If 50%–99% reduction in symptoms, considered "Partial response" ■ If 100% reduction in symptoms, considered "Complete response" ■ If >1 symptom reoccurs per month, considered as "Relapse" ■ No relapse for 6 months after treatment stopped is considered "Continued success" ■ If no relapse after 2 years of treatment stopped, considered "Complete success"

(continues)

Table 15-4 Management of Daytime and Nighttime Urinary Incontinence* *(continued)*

Step	Recommendation	Comments
	Anticholinergic and antispasmodic medication (daytime incontinence or non-monosymptomatic enuresis despite timed voiding) (Table 15-5)	Use as adjunct to strict timed voiding for those with uninhibited bladder spasms and potentially increased functional bladder capacity. May consider: ■ Oxybutynin ■ Tolterodine Second line of treatment for monosymptomatic enuresis or in conjunction with desmopressin acetate (DDAVP).
	Bed alarm system (monosymptomatic enuresis)	Consider for children greater than 6 years of age. Choose loud sensor (sound/lights/vibration) to wake child up at the beginning of accident at night; not the same as setting an alarm at a specific time of the night. Sensor is attached to underwear and is activated by the wetting of the underwear. Child needs to get up (or to be woken up) at the time of alarm activation to void, then reattach alarm. Should follow-up on results in 2–3 weeks; overall regimen for 2–3 months. If not effective, can consider pharmacologic regimen. Pro: conditioning regimen; effective when used correctly in a motivated child and family (80%). Con: wakes up entire family with the loud sound; if soft, then does not wake child up to void; relapse may occur after discontinuation.
	Antidiuretic: DDAVP (monosymptomatic enuresis) (Table 15-5)	First line of pharmacologic treatment for monosymptomatic enuresis.
	Tricyclic antidepressant: imipramine (Tofranil) (Table 15-5)	Third line of pharmacologic treatment for enuresis related to safety concerns.
	Additional modalities: biofeedback	Consider biofeedback therapy to learn to relax sphincter and empty to completion; limited by child's ability to cooperate and follow directions; "bladder-stretching" exercises are not useful.
	Other modalities (less evidence in the literature)	Alpha-blocker therapy for overactive bladder Hypnosis Acupuncture Chiropractor Extracorporeal magnetic innervation therapy Botulinum A toxin for overactive bladder or sphincter dyssynergia
	Timed voiding and stooling regimen	Continue strict timed voiding and stooling along with medication trial.
	Follow-up	Return in 1–2 months for follow-up and minor adjustments. Continued support for patient and family. Provide motivation in compliance with regimen. Reminder regarding length of time required for full recovery.
Step 3: Without improvement despite treatment compliance	Referral for further workup	Pediatric gastroenterology if severe encopresis or stool retention. Pediatric urology if recurrent urinary tract infection, persistent daytime or nighttime wetting, or suspicion of neurogenic bladder (require full workup of renal bladder ultrasound, urodynamic study, spinal magnetic resonance imaging). Psychotherapy for emotional stressors to be assessed and treated.

* Includes treatment, consultation, referral, and follow-up care.

Table 15-5 Common Urologic and Bowel Regimen Medication

Category	Indication/Mechanism of Action	Name	Dosage	Side Effects	Comments
Anticholinergic	Treat daytime incontinence caused by bladder overactivity (uninhibited contractions) Second line of treatment for monosymptomatic enuresis or in conjunction with desmopressin acetate (DDAVP)—must rule out constipation and daytime voiding dysfunction first	Oxybutynin	Daytime: 5 mg PO BID or TID dosing; or XL 10 mg PO daily Nighttime wetting: 5 mg PO QHS Immediate-release, extended-release, and transdermal forms available Max dose 0.4 mg/kg	Dry mouth, constipation, occasional initial drowsiness; do not use in hot weather because of reduced perspiration, which leads to facial flushing; possible mood changes	Contraindication: incomplete emptying
		Tolterodine	2 mg PO QHS or 1 mg PO BID		
Antidiuretic	Synthetic antidiuretic hormone to reduce urine output at night Consider for children >6 years of age 30% respond fully; 40% partial response May use only for sleepovers or camp	DDAVP	Dose: 0.2-mg tablet 1-3 tablets PO QHS (1 hour before bedtime); may use higher dose then taper down	Risk of hyponatremia (rare) with mostly nasal spray formulation (longer half-life); limit fluids after dinner	Contraindication: excessive fluid intake in evening, (+) headache, nausea, or vomiting
Antidepressant	Mechanism unknown; used rarely; 50% response rate	Imipramine	0.5–1.5 mg/kg/d given 1–2 hours before bedtime OR 25–50 mg PO QHS (50 mg for children >9 years of age)	Daytime sedation, anxiety, insomnia, dry mouth, nausea, and personality changes	Overdose can cause fatal cardiac arrhythmias, hypotension, respiratory distress, and convulsions.

(continues)

Table 15-5 Common Urologic and Bowel Regimen Medication *(continued)*

Category	Indication/Mechanism of Action	Name	Dosage	Side Effects	Comments
Osmotic laxative	Induce catharsis by strong electrolyte and osmotic effect	Polyethylene glycol (Miralax)	Cleanout: 1.5 g/kg/d for 3 days (may split to BID dose) followed by daily maintenance dose and daily sit Maintenance: 2–11 years of age: 8.5 g (1/2 cap) in 4 oz. of water per day >12 years of age: 17 g (1 cap) in 8 oz. of water per day; or 0.26–0.84 g/kg/d (titrate accordingly for daily soft stool)	Nausea, vomiting, cramps	If no stooling, return to cleanout procedure and then maintenance Parents will titrate depending on stool output, consistency, and staining
Antibiotic	Treatment of UTI; daily low-dose prophylaxis for prevention of UTIs	Trimethoprim (TMP)–sulfamethoxazole	UTI prophylaxis: 2 mg/kg/dose of TMP daily	Nausea, vomiting, Stevens–Johnson syndrome, rash	Contraindication: hypersensitivity to sulfa drug, trimethoprim, or components
		Nitrofurantoin	UTI prophylaxis: 1–2 mg/kg/d as single daily dose; maximum 100 mg/d	Nausea, vomiting, anorexia, Stevens–Johnson syndrome, rash Avoid suspension; use capsule instead and sprinkle on yogurt or ice cream Administer with food or milk	

UTI, urinary tract infection.
Data from Walia, R., Mahajan, L., & Steffen, R. (2009). Recent advances in chronic constipation. Current Opinion in Pediatrics, 21, 661–666.

d. Valsalva voiding habits should be referred to pediatric urology for consultation and workup.
2. Nighttime incontinence
   a. Non-monosymptomatic: Start with treatment for daytime incontinence and address any other comorbid factors (e.g., stooling) before achieving nighttime continence.
   b. Monosymptomatic primary nocturnal enuresis: following daytime urotherapy and ruling out of stool retention, choice of bed alarm or medication if appropriate
   c. Secondary non-monosymptomatic nocturnal enuresis: Following daytime urotherapy and ruling out of stool retention, if unresponsive, refer to pediatric urology for full workup, possibly with renal bladder ultrasound, urodynamics, and/or spinal magnetic resonance imaging to rule out neurogenic bladder caused by possible tethered cord or other etiologies.

D. Client education
1. Information
   Provide verbal and, preferably, written information regarding the following:
   a. Normal bladder and bowel functions, coordination of detrusor muscle with external sphincter muscle, and relationship between bladder and bowel functions
   b. The disease process, including but not limited to signs and symptoms and underlying etiologies. Emphasize that this condition is neither the child's nor parent's fault and that the healthcare provider will work together with the family to resolve issues. Provide encouragement and motivation throughout the recovery process (average 3–6 months or as long as the length of dysfunction).
   c. Diagnostic tests, including a discussion about preparation, cost, the actual procedures, and aftercare
   d. Management (rationale, action, use, side effects, associated risks, and cost of therapeutic interventions; need for adhering to long-term treatment plans)
2. Counseling
   a. Recommended if symptoms have contributed to emotional distress or social isolation
   b. If underlying issues contribute to the incontinence and encopresis, counseling or other psychotherapy may assist in addressing and correcting the issues.

VI. Resources
A. Provider resources
1. A number of validated tools are available to measure the psychological and behavioral effects of incontinence, such as the Child Behavioral Check List (CBCL) or the PINQ, a cross-cultural continence-specific pediatric quality-of-life measurement tool (Thibodeau et al., 2013).
2. International Children's Continence Society (http://i-c-c-s.org/)

B. Patient and client education websites
1. http://www.Kidshealth.org
   Part of Nemours Foundation's Center for Children's Health Media, Kidhealth.org is a website dedicated to providing health and safety information and helpful tips, in both English and Spanish. Content is designed to specifically address parents, kids, and teenagers. Search "bedwetting" to retrieve helpful information.
2. http://www.Healthychildren.org
   Sponsored by the American Academy of Pediatrics. Contains health topics ranging from regular development to conditions such as enuresis and constipation.
3. http://www.i-c-c-s.org
   International Children's Continence Society official website. Includes resources for providers and patients on bladder and bowel dysfunction.
4. http://www.Bedwettingstore.com
   Offers both resources and products to help manage daytime and nighttime urinary incontinence.

References

Aetna. (2022). *Nocturnal enuresis treatments*. http://www.aetna.com/cpb/medical/data/400_499/0431.html

Arnhym, A. (2018). Nocturnal enuresis. In L. S. Baskin, B. A. Kogan, & J. A. Stocks (Eds.), *Handbook of pediatric urology* (3rd ed., pp. 107–113). Wolters Kluwer Health.

Austin, P. F., Bauer, S. B., Bower, W., Chase, J., Franco, I., Hoebeke, P., Rittig, S., & Walle, J. V. (2016). The standardization of terminology of lower urinary tract function in children and adolescents: Update report from the Standardization Committee of the International Children's Continence Society. *Neurourology and Urodynamics*, 35(4), 471–481. doi:10.1002/nau.22751

Bernal, C. J., Dole, M., & Thame, K. (2018). The role of bowel management in children with bladder and bowel dysfunction. *Current Bladder Dysfunction Reports*, 13(2), 46–55. doi:10.1007/s11884-018-0458-3

Bogaert, G., Stein, R., Undre, S., Nijman, R. J. M., Quadackers, J., 't Hoen, L., Kocvara, R., Silay, S., Tekgul, S., Radmayr, C., & Dogan, H. S. (2020). Practical recommendations of the EAU-ESPU Guidelines Committee for monosymptomatic enuresis—bedwetting. *Neurourology and Urodynamics*, 39(2), 489–497. doi:10.1002/nau.24239

Burgers, R. E., Mugie, S. M., Chase, J., Cooper, C. S., von Gontard, A., Rittig, C. S., Homsy, Y., Bauer, S. B., & Benninga, M. A. (2013). Management of functional constipation in children with lower urinary tract symptoms: Report from the Standardization Committee of the International Children's Continence Society. *Journal of Urology*, *190*(1), 29–36. doi:10.1016/j.juro.2013.01.001

Butler, R., & Heron, J. (2008). An exploration of children's views of bed-wetting at 9 years. *Child: Care, Health and Development*, *34*(1), 65–70. doi:10.1111/j.1365-2214.2007.00781.x

Butler, R., Heron, J., & ALSPAC Study Team. (2006). Exploring the differences between mono- and polysymptomatic nocturnal enuresis. *Scandinavian Journal of Urology and Nephrology*, *40*(4), 313–319. doi:10.1080/00365590600750144

Champeau, A. (2018). Daytime urinary incontinence/bladder and bowel dysfunction (in the otherwise healthy child). In L. S. Baskin, B. A. Kogan, & J. A. Stocks (Eds.), *Handbook of pediatric urology* (3rd ed., pp. 91–106). Wolters Kluwer Health.

Dos Santos, J. (2014). Recommendations for the management of bladder bowel dysfunction in children. *Pediatrics & Therapeutics*, *4*, 1. doi:10.4172/2161-0665.1000191

Dos Santos, J., Lopes, R. I., & Koyle, M. A. (2017). Bladder and bowel dysfunction in children: An update on the diagnosis and treatment of a common, but underdiagnosed pediatric problem. *Canadian Urological Association Journal*, *11*(Suppl. 1–2), 64. doi:10.5489/cuaj.4411

Feldman, A., & Bauer, S. (2006). Diagnosis and management of dysfunctional voiding. *Current Opinion in Pediatrics*, *18*(2), 139–147. doi:10.1097/01.mop.0000193289.64151.49

Glassberg, K., & Combs, A. (2009). Nonneurogenic voiding disorders: What's new? *Current Opinion in Urology*, *19*(4), 412–418. doi:10.1097/MOU.0b013e32832c90d9

Greenfield, S., & Cooper, C. (2019). *Pediatric urology for primary care*. American Academy of Pediatrics.

Joinson, C., Heron, J., von Gontard, A., Butler, U., Golding, J., & Emond, A. (2008). Early childhood risk factors associated with daytime wetting and soiling in school-age children. *Journal of Pediatric Psychology*, *33*(7), 739–750. doi:10.1093/jpepsy/jsn008

Joinson, C., Sullivan, S., von Gontard, A., & Heron, J. (2016). Early childhood psychological factors and risk for bedwetting at school age in a UK cohort. *European Child & Adolescent Psychiatry*, *25*(5), 519–528. doi:10.1007/s00787-015-0756-7

Maternik, M., Krzeminska, K., & Zurowska, A. (2015). The management of childhood urinary incontinence. *Pediatric Nephrology*, *30*(1), 41–50. doi:10.1007/s00467-014-2791-x

Middleton, T., & Ellsworth, P. (2019). Pharmacologic therapies for the management of non-neurogenic urinary incontinence in children. *Expert Opinion on Pharmacotherapy*, *20*(18), 2335–2352. doi:10.1080/14656566.2019.1674282

Thibodeau, B. A., Metcalfe, P., Koop, P., & Moore, K. (2013). Urinary incontinence and quality of life in children. *Journal of Pediatric Urology*, *9*(1), 78–83. doi:10.1016/j.jpurol.2011.12.005

Yang, S., & Chua, M. E. (2018). Diagnosis and management of bladder bowel dysfunction in children with urinary tract infections: A -position statement from the International Children's Continence Society. *Pediatric Nephrology*, *33*(12), 2207. doi:10.1007/s00467-017-3799-9

SECTION III

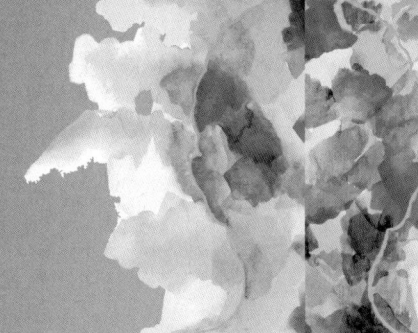

Common Sexual and Reproductive Health Presentations

CHAPTER 16	Abnormal Uterine Bleeding	173
CHAPTER 17	Abortion Care in the Primary Care Setting	187
CHAPTER 18	Amenorrhea and Polycystic Ovary Syndrome	211
CHAPTER 19	Benign Prostatic Hyperplasia	223
CHAPTER 20	Early Pregnancy Loss	231
CHAPTER 21	Contraception	243
CHAPTER 22	Menopause Transition	275
CHAPTER 23	Chronic Pelvic Pain in Persons Assigned Female at Birth	289
CHAPTER 24	Sexual Dysfunction	301
CHAPTER 25	Urinary Incontinence in Persons Assigned Female at Birth	309

CHAPTER 16

Abnormal Uterine Bleeding

Pilar Bernal de Pheils, Lisa Mihaly, and Sarah Nathan

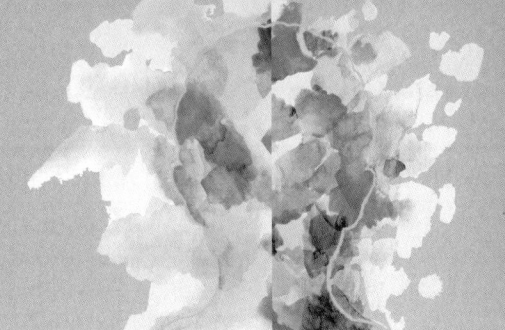

I. Introduction and general background

Abnormal vaginal bleeding is one of the most common reasons that people present for healthcare evaluation. The origin of genital bleeding is most often uterine, in which case it is called *abnormal uterine bleeding* (AUB). It can also arise from other parts of the genital tract and can be caused by systemic illness. Estimates of AUB prevalence range from 3% to 30% (Munro et al., 2018). In the United States, heavy or prolonged menstrual bleeding (previously called *menorrhagia*) alone has been noted as the primary cause for 30% of referrals to gynecological specialty practices (Miller et al., 2015). Changes in the menstrual cycle accounted for 19.1% of the 20.1 million visits to healthcare providers for gynecological conditions observed in a 2-year study (Nicholson et al., 2001).

Menstruation, ovulation, and the coordinated sequence of endocrine signals that comprise the menstrual cycle are the foundation for the regularity, predictability, and consistency of menstrual bleeding (Fritz & Speroff, 2011). Although an extensive review of the endocrinology of the menstrual cycle is beyond the scope of this chapter, an overview of the normal menstrual cycle provides important background and context for understanding AUB.

A normal menstrual cycle consists of three distinct phases: the follicular phase, ovulation, and the luteal phase. All of these phases are managed by the complex feedback loop of the hypothalamic–pituitary–ovarian (HPO) axis (Fritz & Speroff, 2011). During the follicular phase, increasing levels of follicle-stimulating hormone (FSH) from the pituitary cause the development and maturation of a dominant ovarian follicle, which in turn leads to increased production of estrogen by the follicle and the proliferation of the endometrium. Increasing levels of estrogen also stimulate a surge of luteinizing hormone (LH) from the pituitary; ovulation occurs in response. After ovulation, the corpus luteum, which develops from the dominant ovarian follicle, continues to produce estrogen and also begins to produce progesterone. As this luteal phase progresses, the corpus luteum continues to enlarge, producing greater levels of progesterone and estrogen, and the endometrium becomes more organized in preparation for implantation. If conception does not occur, the corpus luteum regresses spontaneously on a predictable and stable timetable. With this regression, estrogen and progesterone levels drop rapidly, and menstruation begins again.

Newer terminology has been adapted to define clinical presentations of AUB (Munro et al., 2012). Terms such as "menorrhagia" and "metrorrhagia" have been replaced by "heavy or prolonged menstrual bleeding" for the former and "irregular bleeding" for the latter. See **Table 16-1** for a description of new terminology as well as the characteristics of the normal limits of the menstrual cycle/bleeding.

Etiologies of AUB are classified as related or unrelated to uterine structural abnormalities, categorized with the acronym PALM-COEIN (Munro et al., 2012). Structural abnormalities (PALM) are polyps, adenomyosis, leiomyomas, and malignancy/hyperplasia; nonstructural abnormalities (COEIN) are coagulopathy, ovulatory dysfunction, endometrial dysfunction, iatrogenic, and not otherwise classified (**Table 16-2**).

AUB can manifest as acute or chronic. *Acute* refers to bleeding in a reproductive-age patient "who is not pregnant, that, in the opinion of the provider is of sufficient quantity to require immediate intervention to prevent further blood loss" (Munro et al., 2012, p. 261). A patient's perception of menstrual blood loss may differ significantly from the measured amount of blood loss (Hallberg et al., 1966). The British National Collaborating Centre for Women's and Children's Health offers a description that addresses patient concerns: "heavy menstrual bleeding" is defined as "excessive menstrual blood loss which interferes with the [patient's] physical, emotional, social and material

Table 16-1 Clinical Presentations of Abnormal Uterine Bleeding

Clinical Presentation	Descriptive Terms—New Terminology: International Federation of Gynecology and Obstetrics (FIGO) (Munro et al., 2012)	Descriptive Terms—Old Terminology	Frequency of Menses Normal Limits
Frequency of menses	Normal		24–38 days
	Frequent	Polymenorrhea	<21–24 days
	Infrequent	Oligomenorrhea	>38 days
	Absent	Amenorrhea	No menses × 3 regular cycles
Regularity of menses, cycle-to-cycle variation over 12 months (timing)	Regular	Regular	(2–20 days, FIGO)
	Irregular	Metrorrhagia	Variation > 20 days acyclical
Duration of flow	Prolonged	Menorrhagia	>8.0 days
	Normal	Normal	4.5–8 days
	Shortened	Hypomenorrhea	<4.5 (2 days)
Volume of monthly blood loss	Heavy	Menorrhagia	>80 cc
	Normal	Normal	5–80 cc
	Light	Hypomenorrhea	<5 cc

Data from Munro, M G, Critchley, H O, & Fraser, I S. (2012). American journal of obstetrics and gynecology, 207(4), 259-65.

Table 16-2 Abnormal Uterine Bleeding Etiologies Outside of Pregnancy

Classification	Likely Etiology
PALM (structural-organic and pelvic tract pathology)	Polyps (AUB-P) Adenomyosis (AUB-A) Leiomyomata (AUB-LSM for submucosal myoma or AUB-LO for myomas in other layers) Malignancy (AUB-M)
COEIN (nonstructural-systemic pathology)	Coagulation disorders (AUB-C) Ovulatory dysfunction (AUB-O) Endometrial: AUB-E Iatrogenic (AUB-I) Not yet classified (AUB-N)

Data from Munro, M G, Critchley, H O, & Fraser, I S. (2012). American journal of obstetrics and gynecology, 207(4), 259-65.

quality of life, and which can occur alone, or in combination with other symptoms" (National Collaborating Centre for Women's and Children's Health, 2007, "Definition of HMB" section).

When abnormal bleeding occurs before menarche or after menopause, malignancy is a primary concern. Pregnancy should always be considered in patients in their reproductive years because bleeding in early pregnancy can lead to severe health consequences and may be a result of a ruptured ectopic pregnancy. See Chapter 20: Early Pregnancy Loss for more information.

A. PALM (structural) etiologies: polyps, adenomyosis, leiomyomas, malignancy (Munro et al., 2012). (Unless otherwise noted, all information in this section is from Munro et al. [2012]; see also Table 16-2.)
  1. Definition and overview
     a. Polyps are focal outgrowths of the endometrium, found in the endometrial cavity or in the cervical

canal. Polyps may be asymptomatic and are almost always benign. They are often seen in association with uterine bleeding in premenopausal and postmenopausal patients. If bleeding occurs, it will likely present as intermenstrual bleeding.
  b. Adenomyosis is a benign condition in which the endometrium invades the myometrium, producing a diffusely enlarged uterus. It can cause heavy bleeding and dysmenorrhea, although it may also be asymptomatic. A presumptive diagnosis is made by ultrasound or magnetic resonance imaging (MRI). A definite diagnosis can only be made via uterine pathology after hysterectomy.
  c. Leiomyomas are benign tumors originating mainly from myometrium (smooth muscle of the uterus). They are also called *myomas* and *fibroids*. They are classified as subserosal (originating at the serosal surface of the uterus), intramural (developing from within the uterine wall), or submucosal (originating from the myometrial cells just underneath the endometrium).

  Leiomyomas are typically asymptomatic, and the evaluation of AUB should not necessarily cease with this finding. However, they may present with pelvic pain and heavy and prolonged menstrual bleeding (Khan et al., 2014). Submucosal leiomyomas are more likely to cause AUB, although bleeding can be significant regardless of location and size (Doherty et al., 2014). Growth of leiomyomas is associated with exposure to circulating estrogen; thus, these lesions can grow rapidly in the reproductive years.
  d. Malignancy is most commonly endometrioid endometrial carcinoma and develops out of endometrial hyperplasia (Emons et al., 2015). It must be considered in nearly all patients who present with AUB, especially postmenopausal patients. Obesity, high blood pressure, and diabetes mellitus may increase the risk of endometrial cancer (Aune et al., 2017).
2. Prevalence
  a. Polyps are detected in an estimated 20%–40% of patients with AUB (Lasmar et al., 2008) but are not always the source of bleeding.
  b. Adenomyosis prevalence estimates vary from 5% to 70% in a range of studies (Munro et al., 2012).
  c. During the reproductive years, uterine leiomyomas are the most common solid pelvic tumor, found in between 25% and 40% of patients (Sparic et al., 2016). They are rarely observed before menarche and significantly decrease in size in the postmenopausal years.
  d. About 3.1% of persons assigned female at birth (AFAB) will develop uterine cancer in their lifetimes (National Institutes of Health [NIH], 2022). However, abnormal endometrial histology in premenopausal patients with irregular bleeding is 14% (Fritz & Speroff, 2011).

Approximately one-third of endometrial cancer cases are diagnosed in patients between 55 and 64 years old, and another third are diagnosed in patients between 65 and 74 (NIH, 2022).
B. COEIN etiologies (nonstructural anomalies): *coagulopathy, ovulatory dysfunction, endometrial dysfunction, iatrogenic, not otherwise classified* (Unless otherwise noted, all information in this section is from Munro et al. [2012].)
  1. Definition and overview
    a. Coagulopathy encompasses a variety of systemic disorders of hemostasis that include clotting defects, thrombocytopenia, and platelet/fibrin function defects. The most common coagulopathy is von Willebrand disease (VWD), which is classified as mild, moderate, or severe (American College of Obstetricians and Gynecologists [ACOG], 2013b). Diagnosis usually occurs at menarche, although clinical symptoms can present at any age, with heavy menstrual bleeding being one of the most significant morbidities (ACOG, 2013b; Ng et al., 2015). Other symptoms of coagulopathies include excessive blood loss with dental work, postpartum hemorrhage, surgery-related bleeding, epistaxis one to two times per month, and frequent gum bleeding (ACOG, 2013b).
    b. Ovulatory disorders commonly present with changes in the frequency and flow of menses (Table 16-1). Previously called *dysfunctional uterine bleeding*, it is now called *ovulatory dysfunction*. Terminology for all subtypes of menstrual variation have been updated, as noted in Table 16-1. Patients with anovulatory cycles experience disrupted and unpredictable patterns of hormone production that result in irregular and variable menstrual bleeding. These patients are essentially in a continuous follicular phase because there is no stimulus for ovulation or subsequent luteal phase development. As a result, the endometrium is continually exposed to estrogen, with resulting proliferation. Ultimately, without the organizing support of progesterone produced during the luteal phase, focal areas of the structurally fragile endometrium begin to break down, leading to a pattern of heavy and/or irregular heavy menstrual bleeding (Fritz & Speroff, 2011). Ovulatory dysfunction can be triggered by many factors, including stress, disordered eating, changes in exercise, and recent illness (Fourman & Fazeli, 2015). This phenomenon can be seen in polycystic ovary syndrome (PCOS). It is also associated with obesity and is more common in patients in the first years after menarche and those in the perimenopausal period (Fritz & Speroff, 2011). Anovulation occurs most often at the extremes of reproductive life: soon after menarche due to immaturity

of the hypothalamic–pituitary axis and in the years before menopause due to declining ovarian function (ACOG, 2013a). In both scenarios, bleeding patterns are noncyclic, and the flow may be heavy or light, with few if any moliminal symptoms (breast tenderness, bloating, mood changes, and dysmenorrhea) (Fritz & Speroff, 2011). For more information, see Chapter 18: Amenorrhea and Polycystic Ovary Syndrome.

c. Endometrial etiologies present as heavy menstrual bleeding in the context of regular predictable menstrual cycles (Sriprasert et al., 2017). The etiology may be a disorder of homeostasis, for which there are no available tests (previously called *idiopathic* AUB), or local inflammation or infection (e.g., *Chlamydia trachomatis*) (Goje, 2021; Sriprasert et al., 2017). Other pelvic tract etiologies include infections such as salpingitis, cervicitis, endometritis, myometritis, pelvic inflammatory disease, and tubo-ovarian abscesses (Goje, 2021). Other etiologies include vulvovaginal trauma such as foreign body, abrasions, lacerations, and sexual abuse or assault (Anderson & Paterek, 2022; Russo et al., 2017).

d. Iatrogenic causes include anticoagulants (e.g., warfarin and heparin), anticonvulsants, and certain antibiotics (e.g., rifampin and griseofulvin) (Brenner, 1996; Hapangama & Bulmer, 2016). Because of enhanced hepatic metabolism, cigarette smoking can increase the incidence of breakthrough bleeding in patients using combined hormonal contraceptives (Rosenberg et al., 1996). Systemic medications that interfere with dopamine metabolism, resulting in inhibition of prolactin release (e.g., tricyclic antidepressants and phenothiazines), may lead to absent or infrequent menses (Gordon et al., 2017). See Chapter 18: Amenorrhea and Polycystic Ovary Syndrome for a list of medications causing amenorrhea and oligomenorrhea.

Menstrual cycles are also affected by medications that influence ovulation, particularly hormonal medications, including estrogens, progestins, and androgens (Thorneycroft, 1999). Hormonal contraceptive agents usually result in regular withdrawal bleeding when used in a cyclical manner, although it can be normal for bleeding not to occur in some cycles. Unscheduled bleeding (also called *breakthrough bleeding*) may be related to missed, delayed, or improper use of hormonal contraceptive methods but can also occur with consistent use (Barr, 2010). Breakthrough bleeding is common in the first 3 months of combined hormonal contraceptive use (Barr, 2010). Patients using progestin-only contraceptives, such as the levonorgestrel intrauterine system (IUS), the progestin-only pill, the Depo-Provera injection, or the contraceptive implant, may have unscheduled bleeding (Villavicencio & Allen, 2016). Patients using the copper intrauterine device (IUD) may have increased menstrual flow, especially in the first 3–6 months after insertion (Villavicencio & Allen, 2016). See Chapter 21: Contraception for more information. Hormone therapy in postmenopausal patients may also cause irregular bleeding (see Chapter 22: Menopause Transition).

e. Not-yet-classified etiologies include those conditions that have not been demonstrated conclusively to contribute to AUB or other disorders that have not yet been identified by current diagnostic assays.

2. Prevalence
   a. As many as 20% of patients with AUB have an underlying coagulation disorder, most commonly VWD (ACOG, 2013a).
   b. Ovulatory dysfunction occurs in over a third of reproductive-age patients (Prior et al., 2015).
   c. Endometrial etiologies occur in approximately 2% of patients (Sun et al., 2018).
   d. Iatrogenic etiologies also occur in approximately 2% of patients (Sun et al., 2018).
   e. Not-yet-classified etiologies account for less than 1% of AUB (Sun et al., 2018).

II. Database (may include but is not limited to)
A. *Subjective*
   1. History of present illness. A menstrual calendar (on paper or using phone applications) can be very helpful in collecting this information.
      a. Precipitating factors associated with abnormal bleeding (e.g., coitus, trauma, douching, presence of pessary, recent life stressors)
      b. Date of onset of change in menses: rapid or gradual change
      c. Flow: heavier or lighter than typical (based on patient's report of their own bleeding patterns)
      d. Presence of intermenstrual bleeding, premenarchal or postmenopausal bleeding, and postcoital bleeding
      e. Relieving factors: medications, supplements, or activities that decrease or regulate bleeding
      f. Aggravating factors: medication, supplements, or activities that increase bleeding or change the bleeding pattern
      g. Associated symptoms, such as cramping or molimina
      h. Impact of AUB on life (e.g., sex, exercise, work or school)
   2. Past medical history (Fritz & Speroff, 2011)
      a. Obstetric history
         i. History of postpartum hemorrhage
         ii. History of pregnancy complicated by leiomyoma
         iii. Recent history of pregnancy ending in spontaneous or therapeutic abortion

b. Gynecological history
   i. General bleeding patterns
   ii. Bleeding associated with sexual or physical activity, trauma, infection
   iii. Gynecological surgeries (C-sections, myomectomy, cervical procedures), including evaluation, findings, and treatment
   iv. Previous episodes of AUB, including workup and treatments
   v. Pap test history, including date and results of most recent Pap smear
   vi. History of sexually transmitted infections and upper reproductive tract infection (e.g., pelvic inflammatory disease, tubo-ovarian abscess). Note treatment and partner treatment.
   vii. Menstrual cycle history, including age at menarche, last normal menstrual period, and previous normal menstrual periods (preferably the previous three menses): usual cycle duration, flow, interval length, molimina symptoms that suggest ovulatory cycles
   viii. Contraception history: methods, side effects, concerns
   ix. Future fertility intent and concerns
   x. Sexual history and risk of sexually transmitted infection (STI)
c. General medical history: medical illnesses associated with bleeding changes (see Table 16-2); general medical health, especially thyroid, pelvic disorders (including pelvic inflammatory disease [PID]), and breast or gynecologic cancers
d. Medication history: medications, vitamins, and supplements (see Table 16-2)
e. Physical trauma history: sexual assault or sexual abuse (consider reporting requirements as appropriate)
f. Radiation exposure history (e.g., to breast, thyroid, pelvis)
g. History of pelvic trauma (e.g., motor vehicle accident) or straddle injuries

3. Family history
   a. Gynecological problems: excessive menstrual blood loss; uterine, breast, and ovarian malignancies; endometriosis; adenomyosis; leiomyomata; and diethylstilbestrol exposure
   b. Medical diseases: endocrine dysfunction, blood-clotting disorders

4. Personal and social history
   a. Education history, occupation, social and family support systems, situational life stress, social and personal anxiety level
   b. Habits: tobacco, alcohol, recreational drug use
   c. Nutrition: dietary history, intentional or unintentional weight loss or gain, disordered eating patterns
   d. Exercise history

5. Review of systems
   a. Constitutional signs: fatigue, weight gain or loss, weakness, malaise, hot or cold sensitivity, appetite change
   b. Skin, hair, and nails: hair loss or unwanted hair growth, petechiae, bruising, jaundice, acne, acanthosis nigricans, and unusual sweating
   c. Cardiac: palpitations, edema
   d. Abdomen: nausea and bloating
   e. Genitourinary: pelvic pain, dyspareunia, dysmenorrhea, hot flashes, night sweats, vaginal dryness, vaginal discharge
   f. Hematologic: excessive blood loss with dental work, postpartum hemorrhage or surgery-related bleeding, frequent gum bleeding

B. *Objective (physical examination)*
   1. Vital signs: orthostatic blood pressure, temperature, SpO_2%, total body weight
   2. General: distressed appearance
   3. Hair: texture, hirsutism, pattern of loss if present (axillary, pubic, and scalp hair)
   4. Eyes and ears: stare, lid lag, exophthalmos, and visual field abnormalities
   5. Neck: thyroid nodules or enlargement and lymph nodes
   6. Skin: pallor, jaundice, petechiae, ecchymosis, hematomas, palmar erythema, spider hemangiomata, rough or velvety texture, striae, acanthosis nigricans, acne, color of nailbeds
   7. Extremities: edema, perfusion, wasting
   8. Cardiovascular: tachycardia and murmurs
   9. Lungs: accessory muscle use
   10. Abdomen: striae, ascites, hepatomegaly, splenomegaly, tenderness, inguinal nodes, uterine fundal height if palpable
   11. Genital
       a. External genitalia: pubic hair distribution and developmental stage, clitoromegaly, ulcerations, edema, bruising, trauma, genitourinary syndrome of menopause (GSM)
       b. Vagina: traumatic lesions, bruising, erythema, type of discharge, foreign bodies, GSM
       c. Cervix: polyps, ectopy, ulcerations, inflammation, erythema, mucopurulent discharge, cervical motion tenderness, GSM
       d. Uterus: enlargement, contour, mobility, shape, consistency, tenderness, masses
       e. Adnexa: masses, tenderness
       f. Anus/rectum: masses, bleeding

C. *Assessment*
   1. Ensure the patient is hemodynamically stable. Suspect hemodynamic instability when the patient reports shortness of breath, dizziness, and/or syncope and when blood pressure is low and heart rate is high. Refer to emergency care if patient is unstable.
   2. Determine the appropriate diagnosis.
       a. Establish if the condition is acute or chronic. If the patient has both acute and chronic bleeding,

control acute bleeding while initiating investigation to determine the underlying etiology.
   b. Assess for any conditions that may underlie AUB: PALM (structural) or COEIN (nonstructural) etiologies (see Table 16-2).
   c. Rule out pregnancy and complications of pregnancy as warranted.
   d. Rule out malignancies as indicated.
   3. Assess the severity of AUB and associated conditions.
   4. Assess the significance of AUB to the patient and their support systems.
D. Goals of clinical management
   1. Choose a cost-effective approach for screening and evaluating AUB.
   2. Develop a treatment plan that addresses AUB and associated conditions and returns the patient to stability and optimal health in a safe and effective manner.
   3. Work with the patient to ensure that the treatment plan is manageable and is designed to reduce long-term complications of AUB, such as anemia and endometrial hyperplasia.
   4. When an ovarian cause is found, institute medical treatment to reestablish cycle regularity and provide endometrial protection (ACOG, 2013c).
E. Plan
   1. Diagnostic tests
      The patient's age, reproductive status, and data from the history and physical examination should guide the choice of appropriate diagnostic tests.
      a. Menstrual tracking
         For patients presenting with a history of irregular cycles, menstrual calendars and phone-based applications can be very helpful in establishing bleeding patterns. Number of pads or tampons and degree of saturation are of limited use in the evaluation of blood loss (Hallberg et al., 1966).
      b. Initial testing (**Table 16-3**) should evaluate for pregnancy, STIs, infection, and coagulopathies.

Table 16-3 Essential Initial Testing in the Investigation of Abnormal Uterine Bleeding (AUB)

Test	Definition	Clinical Implications	Comments
Pregnancy test (hCG)	Measures human chorionic gonadotropin hormone (B-hCG); can be run from urine or blood samples	A positive urine pregnancy test warrants ensuring the pregnancy is intrauterine (Fritz & Speroff, 2011; Strickland et al., 2006).	The American College of Obstetricians and Gynecologists (ACOG, 2013a) recommends that a urine pregnancy test should be ordered in all sexually active patients in their reproductive years, even those who have had a tubal ligation.
Complete blood count (CBC) with platelets	To rule out significant anemia and investigate bleeding disorders	Excessive vaginal bleeding can lead to iron-deficiency anemia. CBC and platelet count are also initial tests in the investigation of von Willebrand disease.	
Prothrombin time (PT), activated partial thromboplastin (aPTT)	Initial coagulation disorder testing	Initial testing for most common coagulation disorders may be indicated based on patient history, signs, and symptoms.	Abnormal results should be interpreted in conjunction with hematology (ACOG, 2013b).
Highly sensitive thyroid-stimulating hormone (TSH)	An anterior pituitary hormone that stimulates growth and function of thyroid cells	An elevated TSH is diagnostic of primary hypothyroidism; a low TSH indicates hyperthyroidism (both can be associated with AUB).	Thyroid disease is common in individuals assigned female at birth (AFAB). See Chapter 65: Thyroid Disorders for more information on diagnostic testing and treatment.

Test	Definition	Clinical Implications	Comments
Pap and/or human papillomavirus (HPV) test	To screen for cervical cancer	Early cervical cancer is frequently asymptomatic. Late cervical cancer may manifest as irregular, heavy, or postcoital bleeding (Cohen et al., 2019).	Endocervical and ectocervical sampling are required for accuracy. See Chapter 38: Adult Healthcare Maintenance and Promotion for further discussion.
Testing for *Neisseria gonorrhoeae* (GC) and *Chlamydia trachomatis* (CT)	Gold-standard method to test for GC and CT is nucleic acid amplification test (NAAT).	Cervicitis, caused by GC or CT, can cause postcoital or intermenstrual bleeding.	As indicated for sexually active patients. It can be collected in the endocervix or in the vagina. Patients can collect vaginal samples. First-catch urine (not clean catch) can also be submitted for NAAT testing.
Wet mount of vaginal secretions with normal saline and potassium hydroxide	Evaluate for vaginal infections: trichomoniasis, bacterial vaginosis, and vulvovaginal candidiasis.	Severe trichomoniasis, vulvovaginal candida, or bacterial vaginosis may present with postcoital bleeding.	Useful if vaginitis is suspected.
Transvaginal ultrasonography of the pelvis (TVS)	Ultrasound imaging (most importantly, transvaginal) plays a pivotal role in the evaluation of AUB.	Indicated to rule out anatomical lesions (endometrial polyps, leiomyomas, or adenomyosis), patients with regular cycles but heavy menstrual bleeding or long duration or intermenstrual bleeding (Dueholm, 2006), and when medical management has failed (Fritz & Speroff, 2011). Also used to measure the thickness of the endometrial lining in the postmenopausal patient and in the evaluation of adnexal and ovarian masses.	If the lining is 4 mm or less in a postmenopausal patient, endometrial cancer is very unlikely (Giannella et al., 2014). There is no standard thickness for premenopausal patients (Bignardi et al., 2009).
Endometrial biopsy (EMB)	Office sampling of the endometrium with low-pressure cannula (e.g., Pipelle), evaluates for the presence of endometrial hyperplasia and cancer.	All patients >45 years of age with suspected anovulatory bleeding should be evaluated for endometrial hyperplasia and cancer (after excluding pregnancy). EMB is indicated in patients with high body weight who are experiencing prolonged bleeding. EMB is also indicated in postmenopausal patients who are not on hormone therapy or in those who have been on hormone therapy for 6 months or more with unpredicted and unscheduled bleeding episodes (Fritz & Speroff, 2011).	The pathologic examination of the sample identifies the presence of hyperplasia, atypia, polyps, and other endometrial lesions. The presence of atypia is of particular importance in determining an appropriate treatment plan (Fritz & Speroff, 2011).

c. Secondary and specialty-based testing includes further testing for blood dyscrasias and procedures to evaluate masses, endometrial abnormalities, and skin lesions (**Table 16-4**). These tests are often done by or in consultation with gynecology and reproductive health specialists.

2. Treatment and management
Therapeutic management of AUB depends on the acuity, chronicity, and etiology of the disorder, along with the goals of the patient, including desire for pregnancy and the long-term consequences of any underlying medical conditions. Treatment of AUB

Table 16-4 Second-Line Testing in the Investigation of AUB, Including Tests Where Consultation or Referral Is Suggested

Test	Definition	Clinical Implications	Comments
Von Willebrand panel: von Willebrand Factor (VWF) antigen, VWF activity (ristocetin cofactor), factor VIII activity	Second-line testing when coagulation disorder is suspected.	Abnormal coagulation panel tests indicate coagulopathies.	Tests should be ordered in conjunction with hematology (American College of Obstetricians and Gynecologists [ACOG], 2013b).
Magnetic resonance imaging (MRI)	MRI is a noninvasive imaging technology.	Should be reserved for those patients in whom adenomyosis diagnosis by transvaginal ultrasonography of the pelvis (TVS) is inconclusive (Dueholm, 2006) MRI can help evaluate masses, adenomyosis, and the presence of endometrial polyps.	MRI has a greater cost than TVS. Consult with gynecology.
Saline infusion sonography (sonohysterography)	Visualizes the contours of the uterine cavity.	Indicated when polyps are not clearly identified with TVS.	Safe and highly sensitive; specific imaging used for the diagnosis of endometrial polyps (Radwan et al., 2014).
Hysteroscopy	A small lighted scope is inserted via the cervix into the uterus to visualize the endometrial cavity. Also allows for instrumentation, as described in the next column.	Direct visualization of the endometrium allows for: Assessment of intrauterine adhesions Assessment and removal of submucosal fibroids or endometrial polyps Removal of embedded intrauterine devices (IUDs) Assessment and biopsy of any lesions for pathologic evaluation (Bignardi et al., 2009; Farquhar et al., 2003)	This instrumentation can be performed in the office setting to remove small endometrial lesions.
Punch or forceps biopsy		Indicated for suspicious vulvar, vaginal, or cervical lesion.	
Dilatation and curettage (D&C)		Indicated for severe acute bleeding events where hypovolemia is present or where suspicion of malignancy is high. In the nonacute setting, it is valuable for the removal of endometrial polyps and for histologic diagnosis when endometrial sampling has been unsuccessful or inadequate.	This instrumentation can be performed in the office setting by gynecology specialist, often in conjunction with hysteroscopy. D&C can also be a curative treatment for AUB.

caused by endometrial hyperplasia or carcinoma is beyond the scope of this chapter.
a. Acute hemorrhagic bleeding in the hemodynamically unstable patient
   Patients with acute hemorrhagic bleeding who are hemodynamically unstable (signs of hypovolemia, including orthostatic changes in physical examination) or who have a positive pregnancy test warrant urgent referral to gynecology or an emergency department. Clinical evaluation and management of such patients are beyond the scope of this discussion.
b. Acute heavy bleeding in the hemodynamically stable patient
   i. Hormonal management (combined oral contraceptives and progestins) is effective for most patients (ACOG, 2013a). For nonpregnant patients of reproductive age, the goal of initial therapy is to stabilize the endometrial lining; prevent recurrence; and establish regular, orderly, and synchronous bleeding patterns. Hormonal therapies, including combined oral contraceptive pills and medroxyprogesterone acetate in both oral and intramuscular forms, are equally effective in most cases for the management of acute heavy menstrual bleeding. High-quality data demonstrating ideal dosages are lacking. Existent studies and expert opinion recommend dosages including medroxyprogesterone 10 mg three times daily for 7 days followed by 10 mg daily for an additional 21 days and 35 mcg combined oral contraceptives (COCs) three times daily for 7 days followed by once daily for an additional 21 days (Munro et al., 2006). If desired, the patient may continue with COCs to prevent anovulatory bleeding; otherwise, patients will experience typical withdrawal bleeding when they stop the medication.

   Estrogen is contraindicated for patients over 35 who smoke, patients with evidence of vascular disease, or those with a personal or family history of thromboembolic events (ACOG, 2013c).
c. Chronic bleeding in premenopausal patients
   If pregnancy is desired, the clinician should promptly consult with or refer the patient to an infertility specialist because AUB etiologies and their management may prevent or complicate pregnancy. Otherwise, pharmacologic management can be attempted as the initial treatment and, if successful, as a long-term treatment. Using combined or progestin-only hormonal methods to induce amenorrhea does not result in adverse effects on the endometrium (Hee et al., 2013). Some of the PALM etiologies and intractable heavy bleeding may ultimately be treated with procedures or surgeries.
   i. Progestin-only methods
      a. Levonorgestrel-releasing IUS (Mirena) (52 mg). This IUS has been observed to reduce heavy menstrual bleeding by 75%–95% after 3–12 months of use (Bofill Rodriguez et al., 2019; Doherty et al., 2014). In patients with a maximum 12-week-size uterus without cavity distortion, LNG-IUS is a safe and effective treatment option for heavy menstrual bleeding characteristic of leiomyomas (Doherty et al., 2014). The Mirena has been shown to work well in larger uteruses with cavity distortion; however, placement by an experienced clinician under sonogram guidance is advised. Limited data suggest that the LNG-IUS is equally effective in patients with adenomyosis (Bitzer et al., 2015). Research is ongoing into whether alternative IUSs (with lower progestin doses) are as effective at managing bleeding (Nelson et al., 2013).
      b. Depot medroxyprogesterone acetate (DMPA) and the etonogestrel subdermal implant are contraceptive methods that can also be used to address abnormal bleeding in patients with dysfunction (Melo et al., 2017). In addition, DMPA has been shown to improve bleeding parameters and increase hemoglobin, with a modest reduction in leiomyoma volume (Doherty et al., 2014). DMPA is injected every 12 weeks, although it can be given more frequently if needed (Centers for Disease Control and Prevention [CDC], 2021). The initial recommended duration of the etonogestrel subdermal implant was 3 years, but it appears to have very high efficacy with up to 5 years of use (Ali et al., 2016; Jacobs, 2018). Both methods have high rates of amenorrhea (Jain & Santoro, 2005), with DMPA resulting in amenorrhea in 12% of patients at 3 months and 80% in those who continue for 5 years (Nelson, 2010) and the etonogestrel implant resulting in amenorrhea in 11% of patients at 3 months and up to 40% of patients at 3 years (Jain & Santoro, 2005). See Chapter 21: Contraception for more information on these and other progestin-only methods.
      c. In addition to the progestin-only contraceptive methods listed previously, oral

medroxyprogesterone acetate (MPA), norethindrone acetate (NA), micronized progesterone (MP), and megestrol acetate (MA) may be used to control bleeding. Recommended daily or cyclic (cycle days 5–26) dosages include MPA 2.5–10 mg, NA 2.5–5 mg, MA 40–3,320 mg, or MP 200–400 mg (Bradley & Gueye, 2016). Cyclic dosing may be less effective with ovulatory cycles (Bradley & Gueye, 2016). MPA and MP are not effective as contraceptives (Edwards & Can, 2021). NA and MA have not been studied as a contraceptive but are effective for bleeding management (Dean et al., 2019).

ii. Combined hormonal methods. COCs may reduce heavy menstrual flow by promoting the development of an atrophic endometrium and can increase levels of factor VIII and von Willebrand factor, combating potential underlying coagulopathies (ACOG, 2013b). Oral contraceptive pills will not improve symptoms related to fibroid size. However, they are inexpensive and may be used as first-line therapy in patients with fibroids and heavy menstrual bleeding (Doherty et al., 2014). Daily cyclic use (withdrawal every 28 days), sequential withdrawal (every 90 days), or continuous use may be considered as treatment strategies, and these regimens are particularly helpful for patients with anemia (Powell, 2017). Combined estrogen and progestin contraceptive options include low-dose, monophasic COCs; contraceptive vaginal rings; and transdermal contraceptive patches. See earlier section on COC use in acute bleeding for discussion of contraindications.

iii. Nonsteroidal anti-inflammatories (NSAIDS). NSAIDS have been shown to reduce heavy menstrual flow in several studies, possibly by reducing prostaglandin levels in the endometrium by enzyme (cyclo-oxygenase) inhibition (Fritz & Speroff, 2011; Lethaby et al., 2013). The efficacy of NSAIDs in patients with leiomyomas with heavy bleeding is limited (Bitzer et al., 2015). NSAIDs do not appear to reduce blood loss in patients with myomas but can help to decrease painful menses. Counseling regarding the potential for gastrointestinal side effects should be provided. Options include 600–800 mg ibuprofen every 6–8 hours and meclofenamate 100 mg three times daily (Bradley & Gueye, 2016).

iv. Tranexamic acid (1300 mg three times daily for 5 days) can be useful for patients with contraindications to estrogen and for those who do not seek contraception. It is taken only during menses, making it more convenient for patients who prefer to avoid daily medications (Bradley & Gueye, 2016). It can be used in conjunction with NSAIDs (Matteson et al., 2013). Use with caution in patients also taking estrogen or in those with a history of thrombosis due to a theoretical risk of thrombosis (ACOG, 2013a).

v. Gonadotropin-releasing hormone (GnRH) agonists/antagonists. GnRH agonists, such as depo leuprolide (Lupron), can be useful for short-term management of heavy menstrual bleeding, particularly in the setting of leiomyoma or adenomyosis, because they reduce fibroid and uterine volume (Doherty et al., 2014). However, this therapy is limited to short-term use because of its expense and unpleasant side effects (menopausal vasomotor symptoms and bone loss), which resolve after discontinuation of therapy. Therefore, these medications are most often used as a preoperative adjunctive therapy for patients intending conservative (myomectomy or endometrial ablation) or definitive (hysterectomy) surgery for abnormal bleeding and should be done in close collaboration with a gynecological specialist. Newer GnRH antagonists, including elagolix and relugolix (approved for use in the United States), show promising results for patients with heavy bleeding associated with fibroids (Taylor et al., 2017; Wright et al., 2022). These medications can be delivered orally (depo leuprolide is an injection) and can be used for longer than the agonists, likely up to 2 years (Wright et al., 2022).

vi. Procedures and surgeries
  a. Surgical options are managed by gynecologists and are guided by the diagnosis, which is most often structural (PALM). Hysteroscopy can be used to remove polyps or some submucosal fibroids (Bignardi et al., 2009), and concurrent dilation and curettage may be performed. Dilation and curettage is most commonly considered for acute bleeding.
  b. In the case of asymptomatic leiomyomas, treatment is not mandatory (Bignardi et al., 2009; Fritz & Speroff, 2011). When they are thought to cause bleeding, they can be surgically removed with hysteroscopic or laparoscopic myomectomy or treated with uterine artery embolization (Manyonda et al., 2020).

c. Other procedures include uterine artery embolization for symptomatic fibroids and endometrial ablation (Keung et al., 2018; Munro et al., 2018). Conservative management with endometrial ablation can be done with hysteroscopic guidance or with newer techniques. In all cases, the goal is to prevent further menorrhagia by eliminating the endometrium. Ablation is not indicated for patients who desire further childbearing, who are menopausal, or who are at high risk of endometrial cancer. Because endometrial ablation can be done in the office or an outpatient surgical unit, it is less costly than hysterectomy, involves less risk of surgical complications, and requires less recovery time. It is appropriate for patients with conditions who prefer or need to avoid major surgery (Fritz & Speroff, 2011; Lethaby et al., 2013).

d. Hysterectomy remains the definitive treatment for menorrhagia and all abnormal bleeding patterns (Wouk & Helton, 2019). It may be appropriate for cases where treatment has failed or has been intolerable and where childbearing is not desired.

d. Chronic bleeding in postmenopausal patients
If endometrial sampling shows polyps, removal via hysteroscopy may resolve the bleeding (Nijkang et al., 2019). If sampling reveals benign tissue and the patient is not on hormonal therapy, watchful waiting is reasonable (Auclair et al., 2019). The presence of atypia or hyperplasia mandates specialty consultation for further evaluation and treatment, which may include hysterectomy or treatment with progestins (Reed et al., 2010). For postmenopausal patients on hormone therapy, endometrial biopsy (EMB) findings can guide dose adjustments once endometrial pathology has been excluded (see Chapter 22: Menopause Transition for further information on adjusting hormone therapy).

F. *Additional considerations and follow-up*
1. Anemia: All patients should be evaluated for anemia and treated as needed.
2. Follow-up: Assessment at regular intervals should be established as warranted (e.g., 3–6 months or as needed). Patients with acute bleeding require follow-up soon after initiation of therapy to evaluate for further bleeding or to evaluate for success of treatment. For leiomyomas, evaluation for symptoms and growth may be done every year, although transvaginal ultrasound (TVUS) may not be required if symptoms remain unchanged.
3. Referrals: Specialty referral should be instituted in the following cases:
    a. Patients with suspected coagulation disorders
    b. When medical treatment fails or AUB is persistent or recurrent
    c. Patients with endometrial hyperplasia or carcinoma

G. *Patient education*
1. Counseling: Counseling the patient on treatment approaches and long-term goals improves success. Patient involvement in the decision-making process, inclusion of family members when desired, and consideration of personal preferences are essential for promoting successful treatment. Consider associated issues, such interference with exercise, stress management, total body weight, and management of related chronic disorders. Referral for emotional support may be useful. Counseling should include the following:
    a. Detailed explanation of the etiologies of AUB
    b. Risks, benefits, procedures, and expected outcomes of essential diagnostic tests
    c. All treatment options (medical vs. surgical) and plans to initiate appropriate referrals to specialists or surgeons
    d. Medication side effects, risks versus benefits, and expected outcomes
2. Resources for patients and clinicians
    a. UptoDate (https://www.uptodate.com/contents/search) offers patient education materials at a range of reading levels.
    b. ACOG also provides many educational pamphlets available online.

References

Ali, M., Akin, A., Bahamondes, L., Brache, V., Habib, N., Landoulsi, S., Hubacher, D., & WHO Study Group on Subdermal Contraceptive Implants for Women. (2016). Extended use up to 5 years of the etonogestrel-releasing subdermal contraceptive implant: Comparison to levonorgestrel-releasing subdermal implant. *Human Reproduction, 31*(11), 2491–2498. doi:10.1093/humrep/dew222

American College of Obstetricians and Gynecologists. (2013a). Committee Opinion No. 557: Management of acute abnormal uterine bleeding in nonpregnant reproductive-aged women. *Obstetrics and Gynecology, 121*(4), 891–896. doi:10.1097/01.AOG.0000428646.67925.9a

American College of Obstetricians and Gynecologists. (2013b). Committee Opinion No. 580: von Willebrand disease in women.

Obstetrics and Gynecology, 122(6), 1368–1373. doi:10.1097/01.AOG.0000438961.38979.19

American College of Obstetricians and Gynecologists. (2013c). Practice Bulletin No. 136: Management of abnormal uterine bleeding associated with ovulatory dysfunction. *Obstetrics and Gynecology, 122*(1), 176–185. doi:10.1097/01.AOG.0000431815.52679.bb

Anderson, J., & Paterek, E. (2022). Vaginal foreign body evaluation and treatment. In *StatPearls*. StatPearls Publishing. http://www.ncbi.nlm.nih.gov/books/NBK549794/

Auclair, M.-H., Yong, P. J., Salvador, S., Thurston, J., Colgan, T. J., & Sebastianelli, A. (2019). Guideline No. 390: Classification and management of endometrial hyperplasia. *Journal of Obstetrics and Gynaecology Canada, 41*(12), 1789–1800. doi:10.1016/j.jogc.2019.03.025

Aune, D., Sen, A., & Vatten, L. J. (2017). Hypertension and the risk of endometrial cancer: A systematic review and meta-analysis of case-control and cohort studies. *Scientific Reports, 7*(1), 44808. doi:10.1038/srep44808

Barr, N. G. (2010). Managing adverse effects of hormonal contraceptives. *American Family Physician, 82*(12), 1499–1506.

Bignardi, T., Van den Bosch, T., & Condous, G. (2009). Abnormal uterine and post-menopausal bleeding in the acute gynaecology unit. *Best Practice & Research Clinical Obstetrics & Gynaecology, 23*(5), 595–607. doi:10.1016/j.bpobgyn.2009.05.001

Bitzer, J., Heikinheimo, O., Nelson, A. L., Calaf-Alsina, J., & Fraser, I. S. (2015). Medical management of heavy menstrual bleeding: A comprehensive review of the literature. *Obstetrical & Gynecological Survey, 70*(2), 115–130. doi:10.1097/OGX.0000000000000155

Bofill Rodriguez, M., Lethaby, A., Low, C., & Cameron, I. T. (2019). Cyclical progestogens for heavy menstrual bleeding. *Cochrane Database of Systematic Reviews, 8*, CD001016. doi:10.1002/14651858.CD001016.pub3 check this in text citation and reference

Bradley, L. D., & Gueye, N.-A. (2016). The medical management of abnormal uterine bleeding in reproductive-aged women. *American Journal of Obstetrics and Gynecology, 214*(1), 31–44. doi:10.1016/j.ajog.2015.07.044

Brenner, P. F. (1996). Differential diagnosis of abnormal uterine bleeding. *American Journal of Obstetrics and Gynecology, 175*(3, Part 2), 766–769. doi:10.1016/S0002-9378(96)80082-2

Calhoun, A. H. (2017). Hormonal contraceptives and migraine with aura—is there still a risk? *Headache: The Journal of Head and Face Pain, 57*(2), 184–193. doi:10.1111/head.12960

Centers for Disease Control and Prevention. (2021, May 20). *CDC—injectables—US SPR—reproductive health.* https://www.cdc.gov/reproductivehealth/contraception/mmwr/spr/injectables.html

Cohen, P. A., Jhingran, A., Oaknin, A., & Denny, L. (2019). Cervical cancer. *The Lancet, 393*(10167), 169–182. doi:10.1016/S0140-6736(18)32470-X

Dean, J., Kramer, K. J., Akbary, F., Wade, S., Hüttemann, M., Berman, J. M., & Recanati, M.-A. (2019). Norethindrone is superior to combined oral contraceptive pills in short-term delay of menses and onset of breakthrough bleeding: A randomized trial. *BMC Women's Health, 19*, 70. doi:10.1186/s12905-019-0766-6

Doherty, L., Mutlu, L., Sinclair, D., & Taylor, H. (2014). Uterine fibroids: Clinical manifestations and contemporary management. *Reproductive Sciences, 21*(9), 1067–1092. doi:10.1177/1933719114533728

Dueholm, M. (2006). Transvaginal ultrasound for diagnosis of adenomyosis: A review. *Best Practice & Research. Clinical Obstetrics & Gynaecology, 20*(4), 569–582. do:10.1016/j.bpobgyn.2006.01.005

Edwards, M., & Can, A. S. (2021). Progestin. In *StatPearls*. StatPearls Publishing. https://www.ncbi.nlm.nih.gov/books/NBK563211/

Emons, G., Beckmann, M. W., Schmidt, D., Mallmann, P., & Uterus Commission of the Gynecological Oncology Working Group. (2015). New WHO classification of endometrial hyperplasias. *Geburtshilfe Und Frauenheilkunde, 75*(2), 135–136. doi:10.1055/s-0034-1396256

Farquhar, C., Ekeroma, A., Furness, S., & Arroll, B. (2003). A systematic review of transvaginal ultrasonography, sonohysterography and hysteroscopy for the investigation of abnormal uterine bleeding in premenopausal women. *Acta Obstetricia et Gynecologica Scandinavica, 82*(6), 493–504. doi:10.1034/j.1600-0412.2003.00191.x

Fourman, L. T., & Fazeli, P. K. (2015). Neuroendocrine causes of amenorrhea—an update. *Journal of Clinical Endocrinology and Metabolism, 100*(3), 812–824. doi:10.1210/jc.2014-3344

Fritz, M. A., & Speroff, L. (2011). Abnormal uterine bleeding. In *Clinical gynecologic endocrinology and infertility* (8th ed., pp. 591–620). Lippincott Williams & Wilkins.

Giannella, L., Mfuta, K., Setti, T., Cerami, L. B., Bergamini, E., et al. (2014). A risk-scoring model for the prediction of endometrial cancer among symptomatic postmenopausal women with endometrial thickness >4mm. *BioMedResearch International.* doi:10.1155/2014/130569

Goje, O. (2021). *Pelvic inflammatory disease (PID).* Merck Manuals Professional Edition. https://www.merckmanuals.com/professional/gynecology-and-obstetrics/vaginitis,-cervicitis,-and-pelvic-inflammatory-disease-pid/pelvic-inflammatory-disease-pid

Gordon, C. M., Ackerman, K. E., Berga, S. L., Kaplan, J. R., Mastorakos, G., Misra, M., Murad, M. H., Santoro, N. F., & Warren, M. P. (2017). Functional hypothalamic amenorrhea: An Endocrine Society clinical practice guideline. *Journal of Clinical Endocrinology & Metabolism, 102*(5), 1413–1439. doi.org:10.1210/jc.2017-00131

Hallberg, L., Högdahl, A.-M., Nilsson, L., & Rybo, G. (1966). Menstrual blood loss and iron deficiency. *Acta Medica Scandinavica, 180*(5), 639–650. doi:10.1111/j.0954-6820.1966.tb02880.x

Hapangama, D. K., & Bulmer, J. N. (2016). Pathophysiology of heavy menstrual bleeding. *Women's Health, 12*(1), 3–13. doi:10.2217/whe.15.81

Hee, L., Kettner, L. O., & Vejtorp, M. (2013). Continuous use of oral contraceptives: An overview of effects and side-effects. *Acta Obstetricia et Gynecologica Scandinavica, 92*(2), 125–136. doi:10.1111/aogs.12036

Jacobs, M. (2018). Treatment duration for etonogestrel implant. *American Family Physician, 98*(3). https://www.aafp.org/afp/2018/0801/od3.html

Jain, A., & Santoro, N. (2005). Endocrine mechanisms and management for abnormal bleeding due to perimenopausal changes. *Clinical Obstetrics and Gynecology, 48*(2), 295–311. doi:10.1097/01.grf.0000159537.89102.97

Keung, J. J., Spies, J. B., & Caridi, T. M. (2018). Uterine artery embolization: A review of current concepts. *Best Practice & Research. Clinical Obstetrics & Gynecology, 46*, 66–73. doi:10.1016/j.bpobgyn.2017.09.003

Khan, A. T., Shehmar, M., & Gupta, J. K. (2014). Uterine fibroids: Current perspectives. *International Journal of Women's Health, 6*, 95–114. doi:10.2147/IJWH.S51083

Lasmar, R. B., Dias, R., Barrozo, P. R. M., Oliveira, M. A. P., da Silva Freire Coutinho, E., & da Rosa, D. B. (2008). Prevalence of hysteroscopic findings and histologic diagnoses in patients with abnormal uterine bleeding. *Fertility and Sterility, 89*(6), 1803–1807. doi:10.1016/j.fertnstert.2007.05.045

Lethaby, A., Duckitt, K., & Farquhar, C. (2013). Non-steroidal anti-inflammatory drugs for heavy menstrual bleeding. *Cochrane Database of Systematic Reviews, 1*, CD000400. doi:10.1002/14651858.CD000400.pub3

Manyonda, I., Belli, A.-M., Lumsden, M.-A., Moss, J., McKinnon, W., Middleton, L. J., Cheed, V., Wu, O., Sirkeci, F., Daniels, J. P., &

McPherson, K. (2020). Uterine-artery embolization or myomectomy for uterine fibroids. *New England Journal of Medicine, 383*(5), 440–451. doi:10.1056/NEJMoa1914735

Matteson, K. A., Rahn, D. D., Wheeler, T. L., Casiano, E., Siddiqui, N. Y., Harvie, H. S., Mamik, M. M., Balk, E. M., & Sung, V. W. (2013). Nonsurgical management of heavy menstrual bleeding: A systematic review. *Obstetrics & Gynecology, 121*(3), 632–643. doi:10.1097/AOG.0b013e3182839e0e

Melo, A. S. de, Reis, R. M. dos, Ferriani, R. A., & Vieira, C. S. (2017). Hormonal contraception in women with polycystic ovary syndrome: Choices, challenges, and noncontraceptive benefits. *Open Access Journal of Contraception, 8*, 13–23. doi:10.2147/OAJC.S85543

Miller, J. D., Lenhart, G. M., Bonafede, M. M., Basinski, C. M., Lukes, A. S., & Troeger, K. A. (2015). Cost effectiveness of endometrial ablation with the NovaSure(®) system versus other global ablation modalities and hysterectomy for treatment of abnormal uterine bleeding: US commercial and Medicaid payer perspectives. *International Journal of Women's Health, 7*, 59–73. doi:10.2147/IJWH.S75030

Munro, M. G., Critchley, H. O. D., & Fraser, I. S. (2012). The FIGO systems for nomenclature and classification of causes of abnormal uterine bleeding in the reproductive years: Who needs them? *American Journal of Obstetrics and Gynecology, 207*(4), 259–265. doi:10.1016/j.ajog.2012.01.046

Munro, M. G., Critchley, H. O. D., Fraser, I. S. (2018). The two FIGO systems for normal and abnormal uterine bleeding symptoms and classification of causes of abnormal uterine bleeding in the reproductive years: 2018 revisions. *International Journal of Gynecology & Obstetrics, 143*(3), 393–408. doi:10.1002/ijgo.12666

Munro, M. G., Mainor, N., Basu, R., Brisinger, M., & Barreda, L. (2006). Oral medroxyprogesterone acetate and combination oral contraceptives for acute uterine bleeding: A randomized controlled trial. *Obstetrics & Gynecology, 108*(4), 924–929. doi:10.1097/01.AOG.0000238343.62063.22

National Collaborating Centre for Women's and Children's Health. (2007). *Heavy menstrual bleeding*. RCOG Press. https://www.ncbi.nlm.nih.gov/books/NBK56530/

National Institutes of Health. (2022). *Cancer of the endometrium—cancer stat facts*. SEER. https://seer.cancer.gov/statfacts/html/corp.html

Nelson, A., Apter, D., Hauck, B., Schmelter, T., Rybowski, S., Rosen, K., & Gemzell-Danielsson, K. (2013). Two low-dose levonorgestrel intrauterine contraceptive systems: A randomized controlled trial. *Obstetrics & Gynecology, 122*(6), 1205–1213. doi:10.1097/AOG.0000000000000019

Nelson, A. L. (2010). DMPA: Battered and bruised but still needed and used in the USA. *Expert Review of Obstetrics & Gynecology, 5*(6), 673–686. doi:10.1586/eog.10.60

Ng, C., Motto, D. G., & Di Paola, J. (2015). Diagnostic approach to von Willebrand disease. *Blood, 125*(13), 2029–2037. doi:10.1182/blood-2014-08-528398

Nicholson, W. K., Ellison, S. A., Grason, H., & Powe, N. R. (2001). Patterns of ambulatory care use for gynecologic conditions: A national study. *American Journal of Obstetrics and Gynecology, 184*(4), 523–530. doi:10.1067/mob.2001.111795

Nijkang, N. P., Anderson, L., Markham, R., & Manconi, F. (2019). Endometrial polyps: Pathogenesis, sequelae and treatment. *SAGE Open Medicine, 7*, 2050312119848247. doi:10.1177/2050312119848247

Powell, A. (2017). Choosing the right oral contraceptive pill for teens. *Pediatric Clinics of North America, 64*(2), 343–358. doi:10.1016/j.pcl.2016.11.005

Prior, J. C., Naess, M., Langhammer, A., & Forsmo, S. (2015). Ovulation prevalence in women with spontaneous normal-length menstrual cycles—a population-based cohort from HUNT3, Norway. *PloS One, 10*(8), e0134473. doi:10.1371/journal.pone.0134473

Radwan, P., Radwan, M., Kozarzewski, M., Polac, I., & Wilczyński, J. (2014). Evaluation of sonohysterography in detecting endometrial polyps—241 cases followed with office hysteroscopies combined with histopathological examination. *Videosurgery and Other Miniinvasive Techniques, 9*(3), 344–350. doi:10.5114/wiitm.2014.43024

Reed, S. D., Newton, K. M., Garcia, R. L., Allison, K. H., Voigt, L. F., Jordan, C. D., Epplein, M., Swisher, E., Upson, K., Ehrlich, K. J., & Weiss, N. S. (2010). Complex hyperplasia with and without atypia: Clinical outcomes and implications of progestin therapy. *Obstetrics & Gynecology, 116*(2), 365–373. doi:10.1097/AOG.0b013e3181e93330

Rosenberg, M. J., Waugh, M. S., & Stevens, C. M. (1996). Smoking and cycle control among oral contraceptive users. *American Journal of Obstetrics and Gynecology, 174*(2), 628–632. doi:10.1016/S0002-9378(96)70440-4

Russo, M., Rosa-Rizzotto, M., Giolito, M., Ranzato, C., Facchin, P., & Aprile, A. (2017). Genital trauma and vaginal bleeding: Is it a lapse of time issue? A case report of a prepubertal girl and review of the literature. *International Journal of Legal Medicine, 131*(1), 185–189. doi:10.1007/s00414-016-1440-2

Sparic, R., Mirkovic, L., Malvasi, A., & Tinelli, A. (2016). Epidemiology of uterine myomas: A review. *International Journal of Fertility & Sterility, 9*(4), 424–435. doi:10.22074/ijfs.2015.4599

Sriprasert, I., Pakrashi, T., Kimble, T., & Archer, D. F. (2017). Heavy menstrual bleeding diagnosis and medical management. *Contraception and Reproductive Medicine, 2*(1), 20. doi:10.1186/s40834-017-0047-4

Strickland, J., Gibson, E. J., & Levine, S. B. (2006). Dysfunctional uterine bleeding in adolescents. *Journal of Pediatric and Adolescent Gynecology, 19*(1), 49–51. doi:10.1016/j.jpag.2005.11.007

Sun, Y., Wang, Y., Mao, L., Wen, J., & Bai, W. (2018). Prevalence of abnormal uterine bleeding according to new International Federation of Gynecology and Obstetrics classification in Chinese women of reproductive age: A cross-sectional study. *Medicine, 97*(31), e11457. doi:10.1097/MD.0000000000011457

Taylor, H. S., Giudice, L. C., Lessey, B. A., Abrao, M. S., Kotarski, J., Archer, D. F., Diamond, M. P., Surrey, E., Johnson, N. P., Watts, N. B., Gallagher, J. C., Simon, J. A., Carr, B. R., Dmowski, W. P., Leyland, N., Rowan, J. P., Duan, W. R., Ng, J., Schwefel, B., . . . Chwalisz, K. (2017). Treatment of endometriosis-associated pain with elagolix, an oral GnRH antagonist. *New England Journal of Medicine, 377*(1), 28–40. doi:10.1056/NEJMoa1700089

Thorneycroft, I. H. (1999). Cycle control with oral contraceptives: A review of the literature. *American Journal of Obstetrics and Gynecology, 180*(Suppl. 2), S280–S287. doi:10.1016/S0002-9378(99)70719-2

Villavicencio, J., & Allen, R. H. (2016). Unscheduled bleeding and contraceptive choice: Increasing satisfaction and continuation rates. *Open Access Journal of Contraception, 7*, 43–52. doi:10.2147/OAJC.S85565

Wouk, N., & Helton, M. (2019). Abnormal uterine bleeding in premenopausal women. *American Family Physician, 99*(7), 435–443.

Wright, D., Kim, J. W., Lindsay, H., & Catherino, W. H. (2022). A review of GnRH antagonists as treatment for abnormal uterine bleeding-leiomyoma (AUB-L) and their influence on the readiness of service members. *Military Medicine*, usac078. doi:10.1093/milmed/usac078

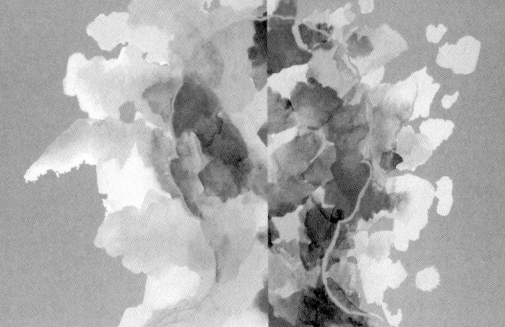

CHAPTER 17

Abortion Care in the Primary Care Setting

Gwendolyn Riddell

"Reproductive justice is the human right to maintain personal bodily autonomy, have children, not have children and parent the children we have in safe and sustainable communities."

— SisterSong Reproductive Justice Collective

I. Introduction and general background

Abortion is a universal phenomenon that has been practiced throughout time. Ancient texts have many references to abortifacients and contraceptives, taken orally or placed in the vagina (Paul et al., 1999). The ability to control family size has allowed for all genders to have more educational and professional options, leading to greater gains in health and welfare for all people (Stover et al., 2016).

Abortion is a complex health topic. The choice to have an abortion and the right to choose to have an abortion are inextricably tied to personal beliefs and the law. Abortion was legal in the United States starting in 1973, when a Supreme Court decision known as *Roe v. Wade* passed. As this chapter goes to press, *Roe v. Wade* has just been overturned. It is estimated that the number of illegal abortions in the United States dropped from 130,000 to 17,000 between 1972 and 1974. Although death is the most extreme and unfortunate consequence of illegal abortions, other complications include infection, hemorrhage, uterine perforation, gut perforations, sepsis, disseminated intravascular coagulation (DIC), and renal failure (World Health Organization [WHO], 2021). It is estimated that globally, depending on the region, 4.7%–13.2% of all maternal deaths are related to unsafe, illegal abortions, which is a 42% drop from the 1990s (WHO, 2021; Singh, 2018). The discovery of mifepristone, the abortion pill, in the 1980s has helped make abortion safer and more accessible (Singh, 2018). Reducing abortion mortality worldwide is directly tied to safe and easy access to legal abortions (Singh, 2018).

Abortion is safe and one of the most common procedures performed today. In fact, it is remarkably safer than carrying a pregnancy to term. It is estimated that the risk of death associated with childbirth is approximately 14 times higher than that of having an abortion (Raymond & Grimes, 2012). In 2014, almost 1 in 5 pregnancies ended in abortion, which means an estimated 1 in 4 U.S. persons assigned female at birth (AFAB) will have an abortion in their lifetime (Jones & Jerman, 2017c). Limiting access to abortion by making laws more restrictive is the only factor that contributes to decreased abortion safety (National Academies of Sciences, Engineering, and Medicine [NASEM], 2018; Upadhyay et al., 2015).

Unintended pregnancy rates are closely tied to abortion rates. Evidence-based, timely, culturally competent, and inclusive sexual and reproductive health care and counseling for all reproductive-age people is essential to preventing unintended pregnancy (Manlove et al., 2015). Information and access to the full range of affordable birth control have been shown to reduce the unintended pregnancy rate significantly (Finer & Zolna, 2016).

A. *Unintended pregnancy rates and abortion*

To understand abortion rates, the larger context of unintended pregnancy rates must be examined. The rate of unintended pregnancy in the United States is about 45%, which has decreased from close to 60% in 1981

(Finer & Zolna, 2016). Despite this drop, large disparities remain in unintended pregnancy rates among people of color, those with low income, and the uninsured.

Disparities in unintended pregnancy rates in these groups can partially be explained by income, lack of insurance, insurance type, access to care, education, and relationship status, but there are many other factors that contribute to these differences (Holliday et al., 2017). Attitudes toward sexuality, pregnancy, and family planning vary by cultural norms and are shaped by and reinforced within communities and individual families (Holliday et al., 2017).

Intimate partner violence (IPV) is also associated with increased unintended pregnancy rates (Holliday et al., 2017). Reproductive coercion (RC) is a behavior within relationships inflicted by IPV that can lead to unintended pregnancy. RC involves pregnancy-coercion behaviors, such as explicit attempts to impregnate a partner against their will or control the outcomes of a pregnancy. It also includes active manipulation of condoms and hormonal contraception to promote a pregnancy, such as breaking condoms on purpose and flushing birth control pills down the toilet (American College of Obstetrics & Gynecologists [ACOG], 2013; Holliday et al., 2017). RC is experienced by about 1 in 4 cisgender persons afab in their lifetime (Holliday et al., 2017). The risk of unintended pregnancy is doubled among those who report both IPV and RC (Miller et al., 2010). About 1 in 4 persons AFAB experience RC in their lifetime, with Black and multiracial persons AFAB having a significantly higher chance (Holliday et al., 2017).

Two major shifts have contributed to the decrease in unintended pregnancies. One is the passage of the Affordable Care Act (ACA) in 2010, which gave a greater part of the population access to insurance that mandated coverage of birth control methods (Guttmacher Institute, 2018b). Another is the increase in the use of long-acting reversible contraceptive (LARC) methods, such as intrauterine devices (IUDs) and contraceptive implants (Kavanaugh et al., 2015). Despite the increase in the use of effective birth control methods, over 50% of patients having an abortion used a contraceptive method during the month they became pregnant (Jones, 2018). This fact illustrates that in spite of a person's best efforts, unintended pregnancies occur, and thus there will always be a need for access to safe abortion care.

As the rate of unintended pregnancies has dropped in the United States, so have the rates of abortion (Guttmacher Institute, 2018b). The number of abortions in the United States fell by 196,000—a 19% decline—from 1,058,000 abortions in 2011 to 862,000 abortions in 2017 (Nash & Dreweke, 2019). One factor in this decrease is the decrease in unintended pregnancies. Other factors include the inability to obtain an abortion due to restrictive abortion laws and the increase in self-managed abortions, which are not included in these statistics (Jones & Jerman, 2017a; Nash & Dreweke, 2019).

B. *Abortion in the sociopolitical context*
Public opinion on abortion has remained remarkably stable over the long term. Polls consistently show that about 80% of Americans support the right to have an abortion in most cases, and attitudes in 2018 were essentially the same as those in the mid-1990s (Durkee, 2021; Nash & Dreweke, 2019). Yet despite this public support, abortion care has become increasingly restricted.

The United States has a dark history of coercive reproductive practices, including forced sterilization of minorities, biased counseling, and lack of equal access to health care (Harris & Wolfe, 2014). Some of these practices continue today and have disproportionately affected people of color; Indigenous people; people whose incomes are below the federal poverty threshold; people who have immigrated; the lesbian, gay, bisexual, transgender, and queer (LGBTQ) community; incarcerated individuals; and those with disabilities. The well-documented practices of RC have shaped the way individuals and communities approach health care, especially reproductive health care (Harris & Wolfe, 2014). Institutional distrust can lead to delayed reproductive health care, which leads to increased gestational age, higher costs, and often, farther travel to obtain abortion care. Unfortunately, the ability to access safe abortion care varies widely based on income, access to health insurance, and location, which are all tied to structural poverty and racism (Baum et al., 2016). Acknowledging and addressing the health consequences of racism is important to eliminating racial health disparities (Chadha et al., 2020).

C. *Barriers to abortion care*
For patients seeking an abortion in the United States, even post-*Roe*, legality does not mean universal access to abortion care. There are many state restrictions and barriers to accessing abortion care (Guttmacher Institute, 2022). Most states have enacted laws that impose gestational limits, restrict funding, allow private insurance companies to decline coverage, allow healthcare providers to refuse to participate in abortion care, restrict who can perform an abortion, require unsubstantiated counseling prior to an abortion, impose waiting periods, and require parental involvement for minors. These restrictions, called *targeted regulation of abortion providers* (TRAP) laws, have led to a decline in providers and clinics offering abortion care in many states. Greater distance to abortion care leads to greater delays in obtaining care, increased expenses, decreased privacy, possible loss of wages, and even loss of employment, as well as the possibility of emergency department follow-up care by providers unfamiliar with abortion care (Baum et al., 2016; Fuentes & Jerman, 2019; Fuentes et al., 2016).

Reproductive health outcomes are directly linked to social injustice and inequity of opportunities to control reproduction. The Turnaway Study followed 1,000 people seeking abortions and found that for those who were denied a wanted abortion and who carried an unwanted pregnancy to term, the odds of living below the federal poverty level were four times greater (Greene Foster, 2020). In addition, the study concluded that those denied an abortion were more likely to experience serious pregnancy complications, including eclampsia and death; more likely to stay involved with an abusive partner; more likely to suffer anxiety and loss of self-esteem in the short term; less likely to have aspirational life plans for the coming year; and more likely to experience poor physical health for years after the pregnancy. Being denied an abortion has serious implications for the children of an unwanted pregnancy, as well as for the existing children in the family. The study conversely found that those who receive a wanted abortion are more financially stable, set more ambitious goals, raise children under more stable conditions, and are more likely to have a wanted pregnancy later (Greene Foster, 2020; McCarthy et al., 2020). It is estimated that 4,000 people are denied wanted abortions every year due to facilities' gestational limits (Upadhyay et al., 2014). As abortion laws become more restricted and abortion care becomes more siloed, many more will be affected.

Roadblocks to abortion care have been well documented and, as the Turnaway Study has shown, have detrimental health outcomes (Greene Foster, 2020; McCarthy et al., 2020). Inaccurate and misleading information provided at crisis pregnancy centers (CPCs) is another barrier to timely abortion care (Bryant & Levi, 2012; Rosen, 2012). These CPCs, also known as *pregnancy support centers* or *limited-service pregnancy centers*, are facilities that offer free services to those facing unintended pregnancies (Bryant & Levi, 2012). These facilities are often staffed by volunteers and employees who lack medical training or licensure, are funded by national antiabortion organizations, belong to evangelical Christian networks, and in some states, outnumber comprehensive reproductive healthcare providers that provide abortion care (Bryant & Levi, 2012; Rosen, 2012). CPCs lure people with the prospect of a free ultrasound, which can be tempting for those without health insurance.

These facilities often distribute unsubstantiated information about abortion in the guise of medical claims, such as statements that abortion is linked to an increased risk of breast cancer, that all abortions make one less likely to be able to get pregnant in the future and increase the risk of ectopic pregnancies, and that abortion has a deleterious effect on long-term mental health (Rosen, 2012). Despite evidence that clearly disproves the link between abortion and breast cancer or infertility, these statements are presented as fact (Bryant & Levi, 2012). High-quality research studies have consistently demonstrated that having an abortion has no negative effect on future fertility or pregnancy outcomes (NASEM et al., 2018). Additional studies have proved that there is no connection between abortion and breast cancer or mental health disorders such as depression, anxiety, and posttraumatic stress disorder (PTSD) (NASEM, 2018). The provision of misinformation in a medical context is contrary to legal and ethical standards of informed consent and poses health risks to the clientele (Rosen, 2012).

D. *Healthcare providers and abortion care*
While discussing abortion care, it is essential to consider that abortion is not in and of itself an adverse outcome (Dehlendorf et al., 2013). A more accurate and inclusive goal is to measure *reproductive autonomy*, defined as the extent to which a person can determine freely whether and when they have children. This shifts the responsibility for achieving greater reproductive autonomy off the shoulders of individuals and onto the healthcare systems responsible for providing reproductive health care (Potter et al., 2019). Although the onus of reproductive autonomy does not fall fully on healthcare providers, they are an important part of the solution to decrease barriers to comprehensive reproductive health care (Anderson et al., 2022; Greene Foster, 2020).

Primary care providers (PCPs) play an important role in mitigating the potentially adverse outcomes of not receiving abortion care when desired (Anderson et al., 2022; Greene Foster, 2020; Holt et al., 2017). When healthcare providers familiarize themselves with local and institutional restrictions, they better understand the barriers that their patients might face when seeking an abortion. Regardless of a provider's bias or belief regarding abortion, the healthcare professional should deliver accurate, nonjudgmental, and evidence-based information, including where to obtain an abortion, and not add more stigma to an already often-difficult life event. Refusal to provide needed and sought abortion care can be harmful to patient welfare (Greene Foster, 2020).

Who can provide an abortion varies by state laws and regulatory bodies. Studies have shown that early abortion care can be provided by certified nurse midwives (CNMs), nurse practitioners (NPs), and physician assistants (PAs) with outcomes equal to those provided by physicians and that patients report high satisfaction during their abortion experience if they are seen by providers they know and trust (National Abortion Federation [NAF], 2020; Taylor et al., 2017; Weitz et al., 2013). Unless the provider works in an organization such as Planned Parenthood or other abortion care organizations that widely employ advance practice nurses (APNs), professional self-study may be the best way to gain skills and increase knowledge in abortion care provision. Further training resources are listed at the end of this chapter.

E. *Who has abortions and when abortion is provided*
The Guttmacher Institute (2018a) estimates that worldwide, about 73 million abortions are performed annually. Approximately 862,320 abortions were performed

in 2017 in the United States (Guttmacher, 2019a). People whose incomes are below the federal poverty threshold and people of color have a higher rate of abortion compared to their counterparts, likely due to decreased access to preventative services (Jerman et al., 2016). Forty-nine percent of abortion patients had family incomes of less than 100% of the federal poverty level, and 26% of patients had incomes that were 100%–199% of the poverty threshold (Jerman et al., 2016). Seventeen percent of abortion patients in 2014 identified themselves as mainline Protestant, 13% as evangelical Protestant, 24% as Catholic, and 8% as some other religious affiliation, and the remaining 38% reported no religious affiliation (Jerman et al., 2016).

The vast majority of abortions worldwide are performed in the first trimester. In the United States in 2013, the majority (66.0%) of abortions were performed by ≤8 weeks' gestation, and nearly all (91.6%) were performed by ≤13 weeks' gestation. Few abortions were performed between 14 and 20 weeks' gestation (7.1%) or ≥21 weeks' gestation (1.3%) (Jatlaoui et al., 2016). Those who seek abortion after 13 weeks are more likely to be young, be a victim of violence, have detected their pregnancy later, feel ambivalent about the abortion decision, and have financial or logistical barriers to abortion care. Some patients present for abortions after the second trimester due to the detection of fetal anomalies or maternal medical complications later in pregnancy that are often diagnosed after 13 weeks (Ipas, 2021; Jones & Jerman, 2017b; Waddington et al., 2015).

Not all people who seek abortions identify as women or heterosexual. Transgender, nonbinary, gender-expansive (TGE) people with intact ovaries and uterus experience undesired pregnancy after transitioning socially, medically, or both and may seek abortion care; they are also more likely to try a self-managed abortion (Light et al., 2014; Moseson et al., 2022). Attempts to better understand the needs of the TGE community in abortion care reveal that due to structural issues, lack of health insurance coverage, legal restrictions, denials of or mistreatment within clinical care, and cost, a high proportion of TGE people have attempted abortion without clinical supervision (Moseson et al., 2022). Creating inclusive and welcoming spaces within healthcare settings for people of all gender identities will help decrease avoidance of care by the TGE community.

F. *Medication abortion*

Medication abortion (MAB), also referred to as *medical abortion*, involves the use of medications rather than uterine aspiration to induce an abortion (ACOG, 2020). There are several medication regimens used, with some being more effective than others. The most widely used and most effective MAB regimen is a combination of mifepristone and misoprostol (Kulier et al., 2011). Medical termination of pregnancy is considered successful if complete expulsion of the products of conception occurs without the need for surgical intervention (Christin-Maitre et al., 2000).

Historically, MAB provision has required the patient to complete an in-person visit to have a pre-abortion ultrasound, evaluation by a provider, and an in-person follow-up visit. With new innovations in health care and the restraints put on the healthcare system due to the COVID-19 pandemic, several new models of MAB provision have been implemented (Aiken et al., 2021). These include "no-test" protocols, mail-order provision, and pharmacy provision. The no-test protocols include recommendations for patient selection, Rh status evaluation and management, the treatment regimen, and follow-up (Aiken et al., 2021). MAB can be provided safely and effectively by telemedicine, with a high level of patient satisfaction, and telemedicine improves access to early abortion care, particularly in areas that lack a healthcare practitioner (Creinin & Grossman, 2020).

Telemedicine involves the use of video and information technology to provide a medical service at a distance. Research indicates these models are safe, effective, and acceptable to patients (Aiken et al., 2021; Grossman & Grindlay, 2017; Guilbert et al., 2020; Raymond et al., 2020). Telemedicine MAB may help reduce delays to care because of barriers to access to abortion in remote areas (Creinin & Grossman, 2020). After MAB through telemedicine was introduced in Iowa, a significant reduction in second-trimester abortion was reported, and patients in remote parts of the state were more likely to obtain an MAB (Creinin & Grossman, 2020). Studies have found that remote MAB is just as effective as an in-person visit, with an overall 0.3% incidence of adverse events (Creinin & Grossman, 2020; Endler et al., 2019).

Prior to qualifying for a telemedicine MAB, a patient must have confirmed the pregnancy with a urine or serum pregnancy test or a prior ultrasound showing an intrauterine pregnancy (Aiken et al., 2021) and must be screened for eligibility. The three key goals of clinical evaluation before a no-test MAB are to confirm that the gestational age is within accepted limits for effective and safe outpatient treatment, exclude ectopic pregnancy, and establish that the patient has no other contraindications to MAB (Aiken et al., 2021). There is growing evidence that these goals can be accomplished via telemedicine alone. The demand for telemedicine abortion will likely rise as access to abortion care is further restricted.

In addition to the increased demand for telemedicine MAB, self-managed MAB, or that conducted outside of the formal health system, has grown in popularity (Aiken et al., 2020, 2022; Baldwin et al., 2022; Donovan, 2018; Fuentes et al., 2020; Kapp et al., 2017). Historically, self-managed abortion has been seen as a last-resort approach to abortion that should only be used when access to abortion is restricted or entirely removed. However, even in areas where abortion is legal, there are multiple reasons why people may seek to self-manage an abortion, and many studies show the safety of this model (Aiken et al., 2020; Harris & Grossman, 2020; Kapp et al., 2017; WHO, 2020). It met the needs of many who might prefer this care, including transgender men, gender-nonconforming people, those who have reason to distrust the medical system, and those who may opt to self-manage abortion for privacy and autonomy (Kapp et al., 2017). Other reasons people may seek self-managed abortion are barriers such as cost; distance to clinics; inability to travel due to childcare, eldercare, work, or school; the desire for privacy or secrecy; and the belief that this approach to abortion is more comfortable (Aiken et al., 2020; Fuentes et al., 2020).

The combination of mifepristone and misoprostol is the most effective for office-based or self-managed abortion. However, due to cost and U.S. Food and Drug Administration (FDA) restrictions on mifepristone, a self-managed abortion may be approached with misoprostol alone (Kapp et al., 2017). Complications are more common if medical abortion regimens are used at gestational ages beyond 10 weeks (Kapp et al., 2017). As the nontraditional models expand, research supporting them will become more robust. In the meantime, providers can support patients by being available for questions and complications if they arise. The management of complications is equivalent to those following office-based MAB or miscarriage, which is reviewed later in this chapter and in Chapter 20: Early Pregnancy Loss. There are many resources for self-managed abortion listed at the end of this chapter.

1. Mifepristone: Mifepristone (Mifeprex) has been used in the United States since 2000 and has been strictly regulated by the FDA in terms of who can prescribe and dispense the medication as well as where the medication can be taken. These restrictions are known as the *Risk Evaluation and Mitigation Strategy* (REMS), and in 2021 they were revised to make it easier for providers to prescribe, including allowing for mail-order provision. The REMS restrictions that remain are that the patient and a certified healthcare provider (who meets certain qualifications) must sign a Prescriber Agreement Form after counseling and prior to the prescription of mifepristone, and pharmacies that dispense mifepristone must be certified (Ehrenreich et al., 2021; FDA, 2023). Information about how to become certified can be found on the FDA website.

    Mifepristone is a glucocorticoid receptor antagonist (Spitz & Bardin, 1993) and an antiprogesterone derivative of norethindrone that inhibits progesterone, the hormone that supports and maintains a pregnancy. The lack of progesterone alters the endometrium directly by affecting the capillary endothelial cells of the decidua, which results in the separation of the trophoblast from the implantation site and decreases secretion of human chorionic gonadotropin (hCG) (Baulieu, 1989; Christin-Maitre et al., 2000). This also increases the release of prostaglandin, a hormone-like substance that can cause the smooth muscle of the uterus to contract and relax. Mifepristone also softens the cervix to allow for expulsion of the product of conception. Mifepristone is not effective in the treatment of extrauterine pregnancy (i.e., ectopic pregnancy), likely due to the lack of progesterone receptor expression in fallopian tubes, where an ectopic pregnancy is usually found (Paul et al., 1999). The claims that patients who change their minds after taking mifepristone can reverse the effects of mifepristone by taking varying doses of progesterone are unsubstantiated (Grossman, et al., 2015).

2. Misoprostol: Misoprostol (Cytotec) is marketed as an oral preparation used to prevent and treat gastroduodenal damage induced by nonsteroidal anti-inflammatory drugs (NSAIDs). Misoprostol is a synthetic prostaglandin E1 analogue that is used off-label for a variety of indications in the practice of obstetrics and gynecology, including MAB, medical management of miscarriage, induction of labor, cervical ripening before surgical procedures, and the treatment of postpartum hemorrhage. Although misoprostol is not approved by the FDA for these indications, in 2002, pregnancy was removed from the label as an absolute contraindication to misoprostol use, although it is still considered off-label to use it during pregnancy. The use of misoprostol up to 48 hours after taking mifepristone is for the purpose of cervical softening, dilation, and uterine contractions, which expel the products of conception (Allen & O'Brien, 2009). Although the evidence is limited, misoprostol can be teratogenic to the fetus and can result in congenital anomalies, such as limb defects with or without Möbius syndrome (i.e., facial paralysis), when used during the first trimester (ACOG, 2020). This is relevant to pre-MAB counseling of patients due to the rare case of an ongoing pregnancy after an MAB. Patients should be made aware of this possible risk prior to taking the medication. MAB using mifepristone and misoprostol is more effective the earlier the gestation age at which the medication is taken. (See **Table 17-1**.)

    Mifepristone is costly and is unavailable in many settings, even in the United States, due to the REMS restrictions (Raymond et al., 2019). Misoprostol alone can be used when mifepristone is not available (ACOG, 2020) and is effective and safe for first-trimester medical abortion (Raymond et al., 2019). Reviews of the efficacy of misoprostol single-agent regimens at gestational ages ≤63 days ranged from 84% to 96% complete abortion (Raymond et al., 2019). This is less effective than the combined regimen of mifepristone and misoprostol (Ngoc et al., 2011). Repeated doses of misoprostol 800 mcg placed vaginally, sublingually, or

Table 17-1 Medication Abortion Regimens and Effectiveness of Each Regimen

Gestational Age and Regimen	Mifepristone Dose	Misoprostol	Efficacy
≤63 days Mifepristone and misoprostol combination	Mifepristone 200 mg PO	Misoprostol 800 mcg buccal 24–48 h, or vaginal 6–72 h after mifepristone	95%–99%
≤63 days Misoprostol only		Misoprostol 800 mcg vaginally or sublingually administered every 3 hours for three doses (with vaginal administration, dosing interval may be as long as 12 hours)	84%–85%
64–70 days Mifepristone and misoprostol combination	Mifepristone 200 mg PO	1st dose misoprostol as with ≤63 days, then consider 2nd dose misoprostol 800 mcg 4 hours.	1 dose: 92%–95% 2 doses: up to 99.6%
71–77 days Mifepristone and misoprostol combination	Mifepristone 200 mg PO	1st dose misoprostol as with ≤63 days, then recommend 2nd misoprostol 800 mcg 4 hours	1 dose: 86.7% 2 doses: 97.6%

Data from Goodman, S., & the TEACH Collaborative Working Group. (2020). TEACH Early Abortion Training Curriculum 6th Edition. UCSF Bixby Center for Global Reproductive Health; National Abortion Federation (NAF). (2020). 2020 Clinical Policy Guidelines. National Abortion Federation. https://prochoice.org/store/clinical-policy-guidelines/; Society of Family Planning (SFP). (2014). Medical management of first-trimester abortion Clinical Guideline. Contraception, 89(3), 148–161.

buccally every 3 hours versus a single dose is more effective. Although most studies typically do not use more than three doses, the WHO does not specify a maximum number of doses (Raymond et al., 2019).

3. Methotrexate: Methotrexate can also be safely used for MAB at up to 56 days of pregnancy and is still used in areas where mifepristone is not available (Creinin et al., 1996). The success rate of complete abortion is 91.7% by 35 days after taking medications (Creinin et al., 1996). Methotrexate in combination with a prostaglandin may be an alternative to the mifepristone/prostaglandin regimen in places where mifepristone is either unaffordable or unavailable, although research is limited (Kulier et al., 2011). Because methotrexate may be used to treat ectopic pregnancies, it may be considered when abortion is desired but the pregnancy is in an unknown location (see Chapter 20: Early Pregnancy Loss, for more information).

G. *Procedural abortion*

Procedural abortion done in the clinic or hospital has historically been termed *surgical abortion*. Different methods have evolved over time, and now the terms *in-clinic* and *in-hospital abortion* are being used more widely because these terms are more accurate and differentiate procedural abortion from medication abortion. The extensive training needed to provide procedural abortion is beyond the scope of this chapter. However, knowledge of techniques can aid in counseling patients who will be referred for these procedures, as well as managing follow-up and complications.

Procedural abortion is safe, with minimal complications (White et al., 2015). Techniques include dilatation and curettage (D&C), power-operated electric vacuum aspiration (EVA), and manual vacuum aspiration (MVA). There are no statistically significant differences in excessive blood loss, blood transfusion, infection, incomplete or repeat uterine evacuation, readmission, postoperative abdominal pain, or therapeutic antibiotic use between MVA, EVA, and D&C (Kulier et al., 2001; White et al., 2015). Prior to an procedural abortion cervical priming (also known as *cervical preparation*) may be considered for all patients with a pregnancy of any gestational age and can be done prior to the procedure with a prostaglandin (usually misoprostol) or with osmotic dilators.

1. EVA or suction is commonly used between 9 and 14 weeks' gestational age. This procedure involves the use of a cannula that is attached by tubing to a bottle and pump, which provides a continuous gentle vacuum. After the cervix is dilated, the cannula is passed into the uterus, the pump is turned on, and the product of conception (POC) is gently removed from the uterus. This procedure requires electric power (Kulier et al., 2001).
2. MVA is a procedure similar to EVA, but it involves a specially designed syringe that is portable and does not require electricity. The syringe is attached to the cannula that has been placed into the uterus after dilation and used to remove the contents of the uterus. It is much quieter than EVA and can be used for up to 12 weeks' gestational age (Ipas, 2014).
3. Dilation and extraction (D&E) is a procedure used to provide second- and third-trimester abortion and in the management of pregnancy loss. An osmotic dilator is often inserted into the cervix prior to the

procedure to allow dilation of the cervix, which reduces the risk of any injury to the cervix during the procedure. This procedure may be safely performed in freestanding clinics, ambulatory surgical centers, and hospitals. The evacuation of the POC is done with a combination of EVA and the use of surgical instruments (curettes and forceps) (Kulier et al., 2001).

II. Database

A. *Subjective*
   1. Options counseling
      PCPs will commonly see a patient who presents to care for pregnancy testing, regardless of appointment type. A pregnancy test should be offered to any sexually active patient with a uterus; with a partner or partners who produce sperm; and who is either not using a birth control method or using birth control inconsistently and reports changes in vaginal bleeding and/or a missed period. When a pregnancy test is positive, a patient may or may not need support in making a decision about how to proceed. Some patients will already know they are pregnant and what their intention is in terms of whether to continue the pregnancy. Some patients will need counseling and time to decide, and some patients will arrive at the clinic having no prior knowledge of the pregnancy. Even if a patient presents requesting an abortion, the full range of pregnancy options should be offered, which includes bias-free information about (1) continuing the pregnancy to term and accessing prenatal care, (2) accessing timely abortion care, and (3) making a plan for adoption. This counseling should be patient centered, using a reproductive-justice framework. This framework upholds patient autonomy in their choice when faced with an unexpected pregnancy.

      Options counseling should do the following:
      - Provide pregnancy tests in a nonjudgmental manner.
      - Deliver the results while sitting at eye level with the patient.
      - Describe the full range of pregnancy options, including gestational limits for abortion.
      - Support patients to choose options consistent with their needs, values, and preferences.
      - Address issues related to indecision, as needed, and help ensure that patients' decisions are informed, voluntary, and free of coercion.
      - Provide information to compare medication and procedural abortion noting that both procedures are safe and effective and neither will affect future fertility (if desired).
      - Use language that is mindful, sensitive, and unassuming; this will support patients through the reaffirmation of their choices during counseling and/or procedures (Goodman & TEACH Collaborative Working Group, 2020).
      - Use language that is understandable to the patient and clarify where necessary. Do not use medical terminology or abbreviations that are not common. Use professional interpreters where necessary. (See **Table 17-2**.)

Table 17-2 Patient-Centered Counseling and Shared Decision Making in Reproductive Care

Support the individual process.	Support each patient's decision-making process by eliciting and being responsive to their unique needs and preferences.
Check assumptions.	Be aware of assumptions you make about a patient's sexual identity, personal situation, communities, feelings about pregnancy, reproductive health, and family planning.
Be aware of bias and avoid assumptions.	Explore how bias may show up in our work, and review strategies for self-reflection. Avoid making assumptions because they often reflect cultural stereotypes and bias.
Be aware of tone.	Be mindful of tone, terminology, and body language.
Use correct pronouns and respect gender identity and sexual identity.	Avoid making assumptions about gender identity, sexual identity, and sexual behavior and practice. Ask each patient for their name and pronouns and, if appropriate, their preferred anatomical terminology. Ensure staff is aware of preferences and that these are reflected accurately in patient records.
Create a safe space.	Use open-ended questions and nonjudgmental listening. Allow time for a patient to think, talk further, and ask additional questions.
Utilize all resources available.	Know when to seek help from more experienced providers or staff in a challenging counseling situation.
Screen for coercion.	Screen for coercion, intimate partner violence, and human trafficking. Provide patients with local resources.

(continues)

Table 17-2 Patient-Centered Counseling and Shared Decision Making in Reproductive Care *(continued)*

Be receptive to patient requests.	Provide an opportunity to see the patient alone, as well as to involve a support person if the patient requests this.
Validate and normalize emotions.	Respect and honor individual emotions surrounding abortion. Some may be conflicted and feel a sense of guilt; others may feel relieved and very determined to end their pregnancy. Follow the patient's lead.
Respect confidentiality and privacy.	Patient information should be confidential and only shared with people directly involved in the patient's care.
Use appropriate language.	Use appropriate translation services if needed to provide the information the patient needs to make the decision.
Counseling people with disabilities appropriately.	Assume intellectual competence unless the patient has a severe cognitive impairment. Conduct sexual health screening without parent/guardian present if possible. Allocate extra time for visits if needed. Elicit how the patient would like to be assisted, if needed.

Reproduced from Goodman, S., & the TEACH Collaborative Working Group. (2020). TEACH Early Abortion Training Curriculum 6th Edition. UCSF Bixby Center for Global Reproductive Health.

2. Counseling patients on the decision between MAB or procedural abortion

   When counseling a patient on whether they will proceed with a medication versus procedural abortion, it is important to help discern what factors are important to them during their abortion experience. Many factors can affect this decision, such as the timing of completion, the amount of bleeding, wanting to avoid instrumentation, and the need for privacy and discretion. It is also important to identify the external factors, such as childcare, eldercare, work or school schedule, and housing situations, that might make one option a better fit over the other. Avoid making assumptions about patients' ability to tolerate pain, and consider this factor when helping them make a decision. Patients who desire quick completion of the abortion process may choose procedural abortion. Patients choosing MAB need to have the ability to follow up to confirm pregnancy termination is complete (by ultrasound or serial hCGs, or a urine pregnancy test at 1 month after the MAB), should have access to emergency care if needed, and must be willing to have an procedural abortion if MAB is unsuccessful (Creinin & Grossman, 2020). (See **Table 17-3**.)

3. Past medical history

   Much of the history is relevant to either method of abortion and can help the provider and patient choose the safest method and location. Although most providers reading this text will not be performing procedural abortion, it is important to understand the needed history to assist with appropriate referrals. A patient must be medically stable in order to receive procedural abortion outside of the hospital setting. Any patient with a condition judged to be so severe that the procedure would pose significant or life-threatening risks must be referred to OB/GYN (Goodman & TEACH Collaborative Working Group, 2020). Hospital-based abortion allows for a wide range of anesthetic options that can be tailored to the medical needs of the patient in a setting in which continuous monitoring of patient status is possible.

   a. Obstetrical history

   i. Details of previous pregnancies and outcomes, including ectopic pregnancy, prior miscarriage or abortion, fetal deaths, live births and mode of delivery, and history of obstetrical hemorrhage requiring transfusion

   ii. If a patient has had two or more cesarean deliveries, may be required to have a hospital-based aspiration due to the increased risk of hemorrhage (Butwick et al., 2017). Patients ≥14 weeks' gestation with a scarred uterus need documentation of the location of the placenta.

   iii. An in-clinic aspiration can be performed for a hydatidiform mole of less than 14 weeks in size (Goodman & TEACH Collaborative Working Group, 2020), but the provider must draw quantitative hCG and either provide follow-up or refer to primary care (Berkowitz & Goldstein, 2009). Patients with moles equal to or more than 14 weeks in size must be referred to OB/GYN. Patients with known or suspected molar pregnancies should not be offered MAB.

   iv. Placenta previa in current pregnancy: Due to the increased risk of hemorrhage, the patient will need to be referred to OB/GYN for in-hospital D&C.

   v. Known or suspected ectopic pregnancy: MAB is contraindicated in patients with a known or suspected ectopic pregnancy. Mifepristone and misoprostol do not treat

Table 17-3 Differences Between Medication Abortion (MAB) and Aspiration, Counseling Patients

	MAB	Procedural Abortion
Brief summary/description of the procedure	"Both work very well, both are safe, and neither changes your chances to get pregnant in the future (if that's what you want)." "You take one pill first, then take a second medicine later, which will cause cramping and bleeding. The pregnancy will usually pass within a few hours."	"Both work very well, both are safe, and neither changes your chances to get pregnant in the future (if that's what you want)." "This is done on an exam table in the office or at a hospital, with instruments inside you. You will be given medicine for pain, and it usually takes 5–10 minutes to complete."
Gestational age	Currently up to 10 weeks in the United States Up to 11 weeks in some countries	Vacuum aspiration to 14–16 weeks Dilation and extraction (D&E) beyond 14–16 weeks
Advantages	Patient has more control over where the abortion takes place Avoids procedure More support options possible May be perceived as more natural, like a miscarriage Options for personalizing the experience	Procedure over in 5–10 minutes Usually less postprocedure bleeding than MAB Options for moderate or deep sedation Leaves the office visit not pregnant Medical staff members with the patient
Disadvantages	Completed in multiple days May experience heavier and longer bleeding and cramps Less control over the time during which bleeding and cramping occur No clinical monitoring May inadvertently see the fetus if ≥ 9 weeks gestational age	Requires clinical setting Risks of instrumentation Risks of anesthesia, if used May be fewer options for support person(s) during the procedure Suction machine may be audible.
Protocol	Take medication at home or in a clinic.	Procedure in office or hospital
Effectiveness	<63 days, 95%–99% 64–77 days, with 2nd miso dose, 99.6% 71–77 days, with 2nd miso dose, 97.6% If the pregnancy does not pass, the patient will need aspiration.	Over 99% of the time May need to repeat the aspiration
Duration	One to several days to complete	One visit; 5- to 10-minute procedure
Pain	Mild to strong cramps after taking misoprostol, lasting a few hours	Mild to strong cramps during and just after the procedure
Bleeding	Possible heavier bleeding with clots during the abortion Light bleeding that may persist on and off for 1–2 weeks or more	Heaviest bleeding during the procedure Light bleeding that may persist on and off for 1–2 weeks or more
Pain management	Oral pain medication	Options of: 1. Oral pain medication 2. Local anesthesia 3. Moderate or deep sedation
Safety	Used safely for >25 years At least 10-fold safer than continuing a pregnancy to term	Used safely for >45 years At least 10-fold safer than continuing a pregnancy to term

Reproduced from Goodman, S., & the TEACH Collaborative Working Group. (2020). TEACH Early Abortion Training Curriculum 6th Edition. UCSF Bixby Center for Global Reproductive Health.

an ectopic pregnancy, and the use of these medications may delay diagnosis and treatment of this life-threatening condition (Danco, 2016).
b. Gynecological history
   i. Menstrual cycle pattern, including menarche, frequency, and length.
   ii. Contraceptive history: Assess for current use and possible method failure versus user error. This will help with accurate dating and will inform counseling of the patient about birth control methods.
   iii. Uterine fibroids: Fibroids may inhibit the ability to complete procedural abortion depending on their size and location in relation to pregnancy. Consider referral to a higher level of care with an experienced provider. MAB may be considered (Creinin & Grossman, 2020).
   iv. Uterine cavity congenital uterine anomalies: MAB may be considered an alternative (Creinin & Grossman, 2020).
   v. Cervical stenosis: A cervical preparation agent such as misoprostol or laminaria may be helpful. Consider the use of an os finder or performing aspiration under ultrasound guidance. MAB may be offered.
   vi. Cervicitis (mucopurulent) or known chlamydia or gonorrhea infection: Initiate treatment per Centers for Disease Control and Prevention (CDC) guidelines prior to procedure.
c. Cardiovascular history
   i. Mild to moderate hypertension (HTN): Refer patient for treatment as needed; mild to moderate HTN does not prevent the patient from having the procedure in the clinic setting or MAB (Guiahi & Davis, 2012).
   ii. Poorly controlled HTN, symptomatic, and/or severe HTN (>160/105) should be treated prior to the procedure or referral for additional management or management of the abortion in the hospital setting (Guiahi & Davis, 2012).
   iii. Heart disease: The state of pregnancy, in itself, increases the risk associated with a history of cardiovascular disease (Davey, 2006). If symptomatic of underlying heart disease, or severe disease, aspiration may be performed in the operating room with monitoring by anesthesia (Goodman & TEACH Collaborative Working Group, 2020). Because clinical trials have excluded patients with angina, valvular disease, arrhythmia, or cardiac failure, MAB is contraindicated in patients with preexisting heart disease (SFP, 2014).
   iv. Ergot drugs, such as methylergonovine maleate (Methergine), should be avoided in those with hypertension. Oxytocin and misoprostol are acceptable uterotonic agents if needed for excessive bleeding (Guiahi & Davis, 2012).
d. Hematological history (bleeding and clotting disorders, anticoagulants, severe anemia)
   i. Anemia: Any patient who has a hemoglobin of less than 9.5–10 g/dL may be at increased risk for blood transfusion should hemorrhage occur, although the transfusion rates associated with MAB are low (less than 0.1%) (Creinin & Grossman, 2020; Guiahi & Davis, 2012). Clinicians must evaluate the patient and determine the appropriate management or referral (Goodman & TEACH Collaborative Working Group, 2020).
   ii. Those using daily anticoagulation medications have an increased risk of blood loss and should be referred for in-clinic aspiration rather than using MAB (Kaneshiro et al., 2011; SFP, 2014). Managing anticoagulation therapy in the context of abortion may require OB/GYN care (Kaneshiro et al., 2011). Anticoagulation medications can be continued for up to 12 weeks, with relatively low risk of additional blood loss (Kaneshiro et al., 2011). Managing patients with an active clotting disorder requires appropriate preparation (intravenous [IV] access, available uterotonics) in an outpatient setting (Kaneshiro et al., 2011).
   iii. Porphyrias are rare metabolic disorders in which genetic mutations alter the body's generation of heme. Theoretically, mifepristone could precipitate an exacerbation caused by an accumulation of protoporphyrin (Guiahi & Davis, 2012).
e. Pulmonary history
   i. Mild, well-controlled asthma does not prevent patients from routine procedural abortion or MAB. Advise the patient to take routine meds before the procedure, even if the lungs are clear to auscultation.
   ii. Patients with poorly controlled asthma will need to delay procedural abortion until asthma is better controlled.
   iii. Active respiratory infection: Consider delaying the procedure. If unable, consider personal protective equipment (PPE) for patients and staff.
   iv. In the context of COVID-19 community transmission, recommend appropriate PPE for both staff and patient (Goodman, 2020).
   v. Because mifepristone also exhibits antiglucocorticoid and weak antiandrogenic activity (Danco, 2016), it can block negative endocrine feedback mechanisms that control cortisol secretion. In patients who

are using long-term corticosteroid therapy for severe or uncontrolled asthma, mifepristone may exacerbate the underlying condition (Sitruk-Ware & Spitz, 2003). Although more studies are needed, one review recommends that increasing the dose of steroid medication can counteract the cortisol-blunting effect of mifepristone. The glucocorticoid dose should be increased for several days before and after mifepristone (Davey, 2006).
   f. Endocrine history
      i. Insulin-dependent diabetes mellitus (IDDM):
         a. Pregnancy can cause hypoglycemia, especially in the first trimester. Hyperemesis, which is common in the first trimester, can also disrupt glycemic control.
         b. Well-controlled IDDM is not a contraindication for MAB.
         c. Patients with IDDM may need to be referred to a physician comfortable with diabetes management.
         d. Consider scheduling the patient for procedural abortion early in the day so that the patient can eat and take their usual dose of insulin after the procedure.
         e. Glucose levels will be evaluated prior to the procedure and will be monitored to adjust the need for insulin. Glucose above 400 mg/dL warrants evaluation for diabetic ketoacidosis (DKA) and requires treatment or referral prior to the procedure (Guiahi & Davis, 2012).
         f. After the procedure, medication requirements may decrease substantially, and thus coordination of care with PCPs may be recommended.
      ii. Hyperthyroidism in pregnancy may present with tachycardia, vomiting, tremulousness, and wide pulse pressure. Mild hyperthyroidism is not contraindicated; however, uncontrolled hyperthyroidism can lead to thyroid storm (Guiahi & Davis, 2012).
      iii. Chronic adrenal failure: In patients with adrenal insufficiency on long-term corticosteroid therapy, mifepristone exposure may exacerbate the underlying condition (Sitruk-Ware & Spitz, 2003).
   g. Renal and hepatic history
      i. Renal and hepatic disease: Adjustments to medications given during aspiration may be necessary. Because mifepristone undergoes hepatic and renal metabolism, MAB with mifepristone is contraindicated.
   h. Neurologic history
      i. Antiseizure medications should be taken as prescribed on the day of aspiration and resumed as usual following the procedure (Goodman & TEACH Collaborative Working Group, 2020).
      ii. Uncontrolled seizure disorder or seizure in the last 2 weeks is a contraindication for in-clinic aspiration (Goodman & TEACH Collaborative Working Group, 2020).
4. Surgical history
   a. Document details of past surgeries, if any, focusing on obstetric, gynecological, and abdominal surgeries.
5. Medications and allergies (daily medication, medications taken in pregnancy, self-abortion attempts)
   a. Use of daily medications, including vitamins and herbal remedies
   b. Allergies to medications and foods, especially shellfish allergy due to cross-reactivity with iodine
6. Assess if self-abortion was attempted. *Self-managed abortion* refers to the practice of attempting to end a pregnancy without the formal supervision of a healthcare professional. This practice will become more common when abortion laws become more restrictive. In locations where abortion is restricted, providers should consider the legal ramifications for their patients of documenting this information.
   a. Ingestion: Some people attempt to self-abort by ingesting herbs, medication, laxatives, quinine, alcohol, detergent, fabric softener, bleach, acid, methylated spirits, castor oil, turpentine, tea brewed with livestock feces, and blood tonics (Singh et al., 2018).
   b. Inserting foreign objects or liquids into the cervix or into the vagina: Some patients may present after having inserted objects or solutions such as saline solutions, concentrated herbal concoctions prepared with water or alcohol, soapy solutions, detergent, or bleach (Singh et al., 2018).
   c. Physical: Another method people use to attempt self-abortion is through physical means, such as manipulating or beating the lower abdomen, or engaging in traumatic or injurious physical activity, such as jumping from the top of the stairs or roof, falling, lifting heavy objects, or exercising excessively (Singh et al., 2018).
7. Family history
   Not relevant to abortion care
8. Psychiatric history
   a. Has a condition that would invalidate informed consent
   b. Many patients who present for abortion care express conflicting emotions, and that is completely normal. It is important to validate and normalize these feelings.
   c. Patients with severe anxiety may need more time to counsel, more staff support and guidance on relaxation, and subtle changes in the clinic atmosphere (lowered lights, use of personal smartphone with headphones, soft music, etc.).

d. Sedation during an procedural abortion may be helpful for patients who face anxiety (Guiahi & Davis, 2012).
e. Document medications used for depression and/or anxiety, encourage patients to take usual doses during the procedure, and ensure patients have access to care as needed.
f. Assess for suicidality if the patient reports severe depression or signals that they are suicidal. Suicidal ideation should be assessed to determine patient safety by asking about suicidal plans, intention, preparations, and prior suicidal attempts. If the clinician ascertains that the safety of the patient is at risk, a warm hand-off to a behavioral health clinician should be made in a timely manner.

9. Personal and social history

When obtaining a patient's social history, it is important to create a safe space for the patient in consideration of the sensitive nature of the visit. Always gather social history directly from the patient in a quiet, private setting without the support person or partner in the room, and make sure the patient consents to referrals as needed. Use professional interpreter services as necessary. It is common to encounter patients who have experienced sexual trauma, IPV, rape, incest, or human trafficking in the reproductive health setting (Goodman & TEACH Collaborative Working Group, 2020). Some groups are at higher risk of sexual assault than others. One in two transgender individuals is sexually abused or assaulted at some point in their lives (Office for Victims of Crime, 2014). Transgender youth, transgender people of color, those involved in the sex trade, unhoused people, and those with disabilities experience much higher rates of sexual assault than the general population (Office for Victims of Crime, 2014).

a. Housing situation: Assess current housing situation. Patients will need a safe place with plumbing during MAB or for recovery after in-clinic aspiration. Unhoused patients may need a hotel room or may be a better candidate for in-clinic aspiration.
b. Support systems: Assessment of support systems, which may include a partner, friend, or family member who will be with the patient during MAB or can help with childcare. Some patients will not have a support person, which is acceptable for MAB if the patient has a safe place to be and understands how to access help if needed. Patients undergoing in-clinic aspiration will need a support person to drive them home if they were given sedating medication.
c. IPV assessment: Assess for current or history of IPV. A reproductive health visit is an important opportunity to assess patients for IPV and patient safety and make referrals as necessary. See Chapter 58: Intimate Partner Violence (Domestic Violence) for more details.
d. History of sexual trauma: Assess patients for history of sexual abuse, rape, incest, or IPV. If a patient is or was underage when the abuse occurred, a child protective services (CPS) report usually must be made, depending on the patient's age, the age of perpetrator, the jurisdiction, local and state laws, and mandated reporting laws. It is common to encounter patients who have experienced sexual trauma and abuse, which will affect patients differently in the reproductive-care setting. Awareness of sexual trauma or abuse should inform the approach to care through recognition of the impact of violence and victimization on coping strategies. Trauma-informed care employs an empowerment model by working to maximize patient choices; creating an atmosphere that is respectful of the survivors' need for safety, respect, and acceptance; and emphasizing the patient's strengths, adaptations, and resilience (Butler et al., 2011). It is important to minimize the possibility of retraumatization, especially during pelvic exams. Victims of rape and incest must be provided referrals for behavioral health if desired, screened for STI, and offered the option to file a police report.
e. History of RC: Asking the patient, "Has anyone tampered with or prevented contraceptive use or pressured you to make a decision about this pregnancy?" elicits this information. If there has been RC and the patient remains in the relationship, offer birth control methods that can be easily hidden and cannot be tampered with by a partner.
f. Screen for human trafficking: Screen for human trafficking and respond to victim identification. Human trafficking, which is estimated to affect 20.9 million people worldwide, is the recruitment, transportation, transfer, harboring, or receipt of persons by means of coercion, abduction, fraud, deception, or abuse of power of a position of vulnerability for the purpose of exploitation (Hemmings et al., 2016; United Nations, 2021). Screening for trafficking should be done by trained individuals with translation as necessary. The National Human Trafficking Resource Center has a one-page algorithm that reviews appropriate questions to ask, such as "Have you been forced to engage in sexual acts for money or favors?" (National Human Trafficking Resource Center, 2010). Individuals who are trafficked may present with unplanned pregnancy due to the high rate of sex trafficking (Tracy & Macias-Konstantopoulos, 2017).
g. Alcohol, opioid, and recreational drug use: Assess patients for a history of or current use of alcohol, opioid dependence, and use of recreational

drugs. Current use of alcohol, opioids, or recreational drugs may influence the patient's ability to give consent. Alcohol-use disorder may require a higher dose of benzodiazepine, if used, due to possible tolerance. Those with opiate-use disorder or those on opioid maintenance therapy may require a larger dose of opiates, if used, due to possible tolerance. NSAIDs may be a good alternative for pain control (Goodman & TEACH Collaborative Working Group, 2020).

10. Other medical conditions
    Occasionally other medical conditions warrant management or referral prior to abortion. Certain medical conditions and patient circumstances may justify recommending a MAB over an procedural abortion. MAB may provide a safer alternative for patients with extremely high total body weight, pelvic tumors that interfere with access to the cervix, or a known history of reactions to anesthetic agents. MAB does not require a lithotomy position and is preferred with patients who have orthopedic conditions or neurological conditions (Guiahi & Davis, 2012).

11. History of present illness (HPI)/history of present condition
    a. Gestational age: If the gestational age is less than 70 days, it is appropriate for most MAB protocols. If a protocol supports providing MAB at 71–77 days' gestational age, the regimen should include a second dose of misoprostol, 800 mcg, 4 hours after the first misoprostol dose (NAF, 2020).
    b. IUD in place: Remove the IUD before starting MAB due to the theoretical risk of uterine perforation from contractions during MAB and the potential risk of infection (Danco, 2016). If an IUD cannot be removed without delaying the MAB, the patient should be offered a uterine aspiration (NAF, 2020). IUDs can be removed during an aspiration procedure.
    c. Breastfeeding: mifepristone can be found in breast milk. Limited data demonstrate undetectable to low levels of the drug in human milk, and it is recommended that breastfeeding need not be interrupted after a single dose of mifepristone 200 mg (Danco, 2016). Misoprostol is also found in breast milk at extremely low levels, and the amounts ingested by the infant are trivial and would not be expected to cause any adverse effects in breastfed infants. No special precautions are required (Drugs and Lactation Database, 2006; Sääv et al., 2010). Depending on the age of the breastfed child, a risk-versus-benefits discussion should be held with the patient, including potential adverse effects on the child from mifepristone and misoprostol versus discontinuing breastfeeding for the duration of the MAB. Other medications sometimes taken during an abortion that may be found in breast milk are antibiotics, benzodiazepines, and opioids. Always consult a reliable resource, such as UpToDate or LactMed, before prescribing medications to those patients who are breastfeeding.

12. Review of systems
    a. Constitutional: fever, chills
    b. Respiratory: shortness of breath, cough
    c. Cardiovascular: loss of consciousness, palpitations
    d. Gastrointestinal: abdominal pain, nausea, vomiting
    e. Genitourinary: dysuria, frequency, vaginal bleeding
    f. Musculoskeletal: back pain, shoulder pain
    g. Neurological: headache, dizziness
    h. Psychiatric: recent changes in mood, anxiety, depression
    i. Bleeding and abdominal pain in early pregnancy are common and must be assessed to determine the cause. Bleeding can be caused by implantation bleeding, which usually occurs at about 5–6 weeks' gestational age, but it can also be worrisome for ectopic pregnancy or early pregnancy loss (EPL). Clinical manifestations of ectopic pregnancy typically appear 6–8 weeks after the last normal menstrual period but may occur later.

B. Objective
Physical exam and laboratory tests prior to abortion vary by practice setting, and telemedicine is changing how MAB is provided. The need for a physical exam is dictated by medical history, patient symptoms, and abortion type. Assessment should be done to ensure the patient is eligible for the chosen procedure, consisting of a focus on pregnancy dating, targeted medical history, and related laboratory testing. These are routinely done prior to procedural abortion, but evolving evidence suggests that many patients can safely undergo telemedicine MAB without the physical exam components.

1. Blood pressure and baseline pulse
   a. Blood pressure screening is recommended for all patients to screen for hypertension and make referrals if necessary (NAF, 2020).
   b. Poorly controlled, severe, or symptomatic hypertension is contraindicated with MAB and warrants treatment prior to an procedural abortion.
2. Lung and heart auscultation
   a. Recommended for patients with underlying conditions such as asthma or heart disease
3. Temperature
   a. Should be done if the patient presents with any symptoms of infection, such as pelvic pain, dysuria, or flank pain

III. Assessment

A. *No contraindications to MAB: Proceed to MAB.*
B. *Contraindications to MAB, or the patient chooses procedural abortion*
Refer the patient in a timely manner to a provider who can perform an procedural abortion. Referrals will be

driven by patient risk factors; gestational age; and scope of practice of the APN, family physician, or OB/GYN. Facilitating this referral by scheduling the appointment will assist the patient in receiving timely care. It is ideal to have an appointment made for the patient before they leave the clinic. If the patient needs to travel to the facility and possibly stay overnight, refer patients, as needed, to resources to assist with costs. There are multiple organizations whose mission is to remove financial and logistical barriers to abortion care, some of which are listed at the end of the chapter in the Resources section.

C. *Ectopic pregnancy*

If an ectopic pregnancy is suspected or confirmed, refer the patient to the emergency department (ED) for immediate treatment. Facilitating this referral by calling the ED and reviewing the clinical findings with the charge nurse or ED provider will help make the transition to care in the hospital more seamless. Counsel the patient on what to expect in the ED, and provide an after-hours number to contact the office if they do not receive appropriate care.

D. *Patient chooses to continue pregnancy*

Refer to prenatal care. Provide a list of prenatal care providers, offer STI screening for early diagnosis and prevention of vertical transmission, provide and/or encourage the patient to start taking prenatal vitamins, and emphasize the importance of entry to prenatal care at or prior to 12 weeks' gestational age. If risk factors such as alcohol or drug use are identified, a facilitative referral to prenatal care and drug and alcohol treatment may be necessary. If the patient has IDDM, inpatient care may be necessary to achieve early glucose control, which dramatically decreases the risk of birth defects.

E. *Patient chooses to continue the pregnancy and take steps toward placing the child up for adoption.*

Refer the patient to adoption agencies and prenatal care. Provide a list of adoption agencies and prenatal care providers, offer STI screening for early diagnosis and prevention of vertical transmission, provide and/or encourage the patient to start taking prenatal vitamins, and emphasize the importance of entry to prenatal care at or prior to 12 weeks' gestational age.

IV. Goals of clinical management

A. *Provide unbiased information in a respectful, nonjudgmental, and safe space for patients to make decisions after reviewing options. Describe the full range of pregnancy options, including gestational limits for abortion. Normalize feelings of sadness, relief, or mixed emotions. Provide referrals for mental health as needed.*

B. *Deliver evidence-based, patient-centered care that supports the patient's preferred approach to treatment of an unwanted pregnancy through shared decision making.*

1. Reassure patients that all options are safe and will not affect future fertility, if desired.

C. *Make timely referrals if abortion care is sought by the patient but not provided by the PCP, directing the patient to available resources if needed. Refer patients to an appropriate provider if the risk factors identified require the patient to receive abortion care in a hospital setting or care provided by a specialist.*

D. *Offer contraception while remaining aware that some patients prefer not to discuss contraception at the time of abortion. Provide a contraceptive method appropriate to the patient's medical history and individual preferences.*

E. *Provide postabortion care that is patient centered and evidence based, if needed.*

V. Plan

A. *Diagnostic testing*

1. Pregnancy testing
   a. Urine: Urine pregnancy tests should be done prior to all abortions, even if the patient is receiving telemedicine abortion care. The use of high-sensitivity urine pregnancy tests (HSPTs) is preferred because these tests are easy to use, are affordable, and can detect a pregnancy as early as cycle day 32–35 (95% of pregnancies) or when hCG concentrations are as low as 20–25 mIU/mL. These tests may remain positive for up to 4 weeks postabortion and can be used in some cases to show completion of MAB if done ≥4 weeks after MAB (Goodman & TEACH Collaborative Working Group, 2020).
   b. Serum: A serum quantitative hCG test must be ordered by a healthcare provider. This test can detect serum levels of hCG as low as 2–10 mIU/mL. It is not appropriate for use in determining the gestational age of the pregnancy. Serial measurements are often used in evaluating suspected ectopic pregnancy, evaluating abortion completion (i.e., when products of conception are not visualized following aspiration), initiating MAB when no IUP is seen on ultrasound, and managing a molar pregnancy (Goodman & TEACH Collaborative Working Group, 2020). There is a rapid decline in hCG levels after a medication abortion (Pocius et al., 2015).

2. Dating the pregnancy
   a. Last menstrual period (LMP): LMP is used to date pregnancies safely and accurately if LMP is certain. The first day of LMP alone (+/– 1 week of certainty) is an accurate means of estimating gestational age, with low rates of under- or overestimation through the mid-first trimester (Bracken et al., 2011; Schonberg et al., 2014). Assess the patient's menstrual cycle for regularity. The average menstrual cycle length can be between 15 and 45 days and varies based on age, total body weight, stress levels, and smoking status (Grieger & Norman, 2020). Dating a pregnancy by LMP alone has been shown to be

accurate with patients who are sure of their LMP if it is within the prior 56 to 63 days (Creinin & Grossman, 2020).

b. Pelvic exam: A pelvic and bimanual exam may not be necessary for patients opting for an MAB. A bimanual exam should only be done by an experienced clinician. This exam, combined with a sure LMP, can improve the estimation of gestational age (Goodman & TEACH Collaborative Working Group, 2020). A bimanual exam should be performed if an ectopic pregnancy is suspected to better identify the location of pain, determine the size of the uterus, and determine if a palpable adnexal mass is present. During a bimanual exam, the adnexa should be palpated gently because excessive pressure may rupture an ectopic pregnancy. This exam can also detect uterine changes due to fibroids. A speculum exam is not necessary for a patient seeking an MAB unless they are symptomatic for cervicitis or present with other symptoms that require an exam to assess.

c. Ultrasound: Ultrasound is not required for MAB or uterine aspiration in the first trimester; however, it is an important tool for dating if LMP is unknown or uncertain. Much of the abortion care provided globally is done without an ultrasound examination (Creinin & Grossman, 2020). Ultrasound should be used for pregnancy dating when gestational age cannot be determined reasonably by other means (NAF, 2020) and if ectopic pregnancy is suspected. Staff members who perform ultrasound exams and clinicians who interpret those exams must either show documentation of proficiency or complete a program of training (NAF, 2020).

Transvaginal ultrasounds (TVUSs) are used to accurately date and determine the location and viability of a pregnancy in the first trimester, and transabdominal ultrasounds are used more often in the second and third trimesters. When performing ultrasounds, it is important to remind the patient of the limitations and purpose of the ultrasound. Ultrasounds done in abortion care settings are limited to determining the dating, location, and viability of the pregnancy. Unless local law requires viewing or describing ultrasound findings, prior to starting the ultrasound, ask the patient if they want to view or not view the images or be informed of ultrasound findings such as multiple gestations or nonviability. Multiple pregnancies make up approximately 2%–3% of all pregnancies and may be a finding on ultrasounds performed during abortion care. A finding of a multiple pregnancy may occasionally change a patient's decision in either direction (Goodman & TEACH Collaborative Working Group, 2020). Do not assume either way that a patient will want to see ultrasound images or know details about the pregnancy beyond eligibility for the procedure. Every person is different. Some patients will ask for a picture, which should be provided only if requested by the patient, unless required by local laws.

An ultrasound must be performed if an ectopic pregnancy is suspected or if the patient is at high risk for an ectopic pregnancy.

See Chapter 20: Early Pregnancy Loss for more information.

3. Rhesus (Rh) testing: Rh testing is an area of evolving evidence. Studies show that Rh testing may not be required in the first trimester of pregnancy (Wiebe et al., 2019). Some institutions are now requiring Rh testing for abortions only after the first trimester. The WHO recently published new recommendations, concluding that overall, the evidence does not favor routine Rh testing in the first trimester; the WHO recommends against it for gestational ages <12 weeks (WHO, 2022).

   a. Rh can be documented by point-of-care testing, by an outside source, or by patient report; if the patient has a donor card, this can be used in lieu of testing.
   b. Patients who are ≥84 days' gestational age and Rh negative should be given a RhoGam injection (WHO, 2022).
   c. If the patient does not desire children in the future or declines testing, Rh testing does not need to be done (Goodman & TEACH Collaborative Working Group, 2020).

4. Hemoglobin/Hematocrit
   a. Point-of-care testing at the time of the procedure with a fingerstick can be done to determine if the patient is anemic, to determine the patient's baseline hemoglobin in case of hemorrhage, and to determine eligibility for MAB or in-clinic procedural abortion (Goodman & TEACH Collaborative Working Group, 2020).
   b. Patients who have severe anemia, defined as hemoglobin 6.5–7.9 g/dL (Badireddy & Baradhi, 2022), should be referred for procedural abortion because of the possible need for transfusion in the case of hemorrhage during the procedure (Guiahi & Davis, 2012).
   c. Moderate or asymptomatic anemia is rarely a reason to delay abortion care.
   d. Prior to administration of methotrexate, a complete blood count (CBC) should be considered for patients with a history of blood dyscrasia (NAF, 2020).
   e. This can be waived if using evidence-based telemedicine protocols that rely on patient history to screen for anemia.

5. STI screening
   a. Chlamydia and gonorrhea (GC/CT) screening: Offer screening to any patient at increased risk

(routine annual screening for any patient under age 26, new or multiple sexual partners in the last year for all age groups).
   b. If cervicitis is noted on pelvic exam, test for GC/CT, and initiate empiric prior to aspiration.
   c. Offer HIV, syphilis, hepatitis C, and hepatitis B screening per risk assessment.
B. *Providing medication abortion*
   1. Ensure no contraindications:
      a. Gestational age is within limits according to practice protocols.
      b. Pregnancy is not suspected to be ectopic.
      c. No medical contraindications to MAB, including heart disease, chronic adrenal failure, hemorrhagic disorder, inherited porphyria, severe anemia, uncontrolled asthma, currently taking anticoagulants, and renal or hepatic disease
      d. IUD must be removed if present.
      e. The patient must understand the process and must agree to an procedural abortion if the MAB is not successful.
      f. Ensure the patient has access to a telephone and the number to call in case of urgent questions, as well as knowledge of the closest ED and a way to get there.
   2. Formulations
      a. Mifepristone and misoprostol:
         i. Mifepristone 200 mg orally once followed by misoprostol taken in one of the following ways:
            a. Up to 10 weeks' gestation: At 24–48 hours after mifepristone, take misoprostol 800 mcg, place buccally for 30 minutes, then swallow any remaining pieces, OR
            b. Up to 9 weeks' gestation: At 6–72 hours after mifepristone, place misoprostol 800 mcg vaginally and lie down for 30 minutes. Vaginal routes enable a patient to complete the MAB process sooner and may be a better option for those who are suffering from severe pregnancy-related nausea. Sometimes the tablets come out when bleeding starts or if the patient is up and about. If the tablets fall out while the patient is bleeding, advise them not to worry. In most cases, enough of the medication will have been absorbed. If the tablets fall out before bleeding starts, the patient may reinsert them or call for instructions on what to do (NAF, 2020). If a patient is seeking care at a facility that may be hostile to abortion, they may consider ensuring that tablets have dissolved before presenting for care or removing any pieces that remain in the vagina.
      b. Misoprostol alone: If mifepristone is contraindicated, a multidose regime of misoprostol alone is an alternative (Creinin & Grossman, 2020). Misoprostol 800 mcg is placed vaginally or sublingually and administered every 3 hours for three doses. If the patient is placing misoprostol vaginally, they may space the doses 12 hours apart.
      c. If using methotrexate (for use up to 63 days' gestational age) plus misoprostol, administer methotrexate 50 mg/m^2 intramuscularly or 50 mg oral. Prescribe or dispense misoprostol 800 mcg per vagina to be used 3–7 days later (Christin-Maitre et al., 2000; Seeber & Barnhart, 2006).
   3. Initiating MAB when a patient has a pregnancy of unknown location (PUL): If it cannot be determined the pregnancy is intrauterine and the risk of ectopic pregnancy is low, the MAB can be initiated if the patient is followed closely with consecutive blood draws of hCGs. Draw hCG on the day the mifepristone is administered and 48–72 hours after misoprostol is taken. If the drop in hCG levels is greater than 50% from baseline, the abortion is complete. If the drop is less than 50% from baseline, the provider should suspect an ectopic pregnancy and immediately refer the patient to the ED to evaluate for ectopic pregnancy (Goodman & TEACH Collaborative Working Group, 2020; Pocius et al., 2015).
   4. If the patient's blood type is Rh negative and the gestational age is ≥84 days, administer Rho(D)-IG 50-mcg dose intramuscularly (IM) within 72 hours of mifepristone (Goodman & TEACH Collaborative Working Group, 2020).
   5. Provide contraception.
      a. Offer contraception while remaining aware that some patients prefer not to discuss contraception at the time of abortion. Patients may feel coerced to use contraception (Brandi et al., 2018).
      b. Provide a contraceptive method appropriate to the patient's medical history and individual preferences, in consideration of RC if present.
      c. While counseling a patient about methods, offer a range of methods through the use of decision aids, and ask the patient if they received what they needed in terms of birth control information and care.
      d. Patients who opt for an IUD will be scheduled for insertion at the follow-up visit after an MAB. Any other birth control method can be initiated during the first MAB visit. An IUD can be placed on the day of an procedural abortion and some patients may choose this method because of this option.
C. *Patient education*
   1. Prepare the patient for what to expect, including side effects:
      a. Bleeding and cramping can occur after taking mifepristone, but this is uncommon (Danco, 2016). Mifepristone may cause spotting about 10% of the time (Danco, 2016), and thus it is important to counsel the patient that even if they experience spotting, this will not be sufficient to pass the pregnancy, and they will still need to take the misoprostol.

b. Nausea (>15%) and vomiting can occur for a short duration, and thus the prescription of an antiemetic is recommended. If vomiting occurs within 1 hour of taking mifepristone, the patient must take a second dose due to possible decreased effectiveness (Bancsi & Grindrod, 2019).
c. Other side effects after taking mifepristone include diarrhea, headache, dizziness, weakness, and fever/chills (Danco, 2016).
d. Patients may experience side effects specific to misoprostol, including a transient, low-level temperature, nausea, and diarrhea (especially if taken orally). Fever and flu-like symptoms are common but should not last longer than 24 hours.
e. Pain due to uterine cramping is expected after taking misoprostol. Discuss pain management with patients and offer to prescribe NSAIDs, such as ibuprofen 800 mg PO Q4–6 hours, as needed. Studies of pain control during an MAB have found that the duration of pain for most patients is no longer than 24 hours after misoprostol administration (Creinin & Grossman, 2020).
f. Bleeding and passing tissue: Bleeding starts within 30 minutes to 48 hours after taking misoprostol and is usually heaviest 4–6 hours after taking misoprostol. Expect heavier bleeding than the usual menstrual period for the first few days, then lighter for 1–2 weeks and spotting up to 4 weeks after MAB (Bancsi & Grindrod, 2019).
g. When prescribing methotrexate, counsel the patient about common side effects, including nausea, vomiting, diarrhea, fever, dizziness, chills, mild stomatitis, and oral ulcers (Christin-Maitre et al., 2000; Seeber & Barnhart, 2006).

2. Ensure the patient has a safe place to be during the MAB.
3. Review the follow-up plan, including if the MAB is unsuccessful.
4. Inform the patient of the teratogenic effect of misoprostol in the case of an ongoing pregnancy after MAB. These risks include the possibility of limb defects with or without Möbius syndrome (i.e., facial paralysis) (ACOG, 2020; Creinin & Grossman, 2020).
5. Patients should be counseled that MAB does not have an adverse effect on future fertility or future pregnancy outcomes (WHO, 2018).
6. Confirm the patient has all the information and supplies needed:
   a. Pain medication
   b. Anti-nausea medication
   c. Additional nonpharmaceutical pain management options that may be helpful include a warm heating pad applied to the lower abdomen.
   d. Maxi pads (not thin pads or pantyliners)
   e. Thermometer
   f. Snacks and nonalcoholic beverages
7. Counsel patient regarding when to call/danger signs:
   a. The patient should call if they do not experience bleeding within 48 hours of taking misoprostol. This may indicate the patient will need a second dose of misoprostol.
   b. Rare possibility of infection, occurring in less than 1% of MABs: Symptoms include a fever over 100.4°F/38°C for more than 4 hours, presenting ≥24 hours after taking misoprostol, and severe, persistent pain lasting more than 24 hours (Danco, 2016).
   c. Heavier-than-expected bleeding, defined as soaking through two thick full-size sanitary pads per hour for 2 consecutive hours, or if concerned about heavy bleeding (Danco, 2016): The need for emergency care is based on how the patient is feeling, baseline hemoglobin or hematocrit level, whether the bleeding seems to be slowing, and the distance from an emergency facility (SFP, 2014).
   d. Passing blood clots larger than the size of a lemon
   e. If the patient experiences heavy bleeding with dizziness, fainting, shortness of breath, or palpitations, they must go directly to the ED.
   f. Vomiting more than 4 hours
   g. Severe cramping felt through pain medications
   h. Feeling sick and weak, with nausea and vomiting, bloating, and/or severe abdominal pain >2 hours
   i. Depression: If a patient is feeling severely depressed, they should be assessed for suicidality and referred appropriately if needed. Hormonal changes may cause a patient to experience mood swings, including sadness. Advise the patient to call if they are experiencing emotions that are more severe than expected. Most patients feel better in the month following an abortion. Several support hotlines are available to help patients through these emotions if needed (see patient resources).
   j. Symptoms of pregnancy that persist more than 1 week after taking MAB medications
8. Schedule follow-up visit in 1–2 weeks to determine that the MAB is complete and to provide contraception if requested. Follow-up after MAB can be done by ultrasound, serum hCG, or evaluation of symptoms (Creinin & Grossman, 2020). Review symptoms and what to expect.
   a. Ultrasound: Return to clinic for a TVUS to determine if the abortion is complete, which is determined by the absence of a gestational sac.
   b. Serum quantitative hCG: Repeat hCG 48–72 hours after misoprostol is taken. If the drop in hCG levels is greater than 50%, the abortion is complete (Pocius et al., 2015).
   c. If follow-up is being done via telemedicine:
      i. An uncomplicated MAB can be assessed for completion via self-assessment using a short series of questions that ask patients whether they have experienced bleeding and cramping, including how much and for how long, and whether they still feel

pregnant or if they think the pregnancy has passed (Creinin & Grossman, 2020).
ii. Remote assessment and self-assessment follow-up can be scheduled by telephone at 1 week after taking medications, with subsequent at-home urine pregnancy testing 4 weeks later (Creinin & Grossman, 2020). Advise the patient that they can expect menses to return in 4–8 weeks. If the patient started a birth control method, the counseling on return to menses should be relevant to the method provided.

D. Complications after MAB
1. Persistent gestational sac seen on ultrasound: If a persistent sac is noted on ultrasound at the follow-up visit, the patient may be offered one of the following:
   a. A second dose of misoprostol 800 mg buccal
   b. Expectant management for up to 4 weeks after initial misoprostol
   c. Scheduled for in-clinic aspiration.
   Studies show that even with a retained sac at 2 weeks after MAB, intervention is not always necessary because expulsion will likely occur in the following weeks. However, some patients may prefer to take a second dose of misoprostol due to bothersome symptoms, such as cramping and prolonged, irregular bleeding (Creinin & Grossman, 2020). More than half of patients with a persistent gestational sac after medical abortion will expel the pregnancy when treated with a second dose of misoprostol (Reeves et al., 2008).
2. Ongoing pregnancy: Continuing pregnancies are reported in less than 1% of patients who begin MAB at or before 63 days of gestation (Kulier et al., 2011). Ongoing pregnancy may be treated with uterine aspiration or a repeat dose of misoprostol (SFP, 2014). Studies have found that treatment with a repeat dose of misoprostol, 800 mcg, resulted in expulsion of the products of conception 36% of the time (Reeves et al., 2008). Patients who take a second dose of misoprostol should be seen for follow-up in 1 week, and if cardiac activity continues to persist at this visit, uterine aspiration should be performed (SFP, 2014).
3. Infection: The incidence of upper genital tract infection after induced abortion is less than 1% in most clinical settings in the United States (Creinin & Grossman, 2020). Patients who present with tachycardia, severe abdominal pain, or general malaise with or without fever that occurs more than 24 hours after misoprostol administration should be examined for genital tract infection and treated for pelvic inflammatory infection per the CDC guidelines (Achilles & Reeves, 2011; Creinin & Grossman, 2020). Endometritis and toxic shock syndrome associated with *Clostridium sordellii* are a rare complication of MAB. Clinical findings include tachycardia, hypotension, edema, hemoconcentration, profound leukocytosis, and absence of fever. These findings and suspicion of *C. sordelli* warrant an immediate referral to the ED (Fischer et al., 2005).
4. Hemorrhage: Overall, large studies demonstrate that less than 1% of patients will need emergency curettage because of excessive bleeding (SFP, 2014).

E. *Aftercare and complications after procedural abortion*
1. PCPs who lack abortion care training may see patients who have had an abortion. This can lead to ordering unnecessary labs and interventions. It can also lead to undertreatment due to a lack of training or personal feelings interfering with care. ED visits after procedural abortion are rare and often not related to the abortion (Upadhyay et al., 2015). Studies reveal that the rate of major complications after an abortion (up to 63 days' gestational age) is very low, about 0.23%, with about 1 in 115 abortions resulting in an ED visit in which the patient receives a diagnosis, treatment, or diagnosis and treatment (Upadhyay et al., 2015). Discharge instructions after an procedural abortion including anticipatory guidance, which helps patients discern between normal symptoms and danger signs, include the following:
   a. Vaginal bleeding can be expected for up to 2 weeks. Bleeding can stop and start for a few weeks after an abortion. Some people have no bleeding for a few days after the procedure and then begin to have bleeding like a period. Other people experience only spotting for a few days and then no bleeding at all. Bleeding may increase when a patient is more active, which is normal. Advise the patient to call if bleeding soaks through more than two large pads per hour for more than 2 hours.
   b. Cramping is expected on and off during the week following an abortion. Recommend taking NSAIDs and using a heating pad for the pain as needed. Advise the patient to call if pain due to cramping increases and is not relieved by pain medication.
   c. Advise patients to call if they experience a temperature higher than 100.4°F/38°C.
   d. Advise the patient that they can expect menses to return in 4–8 weeks. If the patient started a birth control method the day of the abortion, the counseling on return to menses should be relevant to the method provided.
2. Complications:
   a. Excessive bleeding and hemorrhage are rare after aspiration; the incidence is less than 1% (Kerns & Steinauer, 2013; Upadhyay et al., 2015; White et al., 2015; Yonke & Leeman, 2013).
   b. Incomplete abortion is when residual nonviable fetal tissue remains in the uterus, and it usually presents in the days to weeks after aspiration.

The incidence is 0.2%–4.4% (Upadhyay et al., 2015; Weitz et al., 2013; Yonke & Leeman, 2013).
   i. Patients will present with pelvic pain, abnormal bleeding, pregnancy symptoms, and an enlarged or boggy uterus.
   ii. An ultrasound will show persistent IUP or debris.
   iii. Management should be to follow serial hCGs if there is any doubt that the aspiration was complete. The patient can be offered misoprostol or re-aspiration to empty the uterus.
   iv. Re-aspiration should be done if the patient shows signs of infection or has excessive bleeding, severe pain, or significant anemia.
  c. Continuing pregnancy is rare; the incidence is 0.4%–2.3% (Upadhyay et al., 2015).
   i. The patient will present with ongoing pregnancy symptoms or an enlarging uterus.
   ii. Risk factors include early gestational age, uterine anomalies or fibroids, missed multiple gestation, and operator inexperience.
  d. Hematometra (accumulation of blood in uterus following procedure): The incidence is ~2% (Weitz et al., 2013; Yonke & Leeman, 2013).
   i. Hematometra may occur within minutes to hours after aspiration.
   ii. Symptoms include severe lower abdominal or pelvic pain, rectal pressure, minimal to no postprocedural bleeding, hypotension, and vasovagal episode.
   iii. On ultrasound, a large amount of blood or clot may be noted.
   iv. During the pelvic exam, the uterus will feel large and firm.
   v. If the patient presents days to weeks after aspiration, the symptoms may include pelvic pressure or cramping and a low-grade fever.
   vi. Management should be prompt referral for uterine aspiration of blood, which should provide quick relief of symptoms (Goodman & TEACH Collaborative Working Group, 2020).
  e. Postabortal endometritis (pelvic inflammatory disease [PID]): The incidence is 0.09%–2.6% (Achilles & Reeves, 2011; Upadhyay et al., 2015; Yonke & Leeman, 2013).
   i. Patients will present with lower abdominal pain, pelvic pain, fever, and malaise.
   ii. Exam findings include elevated temperature, cervical motion tenderness, pelvic pain, lower abdominal pain, purulent discharge, and elevated white blood cells (WBCs).
   iii. An ultrasound should be performed to assess for retained POC or clot, and re-aspiration may be needed.
   iv. A wet mount may reveal increased WBCs, clue cells, yeast, or trichomoniasis. Collect swabs for gonorrhea and chlamydia on exam.
   v. Treatment is antibiotics for PID per the CDC guidelines
  f. Other rare aspiration complications that usually occur on the day of the procedure and will be managed by the abortion provider (Upadhyay et al., 2015; Weitz et al., 2013; White et al., 2015; Yonke & Leeman, 2013)
   i. Cervical laceration (<0.1%–2.3%)
   ii. Anesthesia-related reactions (0.2%–0.5%)
   iii. Uterine perforation (0.02%–07%)
   iv. Hemorrhage (0.07%–0.4%)

VI. Resources and further learning
A. *For providers*
1. AP Toolkit. A professional guide for APNs, midwives, and PAs in the United States who are either currently providing or would like to offer abortion care. https://aptoolkit.org/becoming-clinically-competent/
2. TEACH Early Abortion Training Workbook. The TEACH Early Abortion Training Workbook is an all-inclusive interactive curriculum with tools to train new reproductive health providers to competence. https://www.teachtraining.org/training-tools/early-abortion-training-workbook/
3. Reproductive Health Access. Mobilizes, trains, and supports clinicians to make reproductive health care accessible to everyone. The website has helpful handouts and training tools. https://www.reproductiveaccess.org/
4. Reproductive Health Education in Family Medicine (RHEDI). The RHEDI website has clinical resources for integrating services and helpful fact sheets. https://rhedi.org/
5. Information on becoming a mifepristone provider/REMS participant on the FDA website can be found here: https://www.accessdata.fda.gov/scripts/cder/rems/index.cfm?event=RemsDetails.page&REMS=390
6. Ipas. Works with partners around the world to advance reproductive justice by expanding access to abortion and contraception. The website has information for both providers and patients, including information on how to self-manage an abortion. https://www.ipas.org/
7. WHO. The WHO provides global technical and policy guidance on the use of contraception to prevent unintended pregnancy and information on abortion care, abortion management (including miscarriage, induced abortion, incomplete abortion, and fetal death), and post-abortion care. https://www.who.int/health-topics/abortion#tab=tab_1
8. Provide. Works to increase access to abortion services by raising awareness. The website contains a curriculum on making referrals, management of EPL, and resources for nurses. https://providecare.org/about/

B. *For patients*
1. National Network of Abortion Funds. Network of independent organizations that provide financial

assistance to patients to pay for abortions. http://www.abortionfunds.org
2. If/When/How—Lawyering for Reproductive Justice. Provides free, confidential legal assistance and information regarding self-managed abortion. https://www.ifwhenhow.org
3. Aid Access. Provides MAB via telemedicine. http://www.aidaccess.org
4. Women on Web. Women on Web's goal is to provide safe, accessible, and affordable online abortion care to women and people around the world. https://www.womenonweb.org/en/i-need-an-abortion
5. Hesperian Health Multilingual Safe Abortion App. Provides comprehensive, accurate abortion information for patients who are seeking an abortion. https://hesperian.org/books-and-resources/our-mobile-applications/safe-abortion-sa/
6. M+A Hotline. Offers support for patients during miscarriage or self-managed abortion. http://www.mahotline.org
7. Plan C. An educational website resource for learning about how people in the United States are accessing abortion pills and safely managing their own abortions. https://www.plancpills.org/
8. National Human Trafficking Resource Center, Polaris Project B 24/7 hotline: 1-888-3737-888 B Text HELP or INFO to BeFree (233733) B. https://polarisproject.org B; https://traffickingresourcecenter.org
9. Abortion support resources for patients:
    a. Exhale: https://exhaleprovoice.org/resources/
    b. All-Options: https://www.all-options.org/
    c. Connect&Breathe: http://www.connectandbreathe.org/
    d. Faith Aloud: https://www.faithaloud.org/

References

Achilles, S. L., & Reeves, M. F. (2011). Prevention of infection after induced abortion. *Contraception*, 83(4), 295–309. doi:10.1016/j.contraception.2010.11.006

Aiken, A., Lohr, P. A., Lord, J., Ghosh, N., & Starling, J. (2021). Effectiveness, safety and acceptability of no-test medical abortion provided via telemedicine: A national cohort study. *BJOG: An International Journal of Obstetrics & Gynaecology*, 128(9), 1464–1474. doi:10.1111/1471-0528.16668

Aiken, A. R. A., Starling, J. E., Gomperts, R., Tec, M., Scott, J. G., & Aiken, C. E. (2020). Demand for self-managed online telemedicine abortion in the United States during the coronavirus disease 2019 (COVID-19) pandemic. *Obstetrics & Gynecology*, 136(4), 835–837. doi:10.1097/aog.0000000000004081

Aiken, A. R. A., Starling, J. E., Scott, J. G., & Gomperts, R. (2022). Association of Texas Senate Bill 8 with requests for self-managed medication abortion. *JAMA Network Open*, 5(2), e221122. doi:10.1001/jamanetworkopen.2022.1122

Allen, R., & O'Brien, B. M. (2009). Uses of misoprostol in obstetrics and gynecology. *Reviews in Obstetrics & Gynecology*, 2(3), 159–168. https://www.ncbi.nlm.nih.gov/pmc/articles/PMC2760893/

American College of Obstetrics and Gynecologists. (2013). Committee Opinion No. 554: Reproductive and sexual coercion. *Obstetrics & Gynecology*, 121(2, Part 1), 411–415. doi:10.1097/01.aog.0000426427.79586.3b

American College of Obstetricians and Gynecologists. (2020). Medication abortion up to 70 days of gestation: ACOG Practice Bulletin, Number 225. *Contraception*, 102(4), 31–47. doi:10.1016/j.contraception.2020.08.004

Anderson, E. M., Cowan, S. K., Higgins, J. A., Schmuhl, N. B., & Wautlet, C. K. (2022). Willing but unable: Physicians' referral knowledge as barriers to abortion care. *SSM—Population Health*, 17, 101002. doi:10.1016/j.ssmph.2021.101002

Badireddy, M., & Baradhi, K. M. (2022). *Chronic anemia.* PubMed. StatPearls Publishing. https://www.ncbi.nlm.nih.gov/books/NBK534803/

Baldwin, A., Johnson, D. M., Broussard, K., Tello-Pérez, L. A., Madera, M., Ze-Noah, C., Padron, E., & Aiken, A. R. A. (2022). U.S. abortion care providers' perspectives on self-managed abortion. *Qualitative Health Research*, 32(5), 788–799. doi:10.1177/10497323221077296

Bancsi, A., & Grindrod, K. (2019). Medical abortion: A practice tool for pharmacists. *Canadian Pharmacists Journal / Revue Des Pharmaciens Du Canada*, 152(3), 160–163. doi:10.1177/1715163519840270

Baulieu, E.-E. (1989). Contragestion and other clinical applications of RU 486, an antiprogesterone at the receptor. *Science*, 245(4924), 1351–1357. doi:10.1126/science.2781282

Baum, S. E., White, K., Hopkins, K., Potter, J. E., & Grossman, D. (2016). Women's experience obtaining abortion care in Texas after implementation of restrictive abortion laws: A qualitative study. *PLOS One*, 11(10), e0165048. doi:10.1371/journal.pone.0165048

Berkowitz, R. S., & Goldstein, D. P. (2009). Molar pregnancy. *New England Journal of Medicine*, 360(16), 1639–1645. doi:10.1056/nejmcp0900696

Bracken, H., Clark, W., Lichtenberg, E., Schweikert, S., Tanenhaus, J., Barajas, A., Alpert, L., & Winikoff, B. (2011). Alternatives to routine ultrasound for eligibility assessment prior to early termination of pregnancy with mifepristone-misoprostol. *BJOG: An International Journal of Obstetrics & Gynaecology*, 118(1), 17–23. doi:10.1111/j.1471-0528.2010.02753.x

Brandi, K., Woodhams, E., White, K. O., & Mehta, P. K. (2018). An exploration of perceived contraceptive coercion at the time of abortion. *Contraception*, 97(4), 329–334. doi:10.1016/j.contraception.2017.12.009

Bryant, A. G., & Levi, E. E. (2012). Abortion misinformation from crisis pregnancy centers in North Carolina. *Contraception*, 86(6), 752–756. doi:10.1016/j.contraception.2012.06.001

Butler, L., Critelli, F., & Rinfrette, E. (2011). Trauma-informed care and mental health. *Directions in Psychiatry*, 31(3), 197–212. https://psycnet.apa.org/record/2011-30401-004

Butwick, A. J., Ramachandran, B., Hegde, P., Riley, E. T., El-Sayed, Y. Y., & Nelson, L. M. (2017). Risk factors for severe postpartum hemorrhage after cesarean delivery. *Anesthesia & Analgesia*, 125(2), 523–532. doi:10.1213/ane.0000000000001962

Chadha, N., Lim, B., Kane, M., & Rowland, B. (2020). *Toward the abolition of biological race in medicine.* Escholarship.org. https://escholarship.org/uc/item/4gt3n0dd

Christin-Maitre, S., Bouchard, P., & Spitz, I. M. (2000). Medical termination of pregnancy. *New England Journal of Medicine, 342*(13), 946–956. doi:10.1056/nejm200003303421307

Creinin, M., & Grossman, D. (2020). Medication abortion up to 70 days of gestation. *Obstetrics & Gynecology, 136*(4), e31–e47. doi:10.1097/aog.0000000000004082

Creinin, M. D., Vittinghoff, E., Keder, L., Darney, P. D., & Tiller, G. (1996). Methotrexate and misoprostol for early abortion: A multicenter trial. I. Safety and efficacy. *Contraception, 53*(6), 321–327. doi:10.1016/0010-7824(96)00080-7

Cunningham, G., Gant, N., Gilstrap, L., Hauth, J., & Westrom, K. (2001). *Williams obstetrics 21st edition*. McGraw-Hill.

Danco. (2016, January 20). *Mifeprex (mifepristone). Prescribing information*. https://bit.ly/37HYECD

Davey, A. (2006). Mifepristone and prostaglandin for termination of pregnancy: Contraindications for use, reasons and rationale. *Contraception, 74*(1), 16–20. doi:10.1016/j.contraception.2006.03.003

Dehlendorf, C., Harris, L. H., & Weitz, T. A. (2013). Disparities in abortion rates: A public health approach. *American Journal of Public Health, 103*(10), 1772–1779. doi:10.2105/ajph.2013.301339

Donovan, M. (2018, October 12). *Self-managed medication abortion: Expanding the available options for U.S. abortion care*. Guttmacher Institute. https://www.guttmacher.org/gpr/2018/10/self-managed-medication-abortion-expanding-available-options-us-abortion-care

Drugs and Lactation Database. (2006). *Misoprostol*. PubMed; National Library of Medicine. https://www.ncbi.nlm.nih.gov/books/NBK501436/

Durkee, A. (2021, November 30). *How Americans really feel about abortion: The sometimes surprising poll results as Supreme Court weighs overturning Roe V. Wade*. Forbes. https://www.forbes.com/sites/alisondurkee/2021/11/30/how-americans-really-feel-about-abortion-the-sometimes-surprising-poll-results-as-supreme-court-weighs-overturning-roe-v-wade/?sh=b4c42ba36c95

Ehrenreich, K., Biggs, M. A., & Grossman, D. (2021). Making the case for advance provision of mifepristone and misoprostol for abortion in the United States. *BMJ Sexual & Reproductive Health, 48*(4), 238–242. doi:10.1136/bmjsrh-2021-201321

Endler, M., Lavelanet, A., Cleeve, A., Ganatra, B., Gomperts, R., & Gemzell-Danielsson, K. (2019). Telemedicine for medical abortion: A systematic review. *BJOG: An International Journal of Obstetrics & Gynaecology, 126*(9), 1094–1102. doi:10.1111/1471-0528.15684

Finer, L. B., & Zolna, M. R. (2016). Declines in unintended pregnancy in the United States, 2008–2011. *New England Journal of Medicine, 374*(9), 843–852. doi:10.1056/nejmsa1506575

Fischer, M., Bhatnagar, J., Guarner, J., Reagan, S., Hacker, J. K., Van Meter, S. H., Poukens, V., Whiteman, D. B., Iton, A., Cheung, M., Dassey, D. E., Shieh, W.-J., & Zaki, S. R. (2005). Fatal toxic shock syndrome associated with *Clostridium sordellii* after medical abortion. *New England Journal of Medicine, 353*(22), 2352–2360. doi:10.1056/nejmoa051620

Fuentes, L., Baum, S., Keefe-Oates, B., White, K., Hopkins, K., Potter, J., & Grossman, D. (2020). Texas women's decisions and experiences regarding self-managed abortion. *BMC Women's Health, 20*(1), 6. doi:10.1186/s12905-019-0877-0

Fuentes, L., & Jerman, J. (2019). Distance traveled to obtain clinical abortion care in the United States and reasons for clinic choice. *Journal of Women's Health, 28*(12),1623-1631. doi:10.1089/jwh.2018.7496

Fuentes, L., Lebenkoff, S., White, K., Gerdts, C., Hopkins, K., Potter, J. E., & Grossman, D. (2016). Women's experiences seeking abortion care shortly after the closure of clinics due to a restrictive law in Texas. *Contraception, 93*(4), 292–297. doi:10.1016/j.contraception.2015.12.017

Goodman, S., & TEACH Collaborative Working Group. (2020). *TEACH early abortion training curriculum* (6th ed.). UCSF Bixby Center for Global Reproductive Health.

Greene Foster, D. (2020). *The Turnaway Study: Ten years, a thousand women, and the consequences of having—or being denied—an abortion*. Scribner.

Grieger, J. A., & Norman, R. J. (2020). Menstrual cycle length and patterns in a global cohort of women using a mobile phone app: Retrospective cohort study. *Journal of Medical Internet Research, 22*(6), e17109. doi:10.2196/17109

Grossman, D., & Grindlay, K. (2017). Safety of medical abortion provided through telemedicine compared with in person. *Obstetrics & Gynecology, 130*(4), 778–782. doi:10.1097/aog.0000000000002212

Grossman, D., White, K., Harris, L., Reeves, M., Blumenthal, P. D., Winikoff, B., & Grimes, D. A. (2015). Continuing pregnancy after mifepristone and "reversal" of first-trimester medical abortion: A systematic review. *Contraception, 92*(3), 206–211. doi:10.1016/j.contraception.2015.06.001

Guiahi, M., & Davis, A. (2012). First-trimester abortion in women with medical conditions. *Contraception, 86*(6), 622–630. doi:10.1016/j.contraception.2012.09.001

Guilbert, E., Costescu, D., Wagner, M., Renner, R., Norman, W., Dunn, S., Fitzsimmons, B., Trouton, K., Bernardin, J., Black, A., Thorne, J., & Gomes, M. (2020). *Canadian protocol for the provision of medical abortion via telemedicine*. Sogc.org, Health Canada. https://sogc.org/common/Uploaded%20files/CANADIAN%20PROTOCOL%20FOR%20THE%20PROVISION%20OF%20MA%20VIA%20TELEMEDICINE.pdf

Guttmacher Institute. (2018a, August 2). *Induced abortion worldwide*. https://www.guttmacher.org/fact-sheet/induced-abortion-worldwide

Guttmacher Institute. (2018b, November 27). *Abortion before and after legalization*. https://www.guttmacher.org/perspectives50/abortion-and-after-legalization

Guttmacher Institute. (2019a, February 14). *Induced abortion in the United States*. https://www.guttmacher.org/fact-sheet/induced-abortion-united-states

Guttmacher Institute. (2022, April 14). *An overview of abortion laws*. https://www.guttmacher.org/state-policy/explore/overview-abortion-laws

Harris, L. H., & Grossman, D. (2020). Complications of unsafe and self-managed abortion. *New England Journal of Medicine, 382*(11), 1029–1040. doi:10.1056/nejmra1908412

Harris, L. H., & Wolfe, T. (2014). Stratified reproduction, family planning care and the double edge of history. *Current Opinion in Obstetrics & Gynecology, 26*(6), 539–544. doi:10.1097/gco.0000000000000121

Hemmings, S., Jakobowitz, S., Abas, M., Bick, D., Howard, L. M., Stanley, N., Zimmerman, C., & Oram, S. (2016). Responding to the health needs of survivors of human trafficking: A systematic review. *BMC Health Services Research, 16*, 320. doi:10.1186/s12913-016-1538-8

Holliday, C. N., McCauley, H. L., Silverman, J. G., Ricci, E., Decker, M. R., Tancredi, D. J., Burke, J. G., Documét, P., Borrero, S., & Miller, E. (2017). Racial/Ethnic differences in women's experiences of reproductive coercion, intimate partner violence, and unintended pregnancy. *Journal of Women's Health, 26*(8), 828–835. doi:10.1089/jwh.2016.5996

Holt, K., Janiak, E., McCormick, M., Lieberman, E., Dehlendorf, C., Kajeepeta, S., Caglia, J., & Langer, A. (2017). Family medicine.

Family Medicine, 49(7). https://www.stfm.org/FamilyMedicine/Vol49Issue7/Holt527

Ipas. (2014). *Steps for performing manual vacuum aspiration (MVA) using the Ipas MVA Plus® and Ipas EasyGrip® cannulae.* https://www.ipas.org/wp-content/uploads/2020/06/PERFMVA-E19.pdf

Ipas. (2021). *Clinical updates archive.* https://www.ipas.org/clinical-update/

Jatlaoui, T. C., Ewing, A., Mandel, M. G., Simmons, K. B., Suchdev, D. B., Jamieson, D. J., & Pazol, K. (2016). Abortion surveillance—United States, 2013. *MMWR. Surveillance Summaries, 65*(12), 1–44. doi:10.15585/mmwr.ss6512a1

Jerman, J., Jones, R., & Onda, T. (2016, June 10). *Characteristics of U.S. abortion patients in 2014 and changes since 2008.* Guttmacher Institute. https://www.guttmacher.org/report/characteristics-us-abortion-patients-2014

Jones, R. K. (2018). Reported contraceptive use in the month of becoming pregnant among U.S. abortion patients in 2000 and 2014. *Contraception, 97*(4), 309–312. doi:10.1016/j.contraception.2017.12.018

Jones, R. K., & Jerman, J. (2017a). Abortion incidence and service availability in the United States, 2014. *Perspectives on Sexual and Reproductive Health, 49*(1), 17–27. doi:10.1363/psrh.12015

Jones, R. K., & Jerman, J. (2017b). Characteristics and circumstances of U.S. women who obtain very early and second-trimester abortions. *PLOS One, 12*(1), e0169969. doi:10.1371/journal.pone.0169969

Jones, R. K., & Jerman, J. (2017c). Population group abortion rates and lifetime incidence of abortion: United States, 2008–2014. *American Journal of Public Health, 107*(12), 1904–1909. doi:10.2105/ajph.2017.304042

Kaneshiro, B., Bednarek, P., Isley, M., Jensen, J., Nichols, M., & Edelman, A. (2011). Blood loss at the time of first-trimester surgical abortion in anticoagulated women. *Contraception, 83*(5), 431–435. doi:10.1016/j.contraception.2010.09.009

Kapp, N., Grossman, D., Jackson, E., Castleman, L., & Brahmi, D. (2017). A research agenda for moving early medical pregnancy termination over the counter. *BJOG: An International Journal of Obstetrics & Gynaecology, 124*(11), 1646–1652. doi:10.1111/1471-0528.14646

Kavanaugh, M. L., Jerman, J., & Finer, L. B. (2015). Changes in use of long-acting reversible contraceptive methods among U.S. women, 2009–2012. *Obstetrics & Gynecology, 126*(5), 917–927. doi:10.1097/aog.0000000000001094

Kerns, J., & Steinauer, J. (2013). Management of postabortion hemorrhage. *Contraception, 87*(3), 331–342. doi:10.1016/j.contraception.2012.10.024

Kulier, R., Cheng, L., Fekih, A., Hofmeyr, G. J., & Campana, A. (2001). Surgical methods for first trimester termination of pregnancy. *Cochrane Database of Systematic Reviews, 2001*(4), CD002900. doi:10.1002/14651858.cd002900

Kulier, R., Kapp, N., Gülmezoglu, A. M., Hofmeyr, G. J., Cheng, L., & Campana, A. (2011). Medical methods for first trimester abortion. *Cochrane Database of Systematic Reviews, 2011*(11), CD002855. doi:10.1002/14651858.cd002855.pub4

Light, A. D., Obedin-Maliver, J., Sevelius, J. M., & Kerns, J. L. (2014). Transgender men who experienced pregnancy after female-to-male gender transitioning. *Obstetrics & Gynecology, 124*(6), 1120–1127. doi:10.1097/aog.0000000000000540

Manlove, J., Fish, H., & Moore, K. A. (2015). Programs to improve adolescent sexual and reproductive health in the US: A review of the evidence. *Adolescent Health, Medicine and Therapeutics, 6*, 47–79. doi:10.2147/ahmt.s48054

McCarthy, M. A., Upadhyay, U., Ralph, L., Biggs, M. A., & Foster, D. G. (2020). The effect of receiving versus being denied an abortion on making and achieving aspirational 5-year life plans. *BMJ Sexual & Reproductive Health, 46*(3), 177–183. doi:10.1136/bmjsrh-2019-200456

Miller, E., Jordan, B., Levenson, R., & Silverman, J. G. (2010). Reproductive coercion: Connecting the dots between partner violence and unintended pregnancy. *Contraception, 81*(6), 457–459. doi:10.1016/j.contraception.2010.02.023

Moseson, H., Fix, L., Gerdts, C., Ragosta, S., Hastings, J., Stoeffler, A., Goldberg, E. A., Lunn, M. R., Flentje, A., Capriotti, M. R., Lubensky, M. E., & Obedin-Maliver, J. (2022). Abortion attempts without clinical supervision among transgender, nonbinary and gender-expansive people in the United States. *BMJ Sexual & Reproductive Health, 48*, e22–e30. doi:10.1136/bmjsrh-2020-200966

Nash, E., & Dreweke, J. (2019, September 6). *The U.S. abortion rate continues to drop: Once again, state abortion restrictions are not the main driver.* Guttmacher Institute. https://www.guttmacher.org/gpr/2019/09/us-abortion-rate-continues-drop-once-again-state-abortion-restrictions-are-not-main

National Abortion Federation. (2020). *2020 Clinical policy guidelines.* https://prochoice.org/store/clinical-policy-guidelines/

National Academies of Sciences, Engineering, and Medicine. (2018). *The safety and quality of abortion care in the United States.* National Academies Press. doi:10.17226/24950

National Academies of Sciences, Engineering, and Medicine, Health and Medicine Division, Board on Health Care Services, & Board on Population Health and Public Health Practice. (2018, March 16). *Long-term health effects.* National Academies Press. https://www.ncbi.nlm.nih.gov/books/NBK507237/

National Human Trafficking Resource Center. (2010). *Medical assessment tool. Polaris Project.* https://humantraffickinghotline.org/sites/default/files/Assessment%20Tool%20-%20Medical%20Professionals.pdf

Ngoc, N. T. N., Blum, J., Raghavan, S., Nga, N. T. B., Dabash, R., Diop, A., & Winikoff, B. (2011). Comparing two early medical abortion regimens: Mifepristone + misoprostol vs. misoprostol alone. *Contraception, 83*(5), 410–417. doi:10.1016/j.contraception.2010.09.002

Office for Victims of Crime. (2014, June). *Sexual assault: The numbers. Responding to transgender victims of sexual assault.* https://ovc.ojp.gov/sites/g/files/xyckuh226/files/pubs/forge/sexual_numbers.html

Paul, M., Lichtenberg, E., Borgatta, Grimes, D., & Stubblefield, P. (1999). *A clinician's guide to medical and surgical abortion.* Churchill Livingstone.

Pocius, K. D., Maurer, R., Fortin, J., Goldberg, A. B., & Bartz, D. (2015). Early serum human chorionic gonadotropin (hCG) trends after medication abortion. *Contraception, 91*(6), 503–506. doi:10.1016/j.contraception.2015.03.004

Potter, J. E., Stevenson, A. J., Coleman-Minahan, K., Hopkins, K., White, K., Baum, S. E., & Grossman, D. (2019). Challenging unintended pregnancy as an indicator of reproductive autonomy. *Contraception, 100*(1), 1–4. doi:10.1016/j.contraception.2019.02.005 https://publicleadershipinstitute.org/abortion-rights/qualified-providers-abortion-act/

Raymond, E. G., & Grimes, D. A. (2012). The comparative safety of legal induced abortion and childbirth in the United States. *Obstetrics and Gynecology, 119*(2, Part 1), 215–219. doi:10.1097/AOG.0b013e31823fe923

Raymond, E. G., Grossman, D., Mark, A., Upadhyay, U. D., Dean, G., Creinin, M. D., Coplon, L., Perritt, J., Atrio, J. M.,

Taylor, D., & Gold, M. (2020). Commentary: No-test medication abortion: A sample protocol for increasing access during a pandemic and beyond. *Contraception, 101*(6), 361–366. doi:10.1016/j.contraception.2020.04.005

Raymond, E. G., Harrison, M. S., & Weaver, M. A. (2019). Efficacy of misoprostol alone for first-trimester medical abortion. *Obstetrics & Gynecology, 133*(1), 137–147. doi:10.1097/aog.0000000000003017

Reeves, M. F., Kudva, A., & Creinin, M. D. (2008). Medical abortion outcomes after a second dose of misoprostol for persistent gestational sac. *Contraception, 78*(4), 332–335. doi:10.1016/j.contraception.2008.06.002

Rosen, J. D. (2012). The public health risks of crisis pregnancy centers. *Perspectives on Sexual and Reproductive Health, 44*(3), 201–205. doi:10.1363/4420112

Sääv, I., Fiala, C., Hämäläinen, J. M., Heikinheimo, O., & Gemzell-Danielsson, K. (2010). Medical abortion in lactating women—low levels of mifepristone in breast milk. *Acta Obstetricia et Gynecologica Scandinavica, 89*(5), 618–622. doi:10.3109/00016341003721037

Schonberg, D., Wang, L.-F., Bennett, A. H., Gold, M., & Jackson, E. (2014). The accuracy of using last menstrual period to determine gestational age for first trimester medication abortion: A systematic review. *Contraception, 90*(5), 480–487. doi:10.1016/j.contraception.2014.07.004

Seeber, B. E., & Barnhart, K. T. (2006). Suspected ectopic pregnancy. *Obstetrics & Gynecology, 107*(2, Part 1), 399–413. doi:10.1097/01.aog.0000198632.15229.be

Singh, S., Remez, L., Sedgh, G., Kwok, L., & Tsuyoshi, O. (2018, December 14). *Abortion worldwide 2017: Uneven progress and unequal access*. Guttmacher Institute. https://www.guttmacher.org/report/abortion-worldwide-2017

Sitruk-Ware, R., & Spitz, I. M. (2003). Pharmacological properties of mifepristone: Toxicology and safety in animal and human studies. *Contraception, 68*(6), 409–420. doi:10.1016/s0010-7824(03)00171-9

Society of Family Planning. (2014). Medical management of first-trimester abortion. Clinical Guideline. *Contraception, 89*(3), 148–161. doi:10.1016/j.contraception.2014.01.016

Spitz, I. M., & Bardin, C. W. (1993). Clinical pharmacology of RU 486—an antiprogestin and antiglucocorticoid. *Contraception, 48*(5), 403–444. doi:10.1016/0010-7824(93)90133-r

Stern, A. M. (2005). Sterilized in the name of public health: Race, immigration, and reproductive control in modern California. *American Journal of Public Health, 95*(7), 1128–1138. doi:10.2105/ajph.2004.041608

Stover, J., Hardee, K., Ganatra, B., García-Moreno, C., & Horton, S. (2016). Interventions to improve reproductive health. In R. Black, R. Laxminarayan, M. Temmerman, & N. Walker (Eds.), *Disease control priorities, third edition (Volume 2): Reproductive, maternal, newborn, and child health* (pp. 95–114). doi:10.1596/978-1-4648-0348-2_ch6

Stulberg, D. B., Dude, A. M., Dahlquist, I., & Curlin, F. A. (2011). Abortion provision among practicing obstetrician–gynecologists. *Obstetrics and Gynecology, 118*(3), 609–614. doi:10.1097/AOG.0b013e31822ad973

Taylor, D., Battistelli, M., Anderson, P., & Arida, J. (2017, August). *HWPP study findings and methods*. Advancing New Standards in Reproductive Health (ANSIRH). https://www.ansirh.org/research/publication/hwpp-study-findings-and-methods

Tracy, E. E., & Macias-Konstantopoulos, W. (2017). Identifying and assisting sexually exploited and trafficked patients seeking women's health care services. *Obstetrics & Gynecology, 130*(2), 443–453. doi:10.1097/aog.0000000000002144

United Nations. (2021). *Human-trafficking*. United Nations, Office on Drugs and Crime. https://www.unodc.org/unodc/en/human-Trafficking/Human-Trafficking.html

Upadhyay, U. D., Desai, S., Zlidar, V., Weitz, T. A., Grossman, D., Anderson, P., & Taylor, D. (2015). Incidence of emergency department visits and complications after abortion. *Obstetrics & Gynecology, 125*(1), 175–183. doi:10.1097/aog.0000000000000603

Upadhyay, U. D., Weitz, T. A., Jones, R. K., Barar, R. E., & Foster, D. G. (2014). Denial of abortion because of provider gestational age limits in the United States. *American Journal of Public Health, 104*(9), 1687–1694. doi:10.2105/ajph.2013.301378

U.S. Food and Drug Administration. (2023). Postmarket drug safety information for patients and providers—Mifeprex (mifepristone) information. https://www.fda.gov/drugs/postmarket-drug-safety-information-patients-and-providers/mifeprex-mifepristone-information

Waddington, A., Hahn, P. M., & Reid, R. (2015). Determinants of late presentation for induced abortion care. *Journal of Obstetrics and Gynaecology Canada, 37*(1), 40–45. doi:10.1016/s1701-2163(15)30361-3

Weitz, T. A., Taylor, D., Desai, S., Upadhyay, U. D., Waldman, J., Battistelli, M. F., & Drey, E. A. (2013). Safety of aspiration abortion performed by nurse practitioners, certified nurse midwives, and physician assistants under a California legal waiver. *American Journal of Public Health, 103*(3), 454–461. doi:10.2105/ajph.2012.301159

White, K., Carroll, E., & Grossman, D. (2015). Complications from first-trimester aspiration abortion: A systematic review of the literature. *Contraception, 92*(5), 422–438. doi:10.1016/j.contraception.2015.07.013

Wiebe, E. R., Campbell, M., Aiken, A. R. A., & Albert, A. (2019). Can we safely stop testing for Rh status and immunizing Rh-negative women having early abortions? A comparison of Rh alloimmunization in Canada and the Netherlands. *Contraception: X, 1*(10), 100001. doi:10.1016/j.conx.2018.100001

World Health Organization. (2018). *Medical management of abortion*. https://apps.who.int/iris/bitstream/handle/10665/278968/9789241550406-eng.pdf

World Health Organization. (2020). *WHO recommendations on self-care interventions: Self-management of medical abortion*. https://apps.who.int/iris/handle/10665/332334

World Health Organization. (2021, November 25). *Abortion*. https://www.who.int/news-room/fact-sheets/detail/abortion

World Health Organization. (2022). *Abortion care guideline*.

Yonke, N., & Leeman, L. M. (2013). First-trimester surgical abortion technique. *Obstetrics and Gynecology Clinics of North America, 40*(4), 647–670. doi:10.1016/j.ogc.2013.08.006

CHAPTER 18

Amenorrhea and Polycystic Ovary Syndrome

Pilar Bernal de Pheils, Sarah Nathan, and Lisa Mihaly

I. Introduction and general background

Amenorrhea is classified as primary or secondary. The overall prevalence of amenorrhea is 3% to 4% (Practice Committee of the American Society of Reproductive Medicine [PCASRM], 2008). Primary amenorrhea is defined as the lack of initiation of menses by age 13 with concomitant lack of growth of secondary sexual characteristics, such as breast development. If growth of secondary sexual characteristics is present, this diagnosis may be delayed until age 15, or within 5 years of breast development, if this happens before age 10 (PCASRM, 2008). Secondary amenorrhea is defined as menstrual cessation for 3 months for those with regular menstrual cycles or 6 months in those individuals with irregular menses (oligomenorrhea) (Deligeoroglou et al., 2010).

Amenorrhea may result from disturbances at the level of the hypothalamus, pituitary, ovaries, uterus, or outflow tract. It may result from chronic illness or other endocrine abnormalities. Polycystic ovarian syndrome (PCOS) is one of the most common causes of amenorrhea, with disturbances that involve the hypothalamic–pituitary–ovarian (HPO) axis. Amenorrhea is physiologic during pregnancy, menopause, and the postpartum period in lactating people. There are also iatrogenic causes, including hormonal contraception, exogenous androgens, or medications.

A. Functional hypothalamic amenorrhea
   1. Definition and overview
      Functional hypothalamic amenorrhea (FHA) is also called *functional hypothalamic gonadotropin-releasing hormone (GnRH) deficiency*. In FHA, there is a decrease in GnRH pulsatile secretion. This causes absent midcycle surges in luteinizing hormone secretion, failure to ovulate, and low serum estradiol concentrations (Gordon, 2010). Low estrogen levels place the patient at risk for osteopenia and osteoporosis. Factors contributing to FHA include nutritional deficiencies, such as marked weight loss, disordered eating, malnutrition, excessive exercise, and severe physical or emotional stress (Couzinet et al., 1999; Warren, 1992).

      Hypothyroidism can lead to hypothalamic amenorrhea (primary or secondary) by decreasing the hypothalamic release of dopamine and increasing prolactin release (Khawaja et al., 2006). Dopaminergic drugs (e.g., phenothiazines, antipsychotics, and antiemetic-gastrointestinal agents) may also be responsible for hypothalamic amenorrhea. Menses usually return to normal after discontinuation of medications. Rarely, hypothalamic amenorrhea may be associated with congenital GnRH deficiency (Kallmann syndrome) if there is associated anosmia or hyposmia (Fritz & Speroff, 2011).
   2. Prevalence and incidence
      FHA is the cause of 25% to 35% cases of secondary amenorrhea and 3% of primary amenorrhea (PCASRM, 2006).

B. Amenorrhea associated with pituitary dysfunction
   1. Definition and overview
      Prolactin-secreting tumors (prolactinomas/lactotroph adenomas) are responsible for most cases of amenorrhea attributed to the pituitary gland. Increased prolactin levels (hyperprolactinemia) lead to anovulation and low ovarian estradiol levels, causing the same problems as seen in FHA. Hyperprolactinemia, unlike FHA, can cause galactorrhea in some patients. Most prolactinomas are microadenomas (<10 mm in diameter), and patients maintain normal pituitary function. Macroadenomas are 10 mm or larger and can exert mass effects, causing headaches and vision changes.

Pituitary functional tumors should be suspected when patients have acromegaly caused by excessive secretion of growth hormone, Cushing disease caused by excessive secretion of adrenocorticotropic hormone, or secondary hyperthyroidism caused by a tumor secreting thyroid-stimulating hormone. These tumors are rare but potential causes of amenorrhea. Most of these tumors are associated with headaches and visual changes (bitemporal hemianopsia/blurred vision) (Fritz & Speroff, 2011).

Hyperprolactinemia can also be caused by decreased clearance of dopamine in patients with chronic renal or liver impairment (Lim et al., 1979). Another disease of the pituitary that can cause amenorrhea is Sheehan syndrome (severe postpartum hemorrhage causing acute infarction and necrosis of the pituitary gland) (Keleştimur, 2003). Hyperprolactinemia may be functional (idiopathic), found in about one-third of patients (Fritz & Speroff, 2011).

2. Prevalence and incidence

Amenorrhea, due to a pituitary dysfunction, is most commonly caused by hyperprolactinemia (Fourman & Fazeli, 2015). Prolactinomas are the most common type of pituitary adenoma (Fourman & Fazeli, 2015). The prevalence of prolactinomas is about 50 per 100,000, and the incidence is 3–5 per 100,000 per year (Chanson & Maiter, 2019).

C. *Amenorrhea originating from disorders of the ovaries*
1. Definition and overview
   a. PCOS (discussed later in this chapter)
   b. Primary ovarian insufficiency (POI), previously known as *premature ovarian failure*, is defined as the cessation of normal ovarian function before the age of 40. People with ovarian insufficiency may have periods of follicular development, ovulation, and menstrual bleeding followed by periods of hypoestrogenemia and anovulation. Causes of POI include autoimmune disorders, such as hypothyroidism, diabetes, and adrenal insufficiency, as well as karyotypic abnormalities (Turner syndrome and mosaicism), fragile X premutations, and idiopathic etiologies. Radiation therapy and chemotherapy can also cause ovarian insufficiency.
   c. Gonadal dysgenesis can present with primary or secondary amenorrhea.
2. Prevalence and incidence
   POI develops in approximately 1% of people with ovaries before the age 40 (Fritz & Speroff, 2011). Chromosomal abnormalities and gonadal dysgenesis are more common causes of primary amenorrhea than secondary amenorrhea (Fritz & Speroff, 2011; Reindollar et al., 1981).

D. *Amenorrhea originating from disorders of the outflow tract or uterus*
1. Definition and overview
   The only disorder of the uterus that causes secondary amenorrhea is Asherman syndrome. Asherman syndrome, manifested clinically by very scant menstrual bleeding or amenorrhea, is due to uterine scarring. Asherman syndrome is usually caused by uterine manipulation, such as dilatation and curettage or other surgical procedures.

   Primary amenorrhea in this category is caused by congenital anomalies that can lead to anatomic alterations in the genital tract. These congenital abnormalities include imperforate hymen, transverse vaginal septum, and müllerian agenesis (absence of the uterus and upper vagina).
2. Prevalence and incidence
   The prevalence of Asherman syndrome is unknown because it is difficult to define the denominator (Berman, 2008). Gonadal dysgenesis, due to congenital abnormalities, is the most common cause of primary amenorrhea, whereas androgen insensitivity is a rare cause with a similarly unknown prevalence (Fritz & Speroff, 2011).

E. *Polycystic ovarian syndrome (PCOS)*
1. Definition and overview
   PCOS is one of the most common causes of anovulation. It is a syndrome, not a disease, reflecting multiple potential etiologies with variable clinical expression. There is likely both an environmental and a genetic component of the syndrome. Hallmarks of the syndrome are ovulatory dysfunction, polycystic ovaries, and hyperandrogenism (Norman et al., 2007). Pathologies commonly found in the syndrome are dysfunction of the hypothalamic–pituitary axis and insulin resistance (Norman et al., 2007). Patients with PCOS are at higher risk of having metabolic syndrome, which poses risks for long-term sequelae, including diabetes and cardiovascular disease (Norman et al., 2007). Among patients with PCOS, 40% to 85% who have Body Mass Indexes (BMIs) over 30 are compared to those of a similar age (Randeva et al., 2012). Depression, anxiety, and obstructive sleep apnea are seen more frequently in patients with PCOS (Jedel et al., 2010; Tasali et al., 2008; Vrbikova & Hainer, 2009).

   The 2003 Rotterdam Criteria, proposed by the European Society of Human Reproduction and Embryology (ESHRE) and the American Society of Reproductive Medicine (ASRM), redefined the diagnosis of PCOS (Rotterdam ESHRE/ASRM-Sponsored PCOS Consensus Workshop Group [REASPCWG], 2004). The Rotterdam Criteria define PCOS as having at least two of the following three criteria: (1) oligo-ovulation or anovulation (irregular cycles), (2) clinical or biochemical markers of hyperandrogenism, and (3) polycystic ovaries on ultrasonography and exclusion of other etiologies (REASPCWG, 2004). The Rotterdam Criteria are the most widely accepted for the diagnosis of PCOS, although alternative definitions exist from other groups (Escobar-Morreale, 2018).

PCOS remains a diagnosis of exclusion and can be diagnosed clinically. In order to confirm the diagnosis, other conditions need to be ruled out, including thyroid disease, hyperprolactinemia, androgen-secreting tumors, and nonclassic congenital adrenal hyperplasia.
2. Prevalence
A systematic review of the prevalence of PCOS found a range of 6% to 10%, depending on the criteria used to define the syndrome (Bozdag et al., 2016).

II. Database
A. Subjective
1. Amenorrhea
a. Past health history
i. Medical illnesses (**Table 18-1**)
ii. Obstetric and gynecological: recent history of severe postpartum hemorrhage or oophorectomy (should also ask about miscarriages and postpartum course); recent history of dilatation and curettage

Table 18-1 Amenorrhea and PCOS: Important Etiologies

Classification	Etiology
Hypothalamic amenorrhea	Functional hypothalamic amenorrhea (common etiology for primary or secondary amenorrhea) ■ Anorexia nervosa ■ Stress ■ Rapid weight loss ■ Excessive exercise ■ Idiopathic Most likely presenting with primary amenorrhea ■ Gonadotropin-releasing hormone deficiency, Kallmann syndrome if associated with anosmia Infiltrative lesions of the hypothalamus
Amenorrhea associated with pituitary dysfunction	Physiologic: breastfeeding Pathologic (pituitary) ■ Pituitary adenomas: functional prolactin-secreting hormone (most common) Other nonfunctional adenomas ■ Adrenocorticotropic hormone–secreting tumor causing Cushing syndrome ■ Thyroid-stimulating hormone–secreting tumor causing hyperthyroidism • Somatotroph adenomas secreting growth hormone and causing acromegaly ■ Other masses (cyst, tuberculosis, sarcoidosis, fat deposits) ■ Renal failure ■ Cirrhosis ■ Sheehan syndrome ■ Empty sella syndrome ■ Medications
Amenorrhea originating from disorders of the ovaries	Physiologic: menopause, constitutional delay Pathologic ■ Polycystic ovary syndrome (caused by internal–external sources)—most likely explanation of secondary amenorrhea ■ Primary ovarian insufficiency (common); supply of oocytes is depleted before age 40; consider autoimmune disorders, karyotype abnormalities Other conditions Local disturbance of ovarian conditions ■ History of infection (tuberculosis, mumps) ■ History of radiation therapy or cytotoxic drugs ■ Problems in gonadal development that can present either with primary or secondary amenorrhea ■ Turner syndrome ■ Mosaicism

(continues)

Table 18-1 Amenorrhea and PCOS: Important Etiologies (continued)

Classification	Etiology
Amenorrhea originating from disorders of the outflow tract	If secondary amenorrhea is present in the setting of a disorder of the outflow tract, it is caused by destruction of the endometrium from dilatation and curettage or other surgery or miscarriage resulting in uterine scarring (Asherman syndrome) Primary amenorrhea, in the setting of a disorder of the outflow tract, is caused by congenital anomalies, leading to anatomic alterations ■ Imperforate hymen, transverse vaginal septum, or cervical atresia ■ Müllerian agenesis (ovaries are present because they are not müllerian structures) ■ Complete androgen insensitivity (testicular feminization)
Pharmacologic	Medications causing dopamine receptor blockade ■ Tranquilizers (phenothiazine derivatives) ■ Antipsychotics (risperidone) ■ Antidepressants (desipramine, monoamine oxidase) ■ Antihypertensive (methyldopa, reserpine, verapamil) ■ Narcotics: opiates and heroin ■ Gastrointestinal medications: metoclopramide (Reglan), cimetidine, domperidone ■ Hormonal contraceptives (high-dose progestin) ■ Danazol (androgen-like medication for endometriosis treatment)
Polycystic ovary syndrome	Unknown etiology. It is a syndrome, not a disease, reflecting multiple potential etiologies with variable clinical expression comprised of anovulation, hyperandrogenism, and insulin resistance.

iii. Exposure history: radiation or chemotherapy directed to the pelvic organs
iv. Medication history: dopamine adrenergic medications or hormonal contraceptives (particularly progestin-only contraceptives and psychiatric medication) (Table 18-1)
b. Family history
  i. Delayed or absent puberty
  ii. POI
  iii. Fragile X syndrome, developmental or intellectual disabilities
  iv. Congenital abnormalities (e.g., Turner syndrome)
  v. Autoimmune disorders
c. Occupational and environmental history
  i. Work-related exposures: radiation
d. Personal and social history
  i. Severe stress, malnutrition, restricting intake, excessive exercise
e. Review of systems
  i. Constitutional symptoms: hot flashes or night sweats
  ii. Skin, hair, and nails: lanugo (anorexia)
  iii. Nose: anosmia (Kallmann syndrome)
  iv. Eyes: blurred vision if pituitary tumor (may be a late symptom in patients with macroadenomas)
  v. Breast: galactorrhea (hyperprolactinemia)
  vi. Genitourinary: oligomenorrhea (may precede amenorrhea), vaginal dryness if hypoestrogenic state, cyclical pelvic pain in primary amenorrhea (imperforate hymen, transverse septum, cervical atresia)
  vii. Endocrine: hot or cold sensitivity (suspect thyroid disease); fatigue, polydipsia, polyphagia (pituitary disease)
  viii. Neurologic: headaches (may be a late symptom in patients with macroadenomas and other pituitary lesions) particularly associated with blurred vision; change in personality, report of marked mood changes (infiltrative pituitary lesions)
2. PCOS
  a. Past health history
    i. Medical illnesses: metabolic syndrome may be present concomitantly or be the result of PCOS
    ii. Obstetric and gynecological history: menstrual irregularities and infertility or pregnancy complications (gestational diabetes and pregnancy-induced hypertension), obstructive sleep apnea
    iii. Mental health diagnoses: depression or anxiety
  b. Family history
    i. PCOS or other endocrinopathies
  c. Review of systems
    i. Constitutional signs and symptoms: fatigue
    ii. Skin and hair: acne, oily skin, acanthosis nigricans (neck, axilla, under breast, or groin), hirsutism, and androgenic alopecia
    iii. Genitourinary: irregular menses or amenorrhea
    iv. Neurologic: depressive or anxious symptoms

Table 18-2 Physical Examination Findings and Likely Etiologies in Amenorrhea and PCOS

Organ or System	Examination Findings	Likely Etiologies
Vitals	Increased blood pressure	High blood pressure may be present in pituitary diseases (e.g., Cushing disease) or karyotype abnormalities (e.g., Turner syndrome) or may be associated with polycystic ovary syndrome (PCOS)
Anthropometric measurements Body mass index	<18.5 kg/m^2—underweight or 25.0–29.9 kg/m^2—overweight and >30 kg/m^2—obesity	Low BMIs may be present in functional hypothalamic amenorrhea (e.g., anorexia nervosa) Higher BMIs may be present in PCOS Waist circumference > 80 cm (31½ in) is predictive of PCOS (Chen et al., 2014) or waist–hip ratio > 0.85 (Fritz & Speroff, 2011)
Height	Short stature: less than 60 inches (152.4 cm)	Consistent with Turner syndrome (Fritz & Speroff, 2011)
General appearance	Mood/affect (depression, anxiety) Change in personality, marked mood changes	Depression associated with PCOS Rare hypothalamic lesions
Hair	Excess terminal (thick, pigmented) body hair in an assigned male at birth distribution, as seen on upper lip, sideburn area, chin, chest, inner thighs, lower back, lower abdomen, and buttocks Thinning of hair Absent axillary and pubic hair Lanugo	PCOS Androgen-secreting tumor Thyroid disease Androgen insensitivity Anorexia
Eyes	Visual field defects Stare, lid lag, exophthalmos	Pituitary tumor Hyperthyroidism
Neck	Thyroid enlargement Webbed neck	Thyroid disease Turner syndrome
Breast	Secretions and galactorrhea expressed from multiple ducts Undeveloped breast in primary amenorrhea	Occurs in 80% of patients with hyperprolactinemia Primary amenorrhea likely caused by karyotype abnormalities
Pelvic examination	Scant/absent hair on mons pubis Vulvar or vaginal atrophy Clitoromegaly Imperforate hymen, transverse vaginal septum, cervical atresia Vaginal pouch (blind or absent vagina), no uterus Enlarged ovaries	Androgen insensitivity Hypoestrogenic state as in primary ovarian insufficiency Virilizing effect as in androgen tumor Congenital developmental abnormalities (primary amenorrhea) Müllerian agenesis (primary amenorrhea) PCOS

B. Objective
1. Physical examination findings (**Table 18-2**). Patient may also have a benign examination.
2. Supporting data from relevant diagnostic tests (Tables 18-3–18-5).

III. Assessment
A. Diagnosis
Diagnosis of amenorrhea is determined by its onset (primary or secondary), significant findings from the history, physical examination, and diagnostic tests (Tables 18-3–18-5). Most common etiologies encountered in primary care are as follows:
1. Primary amenorrhea caused mainly by constitutional delay
2. Primary or secondary amenorrhea caused by:
   a. Hypothalamic etiology, most likely functional hypothalamic
   b. Pituitary etiology, most likely hyperprolactinemia or prolactinoma

c. Ovarian disorders, most likely POI in secondary amenorrhea or ovarian dysgenesis in primary amenorrhea (Turner syndrome and mosaicism)
d. Disorders of the outflow tract, most likely Asherman syndrome in secondary amenorrhea (precipitated by an insult to the endometrium) or müllerian agenesis or complete androgen insensitivity in primary amenorrhea
e. PCOS
3. Other conditions that may explain the patient's amenorrhea or oligomenorrhea and need to be ruled out in the investigation of PCOS are:
   a. Thyroid disease (most likely primary hypothyroidism)
   b. Hyperprolactinemia
   c. Nonclassic congenital adrenal hyperplasia

IV. Goals of clinical management

Select a treatment plan that helps decrease symptoms of hyperandrogenism (acne, hirsutism), prevents endometrial hyperplasia (can occur in the setting of anovulation), provides contraception if the patient does not desire pregnancy, or promotes ovulation if the patient does desire pregnancy.

V. Plan

A. *Diagnostic tests*
Tables 18-3–18-5 provide descriptions of relevant diagnostic studies.
1. All patients late for their menses or with oligomenorrhea should have a urine pregnancy test to rule out pregnancy.
2. Recommended laboratory testing includes prolactin, TSH, and FSH (**Table 18-3**).
3. Some clinicians perform a progesterone withdrawal test in the initial evaluation of amenorrhea to determine endogenous estrogen status; others do not advocate for this test, arguing poor sensitivity and specificity (American College of Obstetricians and Gynecologists [ACOG], 2004; Fritz & Speroff, 2011).
4. Diagnostic workup in the adolescent with primary amenorrhea is based on the presence of breast development, secondary sexual characteristics, and the presence of the uterus and an intact outflow tract, likely determined with an ultrasound. If all are present and FSH is normal, the workup should focus on the etiology of secondary amenorrhea. If there is no breast development and the FSH level is elevated, the probable diagnosis is gonadal dysgenesis.

Table 18-3 Essential Testing in the Investigation of Amenorrhea

Test	Definition	Clinical Implications	Comments
Urine pregnancy test	Measures the beta subunit of human chorionic gonadotropin hormone (HCG)	Pregnancy is the most common cause of amenorrhea. This diagnosis must be ruled out in patients with reproductive capacity.	Pregnancy detection by urine HCG relative to the expected first day of menses (Wilcox et al., 2001): ■ Two days before (79%) ■ Seven days after (97%) ■ Eleven days after (100%)
Prolactin	Prolactin is produced by the lactotrophs of the anterior pituitary. Serum prolactin elevation causes amenorrhea by inhibiting pulsatile gonadotropin-releasing hormone secretion. This inhibits follicle-stimulating hormone (FSH) and luteinizing hormone (LH) secretion, resulting in anovulation and low ovarian estrogen production. Normal prolactin varies from 15 to 20 mcg.	For prolactin levels > 50 ng/mL (or galactorrhea or visual disturbances), order a magnetic resonance imaging (MRI) to rule out pituitary tumors or lesions (some practitioners use 100 ng/mL as cutoff). Prolactin < 100 mcg may be caused by dopamine agonist medications, polycystic ovary syndrome, or hypothyroidism; or may be functional (idiopathic); or may be caused by a microadenoma. Prolactin > 150 most likely indicates a prolactinoma (Casanueva et al., 2006)	Prolactin is best drawn fasting, early in the morning. Pregnancy, stress, intercourse, breast stimulation, and meals can increase levels. Prolactin may be mildly elevated in patients with polycystic ovary syndrome (Casanueva et al., 2006) or with long-standing hypothyroidism (Fritz & Speroff, 2011). If prolactin elevations are mild, repeat on a different day (Casanueva et al., 2006). Medications, primarily psychotropic classes, are a common cause of elevated prolactin.

Test	Definition	Clinical Implications	Comments
Thyroid-stimulating hormone (TSH)	Measurement of TSH: anterior pituitary hormone that stimulates growth and function of thyroid cells	Hypothyroid and hyperthyroid disorders can cause oligomenorrhea or amenorrhea.	
FSH	Measures the amount of FSH produced by the anterior pituitary	FSH ≥ 30 IU/L points to ovarian insufficiency or gonadal dysgenesis. Normal or low FSH: indicates hypothalamic or pituitary etiology, outflow tract disorder, or endocrine disorder	Intermittent follicular development and normalization of FSH values may occur in primary ovarian insufficiency.
Progesterone challenge test	Useful in evaluating the status of estrogen production by administering progestins. Bleeding is expected 2–7 days after discontinuation of the progestin (may bleed up to 15 days later if ovulation triggered). Commonly used: medroxyprogesterone, 10 mg daily for 10 days	Progesterone challenge test is negative in patients who do not bleed after progestin withdrawal, which indicates lack of estrogen or outflow tract disorder. Progesterone challenge test is positive in patients who bleed 2–7 days after progestin withdrawal. This indicates that estrogen is being produced by the ovaries. If a progesterone challenge test is negative, you can give combined oral contraceptives to ensure that Asherman syndrome is not present.	Some clinicians advocate for the progesterone challenge test to help in the interpretation of FSH values and to assist in decision making around the need for estrogen therapy for prevention of bone loss (Fritz & Speroff, 2011). Conflicting recommendations exist for progesterone challenge test because of high rates of false-positive and false-negative results.

A karyotype should then be ordered. If the uterus or outflow tract is not present and the FSH values are normal, then the diagnostic test should be directed to diagnose müllerian agenesis or androgen insensitivity syndrome.

5. Second-line diagnostic tests in the investigation of amenorrhea include tests where consultation and referral are suggested (**Table 18-4**).
6. Magnetic resonance imaging (MRI) is recommended for the evaluation of a pituitary tumor in the setting of hyperprolactinemia, galactorrhea, or headaches and vision field changes. Computerized tomography (CT) scanning, although not the preferred diagnostic due to decreased sensitivity, can be used in areas where MRI is not accessible or cost prohibitive.
7. Karyotype, including fragile X testing, is advised for any patient diagnosed with POI (Fritz & Speroff, 2011) or for patients presenting with primary amenorrhea with no uterus on ultrasound.
8. Hysteroscopy is recommended for the confirmation of intrauterine adhesions present in Asherman syndrome. Hysteroscopy can be used to simultaneously to diagnose, by classification of the lesions, and treat, by removal of the adhesions as indicated (American Association of Gynecologic Laparoscopists, 2017).
9. There are no specific tests for the diagnosis of PCOS. Conditions that can mimic PCOS must first be excluded.
10. Patients diagnosed with PCOS should have testing for the investigation of insulin resistance and metabolic abnormalities, including 2-hour oral glucose tolerance test (GTT) and fasting lipids. Hemoglobin A1C can be used if patients are unable or unwilling to do the GTT (Legro et al., 2013). In addition, they should be screened for mood disorders and obstructive sleep apnea (Legro et al., 2013).
11. Additional testing to consider may be found in **Table 18-5**.

B. Management

Therapeutic management of amenorrhea depends on the etiology; the goals of the patient, including reproductive desires; and the long-term consequences of the condition.

1. Functional hypothalamic amenorrhea
   a. Address the underlying condition and issues related to hypothalamic amenorrhea (e.g., eating disorders or excessive exercise) that may

Table 18-4 Second-Line Testing in the Investigation of Amenorrhea, Including Tests Where Consultation or Referral Is Suggested

Test	Definition	Clinical Implications	Comments
Pelvic ultrasound	Ultrasound imaging to evaluate internal organs, particularly in the case of primary amenorrhea	Absent uterus, vaginal septum, or congenital absence of the vagina	May be useful to confirm the presence of a uterus and ovaries. Absent uterus and vagina is likely caused by müllerian agenesis or androgen insensitivity in primary amenorrhea. If absent uterus, then karyotype, serum total testosterone, and renal ultrasound are indicated. Abnormalities of the urinary tract frequently accompany müllerian anomalies.
Magnetic resonance imaging (MRI) of the sella turcica to evaluate for prolactinomas (prolactin-secreting tumors) or other rare pituitary–hypothalamic tumors	The goal of imaging is to evaluate the possibility of a hypothalamic or pituitary lesion.	In the case of a prolactinoma, the image allows determination of a microadenoma or a macroadenoma (≤ 1 or >1 cm, respectively). Abnormal imaging (or hyperprolactinemia) requires referral to a specialist.	All patients with high serum prolactin values (≥ 50 mcg/L; some practitioners would say >100 mcg/L) should have imaging of the sella turcica (MRI). MRI is also indicated if galactorrhea, headaches, or visual field disturbances are present in the evaluation of amenorrhea. MRI is indicated for delayed puberty and hypogonadism.
Karyotype analysis	To evaluate for chromosomal abnormalities	Turner syndrome is the most common type of sex chromosomal abnormality in patients assigned female at birth (Bondy, 2007).	Karyotype analysis should be performed with patients diagnosed with primary ovarian insufficiency (POI) with or without characteristics of Turner syndrome.
Fragile X premutations	To evaluate fragile X syndrome premutation carriers who are at risk for having a fragile X syndrome (Fritz & Speroff, 2011)	Premutation of fragile X syndrome can result in POI. Indicated when diagnosis of POI is made.	There is an association between POI and premutation in the gene responsible for fragile X syndrome.
Adrenal autoantibodies and antithyroid antibodies	To evaluate autoimmune disorders involved in POI.	Abnormal values for these tests are indicated in the workup for autoimmune disorders causing POI. Patients with POI have increased risk of autoimmune adrenal insufficiency (Betterle et al., 1993) and autoimmune hypothyroidism (Kim et al., 1997).	To test for adrenal insufficiency, order serum adrenal cortical and 21-hydroxylase antibodies. To test for autoimmune hypothyroidism, order thyroid-stimulating hormone and thyroid-peroxidase autoantibodies.
Hysterography	Imaging procedure allows for confirmation of Asherman syndrome.	Presence of intrauterine synechiae.	Hysteroscopic lysis of adhesions is a common method of treatment for intrauterine adhesions.

negatively affect ovulation and interfere with a regular menstrual cycle. Mood disorders should be treated. Cognitive–behavioral therapy, problem-solving strategies, and coping skills to improve healthy eating behaviors have demonstrated improvement in hypothalamic function (Berga et al., 2003).

b. In adolescents and young adult patients who have not had menses resume after 6 to 12 months, initiate estrogen replacement with cyclic progestin

Table 18-5 Additional Tests in the Investigation of Polycystic Ovary Syndrome*

Test	Definition	Clinical Implications	Comments
Total testosterone	Serum testosterone provides an estimate of androgen production.	In patients with hyperandrogenism, serum total testosterone should be ordered. Testosterone values may be normal in patients with polycystic ovary syndrome (PCOS). Total testosterone may be elevated (>60 ng/dL) but is not required for the diagnosis of PCOS. Testosterone twice the upper limit is most likely caused by androgen-producing tumors.	Free testosterone assays are not reliable, so they are not recommended as part of routine care.
Dehydroepiandrosterone sulfate (DHEA)	A direct measurement of adrenal androgen activity. This test may be ordered to rule out androgen-secreting tumor.	This test is not recommended in the evaluation of patients with PCOS, only in patients with severe hyperandrogenism, because it can be elevated in cancer of the adrenal gland.	It is most useful in the evaluation of rapid virilization and not useful in common hirsutism with PCOS (American College of Obstetricians and Gynecologists [ACOG], 2009).
17-Hydroxy-progesterone	Serum blood test that evaluates nonclassic congenital adrenal hyperplasia (caused by 21-hydroxylase deficiency).	Collect sample during the patient's follicular phase: <200 ng/dL excludes nonclassic congenital adrenal hyperplasia.	Sample should be collected in the morning.
Pelvic ultrasound	To evaluate for presence of polycystic ovaries.	There is not consensus on ultrasound criteria: Rotterdam criteria (Rotterdam ESHRE/ASRM-Sponsored PCOS Consensus Workshop Group, 2004) defined polycystic ovaries as 12 or more follicles in one of the ovaries, measuring 2–9 mm in diameter and/or increase in ovarian volume > 10 mL. More recent evidence-based recommendations raised the number to ≥20 in one of the ovaries (Teede et al., 2018).	The appearance of polycystic ovaries is nonspecific. It can also be seen in patients with normal hormonal function or with other androgen excess disorders. Hence it is not recommended solely for the evaluation of PCOS. If done, patients should not be on oral contraceptives because these medications can change the ovarian morphology.

* PCOS is a diagnosis of exclusion. If initial testing for the investigation of amenorrhea and oligomenorrhea is unrevealing, other conditions are advised to rule out other hyperandrogenic conditions.

(Ackerman et al., 2019). An example is transdermal 17-beta E2 patches with cyclic micronized progesterone 200 mg.

    c. Supplement with calcium and vitamin D to strengthen bone health.

    d. Refer to reproductive endocrinology if pregnancy is desired. Some patients may respond to clomiphene citrate.

  2. Amenorrhea associated with pituitary dysfunction

    a. In hyperprolactinemia with pituitary macroadenomas, the treatment goal is to establish normal estrogen secretion, menstrual function, and tumor reduction. Therapy with a dopamine agonist is indicated for all patients with macroadenoma and in most patients with microadenomas, particularly if there are bothersome symptoms, desired fertility, or for the prevention of osteoporosis (Casanueva et al., 2006). Patients with macroadenomas may need transsphenoidal surgery or radiation therapy (Casanueva et al., 2006). Patients desiring fertility may need induction of ovulation, although in many cases pharmacologic management of hyperprolactinemia establishes ovulatory cycles.

Dopamine agonists, such as cabergoline, are the drugs of choice for patients with hyperprolactinemia and prolactinomas. These medications decrease the size of the prolactinomas, restore menstrual function and prolactin levels to normal, and ameliorate galactorrhea. Cabergoline is the best initial choice for microadenomas and macroadenomas (Melmed et al., 2011). Cabergoline 0.25 mg twice a week or 0.5 mg once a week are typical doses.

Dopaminergic treatment reestablishes ovulation. If pregnancy prevention is a goal, contraception may be indicated (Casanueva et al., 2006).
b. Calcium and vitamin D supplementation is advised in the amenorrheic patient for the prevention of osteoporosis.
c. Correct hypothyroidism.
d. Address symptomatic hyperprolactinemia induced by medications. Review the patient medication profile for medications that cause hyperprolactinemia and amenorrhea, such as dopamine agonists and estrogen or danazol. Withdrawal of the medication for 72 hours, if able to do this safely, helps elucidate whether the medication is responsible for hyperprolactinemia. MRI should be considered if this alternative is not feasible, particularly in patients with neurologic symptoms, to rule out a pituitary lesion (Casanueva et al., 2006).

3. Ovarian disorders
   a. Primary amenorrhea: Patients with Turner syndrome or mosaicism need a multidisciplinary approach to management, including the approach for primary or secondary amenorrhea. Individuals with Turner syndrome should be referred to a cardiologist. It is critical to review with a patient in a sensitive manner the consequences of POI, including fertility, bone loss, and cardiovascular complications (Bondy, 2007).
   b. Secondary amenorrhea caused by POI
      i. Order a karyotype for all patients. Malignant tumor formation within the gonad is associated with mosaicism with a Y chromosome. Removal of the gonads in this case is required (Fritz & Speroff, 2011).
      ii. Screen for autoimmune hypothyroidism (Kim et al., 1997).
      iii. Advise all patients with POI to establish standard hormonal therapy with estrogen. Patients are advised to continue at least until age 50 to prevent osteoporosis (Kalantaridou & Nelson, 2000; Ostberg et al., 2007). Progestin should be added to estrogen to protect the endometrium if there is an intact uterus. Hormonal treatment also reduces menopausal symptoms.
      iv. For patients who wish to avoid pregnancy, offer combined hormonal contraception (ACOG, 2017). Estradiol and progestin replacement therapy is not sufficient as a contraceptive.
      v. Refer patients who desire pregnancy to an endocrinology and infertility specialist. Patients with POI are candidates for donated oocytes. Although rare, patients with POI may become pregnant spontaneously (Check & Katsoff, 2006).

4. Disorders of the outflow tract
   a. Primary amenorrhea
      i. Refer patients suspected of or diagnosed with androgen insensitivity to a gynecologist. Patients with this condition need removal of gonads to prevent the development of gonadal neoplasia. Gonadectomy is usually delayed until puberty in patients with complete androgen insensitivity syndrome (Fritz & Speroff, 2011).
      ii. Refer patients diagnosed with müllerian abnormalities or agenesis to a gynecologist. If there is vaginal outlet obstruction, surgery is required to allow passage of menstrual blood (Fritz & Speroff, 2011).
   b. Secondary amenorrhea: Refer patients to a gynecologist if Asherman syndrome is suspected. Final diagnosis is made with hysteroscopy, and lysis of adhesions may be performed during the diagnostic procedure (Fritz & Speroff, 2011).

5. PCOS Treatment goals should be directed to preventing hyperplasia of the endometrium, managing hyperandrogenic manifestations (acne and hirsutism), addressing infertility issues, and reducing risks of diabetes and cardiovascular disease.
   a. Advise weight loss and regular exercise in patients with higher total body weight and PCOS. Weight loss is recommended to decrease hirsutism, induce ovulation, and improve fertility (Conway et al., 2014; Vrbikova & Hainer, 2009). Bariatric surgery is also an option for patients with higher total body weight and has been shown to restore ovulation, improve metabolic abnormalities, and improve fertility (Conway et al., 2014). See "Obesity" (Chapter 63) for more information.
   b. Treatment for menstrual irregularities and hyperandrogenic manifestations:
      i. If no contraindication for combined hormonal contraception, use any low-dose oral contraceptives (ACOG, 2009; Sheehan, 2004). Contraceptive patch and vaginal ring are also alternatives (Legro et al., 2013).
   c. Management of hirsutism:
      i. Combined oral contraceptives (COCs) are the first-line therapy (Martin et al., 2018).
      ii. If there is suboptimal response to a COC, spironolactone can be added after 6 months.
   d. Screen and treat to reduce risk of cardiovascular disease and diabetes.

i. Screen for impaired glucose tolerance with a 2-hour oral GTT at diagnosis of PCOS. If normal, repeat the screen every 2 years, or sooner if additional risks present. If the patient does have impaired glucose tolerance but not diabetes, rescreen every year (Salley et al., 2007).
ii. Screen for cardiovascular risk factors: smoking, higher body weight and increased central fat stores, hypertension, dyslipidemia, diabetes, obstructive sleep apnea, family history of early cardiovascular disease. At diagnosis, a lipid profile should be obtained.
e. Medical therapy for patients with PCOS desiring pregnancy: In terms of ovulation induction medications, letrozole may result in more live births compared to clomiphene citrate (Legro et al., 2013). Discussion of ovulation induction is beyond the scope of this chapter.

C. *Patient education*
Provide verbal and, preferably, written information regarding:
1. Risk-reduction strategies and screening for osteoporosis in patients with hypothalamic and pituitary amenorrhea, metabolic syndrome, and endometrial hyperplasia in patients with PCOS
2. The disease process: signs and symptoms and underlying etiologies
3. Diagnostic tests: preparation, cost, the procedures, and aftercare
4. Medication management: rationale, action, use, side effects, associated risks, cost of therapeutic interventions, and the need for adhering to long-term treatment plans
5. Pregnancy: Patients interested in becoming pregnant should be counseled on possible therapeutic options and referral to reproductive endocrinology specialists.

VI. **Self-management resources and tools**
A. *Patient education*
The Mayo Clinic website has excellent patient information at www.mayoclinic.org. Resources are found under "Health Information"; click on "Diseases and Conditions" and search for "amenorrhea."
B. *Support groups and individual counseling*
Patients may benefit from support groups or individual counseling if they are diagnosed with conditions such as premature ovarian insufficiency.

References

Ackerman, K. E., Singhal, V., Baskaran, C., Slattery, M., Reyes, K. J. C., Toth, A., Eddy, K. T., Bouxsein, M. L., Lee, H., Klibanski, A., & Misra, M. (2019). Oestrogen replacement improves bone mineral density in oligo-amenorrhoeic athletes: A randomised clinical trial. *British Journal of Sports Medicine, 53*(4), 229–236. doi:10.1136/bjsports-2018-099723

American Association of Gynecologic Laparoscopists. (2017). AAGL practice report: practice guidelines on intrauterine adhesions developed in collaboration with the European Society of Gynaecological Endoscopy (ESGE). *Gynecological Surgery, 14*, 1–11. doi:10.1186/s10397-017-1007-3

American College of Obstetrics and Gynecology. (2004). Current evaluation of amenorrhea. *Fertility and Sterility, 82*(Suppl. 1), 266–272. doi:10.1016/j.fertnstert.2004.02.098

American College of Obstetricians and Gynecologists. (2009). ACOG Practice Bulletin No. 108: Polycystic ovary syndrome. *Obstetrics and Gynecology, 114*(4), 936–949. doi:10.1097/aog.0b013e3181bd12cb

American College of Obstetricians and Gynecologists. (2017). Committee Opinion No. 698: Hormone therapy in primary ovarian insufficiency. *Obstetrics and Gynecology, 129*(5), e134–e141. doi:10.1097/aog.0000000000002044

Berga, S. L., Marcus, M. D., Loucks, T. L., Hlastala, S., Ringham, R., & Krohn, M. A. (2003). Recovery of ovarian activity in women with functional hypothalamic amenorrhea who were treated with cognitive behavior therapy. *Fertility and Sterility, 80*(4), 976–981. doi:10.1016/s0015-0282(03)01124-5

Berman, J. M. (2008). Intrauterine adhesions. *Seminars in Reproductive Medicine, 26*(4), 349–355. doi:10.1055/s-0028-1082393

Betterle, C., Rossi, A., Pria, S. D., Artifoni, A., Pedini, B., Gavasso, S., & Caretto, A. (1993). Premature ovarian failure: autoimmunity and natural history. *Clinical Endocrinology, 39*(1), 35–43. doi:10.1111/j.1365-2265.1993.tb01748.x

Bondy, C. A. (2007). Care of girls and women with Turner syndrome: A guideline of the Turner Syndrome Study Group. *Journal of Clinical Endocrinology and Metabolism, 92*(1), 10–25. doi:10.1210/jc.2006-1374

Bozdag, G., Mumusoglu, S., Zengin, D., Karabulut, E., & Yildiz, B. O. (2016). The prevalence and phenotypic features of polycystic ovary syndrome: A systematic review and meta-analysis. *Human Reproduction, 31*(12), 2841–2855. doi:10.1093/humrep/dew218

Casanueva, F., Molitch, M. E., Schlechte, J. A., Abs, R., Bonert, V., Bronstein, M. D., et al. (2006). Guidelines of the Pituitary Society for the diagnosis and management of prolactinomas. *Clinical Endocrinology, 65*(2), 265–273. doi:10.1111/j.1365-2265.2006.02562.x

Chanson, P., & Maiter, D. (2019). The epidemiology, diagnosis and treatment of prolactinomas: The old and the new. *Best Practice & Research Clinical Endocrinology & Metabolism, 33*(2), 101290. doi:10.1016/j.beem.2019.101290

Check, J. H., & Katsoff, B. (2006). Successful pregnancy with spontaneous ovulation in a woman with apparent premature ovarian failure who failed to conceive despite four transfers of embryos derived from donated oocytes. *Clinical and Experimental Obstetrics & Gynecology, 33*(1), 13–15.

Chen, L., Xu, W. M., Zhang, D. (2014). The association of abdominal obesity, insulin resistance, and oxidative stress in adipose tissue in women with polycystic ovary syndrome. *Fertility & Sterility*, 102(4), 1167–1174. doi:10.1016/j.fertnstert.2014.06.027

Conway, G., Dewailly, D., Diamanti-Kandarakis, E., Escobar-Morreale, H. F., Franks, S., Gambineri, A., et al. (2014). The polycystic ovary syndrome: A position statement from the European Society of Endocrinology. *European Journal of Endocrinology*, 171(4), P1–P29. doi:10.1530/eje-14-0253

Couzinet, B., Young, J., Brailly, S., Le Bouc, Y., Chanson, P., & Schaison, G. (1999). Functional hypothalamic amenorrhoea: a partial and reversible gonadotrophin deficiency of nutritional origin. *Clinical Endocrinology*, 50(2), 229–235. doi:10.1046/j.1365-2265.1999.00649.x

Deligeoroglou, E., Athanasopoulos, N., Tsimaris, P., Dimopoulos, K. D., Vrachnis, N., & Creatsas, G. (2010). Evaluation and management of adolescent amenorrhea. *Annals of the New York Academy of Sciences*, 1205(1), 23–32. doi:10.1111/j.1749-6632.2010.05669.x

Escobar-Morreale, H. F. (2018). Polycystic ovary syndrome: Definition, aetiology, diagnosis and treatment. *Nature Reviews Endocrinology*, 14(5), 270–284. doi:10.1038/nrendo.2018.24

Fourman, L. T., & Fazeli, P. K. (2015). Neuroendocrine causes of amenorrhea—An update. *The Journal of Clinical Endocrinology and Metabolism*, 100(3), 812–824. doi:10.1210/jc.2014-3344

Fritz, M. A., & Speroff, L. (2011). *Clinical gynecologic endocrinology and infertility* (8th ed.). Philadelphia, PA: Lippincott Williams & Wilkins.

Gordon, C. M. (2010). Functional hypothalamic amenorrhea. *New England Journal of Medicine*, 363(4), 365–371. doi:10.1056/nejmcp0912024

Jedel, E., Waern, M., Gustafson, D., Landén, M., Eriksson, E., Holm, G., Nilsson, L., Lind, A.-K., Janson, P. O., & Stener-Victorin, E. (2010). Anxiety and depression symptoms in women with polycystic ovary syndrome compared with controls matched for body mass index. *Human Reproduction*, 25(2), 450–456. doi:10.1093/humrep/dep384

Kalantaridou, S. N., & Nelson, L. M. (2000). Premature ovarian failure is not premature menopause. *Annals of the New York Academy of Sciences*, 900, 393–402. doi:10.1111/j.1749-6632.2000.tb06251.x

Keleştimur, F. (2003). Sheehan's syndrome. *Pituitary*, 6(4), 181–188. doi:10.1023/b:pitu.0000023425.20854.8e

Kim, T. J Anasti, J. N., Flack, M. R., Kimzey, L. M., Defensor, R. A., & Nelson, L. M. (1997). Routine endocrine screening for patients with karyotypically normal spontaneous premature ovarian failure. *Obstetrics and Gynecology*, 89(5), 777–779. doi:10.1016/S0029-7844(97)00077-X

Khawaja, N. M., Taher, B. M., Barham, M. E., Naser, A. A., Hadidy, A. M., Ahmad, A. T., et al. (2006). Pituitary enlargement in patients with primary hypothyroidism. *Endocrine Practice*, 12(1), 29–34. doi:10.4158/ep.12.1.29

Legro, R. S., Arslanian, S. A., Ehrmann, D. A., Hoeger, K. M., Murad, M. H., Pasquali, R., et al. (2013). Diagnosis and treatment of polycystic ovary syndrome: An Endocrine Society clinical practice guideline. *Journal of Clinical Endocrinology and Metabolism*, 98(12), 4565–4592. doi:10.1210/jc.2013-2350

Lim, V. S., Kathpalia, S. C., & Frohman, L. A. (1979). Hyperprolactinemia and impaired pituitary response to suppression and stimulation in chronic renal failure: Reversal after transplantation. *Journal of Clinical Endocrinology & Metabolism*, 48(1), 101–107. doi:10.1210/jcem-48-1-101

Martin, K. A., Anderson, R. R., Chang, R. J., Ehrmann, D. A., Lobo, R. A., Murad, M. H., Pugeat, M. M, & Rosenfield, R. L. (2018). Evaluation and treatment of hirsutism in premenopausal women: An Endocrine Society clinical practice guideline. *The Journal of Clinical Endocrinology & Metabolism*, 103(4), 1233–1257. doi:10.1210/jc.2018-00241

Melmed, S., Casanueva, F. F., Hoffman, A. R., Kleinberg, D. L., Montori, V. M., Schlechte, J. A., & Wass, J. A. (2011). Diagnosis and treatment of hyperprolactinemia: An Endocrine Society clinical practice guideline. *Journal of Clinical Endocrinology & Metabolism*, 96(2), 273–288. doi:10.1210/jc.2010-1692

Norman, R. J., Dewailly, D., Legro, R. S., & Hickey, T. E. (2007). Polycystic ovary syndrome. *The Lancet*, 370(9588), 685–697. doi:10.1016/s0140-6736(07)61345-2

Ostberg, J. E., Storry, C., Donald, A. E., Attar, M. J., Halcox, J. P., & Conway, G. S. (2007). A dose-response study of hormone replacement in young hypogonadal women: Effects on intima media thickness and metabolism. *Clinical Endocrinology*, 66(4), 557–564. doi:10.1111/j.1365-2265.2007.02772.x

Practice Committee of the American Society for Reproductive Medicine. (2008). Current evaluation of amenorrhea. *Fertility and Sterility*, 86(5), S148–S155. doi:10.1016/j.fertnstert.2006.08.013

Randeva, H. S., Tan, B. K., Weickert, M. O., Lois, K., Nestler, J. E., Sattar, N., & Lehnert, H. (2012). Cardiometabolic aspects of the polycystic ovary syndrome. *Endocrine Reviews*, 33(5), 812–841. doi:10.1210/er.2012-1003

Reindollar, R. H., Byrd, J. R., & McDonough, P. G. (1981). Delayed sexual development: A study of 252 patients. *American Journal of Obstetrics and Gynecology*, 140(4), 371–380. doi:10.1016/0002-9378(81)90029-6

Rotterdam ESHRE/ASRM-Sponsored PCOS Consensus Workshop Group. (2004). Revised 2003 consensus on diagnostic criteria and long-term health risks related to polycystic ovary syndrome. *Fertility and Sterility*, 81(1), 19–25. doi:10.1016/j.fertnstert.2003.10.004

Salley, K. E., Wickham, E. P., Cheang, K. I., Essah, P. A., Karjane, N. W., & Nestler, J. E. (2007). Glucose intolerance in polycystic ovary syndrome—A position statement of the Androgen Excess Society. *Journal of Clinical Endocrinology and Metabolism*, 92(12), 4546–4556. doi:10.1210/jc.2007-1549

Sheehan, M. T. (2004). Polycystic ovarian syndrome: Diagnosis and management. *Clinical Medicine & Research*, 2(1), 13–27. doi:10.3121/cmr.2.1.13

Tasali, E., Van Cauter, E., & Ehrmann, D. A. (2008). Polycystic ovary syndrome and obstructive sleep apnea. *Sleep Medicine Clinics*, 3(1), 37–46. doi:10.1016/j.jsmc.2007.11.001

Teede, H. J., Misso, M. L., Costello, M. F., Dokras, A., Laven, J., Moran, L., Piltonen, T. & Norman, R. J. (2018). Recommendations from the international evidence-based guideline for the assessment and management of polycystic ovary syndrome. *Human Reproduction*, 33(9), 1602–1618. doi:10.1093/humrep/dey256

Vrbikova, J., & Hainer, V. (2009). Obesity and polycystic ovary syndrome. *Obesity Facts*, 2(1), 26–35. doi:10.1159/000194971

Warren, M. P. (1992). Clinical review 40: Amenorrhea in endurance runners. *Journal of Clinical Endocrinology & Metabolism*, 75(6), 1393–1397. doi:10.1210/jcem.75.6.1464637

Wilcox, A. J., Baird, D. D., Dunson, D., McChesney, R., & Weinberg, C. R. (2001). Natural limits of pregnancy testing in relation to the expected menstrual period. *JAMA*, 286(14), 1759–1761. doi:10.1001/jama.286.14.1759

CHAPTER 19

Benign Prostatic Hyperplasia

Jean N. Taylor-Woodbury and Catherine D. Tanner

I. Introduction and general background

The prostate is a walnut-shaped tubular-alveolar gland located in the lower pelvis of persons assigned male at birth (AMAB), between the bladder and rectum (Aaron et al., 2016). Normally the prostate weighs about 20–25 grams and is about 2 by 4 by 3 centimeters in size. The prostate has three lobes encased by an outer layer of tissue and encircles the neck of the bladder, the urethra, and the ejaculatory duct (Aaron, et al., 2016; National Institutes of Diabetes and Digestion and Kidney Disease [NIDDKH], 2014). The prostate is both fibromuscular and glandular. Previous classification recognized five lobes of the prostate, but current nomenclature divides the prostate into three areas that are anatomically different and histologically specific. These zones are identified as central (base of gland surrounding ejaculatory ducts), transition (area surrounding the urethra), and peripheral (remainder of the gland) (Aaron et al., 2016). The function of the prostate is twofold: to produce seminal fluid, which helps to protect and transport sperm cells, and to aid in expulsion of semen into the urethra.

A. Benign prostatic hyperplasia

1. Definition and overview

    Benign prostatic hypertrophy (BPH) is the most common benign tumor in AMAB persons (Foo, 2019). Specifically, it is stromal and glandular epithelial hyperplasia that occurs in the transition/central zone. Enlargement of the prostate gland increases with age, is most common over the age of 50, and is progressive until death (McCance et al., 2019). There are two growth periods that the prostate experiences. The first stage happens in early puberty, and the second happens in the mid- to late 20s and continues throughout adult life. The second growth phase is when BPH is typically identified It has been proposed that BPH is a result of a "reawakening" and increased cell growth resulting in new ductal architecture in the transition/central zone (Aaron et al., 2016). The exact etiology of BPH is not fully understood. It is likely to encompass tissue changes caused by hormones, specifically dihydrotestosterone, an endogenous androgen sex steroid and hormone related to testosterone (Andriole, 2020). Similarly, higher levels of estrogen within the prostate during this time may encourage prostate cell growth (NIDDKD, 2014).

    Hyperplasia typically begins in the transition zone in a nodular pattern surrounding the urethra. As the prostate enlarges, the gland pushes against the urethra, causing narrowing and lower urinary tract symptoms (LUTSs) (Andriole, 2020). LUTSs may include urinary frequency, hesitancy, nocturia, weak stream, urgency, incomplete bladder emptying, and incontinence or dribbling. However, not all people with BPH exhibit symptoms (Sorenson et al., 2022). Less common complications of an enlarged prostate include obstruction with urinary retention, which may put increased stress on the kidneys. This stress may decrease kidney function if not corrected (Andriole, 2020).

    The association between BPH and prostate cancer remains controversial and complicated. Prostate cancer and BPH do share attributes, such as hormone-dependent growth. However, BPH is generally not considered a premalignant condition (Orsted et al., 2011). BPH's primary symptoms are that of LUTSs, and there are only a small number of people with LUTSs that are directly caused by prostate cancer (Chang et al., 2012). Orsted et al.'s (2011) study of over 3 million AMAB people for 27 years did conclude an association of BPH with prostate cancer; however, their data were inconclusive in inferring direct cause.

2. Prevalence and incidence

    BPH is very common. It has been reported that as many as 14 million people AMAB in the

United States have experienced some symptoms suggestive of BPH ([NIDDKD], 2014). Fifty percent of all people AMAB between the ages of 51 and 60 have BPH, and up to 90% of those over the age of 80 do (NIDDKD, 2014; Sorenson et al., 2021). Studies of disparities in BPH treatment are sparse, although existent research (Patel et al., 2020; Kuznar, 2011) suggests that patients who are African American or Hispanic are undertreated in the outpatient setting.

Prostate enlargement may begin as early as age 45, with development of LUTSs starting by age 60 or 65 (Longo et al., 2014). BPH under the age of 40 is unusual, but if diagnosed and requiring surgical intervention under the age of 60, it may be due to autosomal-dominant traits. First-degree relatives of those with the heritable form of BPH have a fourfold increased relative risk of developing BPH (Sorenson et al., 2021).

Diet, smoking, and exercise can influence BPH progression. The extent of these influences is not well understood. Yet, recent studies have identified that people AMAB with diets higher in starch and red meat have an increased risk of developing BPH (Lim, K.B, 2017). Excessive alcohol intake and metabolic syndrome also increase the risk for and progression of BPH. Likewise, those with diets high in vegetable intake appear to have less severe BPH symptoms (Skinder et al., 2016). Higher body weight is known to increase the risk of BPH, and some studies have shown that diabetes and heart disease might also increase the risk (Mayo Clinic, n.d.). Currently, age and family history remain the strongest predictors of prostate cancer risk (Chang et al., 2012).

II. Database (may include but is not limited to)

A. *Subjective*
  1. BPH
     a. Current symptoms and severity assessment: The American Urological Association (McVary et al., 2011) offers an effective tool for screening symptoms and severity (**Figure 19-1**).
        The possible total runs from 0 to 35 points, with higher scores indicating more severe symptoms. Scores less than 7 are considered mild and generally do not warrant treatment.
     b. Past medical history
        i. System-related medical illnesses: any prostatic disease, renal disease, renal infection, or renal calculi; and any bladder disease, dysfunction, or recurrent infections
        ii. Chronic medical conditions: diabetes mellitus, hypertension, or higher body weight
        iii. Surgical or prior procedure history: bladder, urethral or penile surgeries
        iv. Sexual history, including sexually transmitted infections
        v. Medication history: medications and supplements that may affect urinary flow or retention (e.g., antihistamine and decongestant use). For example, prescription medications such as Minipress, terazosin, Finasteride, and Nitrostat and supplements such as pumpkin seeds and plant sterols. Note any history of use of medications or supplements for treatment of existing or prior genitourinary disorders or diseases or prostate disease.
        vi. History of physical trauma to the bladder or the urethra
        vii. History of neurologic disease or injury
        viii. Trauma history: brain trauma, including infarct or hemorrhagic stroke
        ix. Any history of cancer
        x. Exposure history: any prior chemical or radioactive exposures to the lower genitourinary tract or perineal area, such as cadmium, nickel, and copper metals, or endocrine disruptors, such as phthalates found in items like vinyl flooring, food packaging, toys, and nail polish.
        xi. A history of eye disease or cataracts should also be evaluated. A surgical condition termed *intraoperative floppy iris syndrome* (IFIS) has been observed during phacoemulsification cataract surgery in some patients treated with α_1-blockers, including tamsulosin. Most of these reports were in patients taking the α_1-blocker when IFIS occurred, but in some cases, the α_1-blocker had been stopped before surgery. It is recommended that patients AMAB being considered for cataract surgery, as part of their medical history, be specifically questioned to ascertain whether they have taken tamsulosin or other α_1-blockers. If so, the patient's ophthalmologist should be prepared for possible modifications to their surgical technique that may be warranted should IFIS be observed during the procedure (McVary et al., 2011; Urology Care Foundation, 2021).
     c. Family history
        i. Prostatic disease, particularly in first-degree relatives, including age of onset of disease
        ii. Diabetes
        iii. Neurologic disorders
        iv. Cancer
     d. Occupational and environmental history
        i. Work-related exposures to chemicals (e.g., pesticides or metals like cadmium) or radiation, such as from x-ray exposures and as flight personnel
        ii. Degree of access to appropriate facilities for voiding
     e. Personal and social history
        i. Tobacco use and recreational drugs, including methamphetamines
        ii. Nutrition/diet and caffeine

AUA Symptom Score Questionnaire

The American Urological Association (AUA) has created this symptom index to give you and your physician an understanding of the severity of your enlarged prostate symptoms.

Question	None	Less than 1 time in 5	Less than half the time	About half the time	More than half the time	Almost always	Your score
Incomplete emptying: Over the past month, how often have you had a sensation of not emptying your bladder completely after you finished urinating?	0	1	2	3	4	5	
Frequency: Over the past month, how often have you had to urinate again less than 2 hours after you finished urinating?	0	1	2	3	4	5	
Intermittency: Over the past month, how often have you found that you stopped and started again several times when you urinated?	0	1	2	3	4	5	
Urgency: Over the past month, how often have you found it difficult to postpone urination?	0	1	2	3	4	5	
Weak-stream: Over the past month, how often have you had a weak urinary stream?	0	1	2	3	4	5	
Straining: Over the past month, how often have you had to push or strain to begin urination?	0	1	2	3	4	5	
Nocturia: Over the past month, how many times did you most typically get up to urinate from the time you went to bed at night until the time you got up in the morning?	0	1	2	3	4	5	

Symptom Score
(Add up the points for all questions to determine the severity of your symptoms)

Total score

If you scored 8 points or higher, you should consult your physician.

Symptom Score (Severity) — **0 to 7** (Mild), **8 to 19** (Moderate), **20 to 35** (Severe)

Figure 19-1 American Urological Association symptom score

Reproduced from Urology Care Foundation. For more information, please visit www.UrologyHealth.org

Rate Your Current Satisfaction

These questions are intended to help evaluate your satisfaction with your current enlarged prostate therapy. If you are not completely satisfied, ask your doctor about other treatment options.

How much do you agree or disagree with each of the following statements about your enlarged prostate treatment? Check one answer for each.

Question	Strongly Agree	Agree	Neutral	Disagree	Strongly Disagree
I am completely satisfied with the symptom relief I'm getting with my current enlarged prostate symptoms.					
I do not like the idea of taking daily medications indefinitely to relieve my enlarged prostate symptoms.					
I am bothered by one or more of the side effects of enlarged prostate medications (such as lowered sexual drive, erection problems, dizziness, low blood pressure, nasal congestion).					

Are you interested in learning more about non-medication based treatment options that may improve your BPH symptom relief beyond what you are currently getting?   YES   NO

After you have completed both sides of this form, please present this to your doctor and ask him/her to discuss your enlarged prostate treatment options.

Figure 19-1 (*Continued*)

    f. Review of systems
       i. Abdomen: suprapubic pain (suggestive of acute urinary retention) and flank pain
      ii. Genitourinary: urethral discharge, dysuria, irritative symptoms (urgency, frequency, or nocturia), or obstructive symptoms (hesitancy, decreased or intermittent stream flow, sensation of incomplete void, and dribbling incontinence)
      iii. Neurologic: focal neurologic findings suggestive of neurologic etiology of urinary symptoms, such as lower extremity weakness or radiculopathy or neuropathic symptoms (e.g., saddle anesthesia)

B. Objective
    1. Physical examination
      a. An abdominal examination may demonstrate a palpable, distended bladder, which may be asymptomatic if LUTSs are otherwise mild or absent.
      b. Assess for costovertebral angle pain, which should be absent with uncomplicated BPH.
      c. Assess for urethral discharge or other genital findings that may indicate an infection or a sexually transmitted infection as a source of the LUTSs.

d. A digital rectal examination should be done and may reveal an enlarged prostate, which may be focal or diffuse. However, the size of the prostate correlates poorly with both the symptoms and the signs of BPH.
e. A focused neurologic examination should be performed to investigate neurogenic bladder.
2. Supporting data from diagnostic tests
   a. Urinalysis: dipstick or microscopic for urinary tract infection or hematuria
   b. Screening for prostate cancer via prostate-specific antigen (PSA) remains controversial. The U.S. Preventive Services Task Force (2018) has made the following recommendations:
      - Patients who are 55 to 69 years old should make individual decisions about being screened for prostate cancer with a PSA test.
      - Before making a decision, patients should talk to their provider about the benefits and harms of screening for prostate cancer, including the benefits and harms of other tests and treatments.
      - Those who are 70 years old and older should not be screened for prostate cancer routinely.
   c. PSA levels may be higher than normal in persons with BPH or those with bacterial prostatitis, urinary tract infection, advanced age, recent medical procedures on the prostate, digital rectal exam, or recent ejaculation.

III. Assessment
A. *Determining the diagnosis*
   1. BPH
   2. Prostatitis
   3. Prostatic neoplasm (benign or malignant)
   4. Other conditions that might explain the patient's symptom presentation
      a. Diabetes mellitus
      b. Urethral stricture
      c. Bladder stone
      d. Bladder neck contracture
      e. Neurogenic bladder
B. *Assessing severity of disease*
   1. The American Urological Association's Symptom Index (AUA-SI) International Prostate Symptom Score (IPSS) and the Disease-Specific Quality of Life Questionnaire are helpful tools for assessing the severity of the condition (Figure 19-1).
   2. Assess the significance of the problem to the patient and significant others.

IV. Goals of clinical management
A. *Choose a cost-effective approach for screening or diagnosing BPH.*
B. *Select a treatment plan that alleviates bothersome LUTSs and aids in improving quality of life.*
C. *Select a treatment that also centers on prevention of disease progression and complications.*
D. *Select an approach that maximizes patient adherence.*

V. Plan
A. *Screening*
   1. There are no screening tests for BPH. A prostate examination (digital rectal exam) is usually performed in response to complaints of symptoms because prostate hyperplasia may be detected during an examination.
B. *Diagnostic tests*
   Testing is dependent on patient presentation and may include but is not limited to the following:
   1. Urinalysis: primary step to exclude urinary tract infection (UTI), prostate cancer, renal cancer, prostatitis, cystolithiasis
   2. PSA: remains controversial.
   3. Ultrasound: transabdominal or transrectal—minimally invasive procedure that may be helpful in evaluating size and shape of the prostate gland
   4. Cystoscopy: Internal imaging of urethra and bladder with scope used to assess obstruction. If the predominant symptom is irritation versus obstruction, may assess for bladder carcinoma.
   5. Cross-sectional imaging (computed tomography [CT], magnetic resonance imaging [MRI]): Usually done if surgery is advised. Provides clear image of prostate and surrounding area.
   6. Blood urea nitrogen (BUN) and creatinine: May be helpful in evaluating progressive obstruction and impaired renal function. Not part of initial workup.
   7. Additional and optional assessments for patients with moderate to severe LUTSs include postvoid residual volume test to assess urinary retention and urinary flow test to measure strength of urinary flow. A 24-hour voiding diary may be helpful if predominant urinary output occurs at night.
C. *Management*
   Management and treatment options include active surveillance, prescription medications, minimally invasive surgery, and more invasive surgery. The size of the prostate, overall health, age, and symptom severity should be considered as part of a shared decision model between patients and healthcare providers.
   1. Patients with mild symptoms of LUTSs and AUA-SI/IPSS score of <8 who are not bothered by their symptoms should be managed using a strategy of watchful waiting.
   2. Patients with moderate to severe symptoms of LUTSs and AUA-SI/IPSS score of ≥8 who are bothered by their symptoms should be informed of risks and benefits and consider pharmacological and/or surgical therapy.
   3. Pharmacotherapy includes:
      a. α-blockers: do not use, or stop before cataract surgery (McVary et al., 2011)
         i. Alfuzosin, 10 mg orally daily
         ii. Doxazosin, 1–8 mg orally daily
         iii. Tamsulosin, 0.4 or 0.8 mg orally daily

iv. Terazosin, 1–10 mg orally daily
v. Silodosin, 8 mg orally daily
vi. In using α-blockers, a gradual upward titration is recommended to minimize the risk of orthostatic hypotension that may occur with the use of this class of medications.
b. 5α-Reductase inhibitors (used for individuals with prostates > 40 mL by ultrasonographic examination) (Sorenson et al., 2022)
i. Dutasteride, 0.5 mg orally daily
ii. Finasteride, 5 mg orally daily
iii. Combination therapy: α-blocker and 5α-reductase inhibitor
- Finasteride and doxazosin
- Dutasteride and tamsulosin (available as single tablet)
- α-blockers and antimuscarinics
iv. Phenoxybenzamine, 5–10 mg orally twice daily
v. Prazosin, 0.5–1 mg orally twice daily. According to the current American Urological Association guideline for the management of BPH (McVary et al., 2011), there is insufficient evidence to support the use of either phenoxybenzamine or prazosin for the treatment of LUTSs with BPH.
vi. Phosphodiesterase-5 Inhibitor (PDE5), 5 mg daily for patients with LUTSs/BPH should be considered regardless of erectile dysfunction. According to the American Neurologic Association Guidelines, PDE5 has moderate recommendations with moderate-certainty benefits that will outweigh the risks (Lerner et al., 2021).
c. Dietary supplements
i. Phototherapeutics and other dietary supplements (e.g., saw palmetto [*Serenoa repens*], African prune tree [*Pygeum africanum*], and rye pollen [*Secale cereale*]) are not currently recommended for the treatment of LUTSs with BPH, based on expert panel recommendations and noted in the American Urological Association guideline for the management of BPH (Barry et al., 2011; McVary et al., 2011).
4. If the patient desires surgical therapy (minimally invasive or invasive), refer to urology services. Surgery may be recommended for patients who have renal insufficiency, recurrent UTIs, gross hematuria, or bladder stones related to BPH.
a. The specialist may consider additional optional diagnostic tests, such as pressure flow, urethrocystoscopy, or prostate ultrasound.
b. Minimally invasive surgical options include transurethral laser-induced prostatectomy, prostate urethral lift, transurethral needle ablation of the prostate, and hyperthermia.
c. Conventional surgical therapy includes transurethral resection of the prostate, transurethral incision of the prostate, transurethral electro-vaporization of the prostate, and open simple prostatectomy.
5. Adverse effects of treatment
Regardless of treatment approach, a shared decision-making model should be utilized. Desired and potentially undesired or adverse effects of treatment should be thoroughly discussed. Potential adverse effects depend on treatment course. In the use of α-blockers, patients may experience asymptomatic or symptomatic hypotension. Side effects that warrant urgent medical attention may include hives; swelling of face, lips, tongue, hands, and feet; loss of or blurry vision; painful erection that lasts for hours; shortness of breath; or chest pain. Surgical interventions, whether minimally invasive or invasive, have complications that may include retrograde ejaculation, erectile dysfunction, urinary incontinence, inability to avoid, and urinary tract infections (NIDDKD, 2014; Skinder et al., 2016).

D. *Patient education*
1. Assist the patient and significant others in expressing and coping with concerns and feelings related to the prostate disease process and disease management.
2. Provide oral and, preferably, written information regarding:
a. The disease process, including signs and symptoms and underlying etiologies
b. Diagnostic tests, including a discussion about preparation, cost, the actual procedures, and aftercare
c. Management (rationale, action, use, side effects, and cost of therapeutic interventions; and the need for adhering to long-term treatment plans)
d. Lifestyle modifications: avoiding or reducing caffeine and alcohol; bladder training; reducing intake of fluids prior to sleep or travel; avoiding medications such as decongestants, antihistamines, antidepressants, and diuretics as able; pelvic floor exercises; and preventing and treating constipation
e. Refer to additional resources for self-management/tools, additional education, clinical trials, and support groups.

VI. Self-management resources and tools
A. *Patient education resources*
1. The National Institutes of Health, National Library of Medicine (Medline Plus) provides patient information on prostate disease, including diagnosis and testing. Frequently asked questions and educational handouts are offered in both English and Spanish. Additional links are provided for clinical trials and other resources, including the Mayo Foundation and National Institute of Diabetes and Digestive and Kidney Disease. (https://www.nlm.nih.gov/medlineplus/prostatediseases.html)
2. Johns Hopkins Medicine provides information about BPH and other conditions of the prostate. The

site also offers Health Alerts, electronic subscription services for BPH that provide regular updates on BPH and current treatments. (https://www.hopkinsmedicine.org/search?q=BPH)
3. The Urology Care Foundation website provides health information on BPH, including risk reduction and treatments. The BPH patient guide is available in nine languages. (https://www.urologyhealth.org/search-results?terms=bph)
4. The Merck Manual Consumer Version provides patient education on BPH, symptoms, diagnosis, and treatments. (https://www.merckmanuals.com/home/SearchResults?query=Benign+Prostatic+Hyperplasia+(BPH)&icd9=600)

References

Aaron, L., Franco, O. E., & Hayward, S. W. (2016). Review of prostate anatomy and embryology and the etiology of benign prostatic hyperplasia. *Urologic Clinics of North America*, 43(3), 279–288. doi:10.1016/j.ucl.2016.04.012

Andriole, G. (2020). *Benign prostatic hyperplasia (BPH)*. https://www.merckmanuals.com/home/men-s-health-issues/benign-prostate-disorders/benign-prostatic-hyperplasia-bph?query=Benign%20Prostatic%20Hyperplasia%20(BPH)

Barry, M. J., Meleth, S. S., Lee, J. Y., Kreder, K. J., Avins, A. L., Nickel, J. C., Roehrborn, C. G., Crawford, E. D., Foster, H. E., Kaplan, S. A., McCullough, A., Andriole, G. L., Naslund, M. J., Williams, O. D., Kusek, J. W., Meyers, C. M., Betz, J. M., Cantor, A., & McVary, K. T. (2011). Effect of increasing doses of saw palmetto on lower urinary tract symptoms: A randomized trial. *JAMA*, 306(12), 1344–1351. doi:10.1001/jama.2011.1364

Chang, R. T., Kirby, R., & Challacombe, B. J. (2012). Is there a link between BPH and prostate cancer? *Practitioner*, 256(1750), 13.

Foo, K. T. What is a disease? What is the disease clinical benign prostatic hyperplasia (BPH)? (2019). *World Journal of Urology*, 37, 1293–1296. doi:10.1007/s00345-019-02691

Kuznar, W. (2011). Racial disparities found in treatment of BPH. *Urology Times*, 39(12), 19.

Lerner, L. B. McVary, K. T., Barry, M. J., Bixler, B. R., Dahm, P., Das, A. K., Gandhi, M. C., Kaplan, S. A., Kohler, T. S., Martin, L., Parsons, J. K., Roehrborn, C. G., Stoffel, J. T., Welliver, C., & Wilt, T. J. (2021). Management of lower urinary tract symptoms attributed to benign prostatic hyperplasia: AUA guideline Part I—initial work-up and medical management. *Journal of Urology*, 206(4), 806–817. doi:10.1097/JU.0000000000002183

Lerner, L. B., McVary, K. T., Barry, M. J., Bixler, B. R., Dahm, P., Das, A. K., Gandhi, M. C., Kaplan, S. A., Kohler, T. S., Martin, L., Parsons, J. K., Roehrborn, C. G., Stoffel, J. T., Welliver, C., & Wilt, T. J. (2021). Management of lower urinary tract symptoms attributed to benign prostatic hyperplasia: AUA guideline Part II—surgical evaluation and treatment. *Journal of Urology*, 206(4), 818–826. doi:10.1097/JU.0000000000002184

Lim K. B. (2017). Epidemiology of clinical benign prostatic hyperplasia. *Asian Journal of Urology*, 4(3), 148–151. doi:10.1016/j.ajur.2017.06.004

Longo, D. L., Fauci, A. S., Kasper, D. L., Hauser, S. L., Jameson, J., & Loscalzo, J. (2014). Urinary tract obstruction. In D. L. Longo, A. S. Fauci, D. L. Kasper, S. L. Hauser, J. Jameson, & J. Loscalzo (Eds.), *Harrison's Manual of Medicine* (18th ed.). New York: McGraw-Hill. Retrieved from http://accessmedicine.mhmedical.com/book.aspx?bookID=1140. Mayo Clinic. (n.d.). *Benign prostatic hyperplasia (BPH)*. https://www.mayoclinic.org/diseases-conditions/benign-prostatic-hyperplasia/symptoms-causes/syc-20370087

McCance, K.L, Huether, S.E., Brashers, V. L., Rote, N.S., (2019). The Reproductive Systems.(pp. 846-848) *Pathophsyiology the Biologic Basis for Disease in Adults and Children* (8th edition), Elsivier.

McVary, K. T., Roehrborn, C. G., Avins, A. L., Barry, M. J., Bruskewitz, R. C., Donnell, R. F., Foster, H. E., Jr, Gonzalez, C. M., Kaplan, S. A., Penson, D. F., Ulchaker, J. C., & Wei, J. T. (2011). Update on AUA guideline on the management of benign prostatic hyperplasia. *Journal of Urology*, 185(5), 1793–1803. doi:10.1016/j.juro.2011.01.074

National Institutes of Diabetes and Digestive and Kidney Diseases. (2014). *Prostate enlargement (benign prostatic hyperplasia)*. https://www.niddk.nih.gov/health-information/urologic-diseases/prostate-problems/prostate-enlargement-benign-prostatic-hyperplasia#whatIs

Orstead D., Bojesen, S., Nielsen B., & Nordestegaad, B. (2011). Association of clinical benign prostate hyperplasia with prostate cancer incidence and mortality revisited: A nationwide cohort study of 3,009,258 men. *European Urology*, 60(4), 691–698. doi:10.1016/j.eururo.2011.06.016

Patel, P. M., Sweigert, S. E., Nelson, M., Gupta, G., Baker, M., Modave, F., & McVary, K. T. (2020). Disparities in BPH progression: Predictors of presentation to the emergency department in urinary retention. *Journal of Urology*, 204(2), 332–336. doi:10.1097/JU.0000000000000787

Skinder, D., Zacharia, I., Studin, J., & Covino, J. (2016). Benign prostatic hyperplasia. *Journal of the American Academy of Physician Assistants*, 29(8), 19–23. doi:10.1097/01.JAA.0000488689.58176.0a

Sorensen, M., Walsh, T. J., & Haider M. A. (2022). Urologic disorders. In M. A. Papadakis, S. J. McPhee, M. W. Rabow, & K. R. McQuaid (Eds.), *Current medical diagnosis & treatment 2022* (pp. 952–977). McGraw Hill.

Urology Care Foundation. (2021). *Benign prostatic hyperplasia (BPH) patient guide*. https://www.urologyhealth.org/educational-resources?topic_area=1159%7C&product_format=466%7C&language=1122%7C

U.S. Preventive Services Task Force. (2018). *Final recommendation statement: Prostate cancer: screening*. https://uspreventiveservicestaskforce.org/uspstf/recommendation/prostate-cancer-screening

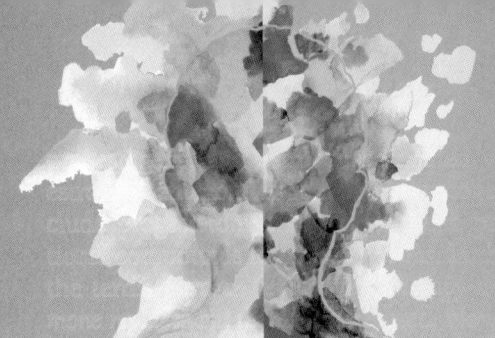

CHAPTER 20

Early Pregnancy Loss

Gwendolyn Riddell

I. Introduction and general background

Early pregnancy loss (EPL) is defined as a nonviable intrauterine pregnancy with either an empty gestational sac or gestational sac containing an embryo without cardiac activity prior to 13 weeks' gestation. The terms *miscarriage*, *spontaneous abortion* (SAB), *EPL*, and *early pregnancy failure* are used interchangeably (Prine & MacNaughton, 2011). **Table 20-1** reviews the common terminology. However, the term *failure* can have a negative connotation, which can make patients feel as if they did something wrong. Primary care providers commonly find this care challenging because of a lack of training (Fernández-Basanta et al., 2020), and thus this care has frequently been shifted to specialty providers. Because it is such a common occurrence, advanced practice nurses (APNs) should be well versed in providing counseling, treatment, and care for those experiencing EPL.

Pregnancy testing should be offered to anyone at risk for pregnancy (even if using reliable contraception) who reports changes in menstrual bleeding, unexplained bleeding with pelvic pain, missed menses, or unprotected sex or pregnancy symptoms such as breast tenderness, nausea, vomiting, or fatigue. Some patients will arrive in care already having performed a home pregnancy test, whereas other patients will not be aware that they are pregnant. Caring for patients with a positive pregnancy test requires sensitivity, active listening, and assessment for desirability of pregnancy (Goodman & TEACH Collaborative Working Group, 2020).

It is estimated that up to 25%–30% of all pregnancies end in SAB, although the majority of these SABs happen before a pregnancy is recognized (American Society for Reproductive Medicine [ASRM], 2012; Prine & MacNaughton, 2011). About 80% of SABs occur in the first 12 weeks of pregnancy, and the rate decreases rapidly thereafter (Cunningham et al., 2001). The etiology of EPL is varied, with chromosomal anomalies accounting for at least half of all EPLs. There are several risk factors associated with EPL, with age (either parent) and prior EPL being the most common (American College of Obstetricians and Gynecologists [ACOG], 2018). The rate of EPL rises with age. The risk is about 9%–17% between the ages of 20 and 30 and rises to approximately 20% at age 35 and 40% at age 40 (ACOG, 2018). The risk of EPL can be as high as 80% in patients who become pregnant at age 45 or older (ACOG, 2018). Other factors that increase the risk of miscarriage are exposure to toxins, having an intrauterine device (IUD) in place, chronic illness, inherited thrombophilia, substance use disorders, infections, heavy caffeine use, trauma, uterine fibroids, and uterine anomalies (ACOG, 2018; Cunningham et al., 2001; Griebel et al., 2019). It is often very difficult to determine the cause of an EPL. Patients who experience multiple EPLs can be evaluated for possible etiologies if pregnancy is desired. A complete workup is not indicated in patients with a single EPL (ACOG, 2018).

There are several different subtypes of EPL (see Table 20-1), which include anembryonic gestation and embryonic or fetal death, inevitable abortion, and incomplete abortion. Determining the correct diagnosis is integral to guiding management decisions.

There are several factors that should guide care and counseling of patients during EPL, including:

- Informing patients about findings in a timely manner.
- Being direct about diagnosis and findings
- Using simple language that the patient can understand

It is important to discuss how the patient feels about the pregnancy, their support systems, and the pregnancy within their life context. This discussion should include the patient's age, information about fertility, previous losses, desirability of future pregnancies, and possible causes such as chronic illness or substance use disorders. This visit can be an opportunity to address some of these issues and make referrals as necessary. It can also be a time to discuss preconception if the patient wishes to discuss

Table 20-1 Early Pregnancy Loss Terminology

	Type of Pregnancy	Presentation	Management Options
Intrauterine pregnancy (IUP)	1st trimester: 0–13 weeks 2nd trimester: 14–26 weeks 3rd trimester: 27–42 weeks	Missed menses, pregnancy forming within the uterus Gestational sac with fetal pole or yolk sac identified on ultrasound	Continue to term, abortion
Nonviable pregnancy	Anembryonic gestation: gestational sac seen on ultrasound but no fetal pole Embryonic demise: fetal pole seen on ultrasound without cardiac activity	Asymptomatic, bleeding in pregnancy Cramping, back pain, and/or loss of pregnancy symptoms	Aspiration, medication management, expectant management
Pregnancy of unknown location (PUL)	Pregnancy of unknown location	Positive pregnancy test, no visible pregnancy seen on ultrasound exam (gestational sac with a yolk sac). A gestational sac alone can be defined as a probable intrauterine pregnancy but must be followed closely.	Follow closely with serial human chorionic gonadotropin (hCG) or ultrasound until a definitive diagnosis can be made.
Ectopic pregnancy (EP)	A fertilized egg that implants outside of the uterus, most commonly in the fallopian tubes but can also be located in the ovary, abdomen, or cervix	Positive pregnancy test, pain, and vaginal bleeding, usually presenting at 6–8 weeks' gestation	Immediate referral for emergency care and management
Spontaneous abortion (SAB)	Spontaneous loss of pregnancy prior to 13 weeks Other terms: miscarriage, early pregnancy failure (not preferred language)	Bleeding, spotting, passing clots, cramping, loss of pregnancy symptoms, fever, malaise	Treatment depends on whether the SAB is complete. If products of conception (POC) remain in the uterus, there are three options for treatment: Expectant management Medication management Aspiration
Threatened abortion	Bleeding during early viable IUP	Bleeding and/or cramping in the first 20 weeks of pregnancy	Follow closely with ultrasound exams.
Missed abortion	IUP in which there is a fetal demise but no uterine activity to expel the POC	Loss of pregnancy symptoms, spotting, cramping but no passage of POC	Options for treatment: Expectant management Medication management Aspiration
Inevitable abortion	Bleeding and cramping with a dilated cervix; passage of tissue is expected.	Bleeding, spotting, passing clots, cramping, loss of pregnancy symptoms, fever, malaise	Options for treatment: Expectant management Medication management Aspiration
Complete abortion	All the POC have passed.	Bleeding, spotting, passing clots, cramping, loss of pregnancy symptoms, fever, malaise	No medical intervention needed if all the POC have passed. Support the patient by offering counseling.
Incomplete abortion	Some of the POC have passed and the cervix is dilated, but some POC remain in the uterus.	Bleeding, spotting, passing clots, cramping, loss of pregnancy symptoms, fever, malaise	Options for treatment: Expectant management Medication management Aspiration
Hydatidiform mole—partial or complete	Molar pregnancy is a premalignant disease that develops in the uterus as a result of a nonviable pregnancy.	Missed menses, spotting, nausea and vomiting, markedly elevated hCG values, "snowstorm" appearance on ultrasound exam	Aspiration, dilation and curettage (D&C), serial hCG levels monitored weekly until levels are undetectable (<5 mIU per milliliter) × 3 weeks, with subsequent monthly testing until levels are undetectable × 6 months (Berkowitz & Goldstein, 2009)

future pregnancies. This conversation should be led by the patient. They may need time to process the current loss before discussing future pregnancies. It is important to reassure the patient that they are not to blame for the pregnancy loss. Some patients may feel relief, and others may feel sadness or guilt, whereas others may have concerns about their health or fertility, so clinicians should not make assumptions about patient reactions. Patients may present with many of these feelings simultaneously (Goodman & TEACH Collaborative Working Group, 2020).

II. Database
A. *Subjective*

Patients with EPL often present with vaginal bleeding, abdominal cramping, or loss of pregnancy symptoms following a missed period or a positive pregnancy test at home. A nonviable pregnancy may also be an incidental finding seen on an early ultrasound, when fetal heart tones are not detected during the first-trimester ultrasound (Goodman & TEACH Collaborative Working Group, 2020).

1. History of presenting illness
   a. Vaginal bleeding: Although bleeding in a desired pregnancy can be alarming to patients, most bleeding in pregnancy is the result of implantation of the pregnancy in the uterus, as the decidua forms and the blastocyst burrows into the uterine lining. Bleeding in the first trimester occurs in up to 30%–40% of pregnancies; more than half of these pregnancies progress normally (Lykke et al., 2010).

   Many etiologies can be the source of bleeding, including cervical anomalies, polyps, trauma, ectopic pregnancy, idiopathic bleeding in a viable pregnancy, infection, molar pregnancy, subchorionic hemorrhage (bleeding beneath the chorion membranes that enclose the embryo in the uterus), or vaginal trauma (Griebel et al., 2019). Ectopic pregnancy should be a top differential diagnosis in any patient who presents with a positive pregnancy test and bleeding. An ectopic pregnancy can also be asymptomatic. Ectopic pregnancies occur in about 1%–2% of all pregnancies (Panelli et al., 2015). Risk factors for ectopic include age (>35), previous ectopic pregnancy, previous tubal surgery, tubal pathology, sterilization, IUD in place, previous sexually transmitted infection (STI), previous pelvic inflammatory disease, history of in utero diethylstilbestrol (DES) exposure, smoking, previous pelvic/abdominal surgery, and previous miscarriage (Ankum et al., 1996; Panelli et al., 2015). Up to 50% of patients diagnosed with ectopic pregnancies have no identifiable risk factors (Panelli et al., 2015).
   b. Abdominal pain, pelvic pain or cramping
   c. Passage of tissue and blood clots
   d. Loss of pregnancy-related symptoms, such as breast tenderness, nausea, fatigue
   e. Constitutional symptoms, such as fever and malaise
   f. Symptoms suspicious of ectopic pregnancy are shoulder pain, urinary symptoms, rectal pressure, and pain on defecation (National Institute for Health Care Excellence [NICE], 2019), in addition to any of the symptoms listed earlier. Pain associated with ectopic pregnancy usually worsens rapidly, is not usually intermittent, and is a medical emergency.
2. Past medical history: In gathering a medical history of a patient experiencing EPL, it is important to gather history that pertains to the treatment plan as well as to help determine the possible preventable risk factors for future pregnancies. Remember that people of all genders and sexual orientations present with EPL, and do not assume that your patient is female or in a heterosexual relationship. Also ask whether the patient used assisted reproductive technology to become pregnant.
   a. Anemia (hematocrit <30% or hemoglobin <10 gm/dL): must evaluate and determine the appropriate management or referral
   b. Allergies to medications or latex
   c. Bleeding disorders: Increases patient risk of SAB (ASRM, 2012). Patients with active clotting diagnoses should be treated with aspiration evacuation (Kaneshiro et al., 2011).
   d. Patients who require daily anticoagulants: Those using daily anticoagulation medications may be at an increased risk of blood loss and may be better candidates for active management of EPL with aspiration evacuation. Anticoagulation medications can be continued with relatively low risk of additional blood loss in EPLs up to 12 weeks' gestation (Kaneshiro et al., 2011).
   e. History of inherited porphyria: Porphyrias are rare metabolic disorders in which genetic mutations alter the body's generation of heme. Theoretically, mifepristone could precipitate an exacerbation caused by an accumulation of protoporphyrin (Guiahi & Davis, 2012). These patients should avoid mifepristone if proceeding with medication management of EPL.
   f. Renal and hepatic disease: Because mifepristone undergoes hepatic and renal metabolism, the use of mifepristone for the treatment of EPL is contraindicated in patients with renal and hepatic disease (Guiahi & Davis, 2012).
   g. Hypertension (HTN): Chronic HTN increases the risk of EPL. Evaluate patients with HTN and refer as needed (Nobles et al., 2018).
   h. Diabetes mellitus (DM): Uncontrolled diabetes is a risk factor for EPL. Patients with DM may need extra testing and care when considering aspiration evacuation of EPL. Consider scheduling the patient

for the procedure early in the day so that the patient can eat and take their usual dose of insulin after the procedure. See Chapter 17, Abortion Care in the Primary Care Setting, for more details.

    i. Thyroid disease: Uncontrolled thyroid disease may be associated with a higher incidence of EPL (ASRM, 2012).

    j. Autoimmune diseases such as celiac disease and antiphospholipid antibody syndrome may be associated with a higher risk of EPL (ASRM, 2012).

    k. Inherited thrombophilia (specifically, factor V Leiden and the prothrombin gene mutations, protein C, protein S, and antithrombin deficiencies) may be associated with an increased risk of EPL (ASRM, 2012).

    l. Infections: Some infections may lead to a higher incidence of EPL: parvovirus B19, malaria, rubella, *Ureaplasma urealyticum*, *Mycoplasma hominis*, *Listeria monocytogenes*, *Toxoplasma gondii*, and cytomegalovirus (ASRM, 2012; Giakoumelou et al., 2015; Prine & MacNaughton, 2011).

    m. Weight: Body mass index (BMI) ≥ 25 is a risk factor for EPL (Metwally et al., 2008; Fedorcsak et al., 2000).

    n. Medications taken: Some medications, such as itraconazole (Sporanox), methotrexate, and retinoids, may increase the risk of EPL (Prine & MacNaughton, 2011), and others may interact with medications used for treatment.

3. Obstetrical history: details of previous pregnancies and outcomes, including gestational age of delivery, live births, fetal demise, and mode of delivery, with a focus on history of previous EPL or ectopic pregnancies (Prine & MacNaughton, 2011)

4. Gynecological history
   a. Uterine fibroids: may increase risk of EPL, depending on type and location (Hartmann et al., 2017)
   b. Uterine anatomical anomalies: Congenital uterine abnormalities (unicornuate, didelphic, bicornuate, septate, or arcuate uteri) are associated with second-trimester pregnancy loss (ASRM, 2012).
   c. STIs and other infections may increase the risk of SAB: bacterial vaginosis, *Ureaplasma*, herpes simplex virus, chlamydia, untreated human immunodeficiency virus (HIV), and syphilis (Giakoumelou et al., 2015).
   d. IUD in place.

5. Surgical history, with a focus on obstetrical, gynecological, and abdominal surgeries.

6. Social history
   a. History of mental health disorders, such as depression and anxiety: Patients who present with EPL and preexisting depression and/or anxiety may need extra time and support and referrals to mental health providers.
   b. History of and current recreational drug use and substance use disorders: The use of cocaine is associated with an increased risk of EPL (Forray, 2016; Ness et al., 1999). Patients with a history of opiate use or dependence may need higher doses of medication for pain control during treatment.
   c. Marijuana use: Because of the increased popularity of marijuana use, several studies have examined the effect of marijuana use on pregnancy outcomes. Overall, the association between marijuana use in pregnancy and stillbirth or miscarriage remains unclear, but studies suggest that there may be some negative effects on pregnancy outcomes, including an increased risk of EPL, preterm delivery, and stillbirth (Thompson et al., 2019). A recent study found that couples with male partners who used marijuana ≥ 1 time per week during preconception had a greater risk of EPL compared with no male marijuana use (Harlow et al., 2019). The reason why is not known, but possible mechanisms include an adverse effect of frequent marijuana use on sperm quality (Harlow et al., 2019).
   d. Current moderate use of alcohol intake of 10 or more drinks/week during conception has been associated with an increased risk of EPL (Henriksen et al., 2004). A partner's use of alcohol can also affect the risk of EPL; studies have shown that increased alcohol found in sperm can increase the risk of EPL (Forray, 2016; Henriksen et al., 2004).
   e. Current cigarette smoking (>10 cigarettes per day) is associated with an increased risk of EPL and ectopic pregnancy (Forray, 2016; Ness et al., 1999; Waylen et al., 2009).
   f. Heavy caffeine use: There may be an increased risk of EPL in those who ingest at least 200–500 mg of caffeine per day versus patients who ingest less than 200 mg per day, but more studies are needed (ACOG, 2010).
   g. Past history of or current sexual abuse, rape, incest, or intimate partner violence (IPV). See Chapter 58, Intimate Partner Violence (Domestic Violence), for more information. Awareness of sexual trauma or abuse should inform the approach to care by recognizing the impact of violence and victimization on coping strategies. Trauma-informed care employs an empowerment model by working to maximize patient choices; creating an atmosphere that is respectful of the survivors' need for safety, respect, and acceptance; and emphasizing the patients' strengths, adaptations, and resilience (Butler et al., 2011). It is important to minimize the possibility of retraumatization, especially during pelvic exams.

B. Objective
   1. Labs prior to the exam: Pregnancy testing should be done to confirm pregnancy.

2. Vitals: Vital signs, including temperature, blood pressure, and pulse (including orthostatics if patient is symptomatic or presents with heavy bleeding). Patients with ectopic pregnancy may present with tachycardia (more than 100 beats per minute), orthostatic hypotension or hypotension (less than 100/60 mmHg), syncope, and lightheadedness (NICE, 2019).
3. General: Observe for pallor. Perform an abdominal exam to rule out other sources of pain or concern for peritoneal signs suggesting blood in the abdomen as a result of a ruptured ectopic pregnancy. Suspicion of ectopic pregnancy should be high in patients with rebound tenderness, peritoneal signs, or abdominal extension (NICE, 2019).
4. Pelvic exam
   a. Perform a bimanual pelvic exam to establish uterine size; evaluate for adnexal tenderness or mass.
   b. A speculum exam should be done to assess the volume of bleeding by noting the quantity of blood in the vagina and the presence or absence of active bleeding or tissue passing through the external os of the cervix. If an IUD is present, it should be removed during this exam.
   c. Ectopic pregnancy should be suspected in patients who, on exam, have cervical motion tenderness (CMT), pelvic or abdominal tenderness, or an enlarged uterus (NICE, 2019).
5. Ultrasound: Ultrasonography, if available, is the preferred modality to expedite diagnosis and management decisions. The staff members who perform ultrasound exams and clinicians who interpret those exams must be sufficiently trained to perform ultrasounds in early pregnancy.
   a. Ultrasound findings in a normal intrauterine pregnancy (IUP) include a decidual reaction, a gestational sac, a yolk sac, and a fetal pole with cardiac activity. When fetal cardiac activity is noted on an ultrasound exam of patients presenting with first-trimester bleeding, the risk of EPL drops to approximately 10% (Prine & MacNaughton, 2011).
   b. Findings on ultrasound exam that are diagnostic of EPL include (Doubilet et al., 2014):
      i. Anembryonic gestation, also referred to as a *blighted ovum*, will appear as a gestational sac without an embryo. Diagnostic criteria include a mean sac diameter (MSD) of ≥ 25 mm and no embryo.
      ii. Embryonic gestation with fetal demise: A gestational sac, yolk sac, and fetal pole are all seen, but no cardiac activity is noted on exam. Cardiac activity should be present in a fetal pole measuring ≥7 mm.
      iii. Absence of embryo with cardiac activity ≥2 weeks after an ultrasound that showed a gestational sac without a yolk sac.
      iv. Absence of an embryo with cardiac activity ≥11 days after an ultrasound that showed a gestational sac with yolk sac.
   c. Finding on ultrasound that is highly suspicious for, but not diagnostic of, EPL include (Doubilet et al., 2014):
      i. Fetal pole measuring 5–7 mm and no cardiac activity.
      ii. Mean gestational sac diameter between 16 and 24 mm and no embryo noted.
      iii. Absence of embryo with cardiac activity 7–13 days after an ultrasound that showed a gestational sac without a yolk sac.
      iv. Absence of embryo with cardiac activity 7–10 days after an ultrasound that showed a gestational sac with a yolk sac.
      v. Absence of embryo ≥6 weeks after sure last menstrual period.
      vi. Small gestational sac in relation to the size of the embryo.
   d. Findings on ultrasound suggestive of hydatidiform mole include a heterogeneous mass in the uterine cavity with multiple anechoic spaces, most commonly referred to as a "snowstorm" appearance (Berkowitz & Goldstein, 2009).
   e. Suspicion of ectopic should be high if the patient reports abdominal pain and vaginal bleeding and the pregnancy cannot be confirmed as intrauterine on ultrasound exam. Ultrasound findings suggestive of ectopic pregnancy are a gestational sac noted outside of the uterus, free fluid in the cul-de-sac, or a pseudosac seen in the uterus. Findings that are definitive of ectopic pregnancy are a gestational sac containing an embryo noted outside of the uterus (Panelli et al., 2015).
   f. A patient with a positive pregnancy test and no visible pregnancy on ultrasound is said to have a pregnancy of unknown location (PUL) (Goodman & TEACH Collaborative Working Group, 2020), which should be suspected as ectopic until laboratory evidence can show otherwise.

III. Assessment

Prior to treatment, it is important to distinguish EPL from other possibly normal early pregnancy symptoms or complications. Incorrectly diagnosing pregnancy loss in a patient with a PUL can prompt interventions that could be detrimental to a normal, desired IUP. Ectopic pregnancy should be a differential diagnosis in all patients presenting with first-trimester bleeding. In addition to confirming the correct diagnosis of EPL and location of the pregnancy, it is important to ensure that the patient is hemodynamically stable.

A. *Spontaneous abortion: incomplete, missed, inevitable, threatened, complete (Table 20-1).*
B. *Ectopic: Although it is important for APNs to be able to recognize the signs and symptoms of and identify ectopic pregnancies, it is not in the APN's scope of practice to*

treat an ectopic pregnancy. When an ectopic pregnancy is suspected or identified, an immediate referral to a provider (often the emergency department) who is able to treat ectopic pregnancies is warranted.

C. Hydatidiform mole/molar pregnancy: Aspiration evacuation is the best management choice (Berkowitz & Goldstein, 2009). See Chapter 17, Abortion Care in the Primary Care Setting, for more information about management and treatment.

IV. Goals of clinical management

A. Deliver evidence-based, patient-centered care that supports the patient's preferred approach to treatment of an EPL through shared decision making. Reassure patients that all treatments of EPL are safe and will not affect future fertility. Studies show that patients do have strong treatment preferences and will have greater satisfaction when treated according to their preferences (Dalton et al., 2006).

B. Provide space for patient grief. Reassure the patient; normalize feelings of sadness, relief, or mixed emotions. Provide referrals for mental health as needed.

C. Review etiology of EPL with patients, focusing on the fact that the majority of EPL causes cannot be determined. Address patient concerns and questions, reassuring patients that they did not cause the pregnancy loss.

D. Identify risk factors for future pregnancies, if desired. Refer patients as needed if risk factors are identified. More than two successive EPLs with the same partner warrants further workup and investigation into potential causes.

V. Review of systems

A. Constitutional: fever, chills.
B. Respiratory: shortness of breath, cough.
C. Cardiovascular: loss of consciousness, palpitations.
D. Gastrointestinal: abdominal pain, nausea, vomiting, rectal pressure, pain on defecation.
E. Genitourinary: dysuria, frequency, vaginal bleeding, pelvic pain, missed menses.
F. Musculoskeletal: back pain, shoulder pain.
G. Neurological: headache, dizziness.
H. Psychiatric: recent changes in mood, anxiety, depression.

VI. Plan

A. Diagnostic tests
  1. Point-of-care hemoglobin level should be done if bleeding is significant. Depending on results, this establishes the need for supplementation, appropriate treatment options, and whether referral is warranted.
  2. For PUL, the clinician will need to draw human chorionic gonadotropin (HCG) levels every 48 hours to diagnose an EPL and differentiate it from an ectopic pregnancy. A normal pregnancy will have a predictable rise (~35%–50% rise over 48 hours). A nonviable pregnancy will have a predictable decline (generally, levels decline 50% in 48 hours). An ectopic pregnancy will have an abnormal rise or fall (Goodman & TEACH Collaborative Working Group, 2020; Silva et al., 2006).
  3. Rhesus (Rh) alloimmunization may jeopardize the health of a subsequent pregnancy (National Abortion Federation [NAF], 2022), and thus Rh testing should be done in patients presenting with a gestational age of >12 weeks. Patients who are >12 weeks gestational age and Rh negative should be given a dose of Rho(D) anti-D immune globulin (Rhogam). There is no evidence to suggest an increased risk of alloimmunization for gestations <12 weeks (NAF, 2022).
  4. STI screening: Chlamydia (CT), gonorrhea (GC), syphilis, HIV, hepatitis C, and hepatitis B screening should be offered to any patient at increased risk or due for routine screening.

B. Treatment and management

Acceptable treatment options of EPL for patients who are hemodynamically stable and for whom an ectopic pregnancy has been ruled out include expectant management (EM), medication treatment, or uterine aspiration. Although these options differ significantly, all are safe and effective and acceptable to patients (ACOG, 2018). The safety and complication rates for all methods are very similar (ACOG, 2018). All options should be reviewed with and offered to patients without medical complications or symptoms requiring urgent uterine aspiration (ACOG, 2018). Management decisions should be driven by patient preference (Dalton et al., 2010). Factors that influence decisions are potential pain and management of pain, time constraints (work, childcare, eldercare, travel), duration of bleeding, personal responsibilities, perceived safety, past experiences, and feelings about the pregnancy (Goodman & TEACH Collaborative Working Group, 2020). Additionally, patients in states where abortion is criminalized may face barriers to accessing care for EPL. There have been isolated cases of providers withholding care for EPL out of fear of violating abortion bans (Felix et al., 2023). It remains to be seen how these laws will influence ongoing care for EPL.

  1. EM can be offered to clinically stable patients who choose to wait for the natural completion of EPL. While the patient is waiting for the pregnancy to pass, they should be followed closely. Studies have shown that most patients pass the pregnancy within 14 days from diagnosis of EPL and that waiting much longer without intervention did not result in a greater chance of successful resolution of the pregnancy (Casikar et al., 2010; Luise, 2002). Success rates for EM in EPL range from 52% and 84% at 2 weeks and differ depending on diagnosis (Casikar et al., 2010; Luise, 2002). Incomplete SABs have been found to be particularly appropriate for EM because of the higher success rates (53% at 7 days, 84% at 14 days, and 91% at 46 days) compared with those who present with missed SAB (30% at 7 days, 59% at 14 days, and 76% at 46 days) or anembryonic pregnancies (25% at 7 days, 52% at 14 days, and 66% at 46 days) (Luise, 2002).

a. Advantages:
   i. Privacy.
   ii. Some patients may prefer EM because it feels like a natural process.
   iii. Patients can be at home.
   iv. No intervention needed if successful.
   v. Support people can be with the patient at all times.
b. Disadvantages:
   i. Uncertainty of when the EPL will resolve, which can cause anxiety to the patient, who might already be experiencing sadness due to the loss of the pregnancy.
   ii. Depending on the diagnosis, the effectiveness can be as low as 66% (Luise, 2002).
c. Candidates:
   i. EM is safe for most patients with a nonviable, incomplete SAB ≤12 gestational weeks who are hemodynamically stable (ACOG, 2018).
   ii. Caution is warranted in patients with severe anemia and those with an IUD in place, which should be removed prior to going home (Nanda et al., 2012).
d. Contraindications: suspicion of ectopic, signs of pelvic infection, sepsis, hemodynamically instability, hemorrhagic disorder, patients taking anticoagulants, fetal demise in second trimester, hydatidiform mole (ACOG, 2018).
e. Additional considerations: patient's ability to access emergency care if needed, such as patients who live in remote areas with limited or no emergency services.
f. Counseling: The patient must be counseled well as to what to expect and given anticipatory guidance regarding time to completion, pain management, and possible complications:
   i. Bleeding:
      a. Patients may experience moderate to heavy bleeding and cramping, and it may happen at an inconvenient time.
      b. Patients may pass large blood clots the size of a small orange, and the fetal tissue might be seen in gestations over 9 weeks.
      c. The patient can wait up to 6–8 weeks from diagnosis of EPL (ACOG, 2018), checking in with a provider every 1–2 weeks.
      d. The need for urgent aspiration is estimated to be up to 10% for excessive bleeding and infection (Nanda et al., 2012).
         i. Pain control: Recommend or prescribe nonsteroidal anti-inflammatory drugs (NSAIDs); advise the patient to use heating pads applied to abdomen for cramping.
   ii. Establish an emergency plan with the patient. Ensure the patient knows how to get in touch with the provider, has a working phone, and knows where the nearest emergency department is located.
   iii. Make a follow-up plan to confirm completion in case of retained tissue or complications.
   iv. Danger signs, when to call: Advise patients to call in or present to emergency department for:
      a. Hemorrhage/excessive bleeding: Define excessive bleeding and when to call (filling two maxi pads in an hour for 2 consecutive hours).
      b. Passing blood clots larger than the size of a lemon.
      c. Rare possibility of infection <1%: Symptoms include fever (>100.4°F/38°C) for ≥4 hours or severe, persistent pain for >24 hours (Danco, 2016).
      d. Feeling sick, weak, nausea and vomiting, bloating, severe abdominal pain >2 hours.
      e. Severe cramping felt through pain medications.
      f. If patient experiences heavy bleeding with dizziness, fainting, shortness of breath, and palpitations, the patient must go directly to the emergency department.
   v. Reassess patients every 1–2 weeks and advise patients that they can change the plan at any time if they tire of waiting.
   vi. Completion can be determined by ultrasound, serial quantitative serum HCG labs, or urine pregnancy tests. HCG levels and urine pregnancy tests may take up to 6 weeks to return to nonpregnant levels. A phone call to review symptoms can also be an acceptable approach to follow up with low-risk patients and with those who have limited access to in-person care (ACOG, 2018).
   vii. If the pregnancy does not pass, a uterine aspiration may be necessary.
g. Complications
   i. Pelvic infection (1%–2%) (Nanda et al., 2012).

ii. Hemorrhage requiring hospitalization or transfusion (0.5%–1.4%) (Nanda et al., 2012).
iii. Incomplete abortion and need for uterine aspiration (~10%) (Luise, 2002; Nanda et al., 2012).

2. Medication management of EPL can be offered to patients without medical complications, infection, or symptoms that require urgent uterine aspiration. Medications used in medical management of EPL are misoprostol and mifepristone. Misoprostol is a synthetic prostaglandin E1 analogue that is used for the purpose of cervical softening, dilation, and uterine contractions, which expel the products of conception (Allen & O'Brien, 2009). Mifepristone is a glucocorticoid receptor antagonist (Spitz & Bardin, 1993) and an antiprogesterone derivative of norethindrone that inhibits progesterone, the hormone that supports and maintains a pregnancy (Christin-Maitre et al., 2000).

   a. Protocol (ACOG, 2018; Prine & MacNaughton, 2011; Zhang et al., 2006):
      i. Incomplete SAB:
         a. Misoprostol 600 mcg placed vaginally, with a repeat dose as needed, no sooner than 3 hours after initial dose
      ii. Missed SAB, anembryonic pregnancy:
         a. Misoprostol 800 mcg placed vaginally, with a repeat dose as needed, no sooner than 3 hours after initial dose (ACOG, 2018). The vaginal or sublingual route avoids the liver first-pass effect, which reduces the bioavailability of the drug (Wu et al., 2017), and is more effective than the oral route (Neilson et al., 2006). Additionally, the vaginal route decreases a common side effect of diarrhea and nausea experienced by patients taking misoprostol orally (Neilson et al., 2006).
      iii. A dose of mifepristone 200 mg orally 24 hours prior to taking misoprostol, if available, increases efficacy to close to 90%–96% by day 8 (Ngoc et al., 2013; Schreiber et al., 2018).
   b. Advantages:
      i. Avoids aspiration evacuation
      ii. Effectiveness of 90%–96% if using mifepristone and misoprostol, depending on original diagnosis (Ngoc et al., 2013). If using misoprostol regimen alone, the effectiveness is about 67%–71% by day 3 and 74%–84% by day 8 (Schreiber et al., 2018; Zhang et al., 2006). Effectiveness is highest in patients with incomplete, inevitable EPL and lowest in anembryonic gestations (Zhang et al., 2006).
   c. Candidates:
      i. Patients who want to shorten time to complete expulsion but prefer to avoid aspiration.
      ii. Medication management is a safe option for most patients with a nonviable, incomplete SAB ≤12 weeks' gestation who are hemodynamically stable.
      iii. Caution is warranted in patients with severe anemia, bleeding disorders, those who are taking anticoagulants, and patients with an IUD in place, which should be removed prior to going home.
      iv. Contraindications: suspicion of ectopic pregnancy, signs of pelvic infection, sepsis, hemodynamically instability, allergies to misoprostol or mifepristone.
      v. Additional considerations: patient's ability to access emergency care if needed, such as patients who live in remote areas with limited or no emergency services.
   d. Counseling:
      i. The counseling for medication management of EPL is similar to the counseling for EM.
      ii. Bleeding pattern:
         a. Passage of tissue may happen 1–7 days after taking medication.
         b. The process is more predictable than EM because bleeding usually starts often within 1–2 hours after taking misoprostol.
         c. Patients may experience moderate to heavy bleeding, heavier than a period, accompanied by moderate to severe cramping.
         d. Define excessive bleeding and when to call (see earlier EM section).
         e. Patients may pass large blood clots the size of a small orange, and the fetal tissue might be seen in gestations over 9 weeks.
      iii. Cramping and pain
         a. Patients may experience stronger uterine cramping than with EM after taking misoprostol.
         b. Recommend or prescribe NSAIDs; advise the patient to use heating pads applied to abdomen for cramping.
         c. Advise patients to take NSAIDs 30 minutes prior to taking misoprostol.
      iv. Danger signs are the same as for EM (see earlier section).
      v. Make a follow-up plan to confirm completion in case of retained tissue or complications.
         a. Reassess patients 1–2 weeks after taking medication.
         b. Completion can be determined by ultrasound, serial quantitative serum HCG labs, or urine pregnancy tests (should

not be done within 6 weeks of pregnancy because it will continue to be positive). A phone call to review symptoms can also be an acceptable approach to follow up with low-risk patients and those who have limited access to in-person care (ACOG, 2018).
- c. If the pregnancy does not pass, an aspiration evacuation is indicated.

vi. Complications:
- a. Pelvic infection (1%–3%) (Schreiber et al., 2018).
- b. Hemorrhage requiring hospitalization or transfusion (0.5%–2%) (Schreiber et al., 2018).
- c. Incomplete abortion and need for uterine aspiration (4%–16%, depending on initial diagnosis and if mifepristone was taken in combination with misoprostol) (Ngoc et al., 2013; Nielsen et al., 2006; Zhang et al., 2005).

3. Uterine aspiration/dilation and curettage (D&C): Because management of EPL with aspiration evacuation has a success rate of 98%–100%, it has been the gold standard for management of EPL until recently (ACOG, 2018; Wu et al., 2017). This has changed more recently as a result of increased education and training, provider comfort with EM and medication management, and patient preferences. Other factors that have contributed to these changes are the increased cost associated with aspiration and complications associated with anesthesia, as well as the wider availability and acceptance of medications used for medication management of EPL. Uterine aspiration is the only treatment option for patients presenting with hemorrhage, hemodynamic instability, or signs of infection, who should be treated urgently. The use of suction curettage, instead of sharp curettage, is the optimal method of aspiration (ACOG, 2018).
  - a. Advantages:
    - i. Success rate is high (ACOG, 2018).
    - ii. More predictable and less follow-up.
    - iii. Patient avoids sight of blood or products of conception.
    - iv. Quick resolution of the miscarriage.
  - b. Candidates:
    - i. Any patient can choose this method of management of EPL.
    - ii. Patients who are hemodynamically unstable and those with medical comorbidities, such as anemia, bleeding disorders, or cardiovascular disease.
    - iii. Patients who have contraindications to mifepristone or misoprostol.
    - iv. Patients who do not have a safe, comfortable place to be during EM or medication management.
    - v. Patients who desire quick resolution of EPL.
  - c. Counseling: Prepare the patient for what to expect during the procedure:
    - i. Pain: Depending on availability and protocol, review options for pain management. Some facilities offer moderate sedation, whereas in a hospital setting, a patient may be able to opt for general anesthesia.
    - ii. The patient will need a support person to drive them home after the procedure if they receive moderate or general anesthesia.
    - iii. Patients will likely be able to return to work within a few days, depending on how they feel.
  - d. Complications:
    - i. Complications are rare, especially when procedures are performed by experienced providers.
    - ii. The safety of aspiration evacuation is equivalent to aspiration abortion, and it can be performed in many outpatient primary care settings by trained providers. See Chapter 17, Abortion Care in the Primary Care Setting.
    - iii. Infection: The risk of infection after aspiration curettage is similar to that of aspiration with induced abortion and slightly higher than that for EM or medication management of EPL. Although there are limited data to support its use, antibiotic prophylaxis should be considered for patients with EPL. A single dose of doxycycline 200 mg prior to the procedure is sufficient to prevent infections.
    - iv. Uterine perforation or bowel damage is a rare complication and can happen if the instruments are passed deeper than expected. Frequency varies from 0.1 to 3 per 1,000, with higher frequencies occurring in training settings and at higher gestational ages (Kerns et al., 2019).
    - v. See Chapter 17, Abortion Care in the Primary Care Setting, for further information on aspiration evacuation.

C. *Provider resources/patient education*
1. Provider resources:
   a. NICE Guidelines: https://www.nice.org.uk/guidance/ng126/resources/ectopic-pregnancy-and-miscarriage-diagnosis-and-initial-management-pdf-66141662244037
   b. Innovative Education in Reproductive Health (IERH) is a program within the University of California, San Francisco (UCSF) Bixby Center for Global Reproductive Health and is a part of the UCSF's Department of Obstetrics, Gynecology & Reproductive Sciences. The IERH has developed educational video series for providers:
      i. EPL diagnosis and counseling: https://bit.ly/2MScxVg
      ii. EPL management: https://bit.ly/3dW7mzg

2. Patient resources:
   a. Reproductive Health Access: patient and provider education, including comprehensive, reprintable fact sheets https://www.reproductiveaccess.org/miscarriage/
   b. March of Dimes: patient education and information about miscarriage https://www.marchofdimes.org/complications/miscarriage.aspx
   c. M+A Hotline: support during miscarriage or abortion www.mahotline.org

References

Allen, R., & O'Brien, B. M. (2009). Uses of misoprostol in obstetrics and gynecology. *Reviews in Obstetrics & Gynecology*, 2(3), 159–168. https://www.ncbi.nlm.nih.gov/pmc/articles/PMC2760893/

American College of Obstetricians and Gynecologists. (2010). *Moderate caffeine consumption during pregnancy*. https://www.acog.org/clinical/clinical-guidance/committee-opinion/articles/2010/08/moderate-caffeine-consumption-during-pregnancy

American College of Obstetricians and Gynecologists. (2018). ACOG Practice Bulletin No. 200. *Obstetrics & Gynecology*, 132(5), e197–e207. doi:10.1097/aog.0000000000002899

American Society for Reproductive Medicine. (2012). Evaluation and treatment of recurrent pregnancy loss: A committee opinion. *Fertility and Sterility*, 98(5), 1103–1111. doi:10.1016/j.fertnstert.2012.06.048

Ankum, W. M., Mol, B. W. J., Van der Veen, F., & Bossuyt, P. M. M. (1996). Risk factors for ectopic pregnancy: A meta-analysis. *Fertility and Sterility*, 65(6), 1093–1099. doi:10.1016/s0015-0282(16)58320-4

Berkowitz, R. S., & Goldstein, D. P. (2009). Molar pregnancy. *New England Journal of Medicine*, 360(16), 1639–1645. doi:10.1056/nejmcp0900696

Butler, L., Critelli, F., & Rinfrette, E. (2011). Trauma-informed care and mental health. *Directions in Psychiatry*, 31(3), 197–210. https://psycnet.apa.org/record/2011-30401-004

Casikar, I., Bignardi, T., Riemke, J., Alhamdan, D., & Condous, G. (2010). Expectant management of spontaneous first-trimester miscarriage: Prospective validation of the "2-week rule." *Ultrasound in Obstetrics and Gynecology*, 35(2), 223–227. doi:10.1002/uog.7486

Christin-Maitre, S., Bouchard, P., & Spitz, I. M. (2000). Medical termination of pregnancy. *New England Journal of Medicine*, 342(13), 946–956. doi:10.1056/nejm200003303421307

Cunningham, G., Gant, N., Gilstrap, L., Hauth, J., & Westrom, K. (2001). *Williams obstetrics* (21st ed.). McGraw-Hill.

Dalton, V. K. Harris, L., Weisman, C. S., Guire, K., Castleman, L., & Lebovic, D. (2006). Patient preferences, satisfaction, and resource use in office evacuation of early pregnancy failure. *Obstetrics and Gynecology*, 108(1), 103–110. doi:10.1097/01.AOG.0000223206.64144.68

Dalton, V. K., Harris, L. H., Gold, K. J., Kane-Low, L., Schulkin, J., Guire, K., & Fendrick, A. M. (2010). Provider knowledge, attitudes, and treatment preferences for early pregnancy failure. *American Journal of Obstetrics and Gynecology*, 202(6), 531.e1–531.e8. doi:10.1016/j.ajog.2010.02.016

Danco. (2016, January 20). *Prescribing Information. Mifeprex. Mifepristone. RU486. Abortion pill. Early option pill*. https://bit.ly/37HYECD

Doubilet, P. M., Benson, C. B., Bourne, T., & Blaivas, M. (2014). Diagnostic criteria for nonviable pregnancy early in the first trimester. *Ultrasound Quarterly*, 30(1), 3–9. doi:10.1097/ruq.0000000000000060

Fedorcsak, P., Storeng, R., Dale, P. O., Tanbo, T., & Åbyholm, T. (2000). Obesity is a risk factor for early pregnancy loss after IVF or ICSI. *Acta Obstetricia et Gynecologica Scandinavica*, 79(1), 43–48. doi:10.1080/j.1600-0412.2000.079001043.x

Felix, M., Sobel, L., & Salganicoff, A. (2023, May 18). *A review of exceptions in state abortion bans: Implications for the provision of abortion bans*. KFF. https://www.kff.org/womens-health-policy/issue-brief/a-review-of-exceptions-in-state-abortions-bans-implications-for-the-provision-of-abortion-services/

Fernández-Basanta, S., Movilla-Fernández, M.-J., Coronado, C., Llorente-García, H., & Bondas, T. (2020). Involuntary pregnancy loss and nursing care: A meta-ethnography. *International Journal of Environmental Research and Public Health*, 17(5), 1486. doi:10.3390/ijerph17051486

Forray, A. (2016). Substance use during pregnancy. *F1000Research*, 5, 887. doi:10.12688/f1000research.7645.1

Giakoumelou, S., Wheelhouse, N., Cuschieri, K., Entrican, G., Howie, S. E. M., & Horne, A. W. (2015). The role of infection in miscarriage. *Human Reproduction Update*, 22(1), 116–133. doi:10.1093/humupd/dmv041

Goodman, S., & TEACH Collaborative Working Group. (2020). *TEACH early abortion training curriculum* (6th ed.). UCSF Bixby Center for Global Reproductive Health.

Griebel, C. P., Halvorsen, J., Golemon, T. B., & Day, A. A. (2019). Management of spontaneous abortion. *American Family Physician*, 72(7), 1243–1250. https://www.aafp.org/afp/2005/1001/p1243.html

Guiahi, M., & Davis, A. (2012). First-trimester abortion in women with medical conditions. *Contraception*, 86(6), 622–630. doi:10.1016/j.contraception.2012.09.001

Harlow, A. F., Wesselink, A. K., Rothman, K. J., Hatch, E. E., & Wise, L. A. (2019). Male marijuana use and spontaneous abortion. *Fertility and Sterility*, 112(3), e3. doi:10.1016/j.fertnstert.2019.07.1333

Hartmann, K. E., Velez Edwards, D. R., Savitz, D. A., Jonsson-Funk, M. L., Wu, P., Sundermann, A. C., & Baird, D. D. (2017). Prospective cohort study of uterine fibroids and miscarriage risk. *American Journal of Epidemiology*, 186(10), 1140–1148. doi:10.1093/aje/kwx062

Henriksen, T. B., Hjollund, N., Jensen, T., Bonde, J., & Andersson, A. (2004). Alcohol consumption at the time of conception and spontaneous abortion. *American Journal of Epidemiology*, 160(7), 661–667. doi:10.1093/aje/kwh259

Kaneshiro, B., Bednarek, P., Isley, M., Jensen, J., Nichols, M., & Edelman, A. (2011). Blood loss at the time of first-trimester surgical abortion in anticoagulated women. *Contraception*, 83(5), 431–435. doi:10.1016/j.contraception.2010.09.009

Kerns, J. L., Ti, A., Aksel, S., Lederle, L., Sokoloff, A., & Steinauer, J. (2019). Disseminated intravascular coagulation and hemorrhage after dilation and evacuation abortion for fetal death. *Obstetrics & Gynecology*, 134(4), 708–713. doi:10.1097/aog.0000000000003460

Luise, C. (2002). Outcome of expectant management of spontaneous first trimester miscarriage: Observational study. *BMJ*, 324(7342), 873–875. doi:10.1136/bmj.324.7342.873

Lykke, J. A., Dideriksen, K. L., Lidegaard, Ø., & Langhoff-Roos, J. (2010). First-trimester vaginal bleeding and complications later in pregnancy. *Obstetrics & Gynecology*, *115*(5), 935–944. doi:10.1097/aog.0b013e3181da8d38

Metwally, M., Ong, K. J., Ledger, W. L., & Li, T. C. (2008). Does high body mass index increase the risk of miscarriage after spontaneous and assisted conception? A meta-analysis of the evidence. *Fertility and Sterility*, *90*(3), 714–726. doi: 10.1016/j.fertnstert.2007.07.1290

Nanda, K., Lopez, L. M., Grimes, D. A., Peloggia, A., & Nanda, G. (2012). Expectant care versus surgical treatment for miscarriage. *Cochrane Database of Systematic Reviews*, *2012*(3), CD003518. doi:10.1002/14651858.cd003518.pub3

National Abortion Federation. (2022). Clinical Policy Guidelines for Abortion Care. https://prochoice.org/wp-content/uploads/2022-CPGs.pdf

National Institute for Health Care Excellence. (2019). *Ectopic pregnancy and miscarriage: Diagnosis and initial management*. National Institute for Health Care Excellence (NICE) Clinical Guidelines, No. 154. https://www.nice.org.uk/guidance/ng126/resources/ectopic-pregnancy-and-miscarriage-diagnosis-and-initial-management-pdf-66141662244037

Neilson, J.P., Hickey, M., & Vazquez, J.C. (2006). Medical treatment for early fetal death (less than 24 weeks). *Cochrane Database of Systematic Reviews*, *2006*(3), CD002253. doi:10.1002/14651858.cd002253.pub3

Ness, R. B., Grisso, J. A., Hirschinger, N., Markovic, N., Shaw, L. M., Day, N. L., & Kline, J. (1999). Cocaine and tobacco use and the risk of spontaneous abortion. *Obstetrical & Gynecological Survey*, *54*(7), 451–452. doi:10.1097/00006254-199907000-00021

Ngoc, N. T. N., Shochet, T., Blum, J., Hai, P. T., Dung, D. L., Nhan, T. T., & Winikoff, B. (2013). Results from a study using misoprostol for management of incomplete abortion in Vietnamese hospitals: Implications for task shifting. *BMC Pregnancy and Childbirth*, *13*(1), 118. doi:10.1186/1471-2393-13-118

Nobles, C. J., Mendola, P., Mumford, S. L., Naimi, A. I., Yeung, E. H., Kim, K., Park, H., Wilcox, B., Silver, R. M., Perkins, N. J., Sjaarda, L., & Schisterman, E. F. (2018). Preconception blood pressure levels and reproductive outcomes in a prospective cohort of women attempting pregnancy. *Hypertension*, *71*(5), 904–910. doi:10.1161/hypertensionaha.117.10705

Panelli, D. M., Phillips, C. H., & Brady, P. C. (2015). Incidence, diagnosis and management of tubal and nontubal ectopic pregnancies: A review. *Fertility Research and Practice*, *1*(1), 15. doi:10.1186/s40738-015-0008-z

Prine, L., & MacNaughton, H. (2011). Office management of early pregnancy loss. *American Family Physician*, *84*(1), 75–82. https://www.aafp.org/afp/2011/0701/p75.html#commenting

Schreiber, C. A., Creinin, M. D., Atrio, J., Sonalkar, S., Ratcliffe, S. J., & Barnhart, K. T. (2018). Mifepristone pretreatment for the medical management of early pregnancy loss. *Obstetric Anesthesia Digest*, *38*(4), 213–214. doi:10.1097/01.aoa.0000547312.79293.b1

Silva, C., Sammel, M. D., Zhou, L., Gracia, C., Hummel, A. C., & Barnhart, K. (2006). Human chorionic gonadotropin profile for women with ectopic pregnancy. *Obstetrics & Gynecology*, *107*(3), 605–610. doi:10.1097/01.aog.0000198635.25135.e7

Spitz, I. M., & Bardin, C. (1993). Mifepristone (RU 486)—A Modulator of Progestin and Glucocorticoid Action. *The New England Journal of Medicine*, *329*(6), 404–412. doi:10.1056/NEJM199308053290607

Thompson, R., DeJong, K., & Lo, J. (2019). Marijuana use in pregnancy. *Obstetrical & Gynecological Survey*, *74*(7), 415–428. doi:10.1097/ogx.0000000000000685

Waylen, A. L., Metwally, M., Jones, G. L., Wilkinson, A. J., & Ledger, W. L. (2009). Effects of cigarette smoking upon clinical outcomes of assisted reproduction: A meta-analysis. *Human Reproduction Update*, *15*(1), 31–44. doi:10.1093/humupd/dmn046

Wu, H., Marwah, S., Wang, P., Wang, Q., & Chen, X. (2017). Misoprostol for medical treatment of missed abortion: A systematic review and network meta-analysis. *Scientific Reports*, *7*(1). doi:10.1038/s41598-017-01892-0

Zhang, J., Gilles, J. M., Barnhart, K., Creinin, M. D., Westhoff, C., & Frederick, M. M. (2006). A comparison of medical management with misoprostol and surgical management for early pregnancy failure. *Obstetrical & Gynecological Survey*, *61*(2), 110–111. doi:10.1097/01.ogx.0000197805.67669.ee

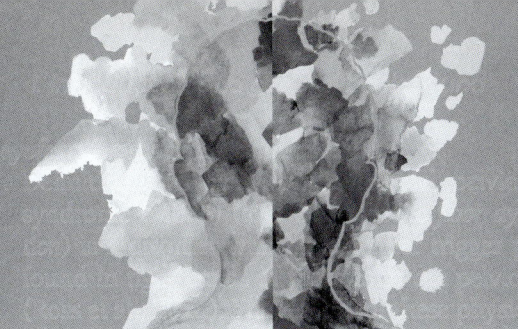

CHAPTER 21

Contraception

Simran Tagore

I. Introduction and general background

Contraception is the deliberate prevention of pregnancy. Planning pregnancy has been shown to help persons assigned female at birth (AFAB) achieve their educational, career and economic goals, increase relationship satisfaction, and decrease anxiety and depression (Sonfield et al., 2013). Use of contraception also reduces maternal mortality, and reduces child and maternal morbidity (American College of Obstetricians and Gynecologists [ACOG], 2015). There are various contraceptive methods available in the United States, most of which are of use by persons AFAB. Persons AFAB have the burden for many reasons, including systemic sexism and the false perception that persons assigned male at birth (AMAB) will not be trusted to provide for contraception (Campo-Engelstein, 2012). Additionally, sperm is produced at a very high rate, leading to difficulties in finding an easy to use pill that can reduce its ability to fertilize an egg (National Institutes of Health, 2023).

Choosing a contraceptive method involves extensive patient education. The patient (and their partner if desired) should be provided with factual and current information about each method and empowered to actively participate in the decision-making process. With adequate education, discussion, and joint decision making, the patient can make a choice that supports their reproductive needs. Because these needs may change over time, contraceptive choices may also change over time. Guiding patients in safe and appropriate decision making is key to safe contraceptive use (Cwiak & Edelman, 2018). Additionally, it is imperative that contraceptive counseling is done within a reproductive justice framework as outlined by ACOG.

The term *reproductive justice* (RJ) was coined by Women of African Descent for Reproductive Justice in the early 1990s and combines reproductive rights and social justice. According to SisterSong (n.d., para. 1), RJ is "the human right to maintain personal bodily autonomy, have children, not have children, and parent the children we have in safe and sustainable communities."

With RJ in mind, the ACOG (ACOG Committee on Health Care for Underserved Women and Committee on Ethics, 2022) encourages patient-centered contraceptive counseling. This counseling acknowledges that people of color and other marginalized communities often have their reproductive desires devalued. It further acknowledges that unconscious or conscious bias on the part of the provider can affect contraceptive counseling and care provision and that work should be undertaken to minimize these biases. Patients' lived experience, values, and preferences should be centered in the counseling interaction. Clinicians may prioritize contraceptive efficacy, length of use, or cost, whereas patients may be considering barriers to reproductive goals, such as difficulty accessing health care, provider behaviors, stigma, discrimination, racism, or intimate partner control or violence. Patients may also be concerned with privacy, ease of use, reversibility, noncontraceptive benefits, menstrual side effects, patient control, invasiveness, or hormone content. The ACOG (ACOG Committee on Health Care for Underserved Women and Committee on Ethics, 2022, p. 351) recommends that providers "explore a person's reproductive goals and contraceptive priorities and preferences while considering the systemic and structural barriers that may impede their ability to do so." Shared decision making allows patients to use clinician expertise to inform a choice that best meets their current needs. Over the course of discussion, patients may disclose a history of trauma, such as sexual violence, that may inform their contraceptive preferences. Clinicians should be prepared to discuss these concerns and place appropriate referrals. See Chapter 58, Interpersonal Violence for more information.

The U.S. Medical Eligibility Criteria for Contraceptive Use (USMEC) provides guidelines for clinicians who assess the potential risk associated with use of a contraceptive method compared with the risk of unintended pregnancy (Curtis, Tepper, et al., 2016). Patients are generally candidates for contraceptive methods when their health risk from contraceptive use is less than the health risk they would face with pregnancy (Cwiak & Edelman, 2018). Medical conditions are assigned categories 1 through 4 based on their safety for a particular method. Category 1 means there are no restrictions for use, Category 2 means the advantages of the method generally outweigh the risks, Category 3 means the risks generally outweigh the advantages, and Category 4 means the risks of the method are unacceptable (Curtis, Tepper, et al., 2016). See **Table 21-1** for a USMEC summary.

Efficacy rate is an important aspect of counseling. The efficacy rate for each method will be reported as a percentage and refers to the number of patients out of 100 who prevent pregnancy in 1 year. "Perfect use" is how effective the method can be when used exactly as directions state

Table 21-1 Summary of Classifications for Hormonal Contraceptive Methods and Intrauterine Devices

Condition	Cu IUD	LNG IUD	Implants	DMPA	POP	CHCs
Personal Characteristics and Reproductive History						
Pregnancy	4*	4*	NA*	NA*	NA*	NA*
Age	Menarche to <20 years: 2; ≥20 years: 1	Menarche to <20 years: 2; ≥20 years: 1	Menarche to <18 years: 1; 18–45 years: 1; >45 years: 1	Menarche to <18 years: 2; 18–45 years: 1; >45 years: 2	Menarche to <18 years: 1; 18–45 years: 1; >45 years: 1	Menarche to <40 years: 1; ≥40 years: 2
Parity						
a. Nulliparous	2	2	1	1	1	1
b. Parous	1	1	1	1	1	1
Post-abortion						
c. First trimester	1*	1*	1*	1*	1*	1*
d. Second trimester	2*	2*	1*	1*	1*	1*
e. Immediate postseptic abortion	4	4	1*	1*	1*	1*
Past ectopic pregnancy	1	1	1	1	2	1
History of pelvic surgery	1	1	1	1	1	1
Smoking						
a. Age < 35 years	1	1	1	1	1	2
b. Age ≥ 35 years						
i. <15 cigarettes per day	1	1	1	1	1	3
ii. ≥15 cigarettes per day	1	1	1	1	1	4
Obesity						
a. BMI ≥ 30 kg/m²	1	1	1	1	1	2
b. Menarche to <18 years and BMI ≥ 30 kg/m²	1	1	1	2	1	2

Condition	Cu IUD	LNG IUD	Implants	DMPA	POP	CHCs
History of bariatric surgery: This condition is associated with an increased risk for adverse health events as a result of pregnancy.						
a. Restrictive procedures: decrease storage capacity of the stomach (vertical banded gastroplasty, laparoscopic adjustable gastric band, or laparoscopic sleeve gastrectomy)	1	1	1	1	1	1
b. Malabsorptive procedures: decrease absorption of nutrients and calories by shortening the functional length of the small intestine (Roux-en-Y gastric bypass or biliopancreatic diversion)	1	1	1	1	3	COCs: 3 Patch and ring: 1
Cardiovascular disease						
Multiple risk factors for atherosclerotic cardiovascular disease (e.g., older age, smoking, diabetes, hypertension, low HDL, high LDL, or high triglyceride levels)	1	2	2*	3*	2*	3/4*
Hypertension: Systolic blood pressure ≥160 mmHg or diastolic blood pressure ≥100 mmHg are associated with an increased risk for adverse health events as a result of pregnancy.						
a. Adequately controlled hypertension	1*	1*	1*	2*	1*	3*
b. Elevated blood pressure levels (properly taken measurements)						
i. Systolic 140–159 mmHg or diastolic 90–99 mmHg	1*	1*	1*	2*	1*	3*
ii. Systolic ≥ 160 mmHg or diastolic ≥ 100 mmHg	1*	2*	2*	3*	2*	4*
c. Vascular disease	1*	2*	2*	3*	2*	4*

(continues)

Table 21-1 Summary of Classifications for Hormonal Contraceptive Methods and Intrauterine Devices *(continued)*

Condition	Cu IUD	LNG IUD	Implants	DMPA	POP	CHCs
History of high blood pressure during pregnancy (when current blood pressure is measurable and normal)	1	1	1	1	1	2
Deep venous thrombosis (DVT)/pulmonary embolism (PE)						
a. History of DVT/PE, not receiving anticoagulant therapy						
i. Higher risk for recurrent DVT/PE (one or more risk factors)	1	2	2	2	2	4
ii. Lower risk for recurrent DVT/PE (no risk factors)	1	2	2	2	2	3
b. Acute DVT/PE	2	2	2	2	2	4
c. DVT/PE and established anticoagulant therapy for at least 3 months						
i. Higher risk for recurrent DVT/PE (one or more risk factors)	2	2	2	2	2	4*
ii. Lower risk for recurrent DVT/PE (no risk factors)	2	2	2	2	2	3*
d. Family history (first-degree relatives)	1	1	1	1	1	2
e. Major surgery						
i. With prolonged immobilization	1	2	2	2	2	4
ii. Without prolonged immobilization	1	1	1	1	1	2
f. Minor surgery without immobilization	1	1	1	1	1	1
Known thrombogenic mutations (e.g., factor V Leiden; prothrombin mutation; and protein S, protein C, and antithrombin deficiencies) This condition is associated with an increased risk for adverse health events as a result of pregnancy.	1*	2*	2*	2*	2*	4*

I. Introduction and general background

Condition	Cu IUD	LNG IUD	Implants	DMPA	POP	CHCs
Superficial venous disorders						
a. Varicose veins	1	1	1	1	1	1
b. Superficial venous thrombosis (acute or history)	1	1	1	1	1	3*
Current and history of ischemic heart disease: This condition is associated with an increased risk for adverse health events as a result of pregnancy.	1	Initiation 2 Continuation 3	Initiation 2 Continuation 3	3	Initiation 2 Continuation 3	4
Stroke (history of cerebrovascular accident): This condition is associated with an increased risk for adverse health events as a result of pregnancy.	1	2	Initiation 2 Continuation 3	3	Initiation 2 Continuation 3	4
Valvular heart disease: Complicated valvular heart disease is associated with an increased risk for adverse health events as a result of pregnancy.						
a. Uncomplicated	1	1	1	1	1	2
b. Complicated (pulmonary hypertension, risk for atrial fibrillation, or history of subacute bacterial endocarditis)	1	1	1	1	1	4
Rheumatic diseases						
Systemic lupus erythematosus: This condition is associated with an increased risk for adverse health events as a result of pregnancy.						
a. Positive (or unknown) antiphospholipid antibodies	Initiation 1* Continuation 1*	3*	3*	Initiation 3* Continuation 3*	3*	4*
b. Severe thrombocytopenia	Initiation 3* Continuation 2*	2*	2*	Initiation 3* Continuation 2*	2*	2*
c. Immunosuppressive therapy	Initiation 2* Continuation 1*	2*	2*	Initiation 2* Continuation 2*	2*	2*
d. None of the above	Initiation 1* Continuation 1*	2*	2*	Initiation 2* Continuation 2*	2*	2*

(continues)

Table 21-1 Summary of Classifications for Hormonal Contraceptive Methods and Intrauterine Devices (*continued*)

Condition	Cu IUD	LNG IUD	Implants	DMPA	POP	CHCs
Rheumatoid arthritis						
a. Receiving immunosuppressive therapy	Initiation 2 Continuation 1	Initiation 2 Continuation 1	1	2/3*	1	2
b. Not receiving immunosuppressive therapy	1	1	1	2	1	2
Neurologic conditions						
Headaches						
a. Nonmigraine (mild or severe)	1	1	1	1	1	1*
b. Migraine						
i. Without aura (This category of migraine includes menstrual migraine.)	1	1	1	1	1	2*
ii. With aura	1	1	1	1	1	4*
Epilepsy: This condition is associated with an increased risk for adverse health events as a result of pregnancy.	1	1	1*	1*	1*	1*
Multiple sclerosis						
a. With prolonged immobility	1	1	1	2	1	3
b. Without prolonged immobility	1	1	1	2	1	1
Depressive disorders						
Depressive disorders	1*	1*	1*	1*	1*	1*
Reproductive tract infections and disorders						
Unexplained vaginal bleeding (suspicious for serious condition) before evaluation	Initiation 4* Continuation 2*	Initiation 4* Continuation 2*	3*	3*	2*	2*
Cervical ectropion	1	1	1	1	1	1
Cervical intraepithelial neoplasia	1	2	2	2	1	2
Cervical cancer (awaiting treatment)	Initiation 4 Continuation 2	Initiation 4 Continuation 2	2	2	1	2

I. Introduction and general background

Condition	Cu IUD	LNG IUD	Implants	DMPA	POP	CHCs
Breast disease: Breast cancer is associated with an increased risk of adverse health events as a result of pregnancy.						
a. Undiagnosed mass	1	2	2*	2*	2*	2*
b. Benign breast disease	1	1	1	1	1	1
c. Family history of cancer	1	1	1	1	1	1
d. Breast cancer						
i. Current	1	4	4	4	4	4
ii. Past and no evidence of current disease for 5 years	1	3	3	3	3	3
Endometrial hyperplasia	1	1	1	1	1	1
Endometrial cancer: This condition is associated with an increased risk for adverse health events as a result of pregnancy.	Initiation 4 Continuation 2	Initiation 4 Continuation 2	1	1	1	1
Ovarian cancer: This condition is associated with an increased risk for adverse health events as a result of pregnancy.	1	1	1	1	1	1
Uterine fibroids	2	2	1	1	1	1
Anatomical abnormalities						
a. Distorted uterine cavity (any congenital or acquired uterine abnormality distorting the uterine cavity in a manner that is incompatible with IUD insertion)	4	4	—	—	—	—
b. Other abnormalities (including cervical stenosis or cervical lacerations) not distorting the uterine cavity or interfering with IUD insertion	2	2	—	—	—	—
Pelvic inflammatory disease (PID)						
a. Past PID						
i. With subsequent pregnancy	Initiation 1 Continuation 1	Initiation 1 Continuation 1	1	1	1	1

(continues)

Table 21-1 Summary of Classifications for Hormonal Contraceptive Methods and Intrauterine Devices *(continued)*

Condition	Cu IUD	LNG IUD	Implants	DMPA	POP	CHCs
ii. Without subsequent pregnancy	Initiation 2 Continuation 2	Initiation 2 Continuation 2	1	1	1	1
b. Current PID	Initiation 4 Continuation 2*	Initiation 4 Continuation 2*	1	1	1	1
Sexually transmitted infections (STIs)						
a. Current purulent cervicitis or chlamydial infection or gonococcal infection	Initiation 4 Continuation 2*	Initiation 4 Continuation 2*	1	1	1	1
b. Vaginitis (including *Trichomonas vaginalis* and bacterial vaginosis)	Initiation 2 Continuation 2	Initiation 2 Continuation 2	1	1	1	1
c. Other factors related to STIs	Initiation 2* Continuation 2	Initiation 2* Continuation 2	1	1	1	1
Human immunodeficiency virus (HIV)						
High risk for HIV	Initiation 2 Continuation 2	Initiation 2 Continuation 2	1	1*	1	1
HIV infection: For patients with HIV infection who are not clinically well or not receiving ARV therapy, this condition is associated with an increased risk for adverse health events as a result of pregnancy.	Initiation — Continuation —	Initiation — Continuation —	1*	1*	1*	1*
a. Clinically well and receiving ARV therapy	Initiation 1 Continuation 1	Initiation 1 Continuation 1	—	—	—	—
b. Not clinically well or not receiving ARV therapy	Initiation 2 Continuation 1	Initiation 2 Continuation 1	—	—	—	—
Malaria	1	1	1	1	1	1
Endocrine conditions						
Diabetes: Insulin-dependent diabetes; diabetes with nephropathy, retinopathy, or neuropathy; diabetes with other vascular disease; or diabetes of >20 years' duration are associated with an increased risk of adverse health events as a result of pregnancy.						
a. History of gestational disease	1	1	1	1	1	1
b. Nonvascular disease						

Condition	Cu IUD	LNG IUD	Implants	DMPA	POP	CHCs
i. Non–insulin dependent	1	2	2	2	2	2
ii. Insulin dependent	1	2	2	2	2	2
c. Nephropathy, retinopathy, or neuropathy	1	2	2	3	2	3/4*
d. Other vascular disease or diabetes of >20 years' duration	1	2	2	3	2	3/4*
Thyroid disorders						
a. Simple goiter	1	1	1	1	1	1
b. Hyperthyroid	1	1	1	1	1	1
c. Hypothyroid	1	1	1	1	1	1
Gastrointestinal conditions						
Inflammatory bowel disease (ulcerative colitis or Crohn disease)	1	1	1	2	2	2/3*
a. Symptomatic						
i. Treated by cholecystectomy	1	2	2	2	2	2
ii. Medically treated	1	2	2	2	2	3
iii. Current	1	2	2	2	2	3
b. Asymptomatic	1	2	2	2	2	2
History of cholestasis						
a. Pregnancy related	1	1	1	1	1	2
b. Past COC related	1	2	2	2	2	3
Viral hepatitis						
a. Acute or flare	1	1	1	1	1	Initiation 3/4* Continuation 2
b. Carrier	1	1	1	1	1	Initiation 1 Continuation 1
c. Chronic	1	1	1	1	1	Initiation 1 Continuation 1
Cirrhosis: Severe cirrhosis is associated with an increased risk for adverse health events as a result of pregnancy.						
a. Mild (compensated)	1	1	1	1	1	1
b. Severe (decompensated)	1	3	3	3	3	4

(continues)

Table 21-1 Summary of Classifications for Hormonal Contraceptive Methods and Intrauterine Devices (continued)

Condition	Cu IUD	LNG IUD	Implants	DMPA	POP	CHCs
Liver tumors: Hepatocellular adenoma and malignant liver tumors are associated with an increased risk for adverse health events as a result of pregnancy.						
a. Benign						
i. Focal nodular hyperplasia	1	2	2	2	2	2
ii. Hepatocellular adenoma	1	3	3	3	3	4
b. Malignant (hepatoma)	1	3	3	3	3	4
Respiratory conditions						
Cystic fibrosis: This condition is associated with an increased risk for adverse health events as a result of pregnancy	1*	1*	1*	2*	1*	1*
Anemias						
Thalassemia	2	1	1	1	1	1
Sickle cell disease: This condition is associated with an increased risk for adverse health events as a result of pregnancy	2	1	1	1	1	2
Iron-deficiency anemia	2	1	1	1	1	1

ARV, antiretroviral therapy; BMI, body mass index; COC, combined oral contraceptive; CHC, combined hormonal contraception; Cu IUD, copper IUD; DMPA, depot medroxyprogesterone acetate; HDL, high-density lipoprotein; IUD, intrauterine device; LDL, low-density lipoprotein; LNG IUD, levonorgestrel IUD; POP, progestin-only pill.
*consult MEC for clarification

and consistently. "Typical use" is how effective the method is during actual, real-life use, which includes inconsistent and incorrect use (Trussel, Aiken, et al., 2018).

A. **Combined hormonal contraception (CHC)**

CHC refers to contraceptive methods that contain estrogen and progesterone. These methods include the combined oral contraceptive pill (COC), the transdermal patch, and the vaginal contraceptive ring. These methods have varying amounts of ethinyl estradiol (EE) as the estrogen component and various types of progestin hormone as the progesterone component. Methods that contain other types of estrogen are available outside of the United States. COCs are the most commonly used reversible contraceptive method in the United States (Daniels et al., 2015).

COCs are available in monophasic or multiphasic formulations. Monophasic formulations contain the same dose of estrogen and progestin throughout the month (Allen, 2022). Multiphasic formulations vary the dose of either or both hormones during the active pill phase and were introduced as a strategy to reduce hormone dose and thus hormone-related side effects and unscheduled bleeding (Allen, 2022). However, there are no data that these preparations have any clinical advantage, and the efficacy rate appears to be similar across all COC types (Allen, 2022). COCs are packaged in a variety of ways; most COCs are available in 28-day packages that contain 21–24 active and 4–7 inert or ferrous fumarate (Fe) tablets (Dickey & Seymour, 2021).

The original COC formulations included hormone-free days to induce a monthly scheduled bleed that patients would interpret as normal menstruation (Read, 2010). Although this scheduled monthly bleed was needed for initial acceptance of the pill, it is now recognized that this scheduled bleeding is not biologically necessary (Edelman, 2002). Progesterone causes atrophy of the endometrial lining, ensuring that no withdrawal bleed is necessary (Read, 2010).

CHCs also include the contraceptive patch and the contraceptive ring. Patients may find the weekly or monthly dosing schedule of the patch or the ring more convenient than the daily COC. There are two types of contraceptive patches available in the United States. The Xulane and Zafemy brands deliver approximately 150 mcg of norelgestromin (N) and 35 mcg of EE daily (National Library of Medicine [NLM], 2022b), and Twirla delivers 120 mcg of levonorgestrel (LNG) and 30 mcg of EE (NLM, 2022a). The patch can be applied to the buttocks, upper arm, lower abdomen, or upper torso (excluding the breasts) and is changed weekly (NLM, 2022a, 2022b).

The vaginal contraceptive rings are the etonogestrel (ENG)/EE (commercial names, NuvaRing, EluRyng) and the segesterone acetate (SA)/EE ring (commercial name, Annovera) (Kerns & Darney, 2020). The ENG/EE releases 120 mcg of ENG and 15 mcg of EE daily (Nanda & Burke, 2018) and is replaced monthly. The SA/EE releases approximately 150 mcg/day of SA and 13 mcg/day of EE over a 21-day period (Baker & Chen, 2022) and may be removed monthly and reused for 1 year. The concentration of EE is lower with ENG/EE vaginal ring compared with other combined hormonal contraceptives (Kerns & Darney, 2020). Fitting by a clinician is not necessary for either ring.

1. Mechanism of action
   CHCs function by suppressing ovulation via inhibition of gonadotropin-releasing hormone (GnRH) from the hypothalamus, as well as inhibition of luteinizing hormone (LH) and follicle-stimulating hormone (FSH) and disruption of the midcycle LH surge (Allen, 2022). EE and progestins have other effects on the reproductive system, but it has not been well substantiated that any of these effects contributes significantly to efficacy (Cwiak & Edelman, 2018). These other effects include slowing of tubal motility, thickening of cervical mucus, endometrial atrophy, changes in the function of endometrial vessels, alterations in the endometrium matrix metalloproteinase content, and localized edema of the endometrium (Cwiak & Edelman, 2018).

2. Efficacy
   The perfect-use efficacy of COC is over 99%, and the typical-use efficacy is 91% (Cwiak & Edelman, 2018). The efficacy rate is 99% for perfect and typical use for the EE/N patch (Smallwood et al., 2001). Efficacy rates for the EE/LNG patch are based on body mass index (BMI); the efficacy rate is 96.5% for a BMI of 18.5 to 24.9, 94.3% for a BMI of 25 to 29.9, and 91.4% for a BMI of 30 and above (Nelson et al., 2021). For the ENG/EE ring, the efficacy rate in the first year of use is 99.7% with perfect use and 91% with typical use (Trussel, 2011). The SA/EE ring has a 97% typical efficacy rate (Archer et al., 2019).

3. Benefits
   See the chapters on amenorrhea and polycystic ovary syndrome (PCOS) (Chapter 18), chronic pelvic pain (Chapter 23), abnormal uterine bleeding (Chapter 16), and menopause (Chapter 22) for more information on the use of CHCs for non-contraceptive benefits. Other benefits not reviewed in those chapters include reducing menstrual migraines, premenstrual syndrome, ovarian cysts, and acne and risk reduction for endometrial and ovarian cancers (Allen, 2022). Additionally, this method is controlled by the patient and may be used without partner knowledge.

4. Side effects and disadvantages
   In one large study, 34% of patients reported that side effects were the main reason for discontinuation of their COC (Westhoff et al., 2007). Common side effects for all CHC methods include bleeding changes, weight changes, mood changes, and changes in libido. Side effects such as nausea, breast tenderness, and headaches are usually minor, often resolve with time, and are less common with the current formulations of CHC contraceptives (Roe et al., 2021). Evidence for weight gain is mixed (Roe et al., 2021).

   Because of differences in types of progestins and amount of EE, each CHC formulation has a different pattern of biologic activity (Dickey & Seymour, 2021). A formulation's endometrial, estrogenic, progestational, and androgenic activities may potentially manifest as some of the side effects listed earlier. For example, breast tenderness, nausea, or mood changes are usually related to estrogen and may be relieved by changing to a pill with greater progestational activity. *Managing Contraceptive Pill Patients and Other Hormonal Contraceptives* (Dickey & Seymour, 2021) is an excellent reference for these clinical challenges and many others.

   Unscheduled bleeding is associated with initial CHC use. The timing of initiation (e.g., whether starting the day the prescription is picked up, the first day of the menses, or the first Sunday after the start of the period) does not change the amount or duration of this bleeding (Brahmi & Curtis, 2013). Unscheduled bleeding affects about one-half of patients during the first month of use but quickly improves over subsequent months (Roe et al., 2021). Extended-cycling formulations with skipped or delayed withdrawal bleed can have a longer duration of unscheduled bleeding, but for most users, bleeding will improve over time (Edelman et al., 2014). Experiencing amenorrhea during the time of a scheduled withdrawal bleed is expected and is normal (Cwiak & Edelman, 2018). This amenorrhea does not signify decreased contraceptive effectiveness in and of itself (Roe et al., 2021).

   The delivery methods of the patch and the ring can cause side effects as well. Some patients may experience transient skin reactions, such as irritation, redness, pigment changes, or a rash at the site of patch application (Nanda & Burke, 2018). Ring users report more vaginal wetness, leukorrhea, and vaginitis compared with COC users (Lopez et al., 2013). Microbiologic evaluation has shown that ring use was associated with an increase in hydrogen peroxide–producing *Lactobacillus*, the predominant species in the healthy human vagina, but no increase in other types of bacteria (Veres et al., 2004).

5. Risks

CHC use has been associated with an increased risk of venous thromboembolism (VTE) and cardiovascular risks such as hypertension, myocardial infarction (MI), and stroke in certain populations (Allen, 2022). The risks vary with estrogen dose and patient factors such as age, body size, and smoking status (Allen, 2022; Cwiak & Edelman, 2018). Although relative risks are increased, the absolute risks are still low for most patients (Han & Jensen, 2015; Shapiro & Dinger, 2010). COCs can rarely cause a mild blood pressure elevation in the range of 3 to 5 mmHg, which is unlikely to be clinically significant in a healthy patient (Allen, 2022). The average overall EE concentration in EE/N patch users is 60% higher than in individuals who use a 35-mcg pill, although data are conflicting as to whether this results in an increased risk of VTE, stroke, or MI (Burkman, 2021).

6. Contraindications

Contraindications include current VTE, history of VTE with high risk of recurrence, cerebrovascular or coronary artery disease, migraine with aura, and current breast cancer (Cwiak & Edelman, 2018). However, a more recent examination of the evidence has led to some discussion that CHCs containing 10–20 mcg of EE may be safer than previously thought (Voedisch & Hindiyeh, 2019). Because of lower efficacy rates, BMI ≥ 30 is considered a contraindication to EE/LNG patch (Burkman, 2021).

B. Progestin-only pills (POPs)

While multiple types of progestin are used for COCs, norethindrone, drosperinone, and norgestrel are the only progestins available as POPs in the United States. The pills are dispensed in packs of 28 pills. The norethindrone and norgestrel POPs are taken continuously and do not include a hormone-free period. (Monterrosa-Castro et al., 2021; Food and Drug Administration [FDA], 2017). The drosperinone-containing POP contains 24 active pills, followed by 4 inert pills (Monterrosa-Castro et al., 2021). The amount of progestin in each POP tablet is lower than the amount in tablets of COC products (Raymond & Grossman, 2018). Unless otherwise noted, the information presented here on POPs primarily applies to norethindrone POPs.

1. Mechanism of action

Norethindrone-containing POPs work by thickening cervical mucus to inhibit sperm migration, suppressing ovulation, lowering the midcycle peaks of FSH and LH, slowing the movement of an egg through the fallopian tubes, and thinning the endometrium (Kaunitz, 2021b). Ovulation is not consistently suppressed with norethindrone POPs; approximately half of users still ovulate (Milsom & Korver, 2008). Therefore, the effects of norethindrone POPs on cervical mucus and endometrium represent the critical factors in the prevention of contraception (Monterrosa-Castro et al., 2021). Norgestrel suppresses ovulation in about two-thirds of users (Glasier et al., 2022). By contrast, drosperinone does suppress ovulation (Kaunitz, 2021b).

2. Efficacy

POPs can be a highly effective contraceptive method when taken as directed (Raymond & Grossman, 2018). The perfect-use efficacy rate for norethindrone POPs is 99.5%, and the typical-use efficacy rate is 95% (NLM, 2018). An initial clinical trial of drosperinone POPs reported an overall pregnancy rate of 1.8% (Kaunitz, 2021b).

3. Benefits

Data suggests that POPs appear not to be associated with an overall clinically important increase in the risk of hypertension, cardiovascular disease, stroke, breast cancer, or blood clots (Raymond & Grossman, 2018). POPs generally have fewer contraindications and can be safely used by almost all patients (Monterrosa-Castro et al., 2021). They have a simple, fixed daily regimen; provide immediate return to fertility; and may improve menstrual symptoms for some patients (Raymond & Grossman, 2018). Daily use of a progestin also protects against the development of endometrial cancer (Weiderpass et al., 1999).

4. Side effects and disadvantages

Unscheduled bleeding and changes in menses are the most common side effects associated with POPs (Kaunitz, 2021b). These changes are unpredictable and may include irregular periods, short cycles, intermenstrual bleeding and spotting, and less commonly, amenorrhea or prolonged bleeding (Raymond & Grossman, 2018). POPs do not appear to be associated with significant weight gain and are not likely to increase headache frequency (Lopez et al., 2016; MacGregor, 2013). Unlike COCs, which inhibit ovarian activity and reduce the risk of functional ovarian cysts, POPs may be associated with an increased incidence of functional ovarian cysts or persistent follicles (Raymond & Grossman, 2018). These follicular changes tend to increase and regress over time and require no intervention other than reassurance in asymptomatic patients (Kaunitz, 2021b).

5. Risks

The drosperinone-containing POP contains antimineralocorticoid activity comparable to a 25-mg dose of spironolactone (Kaunitz, 2021b). Patients at risk for hyperkalemia should use drosperinone with caution (Kaunitz, 2021b). Norethindrone-containing POPs, along with drosperinone-containing POPs, represent a safe contraceptive choice for patients with high risk of, or known, coronary artery disease, cerebrovascular disease, venous thromboembolic disease, hypertension, or other conditions in which use of contraceptive doses of estrogen are contraindicated (ACOG Committee on Practice Bulletins—Gynecology, 2019).

6. Contraindications

Almost all patients can safely use POPs, including most patients who are not eligible to take COCs (Raymond & Grossman, 2018). Current breast cancer is the only condition for which the USMEC states that POPs pose an unacceptable health risk (Raymond & Grossman, 2018).

C. Injectable progestins

Depot medroxyprogesterone acetate (DMPA; brand name, Depo-Provera) is an injectable progestin-only contraceptive. DMPA is available in two formulations, each given every 13 weeks: 150 mg/1 mL for intramuscular injection (IM) and 104 mcg/0.65 mL for subcutaneous (SQ) injection (Mishell, 1996). The efficacy and side-effect profiles of both are similar, and patients who are eligible for progestin injectables may choose either formulation (Dragoman & Gaffield, 2016). Injections are effective when given up to 15 weeks apart, although that interval may be extended to 17 weeks in low-resource settings where pregnancy tests are not available and in patients at lower risk of pregnancy (Kaunitz, 2022).

1. Mechanism of action

DMPA suppresses levels of FSH and LH, eliminates the LH surge, thickens and decreases cervical mucus to prevent sperm penetration, and atrophies the endometrium (Wu & Bartz, 2018).

2. Efficacy

In the first year, perfect-use efficacy is 99.8%, and typical-use efficacy is 96% (Trussel, 2011). Because DMPA use results in high progestin levels, efficacy is not reduced by high body weight or the use of other medications (Segall-Guttierez et al., 2010).

3. Benefits

High amenorrhea rates with ongoing DMPA use make it a suitable choice for patients with heavy menstrual bleeding, dysmenorrhea, or iron-deficiency anemia (Kaunitz, 2021a). DMPA has also been shown to reduce pain associated with endometriosis (Wu & Bartz, 2018). The thickened cervical mucus produced by DMPA may prevent the ascent of cervical pathogens to the upper genital tract and decrease the risk for pelvic inflammatory disease (PID) (Baeten et al., 2001). DMPA use decreases the risk of endometrial cancer by up to 80% and the risk of epithelial ovarian cancer by 39% (up to 80% with 3 years of use) (Wu & Bartz, 2018). Sickle cell crises appear to be improved as well (De Ceulaer et al., 1982). DMPA contains no estrogen and can be safely used in patients with contraindications to estrogen or who choose not to use estrogen-containing contraception. Lastly, DMPA has few drug interactions and has an infrequent dosing schedule.

4. Side effects and disadvantages

During the first months of use, episodes of unpredictable bleeding and spotting lasting for 7 days or longer are common (Kaunitz, 2021a). Generally, the bleeding improves over time (Wu & Bartz, 2018). Approximately 50% of patients will achieve amenorrhea after 1 year of use, and over 70% will report amenorrhea with a longer duration of use (Arias et al., 2006). Studies have reported variable effects of DMPA on weight gain (Jacobstein & Polis, 2014). Overall, the data suggest that in both adult and adolescent DMPA users, there may be a subset of patients with rapid weight gain in the first 6 months of DMPA use who are at greatest risk for continued weight gain (Wu & Bartz, 2018). Weight gain can be of great concern to patients, and it is reasonable to discuss weight gain prior to starting this method. Data on the impact of DMPA on mood are also limited and conflicting (Wu & Bartz, 2018). Progestins may cause or exacerbate depressive symptoms in certain groups of patients, including those with a history of premenstrual syndrome or mood disorders (Kaunitz, 2021a). A history of depression should not be a contraindication to DMPA use, but patients on DMPA who experience symptoms suggestive of depression or have worsening of depressive symptoms should be screened, and discontinuation should be considered on a case-to-case basis (Wu & Bartz, 2018). After discontinuing DMPA, the average time to conception is 9 to 10 months, which is longer than for other hormonal contraceptive methods (Mishell, 1996). Because of this delay in return to fertility, it is reasonable for clinicians to counsel patients to discontinue DMPA use 12 to 18 months prior to when they desire conception.

5. Risks

Concerns regarding DMPA use and its impact on bone mineral density have been controversial. DMPA is associated with a decrease in bone mineral density that is generally temporary and reversible (Cundy et al., 1994). The greatest loss in bone mineral density occurs in the first 1–2 years of use and generally plateaus after 4–5 years (Scholes et al., 2002). There is a U.S. FDA black-box warning regarding the loss of bone mineral density. Given this black-box warning and the evidence, it is encouraged to counsel patients on the risks and benefits of using DMPA. ACOG, the Centers for Disease Control and Prevention (CDC), the Society for Adolescent Health and Medicine (SAHM), and the World Health Organization (WHO) all agree that the advantages of DMPA use as a contraceptive generally outweigh the theoretical concerns regarding skeletal harm (Kaunitz, 2021a).

6. Contraindications: For patients with multiple risk factors for cardiovascular disease and those with a history of stroke or ischemic heart disease, the WHO and the CDC classify DMPA as Category 3 (Curtis, Tepper, et al., 2016).

D. **Implant (Nexplanon)**

The etonogestrel implant is a single-rod contraceptive placed subdermally in the inner upper arm for long-acting, reversible contraception (Darney, 2021). Nexplanon is the only contraceptive implant currently available in the United States (Nelson et al., 2018). It is a single-rod system that measures 4 cm in length and 2 mm in diameter (Nelson et al., 2018). The semi-flexible white rod is made up of an ethylene vinyl acetate core that contains 68 mg of ENG (Nelson et al., 2018). This rod is radiopaque and can be identified with high-resolution sonography, plain radiograph, computed topography, or magnetic resonance imaging (Darney, 2021). All clinicians who wish to provide the ENG contraceptive implant must attend an FDA-approved, company-sponsored training program and have their competency in placement and removal of implants in artificial models certified by the course faculty (Creinin et al., 2017). Information on initial training or repeat training can be found on the manufacturer's website (www.nexplanontraining.com).

The ENG implant is labeled for 3 years of use. However, observational and trial data indicated that it is at least as effective as the copper intrauterine device and levonorgestrel implants for up to 5 years of use (McNicholas et al., 2015).

1. Mechanism of action

   Progestins such as ENG cause changes in cervical mucus and tubal motility that are unfavorable to sperm migration, thus inhibiting fertilization (Darney, 2021). At high doses, such as that in the implant, progestins also inhibit gonadotropin secretion, which inhibits follicular maturation and ovulation (Darney, 2021). ENG also suppresses endometrial activity, which makes the endometrium unreceptive to implantation (Darney, 2021).

2. Efficacy

   The ENG implant has a failure rate of 0.38% (NLM, 2021c).

3. Benefits

   Virtually every patient seeking contraception is eligible for use of the ENG implant (Curtis & Peipert, 2017). It provides pregnancy protection that is superior to the protection provided by any IUD or even permanent contraception. Additionally, the method is discreet and convenient. Among users with baseline dysmenorrhea, 75% showed improvement with implant use (Mansour et al., 2008). There is also a rapid return to fertility once discontinued, and efficacy is not affected by a patient's weight (Nelson et al., 2018).

4. Side effects and disadvantages

   The most common side effect of the ENG implant is unscheduled or irregular uterine bleeding (Darney, 2021). The number of unscheduled bleeding days was the highest in the first 3 months of use, decreased during the first year of use, then plateaued for the second and third years of use (Darney, 2021). Users may also experience headache, weight gain, acne, and mood changes (Nelson et al., 2018). The ENG implant does require minor office-based procedures for placement and removal. Implant-site reactions were reported by nearly 9% of patients. These included erythema, hematoma, swelling, bruising, and pain (Darney, 2021).

5. Risks

   There are very few risks associated with the ENG implant. There are some procedure-related risks, as discussed previously. Distant migration of the contraceptive implant is rare (Nelson et al., 2018).

6. Contraindications

   Most patients are candidates for the ENG implant. Only current or recent (<5 years) breast cancer is Category 4 in the USMEC (Curtis, Tepper, et al., 2016). There are a few medical conditions where the risk of the method exceeds the benefit, such as systemic lupus erythematosus (SLE) with positive or unknown antiphospholipid antibodies, unexplained abnormal vaginal bleeding, and past breast cancer (Curtis, Tepper, et al., 2016).

E. **Levonorgestrel intrauterine device (LNG IUD)**

The LNG IUDs (also called *intrauterine systems* [IUSs] or *intrauterine contraception* [IUC]) are T-shaped devices that release LNG. There are currently four LNG IUDs available in the United States: Mirena (52 mg), Liletta (52 mg), Kyleena (19.5 mg), and Skyla (13.5 mg), which release a varying amount of LNG (Madden, 2021). All have a T-shaped frame with a reservoir containing LNG and polyethylene threads attached to the base to assist with removal (Dean & Schwarz, 2018). They contain barium in the frame to make them detectable by radiograph, and the 19.5-mg and 13.5-mg versions also contain a silver ring at the top of the stem to distinguish them on ultrasound (NLM, 2021a, 2021e). Clinician training is needed to insert LNG IUDs. Clinicians should be trained on each type of LNG IUD because packaging and loading technique may vary.

The 52-mg LNG IUDs have an initial release of approximately 20 mcg per day, which declines to an average 10 mcg/day at 5 years (Madden, 2021). Liletta is approved for 6 years of use, and Mirena is approved for 8 years of use. Each frame is 32 by 32 mm, and the insertion tube diameter is 4.4 mm for Mirena and 4.8 mm for Liletta (NLM, 2020b).

The 19.5-mg LNG IUD initially releases 17.5 mcg per day, which declines to 7.4 mcg per day at 5 years (NLM, 2021a). It is FDA approved for 5 years of use. The 13.5-mg LNG IUD initially releases 14 mcg per day, which declines to 5 mcg per day at 3 years (NLM, 2021e). It is FDA approved for 3 years of use. The LNG 19.5 and LNG 13.5 each have a smaller frame

(28 by 30 mm) and a smaller insertion device diameter (3.8 mm) (NLM, 2021a, 2021e).

1. Mechanism of action

   IUDs work primarily by preventing fertilization via multiple mechanisms (Rivera et al., 1999). When the uterus is exposed to the foreign body of the frame, a sterile inflammatory reaction occurs, which is toxic to sperm and ova (Alvarez et al., 1988). The production of cytotoxic peptides and activation of enzymes lead to inhibition of sperm motility, reduced sperm capacitation and survival, and increased phagocytosis of sperm (Ammälä et al., 1995; Sagiroglu, 1971). LNG thickens cervical mucus, suppresses the endometrium by reducing uterine artery blood flow, and impairs sperm function by changing the uterine immune microenvironment (Dean & Schwarz, 2018). Multiple studies suggest that IUDs do not stop implantation (Dean & Schwarz, 2018).

2. Efficacy

   The cumulative pregnancy rates for the 52 LNG IUDs are 0.1%–0.2% (first year), 0.5%–1.1% (at 5 years), and 0.5% (at 7 years) (Dean & Schwarz, 2018). The cumulative pregnancy rate for the 19.5-mg LNG IUD is 0.16% at 1 year of use and 0.37% at 5 years (Dickey & Seymour, 2021). The 1-year and 3-year cumulative pregnancy rates for the 13.5-mg IUD are 0.4% and 0.9%, respectively (Dickey & Seymour, 2021).

3. Benefits

   This method is highly effective at pregnancy prevention; does not require regular user adherence to maintain high effectiveness; is reversible, long acting, and cost-effective; has few side effects; is private and discreet; and is safe for most patients (Madden, 2021). There are noncontraceptive benefits from LNG IUD use as well. There is a reduced risk of cervical, endometrial, and ovarian cancers (Creinin et al., 2017; Soini et al., 2014; Wheeler et al., 2019). LNG IUD use is associated with a reduction in heavy menstrual bleeding, anemia, dysmenorrhea, endometriosis-related pain, endometrial hyperplasia, and PID (Madden, 2021). The FDA has approved the use of LNG IUDs for the treatment of heavy menstrual bleeding (NLM, 2021b).

4. Side effects and disadvantages

   Common side effects of the LNG IUD include changes in menstrual patterns, pain or discomfort at the time of insertion, cramping, and hormonal side effects. Irregular bleeding or spotting is the norm in the early months of using an LNG IUD, with considerable improvement after the first 3 months (Diedrich et al., 2015). Overall, LNG IUDs are associated with a reduction in menstrual blood loss and may result in amenorrhea. Amenorrhea develops in 20% of LNG 52-mg users by 1 year, 12% of LNG 19.5-mg users, and 6% of LNG 13.50-mg users (Dickey & Seymour, 2021). Counseling regarding expected bleeding changes prior to LNG IUD insertion may improve patients' expectations and satisfaction (Pocius & Bartz, 2021). Hormonal side effects of breast tenderness, mood changes, hair loss, and acne may be reported, although systemic levels of LNG are far lower than with other hormonal methods (Dean & Schwarz, 2018).

5. Risks

   Serious complications with LNG IUD use are rare and include expulsion, PID, perforation, and ectopic pregnancy if contraceptive failure does occur (Pocius & Bartz, 2021). The risk of LNG IUD expulsion in the first year of use is 3%–6% (Dean & Schwarz, 2018). Risk factors include prior expulsion, history of heavy menstrual bleeding or severe dysmenorrhea, and immediate and delayed insertion postpartum or post–second-trimester abortion (Pocius & Bartz, 2021). Historically, there have been concerns that IUD use increases the risk of PID. However, extensive epidemiologic studies do not support this concern (Harper et al., 2008). Although PID resulting from IUD insertion is rare, clinicians should have a low threshold for empiric treatment of PID in patients who have recently undergone IUD insertion, given the possible serious sequelae of PID (Pocius & Bartz, 2021). Prophylactic antibiotic use is not warranted prior to IUD insertion (Grimes & Schulz, 2001). Patients who have an IUD in situ and who are diagnosed with PID do not require IUD removal (Curtis, Tepper, et al., 2016). Additionally, it is a safe method for adolescents, nulliparous patients, patients who have multiple partners, patients who have a history of ectopic pregnancies, and patients who have had a history of PID (Dean & Schwarz, 2018).

6. Contraindications

   USMEC contraindications include post-abortion or puerperal sepsis, unexplained vaginal bleeding, persistent elevated human chorionic gonadotropin (HCG) levels or malignant disease, untreated cervical cancer, endometrial cancer, uterine cavity distortion or anatomical abnormalities, current PID, current purulent cervicitis, current chlamydia or gonorrhea infection, and pelvic tuberculosis (Curtis, Tepper, et al., 2016).

F. *Copper T 380A Intrauterine Contraception (IUC) (ParaGard)*

The Copper T 380A IUC was introduced in the United States in 1988 and is now available in most countries around the world (Dean & Schwarz, 2018). The Copper T 380A IUC is inserted into the uterine cavity by a trained healthcare professional. It consists of a T-shaped polyethylene frame that is wrapped in fine copper wire (Cooper Surgical, 2022). A 3-mm ball at the base of the vertical stem decreases the risk of perforation, and two white monofilament strings are knotted through this ball and aid in removal (Cooper Surgical, 2022).

The Copper T 380A is labeled for 10 years of use by the FDA, although data indicate high effectiveness for 12 years (Ti et al., 2020).

1. Mechanism of action

   As with the LNG IUD, the copper IUC prevents sperm from fertilizing ova. When the uterus is exposed to a foreign body, a sterile inflammatory reaction occurs, which is toxic to ova and sperm (Alvarez et al., 1988). The production of cytotoxic peptides and activation of enzymes lead to inhibition of sperm motility, reduced sperm capacitation and survival, and increased phagocytosis of sperm (Ammälä et al., 1995; Sagiroglu, 1971). The addition of copper enhances the cytotoxic inflammatory response within the endometrium and impairs sperm mobility viability (Ortiz et al., 1996; Stanford & Mikolajczyk, 2002). Ovulation is not affected by the Copper T 380A IUC. Multiple studies suggest that IUCs do not stop implantation (Dean & Schwarz, 2018).

2. Efficacy

   Because of the mechanism of action of the copper IUD, the rates of efficacy for perfect and typical use are similar. The efficacy is 99.4% with perfect use and 99.2% with typical use in the first year (Heinemann et al., 2015).

3. Benefits

   Once the Copper T 380A is inserted, the method is immediately effective and does not require further action by the patient. It is highly effective, reversible, and cost-effective. The Copper T 380A does not contain hormones, and as a result, it does not cause anovulation or amenorrhea, which may be attractive to some patients (Dean & Schwarz, 2018).

4. Side effects and disadvantages

   IUC can cause heavier menstrual periods and increased cramping during and outside of menses. There are rare insertion risks of perforation, infection, and possible spontaneous expulsion (Madden, 2021).

5. Risks

   Risks are similar to those of the LNG IUD, including the rare risks of expulsion, PID, perforation, and ectopic pregnancy if contraceptive failure does occur. Specific to the copper IUD, clinically relevant allergy to copper is extremely rare (Fage et al., 2014). Although serum copper levels are higher in Copper T 380A users compared with nonusers, this increase in circulating copper has not been found to cause adverse clinical effects unless the patient has an allergy to copper or has Wilson disease (De la Cruz et al., 2005).

6. Contraindications

   Contraindications to the copper IUC are similar to those for the LNG IUD. Additionally, patients with Wilson disease or copper allergy should avoid use of the copper IUC (Curtis, Tepper, et al., 2016).

G. Emergency contraception (EC)

Emergency contraceptives are methods that can be used after intercourse to prevent pregnancy. EC does not interrupt an existing pregnancy and does not cause abortion (Turok, 2021). These methods can be used after intercourse when no contraception was used, when a method was used incorrectly, or in cases when sex was forced without the use of contraception (Turok, 2021). EC must be initiated within a specific time frame, and the time intervals vary by product.

In the United States, there are two types of dedicated emergency contraceptive pills (ECPs), 30-mg ulipristal acetate (UPA) and 1.5-mg LNG (Trussel & Cleland, et al., 2018). The copper and 52-mg LNG IUDs and the less effective high-dose COC (called the *Yuzpe method*) may also be used (Trussel & Cleland, et al., 2018; Turok et al., 2021). The IUDs with less progesterone have not been studied and should not be used as EC. UPA is a 30-mg pill that should be taken as soon as possible, within 120 hours (5 days) of unprotected intercourse (NLM, 2020a). Progestin-containing contraceptives should not be used with UPA or for 5 days after UPA administration because of concerns that the progestin contraception will interfere with the UPA action (Hsiang & Dunn, 2016; NLM, 2020a). Oral LNG 1.5 mg is licensed for use up to 72 hours after unprotected intercourse, although it is used off-label beyond that time frame with established efficacy up to 120 hours (Piaggo et al., 2011). The IUDs should be inserted within 5 days of unprotected intercourse (Turok, 2021). The Yuzpe method (COCs and LNG contraceptive pills) is an alternative method of oral EC. To provide EC using the Yuzpe method, the initial dose must contain the equivalent of 100–120 mcg of EE and 0.5–0.6 mg of LNG (or the equivalent) (Trusell & Cleland, et al., 2018). The same dose is then repeated 12 hours after the first dose.

1. Mechanism of action

   The UPA and LNG EC regimens work by preventing ovulation (Brache et al., 2013). LNG prevents ovulation if taken in the pre-ovulatory period by blocking the LH surge, thus inhibiting follicular development and egg release (Turok, 2021). UPA delays ovulation in both the pre-ovulatory period and after the LH surge starts (Turok, 2021). It is this extended period of activity that may explain UPA's greater efficacy in preventing pregnancy when compared with oral LNG (Turok, 2021). When used as a regular or emergency method of contraception, IUDs act primarily to prevent fertilization (Trussel et al., 2018). The mechanisms by which it does this in the case of emergency contraceptive use is not clear. It is plausible that postcoital IUD placement may involve the same mechanisms of action that standard use does (Turok, 2021). When COCs are used, such as in the Yuzpe method, they work by inhibiting or delaying ovulation (Trussel et al., 2018).

2. Efficacy

   There are many factors that affect the calculation of risk of pregnancy, including whether the patient had sex in the fertile window, how many unprotected intercourse exposures the patient had in the cycle, their age, and whether they were also using another contraceptive method (Turok, 2021). The risk of pregnancy following placement of an IUD is less than 1% (Cleland et al., 2012; Turok et al., 2021). Data from trials comparing UPA to oral LNG report pregnancy rates of 1.8% for UPA users versus 2.6% for oral LNG users (Turok, 2021). Importantly, the risk of pregnancy increases with increased weight for both UPA and oral LNG (Glasier et al., 2011). Body weight does not affect the efficacy of the IUD, which in part contributes to its overall high efficacy (Xu et al., 2012). Efficacy for UPA and LNG appears to decrease with increasing weight (Turok, 2021). Effectiveness rates of the Yuzpe method range from 53% to 47% (Trussel et al., 2003).

3. Benefits
   EC can prevent pregnancy after unprotected sexual intercourse or after contraceptive failure or accident (Trussel et al., 2018). Placement of an IUD provides ongoing contraception.

4. Side effects and disadvantages
   Overall, all EC methods are safe and well tolerated. Side effects of the IUD used as EC are similar to those seen after routine placement and may include abdominal discomfort and vaginal bleeding or spotting (Trussel et al., 2018). Nausea, vomiting, menstrual changes, and headaches are commonly reported side effects of oral EC use (Turok, 2021). The most common side effects of the Yuzpe method are nausea and vomiting, which occur more often with this method compared with UPA and LNG (Shen et al., 2019).

5. Risks
   The risks of the IUD, LNG, and Yuzpe methods are the same for EC use as for standard use. There are no known adverse effects on pregnancy from oral EC methods if one were to occur (Trussel et al., 2018). Common side effects from UPA use include headache, abdominal pain, nausea, dysmenorrhea, fatigue, and dizziness (NLM, 2020a).

6. Contraindications
   Contraindications to the Yuzpe method and IUDs are the same as for standard use of those methods. There are no contraindications to the use of any oral ECPs, with the exception of pregnancy (Curtis, Tepper, et al., 2016). ECPs should not be used in pregnancy not because they are dangerous in pregnancy but because they are ineffective (Trussel et al., 2018).

H. Condoms
   The external condom (also known as the *male condom*) is among the most widely available and commonly used contraceptive methods in the United States (Warner & Steiner, 2018). External condoms are made from latex, lamb caecum, and synthetic materials. The internal condom is also known as the *female condom*. FC2, formerly known as *Reality*, is the only internal condom available in the United States (Nelson & Harwood, 2018). The FC2 is a soft, loose-fitting nitrile sheath with two flexible rings (Veru, Inc., n.d.). The internal ring is contained within the closed end of the sheath. This ring serves as an insertion mechanism and internal anchor, and it lies against the cervix (Hoke et al., 2021). The external ring remains outside of the vagina after insertion, holds the condom in place, and covers part of the vulva (Hoke et al., 2021). Silicone-based lubricant lines the inside of the condom, and additional lubricant may be used. The condom is about 17 cm in length, which is similar to that of an external condom (Hoke et al., 2021).

1. Mechanism of action
   Both condoms work by providing a physical barrier to the migration of sperm to the upper reproductive tract, where fertilization occurs (Bartz, 2020). The condom acts as a physical barrier by covering the penile glans and shaft. By blocking the passage of semen, it prevents pregnancy; by covering the major portals of entry and exit for STI pathogens, it prevents infections (Warner & Steiner, 2018).

2. Efficacy
   Perfect-use efficacy for the external condom is 98%, and typical-use efficacy is 87% (Warner et al., 2021). This significant difference in efficacy is a result of the failure to use condoms during every act of intercourse and the failure to use condoms correctly throughout intercourse. The first-year efficacy rates of the FC2 are 95% with perfect use and 79% with typical use (Nelson & Harwood, 2018).

3. Benefits
   Advantages of condoms include protection against STIs, reversibility, low cost, accessibility, ability to be discreetly carried, and lack of disruption to fertility (Warner & Steiner, 2018). They may be used during menses and postpartum (Nelson & Harwood, 2018). They are available without a prescription, and some insurance plans may reimburse for them. The FC2 may be used by patients who cannot use external condoms due to issues of erectile dysfunction or because the penis cannot be fitted with any of the currently available male condoms (Cecil et al., 2010). Condoms are also a method that can be controlled by those AMAB.

4. Side effects and disadvantages
   Because condoms are used at the time of coitus, they must be used consistently and correctly, with each act of intercourse, to be effective. Disadvantages of external condoms include reports of decreased sensation by those that use them, requirement for partner cooperation, lack of spontaneity, and breakage or slippage (Warner & Steiner, 2018). Disadvantages specific to the FC2 include the potential for challenging or awkward placement and that it may become dislodged easily. Additionally, the FC2 is visible outside of the vagina, which may be bothersome to some (Nelson & Harwood, 2018). If the

FC2 is not placed properly, it can cause discomfort, pain, or irritation to users (Ramadimetja et al., 2016). External condoms made from lamb caecum do not prevent STIs (Warner & Steiner, 2018). The internal condom should not be used with the external condom. It is possible that the external condom can stick to the FC2, causing one, or both, to slip off or tear.

5. Risks
Latex condoms present a risk of allergy.

6. Contraindications
Latex allergy is the only contraindication to latex condom use. There are no contraindications to condoms made from other materials.

I. FemCap cervical cap

The FemCap is the only cervical cap available in the United States. It is a reusable silicone cup kept in place by a variable-size brim that stabilizes the unit against the vaginal walls and a rim that fits high into the vaginal vault. There is a thin loop of silicone over the bowl that facilitates removal of the cap (Nelson & Harwood, 2018). The cervical cap comes in three different sizes: small (22 mm) for patients who have never been pregnant, medium (26 mm) for patients who have had an abortion or cesarean delivery, and large (30 mm) for patients who have had a full-term vaginal delivery (FemCap, 2020). Fitting by a trained clinician is not required, but it is preferred and encouraged because sizing and anatomy can vary regardless of parity. Additionally, the clinician can teach correct insertion and removal.

The FemCap should be placed at least 15 minutes in advance of coitus and must be used along with a spermicidal jelly. About one-half teaspoon of spermicide should be placed into the inside of the bowl and one-quarter teaspoon in the groove between the brim and the outside of the bowl, then spread over the brim (Nelson & Harwood, 2018). The FemCap is then placed inside the vagina with the concave side directly over the cervix. The FemCap must remain in place for 6 hours after the last intercourse but should not be used for longer than 48 hours for any one use (FemCap, 2020).

1. Mechanism of action
Cervical caps hold spermicide against the cervix to kill sperm and also prevent fertilization by blocking sperm transport into the upper genital tract (Nelson & Harwood, 2018).

2. Efficacy
The FemCap is 86% effective for patients who have never given birth and 79% effective for patients who have given birth (Planned Parenthood [PP], 2022b).

3. Benefits
The FemCap is well tolerated and easy to fit. It can be placed in advance, can be used for multiple acts of intercourse, is reusable and easy to clean, and can be used with other methods (Nelson & Harwood, 2018).

4. Side effects and disadvantages
Disadvantages include the recommendation for a clinician exam, it may not fit all users, users need to be willing and able to place the device vaginally, resizing may be needed, use may interrupt sex, it may be difficult to remove, and there may be discomfort or trauma to the cervix with use (Nelson & Harwood, 2018).

5. Risks
Use of the FemCap does not pose any significant health risks.

6. Contraindications
The FemCap should not be used during the immediate postpartum period (about 6 weeks) or if the patient has cervicitis, PID, or a history of toxic shock syndrome (TSS) (Nelson & Harwood, 2018).

J. Diaphragm

The diaphragm is a reusable contraceptive device consisting of a dome-shaped cup with a flexible rim. The diaphragm acts as a physical barrier that covers the cervix, preventing sperm from fertilizing an egg. Diaphragms are available in single-size options and multisize options (Bartz, 2020). In the United States, diaphragms are made of silicone, but latex options may be available in other countries. In the Unites States, the silicone single-size diaphragm, commercially named Caya, has largely replaced the original silicone multisize wide-seal diaphragms (Nelson & Harwood, 2018).

The Caya diaphragm is 75 mm long by 67 mm wide and does not require a pelvic examination for fitting (HPSRx, 2018). Its spring enables Caya to be used for a variety of vaginal and cervical sizes and in users who have different degrees of vaginal support. The device fits about 80% of individuals (Nelson & Harwood, 2018). It is available at most pharmacies or directly through the manufacturer with a prescription (HPSRx, 2018). Prior to insertion, the user should hold the diaphragm up to the light, ensuring that the dome of the diaphragm is intact and that there are no tears or holes. The Caya diaphragm is used with spermicide (Mauck et al., 2017). One teaspoon of spermicide should be put into the larger cup and spread around the rim just before placement (HPSRx, 2018). The user pinches the diaphragm in half and places it deeply inside the vagina, ensuring that the cervix is completely covered (HPSRx, 2018). Although the Caya diaphragm does not require a fitting, the patient should see a clinician for examination to ensure proper placement and fitting and to review the best positions for insertion and removal (Nelson & Harwood, 2018).

Ideally, the diaphragm is placed in the vagina less than 1 hour prior to sexual intercourse. If the diaphragm has been left in the vagina for more than 1 hour prior to intercourse, an additional application of spermicide should be applied (Bartz, 2020). The diaphragm must be left in the vagina for 6 hours after intercourse and not more than 24 hours

(HPSRx, 2018). If additional acts of coitus are anticipated, the Caya diaphragm should be kept in place and additional spermicide should be added into the vagina (HPSRx, 2018).

1. Mechanism of action
   The diaphragm prevents fertilization by blocking sperm transport into the upper genital tract. The addition of spermicide to the diaphragm adds another mechanism of action (see Spermicides section).
2. Efficacy
   In the Caya clinical trial, the efficacy rate was 89.6% (Schwartz et al., 2015).
3. Benefits
   The diaphragm is reusable, and the Caya diaphragm may be reused for 2 years (HPSRx, 2018). The Caya diaphragm can be used with other contraceptive methods, is easy to clean, can be used with multiple acts of intercourse, and is generally not detected by the partner (Nelson & Harwood, 2018). Diaphragms have been associated with lower risks for transmitting cervical infections, such as gonorrhea and chlamydia, but no confirmation of that protection with the new diaphragms has been published (D'Oro et al., 1994).
4. Side effects and disadvantages
   Proper placement is required for efficacy, which may require practice and comfort in placing it vaginally (Nelson & Harwood, 2018). Caya cannot be worn for more than 24 hours and should not be used until at least 6 weeks postpartum (HPSRx, 2018). It requires placement prior to sexual contact, and spermicide use may cause local irritation or allergy (Nelson & Harwood, 2018).
5. Risks
   There is a potential risk of TSS, so it is recommended that patients do not use it during menses (Nelson & Harwood, 2018).
6. Contraindications
   It is not an ideal method for those who have repeated urinary tract infections (UTIs), a history of TSS, or significant pelvic relaxation or congenital anatomical anomalies of the reproductive tract that interfere with proper placement (Bartz, 2020). If the patient has an allergy to spermicide or any component of the diaphragm, this method should not be used.

K. **Spermicides**
Spermicides are available as gels, creams, suppositories, foams, films, and sponges. All spermicides currently available in the United States use Nonoxynol-9 (N-9) as their active ingredient and are available over the counter (Nelson & Harwood, 2018). Improper use can alter efficacy. Spermicidal gels, creams, and foams are commonly marketed for use with a diaphragm but can also be used alone or with a condom (Nelson & Harwood, 2018). Spermicidal films and suppositories can be used alone for contraception or with condoms. Rarely are they used with diaphragms or cervical caps.

Each sheet must be introduced into the vagina on or near the cervix at least 15 minutes before intercourse to allow time for the film to melt and disperse (Nelson & Harwood, 2018). All spermicides except the sponge require reinsertion after 1 hour and after each act of intercourse.

The contraceptive sponge is a single-use vaginal spermicide known commercially as the Today Sponge (PP, 2020a). At the time of writing, manufacturing of the sponge had been discontinued, with no available information about plans to restart (Mayer Labs, n.d.).

1. Mechanism of action
   N-9 disrupts the membranes of sperm's flagella and body to immobilize or destroy it (Nelson & Harwood, 2018). Additionally, the sponge fits snugly against the cervix, blocking the entrance to the uterus (PP, 2020a).
2. Efficacy
   With correct and consistent use, spermicides as a single agent have a first-year efficacy rate of 84% and a typical-use efficacy rate of 79% (Nelson & Harwood, 2018).
3. Benefits
   Advantages include availability, lower cost margin, and provision of lubrication (Nelson & Harwood, 2018). Additionally, they have a rapid onset of activity and can enable multiple acts of intercourse (PP, 2020a).
4. Side effects and disadvantages
   Disadvantages include high failure rate, messiness, and risk of causing local skin irritation or breakdown (Nelson & Harwood, 2018). Breakdown of the epithelial cells of the vagina, cervix, and rectum can increase the transmission of human immunodeficiency virus (HIV) (Roddy et al., 2002).
5. Risks
   The primary risk of spermicide use is allergy or sensitivity to product components (Bartz, 2020), as well as a potential increased risk of HIV transmission (Kreiss et al., 1992; Roddy et al., 2002).
6. Contraindications
   Patients at high risk for HIV should not use spermicides alone or in combination with other methods (CDC, 2002).

L. **Vaginal pH regulator gel**
A vaginal pH regulator gel, commercially known as Phexxi, contains lactic acid, citric acid, and potassium bitartrate and was approved for contraceptive use in 2020 (Thomas et al., 2020). This product provides on-demand contraception and must be inserted into the vagina prior to intercourse. The bioadhesive and viscosity-retaining properties allow this gel to coat the vagina and stay in place for up to 10 hours (Bartz, 2020). Phexxi is supplied in single-dose, prefilled vaginal applicators containing 5 mg of gel administered intravaginally no more than 1 hour before each act of vaginal intercourse (Steinberg & Lynch, 2021). Dosing should be repeated if additional acts of intercourse

occur within 1 hour (Steinberg & Lynch, 2021). Phexxi can be used with other forms of contraception but should not be used with the vaginal contraceptive ring (PP, 2022c).

1. Mechanism of action
The vaginal pH regulator gel creates an acidic environment in the vagina, which immobilizes and incapacitates sperm (Baker & Chen, 2022).
2. Efficacy
Perfect-use efficacy is 96%, and actual-use efficacy is 86%–89% depending on the study (Steinberg & Lynch, 2021).
3. Benefits
The vaginal pH regulator spermicide supports vaginal defense systems, and this may provide protection against vaginal infections and microbial imbalances (Keller et al., 2012). The lactic acid component of the vaginal pH regulator decreases the risk of acquisition of chlamydia or gonorrhea (Chappell et al., 2021).
4. Side effects and disadvantages
Vaginal and penile irritation are reported with vaginal pH regulator gel use (Steinberg & Lynch, 2021).
5. Risks
The initial trial of the pH regulator gel found that more than 5% of users reported bacterial vaginosis (Evofem Biosciences, 2021). Genitourinary tract infections were reported in 5.7% of study participants (Baker & Chen, 2022).
6. Contraindications
Patients with allergy or sensitivity to the components in the product should not use Phexxi. It should not be used in patients with urinary tract abnormalities or a history of recurrent UTIs (Steinberg & Lynch, 2021).

M. *Natural family planning (NFP)*
NFP methods help patients understand when they are fertile so that they can avoid vaginal intercourse or use another method. NFP methods include the fertility awareness method (FAM) and the lactational amenorrhea method (LAM). Extensive patient education is vital to helping patients understand and track these changes. FAM methods are best taught by a well-trained clinician. The summaries that follow serve as an overview only.

FAM involves identifying the fertile days of the menstrual cycle. This can be done by observing, recording, and interpreting the body's fertility signs and by keeping track of menstrual cycle days to understand which days are most likely to be fertile (Jennings & Polis, 2018). Studies using lab tests that measured estrogen and progesterone metabolites in urine and ultrasound images of ovarian follicle rupture have established that people are fertile from 5 days before ovulation to 24 hours after ovulation (Wilcox et al., 1998). Thus, there are only about 6 days during the cycle when unprotected intercourse can actually result in pregnancy, related to the lifespan of the gametes (Wilcox et al., 1998, 2000). An ovum is viable for 12–24 hours after release, and sperm live for 3–4 days in the genital tract (Jennings & Polis, 2018). In 95% of menstrual cycles, ovulation occurs in the 4 days before or after the midpoint of the cycle, and in approximately 30% of cycles, ovulation occurs at the exact midpoint of the cycle (Jennings, 2020). Even though ovulation does not occur on the same day of each cycle, in cycles that range between 26 and 32 days long, the fertile window is highly likely to fall within cycle days 8–19 (Arévalo et al., 1999).

Observing the changes in vaginal discharge that occur over a typical 28-day menstrual cycle helps predict ovulation. See **Table 21-2** for a summary of the changes.

The TwoDay Method is a more simplified tracking method based only on the presence or absence of cervical secretions (Sinai et al., 1999). The user monitors their vaginal discharge and then asks themselves two questions: "Did I have any secretions today?" and "Did I have any secretions yesterday?" (Sinai et al., 1999). If any secretions are noted today or yesterday, then today is a potentially fertile day (Sinai et al., 1999). Additionally, basal body temperature (BBT) changes over the course of the menstrual cycle. It is lower in the first half of the cycle and begins to rise around the time of ovulation (Freundl et al., 2010). The symptothermal method uses both BBT and cervical secretions. Some users also track cervical length and position (Jennings & Polis, 2018).

Some FAM methods track menstrual cycles. The Standard Day Method is an option for people with menstrual cycles between 26 and 32 days (Jennings & Polis, 2018). This is done by counting the first day of menstrual bleeding as day 1. Unprotected intercourse is permitted on days 1 to 7 and from day 20 to the end of the cycle (Jennings & Polis, 2018). Many patients who use this method use CycleBeads, a string of colored beads used to help keep track of the days of the menstrual cycle.

There are many computer and smartphone applications to support FAMs. Some apps are essentially digital platforms that support the use of an existing

Table 21-2 Typical Pattern for Vaginal Secretions in Ovulatory Cycles (Jennings, 2020)

Menses
No secretions for 3 to 4 days
Scant, cloudy sticky secretions for 3–5 days
Abundant, clear, wet, stretchy secretions for the 3–4 days immediately before, during, and immediately after ovulation
No secretions for 11–14 days
Menses

FAM, such as the sympothermal method or CycleBeads (Jennings, 2020). These apps replace paper charts and graphs with digital ones. Not all these apps have been empirically studied, so it is important to proceed with some caution (Jennings & Polis, 2018). It is also important to review privacy policies because these apps may sell data about patients' menstrual cycles.

The LAM is the use of exclusive breastfeeding to suppress ovulation in an amenorrheic patient for up to 6 months after delivery (Jennings, 2020). Users must be amenorrheic, nursing at least every 3 hours, and within the first 6 months of delivery. LAM requires nearly full breastfeeding to maximize the amount of suckling, which disrupts GnRH, leading to anovulation (McNeilly, 2001; McNeilly et al., 1994). Formula supplementation should be given only infrequently, in small amounts, and not by bottle (Kennedy & Goldsmith, 2018). Milk expression by hand or pump is not a substitute for breastfeeding (Kennedy & Goldsmith, 2018).

1. Mechanism of action
   Mechanisms of action are described earlier.
2. Efficacy
   The perfect-use efficacy of various FAMs ranges from 94% to 98%, although estimates are hard to gather, given that education on these methods is inconsistent (Jennings & Polis, 2018). Typical-use efficacy ranges from 80% to 88% (Jennings & Polis, 2018). LAM provides more than 98% efficacy in the first 6 months following a birth (Kennedy & Goldsmith, 2018).
3. Benefits
   There are no health risks or side effects. Some patients with religious beliefs that do not allow for the use of other methods of contraception may use FAMs (Jennings & Polis, 2018). Additionally, they are low to no cost.
4. Side effects and disadvantages
   These methods can be an obstacle for patients who do not have their partner's cooperation (Jennings & Polis, 2018). FAMs may prove challenging for those with irregular cycles. LAM cannot be used by patients who need to return to work outside the home or who are not breastfeeding exclusively.
5. Risks
   There are no health risks associated with these methods.
6. Contraindications
   There are no contraindications.

N. **Permanent contraception**
Permanent contraception is one of the safest, most effective, and most cost-effective contraceptive methods available (Hou & Roncari, 2018). Although terms used to describe permanent contraception for persons AFAB include *tubal ligation* and *sterilization*, this chapter uses the term *tubal surgery*. Hysterectomy also provides permanent contraception, although the risks are too high to recommend this surgery solely for contraception (Hou & Roncari, 2018). Tubal surgery is the world's most commonly used method of family planning; in 2019, it was used by 23.7% of all contraceptive users, for a total of 219 million persons worldwide (United Nations, Department of Economic and Social Affairs, 2019). When patients are considering permanent contraception, they should be counseled to discuss vasectomy with their partner, if applicable. Vasectomy carries fewer risks and has greater efficacy than tubal surgery (ACOG Committee on Ethics [COE], 2017), but a full discussion is beyond the scope of this chapter. Although these surgeries will not be performed by advanced practice nurses, it is important that all clinicians counsel patients appropriately before providing referrals for the procedure.

Tubal surgery is indicated for patients who are certain they have completed their childbearing and who do not wish to use a reversible contraceptive method. Techniques include electrocoagulation, mechanical occlusion, ligation, or removal of the fallopian tubes (Hou & Roncari, 2018).

A hysteroscopic approach to sterilization called *Essure* is no longer available in the United States. Essure was approved by the FDA in 2002 and involved the placement of nickel-titanium micro inserts in the fallopian tubes, which, over 12 weeks, caused fibrosis and occlusion of the fallopian tubes (Loder & Flaum, 2019). Increasing reports about side effects led to safety concerns about the device. One study found that the most reported symptoms following Essure placement were abdominal pain, back pain, fatigue, leg and hip pain, dysmenorrhea, and heavy menstrual bleeding (Maassen et al., 2019). A black-box warning was placed on the device in 2015 by the FDA, and the subsequent decrease in sales led to the manufacturer removing it from the market (Loder & Flaum, 2019). If a patient still has Essure and is without symptoms, removal is not required. However, if a patient is having symptoms, a detailed physical exam with a pelvic exam and discussion about the risks and benefits of removal is warranted (Loder & Flaum, 2019).

1. Mechanism of action
   Tubal surgery blocks fertilization by cutting, occluding, or removing the fallopian tubes to prevent the sperm and egg from uniting (Hou & Roncari, 2018).
2. Efficacy
   Tubal surgery is far more effective than short-term user-dependent reversible contraceptive methods (Hou & Roncari, 2018). The cumulative 10-year failure rate of permanent contraception for persons AFAB is 1%–2% (Peterson et al., 1996).
3. Benefits
   Tubal surgeries are highly effective, are safe, lack significant long-term side effects, have a short recovery period, are cost-effective, and are private and discreet (Hou & Roncari, 2018). Tubal surgery appears to have a protective effect against ovarian cancer that

persists over many years (Green et al., 1997; Irwin et al., 1991; Kjaer et al., 2004). Although occlusive techniques are estimated to lower a patient's lifetime risk of ovarian cancer by 24%–36%, bilateral salpingectomy may create an overall 49% reduction in ovarian cancer (Cibula et al., 2011; Yoon et al., 2016). For this reason, the use of salpingectomy for tubal sterilization is increasing (Powell et al., 2017).

4. Side effects and disadvantages
Restoring fertility after permanent contraception is difficult. It is expensive and requires costly assisted reproductive technology (ACOG COE, 2017). Patients who use Medicaid funds must be age 21 or older, and they must wait 30 days after signing a consent document before undergoing the procedure (ACOG COE, 2017). Lastly, patients who undergo tubal surgery at age 30 or younger are at greater risk for regret (Hillis et al., 1999; Jamieson et al., 2002; Schmidt et al., 2000).

5. Risks
All surgical procedures carry some risk specific to the nature of the surgery and anesthetic used (Hou & Roncari, 2018). If the method fails, there is a higher probability of the subsequent pregnancy being an ectopic pregnancy (Peterson et al., 1996).

6. Contraindications
Although there are no absolute medical contraindications, some patients may be at higher risk for surgical complications from these surgical procedures and the necessary anesthesia (Braaten & Dutton, 2022). These groups include patients with a history of complicated abdominal surgery, significantly higher weight, significant medical comorbidity, or severe respiratory disease (Hou & Roncari, 2018).

O. Withdrawal method (coitus interruptus)
The withdrawal method, formally known as *coitus interruptus*, is a nonhormonal method that relies on the penis being withdrawn out of the vagina and away from the external genitalia before ejaculation. The number of patients reporting ever having used the withdrawal method has increased over the last three decades, from 25% in 1982 to 60% in 2010 (Daniels & Mosher, 2013). Many patients do not consider withdrawal to be a legitimate method of contraception and fail to report use unless specifically asked about it (Artega & Gomez, 2016; Frohwirth et al., 2016; Whittaker et al., 2010).

1. Mechanism of action
Withdrawal keeps sperm out of the vagina and thus inhibits fertilization by preventing contact between spermatozoa and the ovum (Jones, 2018). Penile–vaginal intercourse occurs until ejaculation is impending, at which time the penis is withdrawn from the vagina and away from the external genitalia of the partner (Jones, 2018).

2. Efficacy
The probability of pregnancy during the first year of typical use with the withdrawal method is around 20% (Sundaram et al., 2017).

3. Benefits
Despite lower efficacy, the withdrawal method has a few advantages. It requires no devices, no chemicals or hormones are involved, it is readily available, and it has virtually no cost. Some patients will choose this method because it does not require a physical examination or contact with a clinic or pharmacy (Rogow & Horowitz, 1995).

4. Side effects and disadvantages
There are no known side effects. One disadvantage of this method is that the pre-ejaculate fluid contains spermatozoa and could theoretically fertilize an egg (Killick et al., 2011; Pudney et al., 1992). This method has a relatively low efficacy rate. This method relies on the partner to be aware of their own sensations to determine when ejaculation will occur, and this may be difficult for some partners (Jones, 2018).

5. Risks
There are no known risks.

6. Contraindications
There are no absolute contraindications to this method.

II. Database
A. Subjective
Much of the Database section is relevant for all methods; after the initial section, additional subjective information will be reviewed by method as indicated.

1. For all methods
   a. Medical history
   b. Allergies
   c. Desire for future pregnancy and ideal timing, if desired
   d. Obstetrical history: recent delivery, pregnancy, abortion, breastfeeding. See Chapter 29, The Postpartum Visit, for more information on providing contraception after delivery.
   e. Sexual history: recent unprotected intercourse, STI risk, types of sexual activity, gender and sex assigned at birth of partners
   f. Current or past history of IPV
   g. Risk of current, undetected pregnancy
   h. Contraceptive history: recent use of contraception, prior use, satisfaction, adherence
   i. Preference for and comfort with different methods
   j. Side effects: tolerance and acceptance of various side effects
   k. Current medication use
   l. Menstrual history: date of last menstrual period, regularity, concerns regarding pain or heavy bleeding
   m. Financial concerns

2. CHC
   a. Family history of blood clot or clotting disorder; breast, uterine, or ovarian cancer
   b. Smoking status

3. Emergency contraception
   a. Intimate partner violence (IPV): EC should be offered in cases of sexual assault or nonconsensual act within the EC provision window.

4. Barrier methods and spermicide (external condom, internal condom, FemCap cervical cap, diaphragm, vaginal pH regulator gel, and contraceptive sponge)
   a. Medical history: history of PID or TSS (FemCap and diaphragm), congenital anatomical anomalies of the reproductive tract (diaphragm), allergies to latex and nonoxynol-9 (condoms, diaphragm, FemCap, and spermicide), allergy or sensitivity to the components in Phexxi, patients with urinary tract abnormalities or a history of recurrent UTIs (Phexxi)
5. Intrauterine contraception
   a. Medical history: unexplained vaginal bleeding; cervical or endometrial cancer; current post-abortion sepsis; current puerperal sepsis; current gestational trophoblastic disease; uterine cavity distortion; current PID, current purulent cervicitis; current chlamydia, gonorrhea, or pelvic tuberculosis; Wilson disease
   b. Sexual history: unprotected intercourse in the last 5 days (copper IUC and 52-mg LNG IUD EC use)
   c. Perceived ability to tolerate insertion procedure
6. NFP (FAM and LAM)
   a. Medical history: menstrual history, including cycle length, menstrual irregularities
   b. Obstetric history: recent delivery
   c. Breastfeeding status and ability to exclusively breastfeed
7. Tubal surgeries
   a. History of abdominal or pelvic surgeries
8. Withdrawal
   a. Discuss partner's ability to sense when ejaculation is about to occur, which is necessary for this method.

B. *Objective*

Much of the Database is relevant for all methods; after the initial section, additional objective information will be reviewed by method as indicated.
1. All methods
   a. Pregnancy test if clinically indicated
   b. STI screening if clinically indicated
2. CHC
   a. Blood pressure (BP): BP measurement prior to initiation of CHC is recommended but may be prescribed if measurement is not available (Curtis, Tepper, et al., 2016).
   b. Weight
3. IUDs
   a. Bimanual exam: to evaluate size/shape of uterus and position of uterus
4. EC
   a. BMIt
5. Barrier methods and spermicide (external condom, internal condom, FemCap cervical cap, diaphragm, vaginal and contraceptive sponge)
   a. Pelvic exam: fitting for FemCap and diaphragm
6. Tubal surgery: Objective data should be collected by facility performing procedure.

III. Assessment

Many assessments are relevant for all methods; after the initial section, additional assessments will be reviewed by method as indicated.
1. For all methods:
   a. No medical contraindications to the method
   b. Efficacy accepted by patient
   c. No lifestyle or personal barriers to using the method correctly and consistently
2. Side effects acceptable to patient
3. CHC
   a. If BP available, patient normotensive
4. ECP
   a. Timing within window of effective use
   b. Future contraceptive needs addressed
5. Tubal surgery
   a. Meets criteria delineated by applicable laws and insurance regulations
   b. Completed counseling and informed consent

IV. Goals of clinical management

A. *Contraceptive needs met and patient provided with contraceptive method that supports their contraceptive needs while considering future childbearing goals*
B. *Gynecological concerns, cervical cancer screening, STI testing addressed as indicated*
C. *Method chosen maximizes patient adherence and satisfaction*

V. Plan

A. *Screening and diagnostic tests*

There are no diagnostic tests needed before provision of contraception. Patients who are overdue for screening tests, including cervical cancer screening, should not be denied contraception. STI screening should be offered to patients per CDC screening guidelines. These are updated often; see the CDC website for the latest recommendations. Patients utilizing spermicides may be at higher risk for STIs, so it is particularly important to review the STI risk factors of those patients (Roddy et al., 2002).

B. *Method provision and patient education*
1. Ensure patient is not pregnant.
   All methods can be started or used at any time in the menstrual cycle if the clinician can be reasonably certain that the patient is not pregnant. Except for the IUC, none of the contraception methods will pose harm to an early pregnancy. The provider can be reasonably certain that the patient is not pregnant if the patient has no symptoms or signs of pregnancy and meets *any* of the following criteria (Allen, 2022):
   a. The patient has not had intercourse since last normal menses.
   b. The patient has been correctly and consistently using a reliable method of contraception.
   c. The patient is within 7 days from the first day of menstrual bleeding.

Table 21-3 General Guidelines for Starting Contraceptive by Method

Contraceptive Method	When to Start (If the Provider Is Reasonably Certain That the Patient Is Not Pregnant)	Additional Contraception (i.e., Backup) Needed
Copper-containing intrauterine device (IUD)	Anytime	Not needed
Levonorgestrel-releasing IUD	Anytime	If >7 days after menses started, use backup method or abstain for 7 days.
Implant	Anytime	If >5 days after menses started, use backup method or abstain for 7 days.
Injectable	Anytime	If >7 days after menses started, use backup method or abstain for 7 days.
Combined hormonal contraceptive	Anytime	If >5 days after menses started, use backup method or abstain for 7 days.
Progestin-only pill	Anytime	If >5 days after menses started, use backup method or abstain for 2 days.

   d. The patient is within 4 weeks postpartum (for nonlactating patients).
   e. The patient is within the first 7 days post-abortion or post-miscarriage.
   f. The patient is fully or nearly fully breastfeeding, amenorrheic, and fewer than 6 months postpartum.
2. Advise when to start the method. See **Table 21-3** for general guidelines for starting methods, with the exception of the following clinical scenarios:
   a. Pregnancy loss or abortion: Contraception can be initiated anytime after an abortion or pregnancy loss. If a hormonal method was initiated, backup contraception is not needed if initiated within 5 days of the abortion or pregnancy loss (Nippita & Paul, 2018).
   b. After implant removal: If a patient has their contraceptive implant removed and wishes to start a CHC instead, they should start their CHC method that same day (Curtis, Tepper, et al., 2016). If they are not within the first 5 days of their scheduled bleeding, or they have not been having scheduled bleeding, advise them to use a backup method for 7 days.
   c. After IUD removal: Patients who have had recent unprotected intercourse and are more than 5 days from the first day of their menstrual cycle are at risk for unintended pregnancy if the IUD is removed (Cwiak & Edelman, 2018). They can start a new method that day and return in 7 days for IUD removal. They may also abstain for 7 days and return in 7 days for IUD removal and quick start of a desired CHC or other method (Cwiak & Edelman, 2018). They may have the IUD removed, take EC, and start the CHC immediately (if using UPA as EC, they must wait 5 days to start their CHC method) (Cwiak & Edelman, 2018).
3. Provide the method and relevant education.
   a. Education relevant to all methods: Clinicians should review:
      i. Side effects of specific method, including menstrual changes
      ii. Risks and benefits of specific method, addressing patient concerns
      iii. Details of how to use the specific method
      iv. Possible barriers to adherence
      v. EC use in case of method failure
      vi. Backup methods, if applicable
   b. CHC
      i. Select cycling pattern based on patient's desired menstrual pattern and medical history. Patients can use CHCs cyclically, including a placebo or no-hormone time of 4–7 days to induce a withdrawal bleed, or continuously, without such a bleed. Some COC pill packs provide hormone pills for 21 days of a 28-day cycle, followed by 7 days of placebo pills that result in a withdrawal bleed (21/7 regimen), others provide 4 days of placebo or low-dose estrogen pills (24/4), and others provide 84 active days and 7 placebo days (84/7) (Allen, 2022). The shorter the pill-free window, the less likely it is that folliculogenesis will occur (Dinger et al., 2011). Continuous-use (skipping the placebo days altogether) or extended-cycle (allowing a withdrawal bleed less often than monthly) COC regimens allow the

user to choose if and when they will have withdrawal bleeding. Menstrual suppression through these regimens is effective in improving menstrual symptoms and quality of life (Cwiak & Edelman, 2018). Some patients will experience more unpredictable bleeding or spotting events with extended or continuous use of CHCs (Allen, 2022).

    ii. COC: Review the need to take the pill at same time each day and techniques for remembering to take it. For one late or missed pill, advise patients to take one active pill as soon as possible and continue taking their pills daily, which may mean taking two pills in 1 day. If the patient has missed two or more active pills or taken two or more active pills late, advise them to take one active pill as soon as possible and continue taking their pills daily, which may mean taking two pills in 1 day (Cwiak & Edelman, 2018). Patients should use condoms or abstain from vaginal sex until they have taken 7 active pills in a row (Cwiak & Edelman, 2018).

    iii. Patch: Review patch use and placement, rotation of patch site, timing of changing patch, and techniques for remembering to change on schedule. Each contraceptive patch contains enough active hormones for 7 days. Users who wish to have a withdrawal bleed apply a new patch every 7 days for each of 3 weeks, then may have a 7-day patch-free interval to induce a withdrawal bleed (Nanda & Burke, 2018). The patch should not be left on for more than 7 days, and the patch should always be changed/applied on the same day of the week (Burkman, 2021).

    iv. Contraceptive ring: Both the ENG/EE and the SA/EE ring are inserted vaginally and left for 3 weeks (Kerns & Darney, 2020). Patients using the ENG/EE ring cyclically discard the ring after 3 weeks, leave it out for a 7-day interval, and then insert a new ring (Organon, 2022). Patients using the SA/EE ring cyclically remove it, wash it with mild soap and water, dry it with a clean cloth, and then store it in its case until replacing it after 7 days (Kerns & Darney, 2020). The ENG/EE ring contains enough hormone to last for 5 weeks (Kerns & Darney, 2020). If the ENG/EE ring was left in place for more than 5 weeks, advise the patient to remove the ring and use EC if indicated, then insert a new ring and use a backup method for 7 days (Nanda & Burke, 2018). The ring can remain in the vagina during intercourse or be removed. The ENG/EE ring can be left outside the vagina for 3 hours during the 21-day period. If it has been out of the vagina for more than 3 hours during this time, it should be reinserted, and additional contraception should be used for 7 days (Nanda & Burke, 2018). If needed, EC can be used. As with other CHC methods, it is safe to skip the ring-free week and use the method continuously, although no data exist that specifically examined continuous use of the ring.

    v. Advise the patient of warning signs for complications with CHC use. Although rare, the sequelae of complications can be serious and potentially life-threatening (Cwiak & Edelman, 2018). These warning signs are often conveyed to the patient using the mnemonic "ACHES" for Abdominal pain, Chest pain, Headaches, Eye problems, and Severe leg pain (**Table 21-4**).

  c. POP

    i. Discuss adherence to daily pill use and the importance of taking the pill at the same time each day.

    ii. If the norethindrone POP is taken more than 3 hours late or missed on any given day, backup contraception should be used for 2 days (NLM, 2021d). For missed

Table 21-4 ACHES Mnemonic for Warning Signs of Combined Hormonal Contraceptive (CHC) Use

	Symptom	Possible diagnosis
Abdominal pain	Pain, cramping, vomiting, weakness	Blood clot in liver or pelvis
Chest pain	Chest or heart pain, left arm and shoulder pain, coughing, and shortness of breath	Blood clot in lung or vessels of the heart, heart attack, angina
Headache	Blurred vision, spots, zigzag lines, weakness, difficulty speaking, or sudden intellectual impairment	Stroke
Eye problems	Partial or complete vision loss	Stroke or retinal vein thrombosis
Severe leg pain	Pain, swelling, heat, erythema	Deep vein thrombosis

drospirenone pills, follow the same guidance as for missed COC pills (NLM, 2021f). Although no studies have looked at skipping placebo pills with Slynd use, there is no reason to think it would not have the same benefits as skipping placebos with CHC use.
        iii. Review tips for remembering pills daily.
    d. Injectable progestin (medroxyprogesterone acetate, DMPA)
        i. Review injection procedure and protocol.
        ii. Schedule subsequent injections every 13 weeks.
        iii. Manage irregular bleeding with COC or nonsteroidal anti-inflammatory drug (NSAID) use for 1–2 months if no medical contraindications (Nathirojanakun et al., 2006; Said et al., 2006).
        iv. Discuss black-box warning for bone density loss and evidence for safety with use beyond 2 years.
        v. Patients who are more than 2 weeks late for their injection (>15 weeks from the last injection) should have a pregnancy test before the next injection and should use a backup method for 7 days (Kaunitz, 1994).
        vi. There are no restrictions on how early a subsequent injection may be given (Curtis, Jatlaoui, et al., 2016).
    e. Contraceptive implant
        i. Nexplanon can be inserted only by clinicians who have completed the FDA-mandated training.
        ii. Review insertion procedure and aftercare of incision site.
        iii. Review approved duration of use and evidence for extended use.
    f. LNG IUS
        i. Insertion of LNG IUD should be performed by a trained clinician.
        ii. Review insertion procedure.
        iii. Advise to seek care for vasovagal symptoms, heavy bleeding, severe pain, a positive pregnancy test, or concern for IUD expulsion.
        iv. Review duration of use.
    g. Copper IUD
        i. Insertion of copper IUD should be performed by a trained clinician.
        ii. Review insertion procedure.
        iii. Advise patient to seek care for vasovagal symptoms, heavy bleeding, severe pain, or a positive pregnancy test.
        iv. Review approved duration of use and evidence for extended use.
    h. ECP
        i. Review directions for taking ECP and the importance of taking it as soon as possible.
        ii. Discuss possible changes to menstrual pattern.
        iii. Advise pregnancy test if no menses within 3 weeks (Trussel & Cleland et al., 2018).
        iv. If there is any doubt about whether the patient may have become pregnant after previous episodes of unprotected intercourse more than 5 days previous, a pregnancy test may be helpful prior to insertion of the IUD (Trussel & Cleland, et al., 2018).
        v. Elicit desire to seek continued contraceptive method.
        vi. If needed, provide support services and resources for IPV or assault, and report to appropriate agency if indicated.
    i. Barrier methods: external condom, internal condom, FemCap cervical cap, diaphragm, and contraceptive sponge
        i. Provide prescription for method if needed.
        ii. Advise patient to follow up if they have problems placing or removing any method.
        iii. Advise patient that FemCap will need resizing after birth, miscarriage, or abortion.
    j. Spermicide
        i. Review locations for purchase of spermicide; provide prescription if applicable.
        ii. Advise patient to return to clinic if genital irritation, ulceration, or discomfort is experienced.
    k. NFP methods (FAM and LAM)
        i. Ensure that using the method is realistic for the patient's lifestyle.
        ii. Refer to a clinician well trained in FAM methods if this is their preferred method.
        iii. Provide breastfeeding support and referral to lactation consultant as needed.
        iv. Encourage patient to follow up when breastfeeding status changes or if menstrual periods return.
        v. Encourage follow-up for additional teaching, assurance, or if the patient experiences changes to menstrual cycle that may interfere with FAM efficacy.
    l. Tubal sterilization
        i. Patients must be counseled that tubal surgery is a permanent procedure. They should be reasonably certain that they no longer wish to conceive now or in the future, even if circumstances change.
        ii. Counsel that tubal surgery reversal is generally not feasible, is generally expensive, and is not routinely covered by health insurance.
        iii. Patients in the United States with federally funded health insurance must review, sign, and date the federal consent form between 30 and 180 days prior to the procedure. Each provider should be aware of local or institutional policies related to the federal sterilization consent form.

iv. The preoperative counseling and informed consent process should include a detailed discussion of the following, and this discussion should be documented in the medical record:
   a. Permanence
   b. Risk of regret
   c. Efficacy
   d. Risks and benefits of other contraceptive methods
   e. Risk of ectopic pregnancy
   f. Timing and surgical planning
   g. Surgery and anesthesia risks

VI. Patient and provider education resources
1. The Planned Parenthood Federation of America has an excellent website that provides birth control education with clear, concise information that is easy to follow: https://www.plannedparenthood.org/learn/birth-control.
2. Bedsider.org provides contraceptive information and an interactive method explorer.
3. The CDC's *Providing Quality Family Planning Services* (Gavin et al., 2014) provides a framework for improved counseling through a patient-centered approach that solicits reproductive life plan, needs for preventative and preconception services, and needs for STI screening.
4. USMEC is available here: https://apps.who.int/iris/bitstream/handle/10665/181468/9789241549158_eng.pdf?sequence=9. The summary table is found here: https://www.cdc.gov/mmwr/volumes/65/rr/pdfs/rr6503.pdf. There are also applications for handheld devices available via app stores.
5. Additional information about permanent contraception is available at https://www.acog.org/womens-health/faqs/sterilization-for-women-and-men.

References

Allen, R. H. (2022). Combined estrogen-progestin oral contraceptives: Patient selection, counseling, and use. *UpToDate*. https://www.uptodate.com/contents/combined-estrogen-progestin-oral-contraceptives-patient-selection-counseling-and-use

Alvarez, F., Brache, V., Fernandez, E., Guerrero, B., Guiloff, E., Hess, R., Salvatierra, A. M., & Zacharias, S. (1988). New insights on the mode of action of intrauterine contraception in women. *Fertility and Sterility, 49*(5), 768-773.

American College of Obstetricians and Gynecologists, Committee on Ethics. (2017). Committee Opinion No. 695: Sterilization of Women: Ethical Issues and Considerations. *Obstetrics and Gynecology (New York. 1953), 129*(4), e109–e116. doi:10.1097/AOG.0000000000002023

American College of Obstetricians and Gynecologists, Committee on Health Care for Underserved Women. (2015). Committee opinion no. 615: Access to contraception. *Obstetrics and Gynecology, 125*(1), 250–255. doi:10.1097/01.AOG.0000459866.14114.33

American College of Obstetricians and Gynecologists, Committee on Health Care for Underserved Women and Committee on Ethics. (2022, February). *Patient-centered contraceptive counseling*. https://www.acog.org/clinical/clinical-guidance/committee-statement/articles/2022/02/patient-centered-contraceptive-counseling

American College of Obstetricians and Gynecologists, Committee on Practice Bulletins—Gynecology. (2019). ACOG Practice Bulletin No. 206 summary: Use of Hormonal contraception in women with coexisting medical conditions. *Obstetrics and Gynecology, 133*(2), 396–399. doi:10.1097/AOG.0000000000003073

Ammälä, M., Nyman, T., Strengell, L., & Rutanen, E. M. (1995). Effect of intrauterine contraceptive devices on cytokine messenger ribonucleic acid expression in the human endometrium. *Fertility and Sterility, 63*(4), 773–778. doi:10.1016/s0015-0282(16)57480-9

Archer, D. F., Merkatz, R. B., Bahamondes, L. Westhoff, C. L., Darney, P., Apter, D., Jensen, J. T., Brache, V., Nelson, A. L., Banks, E., Bártfai, G., Portman, D. J., Plagianos, M., Dart, C., Kumar, N., Creasy, G. W., Sitruk-Ware, R., & Blithe, D. L. (2019). Efficacy of the 1-year (13 cycle) segesterone acetate and ethinylestradiol contraceptive vaginal system: Results of two multicentre, open-label, single-arm, phase 3 trials. *The Lancet Global Health; 7*(8), e1054–e1064. doi:10.1016/ S2214-109X(19)30265-7

Arévalo, M., Sinai, I., & Jennnings, V. (1999). A fixed formula to define the fertile window of the menstrual cycle as the basis of a simple method of natural family planning. *Contraception, 60*(6), 357–360. doi:10.1016/s0010-7824(99)00106-7

Arias, R. D., Jain, J. K., Brucker, C., Ross, D., & Ray, A. (2006). Changes in bleeding patterns with depot medroxyprogesterone acetate subcutaneous injection 104 mg. *Contraception, 74*(3), 234–238. doi:10.1016/j.contraception.2006.03.008

Artega, S., & Gomez, A. M. (2016). "Is that a method of birth control?": A qualitative exploration of young women's use of withdrawal. *Journal of Sex Research, 53*(4–5), 626–632. doi:10.1080.00224499.2015.1079296

Baeten, J. M., Nyange, P. M., Richardson, B. A., Lavreys, L., Chohan, B., Martin, H. L., Jr Mandaliya, K., Ndinya-Achola, J. O., Bwayo, J. J., & Kreiss, J. K. (2001). Hormonal contraception and risk of sexually transmitted disease acquisition: Results from a prospective study. *American Journal of Obstetrics and Gynecology, 185*(2), 380–385. doi:10.1067.mob.2001.115862

Baker, C. C., & Chen, M. J. (2022). New contraception update—Annovera, Phexxi, Slynd, and Twirla. *Current Obstetrics and Gynecology Reports, 11*(1), 21–27. doi:10.1007/s13669-021-00321-4

Bartz, D. A. (2020). Pericoital contraception: Diaphragm, cervical cap, spermicides, and sponge. *UpToDate*. https://www.uptodate.com/contents/pericoital-contraception-diaphragm-cervical-cap-spermicides-and-sponge

Braaten, K. P., & Dutton, C. (2022). Overview of female permanent contraception. *UpToDate*. https://www.uptodate.com/contents/overview-of-female-permanentcontraception?search=permanent%20contraception&source=search_result&selectedTitle=1~150&usage_type=default&display_rank=1#H20184324

Brache, V., Cochon, L., Deniaud, M., & Croxatto, H. B. (2013). Ulipristal acetate prevents ovulation more effectively than levonorgestrel: Analysis of pooled data from three randomized trials of emergency contraception regimens. *Contraception, 88*(5), 611–618. doi:10.1016/j.contraception.2013.05.010

Brahmi, D., & Curtis, K.M. (2013). When can a woman start combined hormonal contraceptives (CHC's)? A systematic review. *Contraception, 87*(5), 524–538. https://dx.doi.org/10.1016/j.contraception.2012.09.010

Burkman, R. T. (2021). Contraception: Transdermal patches. *UpToDate*. https://www.uptodate.com/contents/contraception-transdermal-contraceptive-patches

Campo-Engelstein, L. (2012). Contraceptive justice: why we need a male pill. *The Virtual Mentor, 14*(2), 146–151. doi:10.1001/virtualmentor.2012.14.2.msoc1-1202

Cecil, M., Nelson, A. L., Trussel, J., & Hatcher, R. (2010). If the condom doesn't fit, you must resize it. *Contraception, 82*(6), 489–490. doi:10.1016/j.contraception.2010.06.007

Centers for Disease Control and Prevention. (2002). Nonoxynol-9 spermicide contraception use—United States, 1999. *Morbidity and Mortality Weekly Report, 51*(18), 389–392.

Chappell, B. T., Mena, L. A., Maximos, B., Mollan, S., Culwell, K., & Howard, B. (2021). EVO100 prevents chlamydia and gonorrhea in women at high risk of infection. *American Journal of Obstetrics and Gynecology, 225*(2), 162.e1–162.e14. doi:10.1016/j.ajog.2021.03.00

Cleland, K., Zhu, H., Goldstuck, N., Cheng, L., & Trussel, J. (2012). The efficacy of intrauterine devices for emergency contraception: A systematic review of 35 years of experience. *Human Reproduction, 27*(7), 1994–2000. https://doi.org/10.1093/humrep/des140

Cibula, D., Widschwendter, M., Zikan, M., & Dusek, L. (2011). Underlying mechanisms of ovarian cancer risk reduction after tubal ligation. *Acta Obstericia et Gynecologica Scandinavica, 90*(6), 559–563. doi:10.1111/j-1600-0412.2011.01114x

Cooper Surgical. (2022). *Resources for your practice: ParaGard intrauterine copper contraceptive.* https://hcp.paragard.com/resources/

Creinin, M. D., Kaunitz, A. M., Darney, P. D., Schwartz, L., Hampton, T., Gordon, K., & Rekers, H. (2017). The US etonogestrel implant mandatory clinical training and active monitoring programs: 6-year experience. *Contraception, 95*(2), 205–210. doi:10.1016/j.contraception.2016.

Cundy, T., Cornish, J., Evans, M.C., Roberts, H., & Reid, I. R. (1994). Recovery of bone density in women who stop using medroxyprogesterone acetate. *BMJ (Clinical Research Ed.), 308*(6923), 247–248. doi:10.1136/bmj.308.6923.247

Curtis, K. M., Jatlaoui, T. C., Tepper, N. K., Zapata, L. B., Horton, L. G., Jamieson, D. J., & Whiteman, M. K. (2016). U.S. selected practice recommendations for contraceptive use, 2016. *Morbidity and Mortality Weekly Report. Recommendations and Reports, 65*(4), 1–66. doi:10.15585/mmwr.rr6504a1

Curtis, K. M., & Peipert, J. F. (2017). Long-acting reversible contraception. *New England Journal of Medicine, 376*(5), 461–468. doi:10.1056/NEJMcp1608736

Curtis, K. M., Tepper, N. K. Jatlaoui, T. C., Berry-Bibee, E., Horton, L. G., Zapata, L. B., Simmons, K. B., Pagano, P., Jamieson, D. J., & Whiteman, M. K. (2016). U.S. medical eligibility criteria for contraceptive use, 2016. *Morbidity and Mortality Weekly Report. Recommendations and Reports, 65*(3), 1–106. doi:10.15585/mmwr.rr6503a1

Cwiak, C., & Edelman, A. (2018). Combined oral contraceptives (COCs). In R. A. Hatcher, A. L. Nelson, J. Trussel, C. Cwiak, P. Cason, M. S. Policar, A. B. Edelman, A. R. A. Aiken, J. M. Marrazzo, & D. Kowal (Eds.), *Contraceptive technology* (21st ed., pp. 263–316). Ayer.

Daniels, K., Daugherty, J., Mosher, W. D., & Daugherty, J. (2015). Current contraceptive use and variation by selected characteristics among women aged 15–44: United States, 2011–2013. *National Health Statistics Reports, 86*, 1–14.

Daniels, K., & Mosher, W. D. (2013). Contraceptive methods women have ever used: United States, 1982–2010. *National Health Statistics Reports, 62*, 1–15.

Darney, P. (2021). Etonogestrel contraceptive implant. *UpToDate*. https://www.uptodate.com/contents/etonogestrel-contraceptive-implant

De Ceulaer, K., Gruber, C., Hayes, R., & Serjeant, G. R. (1982). Medroxyprogesterone acetate and homozygous sickle-cell disease. *Lancet, 2*(8292), 229–331. doi:10.1016/s0140-6736(82)90320-8.

De la Cruz, D., Cruz, A., Arteaga, M., Castillo, L., & Tovalin, H. (2005). Blood copper levels in Mexican users of the T380A IUD. *Contraception, 72*(2), 122–125. doi:10.1016/j.contraception.2005.02.009

Dean, G., & Schwarz, E. B. (2018). Intrauterine devices (IUDs). In R. A. Hatcher, A. L. Nelson, J. Trussel, C. Cwiak, P. Cason, M. S. Policar, A. B. Edelman, A. R. A. Aiken, J. M. Marrazzo, & D. Kowal (Eds.), *Contraceptive technology* (21st ed., pp.157–193). Ayer.

Dickey, R. P., & Seymour, M. L. (2021). *Managing contraceptive pill patients and other hormonal contraceptives* (17th ed.). EMIS, Inc. Medical Publishers.

Diedrich, J. T., Desai, S., Zhao, Q., Secura, G., Madden, T., & Peipert, J. F. (2015). Association of short-term bleeding and cramping patterns with long-acting reversible contraceptive method satisfaction. *American Journal of Obstetrics and Gynecology, 212*(1), 50.e1–50.e8. doi:10.1016/j.ajog.2014.07.025

Dinger, J., Do Minh, T., Buttman, N., & Bardenheuer, K. (2011). Effectiveness of oral contraceptive pills in a large U.S. cohort comparing progesterone and regimen. *Obstetrics and Gynecology, 117*(1), 33–40. doi:10.1097/AOG.0b013e31820095a2

D'Oro, L. C., Parazzini, F., Naldi, L., & La Vecchia, C. (1994). Barrier methods of contraception, spermicides, and sexually transmitted diseases: A review. *Genitourinary Medicine, 70*(6), 410–417. doi:10.1136/sti.70.6.410

Dragoman, M. V., & Gaffield, M. E. (2016). The safety of subcutaneously administered depot medroxyprogesterone acetate (104 mg/0.65 mL): A systematic review. *Contraception 94*(3), 202–215. doi:10.1016/j.contraception.2016.02.003

Edelman, A. (2002). Menstrual nirvana: Amenorrhea through the use of continuous oral contraceptives. *Current Womens Health Reports, 2*(6), 434–438.

Edelman, A., Micks, E., Gallo, M. F., Jensen, J. T., & Grimes, D. A. (2014). Continuous or extended cycle vs. cyclic use of combined hormonal contraceptives for contraception. *Cochrane Database of Systematic Reviews, 2014*(7), CD004695. doi:10.1002/14651858.CD004695.pub3

Evofem Biosciences. (2021). *Phexxi (lactic acid, citric acid, and potassium bitartrate) vaginal gel.* https://www.phexxi.com/pdf/PhexxiUSPI.pdf

Fage, S. W., Faurschou, A., & Thyssen, J. P. (2014). Copper hypersensitivity. *Contact Dermatitis, 71*(4), 191–201. doi:10.1111/cod.12273

FemCap. (2020). *FemCap FAQ.* https://femcap.com/new/faq/

Food and Drug Administration. (2017, August). Opill tablets. https://www.accessdata.fda.gov/drugsatfda_docs/label/2017/017031s035s036lbl.pdf

Freundl, G., Sivin, I., & Batár, I. (2010). State-of-the-art of non-hormonal methods of contraception: IV. Natural family planning. *European Journal of Contraception & Reproductive Health Care, 15*(2), 113–123. doi:10.3109/13625180903545302

Frohwirth, L., Blades, N., Moore, A. M., & Wurtz, H. (2016). The complexity of multiple contraceptive method use and the anxiety that informs it: Implications for theory and practice. *Archives of Sexual Behavior, 45*(8), 2123–2135. doi:10.1007.s10508-016-0706-6

Gavin, L., Moskosky, S., Carter, M., et al. (2014). Providing quality family planning services. Recommendations of CDC and the U.S. office of population affairs. *Morbitity and Mortality Weekly Report, 63*(4), 1–24.

Glasier, A., Cameron, S. T., Blithe, D., Scherrer, B., Mathe, H., Levy, D., Gainer, E., & Ulmann, A. (2011). Can we identify women at risk of pregnancy despite using emergency contraception? Data from randomized trials of ulipristal acetate and levonorgestrel. *Contraception, 84*(4), 363–367. doi:10.1016/j.contraception.2011.02.009

Glasier, A., Edelman, A., Creinin, M. D., Han, L., Matulich, M. C., Brache, V., Westhoff, C. L., & Hemon, A. (2022). Mechanism of action of norgestrel 0.075 mg a progestogen-only pill. I. Effect on ovarian activity. *Contraception, 112*, 37–42. doi:10.1016/j.contraception.2022.03.022

Green, A., Purdie, D., Bain, C., Siskind, V., Russell, P., Quinn, M., & Ward, B. (1997). Tubal sterilisation, hysterectomy, and decreased risk of ovarian cancer. Survey of Women's Health Study Group. *International Journal of Cancer, 71*(6), 948–951. doi:10.1002/(sici)1097-0215(19970611)71:6<948::aid-ijc6>3.0.co;2-y

Grimes, D. A., & Schulz, K. F. (2001). Antibiotic prophylaxis for intrauterine contraceptive device insertion. *Cochrane Database of Systematic Reviews, 2001*(2), CD001327. doi:10.1002/14651858.CD001327.

Han, L., & Jensen, J. T. (2015). Does the progestogen used in combined hormonal contraception affect venous thrombosis risk? *Obstetrics and Gynecology Clinics of North America, 42*(4), 683–698. https://doi:10.1016/j.ogc.2015.07.007.

Harper, C. C., Bum, M., Thiel De Bocanegra, H., Darney, P. D., Speidel, J. J., Policar, M., & Drey, E. A. (2008). Challenges in translating evidence to practice: The provision of intrauterine contraception. *Obstetrics and Gynecology, 111*(6), 1359–1369. doi:10.1097/AOG.0b013e318173fd83

Heinemann, K., Reed, S., Moehner, S., & Minh, T. D. (2015). Comparative contraceptive effectiveness of levonorgestrel-releasing and copper intrauterine devices: The European Active Surveillance Study for Intrauterine Devices. *Contraception, 91*(4), 280–283. doi:10.1016/j.contraception.2015.01.011

Hillis, S. D., Marchbanks, P. A., Tylor, L. R., & Peterson, H. B. (1999). Poststerilization regret: Findings from the United States Collaborative Review of Sterilization. *Obstetrics and Gynecology, 93*(6), 889–895. doi:10.1016/s0029-7844(98)00539-0

Hoke, T., Stone, K. M., Steiner, M. J., & Warner, L. (2021). Internal (formerly female) condoms. *UpToDate.* https://uptodate.com/contents/internal-formerly-female-condoms

Hou, M. Y., & Roncari, D. (2018). Permanent contraception. In R. A. Hatcher, A. L. Nelson, J. Trussel, C. Cwiak, P. Cason, M. S. Policar, A. B. Edelman, A. R. A. Aiken, J. M. Marrazzo, & D. Kowal (Eds.), *Contraceptive technology* (21st ed., pp. 459–486). Ayer.

HPSRx. (2018). *Caya provider catalog.* https://www.caya.us.com/_files/ugd/c2abb7_178534de373649d9b239af3527625731.pdf

Hsiang, D., & Dunn, S. (2016). Emergency contraception. *CMAJ: Canadian Medical Association Journal, 188*(17–18), E536. doi:10.1503/cmaj.160720

Irwin, K. L., Weiss, N. S., Lee, N. C., & Peterson, H. B. (1991). Tubal sterilization, hysterectomy, and the subsequent occurrence of epithelial ovarian cancer. *American Journal of Epidemiology, 134*(4), 362–369. doi:10.1093/oxfordjournals.aje.a116098

Jacobstein, R., & Polis, C. B. (2014). Progestin-only contraception: Injectables and implants. *Best practice & research. Clinical Obstetrics & Gynaecology, 28*(6), 795–806. doi:10.1016/j.bpobgyn.2014.05.003

Jamieson, D. J., Kaufman, S. C., Costello, C., Hillis, S. D., Marchbanks, P. A., Peterson, H. B., & U.S. Collaborative Review of Sterilization Working Group. (2022). A comparison of women's regret after vasectomy versus tubal sterilization. *Obstetrics and Gynecology, 99*(6), 1073–1079. doi:10.1016/s0029-7844(02)10981-6

Jennings, V. (2020). Fertility awareness-based methods pregnancy prevention. *UpToDate.* https://www.uptodate.com/contents/fertility-awareness-based-methods-of-pregnancy-prevention

Jennings, V. H., & Polis, C. B. (2018). Fertility awareness-based methods. In R. A. Hatcher, A. L. Nelson, J. Trussel, C. Cwiak, P. Cason, M. S. Policar, A. B. Edelman, A. R. A. Aiken, J. M. Marrazzo, & D. Kowal (Eds.), *Contraceptive technology* (21st ed., pp. 395–416). Ayer.

Jones, R. K. (2018). Coitus interruptus (withdrawal, pulling out). In R. A. Hatcher, A. L. Nelson, J. Trussel, C. Cwiak, P. Cason, M. S. Policar, A. B. Edelman, A. R. A. Aiken, J. M. Marrazzo, & D. Kowal (Eds.), *Contraceptive technology* (21st ed., pp. 451–457). Ayer.

Kaunitz, A. M. (1994). Long-acting injectable contraception with depot medroxyprogesterone acetate. *American Journal of Obstetrics and Gynecology, 170*(5, Pt. 2), 1543–1549.

Kaunitz, A. M. (2021a). Depot medroxyprogesterone acetate (DMPA): Efficacy, side effects, metabolic impact, and benefits. *UpToDate.* https://www.uptodate.com/contents/depot-medroxyprogesterone-acetate-dmpa-efficacy-side-effects-metabolic-impact-and-benefits

Kaunitz, A. M. (2021b). Progestin-only pills (POPs) for contraception. *UpToDate.* https://www.uptodate.com/contents/progestin-only-pills-pops-for-contraception

Kaunitz, A. M. (2022). Depot medroxyprogesterone acetate (DMPA): Formulations, patient selection and drug administration. *UpToDate.* https://www.uptodate.com/contents/depot-medroxyprogesterone-acetate-dmpa-formulations-patient-selection-and-drug-administration

Keller, M. J., Carpenter, C. A., Lo, Y., Einstein, M. H., Liu, C., Fredricks, D. N., & Herold, B. C. (2012). Phase I randomized safety study of twice daily dosing of acidform vaginal gel: candidate antimicrobial contraceptive. *PloS One, 7*(10), e46901. doi:10.1371/journal.pone.0046901

Kennedy, K. I., & Goldsmith, C. (2018). Contraception after pregnancy. In R. A. Hatcher, A. L. Nelson, J. Trussel, C. Cwiak, P. Cason, M. S. Policar, A. B. Edelman, A. R. A. Aiken, J. M. Marrazzo, & D. Kowal (Eds.), *Contraceptive technology* (21st ed., pp. 511–541). Ayer.

Kerns, J., & Darney, P. D. (2020). Contraception: Hormonal contraceptive vaginal rings. *UpToDate.* https://www.uptodate.com/contents/contraception-hormonal-contraceptive-vaginal-rings

Killick, S. R., Leary, C., Trussel, J., & Guthrie, K. A. (2011). Sperm content of pre-ejaculatory fluid. *Human Fertility, 14*(1), 48–52. doi:10.3109/14647273.2010.520798

Kjaer, S. K., Mellemkjaer, L., Brinton, L. A., Johansen, C., Gridley, G., & Olsen, J. H. (2004). Tubal sterilization and risk of ovarian, endometrial, and cervical cancer. A Danish population-based follow-up study of more than 65,000 sterilized women. *International Journal of Epidemiology, 33*(3), 596–602. doi:10.1093/ije/dyh046

Kreiss, J., Ngugi, E., Holmes, K., Ndinya-Achola, J., Waiyaki, P., Roberts, P.L., Ruminjo, I., Sajabi, R., Kimata, J., & Fleming, T. R. (1992). Efficacy of nonoxynol-9 contraceptive sponge use in preventing heterosexual acquisition of HIV in Nairobi prostitutes. *JAMA, 268*(4), 477–482.

Loder, C., & Flaum, S. (2019). What to consider when discussing Essure removal. *Contemporary Ob/Gyn, 64*(7), 25–29.

Lopez, L. M., Grimes, D. A., Gallo, M. F., Stockton, L. L., & Schulz, K. F. (2013). Skin patch and vaginal ring versus combined oral contraceptives for contraception (review). *Cochrane Database of Systematic Reviews, 2013*(4), CD003552. https://doi:10.1002/14651858.CD003552.pub4.

Lopez, L. M., Ramesh, S., Chen, M., Edelman, A., Otterness, C., Trussell, J., & Helmerhorst, F. M. (2016). Progestin only contraceptives: Effects on weight. *Cochrane Database of Systematic Reviews*, *2016*(8), 1–86, CD008815. doi:10.1002/14651858.CD008815.pub4

Maassen, L. W., van Gastel, D. M., Haveman, I., Bongers, M. Y., & Veersema, S. (2019). Removal of Essure sterilization devices: A retrospective cohort study in the Netherlands. *Journal of Minimally Invasive Gynecology*, *26*(6), 1056–1062. doi:10.1016/j.jmig.2018.10.009

MacGregor, E. A. (2013). Contraception and headache. *Headache: The Journal of Head and Face Pain*, *53*(2), 247–276. doi:10.1111/head.12035.

Madden, T. (2021). Intrauterine contraception: Background and device types. *UpToDate*. https://www.uptodate.com/contents/intrauterine-contraception-background-and-device-types

Mansour, D., Korver, T., Marintcheva-Petrova, M., & Fraser, I. S. (2008). The effects of Implanon on menstrual bleeding patterns. *European Journal of Contraception & Reproductive Health Care*, *13*(S1), 13–28. doi:10.1080/13625180801959931

Mauck, C. K., Brache, V., Kimble, T., Thurman, A., Cochon, L., Littlefield, S., Linton, K., Doncel, G. F., & Schwartz, J. L. (2017). A phase I randomized postcoital testing and safety study of the Caya diaphragm used with 3% Nonoynol-9 gel, Contra-Gel, or no gel. *Contraception*, *96*(2), 124–130. doi:10.1016/j.contraception.2017.05.016

Mayer Labs. (n.d.). *Today Sponge*. http://www.todaysponge.com/purchase.html

McNeilly, A. S. (2001). Neuroendocrine changes and fertility in breast-feeding women. *Progress in Brain Research*, *133*, 207–214. doi:10.1016/s0079-6123(01)33015-7

McNeilly, A. S., Tay, C. C., & Glasier, A. (1994). Physiologic mechanisms underlying lactational amenorrhea. *Annals of the New York Academy of Sciences*, *709*, 145–155. doi:10.1111/j.1748-6632.1994.tb30394.x

McNicholas, C., Maddipatti, R., Zhao, Q., Swor, E., & Peipert, J. (2015). Use of the etonogestrel implant and levonorgestrel intrauterine device beyond the U.S. Food and Drug Administration-approved duration. *Obstetrics and Gynecology*, *125*(3), 599–604. doi:10.1097/AOG.0000000000000690.

Milsom, I., & Korver, T. (2008). Ovulation incidence with oral contraceptives: A literature review. *Journal of Family Planning and Reproductive Health Care*, *34*(4), 237–246. doi:10.1783/147118908786000451.

Mishell, D. R., Jr (1996). Pharmacokinetics of depot medroxyprogesterone acetate contraception. *Journal of Reproductive Medicine*, *415*(Suppl. 5), 381–390.

Monterrosa-Castro, A., Redondo-Mendoza, V., & Monterrosa-Blanco, A. (2021). Current knowledge of progestin-only pills. *Electronic Journal of General Medicine*, *18*(6), em320. doi:10.29333/ejgm/11217

Nanda, K., & Burke, A. (2018). Contraceptive patch and vaginal contraceptive ring. In R. A. Hatcher, A. L. Nelson, J. Trussel, C. Cwiak, P. Cason, M. S. Policar, A. B. Edelman, A. R. A. Aiken, J. M. Marrazzo, & D. Kowal (Eds.), *Contraceptive technology* (21st ed., pp. 263–316). Ayer.

Nathirojanakun, P., Taneepanichskul, S., & Sappakitkumjorn, N. (2006). Efficacy of selective COX-2 inhibitor for controlling irregular uterine bleeding in DMPA users. *Contraception*, *73*(6), 584–587. doi:10.1016/j.contraception.2005.09.013

National Library of Medicine. (2018, May 29). *Camila—norethindrone tablet*. https://www.dailymed.nlm.nih.gov/dailymed/drugInfo.cfm?setid=052bfe45-c485-49e5-8fc4-51990b2efba4

National Library of Medicine. (2020a, January 27). *Ella—ulipristal acetate tablet*. https://www.dailymed.nlm.nih.gov/dailymed/drugInfo.cfm?setid=052bfe45-c485-49e5-8fc4-51990b2efba4

National Library of Medicine. (2020b, April 1). *Liletta—levonorgestrel intrauterine device*. https://dailymed.nlm.nih.gov/dailymed/drugInfo.cfm?setid=aaf0eb2a-f88a-4f26-a445-0fd30176c326

National Library of Medicine. (2021a, July 8). *Kyleena—levonorgestrel intrauterine device*. https://dailymed.nlm.nih.gov/dailymed/drugInfo.cfm?setid=2e07c155-21e1-4781-9633-ce8bddd47080

National Library of Medicine. (2021b, August 11). *Mirena—levonorgestrel intrauterine device*. https://dailymed.nlm.nih.gov/dailymed/drugInfo.cfm?setid=dcbd6aa2-b3fa-479a-a676-56ea742962fc

National Library of Medicine. (2021c, July 8). *Nexplanon—etonogestrel implant*. https://dailymed.nlm.nih.gov/dailymed/drugInfo.cfm?setid=487f8a62-e142-457c-97cc-2e398fde7594

National Library of Medicine. (2021d, October 18). *Nora-Be—norethindrone tablet*. https://www.dailymed.nlm.nih.gov/dailymed/drugInfo.cfm?setid=a9241f0b-e1d0-4782-98e6-7f1eaf9ccc85

National Library of Medicine. (2021e, July 8). *Skyla—levonorgestrel intrauterine device*. DailyMed. https://dailymed.nlm.nih.gov/dailymed/drugInfo.cfm?setid=9f44ff35-e052-49cd-a1c2-0bfd87d49309

National Library of Medicine. (2021f, January 19). *Slynd—drospirenone tablet, film coated*. https://www.dailymed.nlm.nih.gov/dailymed/drugInfo.cfm?setid=db32bc55-f295-4d87-9dbb-0a2f45573dcf#section-2.3

National Library of Medicine. (2022a, April 29). *Twirla—levonorgestrel and ethinyl estradiol patch*. https://dailymed.nlm.nih.gov/dailymed/drugInfo.cfm?setid=bcaf8db0-1750-425d-b008-255b5e7a9cc6

National Library of Medicine. (2022b, March 4). *Xulane—norelgestromin and ethinyl estradiol patch*. https://dailymed.nlm.nih.gov/dailymed/drugInfo.cfm?setid=f7848550-086a-43d8-8ae5-047f4b9e4382

Nelson, A., & Harwood, B. (2018). Vaginal barriers and spermicides. In R. A. Hatcher, A. L. Nelson, J. Trussel, C. Cwiak, P. Cason, M. S. Policar, A. B. Edelman, A. R. A. Aiken, J. M. Marrazzo, & D. Kowal (Eds.), *Contraceptive technology* (21st ed., pp. 367–394). Ayer.

Nelson, A. L., Kaunitz, A. M., Kroll, R., Simon, J. A., Poindexter, A. N., Castaño, P. M., Ackerman, R. T., Flood, L., Chiodo, J. A., & Garner, E. I. (2021). Efficacy, safety, and tolerability of a levonorgestrel/ethinyl estradiol transdermal delivery system: Phase 3 clinical trial results. *Contraception*, *103*, 137–143. doi:10.1016/j.contraception.2020.11.011

Nelson, A. L., Sokol, D. C., & Grentzer, J. (2018). Contraceptive implant. In R. A. Hatcher, A. L. Nelson, J. Trussel, C. Cwiak, P. Cason, M. S. Policar, A. B. Edelman, A. R. A. Aiken, J. M. Marrazzo, & D. Kowal (Eds.), *Contraceptive technology* (21st ed., pp. 263–316). Ayer.

Nippita, S., & Paul, M. (2018). Abortion. In R. A. Hatcher, A. L. Nelson, J. Trussel, C. Cwiak, P. Cason, M. S. Policar, A. B. Edelman, A. R. A. Aiken, J. M. Marrazzo, & D. Kowal (Eds.), *Contraceptive technology* (21st ed., pp. 779–827). Ayer.

Organon. (2022). *Nuva Ring prescribing information*. https://www.organon.com/product/usa/pi_circulars/n/nuvaring/nuvaring_pi.pdf

Ortiz, M. E., Croxatto, H. B., & Bardin, C. W. (1996). Mechanisms of action of intrauterine devices. *Obstetrics and Gynecological Survey*, *51*(Suppl. 12), S42–S51. doi.org/10.1097/00006254-199612000-00014

Peterson, H. B., Xia, Z., Hughes, J. M, Wilcox, L. S., Tylor, L. R., & Trussel, J. (1996). The risk of pregnancy after tubal sterilization: Findings from the U.S. Collaborative Review of Sterilization. *American Journal of Obstetrics and Gynecology*, *174*(4), 1161–1170. doi:10.1016/s0002-9378(96)70658-0

Piaggo, G., Kapp, N., & von Herzen, H. (2011). Effect on pregnancy rates of the delay in the administration of levonorgestrel for emergency contraception: A combined analysis of four WHO trials. *Contraception, 84*(1), 35–39. doi:10.1016/j.contraception.2010.11.010

Planned Parenthood. (2022a). *Birth control sponge*. https://www.plannedparenthood.org/learn/birth-control/birth-control-sponge

Planned Parenthood. (2022b). *Cervical cap*. https://www.plannedparenthood.org/learn/birth-control/cervical-cap.

Planned Parenthood. (2022c). *Phexxi*. https://www.plannedparenthood.org/learn/birth-control/spermicide/phexxi

Pocius, K. D., & Bartz, D. A. (2021). Intrauterine contraception: Management of side effects and complications. *UpToDate*. https://www.uptodate.com/contents/intrauterine-contraception-management-of-side-effects-and-complications

Powell, C.B., Alabaster, A., Simmons, S., Garcia, C., Martin, M., McBride-Allen, S., & Littell, R. D. (2017). Salpingectomy for sterilization: Change in practice in a large integrated health care system, 2011–2016. *Obstetrics and Gynecology, 130*(5), 961–967. doi:10.1097/AOG.0000000000002312

Pudney, J., Oneta, M., Mayer, K., Seage, G., 3rd, & Anderson, D. (1992). Pre-ejaculatory fluid as potential vector for sexual transmission of HIV-1. *Lancet, 340*(8833), 1470. doi:10.1016/1040-6736(92)92659-4

Ramadimetja, M., Mulaudzi, F. M., Peu, M. D., Mataboge, M. S., Ngunyulu, R., & Phiri, S. S. (2016). The constraints and concerns regarding the size and/or shape of the second generation female condom: The narratives from healthcare providers. *African Journal of Primary Health Care & Family Medicine, 8*(2), e1–e7. doi:10.4102.phcfm.v8i2.1146

Raymond, E. G., & Grossman, D. (2018). Progestin-only pills. In R. A. Hatcher, A. L. Nelson, J. Trussel, C. Cwiak, P. Cason, M. S. Policar, A. B. Edelman, A. R. A. Aiken, J. M. Marrazzo, & D. Kowal (Eds.), *Contraceptive technology* (21st ed., pp. 263–316). Ayer.

Read, C. (2010). New regimens with combined oral contraceptive pills—Moving away from traditional 21/7 cycles. *European Journal of Contraception & Reproductive Health Care, 15*(S2), S32–S41. doi:10.3109/13625187.2010.529969

Rivera, R., Yacobsen, I., & Grimes, D. (1999). The mechanism of action of hormonal contraceptives and intrauterine contraceptive devices. *American Journal of Obstetrics and Gynecology, 181*(5, Pt. 1), 1263–1269. doi:10.1016/s0002-9378(99)70120-1

Roddy, R. E., Zekeng, L., Ryan, K. A., Tamoufé, U., & Tweedy, K. G. (2002). Effect of nonoxynol-9 gel on urogenital gonorrhea and chlamydial infection: A randomized controlled trial. *JAMA, 287*(9), 1117–1122. doi:10.1001/jama.287.9.1117

Roe, A., Bartz, D. A., & Douglas, P. S. (2021). Combined estrogen-progestin contraception: Side effects and health concerns. *UpToDate*. https://www.uptodate.com/contents/combined-estrogen-progestin-contraception-side-effects-and-health-concerns

Rogow, D., & Horowitz, S. (1995). Withdrawal: A review of the literature and an agenda for research. *Studies in Family Planning, 26*(3), 140–153.

Sagiroglu, N. (1971). Phagocytosis of spermatozoa in the uterine cavity of women using intrauterine device. *International Journal of Fertility, 16*(1), 1–14.

Said, S., Sadek, W., Rocca, M., Koetsawang, S., Kirwat, O., Piya-Anant, M., Dusitsin, N., Sethavanich, S., Affandi, B., Hadisaputra, W., Kazi, A., Ramos, R. M., d'Arcangues, C., Belse, E. M., Noonan, E., Olayinka, I., & Pinol, A. (2006). Clinical evaluation of the therapeutic effectiveness of ethinyl estradiol and oestrone sulphate on prolonged bleeding in women using depot medroxyprogesterone acetate for contraception. World Health Organization, Special Programme of Research, Development and Research Training in Human Reproduction, Task Force on Long-Acting Systemic Agents for Fertility Regulation. *Human Reproduction, 11*(Suppl. 2), 1–13. doi:10.1093/humrep/11.suppl_2.1

Schmidt, J. E., Hillis, S. D., Marchbanks, P. A., Jeng, G., & Peterson, H. B. (2000). Requesting information about and obtaining reversal after tubal sterilization: findings from the U.S. Collaborative Review of Sterilization. *Fertility and Sterility, 74*(5), 892–898. doi:10.1016/s0015-0282(00)01588-2

Scholes, D., LaCroix, A. Z., Ichikawa, L. E., Barlow, W. E., & Ott, S. M. (2002). Injectable hormone contraception and bone density: Results from a prospective study. *Epidemiology, 13*(5), 581–587. doi:10.1097.00001648-200209000-00015

Schwartz, J. L., Weiner, D. H., Lai, J. J., Frezieres, R. G., Creinin, M. D., Archer, D. F., Bradley, L., Barnhart, K. T., Poindexter, A., Kilbourne-Brook, M., Callahan, M. M., & Mauck, C. K. (2015). Contraceptive efficacy, safety, fit, and acceptability of a single-size diaphragm developed with end-user input. *Obstetrics and Gynecology, 125*(4), 895–903. doi:10.1097/AOG.0000000000000721

Segall-Gutierrez, P., Taylor, D., Liu, X., Stanzcyk, F., Azen, S., & Mishell, D. R., Jr (2010). Follicular development and ovulation in extremely obese women receiving depo-medroxyprogesterone acetate subcutaneously. *Contraception, 81*(6), 487–495. doi:10.1016/j.contraception.2010.01.021

Shapiro, S., & Dinger, J. (2010). Risk of venous thromboembolism among users of oral contraceptives: a review of two recently published studies. *Journal of Family Planning and Reproductive Health Care, 36*(10), 33–38. doi:10.1783/147118910790291037

Shen, J., Che, Y., Showell, E., Chen, K., & Cheng, L. (2019). Interventions for emergency contraception. *Cochrane Database of Systematic Reviews, 2019*(1), CD001324. doi:10.1002/14651858.CD001324.pub6

Sinai, I., Jennings, V., & Arévalo, M. (1999). The TwoDay Algorithm: A new algorithm to identify the fertile time of the menstrual cycle. *Contraception, 60*(2), 65–70. doi:10.1016/s0010-7824(99)00072-4

SisterSong. (n.d.). *Reproductive justice*. https://www.sistersong.net/reproductive-justice

Smallwood, G. H., Meador, M. L., Lenihan, J. P., Shangold, G. A., Fisher, A. C., & Creasy, G. W. (2001). Efficacy and safety of a transdermal contraceptive system. *Obstetrics & Gynecology, 98*(5), 799–805. doi:10.1016/s0029-7844(01)01534-4

Soini, T., Hurskainen, R., Grénman, S., Mäenpää, J., Paavonen, J., & Pukkala, E. (2014). Cancer risk in women using the levonorgestrel releasing intrauterine system in Finland. *Obstetrics and Gynecology, 124*(2, Pt. 1), 292–299. doi:10.1097/AOG.0000000000000356

Sonfield, A., Hasstedt, K., Kavanaugh, M.L., & Anderson, R. (2013, March). *The social and economic benefits of women's ability to determine whether and when to have children*. Guttmacher Institute. https://www.guttmacher.org/sites/default/files/pdfs/pubs/social-economic-benefits.pdf

Stanford, J. B., & Mikolajczyk, R. T. (2002). Mechanisms of action of intrauterine devices: update and estimation of postfertilization effects. *American Journal of Obstetrics and Gynecology, 187*(6), 1699–1708. https://doi.10.1067.mob.2002.128091

Steinberg, J., & Lynch, S. E. (2021). Lactic acid, citric acid, and potassium bitartrate (Phexxi) vaginal gel for contraception. *American Family Physician, 103*(10), 628–629.

Sundaram, A., Vaughan, B., Kost, K., Bankole, A., Finer, L., Singh, S., & Trussel, J. (2017). Contraceptive failure in the United States: Estimates from the 2006–2010 National Survey of Family Growth. *Perspectives on Sexual and Reproductive Health, 49*(1), 7–16. doi:10.1363/psrh.12017

Thomas, M. A., Chappell, B. T., Maximos, B., Culwell, K. R., Dart, C., & Howard, B. (2020). A novel vaginal pH regulator: Results from the phase 3 AMPOWER contraception clinical trial. *Contraception: X, 2*, 10031. doi:10.1016/j.conx.2020.100031

Ti, A. J., Roe, A. H., Whitehouse, K. C., Smith, R. A., Gaffield, M. E., & Curtis, K. M. (2020). Effectiveness and safety of extending intrauterine device duration: A systematic review. *American Journal of Obstetrics and Gynecology*, 223(1), 24–35.e3. doi:10.1016/j.ajog.2020.01.014

Trussel, J. (2011). Contraceptive failure in the United States. *Contraception*, 83(5), 397–404. doi:10.1016/j.contraception.2011.01.021.

Trussel, J., Aiken, A., Micks, E., & Guthrie, K. A. (2018). Efficacy, safety, and personal considerations. In Hatcher, A. L. Nelson, J. Trussel, C. Cwiak, P. Cason, M. S. Policar, A. B. Edelman, A. R. A. Aiken, J. M. Marrazzo, & D. Kowal (Eds.), *Contraceptive technology* (21st ed., pp. 329–365). Ayer.

Trussel, J., Cleland, K., & Schwarz, E. B. (2018). Emergency contraception. In R. A. Hatcher, A. L. Nelson, J. Trussel, C. Cwiak, P. Cason, M. S. Policar, A. B. Edelman, A. R. A. Aiken, J. M. Marrazzo, & D. Kowal (Eds.), *Contraceptive technology* (21st ed., pp. 329–365). Ayer.

Trussel, J., Ellertson, C., von Hertzen, H., Bigrigg, A., Webb, A., Evans, M., Ferden, S., & Leadbetter, C. (2003). Estimating the effectiveness of emergency contraceptive pills. *Contraception*, 67(4), 259–265. doi:10.1016/s0010-7824(02)00535-8

Turok, D. (2021). Emergency contraception. *UpToDate*. https://www.uptodate.com/contents/emergency-contraception

Turok, D. K., Gero, A., Simmons, R. G., Kaiser, J. E., Stoddard, G. J., Sexsmith, C. D., Gawron, L. M., & Sanders, J. N. (2021). Levonorgestrel vs. copper intrauterine devices for emergency contraception. *New England Journal of Medicine*, 384(4), 335–344. doi:10.1056/NEJMoa2022141

United Nations, Department of Economic and Social Affairs. (2019). *Contraceptive use by method 2019*. https://www.un.org/en/development/desa/population/publications/pdf/family/ContraceptiveUseByMethodDataBooklet2019.pdf

Veres, S., Miller, L., & Burington, B. (2004). A comparison between the vaginal ring and oral contraceptives. *Obstetrics & Gynecology*, 104(3), 555–563. doi:10.1097/01.AOG.0000136082.59644.13

Veru, Inc. (n.d.). FC2 female condom. http://www.fc2.us.com

Voedisch, A. J., & Hindiyeh, N. (2019). Combined hormonal contraception and migraine: Are we being too strict? *Current Opinion in Obstetrics & Gynecology*, 31(6), 452–458. doi:10.1097/GCO.0000000000000586

Warner, L., & Steiner, M. J. (2018). Male condoms. In R. A. Hatcher, A. L. Nelson, J. Trussel, C. Cwiak, P. Cason, M. S. Policar, A. B. Edelman, A. R. A. Aiken, J. M. Marrazzo, & D. Kowal (Eds.), *Contraceptive technology* (21st ed., pp. 431–450). Ayer.

Warner, L., Steiner, M. J., & Stone, K. M. (2021). External (formerly male) condoms. *UpToDate*. https://www.uptodate.com/contents/external-formerly-male-condoms

Weiderpass, E., Adami, H., Baron, J. A., Magnusson, C., Bergström, R., Lindren, A., Correia, N., & Persson, I. (1999). Risk of endometrial cancer following estrogen replacement with and without progestins. *Journal of the National Cancer Institute*, 91(13), 1131–1137. doi:10.1093/jnci/91.13.1131

Westhoff, C. L., Heartwell, S., Edwards, S., Zieman, M., Stuart, G., Cwiak, C., Davis, A., Robilotto, T., Cushman, L., & Kalmuss, D. (2007). Oral contraceptive discontinuation: Do side effects matter? *American Journal of Obstetrics and Gynecology*, 196(4), 412e1–412e7. doi:10.1016/j.ajog.2006.12.015.

Wheeler, L. J., Desanto, K., Teal, S. B., Sheeder, J., & Guntupalli, S. R. (2019). Intrauterine device use and ovarian cancer risk: A systematic review and meta-analysis. *Obstetrics and Gynecology*, 134(4), 791–800. doi:10.1097/AOG.0000000000003463

Whittaker, P. G., Merkh, R. D., Henry-Moss, D., & Hock-Long, L. (2010). Withdrawal attitudes and experiences: a qualitative perspective among young urban adults. *Perspectives on Sexual and Reproductive Health*, 42(2), 102–109. doi:10.1363/4210210

Wilcox, A. J., Dunson, D., & Baird, D. D. (2000). The timing of the "fertile window" in the menstrual cycle: Day specific estimates from a progressive study. *British Medical Journal*, 321(7271), 1259–1262. doi:10.1136/bmj.321.7271.1259

Wilcox, A. J., Weinberg, C. R., & Baird, D. D. (1998). Post-ovulatory ageing of the human oocyte and embryo failure. *Human Reproduction*, 12(2), 394–397. doi:10.1093/humrep/13/2/394

Wu, W., & Bartz, D. (2018). Injectable contraceptives. In R. A. Hatcher, A. L. Nelson, J. Trussel, C. Cwiak, P. Cason, M. S. Policar, A. B. Edelman, A. R. A. Aiken, J. M. Marrazzo, & D. Kowal (Eds.), *Contraceptive technology* (21st ed., pp. 263–316). Ayer.

Xu, H., Wade, J. A., Peipert, J. F., Zhao, Q., Madden, T., & Secure, G. M. (2012). Contraceptive failure rates of etonogestrel subdermal implants in overweight and obese women. *Obstetrics and Gynecology*, 120(1), 21–26. doi:10.1097/AOG.0b013e318259565a

Yoon, S. H., Kim, S. N., Shim, S. H., Kang, S. B., & Lee, S. J. (2016). Bilateral salpingectomy can reduce the risk of ovarian cancer in the general population: A meta-analysis. *European Journal of Cancer*, 55, 38–46. doi:10.1016.j.ejca.2015.12.003

CHAPTER 22

Menopause Transition

Zaineh Khalil and Joleen D. Bishop

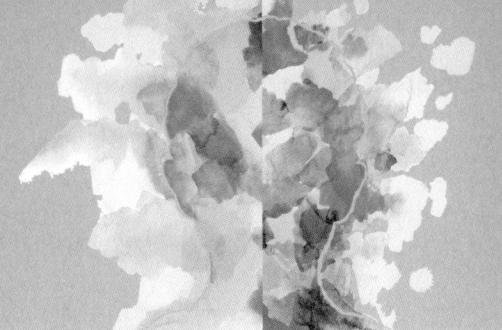

I. Introduction

Menopause is diagnosed when the menstrual cycle has ceased for 12 consecutive months, with no known relation to alternative causes. This occurs as a result of a decrease in follicle activation, with a concurrent depletion in the ovarian reserve (Geraghty, 2021). This process occurs gradually over several years and varies from person to person. About 5 years before the final menstrual period (FMP), people may notice variation in the length of their menstrual cycles, with a slow transition into intervals of amenorrhea for extended periods of time (Geraghty, 2021). The Stages of Reproductive Aging Workshop +10 (STRAW+10) (Harlow et al., 2012) offers a basis for assessing reproductive aging with an understanding of the hypothalamic–pituitary–ovarian axis.

A. Background

Menopause was historically referred to as the *climacteric*, which comes from the Greek root word *klimakter*, literally meaning "rung of a ladder" or figuratively meaning "critical point in life." A true understanding of menopause has only developed as more people are living through and after this stage of life. Only in the last century has there been an increased number of people assigned female at birth (AFAB) who have reached menopause. As of 2021, the life expectancy of people AFAB was 80.5 years in the United States (Arias et al., 2021). This is a significant increase from the 1500s, when AFAB life expectancy was 35 (McKeon, 1988), and even from the 1920s, when it was 55 (Youngs, 1990). With modern advancements in maintaining overall health, AFAB persons who survive until age 50 can expect to live an average of 33 more years, possibly spending almost 40% of their life in nonreproductive years (El Khoudari, 2022). Although strides in understanding have been made during this last century, there was ample opportunity for myths and misinformation about menopause to flourish. Examples of these myths include the belief that menopause is the end of a person's sexual life and that menopause leads to mental illness (McKeon, 1988). Awareness of this historical knowledge gap is integral to understanding why the myths exist. These myths may be significant factors for people in seeking and/or delaying treatment for their symptoms.

B. Demographics

The average (mean) age of menopause varies from 46 to 52 years, depending on the study (Schoenaker et al., 2014). It is estimated that in 2020, there were over 64 million persons AFAB in the United States over age 50 (El Khoudari, 2022).

C. Types of menopause and reproductive aging

In 2001, the Stages of Reproductive Aging Workshop (STRAW) developed and established a standard vernacular and staging system for menopause processes based on menstrual cycle bleeding criteria and follicle-stimulating hormone (FSH) levels. STRAW+10 was refined in 2011 and incorporated new data related to FSH, antral follicle count (AFC), antimullerian hormone (AMH), and inhibin B, as well as evidence regarding postmenopausal symptoms in FSH and estradiol levels (Harlow et al., 2012). STRAW+10 is now the gold standard for understanding the menopause transition. STRAW+10 is a detailed evaluation of the menopause process, dividing this process into seven stages. This staging allows the provider and patient a greater understanding of symptoms and management options at each stage. Each of the STRAW+10's seven stages has specific clinical criteria, endocrine parameters, and characteristic markers of aging. STRAW+10 staging is applicable regardless of demographics, age, weight, and lifestyle. Menstrual cycle criteria cannot be applied to people without regular menstrual cycles or those who have had a hysterectomy or endometrial ablation. In these cases, reproductive aging is assessed after a minimum of 3 months by evaluating endocrine markers (Sokalska & Gracia, 2022).

The FMP is preceded by five stages and followed by two. The reproductive years comprise stages -5 through -3, with few symptoms, but lower anti-mullerian hormone and inhibin levels, and variable FSH levels. The menopause transition comprises stages -2 and -1, with increasing symptoms and FSH levels. Although most people progress from one stage to the next, some may move between stages or skip them altogether (Sokalska & Gracia, 2022). Symptoms of menopause gradually increase as people enter the late reproductive years and progress through the early menopausal transition, but the biggest increase in symptomatology is clearly associated with late transition (Harlow et al., 2012).

In 2005, a National Institutes of Health (NIH) workshop defined four cardinal symptoms of the menopausal transition: menstrual changes, vasomotor symptoms (VMS), sleep disruption, and vaginal dryness/dyspareunia (genitourinary syndrome of menopause [GSM]) (Santoro, 2016). In 2011, STRAW+10 added adverse mood changes. These five cardinal symptoms are addressed in the following sections.

1. Menstrual cycle changes

   All people AFAB will have some type of menstrual changes as a symptom of menopause transition (MT). Pre-transition, an average menstrual cycle is 28 days long, with a follicular phase that lasts for 14 days and a luteal phase that lasts for 14 days. The early MT (STRAW+10 stage −2) is characterized by an increase in cycle irregularity by 7 or more days or periods of amenorrhea lasting up to 60 days (Santoro, 2022). At this time of the transition, estradiol levels are not consistently low, although the prevalence of menopause symptoms begin to increase. By the late transition (STRAW+10 stage −1), follicular depletion drops below a critical threshold. Symptoms often present as irregular menses, absent menses, or persistent abnormal bleeding (AUB). *AUB* is an umbrella term that encompasses heavy menstrual bleeding (previously referred to as *menorrhagia*) and intermenstrual bleeding (previously referred to as *metrorrhagia*). See Chapter 16, Abnormal Uterine Bleeding, for more information.

2. Vasomotor symptoms (VMSs)

   VMSs are described as an acute onset of heat flushing to the upper body, specifically the chest, neck, and face. Daytime VMSs are called *hot flashes*, and overnight VMSs are called *night sweats*. The duration of each episode varies between 1 and 5 minutes, and they may be associated with perspiration, chills, anxiety, and/or heart palpitations. Mild hot flashes include the sensation of heat without sweating, moderate include the sensation of heat with sweating and the ability to continue activity, and severe include the sensation of heat with sweating severe enough to cause the cessation of activity (Thurston, 2022).

   VMSs occur during the MT for up to 80% of people AFAB in the United States, but the daily frequency varies. On average, people report 4–5 hot flashes per day, although some have as many as 20 per day. One in four people report having VMSs every day. Occurrence and intensity are lowest prior to entering the MT. They increase in the early transition and are higher still in the later transition, near the FMP. They may continue to be intense for the first 1–2 years after the last menstrual period. In some patients, VMSs can last for 7–10 years (Thurston, 2022).

   Menopause following an oophorectomy or hysterectomy is often associated with severe and frequent VMSs. VMSs are also rated as more severe in patients following breast cancer treatment (Thurston, 2022).

   The definitive cause of VMSs has yet to be determined. There are multiple physiologic processes that are believed to contribute to these symptoms. Although estradiol levels decline in all persons AFAB, VMSs will not be experienced by all persons AFAB. The degree of change in circulating estradiol levels is associated with VMSs. However, estrogens alone typically do not explain VMSs. It is believed other physiologic mechanisms are also involved (Thurston, 2022).

   Thermoregulatory models of VMSs theorize a change in thermoregulatory function that results in acute heat-dissipation events. The response associated with the distribution of heat is controlled in humans by the hypothalamus (Thurston, 2022). The notable neurotransmitters involved in the thermoregulation of the hypothalamus are norepinephrine (NE) and serotonin (5-HT) (Alexander & Moore, 2007). These neurotransmitters cause vasodilation and vasoconstriction in the cutaneous vessels (Thurston, 2022). According to this model, the thermoneutral zone of patients with menopause is narrowed, and small perturbations in body temperature, particularly over this zone, trigger an acute heat-dissipation event in the form of a hot flash (Randolph et al., 2005). This dysfunction in thermoregulation in the hypothalamic control center, its messengers (norepinephrine and serotonin), or the effectors (cutaneous vessels) is believed to be the underlying process of VMSs (Thurston, 2022).

   Risk factors for VMS include early age at menarche (Zhao et al., 2021), high weight, tobacco and nicotine use, history of premenstrual symptoms, and early perimenopause (Gold et al., 2004). The Study of Women's Health Across the Nation (SWAN) demonstrated differences in the experience of menopausal symptoms between racial and ethnic groups (Santoro & Sutton-Tyrrell, 2011), as well as with socioeconomic status. African American and Hispanic persons have been shown to have a higher odds of reporting VMSs (Gold et al., 2004). Financial strain, social support, and adverse life events as they relate to socioeconomic status have also been shown to influence menopausal symptoms

(Santoro & Sutton-Tyrrell, 2011). Populations historically excluded from health care have been historically misrepresented in the literature, and recent awareness of the structural racism that influences these inequities, such as residential segregation, social deprivation, policy, and economic injustice, have become the correct determinants of health rather than race as a biologic or genetic cause (Julian et al., 2021). As such, we have a greater insight into why many studies have shown racial and ethnic variations in the experience of VMSs.

Given the variations in the prevalence of VMSs, as well as increased awareness of the misclassification of determinants of health, consistent measurement methods of VMSs have been proposed to provide a clearer understanding of the impact of the symptoms on both the patient and the clinician and to allow proper screening and treatment.

3. Genitourinary syndrome of menopause

GSM refers to a group of signs and symptoms associated with estrogen deficiency (Shifren, 2022). This results in thinning of the vaginal tissue and in lower urinary tract symptoms, which can affect the clitoris, labia, vestibule/introitus, vagina, and/or urethra. The diagnosis is based on the patient's reported symptoms and is not based on clinical exam. These symptoms may include vaginal dryness, itching, burning, and discomfort or pain with sexual activity, as well as urinary symptoms such as dysuria, frequency, and urgency (Siegel et al., 2021). In 2014, a consensus conference endorsed the term *GSM* to replace the terms *vulvovaginal atrophy* and *atrophic vaginitis*. The International Society for the Study of Women's Sexual Health (ISSWSH) and the North American Menopause Society (NAMS) believed the older terminology did not encompass the extent of lower urinary tract and vaginal symptoms that many experience (Thurston, 2022). Estimates of GSM in postmenopausal persons range from 27% to 85% (Siegel et al., 2021).

Vaginal symptoms appear relatively early in the transition (Santoro, 2016). Decreased estrogen can cause several changes to genital anatomy that lead to patient discomfort. Diminished blood flow results in the loss of vaginal rugae, thinning of the vagina and shortening of the vaginal vault, loss of elasticity, and narrowing of the introitus. Thinning of the vulvar mucosa may cause vulvar burning, irritation, or constriction of the introitus, resulting in dyspareunia. Narrowing of the vagina and decreased lubrication can cause painful intercourse or coital bleeding. Diminished estrogen may also lead to recurrent urinary tract infections and urinary urgency. Unlike hot flashes and adverse mood, which can improve over time, vaginal dryness is often progressive and does not improve without specific ongoing treatment. In rare cases, the low estrogen levels can result in adhesion of the labia minora, which can present as incomplete bladder emptying, postvoid dribbling, urinary retention, and/or incontinence (Gungor Ugurlucan et al., 2021.)

A cross-sectional, population-based study called the Menopause Epidemiology (MEPI) study found that of the persons AFAB in the United States aged 40 to 65 years, 57% reported symptoms consistent with GSM (Levine et al., 2008). Participants with sexual dysfunction were approximately four times more likely to have GSM symptoms than those without sexual dysfunction. Another study found that the most common symptoms of vaginal discomfort experienced by sexually active menopausal patients were vaginal dryness (85%) and dyspareunia (52%) (Shifren, 2022).

4. Sleep changes

Insomnia disorder, often described by patients as difficulty sleeping, affects about one-third of the general population. It is defined by the American Psychiatric Association as sleep difficulties at least three times per week for at least 3 months that are distressing to the patient due to their effects on the person's daily functioning (Torres, 2020). The 2015 National Health Interview Survey presented data indicating that postmenopausal participants were more likely to report poor sleep quality (defined as waking not feeling well rested). A greater percentage of postmenopausal respondents had trouble falling asleep (27.1%) as well as staying asleep (sleep maintenance) (35.9%) at least four times a week.

Sleep disorders include insomnia, obstructive sleep apnea (OSA), restless leg syndrome (RLS), and periodic limb movement disorder (PLMD). There are many contributing factors to menopausal sleep loss, such as night sweats, stress and psychological factors, medical comorbidities, certain drugs or alcohol, and poor sleep hygiene (Faubion, 2022). Difficulty with sleep often worsens over time, with those in the late menopausal transition and those after surgical menopausal reporting the greatest difficulties (Santoro, 2016). The SWAN study has provided several observations that help clarify the relationships between menopause and sleep. At baseline, 9.8% reported insomnia, and 37.7% reported difficulty sleeping. Sleep difficulty was clearly seen to increase as participants traversed the menopause, with late menopausal transition and surgically induced menopause causing the greatest difficulty (Santoro, 2016).

5. Neuropsychiatric changes

a. Cognition

Cognition encompasses mental skills such as attention and concentration, learning and memory, language, spatial abilities, judgment, problem solving, and reasoning. Many people transitioning through menopause complain of "brain fog," forgetfulness, and difficulty finding words. However, data are still not clear on the effect hormones have on cognition.

Estrogen, progesterone, and testosterone regulate facets of brain function via multiple mechanistic pathways. These same hormones influence neurotransmitter systems, including acetylcholine, serotonin, norepinephrine, glutamate, gamma-aminobutyric acid (GABA), and dopamine. This triggers the formation of synapses to facilitate neuronal communication and results in decreased inflammation, improved blood flow to the brain, and promotion of growth factors that sustain neural function. Clinical studies have shown that sex hormones influence neural networks that are involved in attention, memory, and other cognitive functions. The hippocampus and the prefrontal cortex are rich in estrogen receptors (Maki, 2022). However, longitudinal studies that assess the impact of menopause on cognitive function are scarce. The SWAN study did show impairments in learning new abilities during the transition, followed by a return to premenopausal function in the postmenopausal period (Gava et al., 2019).
   b. Anxiety and depression
   The SWAN study showed that anxiety symptoms were more likely to be reported as people AFAB traverse the MT and may be linked to the onset of major depression. Those individuals with high anxiety at baseline continued to have high anxiety over the course of the menopausal transition, and those with low scores at study enrollment were more likely to become highly anxious as they progressed through menopause (Santoro, 2016).

   At least three large longitudinal cohort studies have examined the prevalence of depressive symptoms in perimenopausal people: SWAN (Sutton-Tyrrell et al., 2014), the Penn Ovarian Aging Study (Freeman & Sammel, 2016), and the Seattle Midlife Women's Health Study (Woods & Mitchell, 2016). These cohort studies followed participants for between 3 and 15 years. Across all studies, there was a notable increase in the occurrence of depressive symptoms. The risk of developing depressive symptoms was also elevated in those with no history of clinical depression. However, most people AFAB experiencing depression during the menopausal transition had a history of experiencing depression in the past (Soares, 2022).
D. *Menopause and long-term health*
   Menopause has also been linked to an increased risk of cardiovascular disease (coronary artery disease and stroke), as well as osteoporosis and some cancers. The earlier a person experiences menopause, the higher the risk of cardiovascular disease or osteoporosis (Nash et al., 2022). Cardiovascular disease is the leading cause of death and disability in postmenopausal people (Abramson et al., 2021). People who experience early-onset menopause or premature menopause are at an increased risk of developing cardiovascular disease (Honigberg et al., 2019). There is also rapid loss of bone mineral density (BMD) during the transition from premenopause to postmenopause (Karlamangla et al., 2022), which increases the risk of fracture. Studies are ongoing into the use of menopausal hormone treatment (MHT) as primary or secondary prevention for cardiovascular disease and colorectal cancer, but at this time, it is not recommended for either (Abramson et al., 2021).

   Although persons with a cervix may no longer need a Pap test after the age of 65 following adequate negative prior screening, a vulvar and vaginal exam continues to be a vital portion of their annual wellness visit. The changes that may occur as a result of untreated vulvar and vaginal atrophy may lead to lichen sclerosis, a precursor to vulvar squamous cell carcinoma (Leis et al., 2022). Therefore, it is important to continue to encourage people with vulvas to see their providers after the age of 65 for any genitourinary concerns, and shared decision making should be used to determine the frequency of screening, if indicated.

II. **Assessment**
A. *Determine diagnosis*
   Utilizing the STRAW+10, determine the stage of the transition.
B. *Other conditions to consider*
   1. Vasomotor symptoms
      a. Medication side effects
      b. Malignancy
      c. Infectious disease(s)
      d. Evaluate patient for endocrine disorders, including hyperthyroidism, pheochromocytoma, carcinoid syndrome, insulinoma, and acromegaly.
   2. Genitourinary syndrome of menopause
      a. Vulvar diseases, including lichen sclerosis, lichen planus, and vulvar cancer
      b. Urinary and anal incontinence
      c. Urinary tract infection
   3. Menstrual cycle changes
      a. Possible alternative causes of secondary amenorrhea: functional hypothalamic amenorrhea, pituitary dysfunction, pregnancy, thyroid disease, Asherman syndrome (see Chapter 18, Amenorrhea and Polycystic Ovary Syndrome)
      b. Possible alternative causes of abnormal vaginal bleeding: endometrial hyperplasia and unopposed estrogen, endometrial or cervical cancer, endometrial polyps, adenomyosis, fibroids, coagulation disorders, inflammation or infection in the uterus, pregnancy, thyroid disease, medication side effects (see Chapter 16, Abnormal Uterine Bleeding)
   4. Mood/Cognition
      a. Dementia and Alzheimer disease (see Chapter 48, Dementia)
      b. Depression and anxiety disorders (see Chapter 42, Anxiety, and Chapter 49, Depression)
      c. Sleep disorders, including OSA and RLS

5. Sexual dysfunction
   a. Sexual trauma history (see Chapter 58, Intimate Partner Violence [Domestic Violence])
   b. Vulvar disease, vulvar pain disorders, pelvic floor muscle dysfunction, vaginal atrophy (see Chapter 23, Chronic Pelvic Pain in Persons Assigned Female at Birth)
   c. Anxiety, depression, disorders of relationship (see Chapter 24, Sexual Dysfunction)

C. *Severity*
Assess severity of the symptoms and the impact on the patient's life. The NAMS Menopause Health Questionnaire can be helpful.

D. *Significance*
1. Assess the significance of the transition to the patient.
2. Determine the patient's strengths and ability to follow treatment plans.

III. Goals of clinical management
A. *Alleviate symptoms and improve quality of life.*
B. *Rule out alternative causes of symptoms.*
C. *Perform routine health screening.*
D. *Determine the patient's goals in seeking diagnoses.*
E. *Determine the patient's treatment goals.*

IV. Plan
A. *Screening and testing based on symptoms*
1. Abnormal bleeding: endometrial biopsy, pelvic ultrasound, complete blood count (CBC), thyroid-stimulating hormone (TSH) (see Chapter 16, Abnormal Uterine Bleeding)
2. Amenorrhea: pregnancy test, prolactin, TSH, FSH (see Chapter 18, Amenorrhea and Polycystic Ovary Syndrome)
3. Changes in mood and cognition: Screening tools include the Patient Health Questionnaire (PHQ-9), General Anxiety Disorder (GAD-7), and Mini-Mental State Exam MMSE (see chapters on depression [Chapter 49], anxiety [Chapter 42], and dementia [Chapter 48]).

B. *Management*
1. Menstrual cycle changes
As persons AFAB approach menopause, they may begin to experience irregularities in their menstrual cycles. Some may report short cycle intervals (<21 days) in the early MT, and others may report longer cycle intervals (>36 days) later in the MT. Because hormonal changes could mask pathologic diagnoses, further evaluation is required to rule out serious diagnoses such as hyperplasia (Delamater & Santoro, 2018). See Chapter 16, Abnormal Uterine Bleeding, for more information.
2. VMSs
   a. Hormone therapy
   Hormone therapy (HT) and *MHT* are used interchangeably and include estrogen therapy (ET), estrogen–progesterone therapy (EPT), progestogens, and estrogen combined with an estrogen antagonist/agonist. Progestogens include progesterone and the synthetic pregestational compounds termed *progestins*. In the past, the terms *estrogen replacement therapy* and *hormone replacement therapy* were used. Now that it is understood that hormone levels are naturally low after menopause, it is no longer appropriate to consider these therapies "replacement." HT, therefore, is intended to be used as a treatment for menopause symptoms. MHT is considered to be a replacement for patients with premature ovarian insufficiency or early surgical menopause (Liu, 2022).

   The U.S. Food and Drug Administration (FDA) has approved HT as a treatment for VMSs and premature hypoestrogenism. Estrogen decreases these symptoms, and progestogens are needed to counter the proliferative effects of estrogen on the endometrium. Without progestogens, there is an increased risk of endometrial neoplasia (Hill et al., 2016). The initiation of ET should involve a shared decision-making process between the clinician and the patient that includes discussion of the effect of symptoms on the patient's life, as well as the risks and benefits of treatment options. Continuous reassessment, especially within the first 8 weeks, can help determine if dose or formulation adjustments are necessary. Ultimately, the goal of therapy is to provide relief with the most appropriate dose, route, duration, and regimen and make adjustments as needed (Liu, 2022).

   In the past, clinicians were encouraged to prescribe the lowest amount of HT for the shortest amount of time. The 2017 NAMS HT position statement (NAMS, 2017) instead recommends that providers work with their patients in shared decision making to "determine the appropriate type, dose, formulation, route of administration, and duration of therapy based on their individual health characteristics and treatment goals" (Pinkerton, 2022, p. 302). Once HT is initiated, patients can continue as long as is needed for symptom relief—while having clear and full understanding of risk as it pertains to their specific regimen and health characteristics (Sherif, 2013).
      i. Estrogen preparations
      Estrogens are available in many prescription preparations, including as single agents in oral preparations, transdermal patches, gels or topical emulsion preparations, vaginal preparations, combination (EPT) preparations, and conjugated estrogen (CE) combined with bazedoxifene (BZA; see further discussion that follows). Intramuscular preparations are

not recommended for HT because serum estrogen levels associated with injections rise to very high levels after administration and may increase the risk for deep vein thrombosis (Liu, 2022). With all oral estrogen products, estrone is the predominant estrogen in circulation because of the first-pass uptake and metabolism in the gastrointestinal (GI) tract and the liver. The hepatic effect with oral ET results in greater stimulation of certain proteins compared with transdermal therapy, including lipoproteins such as high-density lipoprotein cholesterol (HDL-C). Oral estrogen is also associated with a 25% increase in triglycerides, increasing the risk of pancreatitis in those who already have hypertriglyceridemia (Liu, 2022).

Transdermal (patch) or topical (cream) estrogen can be prescribed in lower doses than oral formulations because it is not subjected to absorption through the gut or first-pass hepatic metabolism. Because of this difference in the mechanism of absorption, transdermal and topical administrations of estrogen do not increase triglycerides. However, topical and transdermal ET cannot aid in increasing HDL-C as oral estrogen can. As a result of less liver exposure, transdermal and topical ETs do not affect gallbladder disease and coagulation factors. Serum estrogen levels are more stable in patients who use transdermal rather than oral ET. Therefore, in patients who need stable estrogen levels, transdermal ET is preferred. Additionally, transdermal estrogen may be the clinical choice to avert migraines (Liu, 2022).

Vaginal estrogen preparations are not prescribed for systemic symptoms of menopause, such as VMSs and cognitive concerns. They are reserved for patients with GSM, including vaginal dryness, atrophy, dysuria, and dyspareunia. Although the FDA has required similar labeling for all formulations of estrogen, vaginal estrogen formulations have not been found to result in notable increases in serum estrogen levels (Liu, 2022).

The oral dose of 0.625 mg of CE, available in the United States as conjugated equine estrogen (CEE), is equivalent to 0.005–0.015 mg of ethinyl estradiol (EE). Both are also equivalent to 1 mg of 17β-estradiol (micronized estrogen [ME] or estradiol). These oral doses are equivalent to the transdermal dose of the 0.05-mg estradiol patch and the 1.5-mg/2 metered doses of topical estradiol gel. The doses are equivalent to systemic vaginal formulations of 0.3125 mg of CE and 0.5 mg of 17β-estradiol (Liu, 2022). See **Table 22-1** for comparative doses. There are lower doses available in patch formulations; for example, Menostar is available at 0.014 mg. Some patches are changed twice a week, and others are changed once per week. The choice of administration route is made based on patient preference and ease of use.

ii. Progestogens

The primary menopause-related indication for progestogen use is to prevent endometrial overgrowth and the increased risk of

Table 22-1 Comparative Systemic Estrogen Therapy Doses

Route	Formulation (U.S. Brands)	Standard Dose Equivalent	Doses Available
Oral	Conjugated estrogen (Premarin)	0.625 mg	0.4 mg; 0.45 mg; 0.625mg; 0.9 mg; 1.25 mg
Oral	Esterified estrogen (Menest)	0.625 mg	0.3 mg; 0.625 mg; 1.25 mg
Oral	Ethinyl estradiol (available only as combination with progestin: FemHRT; Jevantique Lo, Jinteli)	0.005–0.015 mg	0.0025 mg; 0.005 mg
Oral	Estradiol (Estrace)	1 mg	0.5 mg; 1 mg; 2 mg
Oral	Estropipate (Ogen)	0.75 mg	0.75 mg; 1.5 mg; 3 mg
Patch	Estradiol (Vivelle-Dot, Climara, Minivelle, Menostar)	0.05 mg	0.014 mg; 0.025 mg; 0.0375 mg; 0.05 mg; 0.06 mg; 0.075 mg; 0.1 mg
Vaginal ring	Estradiol (Femring)	0.5 mg/day	0.5mg/day; 1mg/day

endometrial cancer during unopposed ET use. In the endometrium, progestogens convert estradiol into a weaker estrogen called *estrone*. This results in less endometrial stimulation, therefore preventing hyperplasia (Liu, 2022).

Progestins commonly used include medroxyprogesterone acetate (MPA); norethindrone acetate; and MP, which is bioidentical. Bazedoxifene use with estrogen prevents hyperplasia as well (see following discussion). When adequate progestogen is combined with estrogen, the risk of endometrial neoplasia is not higher than in untreated patients (Liu, 2022).

The most widely studied and commonly prescribed progestogen formulation in the United States for endometrial protection is the synthetic MPA. However, some patients may experience unfavorable side effects, such as mood swings, when taking a synthetic progestin. The clinician and the patient may consider using micronized progesterone (MP), which is bioidentical. MP may have sedating effects, reducing wakefulness without affecting daytime cognitive functions. Thus, bedtime dosing is advised (Liu, 2022).

Progestogen regimens may be classified as continuous-cyclic sequential, continuous-cyclic long cycle, continuous combined, and intermittent combined. Each involves daily estrogen administration. The therapeutic goal of progestogen in EPT is to prevent unopposed estrogen exposure while maintaining estrogen benefits and minimizing unwanted progestogen-induced effects. Research is insufficient to recommend one regimen over another (Liu, 2022).

Continuous-cyclic EPT is the administration of progestogen for 12–14 days of each month. The progestogen can be started on the 1st or 15th day of each month, whichever is easier for the patient to remember. About 80% of patients will experience withdrawal bleeding with this regimen and standard doses of estrogen (CE 0.625 mg or ME 1 mg) (Liu, 2022).

Continuous-cyclic long-cycle EPT is the administration of progestogen every 3–6 months. This regimen reduces the frequency of withdrawal bleeding, although patients may experience heavier and longer bleeding episodes. This regimen remains effective in preventing endometrial hyperplasia as long as the patient uses standard ET (CE 0.3 mg) or less (Liu, 2022). However, the use of 2 mg of 17β- estradiol daily (twice the standard dose) was found to increase the incidence of endometrial hyperplasia when taken with continuous-cyclic long-cycle EPT (Odmark et al., 2005).

Progestogen is taken daily with continuous-combined EPT. This regimen decreases the incidence of withdrawal bleeding. Proper dosing of daily PT in combination with ET is used to prevent endometrial hyperplasia (Liu, 2022). Lastly, intermittent-combined EPT, sometimes referred to as *pulsed-progestogen* or *continuous-pulsed EPT*, is progestogen taken every 3 days. This also reduces the incidence of withdrawal bleeding while avoiding some of the side effects continuous progestogen may cause (Prefest, 2017).

The minimum daily dose of MPA is 5 mg for patients who desire continuous-cyclic EPT or 2.5 mg daily for patients who choose continuous-combined EPT. The minimum daily dose of norethindrone is 0.35–0.7 mg for cyclic EPT regimens versus 0.35 mg daily for continuous EPT regimens. For patients who choose norethindrone acetate, the minimum daily dose is 2.5 mg cyclically or 0.5–1 mg daily. Lastly, in patients who determine that MP is best suited for them, 200 mg is the minimum dose for cyclic regimens, and 100 mg is the minimum dose for daily combined EPT (Liu, 2022).

Estrogen and progestogen together are available in patch and pill formulations. The downside of prescribing combined therapies is the decreased dosing flexibility, although this may not be an issue for some patients who might prefer single-tablet or patch dosing.

Progestin-releasing intrauterine devices (IUDs) have not been approved by the FDA for endometrial protection in postmenopausal patients. However, studies suggest they prevent endometrial hyperplasia. They release progestin directly into the uterus, where it is needed (Depypere & Inki, 2015). Topical or gel formulations of progesterone do not have a sufficient effect on the endometrium. Therefore, they should not be prescribed (Liu, 2022).

Vaginal preparations of estrogen are the most effective treatment for GSM. They can be delivered via creams, rings, tablets, and inserts. All preparations at standard doses have been shown to decrease symptoms of GSM, including dyspareunia, incontinence, and urinary tract infection (UTI) (Rahn et al., 2014). There are two vaginal creams. 17β-estradiol (brand name Estrace) can be used with a starting dose of 2–4 grams per day for 2 weeks, then a maintenance dose of 1 gram twice weekly (Phillips & Bachmann, 2021). Many patients find relief with lower doses such as 0.5 mg. Conjugated estrogen (Brand name Premarin) can be used with a starting dose of 1 gram daily for 2 weeks, then a maintenance dose of 0.5 gram twice weekly (Phillips & Bachmann, 2021). The 17β-estradiol vaginal ring (brand name Estring) is placed vaginally and left for 90 days continuously (Philips & Bachmann, 2021). Estradiol hemihydrate (brand Vagifem) or Estradiol (brand Imvexxy) tablets are inserted vaginally daily for 2 weeks, then 2 times per week for maintenance (Philips & Bachmann, 2021). Non-estrogen treatments include Dehydroepiandrosterone (DHEA)/prasterone suppository (brand Intrarosa), used nightly, and oral Ospemifene (brand Osphena, 60 mg), taken daily (Philips & Bachmann, 2021).

iii. Bazedoxifene and CEE combination

For patients with a uterus who cannot tolerate a progestogen or who have had irregular bleeding and a thickened endometrial stripe with estrogen and progesterone combinations, the BZA/CEE tablet (marketed as Duavee) may be helpful (Liu, 2022). BZA is a selective estrogen receptor modulator, which, at the dose in Duavee, shows enough antagonist effect on endometrial tissue to avoid the proliferative effects of the estrogen. BZA/CEE has also been shown to decrease GSM symptoms (Kagan et al., 2010) and reduce the risk of osteoporosis (Johnson & Hauck, 2016).

iv. Contraindications

HT is contraindicated in patients who present with undiagnosed abnormal vaginal bleeding, who have current or a history of deep vein thrombosis or pulmonary embolism, who have a recent history of arterial thromboembolic disease (within 1 year), who have liver disease, who are pregnant, who are hypersensitive to ET or EPT, or who have a known history of porphyria cutanea tardis. In most cases, ET or EPT is also contraindicated in patients who have a history of breast cancer or estrogen-dependent neoplasia. In select patients, however, ET or EPT may be prescribed while being treated for metastatic disease in consultation with the patient's oncologist (Liu, 2022).

v. Risks

Overall, risks are lower when HT is initiated before the age of 60 and within 10 years of menopause. Studies have shown a rare absolute risk of stroke (<1/1,000) in those who initiated ET and EPT before the age of 60 but an increased risk in those who were taking CE alone within 10 years of their FMP (Manson et al., 2013).

Initial analysis of the Women's Health Initiative (WHI) suggested an increased risk of breast cancer in those taking progestogens. Participants assigned to CE alone had a reduced risk of cancer (hazard ratio [HR], 0.79), whereas participants who were assigned to combined EPT with MPA had a higher risk of new-onset breast cancer (HR, 1.28) (Manson, 2013).

Since the findings of the WHI became public, many studies have continued to evaluate the data. Long-term follow-up of 20.3 years in 98% of participants continues to show a decreased incidence of breast cancer in patients who take CEE alone. Patients can be reassured that taking CEE alone will not elevate their risk of breast cancer over time (Minami & Freedman, 2020).

Furthermore, additional statistical analysis of the WHI sheds light on why a higher incidence of breast cancer in participants assigned to the combined-CEE-with-MPA arm of the study was found: 25% of the participants had started MHT prior to the initiation of the study. An elevated risk of breast cancer was not found in the other 75% of participants receiving CEE with MPA. In addition, the placebo group had a very low incidence of breast cancer, making the numbers appear striking (Kuhl & Stevenson, 2006). Understanding these variances can help the provider properly counsel the patient to provide reassurance before starting HT.

vi. Additional benefits

A Cochrane review (Boardman et al., 2015) found that when HT was initiated within 10 years of menopause, there was a lower risk of coronary heart disease (relative risk [RR], 0.52). The data also showed reduced all-cause mortality. In both trials where women received CE (0.625 mg) with MPA (2.5 mg daily) or CE (0.625 mg) alone, there was a significantly lower rate of diabetes (HR, 0.81). Both trials also found a statistically significant 33% reduction in the incidence of hip fractures. The risk of endometrial cancer was reduced (HR, 0.58) in participants who were on CE with MPA (Manson et al., 2013). Unscheduled bleeding occurring more than 6 months after initiation of HT should be investigated (Liu, 2022).

vii. Side effects

The adverse effects of HT may result in unfavorable effects on quality of life, often

Table 22-2 Coping Strategies for Estrogen Therapy or Estrogen–Progestin Therapy Adverse Events

Adverse Event	Strategy
Fluid retention	Restrict salt; maintain adequate water intake; exercise; try a mild prescription diuretic.
Bloating	Switch to low-dose nonoral continuous estrogen; lower progestogen dose to a level that still protects the uterus; switch to another progestin or to micronized progesterone.
Breast tenderness or enlargement	Lower estrogen dose; switch to another estrogen; restrict salt; switch to another progestin; cut down on caffeine and chocolate.
Headaches	Switch to nonoral continuous estrogen; lower dose of estrogen or progestogen or both; switch to a continuous-combined regimen; switch to progesterone or a 19-norpregnane derivative; ensure adequate water intake; restrict salt, caffeine, and alcohol.
Mood change	Investigate preexisting depression or anxiety; lower progestogen dose; switch progestogen; switch from systemic progestin to the progestin intrauterine system; change to a continuous-combined estrogen–progesterone therapy (EPT) regimen; ensure adequate water intake; restrict salt, caffeine, and alcohol.
Nausea	Advise taking oral estrogen tablets with meals or before bed; switch to another oral estrogen; switch to nonoral estrogen; lower estrogen or progestogen dose.
Bleeding	Lower dose of estrogen or progestogen; switch to nonprogestogen combined therapy.

Reproduced from Table 16, page 301 in Liu, J.H. (2022). Prescription Therapies. In C. Crandall (Ed.), Menopause Practice: A Clinician's Guide (6th ed., pp. 277-312). The Menopause Society.

resulting in cessation of therapy. Dose adjustments and changes in route of administration may be considered to address these side effects. See **Table 22-2**.

viii. Bioidentical HT
The term *bioidentical hormone* was first used as a marketing strategy for custom-compounded hormones. The term now encompasses hormones that are structurally identical to those produced in the human body (Liu, 2022). Estradiol and micronized progesterone fit this definition, which can be reassuring to persons who prefer to use HT they consider bioidentical (Stuenkel, 2021). Custom-compounded hormones are not regulated in the same way commercially available hormones are, so they should be used with caution.

ix. Discontinuation of therapy
Data have not shown there to be a difference in the recurrence of VMSs whether HT is tapered down or stopped abruptly. More than 50% of patients resume HT after 1 year of discontinuation because of the recurrence of symptoms (Lindh-Åstrand et al., 2010).

b. Nonhormonal therapies
Nonhormonal options are indicated for patients who might have contraindications to hormonal therapy or who may prefer them. Low-dose paroxetine is the only nonhormonal medication authorized by the FDA for the treatment of hot flashes. Desvenlafaxine and venlafaxine are appropriate alternatives, especially if a patient is taking tamoxifen, because they do not inhibit the hepatic enzyme responsible for the efficacy of tamoxifen. Other nonhormonal options include gabapentin and clonidine (Hill et al., 2016).

i. Selective serotonin reuptake inhibitors (SSRI) and selective norepinephrine reuptake inhibitors
Paroxetine is the only FDA-approved SSRI for hot flashes. Citalopram and escitalopram have also been shown to reduce hot flashes. In addition, venlafaxine and desvenlafaxine also reduce hot flashes but have been shown to have greater side effects than the others. Fluoxetine and sertraline have not been shown to be beneficial in treating hot flashes (Grady et al., 2007; Suvanto-Luukkonen et al., 2005).

ii. Gabapentin
Night-time use of gabapentin for 4–12 weeks has been shown to reduce the frequency of hot flashes (Shan et al., 2020).

iii. Clonidine
Clonidine is less effective than SSRIs or gabapentin, although it does have a modest effect on hot flashes. It typically has a undesirable side-effect profile, which may include hypotension, dry mouth, dizziness, lightheadedness, headache, and constipation (Sahni et al., 2021).

iv. Neurokinin B (NKB) antagonists
As this text goes to print, the FDA is considering approval of medications in a new class with the indication of reducing menopausal hot flashes. These NKB antagonists are thought to influence the thermoregulatory center of the brain (NAMS, 2022).
c. Complementary and alternative medicine (CAM)
For people who have contraindications for MHT, are unwilling to take MHT, and/or are interested in supplementing treatment with holistic options, there are complementary and alternative modalities. It is important to note that rigorous studies are lacking in understanding the true effect these options have on menopausal symptoms (Mehrnoush et al., 2021).
   i. Acupuncture: Acupuncture can be safe and effective for anxiety, which may accompany menopausal changes (Mehrnoush et al., 2021).
   ii. Yoga: Moderate evidence supports the benefit of yoga on the psychological symptoms of menopause (Mehrnoush et al., 2021).
   iii. St. John's Wort: Studies have shown that the use of St. John's Wort for 8–16 weeks had a significant effect on the severity of depression (Mehrnoush et al., 2021).
   iv. Clinical hypnosis: A randomized control trial of 187 postmenopausal patients showed a reduction in hot flashes of greater than 50% after 12 weeks (Elkins et al., 2013).
   v. Ineffective therapies: Insufficient evidence is available regarding the benefits of boron, zinc, black cohosh, berberine, or dehydroepiandrosterone (DHEA) on bone density. A Cochrane review noted insufficient evidence to support the benefits of herbal therapies for VMSs (Lethaby et al., 2013).
d. Lifestyle strategies
   i. Smoking cessation: Studies have shown that smoking increases the risk of early menopause (Hayatbakhsh et al., 2012). Therefore, smoking cessation should always be part of the treatment plan.
   ii. Plant-based diet: The combination of a low-fat, plant-based diet and whole soybeans has been shown to reduce the frequency and severity of hot flashes and improve quality of life in the vasomotor, psychosocial, physical, and sexual domains (Barnard et al., 2021).
3. GSM
The most effective treatment for GSM is topical estrogen. Prasterone/DHEA vaginal suppositories are also available, as is the oral selective estrogen receptor modulator (SERM) ospemifene.
a. Estrogen treatments
Vaginal preparations of estrogen are the most effective treatment for GSM. They can be delivered via creams, rings, tablets, and inserts. All preparations at standard doses have been shown to decrease symptoms of GSM, including dyspareunia, incontinence, and urinary tract infection (UTI) (Rahn et al., 2014). Adding a progestogen to low-dose vaginal ET is not typically recommended, based on 1-year endometrial safety data (Suckling et al., 2006). Labeling for vaginal estrogens typically includes warnings identical to those for systemic estrogens, but studies have not shown an increase in invasive breast, colorectal, or endometrial cancers; stroke; deep vein thrombosis; or pulmonary embolism (Phillips & Bachmann, 2021). Although systemic estrogen is contraindicated for patients with a history of hormone-responsive cancers (e.g., breast cancer), serum estrogen levels are generally not increased by vaginal estrogens (Rahn et al., 2014). It may be worth consulting with a patient's oncologist if the patient may benefit from estrogen for GSM. Providers should prescribe whichever formulation the patient prefers.
b. Nonestrogen treatments
DHEA and prasterone suppositories are converted via aromatase to androgens and estrogens (Phillips & Bachmann, 2021). They do not increase serum levels of hormones or influence the endometrium. Ospemifene is a SERM that selectively agonizes vaginal tissues without affecting the endometrium or breast (Phillips & Bachmann, 2021). It is the only oral option FDA approved for GSM, and it may cause hot flashes and slightly increases the risk for blood clots.
c. Nonhormonal treatments
Nonhormonal treatments for GSM include nonprescription moisturizers (to be used regularly for prevention of symptoms), such as Replens; hyaluronic acid tablets; and lubricants (to be used during penetrative sexual activity). Moisturizers rehydrate vaginal tissue and lower pH, and lubricants reduce friction (Phillips & Bachmann, 2021). Low-quality studies show that moisturizers and lubricants may work as well as estrogen when patients have a single GSM symptom, such as dyspareunia alone. However, when patients have multiple symptoms, such as dyspareunia and incontinence, vaginal estrogens are superior (Rahn et al., 2014).
4. Osteoporosis
A thorough discussion regarding the prevention and treatment of osteoporosis is beyond the scope of this chapter. However, to offer a brief review, osteoporosis is defined by low BMD and increases in prevalence with age. Between 40% and 50% of postmenopausal people AFAB will experience an

osteoporosis-related fracture in their lifetime. Routine prevention strategies, including adequate calcium and vitamin D intake, regular exercise, and smoking cessation, are recommended for patients who are at risk of developing osteoporosis. However, these measures do not prevent the interval of rapid bone loss that occurs in the first few years of menopause. Oral and transdermal preparations of estrogen have been shown to prevent bone loss in postmenopausal patients (Pinkerton & McClung, 2022). HT is FDA approved for the prevention of osteoporosis, and it can be prescribed for patients in need of osteoporosis treatment who also have VMSs (Pinkerton & McClung, 2022).

V. Patient education

Provide written and verbal information regarding:
1. Normal physiologic decreases in estrogen and resultant signs and symptoms
2. Normal variation in experience of menopause and related symptoms
3. Risks, benefits, and alternatives for treatment of symptoms
4. Follow-up plan, including next planned appointments and when to contact provider between visits

VI. Resources

A. NAMS provides education and resources for patients and providers: https://www.menopause.org/.
B. The NAMS Menopause Health Questionnaire is particularly helpful: https://www.menopause.org/docs/default-document-library/questionnaire.pdf?sfvrsn=90fd425b_0.
C. The WHI is an ongoing research study, and its website provides information about the data and ongoing research: https://www.whi.org/.
D. The American College of Obstetricians and Gynecologists (ACOG) offers resources for patients on many topics, including menopause: https://www.acog.org/womens-health.
E. The Office on Women's Health offers fact sheets for patients on many topics, including menopause: https://www.womenshealth.gov/.

References

Abramson, B. L., Black, D. R., Christakis, M. K., Fortier, M., & Wolfman, W. (2021). Guideline No. 422E: Menopause and cardiovascular disease. *Journal of Obstetrics and Gynaecology Canada, 43*(12), 1438–1443. doi:10.1016/j.jogc.2021.09.010

Alexander, I. M., & Moore A. (2007). Treating vasomotor symptoms of menopause: The nurse practitioner's perspective. *Journal of the American Academy of Nurse Practitioners, 19*(3), 152–162. doi:10.1111/j.1745-7599.2006.00206.x

Arias, E., Tejada-Vera, B., & Ahmad, F. (2021). *Provisional life expectancy estimates for January through June 2020.* Vital Statistics Rapid Release. Centers for Disease Control and Prevention, National Vital Statistics System. https://www.cdc.gov/nchs/data/vsrr/VSRR10-508.pdf

Barnard, N., Kahleova, H., Holtz, D., del Aguila, F., Neola, M., Crosby, L., & Holubkov, R. (2021). The Women's Study for the Alleviation of Vasomotor Symptoms (WAVS): A randomized, controlled trial of a plant-based diet and whole soybeans for postmenopausal women. *Menopause, 28*(10), 1150–1156. doi:10.1097/GME.0000000000001812

Boardman, Hartley, L., Eisinga, A., Main, C., Roqué i Figuls, M., Bonfill Cosp, X., Gabriel Sanchez, R., Knight, B., & Boardman, H. M. (2015). Hormone therapy for preventing cardiovascular disease in post-menopausal women. *Cochrane Database of Systematic Reviews, 2015*(8), CD002229. doi:10.1002/14651858.CD002229.pub4

Delamater, L., & Santoro, N. (2018). Management of the perimenopause. *Clinical Obstetrics & Gynecology, 61*(3), 419–432. doi:10.1097/grf.0000000000000389

Depypere, H., & Inki, P. (2015). The levonorgestrel-releasing intrauterine system for endometrial protection during estrogen replacement therapy: A clinical review. *Climacteric, 18*(4), 470–482. doi:10.3109/13697137.2014.991302

El Khoudari, S. L. (2022). Menopause demographics, staging and terminology. In C. Crandall (Ed.), *Menopause practice: A clinician's guide* (6th ed., pp. 1–3). North American Menopause Society.

Elkins, G. R., Fisher, W. I., Johnson, A. K., Carpenter, J. S., & Keith, T. Z. (2013). Clinical hypnosis in the treatment of postmenopausal hot flashes. *Menopause, 20*(3), 291–298. doi:10.1097/gme.0b013e31826ce3ed

Faubion, S. S. (2022). Disease common in midlife women. In C. Crandall (Ed.), *Menopause practice: A clinician's guide* (6th ed., pp.131–153). North American Menopause Society.

Freeman, E.W., & Sammel, M. D. (2016). Methods in a longitudinal cohort study of late reproductive age women: The Penn Ovarian Aging Study (POAS). *Women's Midlife Health, 2*(1), Article 1. doi:10.1186/s40695-016-0014-2

Gava, G., Orsili, I., Alvisi, S., Mancini, I., Seracchioli, R., & Meriggiola, M. C. (2019). Cognition, mood and sleep in menopausal transition: The role of menopause hormone therapy. *Medicina, 55*(10), 668. doi:10.3390/medicina55100668

Geraghty, P. (2022). Physiology of menopause. In P. Geraghty (Ed.), *Each woman's menopause: An evidence based resource* (pp. 69–90). Springer. doi:10.1007/978-3-030-85484-3_4

Geraghty, P. (2021). *Each Woman's Menopause: For Nurse Practitioners, Advanced Practice Nurses and Allied Health Professionals.* Springer International Publishing AG.

Gold, E. B., Block, G., Crawford, S., Lachance, L., FitzGerald, G., Miracle, H., & Sherman, S. (2004). Lifestyle and demographic factors in relation to vasomotor symptoms: Baseline results from the Study of Women's Health Across the Nation. *American Journal of Epidemiology, 159*(12), 1189–1199. doi:10.1093/aje/kwh168

Gungor Ugurlucan, F., Yasa, C., Tas, I. S., Aslay, I., & Yalcin, O. (2021). Complete labial fusion causing urinary retention in a postmenopausal woman. *American Journal of Clinical and Experimental Urology, 9*(5), 413–415.

Grady, D., Cohen, B., Tice, J., Kristof, M., Olyaie, A., & Sawaya, G. F. (2007). Ineffectiveness of sertraline for treatment of menopausal hot flushes: A randomized controlled trial. *Obstetrics and Gynecology, 109*(4), 823–830. doi:10.1097/01.AOG.0000258278.73505.fa

Harlow, S. D., Gass, M., Hall, J. E., Lobo, R., Maki, P., Rebar, R. W., Sherman, S., Sluss, P. M. & de Villiers, T. J. (2012). Executive summary of the Stages of Reproductive Aging Workshop + 10. *Menopause*, 19(4), 387–395. doi:10.1097/gme.0b013e31824d8f40.

Hayatbakhsh, M. R., Clavarino, A., Williams, G. M., Sina, M., & Najman, J. M. (2012). Cigarette smoking and age of menopause: A large prospective study. *Maturitas*, 72(4), 346–352. doi:10.1016/j.maturitas.2012.05.004

Hill, D. A., Crider, M., & Hill, S. R. (2016). Hormone therapy and other treatments for symptoms of menopause. *American Family Physician*, 94(11), 884–889.

Honigberg, M. C., Zekavat, S. M., Aragam, K., Finneran, P., Klarin, D., Bhatt, D. L., Januzzi, J. L., Scott, N. S., & Natarajan, P. (2019). Association of premature natural and surgical menopause with incident cardiovascular disease. *JAMA*, 322(24), 2411–2421. doi:10.1001/jama.2019.19191

Johnson, K., & Hauck, F. (2016). STEPS: Conjugated estrogens/bazedoxifene (Duavee) for menopausal symptoms. *American Family Physician*, 93(4), 307.

Julian, Z., Mengesha, B., McLemore, M., & Steinauer, J. (2021). Community-engaged curriculum development in sexual and reproductive health equity. *Obstetrics & Gynecology*, 137(4), 723–727. doi:10.1097/AOG.0000000000004324.

Kagan, R., Williams, R. S., Pan, K., Mirkin, S., & Pickar, J. H. (2010). A randomized, placebo- and active-controlled trial of bazedoxifene/conjugated estrogens for treatment of moderate to severe vulvar/vaginal atrophy in postmenopausal women. *Menopause*, 17(2), 281–289. doi:10.1097/gme.0b013e3181b7c65f

Karlamangla, A. S., Shieh, A., Greendale, G. A., Yu, E. W., Burnett-Bowie, S. A. M., Sluss, P. M., Martin, D., Morrison, A., & Finkelstein, J. S. (2022). Anti-mullerian hormone as predictor of future and ongoing bone loss during the menopause transition. *Journal of Bone and Mineral Research*, 37(7), 1224–1232. doi:10.1002/jbmr.4525

Kuhl, H., & Stevenson, J. (2006). The effect of medroxyprogesterone acetate on estrogen-dependent risks and benefits—An attempt to interpret the Women's Health Initiative results. *Gynecological Endocrinology*, 22(6), 303–317. doi:10.1080/09513590600717368

Leis, M., Singh, A., Li, C., Ahluwalia, R., Fleming, P., & Lynde, C. W. (2022). Risk of vulvar squamous cell carcinoma in lichen sclerosus and lichen planus: A systematic review. *Journal of Obstetrics and Gynaecology Canada*, 44(2), 182–192. doi:10.1016/j.jogc.2021.09.023

Lethaby, A., Marjoribanks, J., Kronenberg, F., Roberts, H., Eden, J., Brown, J. (2013). Phytoestrogens for menopausal vasomotor symptoms. *Cochrane Database of Systematic Reviews*, 2013(12), CD001395. doi:10.1002/14651858.CD001395.pub4

Levine, K. B., Williams, R. E., & Hartman, K. E. (2008). Vulvovaginal atrophy is strongly associated with female sexual dysfunction among sexually active postmenopausal women. *Menopause*, 15(4), 661–666. doi:10.1097/gme.0b013e31815a5168

Lindh-Åstrand, L., Bixo, M., Hirschberg, A. L., Sundström-Poromaa, I., & Hammar, M. (2010). A randomized controlled study of taper-down or abrupt discontinuation of hormone therapy in women treated for vasomotor symptoms. *Menopause*, 17(1), 72–79. doi:10.1097/gme.0b013e3181b397c7

Liu, J. H. (2022). Prescription therapies. In C. Crandall (Ed.), *Menopause practice: A clinician's guide* (6th ed., pp. 277–312). North American Menopause Society.

Maki, P. M. (2022). Memory impairment. In C. Crandall (Ed.), *Menopause practice: A clinician's guide* (6th ed., pp. 100–102). North American Menopause Society.

Manson, Chlebowski, R. T., Stefanick, M. L., Aragaki, A. K., Rossouw, J. E., Prentice, R. L., Anderson, G., Howard, B. V., Thomson, C. A., LaCroix, A. Z., Wactawski-Wende, J., Jackson, R. D., Limacher, M., Margolis, K. L., Wassertheil-Smoller, S., Beresford, S. A., Cauley, J. A., Eaton, C. B., Gass, M., … Wallace, R. B. (2013). Menopausal hormone therapy and health outcomes during the intervention and extended poststopping phases of the Women's Health Initiative randomized trials. *JAMA*, 310(13), 1353–1368. doi:10.1001/jama.2013.278040

McKeon, V. A. (1988). Dispelling menopause myths. *Journal of Gerontological Nursing*, 14(8), 26–29. doi:10.3928/0098-9134-19880801-08

Mehrnoush, V., Darsareh, F., Roozbeh, N., & Ziraeie, A. (2021). Efficacy of the complementary and alternative therapies for the management of psychological symptoms of menopause: A systematic review of randomized controlled trials. *Journal of Menopausal Medicine*, 27(3), 115–131. doi:10.6118/jmm.2102

Minami, C. A., & Freedman, R. A. (2020). Menopausal hormone therapy and long-term breast cancer risk: Further data from the Women's Health Initiative trials. *JAMA*, 324(4), 347–349. doi:10.1001/jama.2020.9620

Nash, Z., Al-Wattar, B. H., Davies, M. (2022). Bone and heart health in menopause. *Best Practice & Research Clinical Obstetrics & Gynaecology*, 8, 61–68. doi:10.1016/j.bpobgyn.2022.03.002

North American Menopause Society. (2017). The 2017 hormone therapy position statement of the North American Menopause Society. *Menopause*, 24(7), 728–753. doi:10.1097/gme.0000000000000921

North American Menopause Society. (2022). *What's new and what works in the treatment of hot flashes?* https://www.menopause.org/docs/default-source/press-release/vasomotor-symptom-pharmacologic-treatments-release.pdf

Odmark, I. S., Bixo, M., Englund, D., Risberg, B., Jonsson, B., & Olsson, S.-E. (2005). Endometrial safety and bleeding pattern during a five-year treatment with long-cycle hormone therapy. *Menopause*, 12(6), 699–707. doi:10.1097/01.gme.0000185119.74706.7b

Phillips, N., & Bachmann, G. (2021). The genitourinary syndrome of menopause. *Menopause*, 28(5), 579–588. doi:10.1097/GME.0000000000001728.

Pinkerton, J. V. (2022). Estrogen therapy and estrogen-progestogen therapy. In C. Crandall (Ed.), *Menopause practice: A clinician's guide* (6th ed., pp. 284–304). North American Menopause Society.

Pinkerton, J. V., & McClung, M.R. (2022). Osteoporosis. In C. Crandall (Ed.), *Menopause practice: A clinician's guide* (6th ed., pp. 159–173). North American Menopause Society.

Prefest. (2017). *Teva Women's Health*. Package insert.

Rahn, D. D., Carberry, C., Sanses, T. V., Mamik, M. M., Ward, R. M., Meriwether, K. V., Olivera, C. K., Abed, H., Balk, E. M., & Murphy, M. (2014). Vaginal estrogen for genitourinary syndrome of menopause: A systematic review. *Obstetrics and Gynecology*, 124(6), 1147–1156. doi:10.1097/AOG.0000000000000526

Randolph, J. F., Sowers, M. F., Bondarenko, I., Gold, E. B., Greendale, G. A., Bromberger, J. T., Brockwell, S. E., & Matthews, K. A. (2005). The relationship of longitudinal change in reproductive hormones and vasomotor symptoms during the menopausal transition. *Journal of Clinical Endocrinology & Metabolism*, 90(11), 6106–6112. doi:10.1210/jc.2005-1374

Sahni, S., Lobo-Romero, A., & Smith, T. (2021). Contemporary non-hormonal therapies for the management of vasomotor symptoms associated with menopause: A literature review. *European Endocrinology*, 17(2), 133–137. doi:10.17925/ee.2021.17.2.133

Santoro, N. (2016). Perimenopause: From research to practice. *Journal of Women's Health*, 25(4), 332–339. doi:10.1089/jwh.2015.5556

Santoro, N., & Sutton-Tyrrell, K. (2011). The swan song: Study of women's health across the nation's recurring themes. *Obstetrics and*

Gynecology Clinics of North America, 38(3), 417–423. doi:10.1016/j.ogc.2011.05.001

Santoro, N. F. (2022). Physiology of the menopause transition. In C. Crandall (Ed.), *Menopause practice: A clinician's guide* (6th ed., pp. 7–9). North American Menopause Society.

Schoenaker, D. A. J. M., Jackson, C. A., Rowlands, J. V., & Mishra, G. D. (2014). Socioeconomic position, lifestyle factors and age at natural menopause: A systematic review and meta-analyses of studies across six continents. *International Journal of Epidemiology*, 43(5), 1542–1562. doi:10.1093/ije/dyu094

Shan, D., Zou, L., Liu, X., Shen, Y., Cai, Y., & Zhang, J. (2020). Efficacy and safety of gabapentin and pregabalin in patients with vasomotor symptoms: A systematic review and meta-analysis. *American Journal of Obstetrics and Gynecology*, 222(6), 564–579. doi:10.1016/j.ajog.2019.12.011

Sherif, K. (2013). *Hormone therapy A clinical handbook*. Springer.

Shifren, J. L. (2022). Common genitourinary symptoms in midlife women. In C. Crrandall (Ed.), *Menopause practice: A clinician's guide* (6th ed., pp. 57–75). North American Menopause Society.

Siegel, D., Masten, M., & Santoro, N. (2021). Genitourinary syndrome of menopause: Updated terminology, diagnosis, and treatment. *Topics in Obstetrics & Gynecology*, 41(12), 1–7. doi:10.1097/01.PGO.0000767408.30098.2b.

Soares, C. N. (2022). Depression. In C. Crandall (Ed.), *Menopause practice: A clinician's guide* (6th ed., pp. 138–142). North American Menopause Society.

Sokalska, A., & Gracia, C. R. (2022). Stages of reproductive aging. In C. Crandall (Ed.), *Menopause practice: A clinician's guide* (6th ed., pp. 3–7). North American Menopause Society.

Stuenkel, C. A. (2021). Compounded bioidentical menopausal hormone therapy—a physician perspective. *Climacteric: The Journal of the International Menopause Society*, 24(1), 11–18. doi:10.1080/13697137.2020.1825668

Suckling, J., Lethaby, A., & Kennedy, R. (2006). Local oestrogen for vaginal atrophy in postmenopausal women. *Cochrane Database of Systematic Reviews*, 2006(4), CD001500. doi:10.1002/14651858.CD001500

Sutton-Tyrrell, Selzer, F., Sowers, M., Finkelstein, J., Powell, L., Gold, E., David, G., Weiss, G., Matthews, K., & Brooks, M. M. (2014). Study of Women's Health Across the Nation (SWAN), 2006–2008 Visit 10 dataset (2018th–11th–15th ed.). Inter-university Consortium for Political and Social Research.

Suvanto-Luukkonen, E., Koivunen, R., Sundström, H., Bloigu, R., Karjalainen, E., Häivä-Mällinen, L., & Tapanainen, J. S. (2005). Citalopram and fluoxetine in the treatment of postmenopausal symptoms: A prospective, randomized, 9-month, placebo-controlled, double-blind study. *Menopause*, 12(1), 18–26. doi:10.1097/00042192-200512010-00006

Thurston, R. C. (2022). Vasomotor symptoms. In C. Crandall (Ed.), *Menopause practice: A clinician's guide* (6th ed., pp. 43–55). North American Menopause Society.

Torres, F. (2020). *What are sleep disorders?* American Psychiatric Association. https://www.psychiatry.org/patients-families/sleep-disorders/what-are-sleep-disorders

Woods, N. F., & Mitchell, E. S. (2016). The Seattle Midlife Women's Health Study: A longitudinal prospective study of women during the menopausal transition and early postmenopause. *Women's Midlife Health*, 2(1), 6. doi:10.1186/s40695-016-0019-x

Youngs, D. D. (1990). Some misconceptions concerning the menopause. *Obstetrics & Gynecology*, 75(5), 881–883.

Zhao, W., Smith, J., Yu, M., Crandall, C., Thurston, R., Hood, M., Ruiz-Narvaez, E., Peyser, P., Kardia, S., & Harlow, S. (2021). Genetic variants predictive of reproductive aging are associated with vasomotor symptoms in a multiracial/ethnic cohort. *Menopause*, 28(8), 883–892. doi:10.1097/GME.0000000000001785

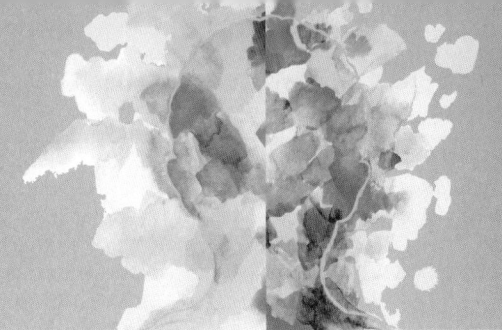

CHAPTER 23

Chronic Pelvic Pain in Persons Assigned Female at Birth

Becca Neuwirth

I. Introduction and general background

Chronic pelvic pain (CPP) in persons assigned female at birth (AFAB) is the reason for 10% of all gynecology office visits, 40% of all laparoscopies, and 12% of all hysterectomies (Lamvu et al., 2021). Prevalence ranges from 2.1% to 26.6%, depending on the study and definition (American College of Obstetricians and Gynecologists [ACOG], 2020, p. 7). The ACOG (2018b) states that CPP

> consists of pain symptoms perceived to originate from pelvic organs or structures typically lasting more than six months. It is often associated with negative cognitive, behavioral, sexual, and emotional consequences and with symptoms suggestive of lower urinary tract, sexual, bowel, pelvic floor, myofascial, or gynecological dysfunction. . . . Cyclical pelvic pain is considered a form of chronic pelvic pain if it has significant cognitive, behavioral, sexual, and emotional consequences.

Patients with CPP often disengage from health care. They may feel that their concerns are not being heard and that their experiences are being invalidated (McGowan et al., 2007). These patients appreciate the space to tell their own stories and feel heard (McGowan et al., 2007). Up to 50% of patients with CPP have a history of sexual or physical abuse (Meltzer-Brody et al., 2007). Therefore, it is vital that the patient be given space to tell their own story, empowered to make their own treatment decisions, and provided with trauma-informed care (see Chapter 58, Intimate Partner Violence).

Further, it is important to keep in mind that patients may have had inequitable access to health care and may have inequitable treatment when they do access care. For example, Newman and Thorne (2022) found that patients with chronic pain and higher levels of disparities (African American or Black, below poverty level, low literacy, unemployed, and/or seeking disability benefits) have poorer functional status. They found that these disparities are likely due to an interplay between biological factors, obstacles in accessing health care, limited resources, racism, sexism, stigma, discrimination, invalidation, and caregiving roles. Most research on disparities in pelvic pain has focused on endometriosis. Because racism has been shown to be a risk factor for many health conditions (Chadha et al., 2020), it is likely that similar racial disparities exist for other CPP conditions. The prevalence of endometriosis varies by racial group (Bougie, Yap, et al., 2019), although there is a documented history of racism resulting in underdiagnosis in Black or African American patients (Bougie, Healey, et al., 2019). When patients are able to access care for their pelvic pain, healthcare disparities continue. Orlando et al. (2022) showed that Black or African American patients were more likely to undergo laparotomy or early oophorectomy, whereas laparoscopy and delayed oophorectomy are generally the standard of care. They further found that Black or African American, Hispanic, Native Hawaiian or Pacific Islander, and American Indian or Alaska Native patients were more likely to experience surgical complications.

Causes of CPP are most often multifactorial, although patients often attribute their pain to their sexual and reproductive organs. Gynecologic etiologies account for only 20% of all CPP etiologies (Lamvu et al., 2021). Many patients have more than one etiology for their pain

Table 23-1 Conditions Seen With Chronic Pelvic Pain Conditions*

Abdominal migraine	Diverticulitis	Nerve entrapment
Abdominal muscular injury	**Dysmenorrhea**	Neuralgia
Abdominal epilepsy	Dyspareunia	Neuropathic pain
Abuse history	Dysthymia	Ovarian mass
Adenomyosis	**Endometriosis**	Ovarian remnant syndrome
Bladder cancer	Fibroids	**Painful bladder syndrome/interstitial cystitis**
Celiac disease	Fibromyalgia	Panic disorder
Central sensitization	Generalized anxiety disorder	Pelvic adhesions
Chronic endometriosis	Inflammatory bowel disease	Postural syndrome
Chronic pelvic inflammatory disease	**Irritable bowel syndrome**	Sleep disorders
Chronic urinary tract infection	Major depressive disorder	Trigger points
Colitis	**Myofascial pelvic pain syndrome**	Vulvodynia
Colon cancer		

*Conditions in **bold** are discussed in this chapter.
Data from American College of Obstetricians and Gynecologists. (2020). ACOG Practice Bulletin No. 218. Chronic pelvic pain. Obstetrics & Gynecology, 135(3), e98–109. https//doi.org/10.1097/AOG.0000000000003716. and Royal College of Obstetricians and Gynaecologists (2012). The initial management of chronic pelvic pain: Green Top Guideline Number 41. Retrieved from https://www.rcog.org.uk/globalassets/documents/guidelines/gtg_41.pdf

(Zondervan et al., 2001), and pain may persist even after initial conditions are treated (ACOG, 2020). A recent review concludes that clinicians should first identify central sensitization syndromes, then identify myalgias and neuralgias, then consider gynecologic and nongynecologic causes (Lamvu et al., 2021). **Table 23-1** reviews many possible causes of pelvic pain. Common etiologies that will be reviewed in this chapter include dysmenorrhea, endometriosis and adenomyosis, painful bladder syndrome/interstitial cystitis (PBS/IC), irritable bowel syndrome (IBS), diverticulitis, musculoskeletal and myofascial pelvic pain syndrome, central sensitization, and comorbid depression and anxiety. Symptom profiles often overlap, and patients may have more than one etiology of their pain.

These overlapping CPPs are explained by the complex interplay between neurological, neuroendocrine, immunological, and neurotransmitter dysfunction in the peripheral and central nervous systems. These systems are often altered by trauma, abuse, psychological disorders, and maladaptive reactions to stress (ACOG, 2020; Turk et al., 2016). Visceral and somatic structures in the pelvis share pathways in the central nervous system, making it difficult for the conscious mind to tell the difference between pain in one region and pain in another. This interconnection also results in viscero-viscero cross-sensitization, where pain in one organ causes hypersensitivity in another organ (Lamvu et al., 2021). Likewise, viscerosomatic convergence results in painful visceral signals causing stimulation of the pain pathways in adjacent somatic regions (Lamvu et al., 2021). Injury to somatic areas can stimulate visceral dysfunction, such as constipation and diarrhea or urinary frequency, urgency, and retention (Rapkin, 2018). Patients with posttraumatic stress disorder (PTSD) may undergo physiologic changes to their central nervous systems, further increasing their risk of CPP (Meltzer-Brody et al., 2007).

Some patients may associate their CPP with the presence of fibroids or ovarian cysts found on imaging. Patients with fibroids often report bulk symptoms, including noncyclic pelvic pain (Lippman et al., 2003). Less commonly, fibroids may necrose or torse, which may cause pain (Gupta et al., 2008). Some studies show higher rates of dysmenorrhea in patients with fibroids (Soliman et al., 2017). However, it is important to note that pain from leiomyoma-associated dysmenorrhea is likely to correlate with heavy menstrual flow and passage of clots rather than with the presence of the fibroids themselves (Stewart & Laughlin-Tommaso, 2021). Likewise, some patients with CPP will be found to have ovarian cysts, but not all cysts are a cause of pelvic pain (Potdar et al., 2020).

Because of the complicated and multifactorial nature of CPP, a multidisciplinary approach leads to the best care for patients. Specialists may include gynecology, primary care, gastroenterology, physical therapy, urology or urogynecology, psychology (including sex therapy), psychiatry, and pain medicine (ACOG, 2020). This chapter will focus on the most common components of CPP in patients AFAB.

A. *Dysmenorrhea*
   1. Definition and overview: Primary dysmenorrhea occurs without known pathology, whereas secondary dysmenorrhea is caused by pelvic pathology, most commonly endometriosis (ACOG, 2018a). Other less common causes of secondary dysmenorrhea include adenomyosis, Mullerian malformations, leiomyomas, pelvic masses, and infection (McKenna & Fogleman, 2021). Empiric treatment can be initiated without determining a specific diagnosis (ACOG, 2010). Patients who do not respond to initial therapy within 3–6 months may have secondary dysmenorrhea.
   2. Prevalence: Rates of dysmenorrhea range from 16% to 91%, depending on the study (AGOG, 2010).
B. *Endometriosis and adenomyosis*
   1. Definition and overview: Endometriosis is the presence, in the pelvic cavity or elsewhere in the body, of cells similar to endometrial cells. Theories of its etiology include retrograde menstruation, blood or lymphatic transport, differentiation of cells from bone marrow, and transformation of the coelomic epithelium (ACOG, 2010). Pathology studies show that endometriosis implants produce prostaglandins as well as other pain-producing chemicals (Rapkin, 2018). Some patients with endometriosis have no symptoms, and there may not be a correlation between severity of endometriosis and severity of symptoms (Abbott et al., 2003). Previously, diagnosis was contingent upon surgical biopsy (ACOG, 2018a). However, the most recent guidelines by the European Society of Human Reproduction and Embryology recommend that a diagnosis of endometriosis be considered in patients with any of the following symptoms: dysmenorrhea, deep dyspareunia, dysuria, dyschezia, painful rectal bleeding or hematuria, shoulder tip pain, catamenial pneumothorax, cyclical cough/hemoptysis/chest pain, cyclical scar swelling and pain, fatigue, and infertility (Becker et al., 2022).

      Similarly, adenomyosis is a disease of ectopic endometrium found in the myometrium, although diagnostic definitions vary. Definitive diagnosis is generally made on surgical pathology after hysterectomy, but clinical diagnosis may be made via ultrasound or magnetic resonance imaging (MRI) findings (Abbot, 2017). Theories of etiology include infolding of the endometrium into the myometrium, damage to the endometrium–myometrium junction from pregnancy or instrumentation of the uterus, and basement membrane damage with tissue factor contributions (Abbott, 2017).
   2. Prevalence: Between 71% and 87% of patients with CPP have endometriosis (ACOG, 2010). Adenomyosis is harder to diagnose because prevalence estimates generally rely on pathology from hysterectomy. Some studies suggest that 20%–35% of persons AFAB have adenomyosis (Abbott, 2017).
C. *Myofascial pelvic pain syndrome*
   1. Definition and overview: Myofascial pelvic pain syndrome (MPPS) (also called *pelvic floor dysfunction*) is a disorder with hard, tender trigger points found in tight bands of muscles in the pelvic floor (Ross et al., 2021). The reason for these physiologic changes is not well understood, but it is thought to be a result of muscle load and/or repeated microtrauma (Ross et al., 2021).
   2. Prevalence: Data are hard to find, but anywhere from 50% to 90% of patients with CPP have MPPS (Lamvu et al., 2021).
D. *Painful bladder syndrome/interstitial cystitis*
   1. Definition and overview: The Society for Urodynamics and Female Urology defines painful bladder syndrome/interstitial cystitis (PBS/IC) as "pain, pressure or other discomfort felt by the patient to be related to the urinary bladder and associated with other lower urinary tract symptoms, lasting for more than 6 weeks, when infection and other possible causes have been ruled out" (Hanno & Dmochowski, 2009). It is unclear whether PBS/IC is a direct result of physical changes to the bladder or whether the bladder symptoms are a result of another process, such as overactive bladder (Hanno et al., 2015). It is primarily a clinical diagnosis. Many patients report urinary urgency and frequency but not incontinence, and severity can change over time (Berry et al., 2011).
   2. Prevalence and incidence: One study found that 84% of patients with CPP also had interstitial cystitis (Parsons et al., 2002). It is estimated that between 3% and 7% of the general population of persons AFAB have PBS/IC (Berry et al., 2011).
E. *IBS*
   1. Definition and overview: See Chapter 59, Irritable Bowel Syndrome.
   2. Prevalence: See IBS, Chapter 59. Parsons et al. (2002) found that 50% of patients with CPP also had IBS.
F. *Central sensitization*
   1. Definition and overview: Central sensitization is "an amplification of neural signaling within the CNS that elicits pain hypersensitivity" (Woolf, 2011, p. 55). The pain response to noxious stimuli increases in amplitude, duration, and area, so a low amount of input can produce a larger pain response (Woolf, 2011). Central sensitization therefore means that patients can experience pain even without the presence of noxious stimuli and that their bodies recognize and process pain as if the noxious stimuli were there. Evidence for central sensitization in patients with CPP comes from studies showing changes to the hypothalamic–pituitary–adrenal axis and increased behavioral response to stimulation of both the pelvic region and somatic areas distal to the pelvis (Brawn et al., 2014).

2. Prevalence and incidence: Data are sparse, but a small study found that 82% of patients with CPP had central sensitization (Stratton et al., 2015). Another study found that 91% of patients with endometriosis had one or more central sensitization diagnoses (Orr et al., 2022).

II. Database

A. *Subjective*
  1. Detailed pain history: when the pain started (because symptoms of endometriosis are less likely to begin in patients over 40 [Gunawardena et al., 2021]); cyclic or random, worse with menses and ovulation (because endometriosis and adenomyosis are more likely to cause cyclic symptoms [Royal College of Obstetricians and Gynaecologists [RCOG], 2012]); location and radiation; quality of pain; duration of pain episodes; character; aggravating and relieving factors; severity; previous treatments, including surgeries (e.g., laparoscopy to diagnose or rule out endometriosis), procedures such as endoscopy/colonoscopy (to diagnose or rule out inflammatory bowel disease [IBD]) or cystoscopy (to diagnose interstitial cystitis); and medications, supplements, diet changes, and procedures
  2. Past medical history (PMH)
      a. Previous surgeries, especially abdominal and pelvic procedures (because these patients are more likely to have MPPS, neuropathic pain, and pelvic adhesive disease)
      b. Current and past medical problems, especially history of other chronic pain conditions such as migraines, fibromyalgia, low back pain, arthritis, autoimmune/rheumatological conditions, temporomandibular joint (TMJ) disorder, chronic fatigue/myalgic encephalomyelitis, or Ehlers–Danlos syndrome (because patients with one chronic pain syndrome are more likely to have others); psychiatric conditions such as anxiety, depression, PTSD; gastrointestinal conditions such as IBS, inflammatory bowel syndrome, diverticulitis, and food sensitivities or allergies; other chronic conditions
      c. Social history: substance use, safety concerns, support systems
      d. Sexual history: sexual practices and whether sex (penetration, orgasm, other activity) worsens pain; history of sexual assault or trauma
      e. Diet: consumption of bladder irritants (acidic foods, caffeine, soda); consumption of foods high in short-chain carbohydrates (fermentable oligosaccharides, disaccharides, monosaccharides and polyols [FODMAPs], other intestinal irritants); consumption of high-fiber foods
  3. ROS
      a. Gastrointestinal: constipation, diarrhea, pain with bowel movements, bowel incontinence, bloating, hematochezia
      b. Urinary: pain with urination, pain with full bladder, urgency, frequency, bladder incontinence, hematuria
      c. Musculoskeletal: joint pain, tenderness of abdominal wall, limitations in movement

B. *Objective, physical exam:* Although a physical exam may be helpful, many patients with CPP have an exam that is grossly "normal."
  1. Physical exam
      a. Vital signs: blood pressure
      b. Observe gait and posture with the patient sitting and standing. Patients with CPP as a result of musculoskeletal structures may have uneven gait and asymmetry and may adjust their position frequently because of pain (Lamvu et al., 2021).
      c. Palpation: Palpate for tenderness of abdomen, lower back, and sacroiliac and pubic symphysis joints (Lamvu et al., 2021). Palpate for abdominal trigger points; Carnett's sign; and flexion, abduction, and external rotation (FABER) test (ACOG, 2020). Positive Carnett's and FABER testing suggest a musculoskeletal component to the pain.
      d. Pelvic exam
          i. Inspection of external structures and light palpation with cotton-tipped swab to investigate allodynia and hyperalgesia (Lamvu et al., 2021)
          ii. Palpate pelvic floor muscles (**Figure 23-1**): Use index finger to palpate levator ani

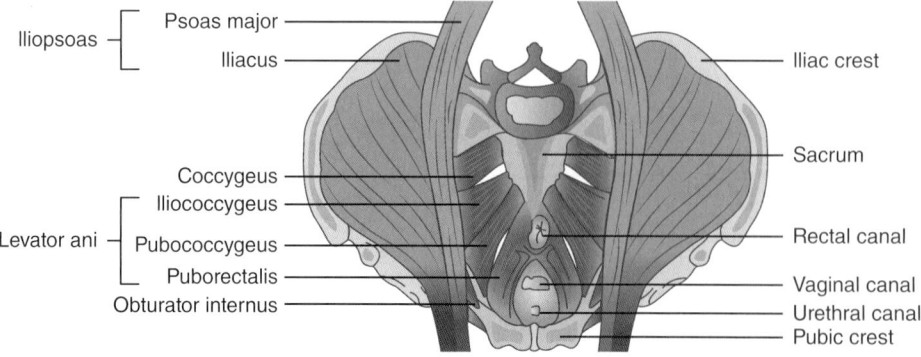

Figure 23-1 Superior View of Pelvic Floor Anatomy

muscles on the lateral vaginal walls, obturator muscles on the anterior vaginal walls, and coccygeus muscles on the posterior vaginal walls on each side. Tenderness, increased tone, or involuntary contractions suggest muscle dysfunction (Lamvu et al., 2021).

  iii. Palpate vagina, uterus, and ovaries. Signs of deeply infiltrating endometriosis include nodularity, especially in posterior fornix; a fixed uterus, especially when retroverted; and ovarian masses (Hickey et al., 2014). A tender, enlarged uterus may indicate adenomyosis. Cervical motion tenderness (CMT) may indicate pelvic inflammatory disease. It may be difficult to differentiate between CMT and generalized tenderness of pelvic floor muscles. Establishing a baseline of the patient's tenderness of the vulva and vagina can help establish any increase with cervical motion.

 e. Rectal exam: Palpate rectovaginal septum for nodularity that may be present with deeply infiltrative endometriosis.

2. Supporting data from relevant diagnostic tests gathered from planning follow.

III. Assessment

A. *Diagnosis:* Determine the diagnosis, including conditions to rule out; most diagnoses are clinical.

B. *Severity of symptoms:* Assess severity of symptoms and how they limit the patient's activities.

C. *Significance to patient:* Assess the meaning of diagnosis to the patient; determine patient's strengths and ability to follow treatment plans.

IV. Goals of clinical management

A. *Determine the patient's goals in seeking diagnosis and their ability to cope if no clear diagnosis is readily available.*

B. *Determine the patient's treatment goals.*

C. *Determine the patient's strengths and areas with room for improvement in terms of ability to adhere to treatment plan.*

V. Plan

A. *Screening:* Lamvu et al. (2021) recommend screening for
 1. Depression (see Chapter 49, Depression)
 2. Anxiety (see Chapter 42, Anxiety)
 3. History of physical and sexual assault/abuse and other trauma (see Chapter 58, Intimate Partner Violence [Domestic Violence])
 4. Distress from pain
 5. Coping strategies

B. *Diagnostic tests*
 1. Laboratory tests
  a. If bladder symptoms (Hanno et al., 2011): urinalysis (UA) and culture, urine cytology if smoking history, frequency and volume chart (see Chapter 25, Urinary Incontinence in Persons Assigned Female at Birth)
  b. Post-void residual if feeling of incomplete emptying (can be done via specialized ultrasound or via catheter)
  c. Chlamydia and gonorrhea cultures if risk factors present
 2. Radiology
  a. Pelvic ultrasound and MRI: Pelvic ultrasound and MRI may show fibroids, ovarian or adnexal cysts, Mullerian anomalies, pelvic adhesions, adenomyosis, and/or advanced endometriosis. Although most early-stage endometriosis is not detectable on imaging, the ability to diagnose advanced-stage endometriosis and adenomyosis is dependent on the facility and the experience of the radiology team (Tavcar et al., 2020). If an ultrasound reveals an endometrioma, consider repeat imaging in 8–12 weeks and yearly if not excised (Andreotti et al., 2020).
  b. Ultrasound, MRI, or computed tomography (CT) scans may note pelvic congestion syndrome, meaning the presence of dilated pelvic veins. However, this diagnosis remains controversial. There is insufficient evidence that the presence of venous congestion causes pelvic pain, and diagnostic criteria are variable (ACOG, 2020). Further research is needed to establish the relationship between pelvic venous congestion and pelvic pain, and patients with this condition noted on radiology should be referred to a pelvic pain specialist for consultation.

C. *Management*

Many treatments for CPP lack robust bodies of evidence, and they are therefore often based on expert opinion (Lamvu et al., 2021). Just as pain etiologies are multifactorial, treatment approaches must be as well. Treatment depends on the symptom patterns of the individual patient and their particular diagnoses. Treatments for different conditions may overlap; for example, amitriptyline may be used for the pain from PBS/IC as well as the pain from endometriosis. Because treatment is so complex and individual, progress should be assessed every 4–8 weeks, and referrals to specialists are made if improvement does not occur after initial treatment trials (Lamvu et al., 2021).

 1. Dysmenorrhea: Less common causes of secondary dysmenorrhea, such as obstructive Mullerian anomalies and cervical stenosis, and pelvic inflammatory disease should be ruled out before starting any of the treatments described next (ACOG, 2018a). See **Table 23-2** for a summary.
  a. Nonsteroidal anti-inflammatory drugs (NSAIDs): NSAIDs taken around the clock starting 1 to 2 days premenstrually (Harel, 2012) are first-line treatments for primary dysmenorrhea.
  b. Hormonal contraceptives: Hormonal contraceptives used to induce amenorrhea are also first-line treatments for primary dysmenorrhea (Harel, 2012). Continuous hormonal regimens

Table 23-2 Medical Treatments for Dysmenorrhea, Endometriosis, and Adenomyosis

Hormones	Nonhormonal Medications
Pills, patches, rings	NSAIDs
5 mg norethindrone acetate	GnRH agonist
Depo medroxyprogesterone acetate	GnRH antagonist
Etonogestrel implant	Aromatase inhibitors
Mirena intrauterine system	
Testosterone	
Danazol	

GnRH, gonadotropin-releasing hormone; *NSAIDs*, nonsteroidal anti-inflammatory drugs.

(i.e., skipping the placebo weeks of pills, patches, or rings) that induce amenorrhea are more likely to help with pain (ACOG, 2018a) than are cyclic regimens that allow for a placebo week and withdrawal bleed. Monophasic formulations are preferred (Lamvu et al., 2021). It may take several trials to find a formulation that works for the individual patient and minimizes side effects because there are many possible side effects.

Five milligrams of norethindrone acetate, although not approved by the U.S. Food and Drug Administration (FDA) as a contraceptive, may work better than lower doses of norethindrone (0.35 mg is available as a progestin-only pill) (ACOG, 2018a) for the treatment of dysmenorrhea. Depot medroxyprogesterone acetate (DMPA) users report amenorrhea rates of 12% after 3 months of use and up to 46% after 1 year of use (Hubacher et al., 2009). DMPA has been shown to decrease menstrual pain (Schlaff et al., 2006). Clinical trials show that etonogestrel implant (Nexplanon) users have a 20% rate of amenorrhea, and 75% of users with dysmenorrhea experience complete resolution (Mansour et al., 2008). The levonorgestrel-releasing Mirena intrauterine system provides 20%–60% of users with amenorrhea and reduces menstrual pain (Petta et al., 2005). In addition to decreasing pain by causing amenorrhea, the progesterone in these medications has been shown to cause pseudodecidualization and atrophy of endometriosis implants (Luciano et al., 1988).

Testosterone is not FDA approved for the treatment of dysmenorrhea, but it induces amenorrhea in almost all patients within 1 year of starting therapy (Ahmad & Leinung, 2017). Few studies have examined the effects of testosterone on dysmenorrhea and CPP, but some patients AFAB who use testosterone for gender affirmation may continue to have pelvic pain in spite of amenorrhea (Shim et al., 2020).

c. Gonadotropin-releasing hormone (GnRH) agonist/antagonist: If hormonal suppression is not effective, GnRH agonists (nafarelin nasal spray, leuprolide acetate depot, goserelin injectable) or antagonists (elagolix) may be used (Lamvu et al., 2021), although they are FDA approved only for the treatment of endometriosis. GnRH agonists and antagonists decrease bone density and may cause menopausal symptoms such as hot flashes, although those effects can be offset with add-back therapy (Zupi et al., 2004). Norethindrone acetate 5 mg is FDA approved as add-back therapy, although estrogen and progesterone may be used as well (ACOG, 2010). GnRH agonists and antagonists are thought to function by inducing a hypogonadotropic, hypogonadal state (Brown et al., 2010).

d. Less common treatments: Other less common treatments include the androgen danazol, which increases androgen levels, decreases ovarian estrogen production, and results in atrophy of endometrial implants (Farquhar et al., 2007). However, side effects include hypoestrogenic effects, such as genitourinary syndrome of menopause and hot flashes, and androgenic effects, such as oily skin and deepening of the voice (Farquhar et al., 2007). Using danazol vaginally is effective and reduces the risk of side effects (Buggio et al., 2017). Transmasculine patients may gain benefit from the androgenic side effects of danazol and prefer it as a first-line treatment.

Aromatase inhibitors (AIs) are also given, although they have a small risk of hypoestrogenic side effects, especially bone density loss (Attar & Bulun, 2006). Before menopause, AIs should be given with progesterone or combined estrogen–progesterone contraceptives to reduce the risks of bone density loss and ovarian cyst formation (Attar & Bulun, 2006). It is reasonable to defer these prescriptions to a specialist.

Complementary therapies: A Cochrane review (Pattanittum et al., 2016) showed low-quality but existent evidence for the ability of fenugreek, fish oil, vitamin B_1, fish oil in combination with vitamin B_1, ginger, valerian, *Zataria*, and zinc to decrease dysmenorrhea.

2. Endometriosis and adenomyosis: Initial medical treatments for endometriosis and adenomyosis are the same as treatments for dysmenorrhea discussed earlier (Becker et al., 2022). The

treatments described next may be used for patients with dysmenorrhea, whether or not it is known to be caused by endometriosis. Interventions for dysmenorrhea caused by adenomyosis are less well studied; however, those studies that have been done suggest that medical treatments for endometriosis work as well for adenomyosis (Abbott, 2017). Patients in whom endometriosis is suspected may be referred for surgical consultation as well (Becker et al., 2022). Patients may also be referred for surgical evaluation if initial therapy of hormones and/or a trial of GnRH agonists/antagonists is insufficient to help dysmenorrhea (ACOG, 2010). Approximately 60%–80% of patients report pain improvement 6 months after laparoscopy for endometriosis (ACOG, 2010), and 32% may need additional surgery (ACOG, 2010). Twenty-three percent of patients need further surgery within 7 years after total hysterectomy with ovarian preservation, and 8% may need further surgery within 7 years after hysterectomy and oophorectomy (Shakiba et al., 2008).

3. MPPS: Pelvic floor physical therapy can be very helpful (ACOG, 2020). Two websites can assist the patient in finding physical therapists (PTs) with training to provide pelvic floor physiotherapy: the Herman & Wallace Pelvic Rehabilitation Institute provides continuing education to pelvic floor PTs and maintains a provider directory at https://pelvicrehab.com/; the American Physical Therapy Association also provides a provider directory, which allows for selecting a Practice Focus of Pelvic Health, at: https://aptaapps.apta.org/APTAPTDirectory/FindAPTDirectory.aspx. Patients should be advised to expect a pelvic exam with their treatment, as well as to expect to have the therapist recommend exercises and stretches to do at home. When physical therapy is not effective, or the patient is unable to tolerate PT, referrals can be made to a gynecologist who performs pelvic floor trigger point or onabotulinumtoxinA injections (Mooney et al., 2021; Ross et al., 2021).

4. PBS/IC: The American Urological Association recommends the following step-wise approach for treating PBS/IC (Hanno et al., 2011, 2015). See **Table 23-3** for a summary. No single treatment has been found to be effective for all patients, and many patients require multiple treatment trials and combination therapies. First-line treatments and second-line medications may be managed by primary care providers.

   a. First-line treatment for PBS/IC includes lifestyle modification such as increasing or decreasing fluids and evaluating whether either affects pain. Patients may also trial eliminating common bladder irritants, such as coffee, tea, and acidic foods (see https://www.ichelp.org/living-with-ic/interstitial-cystitis-and-diet/

Table 23-3 Painful Bladder Syndrome/Interstitial Cystitis (PBS/IC) Initial Treatments

First Line	Second Line
Lifestyle modification	Amitriptyline
Eliminate bladder irritants	Cimetidine
Modify behavioral triggers	Hydroxyzine
Bladder training	Pentosan sulfate (risk of macular eye disease)
	Pelvic floor physical therapy
	Bladder instillations

elimination-diet/least-and-most-bothersome-foods/ for a list) and eliminating or modifying common behavior triggers such as sexual intercourse, wearing tight clothing, and some types of exercise. Other treatments include application of heat or cold, meditation, guided imagery and stress reduction, pelvic floor muscle relaxation, and bladder training and urge suppression (see Chapter 25, Urinary Incontinence in Persons Assigned Female at Birth). Data for episodic use of phenazopyridine, quercetin, and calcium glycerophosphate are lacking, but some patients may find them helpful. Long-term use of phenazopyridine has been associated with methemoglobinemia and renal and liver disease (Singh et al., 2014).

   b. Second-line medications include amitriptyline, cimetidine, hydroxyzine, or pentosan sulfate (PPS). These medications have risks of adverse events, and evidence comes from lower-grade studies. Pentosan sulfate has been linked to macular eye disease with prolonged use (Lindeke-Myers et al., 2022). It is recommended that patients have a retinal exam within 6 months of starting therapy and yearly while continuing treatment (Lindeke-Myers et al., 2022). PPS may also be associated with mild reversible hair loss and elevated liver enzymes. It may take 3–6 months to see results from PPS. Hydroxyzine and cimetidine are thought to help PBS/IC because of the increase in mast cells found in the bladder wall of patients with this condition. They may be associated with drowsiness. Amitriptyline may cause anticholinergic symptoms. Second-line treatments that require referrals include pelvic floor physical therapy (avoiding strengthening exercises such as Kegels) and bladder instillations (placing medications into

Table 23-4 Common Central Sensitization Treatments

Medication	Integrative therapies
Tricyclic antidepressants	Physical activity
Selective serotonin and norepinephrine reuptake inhibitors	Stress management
Gabapentinoids	Meditation
Traditional Chinese medicine	Acupuncture
	Mindfulness
	Cognitive–behavioral therapy
	Sex therapy

the bladder via catheter). PTs trained in pelvic floor techniques can provide treatment for these patients, and urologists or urogynecologists offer bladder instillations. Subsequent treatments, including neurostimulation, cystoscopy with hydrodistension of the bladder, and botulinum toxin injections into the bladder, require referral to a specialist.

5. IBS: See Chapter 59, Irritable Bowel Syndrome, for management.
6. Central sensitization (**Table 23-4**)
   a. Evidence for the use of neuropathic medications for the treatment of CPP is sparse, and the existing evidence shows a modest effect. However, the ACOG does recommend gabapentin and pregabalin and notes that gabapentin and a tricyclic together may decrease pain more than either alone (ACOG, 2020). Selective serotonin and norepinephrine reuptake inhibitors (SNRIs) are also recommended, based on their effectiveness with other pain syndromes such as fibromyalgia (ACOG, 2020). Duloxetine may be superior to venlafaxine (ACOG, 2020).
   b. Patients should be educated about the long-term nature of chronic pain and the importance of physical activity, stress management, meditation, and mindfulness. Cognitive–behavioral therapy has been shown to be effective in fostering coping strategies (Lamvu et al., 2021). Sex therapy may be useful for patients who also have decreased sexual desire or pain with sexual activity (ACOG, 2020).
   c. There is strong evidence that acupuncture helps chronic pain and specifically CPP, and yoga may also be beneficial (ACOG, 2020).
   d. Traditional Chinese herbal medicine has been shown to be as effective as danazol and gestrinone (a progestin not available in the United States), with fewer side effects (Flower et al., 2012).
   e. The ACOG (2020) does not recommend opiate use for chronic pain.
D. *Patient education:* Provide written and verbal information regarding:
   1. Diagnoses, including disease processes and central sensitization
   2. Diagnostic testing, including discussion of possible costs, preparation, procedures, and aftercare
   3. Treatment options, including side effects, risks, possible costs, and length of treatment
   4. Follow-up plan, including next planned appointments and when to contact the provider between scheduled visits
E. *When to refer*
   1. Refer to gynecologist or gynecology advanced practice provider with expertise in endometriosis and/or CPP when patients are not responding to initial treatments of CPP thought to be resulting from dysmenorrhea and/or presumed endometriosis. Some gynecologists may also perform procedures such as a pudendal nerve block or Botox injections into the pelvic floor muscles when pelvic floor dysfunction is not sufficiently helped by physical therapy.
   2. Refer to gynecological surgeon if the patient is interested in laparoscopy for diagnosis of endometriosis. Patients should also be referred for discussion of surgery when initial medical treatment has not improved symptoms. Patients with endometriomas that are larger than 10 cm or enlarging over repeat imaging (Andreotti et al., 2020) should be referred to discuss surgery. Some experts recommend considering removal of endometriomas over 5 cm (Levy & Barbeiri, 2021).
   3. Refer to urogynecology or urology for bladder pain not responding to initial treatments. American Urological Association guidelines recommend referral for further evaluation of patients with PBS/IC symptoms and overactive bladder or incontinence, microscopic or gross hematuria or sterile pyuria, or gastrointestinal or gynecological signs and symptoms (Hanno et al., 2011).
   4. Refer to gastroenterology when gastrointestinal (GI) symptoms are not responding to initial treatments and when warranted for endoscopy. See Chapter 59, Irritable Bowel Syndrome.
   5. Refer to pain medicine when initial treatments are insufficient and central sensitization is suspected or for patients taking chronic opioids. Pain medicine may consider procedures such as hypogastric or pudendal nerve blocks, directed Botox or trigger point injections, and so forth.

6. Refer to psychology or psychiatry if comorbid stress, anxiety, or PTSD are present.
7. Refer to reproductive endocrinologist and infertility (REI) providers in patients desiring future fertility and with recurrent or large endometriomas and/or adnexal surgery to consider egg preservation.

VI. Resources

The following websites provide resources for patients and providers.

A. *International Pelvic Pain Society (IPPS). The IPPS provides training for providers, and the IPPS website includes informational handouts for patients:* https://www.pelvicpain.org/.
B. *Pelvic Pain Education Program (PPEP). The PPEP provides videos and handouts for patient education:* https://www.pelvicpaineducation.com/.
C. *University of Michigan Chronic Pain Guide. This guide provides education and self-management tools for multiple chronic pain conditions:* https://painguide.com/.
D. *Interstitial Cystitis Association (ICA). The ICA provides education and support for patients with PBS/IC:* https://www.ichelp.org/.

References

Abbott, J. A. (2017). Adenomyosis and abnormal uterine bleeding (AUB-A)—Pathogenesis, diagnosis, and management. Best practice & research. *Clinical Obstetrics & Gynaecology, 40,* 68–81. doi:10.1016/j.bpobgyn.2016.09.006

Abbott, J. A., Hawe, J., Clayton, R., & Garry, R. (2003). The effects and effectiveness of laparoscopic excision of endometriosis: A prospective study with 2–5 year follow-up. *Human Reproduction, 18*(9), 1922–1927. doi:10.1093/humrep/deg275

Ahmad, S., & Leinung, M. (2017). The response of the menstrual cycle to initiation of hormonal therapy in transgender men. *Transgender Health, 2*(1), 176–179. doi:10.1089/trgh.2017.0023

American College of Obstetricians and Gynecologists. (2010). ACOG Practice Bulletin No. 114: Management of endometriosis. *Obstetrics & Gynecology, 116*(1), 223–236. doi:10.1097/AOG.0b013e3181e8b073

American College of Obstetricians and Gynecologists. (2018a). ACOG Committee Opinion No. 760: Dysmenorrhea and endometriosis in the adolescent. *Obstetrics & Gynecology, 132*(6), e249–258. doi:10.1097/AOG.0000000000002978

American College of Obstetricians and Gynecologists. (2018b). *reVitalize. Gynecology data definitions (version 1.0).* https://www.acog.org/practice-management/health-it-and-clinical-informatics/revitalize-gynecology-data-definitions

American College of Obstetricians and Gynecologists. (2020). ACOG Practice Bulletin No. 218: Chronic pelvic pain. *Obstetrics & Gynecology, 135*(3), e98–109. doi:10.1097/AOG.0000000000003716.

Andreotti, R. F., Timmerman, D., Strachowski, L. M., Froyman, W., Benacerraf, B. R., Bennett, G. L., Bourne, T., Brown, D. L., Coleman, B. G., Frates, M. C., Goldstein, S. R., Hamper, U. M., Horrow, M. M., Hernanz-Schulman, M., Reinhold, C., Rose, S. L., Whitcomb, B. P., Wolfman, W. L., & Glanc, P. (2020). O-RADS US risk stratification and management system: A consensus guideline from the ACR Ovarian-Adnexal Reporting and Data System Committee. *Radiology, 294*(1), 168–185. doi:10.1148/radiol.2019191150

Attar, E., & Bulun, S. E. (2006). Aromatase inhibitors: The next generation of therapeutics for endometriosis? *Fertility and Sterility, 85*(5), 1307–1318. doi:10.1016/j.fertnstert.2005.09.064

Becker, C. M. Bokor, A., Heikinheimo, O., Horne, A., Jansen, F., Kiesel, L., King, K., Kvaskoff, M., Nap, A., Petersen, K., Saridogan, E., Tomassetti, C., van Hanegem, N., Vulliemoz, N., & Vermeulen, N. (2022). ESHRE guideline: Endometriosis. *Human Reproduction Open, 2022*(2), 1–26. doi:10.1093/hropen/hoac009

Berry, S. H., Elliott, M. N., Suttorp, M., Bogart, L. M., Stoto, M. A., Eggers, P., Nyberg, L., & Clemens, J. Q. (2011). Prevalence of symptoms of bladder pain syndrome/interstitial cystitis among adult females in the United States. *Journal of Urology, 186*(2), 540–544. doi:10.1016/j.juro.2011.03.132

Bougie, O., Healey, J., & Singh, S. S. (2019). Behind the times: Revisiting endometriosis and race. *American Journal of Obstetrics and Gynecology, 221*(1), 35.e1–35.e5. doi:10.1016/j.ajog.2019.01.238

Bougie, O., Yap, M., Sikora, L., Flaxman, T., & Singh, S. (2019). Influence of race/ethnicity on prevalence and presentation of endometriosis: A systematic review and meta-analysis. *BJOG: An International Journal of Obstetrics and Gynaecology, 126*(9), 1104–1115. doi:10.1111/1471-0528.15692

Brawn, J., Morotti, M., Zondervan, K. T., Becker, C. M., & Vincent, K. (2014). Central changes associated with chronic pelvic pain and endometriosis. *Human Reproduction Update, 20*(5), 737–747.

Brown, J., Pan, A., Hart, R. J., & Brown, J. (2010). Gonadotrophin-releasing hormone analogues for pain associated with endometriosis. *Cochrane Library, 2010*(12), CD008475. doi:10.1002/14651858.CD008475.pub2

Buggio, L., Lazzari, C., Monti, E., Barbara, G., Berlanda, N., & Vercellini, P. (2017). "Per vaginam" topical use of hormonal drugs in women with symptomatic deep endometriosis: A narrative literature review. *Archives of Gynecology and Obstetrics, 296*(3), 435–444. doi:10.1007/s00404-017-4448-z

Chadha, N., Lim, B., Kane, M., & Rowland, B. (2020, May 1). *Toward the abolition of biological race in medicine: transforming clinical education, research and practice.* https://www.crg.berkeley.edu/wp-content/uploads/2020/07/TowardtheAbolitionofBiologicalRaceinMedicineFINAL.pdf

Farquhar, C., Prentice, A., Singla, A. A., & Selak, V. (2007). Danazol for pelvic pain associated with endometriosis. *Cochrane Library, 2010*(11), CD000068. doi:10.1002/14651858.CD000068.pub2

Flower, A., Liu, J. P., Lewith, G., Little, P., & Li, Q. (2012). Chinese herbal medicine for endometriosis. *Cochrane Library, 2012*(8), CD006568. doi:10.1002/14651858.CD006568.pub3

Gunawardena, S., Dior, U. P., Cheng, C., & Healey, M. (2021). New diagnosis of endometriosis is less common in women over age forty presenting with pelvic pain. *Journal of Minimally Invasive Gynecology, 28*(4), 891–898.e1. doi:10.1016/j.jmig.2020.08.012

Gupta, S., Jose, J., & Manyonda, I. (2008). Clinical presentation of fibroids. Best practice & research. *Clinical Obstetrics & Gynaecology, 22*(4), 615–626. doi:10.1016/j.bpobgyn.2008.01.008

Hanno, P., & Dmochowski, R. (2009). Status of international consensus on interstitial cystitis/bladder pain syndrome/painful bladder syndrome: 2008 snapshot. *Neurourology and Urodynamics, 28*(4), 274–286. doi:10.1002/nau.20687

Hanno, P. M., Burks, D. A., Clemens, J. Q., Dmochowski, R. R., Erickson, D., FitzGerald, M. P., Forrest, J. B., Gordon, B., Gray, M., Mayer, R. D., Newman, D., Nyberg, L., Jr., Payne, C. K., Wesselmann, U., & Faraday, M. M. (2011). AUA guideline for the diagnosis and treatment of interstitial cystitis/bladder pain syndrome. *Journal of Urology*, 185(6), 2162–2170. doi:10.1016/j.juro.2011.03.064

Hanno, P. M., Erickson, D., Moldwin, R., & Faraday, M. M. (2015). Diagnosis and treatment of interstitial cystitis/bladder pain syndrome: AUA guideline amendment. *Journal of Urology*, 193(5), 1545–1553. doi:10.1016/j.juro.2015.01.086

Harel, Z. (2012). Dysmenorrhea in adolescents and young adults: An update on pharmacological treatments and management strategies. *Expert Opinion on Pharmacotherapy*, 13(15), 2157–2170. doi:10.1517/14656566.2012.725045

Hickey, M., Ballard, K., & Farquhar, C. (2014). Endometriosis. *British Medical Journal*, 348, g1752. doi:10.1136/bmj.g1752

Hubacher, D., Lopez, L., Steiner, M. J., & Dorflinger, L. (2009). Menstrual pattern changes from levonorgestrel subdermal implants and DMPA: Systematic review and evidence-based comparisons. *Contraception*, 80(2), 113–118. doi:10.1016/j.contraception.2009.02.008

Lamvu, G., Carillo, J., Ouyang, C., & Rapkin, A. (2021). Chronic pelvic pain in women: A review. *Journal of the American Medical Association*, 325(23), 2381–2391. doi:10.1001/jama2021.2631

Levi, B. S., & Barbeiri, R. L. (2021). Endometriosis: Management of ovarian endometriomas. *UpToDate*. https://www.uptodate.com/contents/endometriosis-management-of-ovarian-endometriomas

Lindeke-Myers, A., Hanif, A. M., & Jain, N. (2022). Pentosan polysulfate maculopathy. *Survey of Ophthalmology*, 67(1), 83–96. doi:10.1016/j.survophthal.2021.05.005

Lippman, S. A., Warner, M., Sameula, S., Oliva, D., Vercellini, P., Eskenazi, B. (2003). Uterine fibroids and gynecologic pain symptoms in a population-based study. *Fertility and Sterility*, 80(6), 1488–1494. doi:10.1016/S0015-0282(03) 02207-6

Luciano, A. A., Turksoy, R. N., & Carleo, J. (1988). Evaluation of oral medroxyprogesterone acetate in the treatment of endometriosis. *Obstetrics and Gynecology*, 72(3), 323–327.

Mansour, D., Korver, T., Marintcheva-Petrova, M., & Fraser, I. S. (2008). The effects of Implanon on menstrual bleeding patterns. *European Journal of Contraception & Reproductive Health Care*, 13(S1), 13–28. doi:10.1080/13625180801959931

McGowan, L., Luker, K., Creed, F., & Chew, G. C. A. (2007). "How do you explain a pain that can't be seen?" The narratives of women with chronic pelvic pain and their disengagement with the diagnostic cycle. *British Journal of Health Psychology*, 12(2), 261–274. doi:10.1348/135910706X104076

McKenna, K. A., & Fogleman, C. D. (2021). Dysmenorrhea. *American Family Physician*, 104(2), 164–170.

Meltzer-Brody, S., Leserman, J., Zolnoun, D., Steege, J., Green, E., & Teich, A. (2007). Trauma and posttraumatic stress disorder in women with chronic pelvic pain. *Obstetrics & Gynecology*, 109(4), 902–908. doi:10.1097/01.AOG.0000258296.35538.88.

Mooney, S. S., Readman, E., Hiscock, R. J., Francis, A., Fraser, E., & Ellett, L. (2021). Botulinum toxin A (Botox) injection into muscles of pelvic floor as a treatment for persistent pelvic pain secondary to pelvic floor muscular spasm: A pilot study. *Australian & New Zealand Journal of Obstetrics & Gynaecology*, 61(5), 777–784. doi:10.1111/ajo.13396

Newman, A. K., & Thorn, B. E. (2022). Intersectional identity approach to chronic pain disparities using latent class analysis. *Pain*, 163(4), e547–e556. doi:10.1097/j.pain.0000000000002407

Orlando, M. S., Luna Russo, M. A., Richards, E. G., King, C. R., Park, A. J., Bradley, L. D., & Chapman, G. C. (2022). Racial and ethnic disparities in surgical care for endometriosis across the United States. *American Journal of Obstetrics and Gynecology*, 226(6), 824.e1–824.e11. doi:10.1016/j.ajog.2022.01.021

Orr, N. L., Wahl, K. J., Lisonek, M., Joannou, A., Noga, H., Albert, A., & Yong, P. J. (2022). Central sensitization inventory in endometriosis. *Pain*, 163(2), e234–e245. doi:10.1097/j.pain.0000000000002351

Parsons, C. L., Dell, J., Stanford, E. J., Bullen, M., Kahn, B. S., & Willems, J. J. (2002). The prevalence of interstitial cystitis in gynecologic patients with pelvic pain, as detected by intravesical potassium sensitivity. *American Journal of Obstetrics and Gynecology*, 187(5), 1395–400. doi:10.1067/mob.2002.127375

Pattanittum, P., Kunyanone, N., Brown, J., Sangkomkamhang, U. S., Barnes, J., Seyfoddin, V., & Marjoribanks, J. (2016). Dietary supplements for dysmenorrhoea. *Cochrane Library*, 2016(3), CD002124. doi:10.1002/14651858.CD002124.pub2

Petta, C. A., Ferriani, R. A., Abrao, M. S., Hassan, D., Rosa e Silva, J. C., Podgaec, S., & Bahamondes, L. (2005). Randomized clinical trial of a levonorgestrel-releasing intrauterine system and a depot GnRH analogue for the treatment of chronic pelvic pain in women with endometriosis. *Human Reproduction*, 20(7), 1993–1998. doi:10.1093/humrep/deh869

Potdar, N., Pillai, R. N., & Oppenheimer, C. A. (2020). Management of ovarian cysts in children and adolescents. *The Obstetrician & Gynaecologist*, 22, 107–14. doi:10.1111/tog.12648

Rapkin, A. J. (2018). Meaningful endometriosis treatment requires a holistic approach and an understanding of chronic pain. *OBG Management*, 30(12), 26–30.

Ross, V., Detterman, C., & Hallisey, A. (2021). Myofascial pelvic pain: An overlooked and treatable cause of chronic pelvic pain. *Journal of Midwifery & Women's Health*, 66(2), 148–160. doi:10.1111/jmwh.13224

Royal College of Obstetricians and Gynaecologists. (2012). *The initial management of chronic pelvic pain: Green Top Guideline Number 41*. https://www.rcog.org.uk/globalassets/documents/guidelines/gtg_41.pdf

Shakiba, K., Bena, J. F., McGill, K. M., Minger, J., & Falcone, T. (2008). Surgical treatment of endometriosis: A 7-year follow-up on the requirement for further surgery. *Obstetrics and Gynecology*, 111(6), 1285–1292. doi:10.1097/AOG.0b013e3181758ec6

Schlaff, W. D., Carson, S. A., Luciano, A., Ross, D., & Bergqvist, A. (2006). Subcutaneous injection of depot medroxyprogesterone acetate compared with leuprolide acetate in the treatment of endometriosis-associated pain. *Fertility and Sterility*, 85(2), 314–325. doi:10.1016/j.fertnstert.2005.07.1315

Shim, J. Y., Laufer, M. R., & Grimstad, F. W. (2020). Dysmenorrhea and endometriosis in transgender adolescents. *Journal of Pediatric & Adolescent Gynecology*, 33(5), 524–528. doi:10.1016/j.jpag.2020.06.001

Singh, M., Shailesh, F., Tiwari, U., Sharma, S. G., & Malik, B. (2014). Phenazopyridine associated acute interstitial nephritis and review of literature. *Renal Failure*, 36(5), 804–807. doi:10.3109/0886022X.2014.890054

Soliman, A. H., Margolis, M. K., Castelli-Haley, J., Fuldeore, M. J., Owens, C. D., & Coyne, K. S. (2017). Impact of uterine fibroid symptoms on health-related quality of life of US women: Evidence from a cross-sectional survey. *Current Medical Research and Opinion*, 33(11), 1971–1978. doi:10.1080/03007995.2017.1372107

Stewart, E. A., & Laughlin-Tommaso, S. K. (2021). Uterine fibroids (leiomyomas): Epidemiology, clinical features, diagnosis, and natural history. *UpToDate*. from https://www.uptodate.com/contents/uterine-fibroids-leiomyomas-epidemiology-clinical-features-diagnosis-and-natural-history

Stratton, P., Khachikyan, I., Sinaii, N., Ortiz, R., & Shah, J. (2015). Association of chronic pelvic pain and endometriosis with signs of sensitization and myofascial pain. *Obstetrics and Gynecology*, *125*(3), 719–728. doi:10.1097/AOG.0000000000000663

Tavcar, J., Loring, M., Movilla, P. R., & Clark, N. V. (2020). Diagnosing endometriosis before laparoscopy: Radiologic tools to evaluate the disease. *Current Opinion in Obstetrics & Gynecology*, *32*(4), 292–297. doi:10.1097/GCO.0000000000000638

Turk, D. C., Fillingim, R. B., Ohrbach, R., & Patel, K. V. (2016). Assessment of psychosocial and functional impact of chronic pain. *Journal of Pain*, *17*(9), T21–T49. doi:10.1016/j.jpain.2016.02.006

Woolf, C. J. (2011). Central sensitization: Implications for the diagnosis and treatment of pain. *Pain*, *152*(3), S2–S15. doi:10.1016/j.pain.2010.09.030

Zondervan, K. T., Yudkin, P. L., Vessey, M. P., Jenkinson, C. P., Dawes, M. G., Barlow, D. H., & Kennedy, S. H. (2001). Chronic pelvic pain in the community—Symptoms, investigations, and diagnoses. *American Journal of Obstetrics and Gynecology*, *184*(6), 1149–1155. doi:10.1067/mob.2001.112904

Zupi, E., Marconi, D., Sbracia, M., Zullo, F., De Vivo, B., Exacustos, C., & Sorrenti, G. (2004). Add-back therapy in the treatment of endometriosis-associated pain. *Fertility and Sterility*, *82*(5), 1303–1308. doi:10.1016/j.fertnstert.2004.03.062

CHAPTER 24

Sexual Dysfunction

Milan Chavarkar

I. Introduction and general background

Sexual dysfunction (SD) is highly prevalent and often coincides with other chronic conditions (Heiden-Rootes et al., 2017). Approximately 25%–63% of the population reports at least one sexual problem, yet these are rarely addressed in primary care (Chen et al., 2019; Heiden-Rootes et al., 2017; McCabe et al., 2016a). The American Psychiatric Association's (APA) *Diagnostic and Statistical Manual of Mental Disorders* defines SD as a clinically significant disturbance in one's ability to perform sexually or experience sexual pleasure (APA, 2013). SDs are divided into four categories: lack of desire or interest, arousal dysfunction, orgasm and/or ejaculatory dysfunctions, and pain during sexual activities (Holmberg et al., 2019). SD is best understood using the biopsychosocial model, in which there is a complex interplay of neurochemical, psychological, social, and cultural factors that affect sexual response (Harsh & Clayton, 2018; Kingsberg et al., 2017). In caring for the individual, the provider is tasked with universal screening of sexual concerns; reframing the problem; showing empathy, and providing assessment, treatment, education, and/or referrals (Parish et al., 2019). As health care embraces gender-affirming care, it is essential for healthcare providers to embrace a nonbinary gender framework in sexual health care (Eckstrand et al., 2016). In this spirit, this chapter approaches SD with a nonbinary perspective to address the complex needs of sexual health for individuals.

A. Human sexual response

Normal sexual function is an interplay of hormonal, psychogenic, neurogenic, and hemodynamic factors (Chen et al., 2019). Initial studies of sexual response focused on linear models of sexual human response, including desire, arousal, sexual activity, and orgasm/ejaculation (American College of Obstetricians and Gynecologists [ACOG], 2019). Sexual desire was thought to trigger a sexual response like other autonomic responses, such as breathing or sleeping. Newer models of sexual response are nonlinear and have overlapping phases of variable order (Basson, 2015). Desire may not be present upon initial sexual engagement, and sexual excitement can trigger desire and arousal simultaneously (Basson, 2015). Sexual and nonsexual reasons can factor into motivation for participating in partnered sex, depending on the relationship (Basson, 2015). The brain responds to sexual stimuli in a "dual-control" model, in which there are both excitatory and inhibitory mechanisms affecting arousal, and processing of information is both unconscious and conscious (Basson, 2015). Clinical focus on sexual function now emphasizes sexual satisfaction rather than the physical outcomes of lubrication, erection, orgasm, and/or ejaculation (Basson, 2015). By addressing concerns of the relationship, sexual motivation, the brain's response to the sexual environment and stimuli, and the attainment of a satisfying experience, the provider can successfully address SDs.

B. Types of SD

In 2015, The Fourth International Consultation of Sexual Medicine classified sexual dysfunctions based on literature, clinical principles, and consensus of expert opinions (McCabe et al., 2016). Sexual dysfunctions include desire disorders, arousal disorders, orgasmic disorders, ejaculation disorders, pain syndromes. Desire disorder encompasses hypoactive sexual desire dysfunction. Arousal disorders include sexual arousal dysfunction and erectile dysfunction. Orgasmic disorders include orgasmic dysfunction, hypohedonic orgasm, anorgasmia, and post-orgasmic illness syndrome, which is the occurance of negative feelings or symptoms after orgasm. Ejaculation disorders include premature ejaculation, delayed ejaculation, retrograde ejaculation, anhedonic ejaculation, and anejaculation. Pain syndromes include genital-pelvic pain dysfunction, persistent genital arousal disorder, and restless genital syndrome.

C. Prevalence

Studies of the prevalence of SDs are mostly based on self-report, and therefore true prevalence is difficult to assess (Heiden-Rootes et al., 2017). The U.S. National Health and Social Life Survey (NHSLS) interviewed persons assigned female at birth (AFAB) and noted a 43% prevalence of SD in comparison to 31% of those assigned male at birth (AMAB). The most common problems for persons AFAB included desire (33%), orgasm (24%), and lubrication (19%). For persons AMAB, the most common sexual complaints included premature ejaculation (21%), erectile dysfunction (5%), and low desire (5%) (Harsh & Clayton, 2018). The Prevalence of Female Sexual Problems Associated with Distress and Determinants of Treatment Seeking (PRESIDE) study showed similar prevalence rates of sexual complaints at 44.2%. Persons AFAB reported arousal (26.1%) and orgasm (20.5%) as their primary issues. In adjusting for age, those aged 45–64 years had the highest rate (14.8%) of sexual problems in comparison to the lowest rate in those aged 65 years or older (8.9%), with an intermediate rate found in those aged 18–44 years (10.8%). Age clearly is a factor for persons AFAB. Mental health diagnoses also affect the prevalence of sexual complaints; 40% of the participants in the PRESIDE study reported depressive symptoms (Harsh & Clayton, 2018).

Many studies look at SD in the binary model. Now gender identity is viewed as a spectrum, and considerations need to be made for those who identify as nonbinary, gender fluid, transgender, gender queer, transgender masculine, and transgender feminine. Gender dysphoria is the distress associated with gender incongruence and transition and has an impact on sexual function. Research in understanding desire, arousal, orgasm, and discomfort in this population is ongoing (Holmberg et al., 2019).

D. Risk factors

Risk factors for SD include age, single status, low socioeconomic status, pregnancy, postpartum, hysterectomy, perimenopause, hormone use, female genital mutilation/cutting, trauma, prostate surgery, poor general health, chronic disease, heavier body weight, low physical activity, substance use, anxiety, depression, medication use, toxin or endocrine-disruptor exposure, and relationship quality. See **Table 24-1**.

Table 24-1 Medical Conditions and Medications Affecting Sexual Function

System	Medical Condition	Medication
Neurologic	Parkinson disease, multiple sclerosis, spinal cord injury, migraines, traumatic brain injury, and hypothalamic or pituitary damage	Antiepileptic drugs, methyldopa
Urogynecologic	Pregnancy, surgery, adhesions, cancers, prostatectomy, urinary incontinence, benign prostate hyperplasia, Peyronie disease, hysterectomy, complications of vaginal childbirth, radiation therapy, joint disease affecting mobility	5-alpha reductase inhibitors
Endocrine	Diabetes, thyroid disease, hyperprolactinemia, reproductive events (menopause transition, pregnancy, postpartum, premenstrual syndrome), androgen deficiency, Turner syndrome, primary ovarian insufficiency	Oral contraceptives, estrogen, progesterone, aromatase inhibitors, antiandrogens, gonadotropin-releasing hormone (GnRH) agonists
Cardiovascular	Coronary artery disease, heart failure, hypertension, atherosclerosis, stroke	Beta-blockers, alpha-blockers, clonidine, diuretics, lipid-lowering agents, digoxin, thienopyridine drugs (e.g., clopidogrel, ticlopidine, ticagrelor)
Psychiatric	Depression, body image concerns (i.e., visible scar, post-mastectomy, psoriasis or other skin conditions, higher body weight), pain syndrome, anxiety, history of sexual trauma and/or abuse, adverse childhood events, relationship discord	antidepressant medications (e.g., MAOIs, SSRIs, SNRIs, and TCAs), mood stabilizers, antipsychotics, benzodiazepines
Other		Disulfiram, ketoconazole, metronidazole, NSAIDs, antipyretic analgesics, histamine H_2-receptor blockers, anticholinergics, narcotics, pseudoephedrine

MAOI, monoamine oxidase inhibitor; *SSRI*, selective serotonin reuptake inhibitor; *SNRI*, serotonin and norepinephrine reuptake inhibitor; *TCA*, tricyclic antidepressant.

Data from Chen, L., Shi, G. R., Huang, D. D., Li, Y., Ma, C. C., Shi, M., Su, B. X., & Shi, G. J. (2019). Male sexual dysfunction: A review of literature on its pathological mechanisms, potential risk factors, and herbal drug intervention. *Biomedicine & Pharmacotherapy*, *112*, 108585. doi:10.1016/j.biopha.2019.01.046

II. Database

Initial evaluation of SD begins with a thorough medical, surgical, obstetric, gynecologic, urological, social, relationship, and sexual history and a review of the patient's medications. Mental health, trauma, and abuse history are vital to understanding the nature of SD (see Chapter 58, Intimate Partner Violence [Domestic Violence]). An understanding of gender, sexual identity, and sexual orientation is a baseline that guides the exam and treatment (see transgender care in Chapters 7 and 40).

A. *Subjective*
 1. Sexual and genital symptoms
    a. Lack of desire
    b. Lack of response
    c. Change in or lack of orgasm
    d. Lack of sensation
    e. Painful intercourse
    f. Irritation
    g. Dryness
    h. Genital pain
    i. Lesions
 2. Other symptoms
    a. Abdominal pain
    b. Bowel complaints
    c. Bladder or urethral pain
    d. Hernia discomfort
    e. Rectal or perianal pain
    f. Pelvic floor symptoms, including pain and spasms
    g. Perception of pelvic organ prolapse

B. *Objective*
 1. Vital signs, including temperature, weight, pulse, and blood pressure
 2. General physical exam
 3. Abdominal examination
 4. Genital examination, including:
    a. External: mons pubis, skin
    b. Inguinal
    c. Vulva
    d. Bimanual: cervix, uterus, ovaries, vaginal tone, masses
    e. Speculum exam: cervix, vaginal walls, vaginal discharge
    f. Penis
    g. Scrotum/testicles
    h. Urethra
    i. Rectal tone
    j. Prostate
    k. Pelvic floor muscle function

III. Assessment

A. *Determine the diagnosis.*
 The following list of screening questionnaires can determine SD in the areas of desire, arousal, orgasm, and pain. Screening tools for anxiety and depression can also be useful in assessing for underlying mental health symptoms.

 The most common questionnaires include the following:
 1. General: Patient Health Questionnaire-9 (PHQ-9), Generalized Anxiety Disorder, 7-Item (GAD-7) Anxiety
 2. Persons AMAB: Sexual Health Inventory for Men (SHIM)
 3. Persons AFAB: Female Sexual Function Index (FSFI)
 4. There are many other scales available, including those that assess sexual knowledge, multiple domains of sexual dysfunction, drug-related sexual dysfunction in multiple domains, sexual desire, arousal/erection, orgasm, ejaculation, sexual satisfaction, sexual quality of life, vaginismus, and various aspects of marital functioning (Grover and Shouan, 2020). A complete review of those scales is beyond the scope of this chapter, but they are widely accessible.

B. *Severity*
 1. Assess the severity of the condition in each of the areas of desire, arousal, orgasm, and pain.
 2. Assess psychological distress and depression associated with the condition.

C. *Significance*
 1. Assess the significance of the problem to the patient and sexual partner(s).

D. *Motivation and ability*
 1. Determine the patient's goals for treatment.
 2. Determine the patient's preferences for treatment (e.g., behavioral modification, medication, combination of these, or other treatment options).
 3. Determine the patient's willingness and ability to follow the treatment plan.

IV. Goals of clinical management

A. *Screening or diagnosing SD*
 Choose a cost-effective approach for screening or diagnosing SD that is compatible with the patient's goals and preferences.

B. *Treatment*
 Select a treatment plan that achieves the patient's objectives for sexual function in a safe and effective manner.

C. *Patient adherence*
 Select an approach that maximizes patient adherence.

V. Plan

A. *Diagnostic tests*
 Test for other conditions contributing to sexual dysfunction, including infection, chronic disease, and hormonal imbalances.
 1. Genital cultures, sexually transmitted infection (STI) testing, wet mount
 2. Urinalysis
 3. General health lab tests include Hgb A1C, fasting glucose, chemistry panel, liver function testing, kidney function, complete blood count, lipid panel, prostate-specific antigen (PSA), and electrocardiography (ECG/EKG).

4. Hormonal assays include testosterone, estradiol levels, sex hormone binding globulin, prolactin, and thyroid-stimulating hormone. Baseline assessments of testosterone and estradiol are useful if considering hormone therapy.

B. Management
1. Pharmacologic management

There are a growing number of treatments for SD, depending on the symptoms the patient is experiencing. Muscle relaxants and anti-anxiety medications should also be considered for symptom management. See **Table 24-2**.

2. Nonpharmacologic management
   a. Herbal and supplement therapies
      i. ArginMax (Daily Wellness Co, Honolulu, HI, USA) is a proprietary blend of components L-arginine, ginseng, ginkgo, and damiana; B-complex vitamins; vitamins A, C, and E; and minerals iron, calcium, and zinc used to treat SD in persons AFAB and to treat erectile dysfunction. It may have additive effects with anticoagulant, hypertensive, and hypoglycemic drugs.

Table 24-2 Medications for Sexual Dysfunction (SD)

Medication	Dose	Indications (I) and Considerations (C)
Antidepressants and Anxiolytics		
Bupropion	150 mg orally twice daily	I: Improves desire C: Off-label for SD
Amitriptyline	25–100 mg orally at night	I: Neuropathic pain C: Off-label for SD
Buspirone	20–30 mg/day orally divided 2–3×/day	I: Anxiety C: Off-label for SD
Paroxetine	10–40 mg daily	I: Premature ejaculation C: Off-label for SD Meta-analysis data show paroxetine has the strongest ejaculation delay. Other SSRIs can also help with premature ejaculation.
Hormonal Treatments		
Testosterone: Gel 1%–2% Compounded cream 1% Solution 2%	5 mg daily transdermal	I: Improves sexual desire, pleasure, orgasm, and arousal satisfaction in postmenopausal persons AFAB. Improves desire in AMAB. C: Not FDA approved for use in persons AFAB. Supported by multiple societies. Blood CBC, testosterone, and PSA levels should be monitored and maintained within normal values. Check baseline testosterone and after 6 weeks of giving initial dosing; titrate dosing for desired effect without androgenic side effects; once stable, monitor every 4–6 months afterward. Safety of long-term use not established.
Estrogen: Estrogen vaginal 0.625 mg/g Estradiol vaginal Estradiol transdermal	0.5 g vaginally 1–3×/week 10-mcg tablet vaginally 2×/week 1 g cream vaginally 1–3×/week 7.5 mcg per 24 hours/ring placed every 3 months 0.025 to 0.1 mg weekly or twice weekly	I: Sexual desire, arousal, and dyspareunia in postmenopausal persons AFAB C: If given systemically, must be paired with progesterone in patients with an intact uterus.
Prasterone	6.5 mg vaginal at night	I: For vulvovaginal atrophy
Selective Estrogen Receptor Modulator		
Ospemifene	60 mg daily	I: Dyspareunia in postmenopausal patients C: Alternative for persons AFAB with history of hormone-responsive cancers

Medication	Dose	Indications (I) and Considerations (C)
Phosphodiesterase-5 (PDE5) Inhibitors		
Sildenafil	Persons AMAB: 25–100 mg orally 1 hour before intercourse	I: Erectile dysfunction C: Interactions with antidepressants, antifungals, antiretrovirals, nitrites, and antihypertensives. Caution in patients with renal or cardiac disease. Less effective after a high-fat meal. Not FDA approved but in clinical trials for anorgasmia in persons AFAB. Onset: 30–60 minutes Action: 12 hours
Tadalafil	5–20 mg orally 45 minutes before intercourse or 2.5–5 mg daily	Onset: 60–120 minutes Action: 36 hours
Vardenafil	5–20 mg orally 45 minutes before intercourse	Onset: 30–60 minutes Action: 10 hours
Avanafil	50–200 mg orally 15 minutes before intercourse	Onset: 15–30 minutes Action: 6 hours
Serotonin 1A Agonist/2A Antagonist		
Flibanserin	100 mg orally at night	I: Improved sexual desire and quantity of satisfying sexual events and reduced distress in premenopausal AFAB C: Can cause hypotension, not well tolerated with alcohol
Melanocortin Agonists: Hypoactive Sexual Desire Disorder		
Bremelanotide	1.75 mg injected SC per 24 hours; 8 doses/month	I: Increases sexual arousal and sexual desire in premenopausal persons AFAB
Topical Anesthetics		
Lidocaine–prilocaine 2.5%/2.5% Cream or spray	Apply 1–2.5 g to penis glans at least 5 minutes prior to sexual intercourse	I: Premature ejaculation, improved sexual satisfaction in AMAB
Lidocaine 2.5%–5% Gel, cream, spray	Apply a small amount to penis glans 5–20 minutes prior to sexual intercourse	I: Premature ejaculation, improved sexual satisfaction in AMAB

AFAB, assigned female at birth; *AMAB*, assigned male at birth; *CBC*, complete blood count; *FDA*, U.S. Food and Drug Administration; *PSA*, prostate-specific antigen; *SC*, subcutaneous; *SSRI*, selective serotonin reuptake inhibitor.

  ii. Zestra (Innovus Pharmaceuticals, San Diego, CA, USA) is an over-the-counter massage oil of a blend of borage seed oil, angelica extract, evening primrose oil, coleus extract, and vitamins C and E and was designed to increase blood flow to the clitoris, labia, and vaginal opening.
 b. Sexual devices
  i. Eros clitoral therapy devices
   These have been approved by the U.S. Food and Drug Administration (FDA) for female SD. Provides vacuum suction to the clitoris with vibratory sensation. Increases blood flow to pelvic floor, vagina, and clitoris.
  ii. Vibrators
   External or internal devices to stimulate sensitive sexual organs such as the clitoris or frenulum with vibrations.
  iii. Dilators
   A tube-shaped device used to stretch and desensitize the vaginal canal and assist in treating vaginal and pelvic floor pain. Example: Milliforher.com.
  iv. Vaginal exercise devices
   These target the pelvic floor muscles, teaching the body muscle contraction and release and improving strength. Example: Therawand.com.

v. Lubricants
Over-the-counter water- or silicone-based lubricants to reduce pain and increase pleasure associated with sex.
vi. Vacuum devices for erectile dysfunction
An external pump used to assist in maintaining erections. Can be used in conjunction with phosphodiesterase-5 (PDE5) inhibitors.
vii. Occlusive penile ring
Occlusive rings limit venous outflow once erection is obtained to allow for penetration (although they may prevent external ejaculation). Can be used in conjunction with vacuum devices.
viii. Ohnut buffer ring
A stackable external ring applied to penetrative partner to adjust depth of penetration.
3. Psychotherapeutic referrals
Psychotherapeutic referrals should be offered to all patients because of the high association between mental health conditions and SDs. Mental health disparities are particularly significant in lesbian, gay, bisexual, transgender, intersex, queer/questioning, and asexual (LGBTQIA+) patients. Patients can experience mood disorders, anxiety, body image disorders, eating disorders, self-harm, substance use, and trauma, which can affect sexual function (Holmberg et al., 2019; Schulman & Erickson-Schroth, 2017). A combined approach of psychotherapy and pharmacotherapy can be more effective in resolving SDs (Althof et al., 2010).
  a. Cognitive–behavioral therapy (CBT)
  CBT is focused on identifying sexual behaviors and cognitions that contribute to SD and providing education (Kingsberg et al., 2017).
  b. Sex therapy
  Sex therapy is a specialized form of counseling that helps couples with specific techniques to address desire, arousal, orgasm, and pain. It is short term and includes education, couples' exercises, and counseling. The emphasis is on modifying sexual patterns to enhance intimacy and sex (Kingsberg et al., 2017).
  c. Mindfulness-based therapies
  This therapy is focused on present-moment awareness and nonjudgement, with attention and acceptance of the present. Studies show that mindfulness-based therapies are useful for erectile dysfunction and AFAB arousal and desire dysfunctions (Jaderek & Lew-Starowicz, 2019).
4. Specialty referral
  a. Urology: penile Doppler, penile prosthesis, injectable or intraurethral alprostadil for blood vessel expansion in the penis
  b. Cosmetic surgery referrals are common, and some patients find benefit from procedures that they should discuss carefully with their specialist: labiaplasty, vaginoplasty, laser vaginoplasty, perineoplasty, laser rejuvenation, clitoral de-hooding, labia majora augmentation, G-spot amplification, laser treatment of vulvovaginal atrophy, and platelet-rich plasma treatments.
  c. OB/GYN: Trigger point and Botox injections of the pelvic floor may help those with pelvic floor dysfunction. Pelvic floor surgery may be used to treat incontinence or prolapse.
  d. Cardiology: Patients with erectile dysfunction are at high risk for cardiovascular disease and need to be evaluated.
5. Pelvic floor referral
  a. Physical therapy/pelvic floor therapy
  Physical therapists manipulate the pelvic floor muscles to improve function and strength.
  b. Biofeedback
  Biofeedback teaches the patient to control the pelvic floor muscles using visualization to achieve conscious control over the contraction of the pelvic floor and decrease the cycle of spasms.
6. Other specialty referral
  a. Acupuncture
  Acupuncture can help with vulvar pain and premature ejaculation.
C. *Patient education*
  1. Information
  Provide verbal and, preferably, written information regarding:
    a. Sexual health, sexuality, and sexual response
    b. Prevalence, morbidity, cost, and available treatments for SD
    c. Modifiable risk factors for SD, such as higher total body weight, diabetes, and substance use
    d. Management rationale, action, use, side effects, associated risks, and cost of therapeutic interventions; need for adhering to long-term treatment plans
  2. Counseling
    a. Improved diet to facilitate weight loss to improve blood pressure and metabolic diseases such as diabetes
    b. Increased physical activity
    c. Reduction in substance use: alcohol, smoking, drug use
    d. Improving sleep to 7–8 hours nightly
    e. Importance of treatment of chronic disease and mental health conditions
    f. Decision making around surgical procedures and referrals
    g. Use the Permission, Limited Information, Specific Suggestions, and Intensive Therapy (PLISSIT) model to approach sexual topics and counsel patients, depending on the provider comfort level and referral sources available to the provider (Kingsberg et al., 2017).
      i. Permission: Ask patient for permission to discuss sexual function.
      ii. Limited Information: Give information about sexual problems or resources.

iii. Specific Suggestions: Advise patient regarding aids, self-help books, or techniques the patient can try.
iv. Intensive Therapy: Provide or refer to a trained sex therapist.

VI. **Self-management resources and tools**
A. *Patient education websites*
1. American Association of Sexuality Educators, Counselors, and Therapists (https://www.aasect.org)
2. ACOG (https://www.acog.org)
3. American Sexual Health Association (ASHA) (https://www.ashasexualhealth.org)
4. American Urological Association (https://www.auanet.org)
5. Center for Sexual Health (https://www.ucsfhealth.org/clinics/center-for-sexual-health)
6. International Society for Sexual Medicine (ISSM) (https://www.issm.info)
7. International Society for the Study of Women's Sexual Health (ISSWSH) (https://www.isswsh.org)
8. Kinsey Institute (https://kinseyinstitute.org)
9. National Coalition for Sexual Health (https://nationalcoalitionforsexualhealth.org)
10. North American Menopause Society (http://www.menopause.org)
11. Sexual Medicine Society of North America (SMSNA) (https://www.smsna.org)
12. Sexuality Information and Education Council of the United States (https://siecus.org)
13. Society for Sex Therapy and Research (https://sstarnet.org)
14. Society for Scientific Study of Sexuality (https://sexscience.org)

B. *Self-help education*
1. Books
Bibliotherapy can be an accessible, low-cost approach to treating persons with low desire and arousal dysfunctions. Here are some suggested books for patients and providers:
a. *The Joy of Sex*, by Alex Comfort
b. *Becoming Orgasmic: A Sexual and Personal Growth Program for Women*, by Julia Heiman and Joseph Lopiccolo
c. *For Women Only: A Revolutionary Guide to Overcoming Sexual Dysfunction and Reclaiming Your Sex Life*, by Jennifer Berman, Laura Berman, and Elisabeth Bumiller
d. *Getting the Sex You Want: A Woman's Guide to Becoming Proud, Passionate and Pleased in Bed*, by Sandra Leiblum and Judith Sachs
e. *Come as You Are: The Surprising New Science That Will Transform Your Sex Life*, by Emily Nagoski
f. *I [heart] Female Orgasm: An Extraordinary Orgasm Guide*, by Dorian Solot and Marshall Miller
g. *Real Sex for Real Women: Intimacy, Pleasure & Sexual Wellbeing*, by Laura Berman
h. *Hot Monogamy: Essential Steps to More Passionate, Intimate Lovemaking*, by Patricia Love and Jo Robinson
i. *Dr. Ruth's Sex After 50: Revving Up the Romance, Passion & Excitement*, by Ruth Westheimer
j. *Passionate Marriage: Keeping Love and Intimacy Alive in Committed Relationships*, by David Schnarch
k. *Healing Painful Sex: A Woman's Guide to Confronting, Diagnosing, and Treating Sexual Pain*, by Deborah Coady and Nancy Fish

2. Videos
Professional education videos such as those available at Omgyes.com can provide instruction on sexual techniques to increase knowledge and pleasure. The Rosy app, available at meetrosy.com, offers educational videos and other resources for sexual function.

References

Althof, S. E., Abdo, C. H., Dean, J., Hackett, G., McCabe, M., McMahon, C. G., Rosen, R. C., Sadovsky, R., Waldinger, M., Becher, E., Broderick, G. A., Buvat, J., Goldstein, I., El-Meliegy, A. I., Giuliano, F., Hellstrom, W. J., Incrocci, L., Jannini, E. A., Park, K., … Tan, H. M. (2010). International Society for Sexual Medicine's guidelines for the diagnosis and treatment of premature ejaculation. *Journal of Sexual Medicine, 7*(9), 2947–2969. doi:10.1111/j.1743-6109.2010.01975.x

American College of Obstetricians and Gynecologists, Committee on Practice Bulletins—Gynecology. (2019). Female sexual dysfunction: ACOG practice bulletin clinical management guidelines for obstetrician-gynecologists, Number 213. *Obstetrics and Gynecology, 134*(1), e1–e18. doi:10.1097/AOG.0000000000003324

American Psychiatric Association. (2013). *Diagnostic and statistical manual of mental disorders* (5th ed.).

Basson R. (2015). Human sexual response. *Handbook of Clinical Neurology, 130*, 11–18. doi:10.1016/B978-0-444-63247-0.00002-X

Chen, L., Shi, G. R., Huang, D. D., Li, Y., Ma, C. C., Shi, M., Su, B. X., & Shi, G. J. (2019). Male sexual dysfunction: A review of literature on its pathological mechanisms, potential risk factors, and herbal drug intervention. *Biomedicine & Pharmacotherapy, 112*, 108585. doi:10.1016/j.biopha.2019.01.046

Eckstrand, K. L., Ng, H., & Potter, J. (2016). Affirmative and responsible health care for people with nonconforming gender identities and expressions. *AMA Journal of Ethics, 18*(11), 1107–1118. doi:10.1001/journalofethics.2016.18.11.pfor1-1611

Harsh, V., & Clayton, A. H. (2018). Sex differences in the treatment of sexual dysfunction. *Current Psychiatry Reports, 20*(3), 18. doi:10.1007/s11920-018-0883-1

Heiden-Rootes, K. M., Salas, J., Gebauer, S., Witthaus, M., Scherrer, J., McDaniel, K., & Carver, D. (2017). Sexual dysfunction in primary care: An exploratory descriptive analysis of medical record diagnoses. *Journal of Sexual Medicine, 14*(11), 1318–1326. doi:10.1016/j.jsxm.2017.09.014

Holmberg, M., Arver, S., & Dhejne, C. (2019). Supporting sexuality and improving sexual function in transgender persons. *Nature Reviews. Urology, 16*(2), 121–139. doi:10.1038/s41585-018-0108-8

Jaderek, I., & Lew-Starowicz, M. (2019). A systematic review on mindfulness meditation-based interventions for sexual dysfunctions. *Journal of Sexual Medicine, 16*(10), 1581–1596. doi:10.1016/j.jsxm.2019.07.019

Kingsberg, S. A., Althof, S., Simon, J. A., Bradford, A., Bitzer, J., Carvalho, J., Flynn, K. E., Nappi, R. E., Reese, J. B., Rezaee, R. L., Schover, L., & Shifrin, J. L. (2017). Female sexual dysfunction—medical and psychological treatments, Committee 14. *Journal of Sexual Medicine, 14*(12), 1463–1491. doi:10.1016/j.jsxm.2017.05.018

McCabe, M. P., Sharlip, I. D., Lewis, R., Atalla, E., Balon, R., Fisher, A. D., Laumann, E., Lee, S. W., & Segraves, R. T. (2016a). Incidence and prevalence of sexual dysfunction in women and men: A consensus statement from the Fourth International Consultation on Sexual Medicine 2015. *Journal of Sexual Medicine, 13*(2), 144–152. doi:10.1016/j.jsxm.2015.12.034

Parish, S. J., Hahn, S. R., Goldstein, S. W., Giraldi, A., Kingsberg, S. A., Larkin, L., Minkin, M. J., Brown, V., Christiansen, K., Hartzell-Cushanick, R., Kelly-Jones, A., Rullo, J., Sadovsky, R., & Faubion, S. S. (2019). The International Society for the Study of Women's Sexual Health process of care for the identification of sexual concerns and problems in women. *Mayo Clinic Proceedings, 94*(5), 842–856. doi:10.1016/j.mayocp.2019.01.009

Schulman, J. K., & Erickson-Schroth, L. (2017). Mental health in sexual minority and transgender women. *Psychiatric Clinics of North America, 40*(2), 309–319. doi:10.1016/j.psc.2017.01.011

CHAPTER 25

Urinary Incontinence in Persons Assigned Female at Birth

Janis Luft

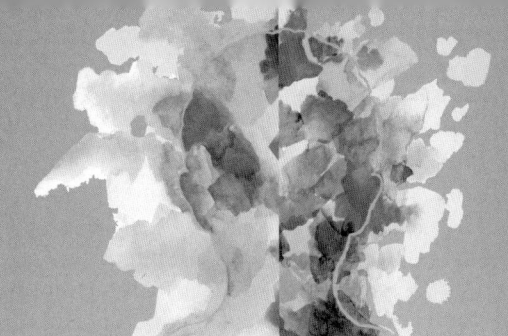

I. Introduction and general background

Involuntary loss of urine, or urinary incontinence (UI), although a common and typically underreported problem affecting adult patients assigned female at birth (AFAB) in the United States, is difficult to quantify. The reasons for this are multiple. Although the definition of UI according to the International Urogynecological Association and the International Continence Society is simply "any involuntary leakage of urine," epidemiological studies may quantify prevalence differently—for example, as daily, weekly, or monthly leakage (Milsom & Gyhagen, 2018). UI rates and reporting may vary across groups studied. In addition, data for patients assigned male and female at birth are often grouped together, although patients AFAB typically have a higher prevalence of UI symptoms, save among the most elderly. Rates of UI rise with increasing age and morbidity. Among noninstitutionalized patients AFAB, half over the age of 65 have reported urinary leakage, and as many as 25% of those of reproductive age have difficulty controlling their bladders (Gorina et al., 2014; Qaseem et al., 2014). Rates of incontinence and treatment for incontinence vary across racial and ethnic groups (Mckellar & Abraham, 2019), suggesting healthcare disparities common to other conditions. UI is associated with a profound adverse impact on quality of life and a higher risk of falls, fractures, nursing home admissions, depression, and social isolation. In 2007, the economic burden of urge UI alone in the United Stated was $65.9 billion (Coyne et al., 2014). Yet, UI is underreported and undertreated (Minassian et al., 2012).

A. Types of UI

UI classification is based on clinical presentation and severity. The primary circumstances leading to leakage of urine determine the type of incontinence. Most patients seen in the ambulatory care setting with UI present with stress, urge, or mixed UI (**Table 25-1**).

1. Stress UI

Stress UI (SUI) is defined as the involuntary loss of urine as a result of physical stress or increased abdominal pressure from coughing, sneezing, straining, or exercise.

Table 25-1 Differential Diagnosis of Urinary Incontinence

Type	Presentation	Timing	Volume
Stress	Leakage associated with greater abdominal pressure from coughing, sneezing, straining, or exercise	Immediate	Small to moderate
Urge	Leakage occurs with a strong urge or need to void	Delayed	Drops to large
Mixed	Combination of stress and urge incontinence; one or the other may predominate	Varies	Varies

2. Urge incontinence and overactive bladder
   a. Urge incontinence (UUI) describes the loss of urine associated with a strong urge or need to void. Urinary frequency and nocturia are frequently part of the clinical presentation of this condition. Some patients report nocturnal enuresis, which is involuntary loss of urine while sleeping.
   b. Patients with overactive bladder (OAB) can be characterized as having wet or dry OAB. Wet OAB includes episodes of UUI. Patients with dry OAB experience frequency, urgency, or nocturia but manage to avoid leaking with various behavioral strategies (e.g., limiting fluids, voiding often, and avoiding dietary bladder irritants). Therefore, an OAB diagnosis does not require incontinence.
3. Mixed incontinence
   Patients with mixed incontinence have symptoms of both stress and urge incontinence, although one or the other condition may predominate.
4. Overflow incontinence
   Bladder outlet obstruction or hypocontractility of the detrusor muscle can cause incomplete bladder emptying. An abnormally full bladder can overspill, resulting in overflow incontinence. This is a less common bladder dysfunction.
5. Functional incontinence
   Functional incontinence is defined as urine loss that occurs because of factors exogenous to the lower urinary tract, such as diminished cognition or limited ambulation. In this case, the bladder and urethra are working normally, and a patient may or may not be aware of the need to urinate but is unable to get to the appropriate location to void.
6. Reflex incontinence or neurogenic bladder
   Reflex incontinence, also known as *neurogenic bladder*, is incontinence associated with neurologic dysfunction (e.g., in cases of multiple sclerosis or spinal cord injury). This can occur without warning or sensory awareness.

B. *Prevalence*
The prevalence of UI types varies according to age and underlying health status. Stress incontinence is more common in younger, ambulatory patients, whereas urge and mixed incontinence increase with age and other health conditions. The proportion of patients with UI varies widely (from 2% to 55%) depending on the definitions researchers used and the populations they surveyed. Researchers in the United States followed 64,000 patients in the Nurses' Health Study (NHS) from 2001 to 2003. The 2-year incidence of UI was 13.7%, but the 2-year remission rate (i.e., the percentage who reported leaking at least once a month at baseline and no leaking on follow-up) was 13.9% (Townsend et al., 2007). But another study using patients enrolled in the NHS and NHSII identified 10,349 participants who reported new-onset UI between 2004 and 2005. These patients were subcategorized as having SUI, UUI, or mixed UI and followed at year 4 and year 8. The researchers found that most patients with incident stress and urgency UI continued to experience similar subtype symptoms over 8 years, but those with severe SUI or UUI were more at risk for progressing to mixed incontinence. A small number in each group with mild to moderate symptoms reported resolution over time, although few with severe symptoms did (Minassian et al., 2020). These results point to the chronic and dynamic nature of UI over time.

C. *Risk factors*
Risk factors include older age, genetics, increased parity, vaginal delivery or other obstetric events, hysterectomy, higher body weight, diabetes, smoking, chronic cough, and constipation. Certain medications may contribute to new-onset UI or increase the severity of UI. These can include diuretics, muscle relaxants, narcotics/hypnotics, and alpha-adrenergic blockers.

II. Initial evaluation
Initial evaluation of UI begins with a thorough medical, surgical, obstetric, and gynecological history and a complete list of the patient's medications. Clinicians can use a three-part screening tool to determine the type of incontinence (Brown et al., 2006). First, patients should be asked if they've leaked even a small amount of urine in the last 3 months. Then they should be asked if the leaking came with physical activity such as lifting or coughing. The third question is whether patients have leaked when they had the urge to urinate but were not able to get to the toilet in time. If they leak most often with physical activity, they have stress incontinence. If they leak most often with urge, they have urge incontinence. If they leak equally with both, they have mixed incontinence, and if they leak but without physical activity or urge, there is another cause. These questions reliably correlate with clinical findings (Brown et al., 2006).

A. *Subjective*
1. Urinary symptoms
   a. Timing, frequency, severity, and precipitants of incontinence episodes
   b. Number of daytime and nighttime urinations
   c. Urinary diary (**Table 25-2**)
2. Amount and nature of fluid intake
3. Bowel habits (e.g., constipation, diarrhea, or straining)

B. *Objective*
Although not a prerequisite to diagnosis and the initiation of nonsurgical treatment for UI, the following may provide data that aid in individualization of treatment or assist in the management of UI refractory to treatment.
1. Assess for genital atrophy. Directed pelvic examination to assess for uterine prolapse or other pathology, such as a pelvic mass.

Table 25-2 Urinary Diary*

Time	Urinate in Toilet	Leaking Accident	Reason for Accident	Fluid Intake	
				Type	Amount
6 a.m.					
7 a.m.					
8 a.m.					
9 a.m.					
10 a.m.					
11 a.m.					
12 noon					
1 p.m.					
2 p.m.					
3 p.m.					
4 p.m.					
5 p.m.					

NOTES
INSTRUCTIONS
1. In the first column, mark an (x) every time you urinate into the toilet.
2. In the second column, mark an (x) every time you accidentally leak urine.
3. If an accident occurred, indicate the reason or circumstances surrounding the accident, for example, "coughed, bent over, sudden urge."
4. Under "Fluid Intake," describe the type (coffee, tea, juice, etc.) and amount (a cup, 1 quart, etc.).
5. Circle the time when you went to bed and when you got up in the morning.
6. Record number and type of pads used.
7. Under "Notes," write any additional information you would like to include. For example, type and dose of medication you may be on for your urinary incontinence.

*Actual diary contains 24 rows labeled for each hour.

   2. Simple neurologic examination: mental status and sensory and motor function of the perineum and lower extremities

III. Assessment
A. *Determine the diagnosis*
   The screening tool can be used to determine the initial diagnosis of UI type (Table 25-1).
B. *Severity*
   Assess the severity of the condition.
   1. Number and types of pads or hygienic products used
   2. Psychological distress and depression associated with the condition (e.g., limitation on travel, time with family, social isolation, fear of odor or accidents, restriction of exercise)
   3. Disruption of sleep
C. *Significance*
   Assess the significance of the problem to the patient and significant others.
   1. Is the patient or caregiver bothered by their symptoms?
   2. Is there an impact on the patient's other medical conditions or health from UI? For example, is there unwillingness or inability to exercise? Is there vulvar or vaginal irritation or skin integrity problems due to constant moisture or pad use?
D. *Motivation and ability*
   1. Determine the patient's goals for treatment (e.g., reduction in incontinent episodes vs. complete dryness, less daytime urination, or less nocturia).
   2. Determine the patient's preferences for treatment (e.g., behavioral modification, medication, combination of these, or other treatment options).

3. Determine the patient's willingness and ability to follow the treatment plan.

IV. Goals of clinical management
1. Choose a cost-effective approach for screening or diagnosing UI that is compatible with the patient's goals and preferences.
2. Select a treatment plan that achieves the patient's objectives for bladder control in a safe and effective manner.
3. Select an approach that maximizes patient adherence.

V. Plan
A. *Screening*
Primary or gynecological providers can effectively screen patients by simply asking about issues of bladder control or using the simple questionnaire.
B. *Diagnostic tests*
   1. Incontinence questionnaire
   2. A urinary diary that the patient keeps for 1–3 days (Table 25-2)
   3. A dipstick urinalysis or culture to rule out underlying infection. Ensure clean specimen collection. A catheterized specimen may be needed for certain patients.
   4. Postvoid residual urine to rule out overflow incontinence. This can be done using a small straight catheter or by bladder ultrasonography within 15 minutes of urination.
   5. Urodynamic testing measures detrusor function, bladder capacity and compliance, and sensation to void. Although such testing may be useful in evaluating patients with complex symptoms or voiding dysfunction, it is not necessary for all patients with incontinence before proceeding to treatment based on clinical presentation.
C. *Management*
   1. Nonpharmacologic management
   Ongoing studies have shown that even simple verbal and written instructions or a one-time group session reviewing nonpharmacologic methods can result in improvement of UI symptoms (Diokno et al., 2018).
      a. Bladder training helps patients reestablish voluntary bladder control in those with UUI or SUI at high volumes. Patients learn how to void on a set schedule, beginning with about 30–60 minutes between voids and then slowly increasing the interval to 3 or 4 hours (**Table 25-3**).

Table 25-3 Bladder Retraining

Bladder retraining is a behavioral treatment for urinary incontinence that uses scheduled toileting to help you relearn normal bladder function. The purpose of bladder retraining is to

a. increase the amount of time between emptying your bladder.
b. increase the amount of fluids your bladder can hold.
c. diminish the sense of urgency and/or leakage associated with your problem.

Keeping a (or this) diary of your bladder activity is very important. This helps us to determine the correct starting interval for you and to monitor your progress throughout your program.

INSTRUCTIONS

1. Empty your bladder as soon as you get up in the morning. This begins your retraining schedule.
2. Go to the bathroom every _____
3. Wait the full amount of time before you urinate again, AND when it is your scheduled time, be sure to empty your bladder even if you feel no urge to urinate. Follow the schedule during waking hours ONLY. During the nighttime, go to the bathroom only if you awaken and find it necessary.
4. A helpful hint: When the urge to urinate is felt before the next designated time, use the "urge-suppression" technique described in the Urge Suppression handout, or try relaxation techniques like deep breathing. Focus on relaxing all other muscles. If possible, sit down until the sensation passes. If the urge is suppressed, adhere to the schedule. If you cannot suppress the urge, wait 5 minutes, and then slowly make your way to the bathroom; then reestablish the schedule. Repeat this process each time an urge is felt.
5. When you have accomplished this goal, gradually increase the time between emptying your bladder by 15-minute intervals. Try to increase your interval each week, but you will be the best judge of how quickly you can advance to the next step. The time between each urination is increased until you reach a 3- to 4-hour voiding interval.
6. It should take between 6 and 12 weeks to accomplish your goal. Don't be discouraged by setbacks. You may find you have good days and bad days. As you continue bladder retraining, you will start to notice more and more good days, so keep practicing.
7. You will hasten your success by doing your pelvic muscle exercises faithfully every day. Your diaries will help you see your progress and identify your problem times.
8. If you need more help, medication or other treatments are available and may be useful.

b. Relaxation and urge-suppression techniques effectively suppress the strong urge to void that is associated with urge UI (**Table 25-4**).
c. Pelvic floor muscle exercises, also known as *Kegel exercises*, strengthen the muscles of the pelvic floor and improve urethral pressure and inhibit involuntary detrusor contractions, thus helping those with SUI but also UUI (Table 25-4). Patients may practice this on their own after education or be referred to a pelvic floor physical therapist.
d. Biofeedback uses electromyography or manometry to help patients learn pelvic floor muscle exercises through directed instructions as they receive feedback in the form of dynamic graphs or tones that reinforces their actions. This modality can help patients isolate pelvic muscles and improve the efficacy of pelvic floor muscle exercises.
e. Weight loss has been shown to improve continence symptoms. As little as 3%–5% weight reduction has been shown to reduce weekly incontinence episodes by 50%–60% (Subak et al., 2009).
f. Diet modification can be helpful. Some patients find that reduction or elimination of "bladder triggers," such as caffeine, alcohol, spicy foods, and concentrated citrus, can improve urinary urgency and frequency. Overhydration and underhydration should be discouraged. Fluid intake sufficient to maintain "lemon juice"–colored urine is ideal, usually 1.5–2 L and modified as needed for chronic conditions (congestive heart failure [CHF], kidney disease).
g. Constipation management and maximizing bowel function will reduce pressure on the bladder from the bowel.

2. Pharmacologic treatment options
Medical treatment of SUI has been largely unsuccessful, and there are no medications approved by the U.S. Food and Drug Administration (FDA) for this indication. However, a growing number of medications are available to treat UUI, urgency, frequency, and nocturia (see **Table 25-5**). Generally, these agents, which inhibit the bladder's contractile activity, have an anticholinergic and/or antimuscarinic effect. Although they provide excellent symptom relief and reduce weekly incontinent episodes by 15%–60%, they may also cause bothersome side effects, such as dry mouth, constipation, drowsiness, and blurred vision. Sustained-release medications may cause fewer side effects. Different anticholinergic medications also vary in their ability to affect specific bladder receptors and in their propensity to cross the blood–brain barrier. There is concern about the possibility of changes in cognitive function with the use of less selective anticholinergic/antimuscarinics, especially in the elderly and those with preexisting dementia. Care should be taken in the selection of appropriate agents in this population. (Kachru et al., 2020). In fact, in 2020, the American Urogynecological Society recommended avoiding anticholinergic medications to treat OAB in patients over age 70 (American Urogynecologic Society, 2021). A quaternary anticholinergic, such as trospium, is less likely to cross the blood–brain barrier and may pose less risk to cognitive function. A newer type of overactive bladder medication is now available. Mirabegron (Myrbetriq) and vibegron (Gemtesa) are the only FDA-approved β3-adrenergic receptor agonists. They act to relax the smooth muscle that surrounds the bladder and help to increase the bladder's ability to store urine. Because mirabegron and vibegron are not anticholinergics, they are

Table 25-4 Urge Suppression

Urge incontinence is the loss of urine when you have a strong desire to urinate and are unable to reach a bathroom in time. The urge is a signal that it is time to urinate. Your goal is to maintain bladder control until you reach a toilet. A normally functioning bladder can wait until the appropriate opportunity to empty; an unstable bladder cannot.
For a person with urge incontinence, rushing to the bathroom when you have a strong urge to urinate can worsen the problem. Rushing causes bladder irritability to increase and interferes with your ability to concentrate on controlling your bladder. When urgency strikes, you should use the "urge-suppression" technique to maintain control.

1. Stop all movement immediately and stand still. Sit down if possible. Remaining still increases your ability to stay in control.
2. Squeeze your pelvic floor muscles quickly and tightly several times. Do not relax the muscles fully between these very quick squeezes. Squeezing your pelvic floor muscles this way signals the bladder to relax and increases your feeling of being in control.
3. Take a deep breath and relax. Shrug your shoulders and let them go limp. Release the tension in the rest of your body.
4. Concentrate on suppressing the urge feeling. Some patients find distraction an effective technique.
5. When the strong urgency subsides, walk slowly and calmly to the bathroom. If the urge begins to build again, repeat these steps. You can also try contracting your muscles as you walk to the bathroom.

Remember: going to the bathroom is not an emergency!

Table 25-5 Medications for Overactive Bladder

Short-acting oral anticholinergics/muscarinic receptor antagonists (MRAs)	Oxybutynin (Ditropan®), 5 mg	0.50–1 tablet two to four times a day
	Tolterodine (Detrol®), 1 and 2 mg	1 tablet twice daily (start with 2 mg and decrease to 1 mg if severe side effects)
	Trospium chloride (Sanctura®), 20 mg	1 tablet twice daily on an empty stomach
Extended-release oral anticholinergics/MRAs	Oxybutynin ER (Ditropan XL®), 5–30 mg	1 tablet daily
	Tolterodine ER (Detrol LA®), 2 and 4 mg	1 capsule daily (start with 4 mg and decrease to 2 mg if severe side effects)
	Trospium chloride (Sanctura®), 60 mg	1 tablet daily on an empty stomach
	Darifenacin (Enablex®), 7.5 and 15 mg	1 tablet daily
	Solifenacin (VesiCare®), 5 and 10 mg	1 tablet daily
	Fesoterodine (Toviaz®), 4 and 8 mg	1 tablet daily
Transdermal anticholinergics/MRAs	Oxybutynin transdermal patch (Oxytrol)®, 3.9 mg/day (over the counter—no prescription needed)	1 patch on dry skin (hip, abdomen, or buttocks) every 3–4 days
	Oxybutynin transdermal gel 10% (Gelnique®), 100 mg/g (individual packet or metered pump)	1 sachet or pump daily to dry, intact skin on the abdomen, upper arms or shoulders, or thighs
Nonanticholinergic medications	Mirabegron (Myrbetriq®) 25 and 50 mg	1 tablet daily
	Vibegron (Gemtesa®) 75 mg	1 tablet daily

Notes for anticholinergic/MRA medications:
Contraindications: Narrow-angle glaucoma, myasthenia gravis, bladder flow obstruction, gastric retention, severe liver or kidney disease.
Cautions: Some studies demonstrate increased risk of cognitive decline and mortality in patients with dementia with the use of nonselective anticholinergics. Consider consulting with a specialist before prescribing these drugs to those with or at high risk of dementia and counseling patients on the associated risk versus overall quality-of-life improvement. Consider reducing the overall anticholinergic burden for patients by using the lowest effective dose and changing or reducing other anticholinergic medications they may be taking.
Lowest brain penetration: trospium > darifenacin > fesoterodine (Callegari et al., 2011)
Side effects: Dry mouth and constipation are the most common. Adjust dose to balance drug effectiveness versus side effects.
Notes for mirabegron and vibegron:
These are β3-adrenergic receptor agonists. Monitor changes in blood pressure after initiation of medication. Mirabegron is contraindicated for patients with uncontrolled hypertension.

presumably safer in regard to a decrease in cognitive function risk. They may also have fewer bothersome side effects, but they have higher cost and require 6–8 weeks to take full effect. Mirabegron has been associated with an increase in blood pressure (Wagg et al., 2014).

A review of studies evaluating the use of vaginal estrogen in postmenopausal patients for the treatment of genitourinary symptoms, including UUI and SUI, concluded that such vaginal estrogen creams, tablets, and rings can be safe and a helpful adjunct to treatment (Rahn et al., 2014).

Treatment of incontinence with oral or transdermal estrogen is not recommended. Two large randomized controlled trials (the Women's Health Initiative and the Heart and Estrogen Replacement Study) demonstrated an increase in the prevalence of UI with the use of both estrogen-only and combined systemic hormone-replacement therapy on stress, urge, and mixed UI (40%–50% over a 4-year

period and 20%–60% at 12 months) (Grady et al., 2001; Hendrix et al., 2005).
3. Treatment usually requiring referral to a continence specialty practice
    a. Pessaries: Well-fit incontinence ring or incontinence dish pessaries can relieve the symptoms of SUI. The pessary compresses the urethra against the upper posterior portion of the symphysis pubis and elevates the bladder neck. This causes an increase in outflow resistance and corrects the angle between the bladder and the urethra. Pessaries can be managed by the patient. If the patient is unable to remove the pessary for cleaning, they should be seen on a regular basis for cleaning and examination of the vaginal mucosa to prevent complications. Common issues of long-term pessary use include mechanical injury to the vaginal epithelium leading to vaginal erosions or bleeding and increased vaginal discharge and odor. Benefits include immediate symptom relief and delay or elimination of the need for surgery.
    b. Electrical stimulation
        i. Vaginal or rectal electrical stimulation uses an internal sensor to deliver electrical currents at preset frequencies. Higher frequency causes involuntary levator ani muscle contractions that improve pelvic floor tone and assist in learning to contract these muscles at will. Lower frequencies are used to blockade the sacral nerve plexus, reducing detrusor irritability.
        ii. Percutaneous tibial nerve stimulation (PTNS) is used to treat OAB. A fine-needle electrode is inserted into the lower, inner aspect of the leg, slightly cephalad to the medial malleolus. The goal is to send stimulation through the tibial nerve. The needle electrode is connected to an external pulse generator that delivers an adjustable electrical pulse that travels to the sacral plexus via the tibial nerve. The treatment protocol requires once-a-week treatments for 12 weeks, roughly 30 minutes per session. If successful, patients are usually switched to a maintenance schedule of about every 4 weeks. Transcutaneous tibial nerve stimulation (TTNS) is also used, in which external electrodes only are used. The recommended treatment protocol and efficacy of this method have not yet been established; however, this method offers a less invasive and potentially patient-managed option for tibial nerve stimulation. Both PTNS and TTNS are overall low-risk options with few contraindications.
    c. Surgical treatments
        Multiple surgical options are available to treat stress incontinence. Discussion of details is beyond the scope of this chapter, but primary care clinicians should be aware of the procedures their patients may undergo.
        i. The most common sling procedure is the midurethral synthetic sling, in which the surgeon places a narrow piece of polypropylene mesh under the midurethra. This can be done by either a retropubic (passed behind the pubic bone through the anterior abdominal wall) or transobturator (passed through the obturator foramen) approach. Recent studies have shown a positive role for surgical treatment of patients with MUI as well. Many patients with MUI who have failed more conservative treatments demonstrate a significant reduction in both stress and urge incontinence. However, some will not improve with surgery, and it is impossible to predict who may or may not benefit from this treatment (Sung et al., 2019).
        ii. Patients whose stress incontinence results from intrinsic sphincter deficiency may benefit from urethral bulking agents, such as Coaptite and Macroplastique, which are injected transurethrally as an outpatient surgery (Kirchin et al., 2017).
        iii. Sacral nerve stimulation, also called *sacral nerve neuromodulation* (InterStim) therapy, is a reversible treatment for people with UUI caused by OAB who do not respond to behavioral treatments or medication. InterStim is a surgically implanted neurostimulation system that sends mild electrical pulses to the S3 sacral nerve root, a nerve that influences bladder control.
        iv. Botulinum toxin A (Botox) injection into the detrusor muscle is an option for neurogenic or idiopathic UUI unresponsive to conservative measures. Botox is injected into numerous sites in the bladder wall using a cystoscope. The toxin works by inactivating proteins involved in neurotransmitter release from nerve terminals. As neurotransmitter levels decrease, underlying muscle spasms may be diminished or ablated.
        v. Bladder augmentation is infrequently used and reserved for people with UUI who do not benefit from bladder retraining or medication. This procedure increases the capacity of a small, hyperactive, or nonresilient bladder by adding bowel segments or by reducing the muscle-squeezing ability of the bladder.
    d. On the horizon
        i. Small studies have shown modest results in trials of benign interventions such as yoga and deep breathing (Huang et al., 2019).
        ii. Gene therapy is being tested as a local intervention aimed at treating OAB with a low risk

of adverse events. Gene therapy is targeted at endogenous physiology in bladder cells in the hopes of restoring normal cell and organ function. Initial studies are underway and show promise for gene therapy as a novel therapy for OAB/UUI (Andersson et al., 2021).

D. Patient education
1. Information
   Provide verbal and, preferably, written information regarding the following:
   a. Prevalence, morbidity, cost, and available treatments for UI
   b. Modifiable risk factors for UI, such as higher body weight, diabetes, and smoking
   c. Management rationale, action, use, side effects, associated risks, and cost of therapeutic interventions; need for adhering to long-term treatment plans
2. Counseling
   a. Weight loss counseling and advice as needed
   b. Management of diabetic glucose levels
   c. Avoidance of constipation
   d. Nonsurgical therapies can be combined to achieve a greater degree of symptom relief and patient satisfaction. Patient education should include encouragement to give these treatment modalities time to evaluate their true effectiveness.
   e. Expectation management regarding outcomes and goals of treatment or therapy

VI. Self-management resources and tools

A. Patient education
1. National Institute of Diabetes and Digestive and Kidney Diseases (NIDDK)
   The NIDDK is a division of the National Institutes of Health. According to the NIDDK website, "the NIDDK conducts and supports research on many chronic and costly diseases affecting the public health. Several diseases studied by the NIDDK are among the leading causes of disability and death in the Nation; all affect seriously the quality of life of those suffering from them." Both patient and provider literature are available on the website (https://www2.niddk.nih.gov).
2. The U.S. Department of Health and Human Services, Office on Women's Health
   This website provides information about UI, pelvic floor prolapse, and treatment options (https://www.womenshealth.gov/).

B. Community support groups
1. National Association for Continence (NAFC)
   Founded in 1982, the NAFC was originally known as Help for Incontinent People. Today, the renamed NAFC is the largest private consumer organization dedicated to educating and advocating for people with bladder and pelvic floor dysfunction. The NAFC provides educational resources, healthcare referrals, public education, and personal support for those with incontinence (https://www.nafc.org or 1-800-BLADDER).
2. The Simon Foundation for Continence
   The mission statement of the Simon Foundation is that of "bringing the topic of incontinence out into the open, removing the stigma surrounding incontinence, and providing help and hope for people with incontinence, their families, and the health professionals who provide their care." The organization provides public education materials (https://www.simonfoundation.org).

C. Mobile apps
   There are a number of mobile phone apps that can help with the behavioral aspects of managing UI, such as keeping a bladder diary (e.g., Bladder Diary by iUFlow), remembering to do pelvic muscle exercises (e.g., Kegel Trainer), or even finding a nearby restroom (e.g., Toilet Finder). Be sure to check if there is a cost associated.

References

American Urogynecologic Society. (2021). AUGS clinical consensus statement: Association of anticholinergic medication use and cognition in women with overactive bladder. *Contemporary OB/GYN*, 66(4), 38–39. doi:10.1097/SPV.0000000000000423

Andersson, K. E., Christ, G. J., Davies, K. P., Rovner, E. S., & Melman, A. (2021). Gene therapy for overactive bladder; a review of BK-channel, α-subunit gene transfer. *Therapeutics and Clinical Risk Management*, 17, 589–599. doi:10.2147/TCRM.S291798

Brown, J. S., Bradley, C. S., Subak, L. L., Richter, H. E., Kraus, S. R., Brubaker, L., Lin, F., Vittinghoff, E., & Grady, D. (2006). The sensitivity and specificity of a simple test to distinguish between urge and stress urinary incontinence. *Annals of Internal Medicine*, 144(10), 715–723. doi:10.7326/0003-4819-144-10-200605160-00005

Callegari, E., Malhotra, B., Bungay, P. J., Webster, R., Fenner, K. S., Kempshall, S., Laperle, J. L., Michel, M. C., & Kay, G. G. (2011). A comprehensive non-clinical evaluation of the CNS penetration potential of antimuscarinic agents for the treatment of overactive bladder. *British Journal of Clinical Pharmacology*, 72(2), 235–246. doi:10.1111/j.1365-2125.2011.03961.x

Coyne, K. S., Wein, A., Nicholson, S., Kvasz, M., Chen, C. I., & Milsom, I. (2014). Economic burden of urgency urinary incontinence in the United States: a systematic review. *Journal of Managed Care and Specialty Pharmacy*, 20(2), 130–140. doi:10.18553/jmcp.2014.20.2.130

Diokno, A. C., Newman, D. K., Low, L. K., & Griebling T. L. (2018). Effect of a group-Administered behavioral treatment on urinary incontinence in older women. *Journal of the American Medical Association Internal Medicine*, 178(10), 1333–1341. doi:10.1001/jamainternmed.2018.3766

Gorina, Y., Schappert, S., Bercovitz, A., Elgadaal, N., & Kramakow, E. (2014). *Prevalence of incontinence among older Americans* (Vital and Health Statistics Series 3, Number 36). Centers for Disease

Control and Prevention. https://www.cdc.gov/nchs/data/series/sr_03/sr03_036.pdf

Grady, D., Brown, J. S., Vittinghoff, E., Applegate, W., Varner, E., Snyder, T., & HERS Research Group. (2001). Postmenopausal hormones and incontinence: The Heart and Estrogen/Progestin Replacement Study. *Obstetrics & Gynecology, 97*(1), 116–120. doi:10.1016/S0029-7844(00)01115-7

Hendrix, S., Cochrane, B., Nygaard, I., Handa, V., Barnabei, V., Iglesia, C., Aragaki, A., Naughton, M. J., Wallace, R. B., & McNeeley, S. G. (2005). Effect of estrogen with and without progestin on urinary incontinence. *Journal of the American Medical Association, 293*(8), 935–948. doi:10.1001/jama.293.8.935

Huang, A. J., Chesney, M., Lisha, A., Vittinghoff, E., Schembri, M., Pawlowsky, S., Hsu, A., &e Subak, L. (2019) A group-based yoga program for urinary incontinence in ambulatory women: Feasibility, tolerability, and change in incontinence frequency over three months in a single-center randomized trial. *American Journal of Obstetrics and Gynecology, 220*(1), 87.e1–87.e13. doi:10.1016/j.ajog.2018.10.031

Kachru, N., Holmes, H. M., Johnson, M. L., Chen, H., & Aparasu, R. R. (2020). Risk of mortality associated with non-selective antimuscarinic medications in older adults with dementia: A retrospective study. *Journal of General Internal Medicine, 35*(7), 2084–2093. doi:10.1007/s11606-020-05634-3

Kirchin, V., Page, T., Keegan, P. E., Atiemo, K. O., Cody, J. D., McClinton, S., & Aluko, P. (2017). Urethral injection therapy for urinary incontinence in women. *Cochrane Database of Systematic Reviews, 2017*(7), CD003881. doi:10.1002/14651858.CD003881.pub4

Mckellar, K., & Abraham, N. (2019). Prevalence, risk factors, and treatment for women with stress urinary incontinence in a racially and ethnically diverse population. *Neurourology and Urodynamics, 38*(3), 934–940. doi:10.1002/nau.23930

Milsom, I., & Gyhagen, M. (2019). The prevalence of urinary incontinence. *Climacteric, 22*(3), 217–222. doi:10.1080/13697137.2018.1543263

Minassian, V. A., Hagan, K. A., Erekson, E., Austin, A. M., Carmichael, D., Bynum, J. P. W., & Grodstein, F. (2020) The natural history of urinary incontinence subtypes in the Nurses' Health Studies. *American Journal of Obstetrics and Gynecology, 222*(2), 163.e1–163.e8. doi:10.1016/j.ajog.2019.08.023

Minassian, V. A., Yan, X., Lichtenfeld, M. J., Sun, H., & Stewart, W. F. (2012). The iceberg of health care utilization in women with urinary incontinence. *International Urogynecology Journal, 23*(8), 1087–1093. doi:10.1007/s00192-012-1743-x

Qaseem, A., Dallas, P., Forciea, M. A., Starkey, M., Denberg, T. D., & Shekelle, P. (2014). Nonsurgical management of urinary incontinence in women: A clinical practice guideline from the American College of Physicians. *Annals of Internal Medicine, 161*(6), 429–440. doi:10.7326/M13-2410

Rahn, D. D., Carberry, C., Sanses, T. V., Mamik, M. M., Ward, R. M., Meriwether, K. V., Olivera, C. K., Abed, H., Balk, E. M., & Murphy, M. (2014). Vaginal estrogen for genitourinary syndrome of menopause: A systematic review. *Obstetrics and Gynecology, 124*(6), 1147–1156. doi:10.1097/AOG.0000000000000526

Subak, L., Wing, R., West, D., Franklin, F., Vittinghoff, E., Creasman, J., Richter, H. E., Myers, D., Burgio, K. L., Gorin, A. A., Macer, J., Kusek, J. W., Grady, D., & PRIDE Investigators. (2009). Weight loss to treat urinary incontinence in overweight and obese women. *New England Journal of Medicine, 360*(5), 481–490. doi:10.1056/NEJMoa0806375

Sung, V. W., Borello-France, D., Newman, D. K., Richter, H. E., Lukacz, E. S., Moalli, P., Weidner, A. C., Smith, A. L., Dunivan, G., Ridgeway, B., Nguyen, J. N., Mazloomdoost, D., Carper, B., & Gantz, M. G. (2019). Effect of behavioral and pelvic floor muscle therapy combined with surgery vs surgery alone on incontinence symptoms among women with mixed urinary incontinence: The ESTEEM randomized clinical trial. *Journal of the American Medical Association, 322*(11), 1066–1076. doi:10.1001/jama.2019.12467

Townsend, M., Danforth, K., Lifford, K., Rosner, B., Curhan, G., Resnick, N., & Grodstein, F. (2007). Incidence and remission of urinary incontinence in middle-aged women. *American Journal of Obstetrics & Gynecology, 197*(2), 167.e1–e5. doi:10.1016/j.ajog.2007.03.041

Wagg, A., Cardozo, L., Nitti, V. W., Castro-Diaz, D., Auerbach, S., Blauwet, M. B., & Siddiqui, E. (2014). The efficacy and tolerability of the β3-adrenoceptor agonist mirabegron for the treatment of symptoms of overactive bladder in older patients. *Age and Ageing, 43*(5), 666–675. doi:10.1093/ageing/afu017

SECTION IV

Obstetric Health Maintenance and Promotion

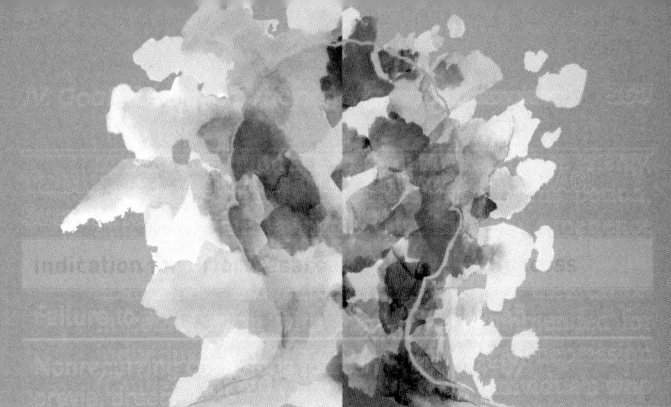

CHAPTER 26	The Initial Prenatal Visit...................................321
CHAPTER 27	Prenatal Genetic Screening and Diagnosis................329
CHAPTER 28	The Return Prenatal Visit....................................337
CHAPTER 29	The Postpartum Visit..345
CHAPTER 30	Guidelines for Medical Consultation, Interprofessional Collaboration, and Transfer of Care During Pregnancy and Childbirth..355

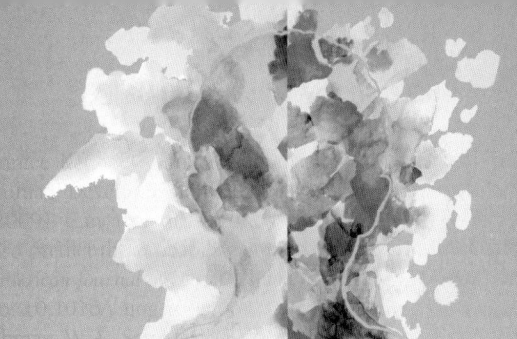

CHAPTER 26

The Initial Prenatal Visit

Rebekah Kaplan

I. Definition and background

Pregnancy is a time of great physical and emotional adjustment in life. Careful, regular monitoring during pregnancy can reassure the parent-to-be and detect variations from a normal pregnancy.

Ideally, prenatal care begins before conception. The basic components of prenatal care include early and continuing risk assessment, health promotion, education, medical and psychosocial interventions, and follow-up. For the patient, pregnancy can be a time to make positive lifestyle changes; prenatal care offers the clinician an opportunity to develop a relationship with a patient over the duration of the pregnancy.

Midwifery-led prenatal care improves birth outcomes, including higher rates of vaginal births, as well as lower rates of preterm birth and fetal loss after 24 weeks, compared to other models of prenatal care (Sandall et al., 2016). The guiding principles of prenatal care should include the following:

- Nonintervention: The reproductive cycle is essentially a healthy process and does not inherently require medical intervention.
- Centering the patient as the most important member of the healthcare team
- Patient-centered provision of education appropriate to age, culture, access to resources, and needs, including anticipatory guidance and nutrition
- Promoting parent's self-esteem and empowerment
- Individualization of care: respecting cultural background, ethnic and/or racial identity, gender identity, sexual orientation, fertility history, pregnancy and birth history, trauma history, and patient priorities

The initial prenatal visit includes a health and psychosocial history and physical exam with a special focus on orienting the patient to the setting's perinatal services, establishing a due date, and identifying risks for complications for both the pregnant person and the fetus. Additional data are gathered through routine laboratory tests and additional ultrasound or diagnostic studies as indicated by findings of history, physical, and/or gestational age.

A. *Addressing social determinants of maternal health*

In the last decades, there has been increasing attention to disparities in the perinatal outcomes of those who are Black, Indigenous, and People of Color (BIPOC) in the United States. These poorer outcomes are especially apparent in Black birthing people. Black people in the United States are more than three times more likely to die in the perinatal period than their White counterparts, even when controlling for education and income. Black people also experience higher rates of preterm birth and small-for-gestational-age infants, and Black infants have a mortality rate two times that of White infants (American College of Obstetricians and Gynecologists [ACOG], 2015; Swanson et al., 2021). Variables posited to explain these inequitable outcomes have included, healthcare access, socioeconomic factors, and/or content of prenatal care; what has become clear is that this disparity is most strongly related to and most directly caused by racism. The impacts of racism take many forms, ranging from individual interactions to systemic inequities in the U.S. healthcare system, our institutional processes, and our legal and social systems. Although this disparity is most prominent in Black birthing people, poorer outcomes are true for any person experiencing racism over time.

Research also demonstrates that BIPOC individuals have a poorer experience of perinatal services than

White people (Altman et al., 2020; Aronson et al., 2013; Green et al., 2021). Implicit bias is believed to be an important influence on how healthcare professionals communicate with and treat Black patients, which leads to some of the disparities in perinatal health (Green, 2021; Howell et al., 2018). Healthcare providers have a mandate to reduce these disparities by reflecting on how their own identities, power, privilege, and bias influence their care and their interactions with patients. It is incumbent on healthcare providers to also increase awareness of the structural determinants of health and incorporate practices that will help to reduce the experience of bias and harm in their care, as well as in the healthcare organizations in which they work. Altman et al. (2020) interviewed women of color and thematically analyzed their recommendations for improving care and building trust, which include the following:

- Spending quality time where patients feel valued and listened to
- Investing time in relationship building and in making meaningful connections
- Providing individualized, person-centered care that values each individual's lived experience and demonstrates respect and dignity, including inquiring about social determinants of health that may affect a family and their care
- True partnership in decision making

At the health systems level, recommendations include the following:

- Continuity of care
- Racial concordance of providers
- Supportive healthcare system structures that include co-located services and referral systems, evening and weekend appointments, and flexibility in appointment times
- Implicit bias training and education to reduce judgment, stereotyping, and discrimination

Implementing these practices will likely benefit all patients receiving prenatal care and are essential for providing quality care to BIPOC individuals and families. Focusing on dismantling institutional policies that disproportionately affect Black birthing people will also help to build trust and reduce inequitable care.

II. Database (may include, but is not limited to)
A. *Subjective*
  1. History of the current pregnancy
      a. Pregnancy symptoms: for example, nausea, vomiting, fatigue, sore breasts, headache, and fetal movement
      b. Problems: for example, vaginal bleeding, excessive vomiting, pelvic pain
      c. Feelings about pregnancy: for example, unplanned, anxious, happy
  2. Information for dating of pregnancy (**Box 26-1**)
      a. Past menstrual history: menarche, cycle interval, length and amount of flow
      b. First day of last normal menstrual period: sureness of date, length of flow, previous menstrual period if last period abnormal and any factors that potentially interfere with duration of cycle or ovulation (e.g., hormonal contraceptives)
      c. Dates and results of home pregnancy testing
      d. Information related to conception: dates of intercourse, use of ovulation predictor, use of reproductive technology
      e. Symptoms of pregnancy, including onset and evolution, as well as fetal movement if present
      f. Previous ultrasound if done
  3. Obstetric history
      a. Total number of pregnancies, including ectopic; abortions (spontaneous and therapeutic); and term, preterm, and living children

---

Box 26-1 Establishing a Due Date

Dating the pregnancy is an essential part of the first prenatal visit. The practitioner must take into consideration all the information for dating the pregnancy and establish a best estimate of the delivery date (EDD). For most pregnant people, a sure and "normal" last menstrual period (LMP) is the most useful method. Calculate the EDD based on LMP by using a gestational wheel, one of many apps, or Naegle's rule (LMP + 7 days − 3 months, based on 28-day cycle). Use an ultrasound EDD if first-trimester ultrasound dates differ by more than 5–7 days or second-trimester dates differ by more than 10 days. (See **Table 28-4** in Chapter 28, The Return Prenatal Visit, for more information on when to change pregnancy dating.)

Accuracy of Dating

- In vitro fertilization ± 1 day
- Ovulation indication ± 3 days
- Single intercourse record/insemination ± 3 days
- Basal body temperature record ± 4 days
- Ultrasound 6–9 weeks (crown–rump length) ± 5 days
- Ultrasound 9–14 weeks (crown–rump length) ± 7 days
- "Regular" and certain LMP with 28-day cycle ± 10–14 days
- Second-trimester ultrasound 10–14 days
- Third-trimester ultrasound 14–28 days
- First-trimester physical examination ± 2 weeks
- Second-trimester physical examination ± 4 weeks
- Third-trimester physical examination ± 6 weeks

Data from Hunter, L. A. (2009). Issues in pregnancy dating: Revisiting the evidence. *Journal of Midwifery & Women's Health, 54*(3), 184–190, doi:10.1016/j.jmwh.2008.11.003; American College of Obstetricians and Gynecologists. (2014). Committee Opinion No. 611: Method for estimating due date. *Obstetrics and Gynecology, 124*(4), 863. doi:10.1097/01.AOG.0000454932.15177.be

b. Deliveries: date, mode of delivery (vaginal birth, cesarean, vacuum or forceps assisted, and indication if operative birth), gestational age, birth weight, length of labor, anesthesia, pregnancy weight gain, spontaneous or induced labor
c. Pregnancy complications, such as preterm labor, gestational diabetes, preeclampsia, gestational hypertension, cholestasis, small- or large-for-gestational-age newborn
d. Delivery complications, such as shoulder dystocia, postpartum hemorrhage, third- or fourth-degree laceration
e. Postpartum complications, such as blood transfusion, infection, wound issues, depression, or mastitis
f. Neonatal or newborn complications and their diagnosis, such as prolonged hospitalization and the reason, jaundice, congenital anomalies, genetic differences

4. Gynecological history
   a. Sexually transmitted infections, including HIV and genital herpes simplex virus of patient or partner
   b. Fibroids or reproductive tract malformations, such as bicornuate uterus
   c. Gynecological surgery, particularly uterine
   d. Abnormal Pap smears and related loop electrosurgical excision procedure or cone procedures
   e. Vulvovaginal disorders or vaginismus

5. Medical history
   a. Present medications: prescriptions, over the counter, supplements
   b. Significant illnesses: asthma, diabetes, hypertension, frequent urinary tract infections, cardiovascular, thyroid, hepatitis, anemia, tuberculosis, seizures, psychiatric diagnoses
   c. Allergies: medications, latex, foods, environmental
   d. Surgeries, hospitalizations, blood transfusions

6. Family history
   a. Significant illnesses with genetic risk: diabetes, hypertension/preeclampsia, renal disease, cardiovascular disease, blood disorders, multiple gestation
   b. Significant illnesses with risk for fetal outcomes: congenital or chromosomal abnormalities, cystic fibrosis, intellectual disability, substance dependence

7. Social history
   a. Country of origin (recent immigrant)
   b. Current living situation
   c. Supports/access to resources
   d. Financial stability, healthcare coverage
   e. Food access
   f. Occupation and work safety (exposure to hazards: chemical, biologic, or physical)
   g. Intimate partner violence
   h. History of trauma and/or sexual abuse
   i. Substance use (cigarettes, alcohol, cannabis, narcotics, current and past use)
   j. Sexually transmitted infection risk factors
   k. Educational history (reading level, years of schooling, how they learn best)

8. Nutritional history
   a. Prepregnancy weight
   b. Weight gain or loss
   c. Current diet: restrictions (vegetarian or lactose intolerant), adequate protein, calcium, grains, fruits, and vegetables

B. Objective
   1. Baseline data: height, weight, basal metabolic index, and blood pressure
   2. Complete physical examination: Pregnancy may be a person's only contact with medical care; hence, it is an opportunity for overall health assessment.
      a. Head, ears, eyes, nose, throat, and teeth
      b. Skin, neck, and thyroid
      c. Breasts, heart, chest, and lungs
      d. Abdomen: including uterine size or fundal height and fetal heart tones (after 10 weeks)
      e. Neurologic: deep tendon reflexes, extremities
      f. Pelvic examination (if indicated for cervical cancer screening, history, or symptoms)
         i. External genitalia
         ii. Vagina: discharge
         iii. Cervix: polyps, dilation of os, length, consistency, and position
         iv. Uterus: size, position, and symmetry
         v. Adnexa: difficult to palpate after 12 weeks
         vi. Rectum: note hemorrhoids

III. Assessment
A. *Estimated gestational age and date of delivery: Size (S)/Dates (D) relationship (S = D, S < D, or S > D)*
B. *Creation of a "problem list" that will guide future care based on issues/risk factors identified from history and physical examination or existing laboratory data—could include:*
   1. Prior cesarean delivery
   2. Rh-negative blood type
   3. Chronic hypertension
C. *Role assessment: need for consultation or collaborative management (see Chapter 30 for guidelines for medical consultation and referral during pregnancy)*

IV. Goals of clinical management
A. *Establish a date of delivery.*
B. *Identify medical, nutritional, and psychosocial problems and risk factors and a plan of care for each problem.*
C. *Provide anticipatory guidance related to pregnancy, birth, parenting, and medical care.*
D. *Individualize care to meet both the family and medical needs and maximize well-being for both the pregnant person and fetus.*

V. Plan
A. *Discuss and order diagnostic and laboratory screening (**Boxes 26-2** and **26-3**).*

Box 26-2 Laboratory Data

Initial routine screening

- Complete blood count with platelets and mean corpuscular volume (MCV): Assess for anemia, low platelets.
- Blood type with antibody screen: Identify rhesus-negative individuals and rule out Rh sensitization.
- Hepatitis B surface antigen: Identify hepatitis B virus (HBV) status and create plan for HBV-positive individuals so as to reduce vertical transmission to fetus.
- Rubella immunity: Identify rubella nonimmune individuals so as to counsel regarding avoidance of infection while pregnant and postpartum immunization.
- Syphilis serology: Identify those with active infection as candidates for treatment to reduce risk of antepartum fetal infection and congenital syphilis.
- HIV antibody with consent: Identify HIV-positive individuals so as to refer for co-management with HIV specialist.
- Urine culture with sensitivities: Identify bacteriuria, including asymptomatic bacteriuria, which should be treated in pregnancy to reduce the risk of pyelonephritis, as risk factor for preterm birth.
- Cervical cancer screening if indicated

Initial risk-based screening based on population or individual risk:

- Hepatitis C antibody: individuals with risk factors for infection or intimate contact with individuals with known risk factors
- Varicella antibody if immunity is unknown
- Purified protein derivative (PPD) tuberculosis (TB) skin test when symptoms, travel history, or country of origin identify risk for active or latent TB
- Toxoplasmosis (immunoglobulin G [IgG], immunoglobulin M [IgM]) when symptoms identify risk of infection or when individual is exposed to cats that are not exclusively indoor pets
- Early glucose load test and/or hemoglobin A1c when individual has risk factors for preexisting diabetes mellitus (see Chapter 33, Gestational Diabetes Mellitus, for more information)
- Tay-Sachs and/or cystic fibrosis carrier status; hemoglobin electrophoresis (see Chapter 28, The Return Prenatal Visit, for more information)
- Wet mount when symptoms or history identify risk for vaginal infection
- Gonorrhea and chlamydia when symptoms or history identify risk
- Thyroid function tests when symptoms or history (including family history) identify risk

---

Box 26-3 Timing of Elective Genetic Diagnostic and Screening Tests Offered to Pregnant People Before 20 Weeks (See Chapter 27 for more information.)

Tests will vary based on location and test availability.
Screening tests:

- First-trimester blood screen (10 weeks–13 weeks and 6 days)
- Nuchal translucency screening ultrasound (11 weeks and 2 days–14 weeks and 2 days weeks)
- Second-trimester or quadruple-marker blood screen (15–20 weeks)
- Noninvasive prenatal testing/cell-free DNA blood test (after 10 weeks)
- Fetal survey/screening ultrasound (18–20 weeks, routine in many practices)

Diagnostic tests:

- Chorionic villus sampling (10–14 weeks)
- Amniocentesis (15–20 weeks)

B. *Discuss and recommend therapeutic interventions and medications.*
  1. Prenatal vitamins
  2. Other vitamins or supplementation as indicated by history or nutritional assessment may include:
     a. Iron, 325 mg every other day if anemic (hemoglobin < 10, hematocrit < 32) (Stoffel et al., 2019)
     b. Calcium if dietary intake less than 1,200 mg daily (Grieger & Clifton, 2014; Hofmeyr et al., 2014)
     c. Vitamin D_3 (Harvey et al., 2014; Kiely et al., 2020; Wei et al., 2013)
     d. Fish oil: omega-3 fatty acids (Mozurkewich & Klemens, 2012)
  3. Prescriptions (assess safety in pregnancy): The provider is responsible for assessing the safety during pregnancy of any medications their patients are taking. The U.S. Food and Drug Administration (FDA) has mandated that drug information must include a pregnancy subsection with a risk summary, clinical considerations, and data on the effects of approved drugs that are prescribed to and used by pregnant people. There is also a lactation subsection that provides

information about using the drug while nursing, such as the amount of drug in breast milk and potential effects on the nursing infant (FDA, 2014).
4. Vaccines
   a. Influenza vaccine recommended for all pregnant people (seasonal)
   b. Tetanus/diphtheria/pertussis (Tdap) recommended for all pregnant people with each pregnancy, between 27 and 36 weeks' gestation (see Chapter 28, The Return Prenatal Visit, for more information)
   c. Hepatitis A and B if at risk (Bridges et al., 2013).
   d. COVID-19 vaccine(s) recommended per Centers for Disease Control and Prevention (CDC) guidelines

C. Patient education (**Figure 26-1**)

Overview	Language preference: Final EDD, by: Preferred delivery provider type (OB or CNM): FOB/partner (if involved): Primary support person: Clinic name: Continuity provider: Centering offered: ** Spanish speaking ❑ Black-identified ❑

General pregnancy info	**Routine PN labs/procedures**
	❑ Routine intake labs complete and reviewed
	❑ Genetic screening summary:
	❑ 20 wk u/s done and reviewed
	❑ Third tri labs (24–28 wks) done and reviewed
	❑ GBS (35–37 wks) done and reviewed
	
	TB Screening (choose one of the following)
	❑ No testing indicated:
	  ■ Low risk TB screen OR
	  ■ Last test was a negative QFT or PPD without new risk factor since last test OR
	  ■ Previous history of LTBI with adequate treatment and no new risk factors
	❑ Positive QFT/PPD and no history of treatment for LTBI:
	  ■ CXR done on ** and results were **
	❑ Testing indicated based on risk factor screen, and no history of prior testing
	
	Specific lab dates/results
	Last pap:
	Blood Rh and type:
	GC/CT:
	RPR: ❑ initial: ❑ third tri:
	HIV: ❑ initial: ❑ third tri:
	Urine cx:
	TB screening status/testing history:
	
	Accepts blood products? ❑ Yes ❑ No
	
	Vaccines
	❑ Flu (Sept.–Mar.):
	❑ TDap (27–36 wks):
	❑ COVID
	
	Referrals made
	❑ Dental
	❑ MSW
	❑ Nutrition
	Other psychosocial – see Social Narrative below

Figure 26-1 Sample flowsheet for "Pregnancy" on electronic medical record (EMR) problem list. (*Continued*)

Social narrative	Narrative of social situation:
	Social needs screening (q trimester)
	    Housing ❑ initial ❑ 2nd tri ❑ 3rd tri
	    Food ❑ initial ❑ 2nd tri ❑ 3rd tri
	    IPV ❑ initial ❑ 2nd tri ❑ 3rd tri
	    Work issues ❑ initial ❑ 2nd tri ❑ 3rd tri
	Depression screening PHQ 2:
	Social referrals made:
	    ❑ MSW
	In care with the following people/agencies for social needs:
	    ❑ Plan of Safe Care completed and in chart:

Baby feeding	Narrative of prior baby feeding experience:
	Patient's barriers to nursing, if any:
	Lactation mentor, if any:
	Education on the importance of the following:
	    ❑ Infant feeding
	    ❑ STS contact
	    ❑ Early initiation
	    ❑ Rooming-in
	    ❑ On-cue feeding
	    ❑ Frequent feeds to maintain supply
	    ❑ Positioning and attachment
	    ❑ Exclusive nursing x 6 months
	    ❑ Risks of human milk substitutes
	    ❑ Nursing after 6 months/introduction of other foods

Family Planning	Narrative of prior contraception use:
	Contraception values and reproductive plan:
	    ❑ Options reviewed:
	    ❑ Postpartum contraception plan:
	If considering sterilization:
	    ❑ Tubal ligation class referred/attended
	Type of sterilization desired:
	    ❑ Consents signed and scanned by 36 wks (date)

Birth preparation	Narrative of prior birth experience, if any:
	Birth values:
	    ❑ Has SisterWeb (Black, Latinx, PI; refer 16–27 wks):
	    ❑ Doula
	    ❑ Childbirth class
	    ❑ Family Birth Center tour
	    ❑ Pain management options reviewed
	    ❑ Birth preferences form completed/reviewed/scanned
	    ❑ s/s labor, danger s/s, and when to go to the hospital

Figure 26-1 (*Continued*)

1. Prenatal care expectations, including where and when to call
2. Common discomforts (see Chapter 32, Common Discomforts of Pregnancy)
3. Physiologic and emotional changes
4. Fetal growth and development
5. Options for prenatal screening and diagnosis offered, reviewed, and discussed
6. Nutrition and exercise
7. Over-the-counter medications
8. Substance use
9. Food safety (e.g., listeria, mercury, and pasteurization)
10. Teratogens
11. Workplace safety and exposure
12. Safer sex
13. Danger signs (specific to gestational age)
14. Community resources such as doula agencies and lactation support

> **Box 26-4 Medical Conditions Requiring Transfer of Care to High-Risk Clinic**
>
> (These may differ in different settings.)
> Medical Conditions
>
> - Chronic hypertension diagnosed before pregnancy
> - Active or uncontrolled seizure disorder
> - Severe asthma (hospitalization or requiring systemic steroids during pregnancy)
> - Cardiac disease (except asymptomatic mitral valve prolapse)
> - Pulmonary hypertension
> - Platelet count less than 100,000
> - Deep vein thrombosis
> - Sickle cell disease
> - Lupus, scleroderma, or any connective tissue disease
> - Cancer
> - Active tuberculosis
> - Active viral hepatitis
> - HIV positive
> - Hyperthyroidism
> - Diabetes: type 1 and type 2
> - Multiple gestation
> - Bariatric surgery

> **Box 26-5 Visit Schedule Guidelines**
>
> Frequency of prenatal visits
>
> - 1–28 weeks—every 4 weeks
> - 28–36 weeks—every 2–3 weeks
> - 36+ weeks—every week
>
> Reduced visit schedule
> One visit during each gestational age or age range (approximately eight visits)
>
> - 6–8 weeks
> - 14–16 weeks
> - 24–28 weeks
> - 32 weeks
> - 36 weeks
> - Weekly from 38 weeks

D. *Consultation and referrals (could include)*
1. Genetic counseling for advanced parturient age; family history of genetic disorder/difference, developmental delays, and cardiovascular defects; as indicated by ethnic background, multiple miscarriages, consanguinity, and exposure to potential teratogens (**Box 26-4**)
2. Ancillary services: social worker, nutritionist, health educator, prenatal classes, psychiatry as needed or desired
3. Community resources (e.g., Women, Infants, and Children nutritional program, public health nurse, smoking cessation, community-based organizations, support groups)
4. Medical consultation and referral

E. *Follow-up*
1. Patient should return per the return visit schedule guidelines. This should be flexible and individualized and depends on parity and risk (**Box 26-5**).
2. Patient should be cared for by an obstetrician if they are assessed to be at high risk per guidelines or for consultation around a specific problem (see Chapter 30, Guidelines for Medical Consultation, Interprofessional Collaboration, and Transfer of Care During Pregnancy and Childbirth).

VI. Internet resources

A. *American College of Nurse-Midwives Consumer Education website*
This site provides information regarding pregnancy, labor and birth, parenting, and reproductive health, including easy-to-use patient education handouts (some in Spanish) from the "Share with Women Series" (http://www.mymidwife.org/).

B. *March of Dimes*
This site provides information for providers and patients in both written and audio/video formats in English and Spanish on pregnancy, birth, and newborn development and care (http://www.marchofdimes.com/).

C. *National Women's Health Information Center*
This is a U.S. Department of Health and Human Services website that provides information on sexual, reproductive, and gender health. There are numerous up-to-date fact sheets on all aspects of reproductive health, including pregnancy, in both Spanish and English (http://www.womenshealth.gov).

D. *Childbirth Connection*
This organization promotes evidenced-based prenatal care and helps pregnant people and providers to make informed decisions. There are numerous patient education, pregnancy, and childbirth resources (http://www.childbirthconnection.org/).

E. *American College of Obstetricians and Gynecologists*
This site offers a limited number of patient education handouts available by provider request (http://www.acog.org/).

F. *SisterSong*
SisterSong's mission is "to strengthen and amplify the collective voices of indigenous women and women of color to achieve reproductive justice by eradicating reproductive oppression and securing human rights" (https://www.sistersong.net/).

G. *Black Mamas Matter Alliance*
The Black Mamas Matter Alliance is a Black women–led cross-sectoral alliance. The alliance centers Black mamas to advocate, drive research, build power, and shift culture for Black maternal health, rights, and justice (https://blackmamasmatter.org).

References

Altman, M. R., McLemore, M. R., Oseguera, T., Lyndon, A., & Franck, L. S. (2020). Listening to women: Recommendations from women of color to improve experiences in pregnancy and birth care. *Journal of Midwifery & Women's Health*, 65(4), 466–473. doi:10.1111/jmwh.13102

American College of Obstetricians and Gynecologists. (2015). ACOG Committee Opinion No. 649: Racial and ethnic disparities in obstetrics and gynecology. *Obstetrics & Gynecology*, 126(6), e130–e134. doi:10.1097/AOG.0000000000001213.

Aronson, J., Burgess, D., Phelan, S. M., & Juarez, L. (2013). Unhealthy interactions: The role of stereotype threat in health disparities. *American Journal of Public Health*, 103(1), 50–56. doi:10.2105/AJPH.2012.300828

Bridges, C. B., Woods, L., & Coyne Beasley, T. (2013). Advisory Committee on Immunization Practices (ACIP) recommended immunization schedule for adults aged 19 years and older—United States, 2013. *MMWR. Surveillance Summaries*, 62(Suppl. 1), 9–19.

Green, T. L., Zapata, J. Y., Brown, H. W., & Hagiwara, N. (2021). Rethinking bias to achieve maternal health equity: Changing organizations, not just individuals. *Obstetrics & Gynecology*, 137(5), 935–940. doi:10.1097/AOG.000000000000436

Grieger, J. A., & Clifton, V. L. (2014). A review of the impact of dietary intakes in human pregnancy on infant birthweight. *Nutrients*, 7(1), 153–178. doi:10.3390/nu7010153

Harvey, N. C., Holroyd, C., Ntani, G, Javid, K., Cooper, P., Moon, R., Cole, Z., Tinati, T., Godfrey, K., Dennison, E., Bishop, N. J., Baird, J., & Cooper, C. (2014). Vitamin D supplementation in pregnancy: A systematic review. *Health Technology Assessment*, 18(45), 1–190. doi:10.3310/hta18450

Hofmeyr, G. J., Lawrie, T. A., Atallah, A. N., & Dully, L. (2014). Calcium supplementation during pregnancy for preventing hypertensive disorders and related problems. *Cochrane Database of Systematic Reviews*, 2014(6), CD001059.

Howell, E. A., Brown, H., Brumley, J., Bryant, A. S., Caughey, A. B., Cornell, A. M., Grant, J. H., Gregory, K. D., Gullo, S. M., Kozhimannil, K. B., Mhyre, J. M., Toledo, P., D'Oria, R., Ngoh, M., & Grobman, W. A. (2018). Reduction of peripartum racial and ethnic disparities: A conceptual framework and maternal safety consensus bundle. *Journal of Obstetric, Gynecologic, & Neonatal Nursing*, 47(3), 275–289.

Hunter, L. A. (2009). Issues in pregnancy dating: Revisiting the evidence. *Journal of Midwifery & Women's Health*, 54(3), 184–190. doi:10.1016/j.jmwh.2008.11.003

Kiely, M. E., Wagner, C. L., Roth, D. E. (2020). Vitamin D in pregnancy: Where we are and where we should go. *Journal of Steroid Biochemistry and Molecular Biology*, 201, 105669. doi:10.1016/j.jsbmb.2020.105669

Mozurkewich, E. L., & Klemens, C. (2012). Omega-3 fatty acids and pregnancy: Current implications for practice. *Current Opinion in Obstetrics & Gynecology*, 24(2), 72–77. doi:10.1097/GCO.0b013e328350fd34

Sandall, J., Soltani, H., Gates, S., Shennan, A., & Devane, D. (2016). Midwife-led continuity models versus other models of care for childbearing women. Cochrane Database of Systematic Reviews. doi:10.1002/14651858.cd004667.pub

Stoffel, N. U., Zeder, C., Brittenham, G. M., Moretti, D., & Zimmermann, M. B. (2019). Iron absorption from supplements is greater with alternate day than with consecutive day dosing in iron-deficient anemic women. *Haematologica*, 105(5), 1232–1239. doi:10.3324/haematol.2019.220830

Swanson, M. L., Whetstone, S., Illangasekare, T., & Autry, A. M. (2021). Obstetrics and gynecology and reparations: The debt we owe (and continue to accumulate). *Health Equity*, 5(1), 353–355. doi:10.1089/heq.2021.0015

U.S. Food and Drug Administration. (2014, December 3). *Pregnancy and lactation labeling (drugs) final rule*. https://www.fda.gov/drugs/labeling-information-drug-products/pregnancy-and-lactation-labeling-drugs-final-rule

Wei, S. Q., Qi, H. P., Luo, Z. C., & Fraser, W. D. (2013). Maternal vitamin D status and adverse pregnancy outcomes: A systematic review and meta-analysis. *Journal of Maternal, Fetal, and Neonatal Medicine*, 26(9), 889–899. doi:10.3109/14767058.2013.765849

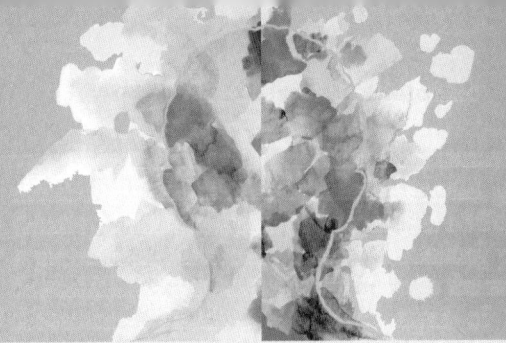

CHAPTER 27

Prenatal Genetic Screening and Diagnosis

Kelly Wong McGrath and Deborah Anderson

I. Introduction and general background

Recent scientific advances in human genetics, combined with new prenatal screening and diagnostic technologies, have resulted in a proliferation of genetic testing options and a concomitant change in the landscape of prenatal genetic testing. All pregnant people now have the option of numerous genetic screening and diagnostic tests.

Screening for aneuploidy should be offered to all pregnant people and may be offered as cell-free DNA screening or first- and second-trimester serum screening with or without nuchal translucency (NT) ultrasound, although serum screening has been phased out by many state programs, due to the improved sensitivity and specificity of cell-free DNA testing. Although cell-free DNA technology was initially reserved for pregnant people greater than 35 years of age, the American College of Obstetricians and Gynecologists (ACOG) now recommends making this test available to all pregnant people regardless of age (ACOG Committee on Practice Bulletins, 2020). Where available, either cell-free DNA screening or serum screening with or without NT measurement may be offered, but both should not be offered simultaneously because this is not cost-effective and can yield conflicting results that are difficult to interpret. Additionally, diagnostic testing may be offered as an option to all pregnant people, regardless of risk factors, after discussing risks and benefits. Carrier screening, traditionally based on an individual's risk based on ethnic and personal background, can and should be made available to all pregnant people and people considering pregnancy based on test availability and personal preference (ACOG Committee on Genetics, 2017a). If patients test positive for these screening tests or have genetic risk factors such as a family history of inherited disorders, advanced age of the birthing parent, a history of offspring with a congenital disorder, or an ethnicity-based risk for autosomal-recessive disorders, they may be referred for genetic counseling and possible genetic diagnostic testing.

As more and more screening and diagnostic tools become available, genetic counselors with requisite knowledge about the multitude of optional genetic tests are key to providing patients with information about all screening and diagnostic options. Included in counseling are the benefits, limitations, and risks of prenatal genetic testing; individualized genetic information; available options; and assistance with interpretation and understanding of test results.

A. *Prenatal genetic screening for trisomies 21, 18, 13; neural tube defects (NTDs); abdominal wall defects; and Smith–Lemli–Opitz syndrome (SLOS)*

Several optional first- and second-trimester screening strategies are available to assess risk for trisomy 21 (Down syndrome), trisomy 18 (Edward syndrome), open NTDs, abdominal wall defects, and SLOS. The tests use serum biochemical markers and fetal ultrasound to refine and improve risk assessment beyond standard population-based risk assessments. Combining these first- and second-trimester serum screening strategies to assess risk, rather than using them as single-method testing, improves accuracy and detection rates for Down syndrome and trisomy 18 (California Department of Public Health, 2021). **Table 27-1** provides the detection rates and timing of these genetic screening strategies.

1. Noninvasive prenatal testing (NIPT) or cell-free fetal DNA testing

Noninvasive prenatal testing screens for trisomy 21 (Down syndrome), trisomy 18 (Edward syndrome), trisomy 13 (Patau syndrome), and some sex chromosome abnormalities. NIPT can also determine fetal sex. The test analyzes the pregnant person's

Table 27-1 Selected Prenatal Screening Strategies, Detection Rates, and Timing of Screening

Timing of Screening (Laboratory Dependent)	Screening Strategy	Detection Rate	Clinical Application
>9 weeks	**Noninvasive prenatal testing or cell-free fetal DNA testing** (gestational parent serum)	Trisomy 21: 99% Trisomy 18: 99% Trisomy 13: 92%	May be used at any point in pregnancy after 9–10 weeks (depending on the lab)
Serum screening and nuchal translucency (NT) ultrasound for the purpose of genetic screening have been phased out of many state programs, including California as of September 2022. The information that follows is provided for programs that still offer this type of testing.			
First-trimester serum: 10–13 weeks, 6 days	**First-trimester serum**		There are no risk assessments for the first trimester as a stand-alone test. (May vary with screening program.) The test combines with the NT and/or the quad marker.
First-trimester serum: 10–13 weeks, 6 days NT: 11 weeks, 2 days–14 weeks, 2 days	**Combined first-trimester screen** (combines gestational parent serum testing results and NT results)	Trisomy 21: 85% Trisomy 18: 60%	Test performed in two steps. If results are positive, first-trimester screening allows for the option of early diagnostic testing and decision making regarding the course of the pregnancy.
15–20 weeks (optimal time 16–18 weeks)	**Quadruple- or quad-marker screen** (gestational parent serum)	Trisomy 21: 80% Trisomy 18: 67% Anencephaly: 97% Open spina bifida: 80% Abdominal wall defects: 85% Smith–Lemli–Opitz: 60%	Can be used alone or combined with first-trimester serum or combined first-trimester screen. Detection rates for trisomy 21 and 18 are improved when combined. May be used in pregnant people with late entry to prenatal care.
First-trimester serum: 10–13 weeks, 6 days Second-trimester serum: 15–20 weeks	**Serum-integrated screen** (combines first-trimester gestational parent serum with quad marker)	Trisomy 21: 85% Trisomy 18: 79% Anencephaly: 97% Open spina bifida: 80% Abdominal wall defects: 85% Smith–Lemli–Opitz: 60%	Test is performed in two steps. Results are only provided after the second-trimester serum analysis is complete.
First-trimester serum: 10–13 weeks, 6 days NT: 11 weeks 2 days–14 weeks, 2 days Second-trimester serum: 15–20 weeks	**Sequential integrated screen** (combines first-trimester serum and NT with quad-marker test results)	Trisomy 21: 90% Trisomy 18: 81% Anencephaly: 97% Open spina bifida: 80% Abdominal wall defects: 85% Smith–Lemli–Opitz: 60%	Patients will receive results in the first trimester and then a modified result in the second trimester.

Data from California Department of Public Health. (2021). *California prenatal screening program.* http://www.cdph.ca.gov/pns

serum for cell-free DNA fragments from the placenta circulating in the gestational parent plasma and has been shown to be highly sensitive and specific, with a >99% detection rate for Down syndrome, a 98% detection rate for trisomy 18, a 99% detection rate for trisomy 13, and a combined false-positive rate of 0.13% (Gil et al., 2017). The ACOG Committee on Practice Bulletins (2020) currently recommends offering NIPT to all pregnant people regardless of the age of the ovum or risk for chromosomal abnormality.

NIPT can result in a "no-call" or failure to report in 1%–3% of cases. In the case of early gestational age (<10 weeks), this may be due to a low fetal fraction of cell-free DNA, and the NIPT may be repeated. Some research has linked no-call results to chromosomal anomalies, preeclampsia, and gestational diabetes (Chan et al., 2017). Based on these data, it is reasonable to treat a no-call result itself as a risk factor, and patients with these results may be referred to genetic counseling for follow-up. There is also a risk of a no-call result with increasing gestational parent body weight (Juul et al., 2020); however, there are currently no clinical guidelines in relation to body mass index, only a need for clinician awareness that the risk of a no-call result is higher in this population and does not necessarily translate into increased risk of genetic disorders. Regardless, any no-call result should result in a referral to a genetic counselor. NIPT is not recommended in patients with a history of organ transplantation. In multi-fetal pregnancies where there has been fetal demise, NIPT should not be used for screening the surviving fetus(es) because cell-free DNA from the nonsurviving fetus may be detected.

Second-trimester serum screening may be offered to those choosing NIPT to report on analyte levels of alpha-fetoprotein (AFP), which can be a marker for open NTDs (e.g., spina bifida). Patients opting for second-trimester serum screening coupled with NIPT will not have risk assessments for trisomies reported but rather analyte levels and their relationship to average values.

2. Combined first-trimester screening: first-trimester gestational parent serum and fetal NT
   Combined first-trimester screening is performed in two steps and determines risk for trisomies 21 and 18. Gestational parent serum testing for pregnancy-associated plasma protein A (PAPP-A) and human chorionic gonadotropin (hCG) is obtained; the serum analyte values are combined with ultrasound examination of fetal NT to determine risk.

   NT refers to a measurement of a clearly demarcated fluid-filled space behind the fetal neck that is present in all fetuses. Skill in obtaining NT measurement requires training for a standardized method of measurement; therefore, this screening tool may not be available in all communities. NT measurement alone has a detection rate for trisomy 21 of 64%–70%, with a 5% false-positive rate (California Department of Public Health, 2021). Detection rates improve and can modify risk assessment when combined with first-trimester serum testing and the quadruple-marker serum screen.

   An increased NT measurement (> 3 mm) is associated with fetal chromosomal abnormalities and cardiac defects. However, the clinical significance of an increased NT measurement is correlated with the degree of increase. For instance, in one population-based study, NT measurements of 3.5–4.4 mm were associated with unaffected children in 70% of cases, whereas NT measurements of 5.5–6.4 mm were associated with unaffected children in only 30% of cases (Ghi et al., 2001). An NT measurement of 3.5 mm or greater is associated with fetal structural anomalies, such as congenital hydrocephalus; agenesis, hypoplasia, and dysplasia of the lung; atresia and stenosis of the small intestine; osteodystrophies; genetic disorders such as Noonan syndrome; and diaphragm anomalies (Baer et al., 2014). Pregnant people found to have an NT result greater than or equal to 3 mm can initially be offered either diagnostic testing and/or NIPT because the residual risk of significant chromosomal abnormality is 2.5% in those who have a normal NIPT result (Norton et al., 2017), followed by genetic counseling and diagnosis, targeted ultrasound, and fetal echocardiogram as determined to be necessary. Alternatively, people with NT results greater than 3 mm may choose to move straight to diagnostic testing, per their preference.

3. Quadruple-marker (quad-marker) serum examination
   The quad marker estimates the risk for trisomies 21 and 18, open NTD, abdominal wall defect, and SLOS. Four biochemical markers are assessed: AFP, hCG, unconjugated estriol (uE3), and dimeric inhibin-A (DIA). It can be used alone, combined with first-trimester serum, or combined with first-trimester screen to improve detection rates.

   Quad-marker serum testing has a detection rate for trisomy 21 of 80%, with a 5% false-positive rate (ACOG Committee on Practice Bulletins, 2020). Patients who have previously received NIPT testing or are otherwise avoiding genetic screening may want to consider quad-marker screening because a number of studies report that abnormal biomarker levels may be associated with poor pregnancy outcomes, including intrauterine growth restriction, preeclampsia, and preterm birth (Huang et al., 2010; Sayin et al., 2008; Xia et al., 2006). Although there are no consensus guidelines available regarding abnormal biomarker levels, some local hospitals and state screening programs report the multiple of the median (MoM) for each analyte and standardized cutoffs based on local population data.

4. Serum-integrated screening: first- and second-trimester serum testing
   Serum-integrated screening combines first-trimester blood test results with quad-marker blood test results. This test may be useful when NT measurements cannot be obtained because of timing or patient wishes or where NT programs are not available.

5. Sequential integrated screening: first- and second-trimester serum testing and NT ultrasound
   Sequential integrated screening combines three tests: first- and second-trimester serum screening and NT. It provides higher detection rates for aneuploidy when compared to combined first-trimester screen or serum-integrated screening.

B. *Carrier screening for recessive conditions*
Carrier screening for recessive conditions should be made available to all pregnant people and people

considering pregnancy. With respect to hemoglobinopathies, a complete blood count with red blood cell indices should be performed for all pregnant people and people considering pregnancy. If red blood cell indices result in a low mean corpuscular hemoglobin or mean corpuscular volume (MCV), hemoglobin electrophoresis should be performed. Hemoglobin electrophoresis should also be performed, regardless of red blood cell indices, if there is a risk for hemoglobinopathies based on ethnicity (African, Mediterranean, Middle Eastern, Southeast Asian, or West Indian descent) (ACOG Committee on Genetics, 2017a). The ACOG currently recommends offering all pregnant people and people considering becoming pregnant carrier screening for spinal muscular atrophy and cystic fibrosis (ACOG Committee on Genetics, 2017b).

Parents with personal or family histories of inherited disorders, such as Tay-Sachs disease, Canavan disease, familial dysautonomia, fragile X syndrome (or a history of intellectual disability), sickle cell anemia, α-thalassemia, and β-thalassemia, should be offered carrier testing along with genetic counseling. In the absence of family history, multiple approaches to carrier screening may be offered to pregnant people, including ethnic-based carrier screening and panethnic screening/expanded carrier screening. In the past, pregnant people and people considering pregnancy have been counseled on specific carrier screening based on ethnic background. However, in our current multiethnic society, predetermined risk for genetic conditions based on ethnicity has lost some predictive value related to the commixture of genetic backgrounds. Therefore, it is also an acceptable approach to offer a set panel of carrier screening tests to all people regardless of ethnic background, also known as *panethnic screening*. A third available option is expanded carrier screening, which can test from a few conditions to several hundred conditions. The ACOG recommends any of these strategies and further recommends that after appropriate counseling, specific carrier testing strategies should be made available based on personal preference (ACOG Committee on Genetics, 2017a).

If a pregnant patient (or patient considering pregnancy) used their own eggs to get pregnant, they should be offered carrier testing. If they are found to be a carrier for a given condition, carrier testing of the other genetic parent/contributor should be considered. In scenarios where both genetic parents are determined to be a carrier for the same condition, the patient should be referred to genetic counseling for further evaluation (ACOG Committee on Genetics, 2017b).

C. *Informed choice and shared decision making*

The choices that are available to families with respect to genetic and carrier screening are many, and it can be hard for families to thoroughly understand the options available to them. It is important for the care provider to fully understand these options, their risks and benefits, and alternatives before discussing options with families. Additionally, it is critical that the care provider present options to families without bias or judgment.

In order to help families begin to understand their testing preferences, it is useful to ask questions about what they would do with the information gained from genetic testing (**Figure 27-1**). Begin by helping families understand the difference between screening tests, which are noninvasive tests that identify an elevated risk of a condition, and diagnostic tests, which are invasive tests that carry additional risk (see following discussion) and confirm the presence or absence of a given condition.

Although the federal Genetic Information Nondiscrimination Act (GINA) bars health insurers from using genetic testing information to make determinations regarding eligibility or coverage, this does not extend to life, disability, or long-term care insurance. Individuals should be informed that genetic testing information from adult genetic parents can affect premium prices and eligibility for these products (ACOG Committee on Genetics, 2017c).

II. **Database**

A. *Subjective*
  1. All pregnant people, regardless of age, should have the option for genetic screening or diagnostic testing (ACOG Committee on Genetics, 2017a; ACOG Committee on Practice Bulletins, 2020). Age of ovum alone is no longer used as a determining factor for who is offered prenatal screening or diagnostic testing but may influence insurance reimbursement for certain tests.
  2. Last menstrual period: If unsure or unreliable, order an ultrasound to determine gestational age. Screening tests for aneuploidy and NTDs are sensitive to gestational age.
  3. Ethnicity
  4. Genetic, obstetric, and family history: Identify any genetic risk factors, such as chromosome abnormalities, inherited genetic disorders, unexplained intellectual disability, primary ovarian insufficiency of unknown etiology, autism, or congenital malformation.
  5. Determine whether the patient desires prenatal testing. Factors to consider with pregnant people when choosing to accept or decline testing include the following:
      a. Gestational age at entry into prenatal care
      b. Ethnicity-based risk factors
      c. Personal, family, genetic, and obstetric history
      d. Number of fetuses
      e. NT availability
      f. Test sensitivity and limitations
      g. Desire for testing
      h. Risks of diagnostic procedures
      i. Options for early termination
      j. Insurance coverage
      k. Patient's desire to know this information in pregnancy

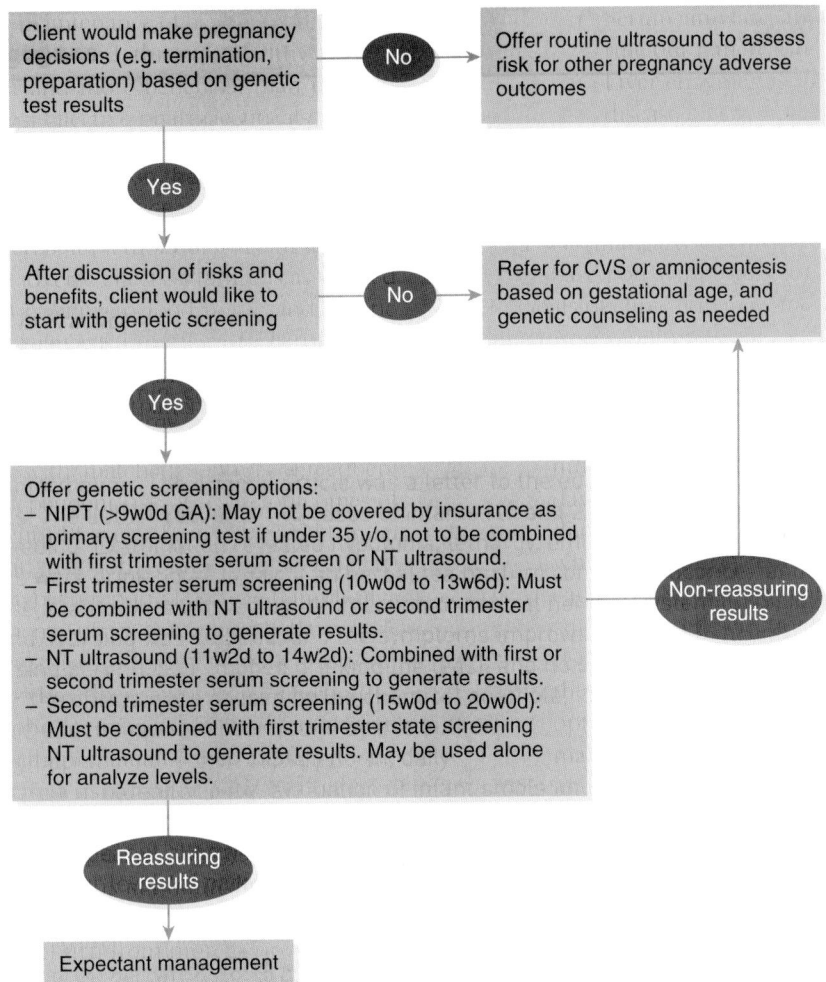

Figure 27-1 Types of genetic testing.

B. Objective
1. Establish expected date of delivery (EDD). Because first- and second-trimester testing is sensitive to gestational age, ultrasound dating of pregnancy reduces rates of false-positive and false-negative results caused by incorrect dating. If the expected date of delivery is changed (**Table 28-4** regarding redating pregnancy) after submission of screening tests, the laboratory must be informed of the new EDD for reinterpretation of test results.
2. Routine laboratory: complete blood count (CBC) with red blood cell indices. Hemoglobin electrophoresis is indicated if risk is identified based on ethnic background or if low mean corpuscular hemoglobin or MCV is identified. Ethnic-based, panethnic/expanded carrier screening should be made available based on patient preference.
3. Genetic screening for fetal chromosomal anomalies: After appropriate counseling, patients should select the options, as discussed earlier, for screening as they desire.
4. Routine ultrasound to assess fetal anatomy at approximately 19–21 weeks' gestation.
5. Weight

III. Assessment
Patient desires/declines prenatal genetic screening tests (specify test) and/or carrier testing.

IV. Goals for clinical management
A. Identify fetuses with specific genetic disorders and/or NTDs prior to birth in requesting families.
B. Establish inherited and/or historical risk for genetic disorders in requesting families.
C. Establish patient desires for genetic screening and diagnostic testing using principles of informed consent and shared decision making.
D. Allow for identification of increased risk for NTDs and genetic disorders and give families the option of diagnostic screening.

V. Plan
A. Counseling regarding tests and results.
  1. All patients are offered screening (NIPT, first- and second-trimester serologic screening, NT ultrasound examination, as available in the area) and/or diagnostic testing and carrier-status testing based on preference and availability.

2. If personal, family, or obstetric history are positive for genetic risk factors such as aneuploidy, inherited genetic disorder, offspring with birth defects, or consanguinity, offer referral to a genetic counselor or a perinatal specialist for counseling and possible prenatal diagnosis.
3. Provide information regarding screening tests in a nondirective, sensitive, and nonjudgmental manner. Include information about the difference between risk assessment and diagnosis, the limitations of the screening tests, the rates and meaning of false positives and negatives, and the difference between carrier traits and diseases. Offer unbiased support for their decisions (Sheets et al., 2011).
4. Document acceptance or refusal of genetic screening tests. Some state-run programs require a standardized signed accept/decline form for first-trimester serum screen, NT, or quad marker.
5. When reviewing results from combined first-trimester, quad-marker, or sequential integrated screen with pregnant people, it is preferred to communicate the numerical risk assessment of the final analysis rather than a "positive" or "negative" result. The numerical risk of a genetic condition can be communicated in both ratios and percentages and may include the chances of having or not having the genetic condition. For example, "There is a 1:50 chance of Down syndrome, which means there is a 49:50 chance that there is not Down syndrome. That equates to a 2% chance of Down syndrome or a 98% chance there is not Down syndrome." It may also be useful to compare their screening risk to their age-related risk.

B. *Laboratory*
1. See **Table 27-1** for the timing of genetic screening tests. The timing of the first-trimester serum screen, NT, and quad-marker testing is limited by gestational age.
2. Fill out the appropriate laboratory forms, including the best dating parameter, current weight, number of fetuses, race, diabetes, and tobacco use. Additional data are used to adjust interpretation of test results.

C. *Consultation and referral*
If the screening test is positive, or if the risk is higher than the procedure-related risk of loss from diagnostic testing, refer to a genetic counselor for further counseling regarding interpretation of results, recommendations for follow-up examinations, possible confirmatory diagnostic testing, and supportive counseling. Patients may also be referred to a genetic counselor if they are not comfortable with their risk estimate and would like more information.

VI. Prenatal genetic diagnosis: Introduction and general background
Invasive prenatal diagnosis allows for the identification of multiple genetic disorders and provides parents with the information necessary to help make well-informed reproductive decisions. Although all pregnant people have the option of prenatal diagnosis, it is most often performed in pregnant people who have known risk factors for heritable genetic diseases or in pregnant people whose prenatal screening tests return positive; age of the ovum is also a known risk factor. Chorionic villus sampling (CVS) and amniocentesis permit a multitude of genetic diagnoses to be made in early pregnancy; preimplantation genetic diagnosis provides genetic diagnosis in an embryo obtained through in vitro fertilization prior to implantation.

A patient's decision to choose prenatal genetic diagnosis includes consideration of the anticipated risk that the fetus will have an abnormality, gestational age of the fetus, previous obstetric history, risk of pregnancy loss from an invasive procedure, feelings about having a child with a chromosomal abnormality, desire for a definitive diagnosis, and beliefs about termination.

A. *Chorionic villus sampling*
Under ultrasound guidance, a small sample of the placenta is obtained through a transcervical or transabdominal route.
1. Timing of test: 10–14 weeks' gestation
2. Benefits
   a. CVS can be done to test for aneuploidy (with karyotype), microdeletions/microduplications (with microarray), and single-gene conditions (if indicated).
   b. Because CVS is generally performed in the first trimester, it allows for early diagnosis and decision making about reproductive choices.
   c. Results are usually available 1–2 weeks after the procedure.
3. Risks
   a. Risk rates approach or may be the same those of as amniocentesis (see amniocentesis discussion).
   b. Amniotic fluid leak or infection, vaginal bleeding, or cell culture failure
   c. Mosaicism that may or may not be confined to the placenta. When mosaicism is detected on CVS, amniocentesis is recommended. There is an approximate 1% change of mosaicism.

B. *Amniocentesis*
Under ultrasound guidance, a small amount of amniotic fluid is aspirated via a transabdominal puncture of the uterus and amnion.
1. Timing of test: 15–20 weeks' gestation
2. Benefits
   a. Amniocentesis can be done to test for aneuploidy (with karyotype), NTDs (with amniotic fluid AFP), microdeletions/microduplications (with microarray), and single-gene conditions (if indicated).
   b. Results are usually available 1–2 weeks after the procedure.
   c. Cytogenetic diagnostic accuracy is greater than 99%.

3. Risks
   a. Procedure-related loss is 0.1%–0.3% in experienced providers (ACOG Committee on Practice Bulletins, 2016).
   b. Amniotic fluid leakage or rupture, transient vaginal spotting, chorioamnionitis, rare needle injury to fetus, and failure of amniotic fluid cell culture
C. *Preimplantation genetic diagnosis*
   Preimplantation genetic diagnosis is performed on cells removed from preimplantation embryos conceived through in vitro fertilization. Single-gene or chromosomal abnormalities can be identified in the embryo, allowing for transfer of only unaffected embryos back to the uterus.
   1. Benefits
      a. Tests for aneuploidy, single-gene disorders, and chromosomal abnormalities, such as deletions and translocations (ACOG Committee on Practice Bulletins, 2016)
      b. Allows for very early reproductive decision making, prior to the establishment of pregnancy
   2. Risks
      a. Requires in vitro fertilization, with its associated risks and expense
      b. False-positive and false-negative test results leading to misdiagnosis. NIPT screening, CVS, or amniocentesis is recommended for pregnancies conceived after prenatal diagnosis.
      c. May decrease the chance of pregnancy, depending on type of testing

VII. Database
A. *Subjective*
   1. Identify genetic indications for prenatal diagnosis.
      a. Chromosomal abnormality in previous offspring, previous fetus, parent, or close relative
      b. Structural anomalies identified by ultrasound examination
      c. Parental carrier of chromosome translocation or chromosome inversion
      d. Parental aneuploidy or mosaicism for aneuploidy
      e. Abnormal prenatal screening test results
      f. Parental carrier of mendelian conditions, such as cystic fibrosis, hemophilia, muscular dystrophy, Tay-Sachs disease, inborn errors of metabolism, or hemoglobinopathies
      g. All pregnant people, regardless of age, should have the option for genetic diagnostic testing if, after reviewing risks and benefits, they elect to do so.
B. *Objective*
   1. Gestational age
   2. Results of prenatal screening tests for aneuploidy, ultrasound evaluations, and carrier screening status of both biological parents
   3. Rh status, hemoglobin electrophoresis, MCV

VIII. Assessment
Patient desires/declines CVS, amniocentesis, or preimplantation genetic diagnosis

IX. Goals for clinical management
A. *Establish patient desires for genetic testing using principles of informed consent and shared decision making.*
B. *Identify fetuses with specific genetic defects and NTDs previous to birth in requesting families.*
C. *Give families information in order to prepare for an affected child or allow for pregnancy termination.*

X. Plan
A. *Diagnosis*
   1. Refer patient for preimplantation genetic diagnosis, CVS, or amniocentesis during appropriate testing window.
B. *Education and counseling*
   1. Review the risks and benefits of procedures; include comparisons to screening tests.
   2. Provide genetic counseling prior to testing; patients should return to their genetic counselors for reporting and interpretation of test results.
   3. A positive diagnosis result is delivered to the patient by a knowledgeable healthcare provider. Provide accurate and balanced information as soon as possible, in the patient's preferred language and in a private setting. Use neutral language in a sensitive and caring manner while avoiding value judgments (Sheets et al., 2011); offer in-person follow-up.
   4. Consider referral to social workers, parent support networks, clergy, and therapeutic counselors for further support and information.
C. *Medication*
   1. Rh-negative nonsensitized pregnant people need Rh (D) immune globulin (Rhogam) administration after CVS or amniocentesis.

References

ACOG Committee on Genetics. (2017a). ACOG Practice Bulletin. Committee Opinion No. 690: Carrier screening in the age of genomic medicine. *Obstetrics and Gynecology*, 129(3), 595–596. doi:10.1097/AOG.0000000000001947

ACOG Committee on Genetics. (2017b). ACOG Committee Opinion No. 691: Carrier screening for genetic conditions. *Obstetrics and Gynecology*, 129(3):e41–e55. doi:10.1097/AOG.0000000000001952

ACOG Committee on Genetics. (2017c). ACOG Committee Opinion No. 693: Counseling about genetic testing and communication of genetic test. *Obstetrics & Gynecology, 129*(4):e96–e101. doi:10.1097/AOG.0000000000004084

ACOG Committee on Practice Bulletins. (2016). ACOG Practice No. 162: Prenatal diagnostic testing for genetic disorders. *Obstetrics and Gynecology, 127*(5), e108–e122. doi:10.1097/AOG.0000000000004084

ACOG Committee on Practice Bulletins. (2020). ACOG Practice Bulletin No. 226: Screening for fetal chromosomal abnormalities. *Obstetrics and Gynecology, 136*(4), e48–e69. doi:10.1097/AOG.0000000000004084

Baer, R. J., Norton, M., Shaw. G., Flessel, M. C., Goldman, S., Currier, R. J., & Jelliffe-Pawlowski, L. L. (2014). Risk of selected structural abnormalities in infants after increased nuchal translucency measurement. *American Journal of Obstetrics and Gynecology, 211*(6), 675–719. doi:10.1016/j.ajog.2014.06.025

California Department of Public Health. (2021). *California prenatal screening program*. Retrieved http://www.cdph.ca.gov/pns.

Chan, N., Smet, M.-E., Sandow, R., da Silva Costa, F., & McLennan, A. (2017). Implications of failure to achieve a result from prenatal maternal serum cell-free DNA testing: A historical cohort study. *BJOG: An International Journal of Obstetrics & Gynaecology, 125*(7), 848–855. doi:10.1111/1471-0528.15006

Ghi, T., Huggon, I. C., Zosmer, N., & Nicolaides, K. H. (2001). Incidence of major structural cardiac defects associated with increased nuchal translucency but normal karyotype. *Ultrasound in Obstetrics & Gynecology, 18*(6), 610–614. doi:10.1046/j.0960-7692.2001.00584.x

Gil, M. M., Accurti, V., Santacruz, B., Plana, M. N., & Nicolaides, K. H. (2017). Analysis of cell-free DNA in maternal blood in screening for aneuploidies: Updated meta-analysis. *Ultrasound in Obstetrics & Gynecology, 50*(3), 302–314. doi:10.1002/uog.17484

Huang, T., Hoffman, B., Meschino, W., Kingdom, J., Okun, N. (2010). Prediction of adverse pregnancy outcomes by combinations of first and second trimester biochemistry markers used in the routine prenatal screening of Down syndrome. *Prenatal Diagnosis, 30*(5), 471–477. doi:10.1002/pd.2505

Juul, L. A., Hartwig, T. S., Ambye, L., Sørensen, S., & Jørgensen, F. S. (2020). Noninvasive prenatal testing and maternal obesity: A review. *Acta Obstetricia et Gynecologica Scandinavica, 99*(6), 744–750. doi:10.1111/aogs.13848

Norton, M. E., Biggio, J. R., Kuller, J. A., & Blackwell, S. C. (2017). The role of ultrasound in women who undergo cell-free DNA screening. *American Journal of Obstetrics and Gynecology, 216*(3), B2–B7. doi:10.1016/j.ajog.2017.01.005

Sayin, N. C., Canda, M. T., Ahmet, N., Arda, S., Sut, N., & Varol, F. G. (2008). The association of triple-marker test results with adverse pregnancy outcomes in low-risk pregnancies with healthy newborns. *Archives of Gynecology and Obstetrics, 277*(1), 47–53. doi:10.1007/s00404-007-0421-6

Sheets, K., Crissman, B., Feist, C., Sell, S. L., Johnson, L. R., Donahue, K. C., Masser-Frye, D., Brookshire, G. S., Carre, A. M., Lagrave, D., & Brasington, C. K. (2011). Practice guidelines for communicating a prenatal or postnatal diagnosis of Down syndrome: Recommendations of the National Society of Genetic Counselors. *Journal of Genetic Counseling, 20*(5), 432–441. doi:10.1007/s10897-011-9375-8

Xia, Y. P., Zhu, M. W., Li, X. T., Zhou, H. P., Wang, J., Lv, J. X., & Zhong, N. (2006). Chromosomal abnormalities and adverse pregnancy outcome with maternal serum second trimester triple screening test for fetal Down syndrome in 4,860 Chinese women. *Journal of Peking University Health Sciences, 38*(1), 49–52.

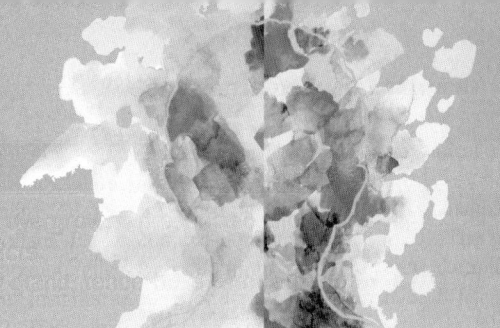

CHAPTER 28

The Return Prenatal Visit

Rebekah Kaplan and Margaret Hutchison

I. Definition and background

The purpose of return prenatal visits is to evaluate the pregnancy through ongoing health, nutritional, and psychosocial assessments. Referrals within the healthcare system and assistance with movement toward positive health behavior changes are also integral parts of the prenatal care process. The frequency and content of prenatal visits can be tailored to the specific needs of each patient (medical risk factors, psychosocial needs, and parity).

The format of care delivery may also vary depending on the site. Most prenatal care in the United States is structured around in-person or telehealth one-on-one visits with a medical care provider. However, there is increasing use of group-based prenatal care models, most notably CenteringPregnancy. For sites using CenteringPregnancy, care is moved out of the examination room and into a group space, and cohorts of 8–12 participants go through pregnancy together. Each of the 10 Centering sessions includes three components: Participants receive medical assessment, health education with interactive learning, and social support within the group space. Randomized controlled trial (RCT) research has shown that pregnant people who participate in CenteringPregnancy, when compared with those in one-to-one care, are less likely to have a premature birth, are more likely to be satisfied with care, and feel more prepared for labor and childbirth (Barger et al., 2015; Byerley & Haas, 2017; Gareau et al., 2016; Ickovics et al., 2007; Mazzoni & Carter, 2017). Numerous other studies support these findings and suggest other positive health outcomes associated with CenteringPregnancy (Baldwin, 2006; Barger et al., 2015; Tilden et al., 2014).

Much of the existing research demonstrates that this impact on preterm birth is even stronger when looking specifically at preterm birth rates among Black-identified patients. The seminal 2007 RCT conducted by Ickovics et al. (2007) demonstrated an overall 33% reduction in preterm birth and a 41% reduction for Black-identified participants. Numerous other studies have had similar findings, most notably a matched cohort study published by Picklesimer et al. in 2012. This study demonstrated a 47% reduction in overall preterm births, with a more marked reduction among Black patients. Significantly, this reduction among Black patients essentially leveled the preterm birth rate for Black and White study participants. Beyond the impact on preterm birth rates, the published evidence also demonstrates a significant impact for Black-identified patients on satisfaction with care, breastfeeding initiation, and numerous other health outcomes.

Thus, CenteringPregnancy has emerged as a way to specifically address racial inequities in perinatal care. The Centering research findings, when coupled with what we have learned from Black, Indigenous, and People of Color (BIPOC) patients about what must be done to mitigate racism in health care, suggest that CenteringPregnancy in and of itself is a powerful antiracism strategy. In summary, this model of care provides high-quality time during the healthcare interaction, opportunities for relationship building, person-centered care that values lived experience and demonstrates respect and dignity, provider continuity, the opportunity for racial concordance with providers (in race-based groups that include concordance with group leaders), and co-location of services (achieved in Centering via its ability to bring services into the group space).

One example of a Centering program developed specifically for the Black community is BElovedBIRTH Black Centering in Oakland, California. This program was designed to honor and celebrate Black birth, Black families, and the Black community and mitigate the racism that increases the risk for birth complications among Black-identified pregnant people:

> We envision a world where Black birthing people have all the support, loving care, and re-sources needed to have happy, healthy, and safe pregnancies, births, and postpartum recov-eries; free from obstetric racism. (Alameda Health System, n.d., para. 1)

This program incorporates an all-Black provider team of midwives, family support advocates, doulas, breastfeeding specialists, doctors, nutritionists, and psychologists, as well as links to other community resources. Participants meet for 2-hour group visits from early pregnancy through the early postpartum period. When patient-provider race concordance and Centering are not available, other options include race-concordant doulas and referral to/participation in community organizations focused on providing services for the BIPOC perinatal community.

For more information on the CenteringPregnancy model, go to www.centeringhealthcare.org/.

Table 28-1 provides a summary of the Essential Elements of CenteringPregnancy.

II. Database
A. *Subjective*
1. Gestational age
2. Estimated delivery date: review dating
3. Problems or concerns since their last visit (e.g., uterine activity, change in vaginal discharge, or psychosocial issues)
4. Follow-up on problems from previous visit (e.g., nausea, back pain, fetal position, psychosocial issues)

Table 28-1 CenteringPregnancy®: Essential Elements

The following are what are considered to be the "Essential Elements" of CenteringPregnancy, with a brief description of the significance of each element. These function as the guiding precepts that make prenatal care conducted in a group setting "centering."

1. Health assessment occurs within the group space.
   Normalizes pregnancy and prenatal care

2. Participants are involved in self-care activities.
   Promotes sense of self-efficacy

3. A facilitative leadership style is used.
   Promotes sense of self-efficacy, supports community building

4. The group is conducted in a circle.
   Supports open, nonhierarchic communications

5. Each session has an overall plan.
   There is an agenda for each session.

6. Attention is given to the core content, although emphasis may vary.
   The facilitative leadership model supports flexibility in discussion content, as dictated by the needs of the group.

7. There is stability in group leadership.
   Group leaders (a provider/nonprovider team) become trusted members of the group.

8. Group conduct honors the contributions of each member.
   Creating a safe group environment supports group cohesion and learning.

9. The composition of the group is stable but not rigid.
   Supports community building and development of trust among participants

10. Group size is optimal to promote the process.
    A group size of 8–12 pregnant participants is recommended to support optimal engagement of participants and sustainable use of staff.

11. Involvement of family support people is optional.
    Support people included as determined by site

12. Opportunity for socializing within the group is provided.
    Supports community building

13. There is ongoing evaluation of outcomes.
    Given challenges inherent in prenatal care system redesign, supports sustainability

Data from materials developed by the Centering Healthcare Institute (used with permission).

Table 28-2 Signs of Pregnancy Complications

Signs listed with condition they may represent in parentheses

First Trimester

- Vaginal bleeding (miscarriage)
- Fever, chills, dysuria (urinary tract infection [UTI] and/or pyelonephritis)
- Persistent nausea and vomiting (hyperemesis gravidarum)

Second and Third Trimesters

- Vaginal bleeding (miscarriage, preterm labor, placental abruption, placenta previa)
- Fever, chills, dysuria, flank pain (UTI and/or pyelonephritis)
- Uterine cramping or contractions (miscarriage, preterm labor, infection)
- Leaking of amniotic fluid
- Decreased fetal movement (fetal compromise, fetal demise)
- Severe headache without relief from analgesics (preeclampsia)
- Visual changes (blurry vision or seeing spots) (preeclampsia)
- Pelvic pressure (preterm labor)
- Continuous pruritus without rash (with affected palms and soles) (intrahepatic cholestasis of pregnancy)

---

5. Follow-up on problems from "problem list" (e.g., Was medication taken for urinary tract infection? Is housing issue resolved?)
6. Danger signs (e.g., signs of spontaneous abortion, preterm labor, urinary tract infection, preeclampsia, cholestasis of pregnancy, or intimate partner violence) (**Table 28-2**)
7. History and health screening review (current pregnancy, obstetric, medical, family, psychosocial—including depression and violence, and nutrition). The Family Violence Prevention Fund recommends screening for intimate partner violence and abuse at each prenatal visit (http://www.cdc.gov/violenceprevention/pdf/ipv/ipvandsvscreening.pdf).
8. Consults: results and management plans. Possible consults include:
    i. Physician, for conditions that require joint or multidisciplinary management (see Chapter 30, Guidelines for Medical Consultation, Interprofessional Collaboration, and Transfer of Care During Pregnancy and Childbirth)
    ii. Social worker for housing or food insecurity or interpersonal violence
    iii. Public health nurse where available when home visits for peripartum support would be helpful

B. Objective
1. Vital signs and urine
    a. Weight
    b. Blood pressure
    c. Urinalysis: if indicated to screen for preeclampsia or urinary tract infection (UTI)
2. Laboratory data
    a. Results for current problems (e.g., urine dip or wet mount)
    b. Are laboratory values up to date (e.g., chest radiograph after a positive purified protein derivative, third-trimester testing for group B streptococcus) (**Figure 28-1**)?
3. Physical examination
    a. General appearance (e.g., new striae or signs of depression)
    b. Abdominal examination
        i. Fundal height: measure by landmarks before 22–24 weeks, then with measuring tape (from the superior border of the symphysis pubis to the fundus). The fundal height should correlate with the number of weeks of gestation. Discrepancies of more than 3 cm should be further investigated, generally by ultrasound (American College of Obstetricians and Gynecologists [ACOG], 2021c).
        ii. Leopold's maneuvers and/or ultrasound for position and presentation after 32–36 weeks
        iii. Estimated fetal weight after 36 weeks
    c. Fetal heart rate
        i. Fetal heart tones can be seen on ultrasound by about 6 weeks.
        ii. Fetal heart rate can be heard via Doppler transabdominally by 9–10 weeks and by fetoscope by 18–20 weeks. Normal fetal heart rate is between 110 and 160 beats per minute.
    d. Other physical examination as indicated by patient presentation or concerns (e.g., costovertebral angle tenderness or vaginal discharge)
4. Testing and procedures:
    a. Screening tests: Figure 28-1 provides a summary. See Chapter 27, Prenatal Genetic Screening and Diagnosis, for details.
    b. 24–28 weeks: complete blood count (CBC) with platelets to screen for anemia. Normal hemoglobin is 11.0 g/dL in the first and third trimesters and 10.5 g/dL in the second. The blood volume increase of 40%–50% during pregnancy results in increased iron needs (ACOG, 2021a).
    c. 24–28 weeks: antibody screen and Rhogam if Rhesus factor (Rh) negative. Rhogam administration prevents the Rh-negative parturient from forming antibodies to the fetus's red blood cells. These antibodies can cause kernicterus and hydrops fetalis (Bowman, 2003).

d. 24–28 weeks: screening for gestational diabetes (see Chapter 33, Gestational Diabetes Mellitus: Early Detection and Management in Pregnancy, for more details)
e. 27–36 weeks: tetanus, diphtheria, and pertussis (Tdap) vaccination for passive transfer of pertussis antibodies to the fetus to reduce the risk of neonatal pertussis (ACOG, 2013b)
f. 35–37 weeks: group B *Streptococcus* (GBS) culture. Genital GBS can be transmitted to a neonate during vaginal delivery and can cause sepsis and pneumonia. Patients who test positive for

8–14 Weeks	15–20 Weeks	20–28 Weeks
LABS/TESTS Sonogram/dating Blood type, Rhesus factor (Rh), antibody screen, complete blood count (CBC), hemoglobin (Hgb) electrophoresis Rapid plasma reagin (RPR), rubella, varicella (by history or titers), HIV, purified protein derivative (PPD), hepatitis B surface antigen Urine culture + sensitivity (C+S), urine dip screening Pap (if due), *Neisseria gonorrhoeae* (GC)/*Chlamydia* per Centers for Disease Control and Prevention (CDC) guidelines	**LABS/TESTS/VACCINES** Sono fetal survey (18–20 weeks) Flu vaccine (October–May)	**LABS/TESTS** CBC Glucose load test (26–28 weeks) HIV, RPR (if indicated)
SELECTIVE TESTING Early glucose load test, fasting glucose and/or hemoglobin A1c Hepatitis C First-trimester genetic screen Nuchal translucency Chorionic villus sampling, noninvasive DNA testing Genetic carrier screening based on family medical history/ethnicity Refusal of blood products consent	**SELECTIVE TESTING** Quadruple-marker screen Amniocentesis Early glucose load test or hemoglobin A1c Chest x-ray (if +PPD) Urine C+S Hepatitis B vaccine Level 2 ultrasound, fetal echo	**SELECTIVE TESTING** 3-hour glucose tolerance test Antibody screen Rhogam at 28 weeks (or with any vaginal bleeding) in Rh-negative person
EDUCATION Orientation to clinic/service Prenatal classes referral Danger signs Common discomforts Nutrition, weight gain, and exercise Genetic screening/testing options Over-the-counter/prescription medicine use Drug, tobacco, and alcohol use Dental services information	**EDUCATION** Infant feeding benefits Exclusive human milk for 6 months Infant feeding class referral Fetal movement and quickening Exercise in pregnancy Common discomforts Danger signs	**EDUCATION** Signs/symptoms of preterm labor (PTL) Contraception Danger signs Fetal movement Vaginal birth after cesarean/trial of labor (VBAC/TOL) discussion Postpartum tubal ligation (PPTL) class referral (PPTL papers can be signed after 17 weeks) Breastfeeding benefits Exercise in pregnancy Attended breastfeeding class Attended prenatal classes
28–32 Weeks	**32–37 Weeks**	**37–41 Weeks**
LABS/TESTS/VACCINES **Optional/Indicated** Antenatal testing Kick counts Tetanus, diphtheria, and pertussis (Tdap) (recommended between 27 and 36 weeks)	**LABS/TESTS/VACCINES** Group B *Streptococcus* (GBS) (35–37 weeks) Tdap **Optional/Indicated** Antenatal testing Disability forms	**LABS/TESTS** **Optional/Indicated** Antenatal testing: nonstress test (NST)/amniotic fluid index (AFI) (after 41 weeks)

IV. Goals of clinical management

8–14 Weeks	15–20 Weeks	20–28 Weeks
EDUCATION Family planning/contraception Planned method _____ Attended PPTL class VBAC/TOL consent Signs and symptoms of PTL Other danger signs Newborn procedures Referral to birth prep class	**EDUCATION** Early initiation of breastfeeding Skin-to-skin contact and rooming in Latch, infant feeding cues Infant feeding and returning to work Colostrum and milk production Infant feeding resources Circumcision Danger signs Signs and symptoms of labor Infant car seat and baby supplies Choosing a pediatric provider Last chance for PPTL papers	**EDUCATION** Labor comfort measures Pain management options Signs and symptoms of labor Managing early labor at home Fetal monitoring options Birth plan/preferences Danger signs Going past due date (induction 41–42 weeks) Attended labor prep class Pain control preference Support system Pediatric provider

Courtesy of Community Health Network of San Francisco, Department of Public Health.

Figure 28-1 Prenatal Care Flow Sheet

GBS should receive antibiotics during labor to reduce these risks (Verani et al., 2010).

III. Assessment
A. *Gestational age/fetal size*
  1. Establish due date using best criteria if not previously done (ACOG, 2014).
  2. Identify any size and date discrepancy.
B. *Differential diagnosis*
  1. Establish for identified abnormal physical examination or laboratory findings (e.g., anemia, preterm labor, or UTI)
C. *Determine appropriateness of weight gain and nutritional status* (**Tables 28-3** and **28-4**).
D. *Determine prenatal educational needs.*
E. *Identify psychosocial issues or needs* (e.g., food insecurity, violence, immigration problems, housing, or social isolation).
F. *Role assessment: Identify the need for consultation or collaborative management with other health team members or referral to community resources* (e.g., race-concordant doula network).

IV. Goals of clinical management
A. *Identify medical, nutritional, and psychosocial problems and risk factors and develop a plan of care for each problem.*
B. *Provide anticipatory guidance related to pregnancy, birth, parenting, and medical care.*
C. *Individualize care to meet both the family and medical needs and maximize the well-being of the pregnant person and fetus.*

Table 28-3 Recommended Pattern of Weight Gain for Pregnancy

First trimester: 1.1–4.4 lb
Rates for second and third trimesters by body mass index (BMI)
- BMI less than 18.5: 1 lb/wk (1–1.3): total weight gain (TWG) 28–40 lb
- BMI 18.5–24.9: 1 lb/wk (0.8–1): TWG 25–35 lb
- BMI 25–29.9: 0.6 lb/wk (0.5–0.7): TWG 15–25 lb
- BMI 30 or greater: 0.5 lb/wk (0.4–0.6): TWG 11–20 lb

Data from Institute of Medicine. (2009). *Report brief. Weight gain during pregnancy: Reexamining the guidelines.* National Academies Press; ACOG. (2013). ACOG Committee Opinion No. 548: Weight gain during pregnancy. *Obstetrics and Gynecology, 121*(1), 210–212.

Table 28-4 Daily Dietary Needs for Normal-Weight Pregnant People

First trimester: No additional caloric needs. Second and third trimesters: Approximately 300 additional calories a day (e.g., 8 oz 1% milk, one hardboiled egg, and one apple)
- Protein: 60 g (teenagers, 75–80 g)
- Grains: 6 oz
- Vegetables: 2.5 cups
- Fruit: 2 cups
- Calcium: 1,000 mg

V. Plan (Figure 28-1)

A. *Laboratory*
1. Laboratory or diagnostic testing (**Figure 28-1**)
2. Other laboratory tests needed related to physical examination findings (e.g., urine culture, chlamydia test, or anemia workup)
3. Follow-up on any previous abnormal laboratory studies

B. *Medication*
1. Refill prenatal vitamins as necessary.
2. Supplementation: calcium, fish oil, vitamin D_3, and iron if deficient
3. Treatment of specific problems (e.g., UTI or vaginitis)

C. *Education and counseling*
1. Patient concerns
2. Current laboratory data
3. Weight gain and diet
4. Teaching appropriate to gestational age and patient needs (**Figure 28-1**; also see **Figure 27-1** in Chapter 27, Prenatal Genetic Screening and Diagnosis)
5. Danger signs of pregnancy (e.g., spontaneous abortion, preterm labor, and preeclampsia)
6. Emotional preparation for parenthood
7. Exercise, stress management, and behavior modification

D. *Refer for consultation or antepartum fetal evaluation*
1. Refer any patients as indicated for physician consultation or transfer of care (see Chapter 30, Guidelines for Medical Consultation, Interprofessional Collaboration, and Transfer of Care During Pregnancy and Childbirth) or for genetics, nutrition, or social services.
2. Initiate and refer for fetal evaluation and antenatal testing if indicated (**Table 28-5**).

E. *Update problem list*
1. Add or resolve any outstanding problems or concerns.

F. *Follow-up visit*
1. This should be flexible and individualized based on patient needs, parity, and risk, following a standard or reduced visit schedule (reviewed in Chapter 26, The Initial Prenatal Visit).
2. Postterm pregnancy (**Table 28-6**)

Table 28-5 Antepartum Fetal Evaluation

Conditions posing risk for fetal compromise include but are not limited to:
- Postterm pregnancy; hypertensive disease; fetal growth restriction; diabetes; previous unexplained stillbirth; decreased fetal movement; abnormal analytes on serum genetic screening tests; increased serum human chorionic gonadotropin; cholestasis of pregnancy; twins with discordant growth; preterm premature rupture of membranes; oligohydramnios; unexplained severe polyhydramnios; Rhesus factor isoimmunization; active substance use disorder; lupus; gastroschisis; and medical problems (e.g., cardiac disease, hyperthyroidism). There is also a linear relationship between total weight of the birthing parent and fetal compromise.

Management
- Review of dating criteria
- Leopold's for estimation of fetal weight and position

Initiation of testing
- Begin testing at the gestational age at which the provider is willing to intervene to save the life of the fetus balanced with the age at which one would expect to detect abnormal testing (generally 34–36 weeks).

Methods of testing (ACOG, 2021b)
- Fetal movement awareness
- Nonstress test (NST): monitoring with external transducer for 20 minutes
- Amniotic fluid index (AFI): measures amount of amniotic fluid in each quadrant of the uterus via transabdominal ultrasound. The deepest vertical pocket (DVP) should measure at least 2 cm, and the pockets of fluid from each quadrant should total at least 5 cm.
- Vibroacoustic stimulation: may be used to stimulate a fetus who is sleeping in order to better evaluate the NST.
- Biophysical profile (BPP): NST combined with an ultrasound to evaluate fetal breathing movements, fetal movements, extension and flexion of a limb or hand, and assessment of amniotic fluid volume
- Modified BPP: NST and DVP
- Contraction stress test: inducing contractions with Pitocin or nipple stimulation and evaluating fetal heart rate in reaction to contractions

First line:
No consistent evidence suggests that formal kick counts decrease the incidence of intrauterine fetal demise, although the method is widely used in practice for higher-risk pregnancies (Darby et al., 2009).

Second line:
Modified biophysical profile:
If modified biophysical profile is not reassuring, consult for biophysical profile, Doppler flow studies, and induction of labor after a contraction stress test.

Table 28-6 Postterm Pregnancy

Definitions

- Term delivery is considered to be between 37–42 weeks.
- Early term: 37 wk + 0 days to 38 wk + 6 days
- Full term: 39 wk + 0 days to 40 wk + 6 days
- Late term: 41 wk + 0 days to 41 wk + 6 days
- Postterm: 42 wk +

Management

- Examine cervix; Bishop's score greater than 5 is favorable for induction of labor.
- Consider sweeping membranes at 38–41 weeks.
- Consider alternative methods of induction.

Education

- Counsel on risks and benefits of induction versus expectant management.

Follow-up

- Biweekly antenatal testing (nonstress test [NST], amniotic fluid index [AFI]) by 41 weeks' gestation
- Kick counts should be initiated at 40–41 weeks.
- Offer induction of labor between 41 and 42 weeks.

Data from American College of Obstetricians and Gynecologists. (2013). ACOG Committee Opinion No. 579: Definition of term pregnancy. *Obstetrics and Gynecology, 122*(5), 1139–1140. doi:10.1097/01.AOG.0000437385.88715.4a

References

Alameda Health System. (n.d.). *BElovedBirth Black Centering.* http://www.alamedahealthsystem.org/family-birthing-center/black-centering/

American College of Obstetricians and Gynecologists. (2013b). ACOG Committee Opinion No. 566: Update on immunization and pregnancy: Tetanus, diphtheria, and pertussis vaccination. *Obstetrics and Gynecology, 121*(6), 1411–1414. doi:10.1097/01.AOG.0000431054.33593.e3

American College of Obstetricians and Gynecologists. (2021a). ACOG Practice Bulletin No. 233: Anemia in pregnancy. *Obstetrics and Gynecology, 138*(2), e55–e64. doi:10.1097/AOG.0000000000004477

American College of Obstetricians and Gynecologists. (2021b). ACOG Practice Bulletin No. 229: Antepartum fetal surveillance. *Obstetrics and Gynecology, 137*(6), e116–e127. doi:10.1097/AOG.0000000000004410

American College of Obstetricians and Gynecologists. (2021c). ACOG Practice Bulletin No. 227: Fetal growth restriction. *Obstetrics and Gynecology, 137*(2), e16–e28. doi:10.1097/AOG.0000000000004251

Baldwin, K. A. (2006). Comparison of selected outcomes of centering pregnancy versus traditional prenatal care. *Journal of Midwifery & Women's Health, 51*(4), 266–272. doi:10.1016/j.jmwh.2005.11.011

Barger, M., Faucher, M. A., & Murphy, P. A. (2015). Part II: The centering pregnancy model of group prenatal care. *Journal of Midwifery & Women's Health, 60*(2), 211–213. doi:10.1111/jmwh.12307

Bowman, J. (2003). Thirty-five years of Rh prophylaxis. *Transfusion, 43*(12), 1661–1666. doi:10.1111/j.0041-1132.2003.00632.x

Byerley, B. M., & Haas, D. M. (2017). A systematic overview of the literature regarding group prenatal care for high-risk pregnant women. *BMC Pregnancy and Childbirth, 17*(1), 329–329. doi:10.1186/s12884-017-1522-2

Darby-Stewart, A. L., Strickland, C., & Jamieson, B. (2009). Do abnormal fetal kick counts predict intrauterine death in average-risk pregnancies? *Journal of Family Practice, 58*(4), 220a–220c.

Gareau, S., Lòpez-De Fede, A., Loudermilk, B. L., Cummings, T. H., Hardin, J. W., Picklesimer, A. H., Crouch, E., & Covington-Kolb, S. (2016). Group prenatal care results in Medicaid savings with better outcomes: A propensity score analysis of CenteringPregnancy participation in South Carolina. *Maternal and Child Health Journal, 20*(7), 1384–1393. doi: 10.1007/s10995-016-1935-y

Ickovics, J. R., Kershaw, T. S., Westdahl, C., Magriples, U., Massey, Z., Reynolds, H., & Rising, S.. (2007). Group prenatal care and perinatal outcomes: A randomized controlled trial. *Obstetrics & Gynecology, 110*(2, Pt. 1), 330–339. doi:10.1097/01.AOG.0000275284.24298.23

Mazzoni, S. E., & Carter, E. B. (2017). Group prenatal care. *American Journal of Obstetrics and Gynecology, 216*(6), 552–556. doi:10.1016/j.ajog.2017.02.006

Picklesimer, A. H., Billings, D., Hale, N., Blackhurst, D., & Covington-Kolb, S. (2012). The effect of CenteringPregnancy group prenatal care on preterm birth in a low-income population. *American Journal of Obstetrics and Gynecology, 206*(5), 415.e1–415.e7. doi:10.1016/j.ajog.2012.01.04

Tilden, E. L., Hersh, S. R., Emeis, C. L., Weinstein, S. R., & Caughey, A. B. (2014). Group prenatal care: Review of outcomes and recommendations for model implementation. *Obstetrical and Gynecological Survey, 69*(1), 46–55. doi:10.1097/OGX.0000000000000025

Verani, J., McGee, L., & Schrag, S. J. (2010). Prevention of perinatal group B streptococcal disease: Revised guidelines from CDC, 2010. *MMWR. Recommendations and Reports, 59*(RR-10), 1–31.

CHAPTER 29

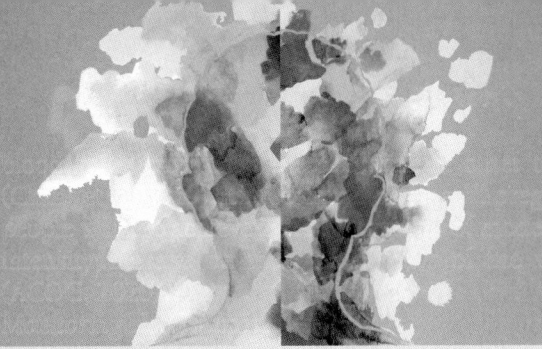

The Postpartum Visit

Jenna Shaw-Battista and Holly Cost

I. Introduction and general background

The postpartum period is a time of tremendous physical and emotional change for new parents. The early-postpartum period is defined as 42 days, although late-postpartum morbidity and mortality can occur in the year after childbirth (World Health Organization [WHO], 2022). Although childbearing persons experience the most profound adaptations during this "fourth trimester," their partners, older children, extended family, and community may also experience significant transitions (American College of Obstetricians and Gynecologists [ACOG], 2018; Declercq et al., 2013). The goals of family-centered postpartum care include the prevention, identification, management, and resolution of abnormal physical, psychologic, and psychosocial adaptations. Postpartum visits include monitoring and education related to parturition complications with short-term or lifelong health implications. They also serve as a transition from obstetric to primary health care with opportunities to initiate or resume routine screening and health maintenance activities.

There is limited research on optimal postpartum care and no evidence to support some routine counseling and recommendations often made by healthcare providers in the postpartum period (Yang et al., 2022). For example, myths persist that stair climbing and lifting should be avoided despite compelling research that physical activity benefits psychological and physical health and can safely be initiated or resumed by 6–8 weeks' postpartum, if not earlier (Evenson et al., 2014). Accurate health education and promotion may be particularly effective in the postpartum period because many new parents have knowledge deficits and are highly motivated to make lifestyle and other changes to improve their health and that of their growing family (Declercq et al., 2013). Postpartum education may include self- and infant care; addressing symptoms that require immediate evaluation; and recommendations for primary care and health-promoting activities, such as exercise, healthful nutrition, breastfeeding, immunizations, sleep hygiene, child safety, contraception, and sexually transmitted infection prevention.

The postpartum period is a key time for education and interventions because perinatal care is often the entry point into health care for communities that experience perinatal disparities due to structural inequities in many facets of life for reproductive-aged persons (DiBari et al., 2014) and who experience disparate adverse perinatal outcomes with lifelong implications. Communities particularly affected include people who experience discrimination based on race, ethnicity, and ability and lesbian, gay, bisexual, transgender, intersex, queer/questioning, asexual (LGBTQIA+) families with childbearing people who do not identify as "mothers," which is why inclusive gender-neutral terms are used. The same communities are more likely to experience bias and mistreatment from perinatal care providers (Greenfield & Darwin, 2021; Vedam et al., 2019), a risk factor for postpartum visit nonattendance (Attanasio et al., 2021), and birth trauma, which occurs in up to 45% of all parturients (Alcorn et al., 2010), with posttraumatic stress disorder observed in 4% of community samples and 18.5% of high-risk groups (Yildiz et al., 2017). It is important to assess for trauma and associated risk factors in the review of the new parent's birth story.

New parents commonly appreciate opportunities to discuss their experience of childbirth and early parenting, although there are scarce data to guide the format or content of these conversations. People who have recently given birth may wish to review clinical details and ask questions to "fill in the blanks" in their childbirth memories to make meaning from the experience (Bastos et al., 2015). They may not have anticipated the intensity of the experience and may benefit from reassurance that their coping behaviors and choices were respected. Postpartum care providers can prioritize sensitive and effective therapeutic communications because vulnerability, changes in self-perception, uncertainty, and disequilibrium are common during the postpartum role transition (Association of Women's Health, Obstetric and Neonatal Nurses [AWHONN], 2020). Ideally, people are provided an opportunity for a postpartum visit conducted by a culturally congruent provider who attended their care in the antepartum and intrapartum to extend or facilitate new continuity of care, allow for exchange of information, and provide feedback (Barimani et al., 2015; Sandall et al., 2015).

The timing, number, and content of postpartum visits vary based on individual risk factors, and visits should be customized for individuals. Newly postpartum individuals are typically followed daily during their inpatient stay and scheduled for outpatient follow-up one or more times during the following 1–12 weeks (Declercq et al., 2013), per individual risk factors and personalized care plans (ACOG, 2018). Those choosing out-of-hospital birth will typically have more frequent postpartum evaluations.

Historically, only a 6-week postpartum visit was standard, based on the understanding that uterine involution is typically complete by then (ACOG, 2018). However, 6 weeks may be too late to detect or prevent some postpartum complications or to provide optimal contraceptive counseling because many people resume sexual intercourse before this time (Sridhar & Salcedo, 2017). For these reasons, contemporary guidelines recommend that all people have contact with their obstetric care providers within 1–2 weeks after childbirth (WHO, 2022) or within the first 3 weeks, with follow-up care as needed, including a comprehensive postpartum visit by 12 weeks' postpartum (ACOG, 2018). Earlier or more frequent examinations may be indicated, and facility-based visits may be supplemented with telephone encounters or home visits, which may increase parental satisfaction with services (Lavender et al., 2013; Yonemoto et al., 2021) and assist with the management of perinatal mood disorders (Guille & Douglas, 2017). The WHO (2022) recommends home visits for all postpartum persons and their newborns.

Earlier and increased postpartum visits should be considered when significant risk factors for adverse postpartum conditions are present; when complications arose prenatally or during the intrapartum and immediate postpartum period; or for other reasons, such as chestfeeding/breastfeeding difficulties, management of chronic or perinatal health conditions, or optimal timing of birth control initiation. For example, persons with hypertensive disorders of pregnancy requiring antihypertensive medication should be seen 3–7 days after birth, whereas those not requiring medication may be seen at 1–2 weeks postpartum if they are provided a home blood pressure cuff for self-monitoring and educated about when to report elevated readings (Druzin et al., 2021). Visits should be scheduled within 1–2 weeks after a cesarean section, with targeted assessments for postoperative complications, including trauma, excessive blood loss, anemia, thrombophlebitis, oliguria, and infection (e.g., surgical wound infections that most commonly present 3–8 days' postpartum) (AWHONN, 2020). A 1–2 week postpartum visit may also be helpful to evaluate parent–infant bonding, mood, risks for discontinuing chestfeeding/breastfeeding, and family support and integration (AWHONN, 2020; Yonemoto et al., 2021). Despite recent updates in postpartum clinical guidelines, many postpartum individuals receive inadequate care and treatment geared toward public health goals, including depression screening for new parents (Office of Disease Prevention and Health Promotion, n.d.). In a recent study of postpartum individuals in California, nearly 1 in 10 had no outpatient postpartum care, and half had only a single visit (Sakala et al., 2018). Outreach to disenfranchised communities is particularly recommended because of socioeconomic and racial disparities in the number and timing of postpartum visits (Sakala et al., 2018). Digital notifications, appointment reminders, and incentives may increase postpartum visit attendance and prove particularly useful in the care of high-risk populations (e.g., adolescents and new parents with a history of mood disorders) (Centers for Medicare and Medicaid Services, 2015; WHO, 2022). Perinatal outcomes may also be improved in vulnerable and high-risk populations with home visits, phone calls, and web-based programs, as well as referrals to postpartum education, fitness classes, and peer support groups, among other interventions (Lavender et al., 2013; Poyatos-León et al, 2017; Wallace et al., 2018; Yonemoto et al., 2021). Counseling, social support facilitation, reinforcement of healthful coping strategies, and discussion of role transition and self-perception alterations may help to reestablish psychologic equilibrium, whether performed by clinicians or community members (Guille & Douglas, 2017; Lassi & Bhutta, 2015), particularly for people who experienced unanticipated obstetrical procedures, emergencies, or trauma related to pregnancy and childbirth (Asadzadeh et al., 2020; Dekel et al., 2017). Parents who experienced perinatal loss, had an infant removed from their custody by child protective services, placed their infant with an adoptive family, or served as a surrogate may require unique or additional supports during their postpartum transition.

In addition to considering each individual's underlying health status, risk factors, and systematic bias, the time elapsed since childbirth informs the type of screening, intervention, education, and referrals provided in postpartum visits. The use of structured visit note templates improves providers' adherence to guidelines for comprehensive care and recommended postpartum visit elements (Grotell et al., 2021); these guidelines are outlined in the next section.

II. Database (may include but is not limited to)

Data may be gleaned from postpartum patient interviews and review of medical records when available.

A. *Subjective data*
   1. History of medical conditions, antenatal, intrapartum, or postpartum complications requiring follow-up, including:
      a. Mental health conditions, including mood and anxiety disorders

b. Endocrine disorders (e.g., thyroid disorder and type 1, type 2, or gestational diabetes mellitus)
c. Hypertension (e.g., chronic or gestational hypertension, preeclampsia, or eclampsia)
d. Infectious processes such as sexually transmitted infections, latent tuberculosis, or chronic hepatitis infection
e. Elevated or low total body weight
f. Tobacco exposure, either first- or second-hand
g. Substance use disorders
h. Intimate partner or family violence
i. Psychosocial stressors, including housing and food insecurity

2. Description of the intrapartum experience, including:
    a. Date and location (e.g., home, hospital, birth center, other) of delivery
    b. Type of delivery: vaginal, assisted, cesarean
    c. Type of anesthesia used, if any
    d. Estimated or quantified blood loss
    e. Complications of delivery, including lacerations and use of catheter
    f. Neonatal Apgar scores and postdelivery course
    g. Postpartum complications, including hemorrhage
    h. The new parent's understanding and feelings about their labor and the infant's birth: Note and explore any traumatic feelings expressed about the experience, which are more likely after obstetrical emergencies, unplanned cesarean or assisted vaginal birth, and situations in which decisions were perceived to have been made for versus with the parturient (Asadzadeh et al., 2020; Dekel et al., 2017).

3. General health, well-being, and psychological status should be assessed, with screening for the following:
    a. Self-care:
        i. What self-care activities are being performed?
        ii. Do they have the opportunity to get exercise or leave the house?
        iii. Can they nap/sleep when the baby sleeps?
        iv. If they sustained a perineal laceration, are they using a peri bottle for hygiene and/or comfort measures such as witch hazel pads, anesthetic spray, or sitz baths at home? How often?
    b. Adjustment, capabilities, and satisfaction with parenting
    c. Perinatal mood disorders, the most common postpartum complication
        i. New parents with depression and/or anxiety frequently present with physical symptoms in primary care–oriented visits during the first 12 months' postpartum, which should prompt careful screening for risk factors and psychological symptoms (Cerimele et al., 2013).
        ii. Risk factors: personal and family history of depression or anxiety, perinatal loss, complications of pregnancy, hyperemesis, multiple gestation, gestational diabetes, major life events unrelated to pregnancy and childbirth, lack of support or resources, and social stigma (e.g., single or adolescent parenthood) (Liu et al., 2021).
        iii. Symptoms: inability to cope with demands of new role, disorganized daily routine, poor sleep hygiene, excessive fatigue that interferes with self- or infant care, depression or mania, anhedonia, frequent crying, insomnia, anxiety, hypervigilance, or thoughts of harming self or infant (Cerimele et al., 2013)
    d. Postpartum psychosis, a medical emergency characterized by disorganized behavior, visual or auditory hallucinations, and delusions (AWHONN, 2020)
    e. Posttraumatic stress disorder, which may recur due to childbirth-related stressors among people with a prior diagnosis or present for the first time as a consequence of trauma experienced during pregnancy and childbirth. Risk factors for new postpartum onset of posttraumatic stress disorder include subjective report of distress during labor, obstetrical emergencies, and unplanned mode of delivery (Dekel et al., 2017).
    f. Substance use or abuse, which frequently co-occurs with perinatal mood disorders and intimate partner violence (AWHONN, 2020)
    g. Screening and referral for depression in the partners of parturients should be considered, given that the incidence of paternal postpartum depression ranges from 1.2% to 25.5%, with significant impacts on family dynamics and well-being (Wang et al., 2021). Risk factors include limited social support, unemployment, a history of personal or partner mental illness, first pregnancy, and low marital satisfaction (Wang et al., 2021).

4. How is the infant?
    a. Any health or growth issues?
    b. Does the infant have a pediatric care provider? Have they been seen recently?
    c. Is the infant in a safe sleeping environment at home and/or in other care situations?
    d. Using a car seat appropriately?
    e. Ask about methods being used to soothe the infant, which may include skin-to-skin contact, swaddling, movement, white noise, singing or other sounds, and sucking (pacifier).

5. Infant feeding
    a. If infant is nursing, assess term used by new parent: *chestfeeding* or *breastfeeding*?
    b. How is nursing going—any questions or concerns?
    c. Determine if chestfeeding/breastfeeding is exclusive or if there is formula supplementation.

d. Does the parent have support for nursing from partner/family/friends?
e. Do they feel milk supply is adequate?
f. How long do they plan to nurse?
g. Do they plan to return to work, and if so, when? Will they have support for pumping and milk storage at work?
h. Do they have information about milk collection and storage? Do they need a breast pump?
i. If supplementing with donor breast milk or formula, how much and why?
   i. Do they have information about how to properly clean bottles and nipples and safely make and store formula and donor milk?
   ii. Do they have or need resources to obtain sufficient formula or donor milk?
6. Community and governmental support programs
   a. Are they utilizing support services or do they qualify for new referrals, such as for the Special Supplemental Nutrition Program for Women, Infants, and Children (WIC), which provides healthy food while chestfeeding/breastfeeding or infant formula?
   b. Have they assessed whether their public or private insurance will cover the cost of donor milk in part or in full for babies with certain medical conditions or who lack access to human milk from an ill or absent parent?
7. Nutrition status, including the following:
   a. Daily nutritional intake, including adequacy of protein, calcium sources, and fruits and vegetables
   b. Do they require additional support or education to obtain a diet appropriate for lactation, iron deficiency, or other common postpartum circumstances?
   c. Nutritional risk factors such as weight outside of the normal range, gestational diabetes, or eating disorders that would benefit from ongoing nutritional support?
   d. Any use of vitamins, minerals, herbs, or other supplements?
   e. Adequate water intake?
8. Medications with dosage and indication, if any
9. Sexual and reproductive health, including the following:
   a. Altered self-perception
   b. Libido and satisfaction
   c. Resumption of sexual activity
   d. Need for contraception
   e. Knowledge of pregnancy-spacing recommendations and preconception self-care practices to promote health of future pregnancy
10. Family, social, and community integration and support
    a. Bonding with infant
    b. What types of physical and emotional support and daily help do they have?
    c. Housing and economic status: Do they have what is needed to care for self and infant?
    d. Any plans to start or return to work outside the home, with impact on infant and self-care?
    e. Relationship conflict or interpersonal violence
    f. Partner adjustment, if applicable
    g. Sibling, grandparent, extended family, and social support network adjustment
    h. Cultural or religious practices in the postpartum period (Dennis et al., 2007)
11. Review of systems
    a. Chest (see Chapter 37, Human Lactation, for more information on infant feeding and chestfeeding/breastfeeding concerns)
       i. Mammary tissue or nipple pain
       ii. Masses or erythema noted
       iii. Concerns about insufficient milk supply or infant feeding
    b. Abdomen
       i. Abdominal or uterine pain or cramping that has increased since birth or is unrelieved with pain medication
       ii. Report of pain, redness, odor, or discharge at the site of a cesarean incision
    c. Pelvis, genitals, and lochia
       i. Pelvic pressure or pain, particularly over the symphysis pubis or coccyx, which may result from injury during childbirth
       ii. Vaginal, vulvar, or perineal pain that has increased since delivery or is unrelieved by pain medication, with or without edema
       iii. Abnormal, excessive, or prolonged bleeding (e.g., fills pad in <1–2 hours, large recurrent clots, lochia serosa or alba that reverts to lochia rubra, or lochia that persists beyond 6 weeks' postpartum)
       iv. Foul-smelling lochia
       v. Resumption of menses
    d. Elimination
       i. Urinary, fecal, or flatus incontinence
       ii. Urinary retention
       iii. Dysuria
       iv. Constipation
    e. Extremities
       i. Calf pain, heat, or redness
       ii. Edema that is unilateral and/or increases or persists beyond 7 days' postpartum

B. *Objective data*
   1. General well-being and psychologic status
      a. Observe affect and appearance.
   2. Family integration
      a. Observe interactions between parent and newborn and any older children or other family members present.
   3. Weight and vital signs
   4. Head and neck
      a. Thyroid gland: Palpate for size and nodularity.
      b. Lymph nodes: Palpate for size and tenderness.

5. Chest
    a. Observe size, color, and symmetry of mammary tissue.
    b. Palpate for tenderness, masses, and warmth.
    c. Examine the nipples and areola for cracks, fissures, bleeding, lesions, and compression stripes.
    d. If possible, observe infant position and latch during chestfeeding/breastfeeding.
6. Abdomen
    a. Inspect and palpate for masses, tenderness, uterine involution, hernias, diastasis recti, and muscle tone.
    b. Check surgical sites for closure, pain, masses, exudate, and erythema if applicable (e.g., cesarean or postpartum tubal ligation).
7. Pelvis, genitals, and lochia
    a. Palpate over symphysis pubis and coccyx if report of pain.
    b. External genitalia and perineum
        i. Inspect for symmetry, excoriation, and varicosities.
        ii. Assess any lacerations for approximation, exudate, and healing.
        iii. Visualize the amount and appearance of lochia.
        iv. Assess for leakage of urine during Valsalva.
    c. Pelvic examination as indicated
        i. Vagina: Assess for uterine prolapse, cystocele, or rectocele; check the strength of pelvic musculature during a Valsalva maneuver and/or Kegel exercise.
        ii. Uterus: Assess position, size, and tenderness.
        iii. Cervix: Assess os appearance and closure.
    d. Rectal exam: Assess for hemorrhoids, fissures, fistulas, masses, and sphincter tone (for third- and fourth-degree lacerations).
8. Extremities
    a. Assess for calf tenderness, heat, or redness on inspection and palpation.
    b. Assess for edema that increases or persists beyond 7 days' postpartum or is unilateral.

III. Assessment

Assessment should incorporate subjective and objective data and address the postpartum person's physical, emotional, and social adaptation, along with any complications noted.

IV. Goals for clinical management

The goals of family-centered postpartum care include skilled support for optimal health during the transition, with the prevention, identification, management, and resolution of abnormal physical, psychologic, and psychosocial adaptations.

A. *Identify persons at risk for postpartum complications, including mood disorders, and individualize care to promote health and minimize harm.*

B. *Assess postpartum adjustment and support families during the postpartum transition period; provide care and referrals as needed.*

C. *Screen for dangers to the birthing person, baby, and family.*

D. *Chestfeeding/breastfeeding support: Provide lactation care, anticipatory guidance, and nutritional counseling.*

E. *Family planning: Provide families access to desired contraception if indicated, and encourage a healthy pregnancy interval with preconception self-care.*

F. *Identify and address health education, maintenance, and primary care needs; provide or refer as indicated by availability of services.*

V. Plan

A. *Diagnostics*
   1. Laboratory testing or imaging if indicated by history or examination, for example:
       a. Urine dipstick to assess for protein or nitrites if hypertensive or symptomatic for urinary tract infection
       b. Urine culture and sensitivity to rule out urinary tract infection if symptomatic
       c. Complete blood count to assess for infectious processes or anemia if symptomatic of infection or if had anemia during pregnancy
       d. Wet mount to assess for vaginitis or infection if symptomatic
       e. Sexually transmitted infection testing if indicated
       f. Ultrasound of mammary tissue if mastitis with progression to abscess is suspected
       g. Postpartum screening of individuals diagnosed with gestational diabetes with a 2-hour, 75-gram oral glucose tolerance test performed 6–12 weeks after delivery (ACOG, 2018)
   2. Primary care health maintenance and screening as indicated by age or health history (see Chapter 38, Adult Healthcare Maintenance and Promotion, for more information)
       a. Pap smear
       b. Occult fecal blood, fecal immunoglobulin testing, or referral for colonoscopy
       c. Mammography (chestfeeding/breastfeeding is not a contraindication for routine mammography)
       d. Lipid profile (results confounded by chestfeeding/breastfeeding)

B. *Treatment and follow-up*
   1. Visit schedule and providers
       a. Daily inpatient postpartum visits by a maternity or primary care provider are standard, with outpatient follow-up one or more times. A visit should be scheduled within 3 weeks of birth, and a comprehensive exam should be performed within 3 months (ACOG, 2018).
       b. Early or repeated outpatient visits, with supplementary home visits or telephone consultations, may be indicated, particularly for people who

experienced obstetrical complications or have adverse health conditions or other risk factors for postpartum complications (Lavender et al., 2013; Yonemoto et al., 2021), including perinatal mood disorders (Guille & Douglas, 2017).
   c. Visits should be conducted by competent and qualified providers, ideally with continuity of care by midwives (WHO, 2022) or other advanced practice nurses with backgrounds in perinatal care. Access to medical records is essential if continuity of care is not feasible or desired by the postpartum person. Visits may be performed by interprofessional team members such as physicians, registered nurses, lactation consultants, nutritionists, social workers, therapists, psychologists or psychiatrists, and health educators in addition to, or instead of, nurse practitioners and nurse-midwives (Lassi & Bhutta, 2015).
2. Medications and therapeutics
   a. Continue daily prenatal vitamins or multivitamin during lactation if diet is lacking in whole foods, variety, and balance.
   b. Other medications as warranted by subjective and objective data (e.g., iron, stool softener, analgesics, or antibiotics)
   c. Consider recommending or supplying vaginal lubricant for the vaginal dryness commonly reported during lactation.
   d. Vaccinations as needed, such as COVID; influenza; tetanus, diphtheria, and pertussis (Tdap; if not given during pregnancy); measles, mumps, and rubella; varicella; or hepatitis A and B vaccines, with reminders and follow-up appointments as required for series
   e. Contraception should be discussed and prescriptions given as indicated. Ovulation may resume as quickly as 3 weeks' postpartum in people who are not chest/breastfeeding (Makins & Cameron, 2020). Conclusive data are lacking, but ACOG and the Society for Maternal-Fetal Medicine (Louis et al., 2019) recommend an interpregnancy interval of at least 6 months because of the risks of subsequent small-for-gestational-age neonates, preterm birth, infant mortality, and malnutrition (Makins & Cameron, 2020). Inter-delivery intervals of fewer than 18 months may increase the risk of uterine rupture in labor after cesarean (Louis et al., 2019). Contraception initiation will depend on the patient's sexual desires, timing of resumption of sexual activity, lactation, and desired method. Because not all patients have partners who produce sperm or engage in intercourse as a sexual practice, clinicians should solicit the contraceptive needs of patients rather than assuming those needs. Contraceptive options and return to fertility are ideally included in antepartum teaching to ensure informed consent and develop a postpartum implementation plan in advance. Due to historical abuse and control of fertility in historically excluded communities, it is critical to ensure that everyone is provided accurate information about all contraceptive options and noncoercive assistance in accessing the method(s) of their choice (ACOG, 2018). See Chapter 21, Contraception, for more detail on all methods; the information that follows is specific to contraception in the postpartum period.
      i. Combined estrogen and progestin hormonal contraception (CHC) is not generally recommended until 6 weeks' postpartum because of the increased risk of venous thromboembolism (VTE) secondary to the resolving hypercoagulable state of pregnancy (Sridhar & Salcedo, 2017). In addition, there are some concerns about estrogen affecting milk supply, although research findings and recommendations are mixed (Sridhar & Salcedo, 2017; Tepper et al., 2015). Those without risk factors for VTE can start CHC at 21 days' postpartum, and those with risk factors should wait until 43 days' postpartum (WHO, 2015).
      ii. Progesterone-only pills and implants may be initiated immediately postpartum regardless of breastfeeding status (WHO, 2015). Injectable progestins such as depo medroxyprogesterone acetate should be avoided in the first 6 weeks' postpartum for patients who are breastfeeding, unless no other alternatives are available (WHO, 2015). Injectable progestins may be initiated immediately postpartum in those who do not breastfeed (WHO, 2015).
      iii. Intrauterine devices (IUDs) may be placed immediately postpartum (including postcesarean) or after 4 weeks, although new research supports their placement at less than 4 weeks' postpartum (Kennedy & Goldsmith, 2018). There may be a higher rate of expulsion between these time frames.
      iv. The lactational amenorrhea method may be used by breastfeeding parents for up to 6 months. See Chapter 21, Contraception, for a detailed description.
      v. Spermicides, condoms, withdrawal: Withdrawal and condoms may be used at any time in the postpartum period. Spermicides should not be used until lochia has stopped (Nelson & Harwood, 2018).
      vi. Diaphragm, cervical cap, and sponge use should be delayed until 6 weeks' postpartum to allow for uterine involution (WHO, 2015). Further, lochia may increase the risk of toxic shock syndrome, and pregnancy and delivery may change diaphragm and cervical cap fit (Kennedy & Goldsmith, 2018).

vii. Tubal contraceptive surgeries may be performed during a cesarean section or before hospital discharge. If not performed within 7 days, it is recommended to delay this procedure until after day 42, due to the VTE risk of surgery (Makins & Cameron, 2020).
viii. A prescription for emergency contraception in case of contraceptive failure may be beneficial. If ulipristal is used, breastfeeding is not recommended for 7 days (WHO, 2015).
f. Therapeutics for postpartum conditions or complications, including the following:
i. Discomfort from genital edema and perineal laceration may be treated with local cooling with ice or gel packs (East et al., 2020; WHO, 2022). There is a lack of data to support the use of topical anesthesia (Hedayati et al., 2005) or complementary therapies commonly employed, such as witch hazel, castor oil, and herbal sitz baths, although hydrotherapy may promote healing and comfort (Aderhold & Perry, 1991; Batten et al., 2017). Compression stockings and hydrotherapy may be considered for symptomatic varicosities.
ii. A pelvic brace or binder may reduce discomfort from pelvic girdle pain or symphysis pubis mobility and separation. In severe cases, a walker or cane may be indicated.

C. *Patient education*
1. Answer questions and address concerns of the postpartum individual and their family, which often include the following:
a. Clarifying questions about the labor and birth experience and any impact of complications or procedures on future health or childbearing (Declercq et al., 2013)
b. Recovery after cesarean birth (AWHONN, 2020)
i. Postoperative self-care and pain management
ii. Alternate infant feeding positions per parental comfort (see Chapter 37, Human Lactation, for more information)
iii. Possible discomforts from surgery or anesthesia (e.g., edema and constipation)
iv. Surgical complications, such as excessive blood loss; thrombophlebitis; oliguria; and infection of the surgical wound, uterus, or urinary tract
v. The choice between vaginal birth after cesarean and elective repeat cesarean birth in future pregnancies is multifactorial and can be deferred in the postpartum period with referral to informational resources and future obstetrical care providers, if applicable. In most cases, individuals with one or two prior cesareans may be counseled to consider vaginal birth after cesarean (ACOG, 2019).
c. Return to normal daily activities, exercise, and work as dictated by physical and mental wellness
d. Infant care, including feeding, soothing, pediatric visits, immunizations, circumcision, and safety measures (e.g., sleeping arrangements and car seats) (see Chapter 1, First Well-Baby Visit; Chapter 3, 0 to 3 Years of Age Interval Visit; and Chapter 37, Human Lactation, for more information)
e. Parturients experience many postpartum physical changes that may be unexpected or concerning and prompt questions about normal versus abnormal symptoms. Individuals should be given warning signs and information about how to seek follow-up care.
i. Excessive bleeding (soaking a large menstrual pad in 1 hour or less)
ii. Mammary tissue pain from engorgement (bilateral) versus mastitis (usually signaled by unilateral mass with fever) (see Chapter 37, Human Lactation, for more information)
iii. Symptoms of preeclampsia (see Chapter 34, Hypertension Disorders in Pregnancy: Gestational Hypertension and Preeclampsia-Eclampsia, for more information about postpartum preeclampsia)
iv. Uterine tenderness, foul-smelling discharge, fever as signs of postpartum endometritis
v. Worsening pain, increasing swelling, or other signs of infection at the site of surgical incision or laceration repair
f. Sexual health and dysfunction, which are critical topics but frequently omitted from postpartum visits (Declercq et al., 2013; Sakala et al., 2018) (see Chapter 24, Sexual Dysfunction, for more information)
i. Dyspareunia, frequently related to genital laceration and insufficient lubrication related to postpartum hormonal changes and chestfeeding/breastfeeding. Consider vaginal estrogen for persistent or concerning dyspareunia.
ii. Postpartum and other changes in psychological aspects of sexuality, including self-perception and partner relationships
iii. Return to menses, which can be highly variable based on the individual
2. Counseling about nutrition and exercise is essential in the postpartum period, may have lifelong impacts on all family members, and should include the following:
a. Basic principles of optimal nutrition and hydration, considering each person's individual cultural postpartum practices
b. Encouragement to achieve and maintain a normal body weight to reduce immediate and long-term health risks (Amorim et al., 2013)

c. Advice that regular exercise may improve health and prevent or reduce depressive symptomatology (Poyatos-León et al., 2017)
d. Continue daily 400–800 mcg folate throughout childbearing years for the prevention of neural tube defects in case of unintended pregnancy; dosage is adjusted according to gestational parent risk factors up to 4–5 mg per day (Gomes et al., 2015).
e. Nutritional supplementation specific to the postpartum period (ACOG, 2018; WHO, 2022)
    i. Routine supplementation is not indicated in the absence of nutritional deficiencies, in which case a multivitamin including calcium and vitamins B and D may be helpful.
    ii. Iron supplementation following postpartum hemorrhage or anemia diagnosis
    iii. Fluid and fiber to support bowel function
    iv. Essential fatty acid intake may minimize the incidence and severity of postpartum depression (Zhang et al., 2020).
f. Nutrition during chestfeeding/breastfeeding (AWHONN, 2020; Jouanne et al., 2021)
    i. A personalized approach to counseling should be provided, with reference to body mass and composition, dietary intake, and individual risk factors.
    ii. The minimal daily caloric intake required for milk production in the average lactating individual is 1,800, with 500 calories typically used for this purpose each day.
    iii. Weight loss of several pounds per month does not typically affect lactation.
    iv. Although common, routine vitamin supplementation is not indicated during lactation if the lactating individual's diet is wholesome, balanced, and varied, in the absence of identified deficiencies.
    v. Essential fatty acid intake may optimize brain development and cognition in nursing infants (Nevins et al., 2021).
3. Additional health maintenance counseling should include the following:
    a. Signs and symptoms that require immediate evaluation
    b. Resumption of routine gynecological and primary care
    c. Self-knowledge and examination (e.g., chest and skin)
    d. Sexual health
    e. Pelvic muscle tone and continence: There is currently insufficient data to advise routine pelvic floor muscle training after childbirth for the prevention of postpartum urinary or fecal incontinence (WHO, 2022). If urinary or fecal incontinence is present, advise that this is commonly reported by 25%–45% of people, particularly those who have experienced pregnancy, labor, and vaginal birth, although the relevance of these risk factors decreases substantially with age as the overall incidence increases (Dumoulin et al., 2018). Pelvic floor muscle training, pessary fitting, and surgical intervention may be discussed and referred if incontinence does not improve within 1–2 months' postpartum (Dumoulin et al., 2018).

D. *Consultation and referral as indicated*
    1. Conditions that warrant medical consultation or referral may include but are not limited to the following:
        a. Endometritis
        b. Infection or dehiscence of surgical site or perineal laceration site
        c. Excessive or prolonged vaginal bleeding
        d. Abscess within the mammary tissue
        e. Postpartum thyroiditis
        f. Chronic medical conditions requiring follow-up, if outside of the advanced practice nurse's scope of practice
        g. Intimate partner violence
        h. Poor parental adaptation
        i. Postpartum depression, anxiety, mania, or psychosis
        j. Substance abuse treatment
        k. Suspected child abuse or neglect (notify pediatrician and child protective services)
        l. Housing, food, and financial assistance programs
    2. Local and web-based resources
        a. Public health programs, visiting nurses' associations, lactation consultants, nutritionists, chestfeeding/breastfeeding and birth trauma support groups, therapists, social workers, psychologists, psychiatrists, and postpartum doulas may have services for the evaluation, monitoring, and treatment of select parental physical and psychosocial problems and infant/chestfeeding/breastfeeding concerns.
        b. New parents can be encouraged to seek support groups and other services for new parents, particularly if they lack family and social support; experienced childbirth-related trauma; or have special circumstances, such as multiples or perinatal loss. Online forums may be a useful adjunctive or primary source of meaningful support if local resources are limited, particularly for patients with unusual diagnoses or infants with rare conditions that are not addressed by programs in the community.
    3. Primary care
    Parents and their families need a medical home for ongoing health maintenance. This might be a practice setting led by a nurse practitioner or midwife, a community clinic, or other primary care location. Postpartum patients may be guided to access ongoing health care elsewhere if they will not remain in your practice beyond the postpartum period.
    Advanced practice clinicians are uniquely situated to have a profound effect on the health of families.

The relationships we establish with our patients in the antepartum period, as we assist them to have the safest and healthiest pregnancies possible, provides the platform for further growth in the postpartum period. Advanced practice nurses can and do have an ongoing positive impact on the lives of our patients and their families, ideally resulting in intergenerational health promotion and improved public health.

References

Aderhold, K. J., & Perry, L. (1991). Jet hydrotherapy for labor and postpartum pain relief. *MCN: The American Journal of Maternal Child Nursing, 16*(2), 97–99. doi:10.1097/00005721-199103000-00013

Alcorn, K. L., O'Donovan, A., Patrick, J. C., Creedy, D., & Devilly, G. J. (2010). A prospective longitudinal study of the prevalence of post-traumatic stress disorder resulting from childbirth events. *Psychological Medicine, 40*(11), 1849–1859. doi:10.1017/S0033291709992224

American College of Obstetricians and Gynecologists. (2018). ACOG Committee Opinion No. 736: Optimizing postpartum care. *Obstetrics & Gynecology, 131*(5), e140–e150. doi:10.1097/AOG.0000000000002633

American College of Obstetricians and Gynecologists. (2019). Practice Bulletin No. 205: Vaginal birth after cesarean delivery. *Obstetrics and Gynecology, 133*(2), e110–e127. doi:10.1097/AOG.0000000000003078

Amorim, A. R., Linne, Y. M., & Lourenco, P. M. (2013). Diet or exercise, or both, for weight reduction in women after childbirth. *Cochrane Database of Systematic Reviews, 2013*(7), CD005627.

Asadzadeh, L., Jafari, E., Kharaghani, R., & Taremian, F. (2020). Effectiveness of midwife-led brief counseling intervention on post-traumatic stress disorder, depression, and anxiety symptoms of women experiencing a traumatic childbirth: A randomized controlled trial. *BMC Pregnancy and Childbirth, 20*(1), 142. doi:10.1186/s12884-020-2826-1

Association of Women's Health, Obstetric and Neonatal Nurses. (2020). *The compendium of postpartum care* (3rd ed.).

Attanasio, L. B., Ranchoff, B. L., & Geissler, K. H. (2021). Perceived discrimination during the childbirth hospitalization and postpartum visit attendance and content: Evidence from the Listening to Mothers in California survey. *PloS One, 16*(6), e0253055. doi:10.1371/journal.pone.0253055

Barimani, M., Oxelmark, L., Johansson, S., & Highland, I. (2015). Support and continuity during the first 2 weeks postpartum. *Scandinavian Journal of Caring Sciences, 29*(3), 409–417. doi:10.1111/scs.12144

Bastos, M. H., Furuta, M., Small, R., McKenzie-McHarg, K., & Bick, D. (2015). Debriefing interventions for the prevention of psychological trauma in women following childbirth. *Cochrane Database of Systematic Reviews, 2015*(4), CD007194. doi:10.1002/14651858.CD007194.pub2

Batten, M., Stevenson, E., Zimmermann, D., & Isaacs, C. (2017). Implementation of a hydrotherapy protocol to improve postpartum pain management. *Journal of Midwifery & Women's Health, 62*(2), 210–214. doi:10.1111/jmwh.12580

Centers for Medicare and Medicaid Services. (2015). *Resources on strategies to improve postpartum care among Medicaid and CHIP populations.*

Cerimele, J., Vanderlip, E., Croicu, C., Melville, J., Russo, J., Reed, S., & Katon, W. (2013). Presenting symptoms of women with depression in an obstetrics and gynecology setting. *Obstetrics & Gynecology, 122*(2), 313–318. doi:10.1097/AOG.0b013e31829999ee

Declercq, E. R., Sakala, C., Corry, M. P., Applebaum, S., & Herrlich, A. (2013). *Listening to mothers III: New mothers speak out.* Childbirth Connection.

Dekel, S., Stuebe, C., & Dishy, G. (2017). Childbirth induced post-traumatic stress syndrome: A systematic review of prevalence and risk factors. *Frontiers in Psychology, 8,* 560. doi:10.3389/fpsyg.2017.00560

Dennis, C. L., Fung, K., Grigoriadis, S., Robinson, G. E., Romans, S., & Ross, L. (2007). Traditional postpartum practices and rituals: A qualitative systematic review. *Women's Health, 3*(4), 487–502. doi:10.2217/17455057.3.4.487

DiBari, J., Yu, S., Chao, S., & Lu, M. (2014). Use of postpartum care: Predictors and barriers. *Journal of Pregnancy, 2014,* 530769. doi:10.1155/2014/530769

Druzin, M., Shields, L., Peterson, N., Sakowski, C., Cape, V., & Morton, C. (2021). *Improving health care response to hypertensive disorders of pregnancy, a California Maternal Quality Care Collaborative quality improvement toolkit.* California Maternal Quality Care Collaborative.

Dumoulin, C., Cacciari, L. P., & Hay-Smith, E. (2018). Pelvic floor muscle training versus no treatment, or inactive control treatments, for urinary incontinence in women. *Cochrane Database of Systematic Reviews, 2018*(10), CD005654. doi:10.1002/14651858.CD005654.pub2

East, C. E., Dorward, E. D., Whale, R. E., & Liu, J. (2020). Local cooling for relieving pain from perineal trauma sustained during childbirth. *Cochrane Database of Systematic Reviews, 2020*(10), CD006304. doi:10.1002/14651858

Evenson, K. R., Mottola, M. F., Owe, K. M., Rousham, E. K., & Brown, W. J. (2014). Summary of international guidelines for physical activity after pregnancy. *Obstetrical & Gynecological Survey, 69*(7), 407–414. doi:10.1097/OGX.0000000000000077

Gomes, S., Lopes, C., & Pinto, E. (2015). Folate and folic acid in the periconceptional period: Recommendations from official health organizations in thirty-six countries worldwide and WHO. *Public Health Nutrition, 19*(1), 176–189. doi:10.1017/S1368980015000555

Greenfield, M., & Darwin, Z. (2021). Trans and non-binary pregnancy, traumatic birth, and perinatal mental health: A scoping review. *International Journal of Transgender Health, 22*(1–2), 203–216. doi:10.1080/26895269.2020.1841057

Grotell, L., Byson, L., Florence, A., & Fogel, J. (2021). Postpartum note template implementation demonstrates adherence to recommended counseling guidelines. *Journal of Medical Systems, 45*(1), 14. doi:10.1007/s10916-020-01692-6

Guille, C., & Douglas, E. (2017). Telephone delivery of interpersonal psychotherapy by certified nurse-midwives may help reduce symptoms of postpartum depression. *Evidence-Based Nursing, 20*(1), 12–13. doi:10.1136/eb-2016-102513

Hedayati, H., Parsons, J., & Crowther, C. A. (2005). Topically applied anaesthetics for treating perineal pain after childbirth.

Cochrane Database of Systematic Reviews, 2005(2), CD004223. doi:10.1002/14651858.CD004223.pub2

Jouanne, M., Oddoux, S., Noël, A., & Voisin-Chiret, A. S. (2021). Nutrient requirements during pregnancy and lactation. *Nutrients, 13*(2), 692. doi:10.3390/nu13020692

Kennedy, K. I., & Goldsmith, C. (2018). Contraception after pregnancy. In R. A. Hatcher, A. L. Nelson, J. Trussell, C. Cwik, P. Cason, M. S. Policar, A. B. Edelman, A. R. A. Aiken, J. M. Marrazzo, & D. Kowal (Eds.), *Contraceptive technology* (21st ed., pp. 511–541). Ayer Company.

Lassi, Z. S., & Bhutta, Z. A. (2015). Community-based intervention packages for reducing maternal and neonatal morbidity and mortality and improving neonatal outcomes. *Cochrane Database of Systematic Reviews, 2015*(3), CD007754. doi:10.1002/14651858.CD007754.pub3

Lavender, T., Richens, Y., Milan, S., Smyth, R., & Dowswell, T. (2013, July 18). Telephone support for women during pregnancy and the first six weeks postpartum. *Cochrane Database of Systematic Reviews, 2013*(7), CD009338. doi:10.1002/14651858.CD009338.pub2

Liu, X., Wang, S., & Wang, G. (2021). Prevalence and risk factors of postpartum depression in women: A systematic review and meta-analysis. *Journal of Clinical Nursing, 31*(19–20), 2665–2677. doi:10.1111/jocn.16121.

Louis, J. M., Bryant, A., Ramos, D., Stuebe, A., & Blackwell, S. C. (2019). Interpregnancy care. *American Journal of Obstetrics and Gynecology, 220*(1), B2–B18. doi:10.1016/j.ajog.2018.11.1098

Makins, A., & Cameron, S. (2020). Post pregnancy contraception. *Best Practice & Research. Clinical Obstetrics & Gynaecology, 66*, 41–54. doi:10.1016/j.bpobgyn.2020.01.004

Nelson, A., & Harwood, B. (2018). Contraception after pregnancy. In R. A. Hatcher, A. L. Nelson, J. Trussell, C. Cwik, P. Cason, M. S. Policar, A. B. Edelman, A. R. A. Aiken, J. M. Marrazzo, & D. Kowal (Eds.), *Contraceptive Technology* (21st ed., pp. 511–541). Ayer Company.

Nevins, J. E. H., Donovan, S. M., Snetselaar, L., Dewey, K. G., Novotny, R., Stang, J., Taveras, E. M., Kleinman, R. E., Bailey, R. L., Raghavan, R., Scinto-Madonich, S. R., Venkatramanan, S., Butera, G., Terry, N., Altman, J., Adler, M., Obbagy, J. E., Stoody, E. E., & de Jesus, J. (2021). Omega-3 fatty acid dietary supplements consumed during pregnancy and lactation and child neurodevelopment: A systematic review. *Journal of Nutrition, 151*(11), 3483–3494. doi:10.1093/jn/nxab238

Office of Disease Prevention and Health Promotion. (n.d.). *Pregnancy and childbirth. Healthy People 2030*. U.S. Department of Health and Human Services. https://health.gov/healthypeople/objectives-and-data/browse-objectives/pregnancy-and-childbirth

Poyatos-León, R., García-Hermoso, A., Sanabria-Martínez, G., Álvarez-Bueno, C., Cavero-Redondo, I., & Martínez-Vizcaíno, V. (2017). Effects of exercise-based interventions on postpartum depression: A meta-analysis of randomized controlled trials. *Birth, 44*(3), 200–208. doi:10.1111/birt.12294

Sakala, C., Declercq, E. R., Turon, J. M., & Corry, M. P. (2018). *Listening to Mothers in California: A population-based survey of women's childbearing experiences, full survey report*. National Partnership for Women & Families.

Sandall, J., Soltani, H., Gates, S., Shennan, A., & Devane, D. (2015). Midwife-led continuity models versus other models of care for childbearing women. *Cochrane Database of Systematic Reviews, 2015*(9), CD004667. doi:10.1002/14651858.CD004667.pub3

Sridhar, A., & Salcedo, J. (2017). Optimizing maternal and neonatal outcomes with postpartum contraception: impact on breastfeeding and birth spacing. *Maternal Health, Neonatology and Perinatology, 3*, 1. doi:10.1186/s40748-016-0040-y

Tepper, N. K., Phillips, S. J., Kapp, N., Gaffield, M. E., & Curtis, K. M. (2015, May 19). Combined hormonal contraceptive use among breastfeeding women: An updated systematic review. *Contraception, 94*(3), 262–274. doi:10.1016/j.contraception.2015.05.006

Vedam, S., Stoll, K., Taiwo, T.K. et al. (2019). The Giving Voice to Mothers study: Inequity and mistreatment during pregnancy and childbirth in the United States. *Reproductive Health 16*, 77. https://doi.org/10.1186/s12978-019-0729-2

Wallace, C., Farmer, J., & McCosker, A. (2018). Community boundary spanners as an addition to the health workforce to reach marginalised people: A scoping review of the literature. *Human Resources for Health, 16*(1), 46. doi:10.1186/s12960-018-0310-z

Wang, Z., Liu, J., Shuai, H. et al. (2021). Mapping global prevalence of depression among postpartum women. *Translational Psychiatry* 11, 543 (2021). https://doi.org/10.1038/s41398-021-01663-6

World Health Organization. (2015). *Medical eligibility criteria for contraceptive use* (5th ed.). https://www.who.int/publications/i/item/9789241549158

World Health Organization. (2022). *Recommendations on maternal and newborn care for a positive postnatal experience*.

Yang, M., Yue, W., Han, X., Hu, C., Sun, X., & Luo, J. (2022). Postpartum care indications and methodological quality: A systematic review of guidelines. *Journal of Public Health, 30*(9), 2261–2275. doi:10.1007/s10389-021-01629-4

Yildiz, P. D., Ayers, S., & Phillips, L. (2017). The prevalence of posttraumatic stress disorder in pregnancy and after birth: A systematic review and meta-analysis. *Journal of Affective Disorders, 208*, 634–645. doi:10.1016/j.jad.2016.10.009

Yonemoto, N., Nagai, S., & Mori, R. (2021, July 21). Schedules for home visits in the early postpartum period. *Cochrane Database of Systematic Reviews, 2021*(8), CD009326. doi:10.1002/14651858.CD009326.pub3

Zhang, M. M., Zou, Y., Li, S. M., Wang, L., Sun, Y. H., Shi, L., Lu, L., Bao, Y. P., & Li, S. X. (2020). The efficacy and safety of omega-3 fatty acids on depressive symptoms in perinatal women: A meta-analysis of randomized placebo-controlled trials. *Translational Psychiatry, 10*(1), 193. doi:10.1038/s41398-020-00886-3

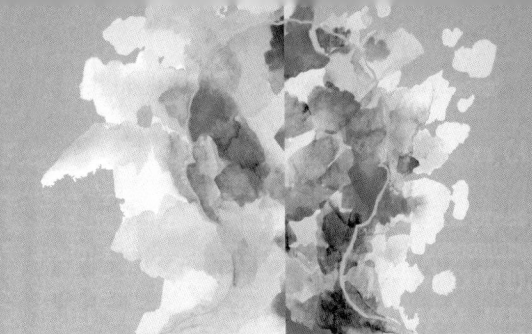

CHAPTER 30

Guidelines for Medical Consultation, Interprofessional Collaboration, and Transfer of Care During Pregnancy and Childbirth

Jenna Shaw-Battista and Annette Fineberg

I. Introduction and general background

Pregnant people are frequently dichotomized as being at "low" or "high" risk for suboptimal perinatal outcomes despite a continuum of medical and obstetric risk. Integrating nurse practitioners, nurse-midwives, and physician assistants into obstetric care provided at any level of risk is a safe and effective way to improve care with appropriate stratification, delineation of scope and responsibilities, and communication between care providers (American College of Nurse-Midwives [ACNM] & American College of Obstetricians and Gynecologists [ACOG], 2011; Smith et al., 2016). Nurse practitioners and midwives provide independent, comprehensive, and holistic care for low-risk pregnancies, with benefits including facilitation of normal term deliveries, less use of obstetric interventions, and high levels of patient satisfaction (ACNM et al., 2013; Renfrew et al., 2014; Sandall et al., 2016). At the other end of the spectrum are pregnancies complicated by high-risk medical conditions affecting either the patient or their fetus(es) and unstable and severe complications of pregnancy and parturition. In these situations, physician care and referral to perinatology or neonatology services are immediately indicated (AGOG, 2019b). In the middle are pregnant people with one or more moderate risk factors, for whom consultation and referral to medical providers by advanced practice clinicians are less clear. This is due to a lack of robust studies to guide many perinatal clinical management decisions, including the selection of healthcare provider type (Brock et al., 2021; Chauhan et al., 2016; Gutierrez et al., 2022).

Gray areas in clinical decision making ethically necessitate partnership with individuals to develop care plans guided by their values, culture, and preferences for providers and care practices (ACOG, 2016). Individual clinicians' experience, skill set, values, and scope of practice influence clinical decisions, including consultations, collaborations, and referrals. Additional influential factors include state and federal regulatory language; institutional policies and interprofessional practice protocols; research findings; community standards; healthcare ethics; and financial considerations (ACNM & ACOG, 2011; AGOG, 2016; Renfrew et al., 2014; Sandall et al., 2016). Within this complex context, nurse practitioners and nurse-midwives frequently collaborate with physician colleagues to care for pregnant people with perinatal risk factors for adverse outcomes and high-risk conditions, including selected disorders of the endocrine, cardiovascular, hematologic, neurologic, musculoskeletal, pulmonary, gastrointestinal, and renal systems and specific psychiatric diagnoses, infectious diseases, malignancies, and abnormal diagnostic testing (ACNM & ACOG, 2011; AGOG, 2016; Office of Technology Assessment, 1986; Renfrew et al., 2014; Sandall et al., 2016).

A. *Perinatal risk factors and complications include but are not limited to the following:*
   1. History of pregnancy or childbirth complications
      a. Gestational diabetes, hypertensive disorder, or other pregnancy complication
      b. Habitual abortion (<12–20 weeks' gestation), stillbirth (≥20 weeks' gestation), or death of a newborn or infant in the first year of life
      c. Large- or small-for-gestational-age infant
      d. Preterm delivery
      e. Dystocia, maternal or neonatal birth injury, postpartum hemorrhage, or other complication of parturition
      f. Previous cesarean section or other uterine surgery
   2. Variants and complications of current pregnancy and parturition
      a. Prenatal diagnosis of minor or major fetal anomaly
      b. Multiple gestation
      c. Nonvertex fetal presentation at term or fetal malpresentation incompatible with vaginal birth
      d. Prolonged pregnancy (41–42 weeks' gestation) or postterm pregnancy (≥42 weeks' gestation)
      e. Preterm labor or ruptured membranes before term (20–36 weeks' gestation)
      f. Prolonged premature rupture of membranes at term
      g. Polyhydramnios or oligohydramnios
      h. Abnormal placentation (e.g., previa or accreta)
      i. Unexplained vaginal bleeding
      j. Rhesus factor sensitization or other immunoglobulin G (IgG) antibody sensitization
      k. Hypertensive disorders (essential or gestational hypertension, or preeclampsia–eclampsia)
      l. Hemolysis, elevated liver enzymes, and low platelets syndrome
      m. Idiopathic thrombocytopenic purpura
      n. Cholestasis of pregnancy
      o. Preexisting or gestational diabetes mellitus
      p. Selected anemias or hemoglobinopathies (e.g., thalassemias and hemoglobin less than 10 g/dL, not responsive to iron therapy)
      q. Sickle cell crisis
   3. Selected gestational parent infections with potential fetal sequelae (e.g., HIV, cytomegalovirus, parvovirus, rubella, syphilis, toxoplasmosis, primary herpes infection, or presence of genital lesions at term)
   4. Additional maternal illnesses (e.g., unstable new or chronic health conditions, severe asthma requiring hospitalization during pregnancy, autoimmune disorders, cardiac disease other than asymptomatic mitral valve prolapse, renal disease, recurrent urinary tract infections, or thyroid disorders)
   5. Psychosocial risk factors (e.g., psychiatric diagnoses, substance abuse, interpersonal violence, social deprivation, poverty, or homelessness)

B. *Intrapartum and postpartum complications and procedures for which medical consultation, co-management, or referral is recommended include the following:*
   1. Preterm labor and delivery
   2. Induction or augmentation of labor
   3. Prodromal or protracted labor or arrest of labor or fetal descent
   4. Abnormal fetal surveillance and variant fetal heart rate tracings (category II and III)
   5. Amnioinfusion
   6. Prolapsed cord
   7. Chorioamnionitis or other intrapartum infection
   8. Abnormal vaginal bleeding in labor
   9. Anticipated or actual shoulder dystocia
   10. Indications for, and occurrence of, operative vaginal delivery or cesarean section
   11. Severe perineal laceration (third or fourth degree) or cervical laceration
   12. Prolonged third stage of labor (>30 minutes), with or without postpartum hemorrhage (>500–1,000 mL)
   13. Unstable genitourinary hematoma
   14. New disease or exacerbation of chronic illness of the pregnant person
   15. Child abuse or neglect, suspected or observed (notify pediatrician and child protective services)
   16. Neonatal health conditions, anticipated or observed

Figure 30-1 contains an algorithm for medical consultation and referral during pregnancy. Interprofessional

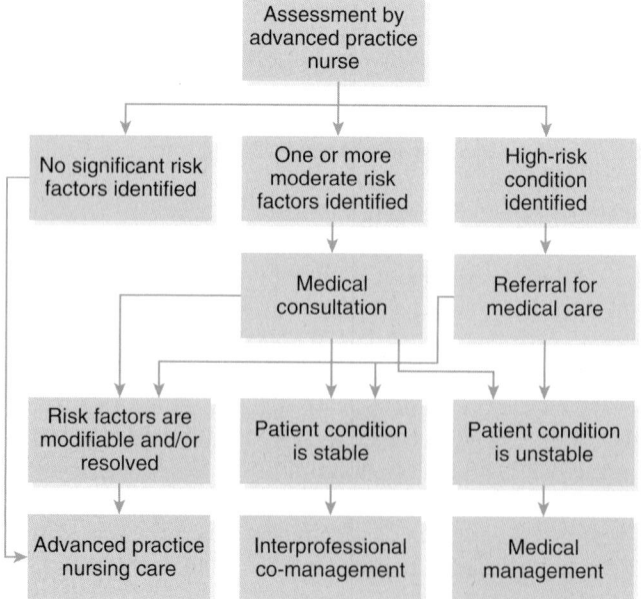

Figure 30-1 Algorithm for medical consultation and referral during pregnancy.

practices benefit from applied algorithms in the form of clinical guidelines and written policies regarding methods and types of consultation and referral in their practice settings. These and other formal and informal strategies to encourage interprofessional communication and standardize collaborations may facilitate mutual understanding of varied scopes of practice and improve care team efficacy and job satisfaction, along with patient outcomes (Hamlin et al., 2021; Hutchison et al., 2011; Reeves et al., 2017; Sandall et al., 2016; Shaw-Battista et al., 2011).

Interprofessional guidelines for maternity care frequently describe consultation and co-management of individuals with specific medical, obstetric, and neonatal risk factors. Varied levels of consultation may be delineated, with or without direct physical assessment and documentation of collaborative management plans required of the medical consultant for specific diagnoses. When pregnant people experience complications that require ongoing medical or obstetric management or co-management, transfer of care to a physician rather than consultation may be indicated. High-risk patients may return to nurse practitioner or nurse-midwife care for pregnancy or childbirth care if their condition stabilizes and collaborative or independent advanced practice nursing care becomes feasible and mutually agreeable.

For many childbearing individuals, risk status and maternity care provider type are determined by the severity and number of risk factors rather than the presence of a specific condition. For example, nurse practitioners and nurse-midwives may independently or collaboratively care for individuals with gestational diabetes who can maintain euglycemia with diet and exercise or oral hypoglycemic agents, but they may comanage care with obstetrician colleagues if insulin becomes necessary or transfer care to physicians if blood sugars are poorly controlled regardless of treatment type (ACOG, 2018b; Qiu et al., 2020). Similarly, collaborative practice guidelines may suggest transfer to physician care when individuals have severe hypertensive disorders of pregnancy or require pharmacological treatment (e.g., antihypertensive medications or magnesium sulfate for seizure prophylaxis) but endorse independent advance practice nursing care or interprofessional co-management of individuals with mild, stable gestational hypertension or preeclampsia (e.g., no pharmacological treatment is required, or the physician provides medication management while the nurse practitioner or nurse-midwife continues other aspects of maternity care) (Shaw-Battista et al., 2011). These details, and other specifics of clinical protocols and collaborative practice agreements, necessarily differ among practice sites. Variation also occurs over time as interprofessional practices evolve in response to changes in clinical team members, patient populations, and supportive data (Reeves et al., 2017). **Table 30-1** contains a sample policy for outpatient obstetric providers and obstetric physician consultants available to accept transfers of care during pregnancy as indicated.

In some cases, obstetrical consultation, collaboration, and referral may not be required for a preexisting physiologic condition or new complication of pregnancy but is instead indicated for a behavioral health and psychosocial concern that warrants further evaluation and treatment. In this case, physician consultation, collaboration, and referral considerations by advanced practice clinicians are largely dictated by the expertise and availability of providers in the region. For example, a high-risk maternal–fetal medicine service may offer comprehensive perinatal substance use treatment within behavioral health services in one community, whereas parturients with these treatment needs in other regions may be best served by nurse-midwives collaborating with behavioral health colleagues in specialized programs offered in public or community healthcare settings. Regardless of treatment referral destination, interprofessional colleagues and collaborative maternity care teams benefit when individual practice guidelines specify consultation, collaboration, or referral by a nurse practitioner or nurse-midwife caring for pregnant persons with significant psychosocial risk factors for adverse perinatal and primary healthcare outcomes.

Among the psychosocial impacts on perinatal care are patients who decline or request obstetric intervention contrary to standards of care and provider recommendations. Examples include pregnant persons who decline recommended testing or expedited delivery and those on the other side of the spectrum of obstetric intervention who request elective cesarean or induction of labor without medical indication. Written policies and procedures are useful to guide interprofessional team members and specify roles and responsibilities related to health education, informed consent, and any required documentation when patients choose care counter to medical advice. In addition to consultation and collaboration among maternity care providers, cases may benefit from the involvement of other care team members as indicated by the particular clinical and psychosocial situation (e.g., pediatrics, social work, psychiatry, ethical review, chaplain).

Requests for elective obstetric interventions should be approached with curiosity about motivating factors and knowledge base, and patients should be provided health education, including the standard to wait until 39 weeks' gestation. The informed consent process best occurs between pregnant persons and their prenatal care providers, including nurse practitioners or midwives and any consulting physician as required by site-specific policies and procedures. The balance of risks versus benefits of elective deliveries is decided by a pregnant person and their care providers, with reference to research and clinical guidance by professional organizations (ACOG, 2009, 2018a, 2019a; National Institutes of Health [NIH], 2006, 2010; Society for Maternal-Fetal Medicine, 2019).

Requests for elective cesareans should trigger comprehensive psychosocial assessment, including trauma, phobias, and conditions that may be responsive to treatment and educational interventions before term in order to limit the primary cesarean birth rate and related morbidity and mortality (ACOG, 2019a; Evans et al., 2022; NIH, 2006). Ultimately, a patient persistently requesting

Table 30-1 Sample Guidelines for Consultation and Referral During Pregnancy

Conditions Requiring Obstetric Physician Consultation

Conditions of the Pregnant Person
- Pelvic mass noted by physical exam or ultrasound
- Uterine malformations
- Patients with large fibroids in the lower uterine segment
- Infections with potential fetal sequelae (e.g., toxoplasmosis, cytomegalovirus)
- Recurrent pyelonephritis
- Nephrolithiasis
- Persistent severe anemia with hematocrit < 9 g/dL) despite iron therapy
- History of thromboembolic disease regardless of etiology
- Hypothyroidism not well controlled with thyroid replacement
- Seizure disorder well controlled with medication
- Extremely low or high body weight, or other significant concern for nutrition or mobility ≥ 45
- Chronic hypertension diagnosed before pregnancy
- Active drug or alcohol use
- Mental illness characterized by the use of psychotropic medication, history of suicide attempts, violence, trauma, or hospitalization for psychiatric problems, with a probability of recurrence

Fetal Conditions
- Intrauterine growth restriction with ultrasound-estimated fetal weight ≤ 10th percentile
- Fetal macrosomia with estimated fetal weight ≥ 95th percentile on ultrasound
- Oligohydramnios
- Polyhydramnios
- Any fetal structural abnormality detected by ultrasound
- Antibodies to C, c, D, Kell, E, e, or Duffy with titers < 1:8 or rising titers

Obstetrical History
- Recurrent pregnancy loss: history of ≥ 3 spontaneous abortions if under age 35, or ≥ 2 if over age 35
- History of uterine cavity surgery other than cesarean birth

Conditions Requiring Transfer of Care to High-Risk Obstetric Service

Conditions of the Pregnant Person
- Hypertension in pregnancy requiring medication
- Active or uncontrolled seizure disorder
- Severe asthma with hospitalization for asthma during pregnancy
- Cardiac disease (except asymptomatic mitral valve prolapse)
- Pulmonary hypertension
- Platelet count less than 100,000
- Deep vein thrombosis
- Sickle cell disease
- Lupus/scleroderma/any connective tissue disease
- Cancer
- Active tuberculosis
- Active viral hepatitis
- HIV positive
- Hyperthyroidism
- Diabetes: type 1, type 2, or poorly controlled gestational diabetes requiring medication
- Hyperemesis gravidarum with hospital admission, until resolved
- Paraplegia or quadriplegia

Fetal Conditions
- Complete placenta previa or partial previa in the third trimester
- Chronic placental abruption diagnosed by hospital admission
- Presence of antibodies to C, c, D, Kell, E, e, or Duffy, with antibody titers ≥ 1:8
- Multiple gestation

Obstetrical History
- Incompetent cervix or history suggestive thereof (i.e., painless cervical dilatation <24 weeks' gestation)

elective cesarean would require referral to a surgeon for further assessment and counseling done on an individual basis that considers the reason for the request, parturient age and parity, plan for future fertility, and any pregnancy complications or preexisting health conditions, with reference to national guidelines that acknowledge significantly greater risks after cesarean among people planning future pregnancies compared to those who do not plan future pregnancies (ACOG, 2019a; NIH, 2006, 2010).

Elective induction of labor is much more common than elective cesarean delivery upon request, particularly since the landmark ARRIVE trial publication

(Grobman et al., 2018), leading to an increase in elective induction of labor rates despite substantial critique of the research, including selection bias and lack of ability to generalize or reproduce study conclusions (Carmichael & Snowden, 2019; Grobman et al., 2018). Site guidelines should specify the informed consent process for elective inductions, which ideally occurs between a pregnant person and their prenatal and intrapartum care providers and includes the risks and benefits of induction of labor, what to expect during the process of cervical ripening and labor induction, and research outcomes of expectant management versus elective inductions of labor at 39–41 weeks' gestation. Pregnant persons who prefer "natural childbirth" without pharmacological pain relief methods should be advised that research shows that induction and augmentation of labor result in more requests for pain medication and regional anesthesia compared to people coping with spontaneous labor (National Collaborating Centre for Women's and Children's Health UK, 2008). Although the ARRIVE trial findings suggested that cesarean deliveries may be decreased with elective labor induction versus spontaneous labor at 39–41 weeks, these findings cannot be generalized to more diverse patient populations than the low-risk study group or to facilities with baseline cesarean rates that are considerably different than the study sites' underlying risk of cesarean, which was slightly less than 1 in every 4 deliveries (Carmichael & Snowden, 2019; Grobman et al., 2018). ARRIVE trial data regarding cesarean sections should be considered alongside other well-established, evidence-based approaches to decreasing the rate of unindicated cesareans, which include midwifery care, continuous labor support, upright positions and activity in labor, and intermittent fetal heart rate monitoring for healthy perinatal populations (ACOG, 2014; Renfrew et al., 2014; Sandall et al., 2016). The complex informed consent conversations about elective induction of labor need not require the participation of an advanced practice clinician's collaborating physician, although discussion and agreement about elective delivery clinical policies and procedures and key components of informed consent are recommended for interprofessional care teams. Physician consultation at the time of patient admission for labor induction initiation by an advanced practice clinicians may be desired by individual obstetricians or required by practice and hospital policies.

Regardless of the indication for collaborative care, co-management must include ongoing communication among providers to ensure patient safety (Reeves et al., 2017). The structure of interprofessional communication varies among sites but typically includes periodic conversations about specific patients to achieve consensus about management plans via electronic medical record, telephone, secure email, or in person, depending on patient acuity and timeliness of necessary decision making. Interprofessional practices may use regularly scheduled meetings to discuss their higher-risk prenatal caseload over time, which formalizes the co-management process and ensures timely review of evolving health conditions to facilitate optimal outcomes. These interprofessional communications about risk assessment and plans of care should be documented in the medical record, along with routine charting following clinical encounters and any written consultant reports. Patients should be kept apprised of changing assessments; participate in formulating and revising care plans; and receive information about healthcare providers' responsibilities and relationships upon initiating care and when consultation, co-management, or transfer of care occurs.

In addition to formal interprofessional relationships, effective communications, and shared clinical guidelines, optimal perinatal outcomes are fostered through collegial interactions that are characterized by mutual respect, professionalism, and trust (ACNM & ACOG, 2011). Shared goals related to high-quality patient-centered care, healthcare education, research, and public health may also strengthen interprofessional practice relations (Avery et al., 2012; Hutchison et al., 2011; King et al., 2012; Shaw-Battista et al., 2011). Interprofessional clinical practices that include nurse practitioners and nurse-midwives contribute to public health by increasing access to safe and effective maternity care with comprehensive physiological and psychosocial support services, facilitation of normal childbirth, and decreased use of unnecessary costly obstetric interventions among childbearing individuals across the spectrum of health and perinatal risk (Hoope-Bender et al., 2014; Renfrew et al., 2014; Sandall et al., 2016). Public health policies and clinical organizations should support nurse- and midwife-led care and interprofessional team-based care as alternatives to conventional physician-led maternity care service models (Hoope-Bender et al., 2014; Renfrew et al., 2014; Sandall et al., 2016).

References

American College of Nurse-Midwives & American College of Obstetricians and Gynecologists. (2011). *Joint statement of practice relations between obstetrician-gynecologists and certified nurse-midwives/certified midwives* [reaffirmed 2021]. American College of Nurse-Midwives.

American College of Nurse-Midwives, Midwives Alliance of North America, & National Association of Certified Professional Midwives. (2013). Supporting healthy and normal physiologic childbirth: A consensus statement by ACNM, MANA, and NACPM. *Journal of Perinatal Education*, 22(1), 14–18. doi:10.1891/1058-1243.22.1.14.

American College of Obstetricians and Gynecologists. (2009). Practice Bulletin No. 107: Induction of labor. *Obstetrics & Gynecology*, 114(2, Pt. 1), 386–397. doi:10.1097/AOG.0b013e3181b48ef5

American College of Obstetricians and Gynecologists. (2014). Safe prevention of the primary cesarean delivery. Obstetric Care

Consensus No. 1. *Obstetrics & Gynecology, 123*(3), 693–711. doi:10.1097/01.AOG.0000444441.04111.1d

American College of Obstetricians and Gynecologists. (2016). Committee Opinion No. 664: Refusal of medically recommended treatment during pregnancy [reaffirmed 2022]. *Obstetrics & Gynecology, 127*(6), e175–182. doi:10.1097/AOG.0000000000001485

American College of Obstetricians and Gynecologists. (2018a). *Practice advisory: Clinical guidance for integration of the findings of the ARRIVE trial: Labor induction versus expectant management in low-risk nulliparous women*. https://www.acog.org/clinical/clinical-guidance/practice-advisory/articles/2018/08/clinical-guidance-for-integration-of-the-findings-of-the-arrive-trial?utm_source=redirect&utm_medium=web&utm_campaign=otn

American College of Obstetricians and Gynecologists. (2018b). Practice Bulletin No. 190: Gestational diabetes mellitus. *Obstetrics & Gynecology, 131*(2), e49–e64. doi:10.1097/AOG.0000000000002501

American College of Obstetricians and Gynecologists. (2019a). Committee Opinion No. 761: Cesarean delivery on maternal request. *Obstetrics & Gynecology, 133*(1), e73–77. doi:10.1097/AOG.0000000000003006

American College of Obstetricians and Gynecologists. (2019b). Obstetric Care Consensus No. 9: Levels of maternal care [reaffirmed 2021]. *Obstetrics & Gynecology, 134*(4), e41–55. doi:10.1097/AOG.0000000000003495

Avery, M. D., Montgomery, O., & Brandl-Salutz, E. (2012). Essential components of successful collaborative maternity care models: The ACOG-ACNM project. *Obstetrics and Gynecology Clinics of North America, 39*(3), 423–434. doi:10.1016/j.ogc.2012.05.010

Brock, C. O., Blackwell, S. C., & Chauhan, S. P. (2021). Assessment of evidence underlying guidelines by the Society for Maternal-Fetal Medicine. *American Journal of Obstetrics and Gynecology, 224*(2), 223, e1–10. doi:10.1016/j.ajog.2020.08.052

Carmichael, S. L., & Snowden, J. M. (2019). The ARRIVE trial: Interpretation from an epidemiologic perspective. *Journal of Midwifery and Women's Health, 64*(5), 657–663. doi:10.1111/jmwh.12996

Chauhan, S., Hammad, I., Weyer, K., & Ananth, C. (2016). False alarms, pseudoepidemics, and reality: A case study with American College of Obstetricians and Gynecologists practice bulletins. *American Journal of Perinatology, 33*(5), 442–448. doi:10.1055/s-0035-1566247

Evans, K., Fraser, H., Uthman, O., Osokogu, O., Johnson, S., & Al-Khudairy, L. (2022). The effect of mode of delivery on health-related quality-of-life in mothers: A systematic review and meta-analysis. *BMC Pregnancy and Childbirth, 22*(1), 149. doi:10.1186/s12884-022-04473-w

Grobman, W. A., Rice, M. M., Reddy, U. M., Tita, A., Silver, R. M., Mallett, G., Hill, K., Thom, E. A., El-Sayed, Y. Y., Perez-Delboy, A., Rouse, D. J., Saade, G. R., Boggess, K. A., Chauhan, S. P., Iams, J. D., Chien, E. K., Casey, B. M., Gibbs, R. S., Srinivas, S. K., . . . Eunice Kennedy Shriver National Institute of Child Health and Human Development Maternal–Fetal Medicine Units Network. (2018). Labor induction versus expectant management in low-risk nulliparous women. *New England Journal of Medicine, 379*(6), 513–523. doi:10.1056/NEJMoa1800566

Gutierrez, R., Bicocca, M., Opara, G., Gupta, M., Bartal, M. F., Chauhan, S. P., & Wagner, S. (2022). Incorporation of randomized controlled trials into organizational guidelines for obstetricians and gynecologists. *European Journal of Obstetrics & Gynecology and Reproductive Biology, 14*, 100142. doi:10.1016/j.eurox.2022.100142

Hamlin, L., Grunwald, L., Sturdivant, R. X., & Koehlmoos, T. P. (2021). Comparison of nurse-midwife and physician birth outcomes in the military health system. *Policy, Politics & Nursing Practice, 22*(2), 105–113. doi:10.1177/1527154421994071

Hoope-Bender, P. T., de Bernis, L., Campbell, J., Downe, S., Fauveau, V., Fogstad, H., Homer, C. S. E., Powell Kennedy, H., Matthews, Z., McFadden, A., Renfrew, M. J., & Van Lerberghe, W. (2014). Improvement of maternal and newborn health through midwifery, *The Lancet, 384*(9949), 1226–1235. doi:10.1016/S0140-6736(14)60930-2

Hutchison, M., Ennis, L., Shaw-Battista, J., Delgado, A., Myer, K., & Cragin, L. (2011). Great minds don't think alike: Collaborative maternity care at San Francisco General Hospital. *Obstetrics & Gynecology, 118*(3), 678–682. doi:10.1097/AOG.0b013e3182297d2d

King, T. L., Laros, R. K., & Parer, J. T. (2012). Interprofessional collaborative practice in obstetrics and midwifery. *Obstetrics and Gynecology Clinics of North America, 39*(3), 411–422. doi:10.1016/j.ogc.2012.05.009

National Collaborating Centre for Women's and Children's Health UK. (2008). 7: Monitoring and pain relief for induction of labour. In *NICE Clinical Guidelines No. 70*. RCOG Press. https://www.ncbi.nlm.nih.gov/books/NBK53623/

National Institutes of Health. (2006). State of the Science Conference: Cesarean delivery on maternal request. *Advances in Neonatal Care, 6*(4), 171–172.

National Institutes of Health. (2010). National Institutes of Health Consensus Development Conference Statement: Vaginal birth after cesarean: New insights March 8–10, 2010. *Seminars in Perinatology, 34*(4), 293–307. doi:10.1053/j.semperi.2010.05.001

Office of Technology Assessment. (1986). *Nurse practitioners, physician assistants, and certified nurse-midwives: A policy analysis* (Health Technology Case Study 37). U.S. Government Printing Office.

Qiu, J., Liu, Y., Zhu, W., & Zhang, C. (2020). Comparison of effectiveness of routine antenatal care with a midwife-managed clinic service in prevention of gestational diabetes mellitus in early pregnancy at a hospital in China. *Medical Science Monitor, 26*, e925991. doi:10.12659/MSM.925991

Reeves, S., Pelone, F., Harrison, R., Goldman, J., & Zwarenstein, M. (2017). Interprofessional collaboration to improve professional practice and healthcare outcomes. *Cochrane Database of Systematic Reviews, 2017*(6), CD000072. doi:10.1002/14651858.CD000072.pub3

Renfrew, M. J., McFadden, A., Bastos, M. H., Campbell, J., Channon, A. A., Cheung, N. F., Audebert Delage Silva, D. R., Downe, S., Powell Kennedy, H., Malata, A., McCormick, F., Wick, L., & Declercq, E. (2014). Midwifery and quality care: Findings from a new evidence-informed framework for maternal and newborn care. *The Lancet, 384*(9948):1129–1145. doi:10.1016/S0140-6736(14)60789-3

Sandall, J., Soltani, H., Gates, S., Shennan, A., & Devane, D. (2016). Midwife-led continuity models versus other models of care for childbearing women. *Cochrane Database of Systematic Reviews, 2016*(4), CD004667. doi:10.1002/14651858.CD004667.pub5

Shaw-Battista, J., Fineberg, A., Skubic, B., Wooley, D., & Tilton, Z. (2011). Collaborative maternity care: A successful model of public health and private practice partnership. *Obstetrics & Gynecology, 118*(3), 663–672. doi:10.1097/AOG.0b013e31822ac86f

Smith, H., Peterson, N., Lagrew, D., & Main, E. (2016). *Toolkit to support vaginal birth and reduce primary cesareans: A quality improvement toolkit*. California Maternal Quality Care Collaborative.

Society for Maternal-Fetal Medicine. (2019). SMFM statement on elective induction of labor in low-risk nulliparous women at term: The ARRIVE trial. *American Journal of Obstetrics and Gynecology, 221*(1), B2–B4. doi:10.1016/j.ajog.2018.08.009

SECTION V

Common Obstetric Presentations

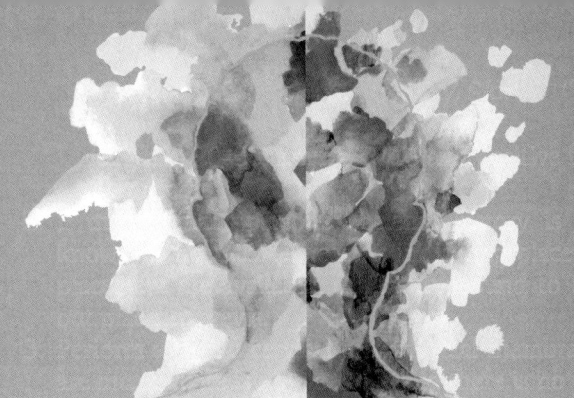

CHAPTER 31	Birth Choices for Pregnant People with a Previous Cesarean Delivery	363
CHAPTER 32	Common Discomforts of Pregnancy	371
CHAPTER 33	Gestational Diabetes Mellitus: Early Detection and Management in Pregnancy	389
CHAPTER 34	Hypertension Disorders in Pregnancy: Gestational Hypertension and Preeclampsia	397
CHAPTER 35	Preterm Labor Management	405
CHAPTER 36	Perinatal Mood and Anxiety Disorders (PMADs)	413
CHAPTER 37	Human Lactation	423

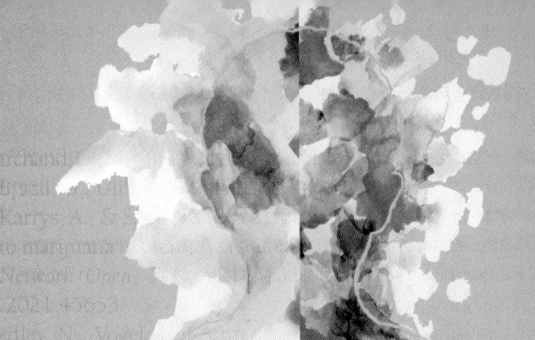

CHAPTER 31

Birth Choices for Pregnant People With a Previous Cesarean Delivery

Rebekah Kaplan

I. Introduction and general background

Currently, almost a third of births in the United States are by cesarean section; with this, increasing numbers of people are faced with the choice of whether to have a repeat cesarean birth or a trial of labor after a cesarean (TOLAC) and attempt a vaginal birth after a cesarean (VBAC). Cesarean delivery rates in the United States rose by almost 60% from a rate of 20.7% in 1996 to a record high of 32.9% in 2009. In 2019, the rate had fallen slightly to 31.7% (Martin et al., 2021).

For most of the 20th century, people who had a primary cesarean were advised to have subsequent cesarean deliveries. In 1980, the National Institute of Child and Human Development and the National Center for Health Care Technology examined the evidence for this practice and outlined recommendations for offering people a TOLAC. From 1980 to 1996, VBAC rates increased from about 5% in 1985 to 28.3% in 1996. With increasing reports of uterine rupture, TOLAC rates decreased, and between 1996 and 2007, rates steadily declined from 28.3% to 8.3%; they subsequently rose to 13.8% in 2019, which was a 4% increase from 2018 (American College of Obstetricians and Gynecologists [ACOG], 2019; Curtin et al., 2015; Martin et al., 2021). Interestingly, for those people who choose to have a TOLAC, the rates of successful VBAC have remained steady at about 74% (Eden et al., 2012; Grobman et al., 2021).

In 2010, the National Institutes of Health (NIH) addressed the issue of safety and outcomes of TOLAC, as well as declining availability and low VBAC rates, at the Consensus Development Conference on Vaginal Birth After Cesarean. The NIH's recommendation was that institutions should offer TOLAC as an option to those with previous low transverse cesarean sections (LTCSs) (NIH, 2010). The American Academy of Family Physicians (King et al., 2015), American College of Nurse-Midwives (2011), and ACOG (2019) have made the same recommendation.

When helping pregnant people and families make the decision about their preferred mode of delivery, the practitioner must incorporate principles of informed consent and shared decision making, including assessing the patient's values and desires, their candidacy for TOLAC, their chances of success, their risk of uterine rupture, and risks and benefits for themselves and their babies (see internet resources at the end of this chapter). It is important that the provider attend to power imbalances by verbally creating a safe environment, inviting contributions from everyone, and avoiding making assumptions (Vedam et al., 2017). Research has demonstrated that communities facing barriers to healthcare are especially vulnerable to power imbalances when making medical decisions, and shared decision-making tools can help to mitigate these disparities (Durand et al., 2014). Additional context and examination of these power imbalances is beyond the scope of this chapter. The literature also shows that prior birth experience, perceived risk, fear and anxiety, opinions of family and friends, desire for planning and control, knowledge of birth options, and perceived provider preference significantly factor into the decision (Bernstein et al., 2012; Shorten et al., 2014). It is also important to meet a patient on their own health comprehension terms. It may be helpful to use visual aids such as an icon array to enhance understanding and reduce provider bias (Cox, 2014; Garcia-Retamero & Dhami, 2013), or use qualitative data and storytelling as opposed to strictly quantitative data. **Figures 31-1** and **31-2** provide guidance on centering the

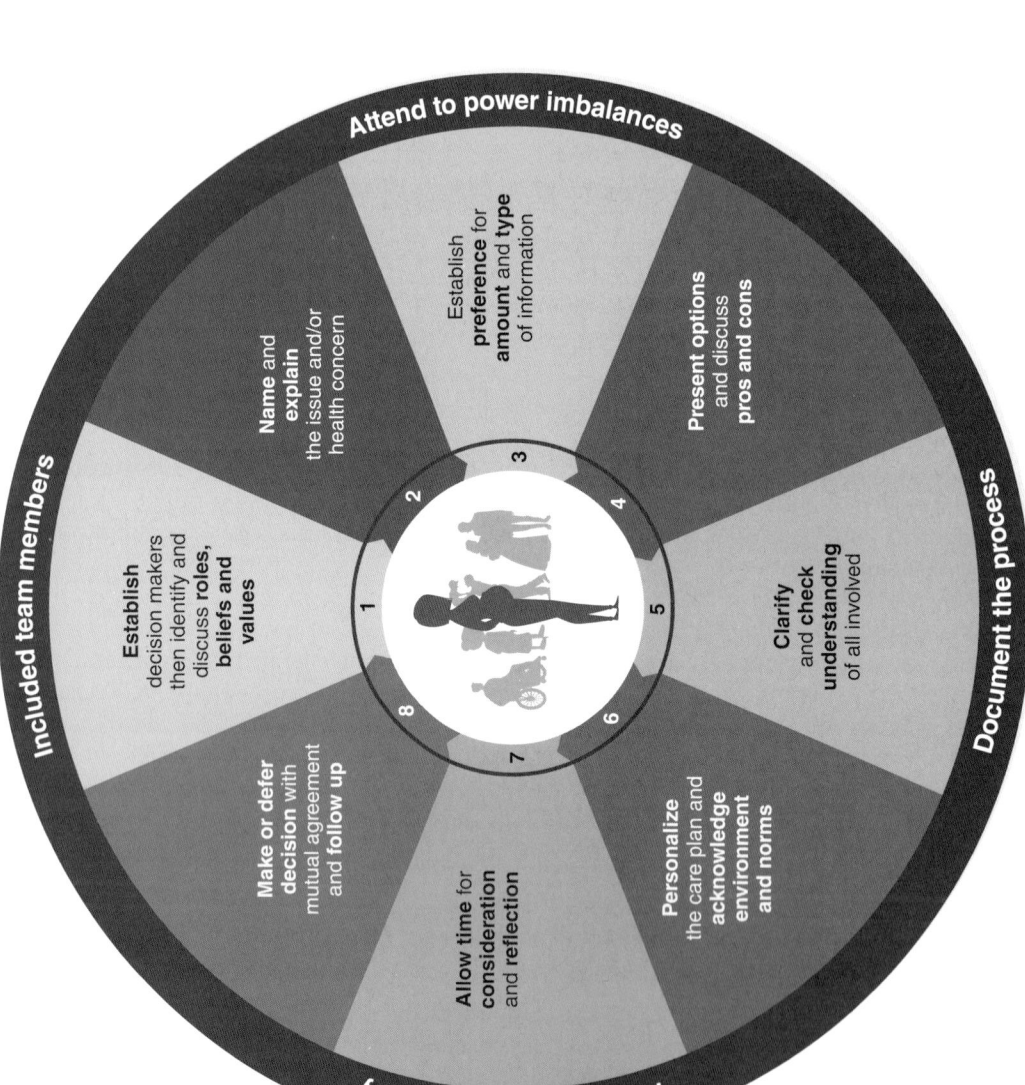

Figure 31-1 Person-centered decision-making model

Developed by Dr. Saraswathi Vedam and her team at the Birth Place Lab, University of British Columbia. https://www.birthplacelab.org/projects/. Stoll, K, Wang, J.J., Niles, P. et al. I felt so much conflict instead of joy: an analysis of open-ended comments from people in British Columbia who declined care recommendations during pregnancy and childbirth. Reprod Health 18, 79 (2021). https://doi.org/10.1186/s12978-021-01134-7

Plan a vaginal birth (VBAC)	How much does it matter to you?	Plan a repeat cesarean birth	How much does it matter to you?
You have a greater chance of having an easier recovery and shorter stay in the hospital.	* * * * *	You know what to expect from having a cesarean.	* * * * *
You have a smaller chance of problems after surgery, such as infection, blood clots, or hysterectomy.	* * * * *	You have a smaller chance of having a tear in the scar of the uterus.	* * * * *
You have a smaller chance of having problems with the placenta in the future.	* * * * *	Your baby has a smaller chance of rare but serious complications of uterine rupture.	* * * * *
You have a greater chance of having your baby with you after the birth (not as many admissions to the NICU).	* * * * *	You have a greater chance of avoiding labor all together.	* * * * *
You have a greater chance of having a vaginal birth.	* * * * *	You can know the date your baby will be born.	* * * * *
Other things you value?	* * * * *	Other things you value?	* * * * *
Total stars	VBAC =		Repeat C/S =

Figure 31-2 Values Clarification Tool: Birth Choices after a Previous Cesarean Birth
Courtesy of Community Health Network of San Francisco, Department of Public Health

patient's desires and helping them identify their own values as it pertains to a birth plan. After a decision is made, the patient should understand that they can revise the plan if desired, and the process should be documented. Choices may be institution specific, and a provider should know who in the birth community offers TOLAC as an option.

II. Risks and benefits of TOLAC versus repeat cesarean birth

Having a VBAC offers the birthing parent the opportunity to experience a vaginal birth as well as other potential benefits. Those who achieve a VBAC avoid major abdominal surgery and have lower rates of thromboembolism, hemorrhage, and infection and a shorter recovery period than parturients who have an elective repeat cesarean birth (ERCB). There are also risks associated with multiple cesarean births, including hysterectomy, bowel or bladder injury, transfusion, infection, and abnormal placentation (e.g., placenta previa and placenta accrete) (ACOG, 2019). However, it is difficult to compare the differences between a VBAC and an ERCB because the risks and benefits may be disproportionately associated with a failed TOLAC (VBAC is associated with fewer complications than ERCB, and failed TOLAC is associated with more complications) (ACOG, 2019). The following section outlines the risks to both the birthing parent and the neonate.

A. *Uterine rupture*

The risk of a uterine rupture for someone choosing a TOLAC is 0.47% (0.2%–0.77%) (Dodd et al., 2013; Guise et al., 2010). If a patient has had a previous vaginal birth either before or after their cesarean birth, this rate drops (Guise et al., 2010). If the prior cesarean was done within 24 months of the birth, the risk of rupture is slightly higher (Landon et al., 2004). People with a history of two prior LTCSs have about a 2% risk of uterine rupture. The ACOG (2019) considers patients who have had two LTCSs candidates for TOLAC. If labor is being induced, the rate of rupture increases to approximately 1.1%–1.5% (NIH, 2010; Rossi & Prefumo, 2015). Labor augmentation with oxytocin does not seem to increase the risk of uterine rupture (NIH, 2010; Ouzounian et al., 2011). There have been no reported parturient deaths caused by uterine rupture (NIH, 2010), although it is possible that this is due to underreporting or failure to indicate rupture as the cause of death. Approximately 6% of uterine ruptures result in neonatal death (NIH, 2010).

Guise et al. (2004) notes that literature on uterine rupture varies based on source and method of review, however, it is estimated that approximately 370 elective cesarean deliveries will need to be performed in order to prevent one.

B. *Risk for future pregnancies*
1. Placenta accreta and hysterectomy
   People with multiple cesareans have an increased rate of placenta accreta and hysterectomy with each subsequent cesarean birth, as evidenced by many

studies (ACOG, 2012; Jauniaux & Bhide, 2017; Marshall et al., 2011). Some of the best evidence comes from Silver et al. (2006), who cited the incidence of placenta accreta from one previous cesarean to five or more as 0.31%, 0.57%, 2.1%, 2.3%, and 6.7%, respectively. The risk of hysterectomy from one previous cesarean to five or more was found to be 0.42%, 0.90%, 2.41%, 3.49%, and 8.99%, respectively (Jauniaux & Bhide, 2017; Marshall et al., 2011; Silver et al., 2006).

2. Placenta previa

The incidence of placenta previa significantly increases with each additional cesarean delivery, occurring in 0.9% of those who have had one prior cesarean delivery, 1.7% of those who have had two prior cesarean deliveries, and 3% in people who have had three or more cesarean deliveries (NIH, 2010). People with placenta previa having their third or greater cesarean have a much greater risk of hysterectomy (0.7%–4% vs. 50%–67%), as well as composite intrapartum and immediate postpartum morbidity (15% vs. 83%) (Marshall et al., 2011).

C. *Parturient mortality*

Overall numeric estimates of intrapartum death are 4 per 100,000 for people who undergo a TOLAC versus 13 per 100,000 for a repeat elective cesarean birth (Dodd et al., 2013; Guise et al., 2010). The ACOG (2019) cites the parturient death rate at 0.0019% for TOLAC and 0.0096% for ERCB (ACOG, 2019).

D. *Parturient morbidity*

Overall, cesarean deliveries are associated with a 10% risk of morbidity, including increased risk of infection (endometritis, urinary tract, or wound), thromboembolism, hysterectomy (2%), greater blood loss and severe postpartum hemorrhage (7.3%), blood transfusion, and surgical injury (e.g., injury to the bladder, ureter, or bowel). People who have a TOLAC have a 4.6% risk of infection versus 3.2% in the ERCB group, although the ERCB group is more at risk for deep vein thrombosis and pulmonary embolism than the TOLAC group. The risks of hysterectomy, blood transfusion, and infection are similar in both groups, although the evidence is confounding (Guise et al., 2010). In people with increasing numbers of cesarean births, the rates of hysterectomy, blood transfusions, adhesions, and surgical injury all continue to increase (Marshall et al., 2011). The long-term effects of urinary incontinence in people who have a VBAC versus cesarean birth are confounding, although mild incontinence may be higher in the short term for people who have a VBAC, and an increase in pelvic organ prolapse has been noted (Sandall et al., 2018). Evidence shows lower rates of parturient morbidity in TOLAC patients, with predicted VBAC success rates of greater than 60%–70% (**Table 31-1**) (ACOG, 2019; Grobman et al., 2009).

E. *Neonatal mortality*

Studies show that the neonatal mortality rate is higher for TOLAC at 1.3 per 1,000 compared to elective repeat cesarean at 0.5 per 1,000. The neonatal mortality rate for all first-time birth parents is 1 per 1,000 (Guise et al., 2010; Smith et al., 2002). Neonatal death rates are higher in settings where rapid emergent cesarean sections cannot be performed (ACOG, 2019).

F. *Neonatal morbidity*

Evidence indicates that infants born by cesarean have higher rates of respiratory distress syndrome, persistent pulmonary hypertension, transient tachypnea of the newborn, and need for oxygen and ventilator support than do infants born vaginally (NIH, 2010). Rates of hypoxic–ischemic encephalopathy in one study were 0.08% in the TOLAC group and none in the ERCB group (Landon et al., 2004), whereas the ACOG (2019) reported a rate of 0%–0.32% in the ERCB group and 0%–0.89% in the TOLAC group (ACOG, 2019).

G. *Long-term consequences in offspring*

Evidence suggests that exposure to vaginal flora at birth is associated with the development of a healthy immune response. This is thought to be caused by microflora colonization of the neonatal intestinal tract, adaptive stress of labor and birth, and epigenetic regulation of gene expression, each of which is altered in cesarean birth (Cho & Norman, 2013; Fouhy et al., 2019). Children and adults born by cesarean have a 20% increased risk of developing asthma and a 23% increased risk of developing type 1 diabetes (Cho & Norman, 2013; Chu et al., 2017). There is also a greater prevalence of allergic rhinitis, food allergies, celiac disease, and inflammatory bowel disease and increased hospitalization for gastroenteritis in these children (Bager et al., 2012; Cho & Norman, 2013; Decker et al., 2011; Sandall et al., 2018). An association between cesarean birth and high body weight in childhood and young adulthood has also been cited in many studies (Li et al., 2013; Mesquita et al., 2013; Sandall et al., 2018). In addition, a large longitudinal study found that among siblings born to the same parent, one by cesarean and one by VBAC, the VBAC offspring had 31% less risk of developing high body weight as an adult (Yuan et al., 2016).

Infants born by cesarean are also more likely to have antibiotic exposure during birth, which may subtly alter the infant's physiology and immune development and microbiome diversity (Sandall et al., 2018). Preliminary research shows that vaginal seeding, or swabbing the newborn born by cesarean with the birthing person's vaginal secretions, may help to restore the infant's microbiome (Mueller et al., 2016).

H. Postpartum period

People recover more quickly, have less postpartum pain, and have shorter hospital stays after a vaginal birth versus an operative birth. Birthing parents who have cesareans not only have a longer recovery but also delayed infant interaction, lower rates of breastfeeding, and more difficulty establishing breastfeeding. People with cesarean births have less perineal or vaginal trauma and decreased urinary incontinence and organ prolapse in the postpartum period. The rehospitalization rate within 30 days is 2.3 times higher in people with a cesarean birth (Declercq et al., 2007). According to Silver (2012), almost 20% of people reported chronic pain 3 months after their surgery and 12% a year after, and 33% had daily incisional pain at their surgery site 2 years after surgery. Pain, as well as other morbidity, increased with additional numbers of cesarean births (Miller et al., 2013; Silver, 2012).

III. Data collection

A. *Subjective: First visit*
  1. Document the reason for previous cesarean and events surrounding the birth. These include:
     a. Reason for prior cesarean (e.g., cesarean birth for non-reassuring fetal heart tracing, placenta previa, arrest of dilation or descent, breech presentation)
     b. Emergent versus nonemergent surgery (emergent more likely to have a classical incision)
     c. Gestational age and fetal weight (early preterm more likely to have a classical incision)
     d. Stage of labor (cervical dilation and station) and length of labor
     e. Fetal position, if possible (e.g., posterior)
     f. Where surgery was performed (e.g., small community or major urban hospital)
     g. Type of physician performing surgery (obstetrician/gynecologist, or general practitioner)
     h. Future TOLAC: Did the physician advise the patient whether they could attempt a TOLAC in the future?
     i. Patient's experience of previous labor and birth
  2. Note desired family size.

B. *Objective*
  1. Assess type of scar: On physical abdominal examination, assess transverse or vertical skin scar, although skin incision does not reflect uterine incision.

IV. Goals for clinical management/assessment

A. *Establish if the patient is a candidate for TOLAC.*
B. *Individualize predicted success rate* (**Tables 31-1** and **31-2**).
  1. The use of the VBAC calculator, which was first published by the Maternal-Fetal Medicine Units Network (MFMU) in 2007 (Grobman et al., 2007), has

Table 31-1 Vaginal Birth After Cesarean (VBAC) Success Rates

Indication for Prior Cesarean	% Success
Failure to progress	60–65
Nonrecurring conditions (placenta previa, breech)	74–89
Fetal intolerance of labor	69–73
Body mass index > 40	52–70

See Internet VBAC success calculator (2021) for individual risk: https://mfmunetwork.bsc.gwu.edu/web/mfmunetwork/vaginal-birth-after-cesarean-calculator

Table 31-2 Factors for Vaginal Brith After Cesarean (VBAC) Success

Positive factors
- Age < 40
- Prior vaginal delivery (especially VBAC)
- Favorable cervical factors
- Presence of spontaneous labor
- Nonrecurring indication for previous cesarean (e.g., breech, placenta previa)
- Greater gestational parent height

Negative factors
- Increased number of prior cesarean deliveries
- Gestational age > 40 weeks
- Birth weight > 4,000 g
- Induction or augmentation of labor (63% success)
- Increasing total body weight
- Increased interpregnancy weight gain
- Increased risk of rupture with short interpregnancy interval
- Gestational diabetes
- Chronic disease (e.g., hypertension)

Data from ACOG Practice Bulletin No. 205: Vaginal Birth After Cesarean Delivery. Obstetrics and Gynecology. 2019 Feb;133(2):e110-e127. DOI: 10.1097/aog.0000000000003078. PMID: 30681543. Data from: Vaginal birth after previous cesarean deliv-ery. National Institutes of Health Consensus Development Conference statement: Vaginal birth after cesarean: New insights. March 8–10, 2010.8

come under criticism for continuing to perpetuate existing health inequities in perinatal care (Thornton, 2018; Vyas et al., 2018). By the inclusion of race and ethnicity, which are social, not biological, constructs, this calculator underestimated VBAC success in Black and Latinx patients, which may have resulted in those patients being unnecessarily discouraged from TOLAC and, furthermore, the perpetuation of disparities in cesarean section rates, as well as leading to disparities in parturient morbidity and mortality. In 2021, the calculator was updated to exclude race and ethnicity as variables (Grobman et al., 2021). The calculator continues to be far from perfect. Relevant variables, such as provider attitudes and institutional differences, are not accounted for, and providers should be mindful and transparent about calculator limitations when counseling patients if they are using this tool (Thornton, 2018).

C. Establish patient's choice using principles of shared decision making.

V. Plan

A. Attempt to obtain an operative report (**Table 31-3**).
   1. TOLAC is not contraindicated with an unknown uterine incision unless there is a high clinical suspicion of a classical scar (ACOG, 2019; Smith et al., 2015).
B. Educate on risks and benefits of repeat cesarean versus TOLAC. Consider patient values, desires, factors for success, and previous experience.
C. Establish the patient's understanding of benefits and risks.
D. Use principles of shared decision making to ascertain patient's choice. See "Six Steps of Shared Decision Making for Health Care Providers" in the resources section at the end of the chapter.
E. Engage in values clarification (Figure 31-1).
F. Have the patient sign consent for their birth choice if institutional policy.
G. If the patient has an unknown scar, a consultation with a physician may be indicated at your site.
H. For those choosing TOLAC
   Discuss with the patient the care during their birth (continuous fetal monitoring, intravenous or saline lock). Consult per site guidelines. With induction of labor, the risk of uterine rupture increases and VBAC success decreases. If induction is indicated, the patient needs to be recounseled.
I. For patients choosing a cesarean delivery
   1. Consult with the physician obstetric team to schedule a cesarean at 39 weeks except for those with prior classical scars.
      a. Good dating: 39 weeks
      b. Two prior cesareans: 39 weeks
      c. Known classical scar: early term delivery

Table 31-3 Contraindications for Trial of Labor

- Previous cesarean birth with a uterine incision in the upper part of the uterus ("classical" incision) or low transverse uterine incision with an extension into the upper part of the uterus (active segment)
- Previous transfundal uterine surgery
- Previous uterine rupture
- Medical or obstetric complication that precludes vaginal birth
- Inability to perform emergency cesarean birth

VI. Internet resources for providers, patients, and families

A. VBAC Success Calculator
   https://mfmunetwork.bsc.gwu.edu/web/mfmunetwork/vaginal-birth-after-cesarean-calculator
   Enter data—age, height, weight, vaginal birth history, if previous cesarean for arrest of descent, treatment for chronic hypertension—to calculate the predicted chance of VBAC (based on Grobman et al., 2021).

B. Childbirth Connection
   http://www.childbirthconnection.org/
   Organization promoting evidence-based maternity care and helping people and providers make informed decisions. Several sections regarding TOLAC decision making.

C. Informed Medical Decisions Foundation: "Six Steps of Shared Decision Making for Health Care Providers" (Wexler, 2012)
   http://www.slideshare.net/fimdm/six-steps-of-shared-decision-making

D. The Birth Place Lab (BPL) in the Faculty of Medicine at the University of British Columbia
   https://www.birthplacelab.org/projects/
   The BPL facilitates community-based participatory research and knowledge translation around equitable access to high-quality maternity health care. Lead investigators Dr. Saraswathi Vedam and Dr. Kathrin Stolaci, in response to findings from their patient-oriented research, have engaged community members to co-develop instruments and accountability tools that they can use to report on their experiences of autonomy, respect, and mistreatment when interacting with the healthcare system. This includes a person-centered decision-making model.

References

American College of Nurse-Midwives. (2011). Care for women desiring vaginal birth after cesarean. *Journal of Midwifery Women's Health*, 56(5), 517–525. doi:10.1111/j.1542-2011.2011.00112.x

American College of Obstetricians and Gynecologists. (2012). ACOG Committee Opinion No. 529: Placenta accreta. *Obstetrics & Gynecology*, 120(1), 207–211. doi:10.1097/AOG.0b013e318262e340

American College of Obstetricians and Gynecologists. (2019). Practice Bulletin No. 205: Vaginal birth after cesarean delivery. *Obstetrics & Gynecology*, 133(2), 110–127. doi:10.1097/AOG.0000000000003078

Bager, P., Simonsen, J., Nielsen, N. M., & Frisch, M. (2012). Cesarean section and offspring's risk of inflammatory bowel disease: A national cohort study. *Inflammatory Bowel Diseases*, 18(5), 857–862. doi:10.1002/ibd.21805

Bernstein, S. N., Matalon Grazi, S., & Rosenn, B. M. (2012). Trial of labor versus repeat cesarean: Are clients making an informed decision? *American Journal of Obstetrics and Gynecology, 207*(3), 204–206. doi:10.1016/j.ajog.2012.06.057

Cho, C. E., & Norman, M. (2013). Cesarean section and development of the immune system in the offspring. *American Journal of Obstetrics and Gynecology, 208*(4), 249–254. doi:10.1016/j.ajog.2012.08.009

Chu, S., Chen, Q., Chen, Y., Bao, Y., Wu, M., & Zhang, J. (2017). Cesarean section without medical indication and risk of childhood asthma, and attenuation by breastfeeding. *PLoS One, 12*(9), e0184920. doi:10.1038/s41598-017-10206-3

Cox, K. J. (2014). Counseling women with a previous cesarean birth: Toward a shared decision-making partnership. *Journal of Midwifery & Women's Health, 59*(3), 237–245. doi:10.1111/jmwh.12177

Curtin, S. C., Gregory, K. D., Korst, L. M., & Uddin, S. F. G. (2015). Maternal morbidity for vaginal and cesarean deliveries, according to previous cesarean history: New data from the birth certificate, 2013. *National Vital Statistics Reports, 64*(4), 1–13.

Decker, E., Hornef, M., & Stockinger, S. (2011). Cesarean delivery is associated with celiac disease but not inflammatory bowel disease in children. *Gut Microbes, 2*(2), 91–98. doi: 10.1542/peds.2009-2260

Declercq, E., Barger, M., Cabral, H. J., Evans, S. R., Kotelchuck, M., Simon, C., Weiss, J., & Heffner, L. J. (2007). Maternal outcomes associated with planned primary cesarean births compared with planned vaginal births. *Obstetrics & Gynecology, 109*(3), 669–677. doi:10.1097/01.AOG.0000255668.20639.40

Dodd, J. M., Crowther, C. A., Huertas, E., Guise, J. M., & Horey, D. (2013). Planned elective repeat caesarean section versus planned vaginal birth for women with a previous caesarean birth. *Cochrane Database of Systematic Reviews, 2013*(12), CD004224. doi:10.1002/14651858.CD004224.pub3

Durand, M., Carpenter, L., Dolan, H., Bravo, P., Mann, M., Bunn, F., & Elwyn, G. (2014). Do interventions designed to support shared decision-making reduce health inequalities? A systematic review and meta-analysis. *PLoS One, 9*(4), e94670–e94670. doi:10.1371/journal.pone.0094670

Eden, K. B., Denman, M. A., Emeis, C. L., McDonagh, M. S. Fu, R., Janik, R. K., Broman, A. R., & Guise, J. M. (2012). Trial of labor and vaginal delivery rates in women with a prior cesarean. *Journal of Obstetric, Gynecologic, and Neonatal Nursing, 41*(5), 583–596. doi:10.1111/j.1552-6909.2012.01388.x

Fouhy, F., Watkins, C., Hill, C. J., O'Shea, C., Nagle, B., Dempsey, E. M., O'Toole P.W., Ross R. P., Ryan C. A., & Stanton, C. (2019). Perinatal factors affect the gut microbiota up to four years after birth. *Nature Communications, 10*(1), 1517. doi:10.1038/s41467-019-09252-4

Garcia-Retamero, R., & Dhami, M. K. (2013). On avoiding framing effects in experienced decision makers. *Quarterly Journal of Experimental Psychology, 66*(4), 829–842. doi:10.1080/17470218.2012.727836

Grobman, W. A., Lai, Y., Landon, M. B., Spong, C. Y., Leveno, K. J., Rouse, D. J., Varner, M.W., Moawad, A. H., Caritis, S. N., Harper, M., Wapner, R. J., Sorokin, Y., Miodovnik, M., Carpenter, M., O'Sullivan, M. J., Sibai, B. M., Langer, O., Thorp, J. M., Ramin, S. M., Mercer, B. M., & National Institute of Child Health and Human Development (NICHD) Maternal-Fetal Medicine Units Network (MFMU). (2007). Development of a nomogram for prediction of vaginal birth after cesarean delivery. *Obstetrics & Gynecology, 109*(4), 806–812. doi:10.1097/01.AOG.0000259312.36053.02

Grobman, W. A., Lai, Y., Landon, M. B., Spong, C. Y., Leveno, K. J., Rouse, D. J., Varner, M. W., Moawad, A. H., Caritis, S. N., Harper, M., Wapner, R. J., Sorokin, Y., Miodovnik, M., Carpenter, M., O'Sullivan, M. J., Sibai, B. M., Langer, O., Thorp, J. M., Ramin, S. M., ... Eunice Kennedy Shriver National Institute of Child Health and Human Development Maternal-Fetal Medicine Units Network. (2009). Can a prediction model for vaginal birth after cesarean also predict the probability of morbidity related to a trial of labor? *American Journal of Obstetrics and Gynecology, 200*(1), 56e1–56e6. doi:10.1016/j.ajog.2008.06.039

Grobman, W. A., Sandoval, G., Rice, M. M., Bailit, J. L., Chauhan, S. P., Costantine, M., Gyamfi-Bannerman, C., Metz, T. D., Parry, S., Rouse, D. J., Saade, G. R., Simhan, H. N., Thorp, J. M., Jr., Tita, A. T. N., Longo, M., Landon, M. B., & Eunice Kennedy Shriver National Institute of Child Health and Human Development Maternal-Fetal Medicine Units Network. (2021). Prediction of vaginal birth after cesarean delivery in term gestations: A calculator without race and ethnicity. *American Journal of Obstetrics and Gynecology, 225*(6), 664.e1–664.e7. doi:10.1016/j.ajog.2021.05.021

Guise, J., Denman, M. A., Emeis, C., Marshall, N., Walker, M., Fu, R., Janik, R., Nygren, P., Eden, K. B., & McDonagh, M. (2010). Vaginal birth after cesarean: New insights on maternal and neonatal outcomes. *Obstetrics and Gynecology, 115*(6), 1267–1278. doi:10.1097/AOG.0b013e3181df925f

Guise, J. M., McDonagh, M. S., Osterweil, P., Nygren, P., Chan, B. K., & Helfand, M. (2004). Systematic review of the incidence and consequences of uterine rupture in women with previous caesarean section. *British Medical Journal, 329*(7456), 19–25. doi:10.1136/bmj.329.7456.19

Jauniaux, E., & Bhide, A. (2017). Prenatal ultrasound diagnosis and outcome of placenta previa accreta after cesarean delivery: A systematic review and meta-analysis. *American Journal of Obstetrics and Gynecology, 217*(1), 27–36. doi:10.1016/j.ajog.2017.02.050

King, V. J., Fontaine, P. L., Atwood, L. A., Powers, E., Leeman, L., Ecker, J. L., Avery, M. D., Sakala, C., Campos-Outcalt, D., Jeffcott-Pera, M., & Schoof, B. (2015). Clinical practice guideline executive summary: Labor after cesarean/planned vaginal birth after cesarean. *Annals of Family Medicine, 13*(1), 80–81. doi:10.1370/afm.1738

Landon, M. B., Hauth, J. C., Leveno, K. J., Spong, C. Y., Leindecker, S., Varner, M., Moawad, A. H., Caritis, S. N., Harper, M., Wapner, R. J., Sorokin, Y., Miodovnik, M., Carpenter, M., Peaceman, A. M., O'Sullivan, M. J., Sibai, B., Langer, O., Thorp, J. M., Rami, S. M., ... National Institute of Child Health and Human Development Maternal-Fetal Medicine Units Network. (2004). Maternal and perinatal outcomes associated with a trial of labor after prior cesarean delivery. *New England Journal of Medicine, 351*(25), 2581–2589. doi:10.1056/NEJMoa040405

Li, H. T., Zhou, Y. B., & Liu, J. M. (2013). The impact of cesarean section on offspring overweight and obesity: A systematic review and meta-analysis. *International Journal of Obesity, 37*(7), 893–899. doi:10.1038/ijo.2012.195

Marshall, N. E., Fu, R., & Guise, J. (2011). Impact of multiple cesarean deliveries on maternal morbidity: A systematic review. *American Journal of Obstetrics and Gynecology, 205*(3), 262–268. doi:10.1016/j.ajog.2011.06.035

Martin, J. A., Hamilton, B. E., Osterman, M. J. K., & Driscoll, A. K. (2021). Births: Final data for 2019. *National Vital Statistics Report, 70*(2), 1–51.

Mesquita, D. N., Barbieri, M. A., Goldani, H. A., Cardoso, V. C., Goldani, M. Z., Kac, G., Silva, A. A., & Bettiol, H. (2013). Cesarean section is associated with increased peripheral and central adiposity in young adulthood: Cohort study. *PLoS One, 8*(6), e66827. doi:10.1371/journal.pone.0066827

Miller, E. S., Hahn, K., & Grobman, W. A. (2013). Consequences of a primary elective cesarean delivery across the reproductive life. *Obstetrics and Gynecology, 121*(4), 789–797. doi:10.1097/AOG.0b013e3182878b43

Mueller, N. T., Dominguez Bello, M. G., Appel, L. J., & Hourigan, S. K. (2020). "Vaginal seeding" after a caesarean section provides benefits to newborn children: FOR: Does exposing caesarean-delivered newborns to the vaginal microbiome affect their chronic disease risk? The critical need for trials of "vaginal seeding" during caesarean section. *BJOG, 127*(2), 301. doi:10.1111/1471-0528.15979

National Institutes of Health. (2010). NIH Consensus Development Conference statement on vaginal birth after cesarean: New insights. March 8–10, 2010. *Obstetrics & Gynecology, 115*(6), 1279–1295. doi:10.1097/AOG.0b013e3181e459e5

Ouzounian, J. G., Miller, D. A., Hiebert, C. J., Battista, L. R., & Lee, R. H. (2011). Vaginal birth after cesarean section: Risk of uterine rupture with labor induction. *American Journal of Perinatology, 28*(8), 593–596. doi:10.1055/s-0031-1275386

Rossi, A. C., & Prefumo, F. (2015). Pregnancy outcomes of induced labor in women with previous cesarean section: A systematic review and meta-analysis. *Archives of Gynecology and Obstetrics, 291*(2), 273–280. doi:10.1007/s00404-014-3444-9

Sandall, J., Tribe, R. M., Avery, L., Mola, G., Visser, G. H., Homer, C. S., Gibbons, D., Kelly, N. M., Kennedy, H. P., Kidanto, H., Taylor, P., & Temmerman, M. (2018). Short-term and long-term effects of caesarean section on the health of women and children. *The Lancet, 392*(10155), 1349–1357. doi:10.1016/S0140-6736(18)31930-5

Shorten, A., Shorten, B., & Kennedy, H. P. (2014). Complexities of choice after prior cesarean: A narrative analysis. *Birth, 41*(2), 178–184. doi:10.1111/birt.12082

Silver, R. M. (2012). Implications of the first cesarean: Perinatal and future reproductive health and subsequent cesareans, placentation issues, uterine rupture risk, morbidity, and mortality. *Seminars in Perinatology, 36*(5), 315–323. doi:10.1053/j.semperi.2012.04.013

Silver, R. M., Landon, M. B., Rouse, D. J., Leveno, K. J., Spong, C. Y., Thom, E. A., Moawad, A. H., Caritis, S. N., Harper, M., Wapner, R. J., Sorokin, Y., Miodovnik, M., Carpenter, M., Peaceman, A. M., O'Sullivan, M. J., Sibai, B., Langer, O., Thorp, J. M., Ramin, S. M., . . . National Institute of Child Health and Human Development Maternal-Fetal Medicine Units Network. (2006). Maternal morbidity associated with multiple repeat cesarean deliveries. *Obstetrics & Gynecology, 107*(6), 1226–1232. doi:10.1097/01.AOG.0000219750.79480.84

Smith, D., Stringer, E., Vladutiu, C. J., Zink, A. H., & Strauss R. (2015). Risk of uterine rupture among women attempting vaginal birth after cesarean with an unknown uterine scar. *American Journal of Obstetrics and Gynecology, 213*(1), 80. doi:10.1016/j.ajog.2015.01.056

Smith, G. C., Pell, J. P., Cameron, A. D., & Dobbie, R. (2002). Risk of perinatal death associated with labor after previous cesarean delivery in uncomplicated term pregnancies. *Journal of the American Medical Association, 287*(20), 2684–2690. doi:10.1001/jama.287.20.2684

Thornton, P. (2018). Limitations of vaginal birth after cesarean success prediction. *Journal of Midwifery & Women's Health, 63*(1), 115–120. doi:10.1016/j.ijnurstu.2022.10435

Vedam, S., Stoll, K., Martin, K., Rubashkin, N., Partridge, S., Thordarson, D., Jolicoeur, G., & Changing Childbirth in BC Steering Council. (2017). The Mother's Autonomy in Decision Making (MADM) scale: Patient-led development and psychometric testing of a new instrument to evaluate experience of maternity care. *PLoS One, 12*(2), e0171804. doi:10.1371/journal.pone.0171804

Vyas, D. A., Jones, D. S., Meadows, A. R., Diouf, K., Nour, N. M., & Schantz Dunn, J. (2019). Challenging the use of race in the vaginal birth after cesarean section calculator. *Women's Health Issues, 29*(3), 201–204. doi:10.1016/j.whi.2019.04.007

Wexler, R. (2012). *Six steps of shared decision making for health care providers. Shared slides.* Informed Medical Decisions Foundation. http://www.slideshare.net/fimdm/six-steps-of-shared-decision-making.

Yuan, C., Gaskins, A. J., Blaine, A. I., Zhang, C., Gillman, M. W., Missmer, S. A., Field, A. E., & Chavarro, J. E. (2016). Association between cesarean birth and risk of obesity in offspring in childhood, adolescence, and early adulthood. *JAMA Pediatrics, 170*(11), e162385. doi:10.1001/jamapediatrics.2016.2385

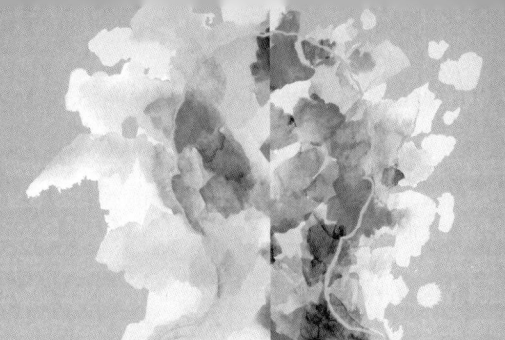

CHAPTER 32

Common Discomforts of Pregnancy

Jamie Meyerhoff and Cynthia Belew

I. Introduction to common discomforts of pregnancy

The common discomforts discussed in this chapter result from the profound physiologic changes of pregnancy. Although rarely posing a risk to the well-being of the fetus, they result in real suffering for the pregnant person. Symptoms range from mild to severe. For the classic common discomforts of pregnancy, diagnosis centers on the subjective. Thus, a provider's commitment to understanding an individual's own words and a provider's ability to listen with humility and respect are core to communication and care.

Pregnant people calling the Motherisk Helpline reported that providers trivialize when attempting to normalize common pregnancy discomforts (Madjunkova et al., 2013). In cases of mild discomfort, providers tend to estimate pain accurately and respond appropriately; in contrast, when people report severe symptoms, providers are more likely to underestimate and underrespond (Tait & Chibnall, 2014). Thoroughness, humility, and high-quality communication are requisite. Offer a provider or interpreter who shares the patient's language and culture. Tait and Chibnall (2014) found that people tended to share the depth and severity of discomfort more with a provider they perceived as race and culture concordant. In the absence of a language and culture concordant provider, professional interpreters do not simply translate but offer a necessary bridge for both language and cultural barriers (Clarke et al., 2019).

As healthcare providers, we cannot manage care as though patient health exists in an isolated, separate health equation. We partner because we are a part of the equation. The benefits of a provider listening and learning with respect are immediate: pregnant people reported feeling increased confidence when perceiving the provider listening to concerns and treating them with respect (Avery et al., 2014). Confidence is a happy success. Growing confidence and understanding of one's own changing pregnant body, confidence in one's own knowledge, is the embodied work of growing into parenthood. Confidence in relationship with the provider opens doors for future work together to support optimal health. Through a partnership approach to clinical care, the provider supports the pregnant person's confidence and self-efficacy in their work of listening to and understanding their symptoms.

When assessing common discomforts, strive to understand the context of prenatal symptoms. Providers must ask about stress and stressors. The severity of symptoms in common discomforts of pregnancy is associated with increasing stress levels (Kamysheva et al., 2009; McDaid et al., 2019). For example, low back pain in pregnancy affects at least 60% of pregnant people. Stress does not cause low back pain in pregnancy; however, stress is an independent risk factor for increased severity of lower back pain in pregnancy (Backhausen et al., 2019).

Despite the complexity of causal factors—such as pregnancy's increased weight and changing posture and center of gravity, stressors, previous injuries, and demands of work and home—exercise is consistently associated with a reduction in low back pain in pregnancy (Shiri et al., 2018). Neighborhood health determines opportunities for physical activity (Gianfredi et al., 2021). Accessible urban green space (and even an increasing number of trees) was directly correlated with increased exercise, decreased stress, and improved health across dozens of health markers in a systematic review and meta-analysis of 134 studies (Gianfredi et al., 2021; Twohig-Bennett & Jones, 2018). In contrast, neighborhood stress and poverty are associated with barriers to exercise, increased stress, inability to find healthy food options (Hawes et al. 2019; Karpyn et al., 2019), and inadequate sleep (Mellman et al., 2018).

After assessment of symptoms, context, and coming to a diagnosis, the next step is the care plan: the act of responding when change is needed. Responding authentically and creatively is part of the dynamic living equation that is health care. An individual's health is an equation of connected factors, encompassing water, food, and neighborhood health (Karpyn et al., 2019; Twohig-Bennett & Jones, 2018). First-line approaches to remedy common discomforts of pregnancy consistently correlate with optimal health, such as a whole-foods diet, addressing stressors, and regular physical activity.

A series of themed discussions brought together policymakers, Indigenous elders, researchers, and healthcare providers on subjects such as health determinates, COVID-19 impacts, policies and practices that amplify or undermine health equity and justice, and community response. Together, they identified goals, including the following: recognize the interconnectedness of all planetary elements; invest in the ecological and social determinants of health for all communities; transform health and social systems to better account for equity; and develop approaches grounded in an ethic of care, compassion, trust building, and togetherness (Ndumbe-Eyoh et al., 2021).

To achieve health, providers should partner with communities toward change. Health is a weighted equation in which we are all factors; it is simultaneously an equation of individual, community, and ecological health. Creativity and change are required to balance the equation and move toward health. We do it together because we are in it together.

Prenatal care for common discomforts is an opportunity to work together toward optimal health over time through listening, learning, and reflecting on needs and priorities; sharing information and evidence-based approaches; identifying goals; creating an evolving care plan together; and staying in a relationship supportive of health.

II. Poor quality of sleep

Most pregnant people report poor sleep quality (Kizilirmak et al., 2012). Through careful subjective history, the provider differentiates normal altered sleep in pregnancy (discussed in detail later in this section) and actual lack of adequate sleep and sleep disorders. Lack of adequate sleep and sleep disorders are associated with depression, preterm birth, and serious neonatal and maternal complications (Brown et al., 2018; Querejeta Roca et al., 2020). A large meta-analysis of 65 studies correlated sleep disorders (obstructive sleep apnea, snoring, excessive sleep, and inadequate sleep) with multiple complications, including preeclampsia, gestational diabetes, cesarean birth, and depression (Yang et al., 2020). Societal factors and socioeconomic stressors are not to be underestimated: neighborhood stress and violence correlate directly to the duration of a pregnant person's sleep (Mellman et al., 2018).

Many factors may contribute to altered sleep and poor quality of sleep during pregnancy: safety, life stressors, musculoskeletal pain, fetal movement, increased frequency of voids, hunger, and nausea. Individuals report poor sleep quality in every trimester of pregnancy, including difficulty falling asleep and staying asleep and frequent waking.

After thorough history and diagnosis of benign pregnancy sleep alterations, sharing information about natural, beneficial alterations in sleep during pregnancy may help reframe mild discomfort. For example, restless sleep and multiple nocturnal voids have beneficial effects: research suggests they protect from stillbirth. In a prospective case-control study, pregnant people reported having voided only once or less the night before a stillbirth (Heazell et al., 2018). Light, restless, broken sleep patterns also appear to be protective for the fetus. A review of case-control studies found that restless sleep was associated with decreasing odds of stillbirth (Cronin et al., 2020). Nunn et al. (2016) suggest that a biphasic sleep pattern with a "first sleep" followed by a period of wakefulness and a "second sleep" has been part of the human sleep pattern throughout evolution. Understanding the normalcy of nighttime waking is a perspective change: the goals are to focus on obtaining adequate sleep overall and the ability to fall back to sleep and address discomforts and mental and physical health needs in the night.

A. *Subjective*
  1. Timing and severity of sleep disturbances, with particular attention to inadequate or excessive sleep
  2. Perceptions and expectations
  3. Sleep positions
  4. Screening for anxiety and posttraumatic stress disorder (PTSD)
  5. Sources of stress
  6. Pain
  7. Nighttime disturbances: noises, neighborhood, pets, family members, work hours
  8. Breathing, screening for obstructive sleep apnea, disordered breathing, snoring
  9. Impact on daily functioning
  10. Caffeine and other stimulant intake
  11. Daily habits, including daily exercise
  12. Evening routine and screen time
  13. Self-treatment
  14. Use of any dietary supplements, herbs, or medications for sleep

B. *Goals for clinical management*
  1. Assess quantity and quality of sleep and perceptions regarding sleep.
  2. Provide support to identify and address stressors and disturbances.
  3. Differentiate between normal altered sleep in pregnancy and lack of adequate sleep. As appropriate, provide information regarding sleep hygiene, circadian rhythms, and measures to improve sleep.
  4. Support the pregnant person in choosing and moving toward their goals for sleep.

C. *Management*
  Once expected and normal alterations in sleep patterns during pregnancy are differentiated from true primary insomnia or secondary insomnia, treatment focuses on individual causes and individual needs. Sleep experts recommend avoiding caffeine intake within a minimum

of 8–10 hours before bedtime (Huberman, 2021). Robust evidence in broader demographic groups supports cognitive–behavioral therapy for true insomnia (Baglioni et al., 2020). Moderate exercise, such as daily brisk walking, has also been an effective treatment in other demographic populations (King et al., 1997).

Sleep is crucial to health, and sleep in the second half of pregnancy is challenging for most. Exploration of sleep hygiene as a treatment plan may be helpful. Sleep hygiene includes the creation of an evening rhythm that is performed every night before going to sleep. The pregnant person notes factors that help them feel drowsy, safe, and relaxed. Explore barriers to self-care and relaxation. Evening relaxation therapies include massage, warm baths, showers, low light, warm bedroom, strolling outside, avoiding activating or disturbing stimuli, calming music and scents, reading children's bedtime stories, and singing lullabies and humor. Chamomile contains apigenin, a flavonoid associated with improved sleep quality, and chamomile itself improves sleep quality and is safe, as reported in a meta-analysis of 12 randomized controlled trials (Godos et al., 2020; Hieu et al., 2019).

Exposure to the light of screens on computers, tablets, and cell phones is associated with poor sleep quality (Salfi et al., 2021), suppresses melatonin production, disrupts sleep quality, and leads to decreased alertness the following day (Sroykham & Wongsawat, 2013; West et al., 2011). Reducing late-evening blue-light exposure by wearing amber glasses reduces insomnia (Shechter et al., 2018) and improves sleep quality and mood (Burkhart & Phelps, 2009). Although avoiding evening exposure to blue light from screens is necessary for optimal sleep, bright light and overhead light of any color suppress melatonin. In contrast, low lighting, such as candles or desk or table lamps rather than bright overhead lamps, after 10 p.m. promotes quality sleep (Huberman, 2021).

Sleep pattern is determined by light exposure; the types of orange-hued light seen at sunrise and sunset provide key stimuli for setting circadian rhythm daily (Rivera & Huberman, 2020). People exposed to greater amounts of bright light in the early morning fall asleep more quickly and have fewer sleep disturbances during the night compared to those exposed to low light in the morning (Figueiro et al., 2017). Neuroscientist Andrew Huberman and sleep expert Matthew Walker recommend early-morning and late-evening sunlight exposure as among the most effective interventions for sleep. They recommend exposure to bright light within 30–60 minutes of waking. Even on a cloudy day, sunlight provides a much greater light intensity than a lightbox or any type of indoor lighting. Twenty to 60 minutes of sun exposure is optimal, but lesser durations of time and the use of lightboxes can be a helpful alternative (Huberman, 2021). Other sleep researchers focus on the correlation between lower vitamin D levels and poor quality sleep and shorter sleep duration (Muscogiuri et al., 2019). Studies suggest that vitamin D supplements improve sleep quality (Chan & Lo, 2021).

A higher intake of vegetables and fruits is also associated with better sleep quality, shorter time to fall asleep, and better-quality sleep (Jansen et al., 2021). In young people with low fruit and vegetable intake, an increase of three or more servings led to a decrease in insomnia compared to those with no change or a more minor increase in fruit and vegetable intake (Jansen et al., 2021).

In small case-controlled trials on acupuncture for sleep in pregnancy, acupuncture significantly improved sleep scores (Foroughinia et al., 2020). Studies in nonpregnant populations suggest that acupuncture may be an effective, safe treatment for insomnia (Lan et al., 2015). In a blinded randomized clinical trial using the "double dummy" technique, the acupuncture cohort slept more and reported significantly better daytime functioning and return of their full energetic state; this concords with Chinese medical theory that "energetic daytime function" and "powerful nocturnal sleep" form a circle. Rupture of this cycle leads to "daytime low spirit" and "nighttime hyperarousal state" (Guo et al., 2013). Some communities have the availability of low-cost treatment through community acupuncture clinics (https://www.pocacoop.com).

Pharmacologic treatment of insomnia is discouraged in pregnancy because of inadequate safety data and side effects. However, pharmacologic treatment has been shown in a meta-analysis to be no superior to behavioral therapy in treating insomnia (Mitchell et al., 2012).

III. Musculoskeletal

Musculoskeletal discomforts are experienced by many pregnant people, with over 60% incidence of back pain in pregnancy. The majority of these cases are new onset (Wang et al., 2004). Hormonal changes of pregnancy cause the relaxation of ligaments throughout the body. The resulting increased mobility of pelvic joints and widening of the sacroiliac and symphyseal joints facilitate childbirth but may lead to pelvic instability and pain. Biomechanical factors contribute to pain. The growing uterus moves the center of gravity forward, pulls the spine into lordosis, and strains the lower back. In most cases, the pain resolves within 4 weeks after delivery.

Two distinct sites of lumbopelvic pain are common during pregnancy: low back pain (LBP) in the lumbar spine area and pelvic girdle pain (PGP) in the sacroiliac area, the symphysis pubis, or the gluteal area, possibly with radiation to the posterior thigh. LBP and PGP may occur concurrently (Vermani et al., 2009). Both LBP and PGP may be provoked by any sustained posture or activity, including prolonged sitting, standing, or walking. PGP generally is more debilitating than LBP (Gutke et al., 2006). Individuals with PGP may report a "catching" sensation in the leg while walking and may report that pain is aggravated by twisting, standing on one leg, climbing stairs, and turning in bed.

Many treatments target both LBP and PGP; differences in approach are specified next and in **Table 32-1**.

Table 32-1 Differential Diagnosis and Management of Pelvic Pain and Low Back Pain in Pregnancy

	Subjective	Physical Exam	Imaging	Treatment
Low back pain	Lumbar pain, worse with forward flexion	Negative posterior pelvic pain provocation test	Not indicated	Water aerobics Group exercise for abdominal, back, and pelvic strength Acupuncture Osteopathic manipulation Exercise: pelvic tilt Abdominal support garments
Pelvic girdle pain	Sacroiliac pain May radiate to the posterior thigh May involve symphysis pubis or gluteal area	Positive posterior pelvic pain provocation test	Not indicated	Nonelastic pelvic belt to increase stability of the sacroiliac joint Individualized pelvic stabilizing and core strengthening exercises
Cauda equina syndrome (severe nerve compression)	Rapid onset of bilateral radiating pain Lower extremity numbness and weakness Numbness of perineum, inner thigh, back of legs Bladder or bowel dysfunction	Supine straight leg raise elicits radiating pain to ipsilateral foot on hip flexion.	Immediate magnetic resonance imaging	Orthopedic consultation If stable: bed rest and muscle relaxants If deteriorating: surgery

Data from Smith, M. W., Marcus, P. S., & Wurtz, L. D. (2008). Orthopedic issues in pregnancy. *Obstetrical & Gynecological Survey, 63*(2), 103–111. doi:10.1097/OGX.0b013e318160161c; Vermani, E., Mittal, R., & Weeks, A. (2009). Pelvic girdle pain and low back pain in pregnancy: A review. *Pain Practice, 10*(1), 60–71. doi:10.1111/j.1533-2500.2009.00327.x

A. *Prevention*

Regular moderate exercise before and throughout pregnancy is strongly recommended. Canadian guidelines promote a total 150 minutes of moderate exercise weekly (Mottola et al., 2018). Regular exercise decreases LBP (Backhausen et al., 2019) and reduces the severity but not the incidence of LBP and PGP (Davenport et al., 2019).

Workplace restrictions may significantly affect an individual's risk. Because sustained sitting and standing may provoke pain, a pregnant person benefits from the freedom to change activities and positions frequently. Research shows that pregnant people who have job autonomy and the ability to take breaks at work experience less back pain, whereas those working in jobs that necessitate staying in a confined area experience more back pain (Cheng et al., 2009).

Disruptions in the intestinal microbiome (dysbiosis) and the associated impaired barrier function of the intestinal mucosa (leaky gut) lead to central sensitization and neuroinflammation and are linked with many types of chronic pain, including LBP (Dekker et al., 2020; Dworsky-Fried et al., 2020) A whole-foods diet with an abundance and variety of vegetables and fruits to provide polyphenols and fibers may decrease the risk of musculoskeletal pain, as well as improve overall health. Polyphenols and fiber are necessary for a healthy intestinal microbiome and reduction of inflammation. In addition, polyphenols have anti-nociceptive effects and attenuate neuropathic and inflammatory pain (Deledda et al., 2021). An anti-inflammatory diet, as described by the Dietary Inflammatory Index score, correlates with less pain sensitivity and a lower prevalence of LBP (Association of Academic Physiatrists, 2021; Correa-Rodríguez et al., 2020).

In a review of 81 studies, low vitamin D levels correlated with the prevalence of various types of chronic pain (Wu et al., 2018). Researchers have demonstrated that vitamin D supplementation reduces widespread chronic pain (Yong et al., 2017), nonspecific musculoskeletal pain (Le Goaziou et al. 2013), and LBP (Ghai et al., 2017). In addition, labor pain is more intense for those with low intrapartum vitamin D levels (Koyucu & Özcan, 2021).

Researchers have described inaccuracies in the Institute of Medicine analysis that underestimated the required daily intake (Vieth & Holick, 2018). Recommended daily intake is 600 IU for the pregnant person (Office of Dietary Supplements [ODS], 2021). Supplementation of 1,000 IU daily for 2 months was insufficient to raise blood levels to at least 30 ng/mL in those with mild insufficiency (Biancuzzo et al., 2013). In an analysis of 108 studies, researchers concluded that a daily intake of 2,909 IU is needed to achieve 25(OH)D concentrations of 20 ng/mL in 97.5% of healthy adults (Veugelers et al., 2015). The tolerable upper intake level for pregnant and nonpregnant adults is 4,000 IU (100 mcg) (ODS, 2021). Research is unclear whether higher doses of vitamin D in conjunction with calcium supplementation may be associated with kidney stones over time (Giustina et al., 2020).

B. Database

The distribution of pain is the most helpful history item for diagnosis. The presence of "red-flag" signs and symptoms indicates the possibility of disk herniation and requires immediate consultation and possibly magnetic resonance imaging (MRI) of the spine (**Table 32-2**).

1. Subjective
   a. Signs or symptoms of preterm labor: regular rhythmic pain, with or without increased pelvic pressure, leaking of vaginal fluid, vaginal bleeding
   b. Signs or symptoms of pyelonephritis: midback or flank pain, fever, malaise, nausea and vomiting, dysuria, suprapubic pain
   c. Events preceding onset
      i. Recent or past history of physical trauma
      ii. History of similar pain
      iii. Anxiety or depression
      iv. Patterns of activity throughout the day
   d. Location and characteristics of pain
      i. Radiation: bilateral or unilateral to thigh or foot
      ii. Pattern of pain: intermittent or constant
      iii. Postures or movements that provoke or alleviate pain
      iv. Quality: sharp, aching, dull; intensity
      v. Level of impact on function and patterns of pacing activity during the day
      vi. Self-treatment, coping strategies, pain beliefs, remedies, and over-the-counter medications
2. Objective
   a. In the setting of rhythmic LBP, consider cervical examination as part of preterm labor assessment (see Chapter 35, Preterm Labor Management).
   b. In the setting of flank (midback pain), evaluate costovertebral angle tenderness to rule out pyelonephritis.
   c. Observe gait and ability to change positions; observe distress level.
   d. Palpate over the sacroiliac, lumbar, and symphysis regions. This may help identify pain distribution to differentiate between LBP and PGP and rule out structural abnormalities.
   e. Do a posterior pelvic pain provocation test to differentiate PGP from LBP.
      i. The patient lies supine with hips flexed to 90 degrees.
      ii. The examiner applies pressure on the flexed knee in the longitudinal axis of the femur while stabilizing the pelvis with the other hand resting on the opposite anterior superior iliac spine.
      iii. If this maneuver produces deep pain in the gluteal region, the test is positive and supports a diagnosis of PGP.
   f. Perform the supine active straight leg raise (SLR) test to identify the possibility of disk herniation with nerve compression. If the SLR elicits pain radiating in a dermatomal pattern or numbness or leg weakness, carry out the following tests: reflexes (Achilles or knee), sensation of lateral and medial sides of feet and toes, and strength testing of the big toe during extension.
   g. Imaging studies, such as MRI, are recommended only when in the setting of multiple red flags (Albert et al., 2008).
3. Differential diagnosis
   a. Pregnancy-related LBP or PGP
   b. Preterm labor
   c. Pyelonephritis
   d. Muscle strain caused by trauma
   e. Sciatica

Table 32-2 Musculoskeletal Red-Flag Symptoms Requiring Consultation or Referral

- Sudden onset of incapacitating back or leg pain, especially pain radiating from the spine along a dermatome bilaterally
- Numbness of perineum, inner thighs, or backs of legs
- Bladder or bowel dysfunction; decreased rectal sphincter tone
- Localized neurologic symptoms: symptoms limited to one nerve root dermatome
- Decreased muscle strength and sensitivity
- Structural deformity
- Altered deep tendon reflexes

4. Goals for clinical management
   a. Decrease daily pain
   b. Physical fitness for reduction of musculoskeletal pain
      i. PGP is less likely than LBP to respond to exercise classes. The abdominal lift garment may be the most beneficial maternity support garment for LBP (Albert et al., 2008).
      ii. Workplace modification: a provider's letter to the employer recommending regular rest breaks and movement outside of confined working areas may benefit some individuals.
   c. Medication for pregnancy-related LBP and PGP
      i. Acetaminophen may not be more effective than a placebo for LBP and PGP of pregnancy (Vermani et al., 2009).
      ii. Nonsteroidal anti-inflammatory drugs such as ibuprofen are not recommended in the last trimester of pregnancy because of risks of premature closure of the ductus arteriosus and oligohydramnios.
      iii. Opioids: Occasional use of small doses of opioids (e.g., codeine) is sometimes indicated in severe pain cases. Opioid use in late pregnancy can cause respiratory depression in the newborn and, with long-term use, withdrawal effects in the newborn (Vermani et al., 2009).
      iv. Curcumin, a component of turmeric, is a dietary supplement with an analgesic and anti-inflammatory effect similar to that of ibuprofen, without the adverse effects (Marton et al., 2020). In 2018 the U.S. Food and Drug Administration (FDA) granted curcumin the status of "Generally Recognized as Safe" (FDA, 2018). The European Food Safety Authority (EFSA, 2010) reports no concerns about genotoxicity. Several authors have reviewed a large body of preclinical evidence supporting the use of curcumin for the prevention and management of pregnancy complications such as gestational diabetes, preeclampsia, depression, fetal growth restriction, and preterm birth (Filardia et al., 2020; Ghaneifar et al., 2020; Tossetta et al., 2021).
      Curcumin is used in divided doses of 1 g daily for chronic pain and up to 1.5–2.0 g daily for acute pain. Doses of 2 g daily may cause gastric upset; lower doses are well tolerated.
      v. Vitamin D supplementation
5. Referrals and self-management resources
   a. European guidelines consider the evidence sufficient to recommend the following for PGP: gentle exercise, individualized physical therapy, massage, acupuncture, osteopathic manipulation, and chiropractic care (Albert et al., 2008).
   b. Pelvic Partnership (http://www.pelvicpartnership.org.uk/).
6. Patient education (adapted from www.acpwh.org)
   a. Be as active as possible within the limits of pain. Staying active can reduce pain and improve function (Davenport et al., 2019; Krismer & van Tulder, 2007).
   b. Regular exercise decreases LBP (Backhausen et al., 2019) and reduces the severity but not the incidence of LPB and PGP (Davenport et al., 2019).
   c. Some studies report that craniosacral therapy and acupuncture reduce PGP pain (Liddle & Pivnick, 2015).
   d. For PGP, pelvic stabilizing exercises given by a physical therapist are effective (Vleeming et al., 2008).
   e. Identify and modify activities that worsen the pain. Advise supportive shoes and avoidance of heels.
   f. Maternity support garments as needed:
      i. For PGP, a nonelastic pelvic belt stabilizes the sacroiliac joints and may provide pain relief (Damen et al., 2006). It is most effective when at the level of the greater trochanter.
      ii. Physiotherapists recommend that pelvic support belts be worn for short periods of time rather than continuously (Albert et al., 2008; Chow et al., 2009).
      iii. Place one or more pillows between the knees and one under the abdomen when sleeping side-lying. The exaggerated Simms position is ideal for the end of pregnancy. A demonstration or showing images is necessary to teach exaggerated Simms.
   g. Posture exercises for pregnancy (Johns Hopkins Medicine, n.d.):
   Stand with back to a wall, knees slightly bent, feet hip-width apart. Gently and slowly tilt and circle pelvis and hips to find the relaxed spot where the low back is not affected. Gently bring the low back toward the wall.
   Imagine a line going up from the top and back of the head, drawing it up (like the stem at the top of a hanging pear). Try slightly tipping the chin downward. Do not force the shoulders back. Instead, play with the exercises just described while feeling for a release in the low back, shoulders, hips, and jaw. Wait for the in-breath. Pretend to be a pear: feel the in-breath fill the low belly and back.
   Cat–cow exercise: On hands and knees, slowly and gently tip pelvis while lower back straightens and rounds. Do not overextend; come to flat back and repeat. Breathe slowly.

IV. Gastrointestinal tract
Elevated levels of hormones support the pregnancy itself by relaxing the uterine muscle and have the consequence

of relaxing other smooth muscles throughout the body (Amazu et al., 2020). Smooth muscle relaxation decreases gastric and intestinal motility and contributes to nausea, heartburn, and constipation. Internal pressure from the growing uterus additionally contributes to heartburn.

Treatment approaches to common gastrointestinal tract discomforts of pregnancy, such as nausea, heartburn, and constipation, proceed in a stepwise algorithm beginning with lifestyle and dietary modifications and gentle natural remedies, with prescription pharmaceutical treatment reserved for severe symptoms.

A. *Nausea and vomiting of pregnancy*
  1. Definition and clinical implications
     Nausea and vomiting of pregnancy (NVP) are considered to be a result of hormonal changes. The reported incidence of NVP is 50%–85% of all pregnant people. The term "morning sickness" is misleading; research has found that nausea of pregnancy peaks in the morning, continues throughout the day, and peaks again in the evening (Gadsby et al., 2020). Typically, symptom onset is around 5–7 weeks from the last menstrual period, with resolution at 11–14 weeks' gestation. In a subset of individuals, symptoms may persist until 18 weeks, and 5% of pregnant people have nausea throughout pregnancy. Hypoglycemia or extreme fatigue can precipitate nausea in any trimester. Some individuals experience a return of mild nausea of pregnancy in the final weeks.

     The presence of first-trimester nausea is protective against miscarriage (DeVilbiss et al., 2020). Reduced maternal nutrient intake, as commonly occurs during the first trimester in individuals with NVP, seems to trigger complex hormonal and metabolic changes that enhance placental growth (Huxley, 2000). It is also proposed that NVP serves a protective evolutionary function, causing people to avoid foods that could cause harm to the embryo (Sherman & Flaxman, 2002).

     Individuals presenting with NVP must be screened for hyperemesis gravidarum (HG), which has an incidence of 0.3%–1% of pregnancies (Boelig et al., 2018). On the continuum from severe NVP to HG, HG is defined as symptoms that lead to weight loss of more than 5% of prepregnancy body weight, hypokalemia, and dehydration or ketonuria. HG may require hospitalization. It can be associated with severe sequelae, such as micronutrient deficiency or Wernicke encephalopathy (Dodds et al., 2006; Holmgren et al., 2008). HG requires medical management.

     Explore self-treatment when an individual presents with NVP. Hollyer et al. (2002) report that 61% of individuals with NVP report using complementary and alternative remedies, but only 8% of individuals had discussed these remedies with their healthcare provider.

B. *Database*
  1. Subjective data
     a. Timing of onset, pattern, and frequency of nausea and vomiting
        i. The Pregnancy-Unique Quantification of Emesis and Nausea (PUQE) index may be used to evaluate severity. The individual's subjective experience of the impact of symptoms on their life is an important consideration and may override the PUQE score (King & Murphy, 2009) (**Table 32-3**).

Table 32-3 Pregnancy-Unique Quantification of Emesis and Nausea Index

1. On an average day, for how long do you feel nauseated or sick to your stomach?				
>6 hr	4–6 hr	2–3 hr	≤1 hr	Not at all
(5 points)	(4 points)	(3 points)	(2 points)	(1 point)
2. On an average day, how many times do you vomit or throw up?				
≥7	5–6	3–4	1–2	None
(5 points)	(4 points)	(3 points)	(2 points)	(1 point)
3. On an average day, how many times do you have retching or dry heaves without bringing anything up?				
≥7	5–6	3–4	1–2	None
(5 points)	(4 points)	(3 points)	(2 points)	(1 point)

Total score (sum of replies to 1, 2, and 3): mild NVP, ≤6; moderate NVP, 7–12; severe NVP, ≥13.

Reprinted from Lacasse, A., Rey, E., Ferreira, E., Morin, C., & Bérard, A. (2008). Validity of a modified Pregnancy-Unique Quantification of Emesis and Nausea (PUQE) scoring index to assess severity of nausea and vomiting of pregnancy. *American Journal of Obstetrics and Gynecology*, 198(1), 71.e3. doi:10.1016/j.ajog.2007.05.051; with permission from Elsevier.

b. Triggers and coexisting gastric reflux
c. Eating habits and self-treatment
d. Red flags for gallbladder disease and hemolysis, elevated liver enzymes, and low platelets (HELLP) syndrome, which may present with nausea and emesis
    i. Epigastric pain, right upper quadrant pain, or coffee grounds emesis
    ii. Upper abdominal pain in a pattern of biliary colic (episodes of sharp, intense pain after meals or at night lasting 30 minutes to 3 hours, or radiation to back or right shoulder) may indicate gallbladder disease.
2. Objective data
    a. Weight loss
    b. Urinalysis: ketones and specific gravity
    c. Signs of dehydration: tachycardia, dry mucosa, and sunken eyes
    d. If severe symptoms are present: Order an electrolyte panel and an obstetric ultrasound to rule out twin gestation or trophoblastic disease (molar pregnancy).
    e. If the onset of symptoms occurs in the third trimester: Rule out HELLP syndrome with complete blood count (CBC) and platelets, even if symptoms are not severe.
    f. If symptoms suggest gallbladder disease: CBC, lipase, liver enzymes, and abdominal ultrasound
3. Differential diagnosis
    a. Dehydration
    b. Ketonuria
    c. Electrolyte imbalance
    d. Hyperemesis gravidarum
    e. Gallbladder, liver, or pancreatic disease
    f. HELLP syndrome (third trimester)
    g. Fatty liver of pregnancy (rare)
4. Goals for clinical management
    a. Differentiate normal NVP from hyperemesis and other serious pathology.
    b. Provide comprehensive education for individuals with NVP about dietary and lifestyle changes to minimize symptoms.
    c. Provide evidence-based information about safe alternative and complementary treatments for NVP.
    d. Provide evidence-based pharmacotherapy for the treatment of NVP.
    e. Assess results of treatment and provide intravenous rehydration as needed.
5. Treatment
   People commonly find that one therapeutic measure works well for a few days but becomes less effective. Knowledge of multiple treatments is beneficial to switch tactics as needed. If heartburn exists concurrent with NVP, treatment of the heartburn is shown to decrease symptoms of NVP (Gill et al., 2009).
6. Education
   Reassure that mild to moderate symptoms do not harm fetal growth and development. Discuss dietary and lifestyle changes.
7. Hydration and nutrition
    a. Avoid dehydration by sipping small amounts of water frequently (as little as an ounce every 15 minutes). Large volumes of fluid may provoke nausea.
    b. Drink cold fluids between meals instead of with meals.
    c. Eat small amounts of food that include protein every 1–2 hours. Low blood sugar provokes nausea. Eat a high-protein snack at bedtime.
    d. Keep dry crackers at the bedside and eat a few before rising in the morning.
    e. Avoid spicy or fatty foods.
8. Trigger avoidance: Triggers are highly individual but may include the following:
    a. Strong odors and stuffy rooms
    b. The sight or smell of certain foods
    c. Brushing teeth and toothpaste: Avoid brushing teeth within 1–2 hours after eating. Use a child's size toothbrush and small amounts of low-foaming toothpaste or natural toothpaste, or brush without toothpaste.
    d. Multivitamins: Continue to take a multivitamin if possible because it may decrease symptoms, but if taking a multivitamin aggravates nausea, discontinue and replace with 600 mcg of folic acid—resume multivitamin at a later gestational age when NVP resolves. A multivitamin without iron may be more easily tolerated.
9. Therapeutic
    a. Alternative and complementary: Ginger, chamomile, fennel seed, raspberry leaf, and mint are traditionally used in a tea or tincture for gastric upset. These herbs are regarded as safe by the Canadian Motherisk group (Mills et al., 2006) and the German Commission E (Blumenthal et al., 2000).
    b. Evidence exists supporting the effectiveness and safety of the following therapies:
        i. Acupressure wrist bands (Seabands, Travel-Eze) worn continuously over the P6 acupuncture point (Can Gürkan & Arslan, 2008)
        ii. Ginger capsules, 250 mg orally four times a day: Systematic reviews and meta-analyses conclude that ginger is safe and effective for reducing nausea in pregnancy (Hu et al., 2022; Sharifzadeh et al., 2018; Stanisiere et al., 2018).
        iii. Vitamin B_6, 25 mg orally three times a day, was not more effective than ginger (Hu et al., 2022). Avoid excessive doses of vitamin B_6 because it may cause peripheral neuropathy (Keller et al., 2008).

c. Intravenous fluid therapy: Intravenous fluid therapy with normal saline, alone or in combination with pharmaceuticals, typically improves symptoms for several days. Some people choose it as a primary management strategy, receiving hydration every few days as needed (King & Murphy, 2009). Avoid dextrose-containing fluids; they may precipitate Wernicke's encephalopathy, a rare but serious complication, in a person with thiamine deficiency. The addition of thiamine is recommended for the prevention of Wernicke encephalopathy. Potassium chloride may be added as needed. Consultation is necessary for persistent nausea and vomiting with dehydration, and intravenous vitamins and minerals may be required.

10. Pharmacotherapy (**Table 32-4**)

    a. Antihistamines

    Diclegis, delayed release (doxylamine 10 mg, combined with pyridoxine 10 mg), is the only drug approved by the FDA for NVP (Nuangchamnong & Niebyl, 2014). Diclegis is taken as a daily dose rather than as needed.

Table 32-4 Pharmacotherapy for NVP

Generic Name (trade name)	Dosage	Major Side Effects
Antihistamines		
Doxylamine succinate-pyridoxine hydrochloride (Diclegis®)	10 mg doxylamine combined with 10 mg of pyridoxine, delayed release Four tablets daily: 2 at night, 1 in the morning, 1 in the afternoon	Mild drowsiness
Diphenhydramine	50–100 mg q 4–6 hr PO/IM/IV For treatment of dystonic reaction: 50 mg IV	Drowsiness
Trimethobenzamide	200 mg IM/PR q 6–8 hr	Drowsiness
Dopamine antagonists		
Metoclopramide	1–2 mg/kg IV (dilute in 50 mL IVF) or 5–10 mg q 8 hr PO/PR/IM	Agitation, anxiety, acute dystonic reactions*
Prochlorperazine	5–10 mg PO/IV/IM q 6–8 hr or 25 mg rectal suppository BID/PRN for breakthrough vomiting with other medications	Sedation, anticholinergic effects, EPS
Promethazine	12.5–25 mg PO/IV/IM/PR q 4–6 hr	Sedation, anticholinergic effects, dystonic reactions*
Serotonin (5-HT3) antagonists		
Ondansetron	4–8 mg PO q 6–8 hr 4–8 mg IV q 12 hr, given over 15 min	Headache Avoid use before 10 weeks due to possible fetal cleft palate and cardiac anomalies
Other		
Pyridoxine (vitamin B$_6$)	25 mg TID Consider combining with doxylamine	
Zingiber officinale (ginger)	Capsules: 250–500 mg TID-QID Not to exceed 1.5 g in 24 hr	

* Give 50 mg diphenhydramine before dose to prevent extrapyramidal reactions.

BID, twice daily; EPS, extrapyramidal symptoms; IM, intramuscular; IV, intravenous; IVF, intravenous fluid; PO, by mouth; PR, per rectum; PRN, as needed; QID, four times daily; TID, three times daily.

Data from King, T. L., & Murphy, P. A. (2009). Evidence-based approaches to managing nausea and vomiting in early pregnancy. *Journal of Midwifery & Women's Health*, 54(6), 435. doi: 10.1016/j.jmwh.2009.08.005; with permission from Elsevier.

b. Dopamine antagonists
Metoclopramide has been a drug of choice for many providers in treating severe NVP and HG. Recent research examining more than 3,400 first-trimester exposures found no association with any of several adverse outcomes (Matok et al., 2009). Comparing promethazine and metoclopramide, Tan and colleagues (2010) found similar efficacy, but metoclopramide had fewer side effects. In a small study on the treatment of HG, metoclopramide had similar efficacy compared to ondansetron but with increased side effects (Abas et al., 2014). Metoclopramide was associated with increased dizziness, dry mouth, headache, diarrhea, and palpitations.

c. 5-Hydroxytryptamine 3-receptor antagonists
Ondansetron is used increasingly off-label in the treatment of NVP. It is effective and has high patient satisfaction. Its use has been accompanied by controversy regarding safety. Small associations with fetal cardiac anomalies have been found in some studies with the use of ondansetron in the first trimester (Andrade, 2020; Danielsson et al., 2014), whereas a large retrospective study including 1,816,414 pregnancies, 88,467 with first-trimester ondansetron use, found no association between ondansetron use in the first trimester and newborns with cardiac anomalies (Huybrechts et al., 2018). Other authors report no cardiac anomalies but concur in reporting small associations between first-trimester use and birth anomalies, such as renal agenesis-dysgenesis and cleft palate (Huybrechts et al., 2018; Parker et al., 2018), and small-for-gestational-age babies at birth (Suarez et al., 2021).

Other concerns exist. The FDA has issued warnings about serious maternal dysrhythmias associated with the use of ondansetron (Koren, 2014). Additionally, there have been 33 case reports of rare but life-threatening intestinal obstruction in which ondansetron was the sole associated pharmaceutical, one of which was in a pregnant patient (Cohen et al., 2014).

d. Phenothiazines
Promethazine and prochlorperazine may be as effective as ondansetron and have no evidence of being teratogenic, although there is less human data than for metoclopramide and Diclegis (Briggs et al., 2015). These drugs cause significant sedation, making them difficult for individuals to tolerate.

11. Follow-up
a. Advise going to labor and delivery for rehydration and medication as needed for persistent emesis and inability to keep down fluids or foods.
b. Consider increasing the frequency of prenatal visits until moderate to severe symptoms diminish.

V. **Heartburn**
A. *Definition and discussion*

Heartburn is common during pregnancy. It is characterized by pain in the epigastric region. Symptoms are usually mild to moderate. Pregnancy seems to be protective against esophagitis and gastric ulcer disease, and these conditions are uncommon during pregnancy (Kang et al., 2020). Even severe heartburn of pregnancy typically resolves with birth.

A stepwise approach is recommended for treatment (Katz et al., 2022). Healthy lifestyle and dietary modifications are first-line approaches and resolve symptoms for many individuals: small healthy meals throughout the day, instead of a large evening meal, and longer intervals between eating and lying down (Quach et al., 2021). Dietary fiber, such as flax (psyllium), vegetables, whole grains, and legumes, is associated with decreased symptoms (Morozov et al., 2018). Individual heartburn triggers may be identified and avoided. Typical food triggers precipitating heartburn include tomato products, peppermint tea, citrus, soda, alcohol, tobacco, and fried food. Many midwives report that their patients find heartburn relief from slowly chewing raw almonds throughout the day.

If symptoms persist, the next step in the stepwise approach is safe home remedies and simple calcium or magnesium antacids to provide immediate relief for heartburn of pregnancy. Avoid Alka-Seltzer in pregnancy. Garden of Life's Vitamin Code Raw Cal-Mag is a safe food-based option. Ginger (*Zingiber officinale*), marshmallow root (*Althaea officinalis*), and the inner bark of slippery elm (*Ulmas rubra*) provide soothing relief for heartburn and gastritis (Romm, 2010). These herbs are considered generally regarded as safe for consumption (GRAS). Marshmallow root and slippery elm contain mucilage (insoluble polysaccharides) that soothes irritated or inflamed mucosa (Deters et al., 2010).

If pharmaceutical treatment is needed, current guidelines recommend daily Sucralfate or alginates such as Gaviscon as the first-line treatment for pregnancy heartburn (Katz et al., 2022). Both of these protect the esophagus locally rather than by systemic action. Sucralfate contains aluminum, which is minimally absorbed. Sucralfate's aluminum absorption into the bloodstream increases with multivitamin use; its dosing must be separated. Sucralfate will decrease the absorption of levothyroxine and certain antibiotics, including ciprofloxacin. The alginate Gaviscon is entirely different: it combines a low dose of antacid with sodium alginate, derived from a seaweed, which forms a mechanical barrier to reflux and protects the esophagus; research shows it be effective in treating heartburn in pregnancy that does not respond to simple antacids (De Ruigh et al., 2014; Quartarone, 2013).

Reserve histamine-2 receptor antagonists (H2RAs) for severe symptoms and proton pump inhibitors (PPIs) for the most persistent, severe cases. Stomach acid is necessary for the absorption of essential nutrients, destruction of ingested pathogens, and maintenance of a beneficial gastrointestinal microbiome: all of these are key functions for the maintenance of health in pregnancy. If symptoms can be relieved through healthy dietary changes, this is safer and more beneficial than medication. PPIs are the most effective pharmaceuticals for gastroesophageal reflux disease (GERD), providing profound and lasting suppression. They are not an appropriate first-line treatment for the benign heartburn of pregnancy because of safety concerns: a plethora of ongoing research associates PPIs with adverse effects. PPI use is associated with increased susceptibility to food-borne and enteric infection, including *Salmonella*, invasive *Escherichia coli*, *Listeria*, and *Clostridium difficile* infection (Hafiz et al., 2018; Trifan et al., 2017). Outpatients prescribed PPIs have as much as a threefold increased risk of *C. difficile* infection compared with matched controls (Freedberg et al., 2014). An independent risk of severe outcomes of COVID-19 for current PPI users (Lee et al., 2021) and a PPI dose-dependent risk of contracting COVID-19 (Almario, 2020) have been reported. Research implicates PPI use in iron deficiency (Tran-Duy et al., 2019).

Acid-suppressing drugs rapidly alter the gastrointestinal microbiome (Freedberg et al., 2014). The disruption in the microbiome may explain the association of pregnant individuals' prenatal use of acid-suppressive drugs with an increased risk of allergic disease in their children (Mulder et al., 2014). The FDA recommends limiting PPI use to no more than 2 weeks (FDA, 2021).

B. *Database (may include but is not limited to)*
Red-flag symptoms and signs (listed in Section 1b) differentiate benign heartburn from more serious medical conditions. Gallbladder disease, pancreatitis, and in the third trimester, HELLP syndrome and preeclampsia must be ruled out. Red-flag symptoms and signs require immediate medical evaluation.
   1. Subjective
      a. Typical symptoms of gastric acid reflux during pregnancy include the following:
         i. Transitory burning in the upper abdomen or mid-chest
         ii. Discomfort associated with eating or with a recumbent position
         iii. Relieved by antacids
      b. Red-flag symptoms include:
         i. Gallbladder disease: episodes of biliary colic
         ii. HELLP: Third-trimester persistent right upper quadrant, mid-epigastric, or retrosternal pain; possibly accompanied by generalized edema, nausea, vomiting, and malaise. HELLP may occur with or without hypertension.
         iii. Pancreatitis: acute onset of persistent, severe epigastric pain
   2. Objective
      a. Physical examination
         i. Assess for red-flag signs.
         ii. Right upper quadrant or mid-epigastrium tenderness
      b. Laboratory tests for persistent, as opposed to transitory, symptoms
         i. Serum amylase and lipase as indicated to rule out pancreatitis
         ii. Liver enzymes as indicated to rule out liver disease
         iii. Liver enzymes and platelets as indicated to rule out HELLP
   3. Assessment
      a. Normal gastric reflux of pregnancy: Diagnosis is based on symptoms alone.
   4. Goals of clinical management
      a. Assess reflux during pregnancy and rule out serious pathology.
      b. Discuss approaches, including lifestyle and dietary changes. Identify personal triggers. Eat multiple small, healthy meals throughout the day. Eat 3 hours before lying down. Increase dietary fiber through whole foods, such as flax, whole grains, vegetables, and legumes. Address causes of stress. Try natural remedies. Provide support in self-selection of the best treatment.
      c. If medication is needed, educate patients about the benefits and adverse effects of medication options. Begin with treatments that have minimal risks and maximal health benefits. Proceed in a stepwise approach.
   5. Management (**Table 32-5**)
   6. Follow-up
      a. Increase frequency of visits based on response to treatment
      b. Nutritionist referral
      c. Educate regarding danger signs: Heartburn and indigestion are not common postpartum symptoms; it is critical to seek care if epigastric pain occurs postpartum. Return to care promptly during pregnancy for persistent pain unresponsive to treatment for evaluation and workup for other causes (liver, gallbladder, pancreas).
      d. Physician consultation for persistent severe symptoms

VI. Constipation

As with nausea and heartburn, the hormones of pregnancy contribute to constipation. Forty percent of pregnant people report constipation during pregnancy, and more than half experience it in the postpartum, at rates two to three times higher than those of nonpregnant people (Kuronen et al., 2021). Almost half of people suffer from hemorrhoids during pregnancy or postpartum (Poskus et al., 2014). Prevention of constipation is the best prevention for hemorrhoids.

A. *Database*
   1. Subjective
      a. Frequency, discomfort, and most recent bowel movements, including pain and hardness
      b. Symptoms of hemorrhoids: pain, bulging, itching, bleeding
      c. Physical activity
      d. Review of hydration
      e. Detailed diet review

Table 32-5 Management for Heartburn During Pregnancy

Lifestyle Modifications

- Eat small frequent meals rather than two large meals (Jarosz & Taraszewska, 2014).
- Avoid frequent consumption of mint tea (Jarosz & Taraszewska, 2014).
- Do not drink large amounts of liquid with meals.
- Take a walk after dinner (Karim et al., 2011).
- Do not recline after meals (Karim et al., 2011).
- Do not gain more than the recommended weight during pregnancy.
- Eat in a slow and relaxed manner (Yamamichi et al., 2012).
- Identify and avoid triggers, which may include tomatoes, peppermint tea, citrus, carbohydrates, tobacco, alcohol, soda, and chocolate.

Remedies (Romm, 2010)

- Raw almonds (8–10 at a time) chewed slowly, as frequently as needed
- Ginger chews, a candy variety. Suck, do not chew, to treat symptoms PRN.
- Slippery elm lozenges 2–4 PRN, or slippery elm powder (1 teaspoon stirred into applesauce, juice, or water)
- Marshmallow root: 1 ounce of dried herb steeped for at least 30 minutes in 1 quart of hot water; strain, sip throughout the day as needed, up to 3 cups daily.
- Strong tea of chamomile, fennel, ginger, linden, alone or in combination
- Dandelion root tea (1–3 cups sipped throughout the day) or tincture (20–40 drops diluted in a small amount of water three times daily); contraindicated if there are painful gallstones (acute biliary colic) or cholecystitis

Antacids

Avoid magnesium trisilicate, sodium bicarbonate, bismuth, and Alka-Seltzer (Mahadevan & Kane, 2006).

Medication	Considerations
Gaviscon (Quartarone, 2013)	■ Avoid high doses in pregnancy. ■ Generally well tolerated ■ For maximum effect, take 30 minutes after meals and maintain an upright position.
Calcium- or magnesium-containing antacids (Tytgat et al., 2003)	■ Excessive use of calcium carbonate (> 2 g/day) can result in milk-alkali syndrome (hypercalcemia and alkalosis, which can cause renal damage). ■ Magnesium-containing antacids may cause diarrhea. ■ Avoid excessive doses of aluminum salts. ■ Although some advocate the benefits of calcium carbonate as an antacid because it also provides supplemental calcium, in reality, calcium carbonate contains only 40% elemental calcium and has poor bioavailability (Sipponen & Härkönen, 2010).
Sucralfate	Adverse effects unlikely

Histamine-2 receptor antagonists (H2RAs)

Cimetidine or ranitidine is preferred (Mahadevan & Kane, 2006).	■ A decrease in effectiveness of H2RA treatment may occur within 2–6 weeks of initiation of therapy (Komazawa et al., 2003). ■ The safety of H2RAs during the first trimester has not been established (Gilboa et al., 2014).

Proton pump inhibitors (PPIs)

Omeprazole (Prilosec®) is recommended as the PPI of choice (Mahadevan & Kane, 2006).	■ The use of PPIs during pregnancy is not associated with an increased risk of birth defects, perinatal mortality, or morbidity (Matok et al., 2012). ■ Adverse effects of PPIs include impaired nutrient absorption; increased risk of enteric infections, including gastroenteritis and *Clostridium difficile* infection; increased risk of community-acquired pneumonia; disrupted gastrointestinal microbiome; and an association with increased risk of allergic disease in the offspring (see text).

2. Objective
   a. Physical exam for assessment of hemorrhoids as needed
   b. Signs of mild dehydration: elevated pulse, dry lips, dry skin
   c. Elevated uterine fundal height on abdominal exam
3. Assessment
   a. Uncomplicated constipation of pregnancy
4. Goals of clinical management
   a. One or two normal, nonpainful bowel movements daily
   b. Maintain hydration status
5. Management
   a. Education: Hydration is critically essential to fetal and maternal health. Constipation is a helpful sign for the pregnant person to increase hydration. Adequate hydration can prevent complications for the pregnant person and their baby, such as maternal urinary tract infections, pyelonephritis, oligohydramnios, fetal cord compression, and painful maternal hemorrhoids.
   b. Adjust daily diet. At each meal and snack, include foods that help with constipation, such as:
      Fiber, such as green leafy vegetables or broccoli; whole grains; legumes like lentils, black beans, and chickpeas; chia; psyllium
      Flax: a unique source of fiber and fats
      Fats: avocado, olive oil, coconut oil, butter
      Fluids: Water throughout the day. Coffee is also a laxative.
      Fruits: Kiwi, papaya, and prunes are especially beneficial for gut health. Research suggests six prunes twice daily are more effective than psyllium supplements (Metamucil) (Attaluri et al., 2011).
      Flora: prebiotic and probiotic supplements and foods
   c. Lifestyle changes: Daily exercise combined with hydration helps prevent constipation.
   d. A bowel movement is an opportunity to prevent hemorrhoids and practice for the second stage of labor. Instead of straining while holding the breath, practice relaxing to aid the passage of a bowel movement. This practice can help individuals who have birthed rapidly in the past prepare for a gentler birth of the baby's head, and it may help prevent hemorrhoids during birth and bowel movements.
   e. Only when hydration, lifestyle, and dietary changes are inadequate is medication considered. Bulk-forming laxatives, such as the supplements ground flax or Metamucil (psyllium), are first-line pharmaceutical treatments for constipation during pregnancy. They are safe. Lactulose and bisacodyl have minimal absorption from the intestines, so they are theoretically safe. Other medications are used as needed for severe and persistent constipation, such as magnesium hydroxide, lactulose, and bisacodyl. Garden of Life's Vitamin Code Raw Cal-Mag is another natural alternative. Advise the pregnant person to start with small doses, less than recommended on the bottle, to discover the dosage that works for their body.
   f. Probiotics and prebiotics contribute to health (Hughes et al., 2022). The Clinical Guide to Probiotic Products Available in the USA is an evidence-based smartphone app designed for easy use to identify the scientific evidence for probiotics and the appropriate product, dose, and formulation for specific indications (Skokovic-Sunjic, 2022). This resource lists functional foods with added probiotic organisms as effective for constipation, including Activia and Yakult and several specific strains of bacteria used in probiotic supplements. Inulin, a prebiotic fiber available as an inexpensive supplement, is found in onion-family plants and chicory and dandelion roots. As a prebiotic, it improves the composition of the intestinal microbiome and modulates inflammation, with demonstrated benefits for insulin sensitivity, mineral absorption, and satiety (Hughes et al., 2022). It improves stool frequency and consistency in adults with constipation (Collado Yurrita et al., 2014), as well as in those with constipation related to inflammatory bowel disease (Bărboi et al., 2020). The addition of any new dietary or supplemental fiber or prebiotic can cause uncomfortable intestinal symptoms at first until the microbiome adjusts to the new substrate. Initial dosing of any prebiotic should be low. Inulin dosing should start at not more than 1–3 g a day for the first 1–2 weeks, gradually increasing the dose as tolerated up to 10–20 g/day. Some people may be unable to adjust to inulin supplement intake (Rezende et al., 2021).

References

Abas, M. N., Tan, P. C., Azmi, N., & Omar, S. Z. (2014). Ondansetron compared with metoclopramide for hyperemesis gravidarum: A randomized controlled trial. *Obstetrics and Gynecology, 123*(6), 1272–1279. doi:10.1097/AOG.0000000000000242

Albert, H. B., Ostgaard, H. C., Sturesson, B., Stuge, B., & Vleeming, A. (2008). European guidelines for the diagnosis and treatment of pelvic girdle pain. *European Spine Journal, 17*(6), 794–819. doi:10.1007/s00586-008-0602-

Almario, C. V., Chey, W. D., & Spiegel, B. (2020). Increased risk of COVID-19 among users of proton pump inhibitors. *American Journal of Gastroenterology, 115*(10), 1707–1715. doi:10.14309/ajg.0000000000000798

Amazu, C., Ma, X., Henkes, C., Ferreira, J. J., Santi, C. M., & England, S. K. (2020). Progesterone and estrogen regulate NALCN expression in human myometrial smooth muscle cells. *American Journal of Physiology. Endocrinology and Metabolism, 318*(4), E441–E452. doi:10.1152/ajpendo.00320.2019

Andrade C. (2020). Major congenital malformation risk after first trimester gestational exposure to oral or intravenous ondansetron. *Journal of Clinical Psychiatry, 81*(3), 20f13472. doi:10.4088/JCP.20f13472

Association of Academic Physiatrists. (2021, February 10). Pro-inflammatory diet associated with low back pain prevalence in U.S. adults. *Newswise.* https://www.newswise.com/articles/pro-inflammatory-diet-associated-with-low-back-pain-prevalence-in-u-s-adults?sc=dwhr&xy=10007438

Attaluri, A., Donahoe, R., Valestin, J., Brown, K., & Rao, S. S. (2011). Randomised clinical trial: dried plums (prunes) vs. psyllium for constipation. *Alimentary Pharmacology & Therapeutics, 33*(7), 822–828. doi:10.1111/j.1365-2036.2011.04594.x.

Avery, M. D., Saftner, M. A., Larson, B., & Weinfurter, E. V. (2014). A systematic review of maternal confidence for physiologic birth: Characteristics of prenatal care and confidence measurement. *Journal of Midwifery & Women's Health, 59*(6), 586–595. doi:10.1111/jmwh.12269

Backhausen, M. G., Bendix, J. M., Damm, P., Tabor, A., & Hegaard, H. K. (2019). Low back pain intensity among childbearing women and associated predictors. A cohort study. *Women and Birth: Journal of the Australian College of Midwives, 32*(4), e467–e476. doi:10.1016/j.wombi.2018.09.008

Baglioni, C., Bostanova, Z., Bacaro, V., Benz, F., Hertenstein, E., Spiegelhalder, K., Rücker, G., Frase, L., Riemann, D., & Feige, B. (2020). A systematic review and network meta-analysis of randomized controlled trials evaluating the evidence base of melatonin, light exposure, exercise, and complementary and alternative medicine for patients with insomnia disorder. *Journal of Clinical Medicine, 9*(6), 1949. doi:10.3390/jcm9061949

Bărboi, O. B., Ciortescu, I., Chirilă, I., Anton, C., & Drug, V. (2020). Effect of inulin in the treatment of irritable bowel syndrome with constipation (review). *Experimental and Therapeutic Medicine, 20*(6), 185. doi:10.3892/etm.2020.931

Biancuzzo, R. M., Clarke, N., Reitz, R. E., Travison, T. G., & Holick, M. F. (2013). Serum concentrations of 1,25-dihydroxyvitamin D2 and 1,25-dihydroxyvitamin D3 in response to vitamin D2 and vitamin D3 supplementation. *Journal of Clinical Endocrinology Metabolism, 98*(3), 973–979. doi:10.1210/jc.2012-2114

Blumenthal, M., Goldberg, A., & Brinckmann, J. (2000). *Herbal medicine: Expanded Commission E monographs.* Integrative Medicine Communications.

Boelig, R. C., Barton, S. J., Saccone, G., Kelly, A. J., Edwards, S. J., & Berghella, V. (2018). Interventions for treating hyperemesis gravidarum: A Cochrane systematic review and meta-analysis. *Journal of Maternal-Fetal & Neonatal Medicine, 31*(18), 2492–2505. doi:10.1080/14767058.2017.1342805

Briggs, G. G., Freeman, R. K., & Yaffe, S. J. (2015). *Drugs in pregnancy and lactation: A reference guide to fetal and neonatal risk* (10th ed.). Wolters Kluwer/Lippincott Williams & Wilkins Health.

Brown, N. T., Turner, J. M., & Kumar, S. (2018). The intrapartum and perinatal risks of sleep-disordered breathing in pregnancy: A systematic review and metaanalysis. *American Journal of Obstetrics and Gynecology, 219*(2), 147–161.e1. doi:10.1016/j.ajog.2018.02.004

Burkhart, K., & Phelps, J. R. (2009). Amber lenses to block blue light and improve sleep: A randomized trial. *Chronobiology International, 26*(8), 1602–1612. doi:10.3109/07420520903523719

Can Gürkan, O., & Arslan, H. (2008). Effect of acupressure on nausea and vomiting during pregnancy. *Complementary Therapy Clinical Practice, 14*(1), 46–52. doi:10.1016/j.ctcp.2007.07.002

Chan, V., & Lo, K. (2021). Efficacy of dietary supplements on improving sleep quality: A systematic review and meta-analysis. *Postgraduate Medical Journal, 98*(1158), 285–293. doi:10.1136/postgradmedj-2020-139319

Cheng, P. L., Pantel, M., Smith, J. T., Dumas, G. A., Leger, A. B., & Plamondon, A. (2009). Back pain of working pregnant women: Identification of associated occupational factors. *Applied Ergonomics, 40*(3), 419–423. doi:10.1016/j.apergo.2008.11.002

Chow, D. H., Chung, J. W., Ho, S., Lao, T., Li, Y., & Yu, W. (2009). Effectiveness of maternity support belts in reducing low back pain during pregnancy: A review. *Journal of Clinical Nursing, 18*(11), 1523–1532. doi:10.1111/j.1365-2702.2008.02749.x

Clarke, S., Jaffe, J., & Mutch, R. (2019). Overcoming communication barriers in refugee health care. *Pediatric Clinics of North America, 66*(3), 669–686. doi:10.1016/j.pcl.2019.02.012

Cohen, R., Shlomo, M., Dil, D. N., Dinavitser, N., Berkovitch, M., & Koren, G. (2014). Intestinal obstruction in pregnancy by ondansetron. *Reproductive Toxicology, 50*, 152–153. doi:10.1016/j.reprotox.2014.10.014

Collado Yurrita, L., San Mauro Martín, I., Ciudad-Cabañas, M. J., Calle-Purón, M. E., & Hernández Cabria, M. (2014). Effectiveness of inulin intake on indicators of chronic constipation; a meta-analysis of controlled randomized clinical trials. *Nutricion Hospitalaria, 30*(2), 244–252. doi:10.3305/nh.2014.30.2.7565

Correa-Rodríguez, M., Casas-Barragán, A., González-Jiménez, E., Schmidt-RioValle, J., Molina, F., & Aguilar-Ferrándiz, M. E. (2020). Dietary inflammatory index scores are associated with pressure pain hypersensitivity in women with fibromyalgia. *Pain Medicine, 21*(3), 586–594. doi:10.1093/pm/pnz238

Cronin, R. S., Wilson, J., Gordon, A., Li, M., Culling, V. M., Raynes-Greenow, C. H., Heazell, A., Stacey, T., Askie, L. M., Mitchell, E. A., Thompson, J., McCowan, L., & O'Brien, L. M. (2020). Associations between symptoms of sleep-disordered breathing and maternal sleep patterns with late stillbirth: Findings from an individual participant data meta-analysis. *PloS One, 15*(3), e0230861. doi:10.1371/journal.pone.0230861

Damen, L., Mens, J. M., Snijders, C. J., & Stam, H. J. (2006). The mechanical effect of a pelvic belt in patients with pregnancy-related pelvic pain. *Clinical Biomechanics, 21*(2), 122–127. doi:10.1016/j.clinbiomech.2005.08.016

Danielsson, B., Wikner, B. N., & Källén, B. (2014). Use of ondansetron during pregnancy and congenital malformations in the infant. *Reproductive Toxicology, 50*, 134–137. doi:10.1016/j.reprotox.2014.10.017

Davenport, M. H., Marchand, A. A., Mottola, M. F., Poitras, V. J., Gray, C. E., Jaramillo Garcia, A., Barrowman, N., Sobierajski, F., James, M., Meah, V. L., Skow, R. J., Riske, L., Nuspl, M., Nagpal, T. S., Courbalay, A., Slater, L. G., Adamo, K. B., Davies, G. A., Barakat, R., & Ruchat, S. M. (2019). Exercise for the prevention and treatment of low back, pelvic girdle and lumbopelvic pain during pregnancy: A systematic review and meta-analysis. *British Journal of Sports Medicine, 53*(2), 90–98. doi:10.1136/bjsports-2018-099400

De Ruigh, A., Roman, S., Chen, J., Pandolfino, E., & Kahrilas, P. J. (2014). Gaviscon Double Action Liquid (antacid & alginate) is more effective than antacid in controlling post-prandial oesophageal acid exposure in GERD patients: A double-blind crossover study. *Alimentary Pharmacology & Therapeutics*, *40*(5), 531–537. doi:10.1111/apt.12857

Dekker N., M., Mousa, A., Barrett, H. L., Naderpoor, N., & de Courten, B. (2020). Altered gut microbiota composition is associated with back pain in overweight and obese individuals. *Frontiers in Endocrinology*, *11*, 605. doi:10.3389/fendo.2020.00605

Deledda, A., Annunziata, G., Tenore, G. C., Palmas, V., Manzin, A., & Velluzzi, F. (2021). Diet-derived antioxidants and their role in inflammation, obesity and gut microbiota modulation. *Antioxidants*, *10*(5), 708. doi:10.3390/antiox10050708

Deters, A., Zippel, J., Hellenbrand, N., Pappai, D., Possemeyer, C., & Hensel, A. (2010). Aqueous extracts and polysaccharides from Marshmallow roots (Althea officinalis L.): Cellular internalisation and stimulation of cell physiology of human epithelial cells in vitro. Journal of Ethnopharmacology, 127(1), 62–69. doi:10.1016/j.jep.2009.09.050

DeVilbiss, E. A., Naimi, A. I., Mumford, S. L., Perkins, N. J., Sjaarda, L. A., Zolton, J. R., Silver, R. M., & Schisterman, E. F. (2020). Vaginal bleeding and nausea in early pregnancy as predictors of clinical pregnancy loss. *American Journal of Obstetrics and Gynecology*, *223*(4), 570.e1–570.e14. doi:10.1016/j.ajog.2020.04.002

Dodds, L., Fell, D. B., Joseph, K. S., Allen, V. M., & Butler, B. (2006). Outcomes of pregnancies complicated by hyperemesis gravidarum. *Obstetrics & Gynecology*, *107*(2), 285–292. doi:10.1097/01.AOG.0000195060.22832.cd

Dworsky-Fried, Z., Kerr, B. J., & Taylor, A. (2020). Microbes, microglia, and pain. *Neurobiology of Pain*, *7*, 100045. doi:10.1016/j.ynpai.2020.100045

European Food Safety Authority. (2010). Scientific opinion on the re-evaluation of curcumin (E 100) as a food additive. *EFSA Journal*, *8*(9), 1679.

Figueiro, M. G., Steverson, B., Heerwagen, J., Kampschroer, K., Hunter, C. M., Gonzales, K., … Rea, M. S. (2017). The impact of daytime light exposures on sleep and mood in office workers. Sleep Health, 3(3), 204–215. doi:10.1016/j.sleh.2017.03.005

Filardi, T., Varì, R., Ferretti, E., Zicari, A., Morano, S., & Santangelo, C. (2020). Curcumin: Could this compound be useful in pregnancy and pregnancy-related complications? *Nutrients*, *12*(10), 3179. doi:10.3390/nu12103179

Foroughinia, S., Hessami, K., Asadi, N., Foroughinia, L., Hadianfard, M., Hajihosseini, A., Pirasteh, N., Vossoughi, M., Vafaei, H., Faraji, A., Kasraeian, M., Doroudchi, M., Rafiee Monjezi, M., Roozmeh, S., & Bazrafshan, K. (2020). Effect of acupuncture on pregnancy-related insomnia and melatonin: A single-blinded, randomized, placebo-controlled trial. *Nature and Science of Sleep*, *12*, 271–278. doi:10.2147/NSS.S247628

Freedberg, D. E., Lebwohl, B., & Abrams, J. A. (2014). The impact of proton pump inhibitors on the human gastrointestinal microbiome. *Clinics in Laboratory Medicine*, *34*(4), 771–785. doi:10.1016/j.cll.2014.08.008

Gadsby, R., Ivanova, D., Trevelyan, E., Hutton, J. L., & Johnson, S. (2020). Nausea and vomiting in pregnancy is not just "morning sickness": Data from a prospective cohort study in the UK. *British Journal of General Practice*, *70*(697), e534–e539. doi:10.3399/bjgp20X710885

Ghai, B., Bansal, D., Kanukula, R., Gudala, K., Sachdeva, N., Dhatt, S. S., & Kumar, V. (2017). Vitamin D supplementation in patients with chronic low back pain: An open label, single arm clinical trial. *Pain Physician*, *20*(1), E99–E105.

Ghaneifar, Z., Yousefi, Z., Tajik, F., Nikfar, B., Ghalibafan, F., Abdollahi, E., & Momtazi-Borojeni, A. A. (2020). The potential therapeutic effects of curcumin on pregnancy complications: Novel insights into reproductive medicine. *IUBMB Life*, *72*(12), 2572–2583. doi:10.1002/iub.2399

Gianfredi, V., Buffoli, M., Rebecchi, A., Croci, R., Oradini-Alacreu, A., Stirparo, G., Marino, A., Odone, A., Capolongo, S., & Signorelli, C. (2021). Association between urban greenspace and health: A systematic review of literature. *International Journal of Environmental Research and Public Health*, *18*(10), 5137. doi:10.3390/ijerph18105137

Gilboa, S. M., Ailes, E. C., Rai, R. P., Anderson, J. A., & Honein, M. A. (2014). Antihistamines and birth defects: A systematic review of the literature. *Expert Opinion on Drug Safety*, *13*(12), 1667–1698. doi:10.1517/14740338.2014.970164

Gill, S. K., Maltepe, C., Mastali, K., & Koren, G. (2009). The effect of acid-reducing pharmacotherapy on the severity of nausea and vomiting of pregnancy. *Obstetrics and Gynecology International*, 585269. doi:10.1155/2009/585269

Giustina, A., Adler, R. A., Binkley, N., Bollerslev, J., Bouillon, R., Dawson-Hughes, B., Ebeling, P. R., Feldman, D., Formenti, A. M., Lazaretti-Castro, M., Marcocci, C., Rizzoli, R., Sempos, C. T., & Bilezikian, J. P. (2020). Consensus statement from 2nd International Conference on Controversies in Vitamin D. *Reviews in Endocrine & Metabolic Disorders*, *21*(1), 89–116. doi:10.1007/s11154-019-09532-w

Godos, J., Currenti, W., Angelino, D., Mena, P., Castellano, S., Caraci, F., Galvano, F., Del Rio, D., Ferri, R., & Grosso, G. (2020). Diet and mental health: Review of the recent updates on molecular mechanisms. *Antioxidants*, *9*(4), 346. doi:10.3390/antiox9040346

Guo, J., Wang, L. P., Liu, C. Z., Zhang, J., Wang, G. L., Yi, J. H., & Cheng, J.-L. (2013). Efficacy of acupuncture for primary insomnia: A randomized controlled clinical trial. *Evidence-Based Complementary and Alternative Medicine*, 163850. doi:10.1155/2013/163850

Gutke, A., Oberg, B., & Ostgaard, H. C. (2006). Pelvic girdle pain and lumbar pain in pregnancy: A cohort study of the consequences in terms of health and functioning. *Spine*, *31*(5), e149–e155. doi:10.1097/01.brs.0000201259.63363.e1

Hafiz, R. A., Wong, C., Paynter, S., David, M., & Peeters, G. (2018). The risk of community-acquired enteric infection in proton pump inhibitor therapy: Systematic review and meta-analysis. *Annals of Pharmacotherapy*, *52*(7), 613–622. doi:10.1177/1060028018760569

Hawes, A. M., Smith, G. S., McGinty, E., Bell, C., Bower, K., Lavish, T. A., Gaskin, D. J., & Thorpe, R. J., Jr. (2019). Disentangling race, poverty, and place in disparities in physical activity. *International Journal of Environmental Research and Public Health*, *16*(7), 1193. doi:10.3390/ijerph16071193

Heazell, A., Li, M., Budd, J., Thompson, J., Stacey, T., Cronin, R. S., Martin, B., Roberts, D., Mitchell, E. A., & McCowan, L. (2018). Association between maternal sleep practices and late stillbirth—findings from a stillbirth case-control study. *BJOG*, *125*(2), 254–262. doi:10.1111/1471-0528.14967

Hieu, T. H., Dibas, M., Surya Dila, K. A., Sherif, N. A., Hashmi, M. U., Mahmoud, M., Trang, N., Abdullah, L., Nghia, T., Y, M. N., Hirayama, K., & Huy, N. T. (2019). Therapeutic efficacy and safety of chamomile for state anxiety, generalized anxiety disorder, insomnia, and sleep quality: A systematic review and meta-analysis of randomized trials and quasi-randomized trials. *Phytotherapy Research: PTR*, *33*(6), 1604–1615. doi:10.1002/ptr.6349

Hollyer, T., Boon, H., Georgousis, A., Smith, M., & Einarson, A. (2002). The use of CAM by women suffering from nausea and vomiting during pregnancy. *BMC Complementary and Alternative Medicine, 2*, 5. doi:10.1186/1472-6882-2-5

Holmgren, C., Aagaard-Tillery, K. M., Silver, R. M., Porter, T. F., & Varner, M. (2008). Hyperemesis in pregnancy: An evaluation of treatment strategies with maternal and neonatal outcomes. *American Journal of Obstetrics and Gynecology, 198*(1), 56.e1–e4. doi:10.1016/j.ajog.2007.06.004

Hu, Y., Amoah, A. N., Zhang, H., Fu, R., Qiu, Y., Cao, Y., Sun, Y., Chen, H., Liu, Y., & Lyu, Q. (2020). Effect of ginger in the treatment of nausea and vomiting compared with vitamin B6 and placebo during pregnancy: A meta-analysis. *Journal of Maternal-Fetal & Neonatal Medicine, 35*(1), 187–196. doi:10.1080/14767058.2020.1712714

Huberman, A. (2021). *Toolkit for sleep*. Huberman Lab at Stanford School of Medicine. https://hubermanlab.com/toolkit-for-sleep/.

Hughes, R. L., Alvarado, D. A., Swanson, K. S., & Holscher, H. D. (2022). The prebiotic potential of inulin-type fructans: A systematic review. *Advances in Nutrition, 13*(2), 492–529. doi:10.1093/advances/nmab119.

Huxley, R. (2000). Nausea and vomiting in early pregnancy—its role in placental development. *Obstetrics & Gynecology, 95*(5), 779–782. doi:10.1016/s0029-7844(99)00662-6

Huybrechts, K. F., Hernández-Díaz, S., Straub, L., Gray, K. J., Zhu, Y., Patorno, E., Desai, R. J., Mogun, H., & Bateman, B. T. (2018). Association of maternal first-trimester ondansetron use with cardiac malformations and oral clefts in offspring. *JAMA, 320*(23), 2429–2437. doi:10.1001/jama.2018.18307

Jansen, E. C., She, R., Rukstalis, M., & Alexander, G. L. (2021). Changes in fruit and vegetable consumption in relation to changes in sleep characteristics over a 3-month period among young adults. *Sleep Health, 7*(3), 345–352. doi:10.1016/j.sleh.2021.02.005

Jarosz, M., & Taraszewska, A. (2014). Risk factors for gastroesophageal reflux disease: The role of diet. *Przeglad Gastroenterologiczny, 9*(5), 297–301. doi:10.32394/rpzh.2021.0145

Johns Hopkins Medicine. (n.d.). *Pregnancy and posture*. https://www.hopkinsmedicine.org/health/conditions-and-diseases/staying-healthy-during-pregnancy/pregnancy-and-posture

Kamysheva, E., Wertheim, E. H., Skouteris, H., Paxton, S. J., & Milgrom, J. (2009). Frequency, severity, and effect on life of physical symptoms experienced during pregnancy. *Journal of Midwifery & Women's Health, 54*(1), 43–49. doi:10.1016/j.jmwh.2008.08.00

Kang, A., Khokale, R., Awolumate, O. J., Faye, H., & Cancarevic, I. (2020). Is estrogen a curse or a blessing in disguise? Role of estrogen in gastroesophageal reflux disease. *Cureus, 12*(10), e11180. doi:10.7759/cureus.1118

Karim, S., Faryal, A., Majid, S., Majid, S., Salih, M., Jafri, F., Hamid, S., Shah, H. A., Nawaz, Z., & Tariq U. (2011). Regular post dinner walk; can be a useful lifestyle modification for gastroesophageal reflux. *Journal of the Pakistan Medical Association, 61*(6), 526–530.

Karpyn, A. E., Riser, D., Tracy, T., Wang, R., & Shen, Y. E. (2019). The changing landscape of food deserts. *UNSCN Nutrition, 44*, 46–53.

Katz, P. O., Dunbar, K. B., Schnoll-Sussman, F. H., Greer, K. B., Yadlapati, R., & Spechler, S. J. (2022). ACG clinical guideline for the diagnosis and management of gastroesophageal reflux disease. *American Journal of Gastroenterology, 117*(1), 27–56. doi:10.14309/ajg.0000000000001538

Keller, J., Frederking, D., & Layer, P. (2008). The spectrum and treatment of gastrointestinal disorders during pregnancy. *Nature Clinical Practice Gastroenterology & Hepatology, 5*(8), 430–443.

King, A. C., Oman, R. F., Brassington, G. S., Bliwise, D. L., & Haskell, W. L. (1997). Moderate-intensity exercise and self-rated quality of sleep in older adults. A randomized controlled trial. *JAMA, 277*(1), 32–37.

King, T. L., & Murphy, P. A. (2009). Evidence-based approaches to managing nausea and vomiting in early pregnancy. *Journal of Midwifery & Women's Health, 54*(6), 430–444. doi:10.1016/j.jmwh.2009.08.005.

Kizilirmak, A., Timur, S., & Kartal, B. (2012). Insomnia in pregnancy and factors related to insomnia. *Scientific World Journal*, 197093. doi:10.1100/2012/197093

Komazawa, Y., Adachi, K., Mihara, T., Ono, M., Kawamura, A., Fujishiro, H., & Kinoshita, Y. (2003). Tolerance to famotidine and ranitidine treatment after 14 days of administration in healthy subjects without *Helicobacter pylori* infection. *Journal of Gastroenterology and Hepatology, 18*(6), 678–682. doi:10.1046/j.1440-1746.2003.03041.x

Koren, G. (2014). Treating morning sickness in the United States—changes in prescribing are needed. *American Journal of Obstetrics and Gynecology, 211*(6), 602–606. doi:10.1016/j.ajog.2014.08.017

Koyucu, R. G., & Özcan, T. (2021). Effect of intrapartum vitamin D levels on labor pain. *Journal of Obstetrics and Gynaecology Research, 47*(11), 3857–3866. doi:10.1111/jog.14960

Krismer, M., & van Tulder, M. (2007). Strategies for prevention and management of musculoskeletal conditions: Low back pain (non-specific). *Best Practice & Research Clinical Rheumatology, 21*(1), 77–91. doi:10.1016/j.berh.2006.08.004

Kuronen, M., Hantunen, S., Alanne, L., Kokki, H., Saukko, C., Sjövall, S., Vesterinen, K., & Kokki, M. (2021). Pregnancy, puerperium and perinatal constipation—an observational hybrid survey on pregnant and postpartum women and their age-matched non-pregnant controls. *BJOG, 128*(6), 1057–1064. doi:10.1111/1471-0528.16559

Lan, Y., Tan, H. J., Xing, J. J., Wu, N., Xing, J. J., Wu, F. S., Zhang, L. X., & Liang, F. R. (2015). Auricular acupuncture with seed or pellet attachments for primary insomnia: A systematic review and meta-analysis. *BMC Complementary and Alternative Medicine, 15*, 103. doi:10.1186/s12906-015-0606-7

Lee, S. W., Ha, E. K., Yeniova, A. Ö., Moon, S. Y., Kim, S. Y., Koh, H. Y., Yang, J. M., Jeong, S. J., Moon, S. J., Cho, J. Y., Yoo, I. K., & Yon, D. K. (2021). Severe clinical outcomes of COVID-19 associated with proton pump inhibitors: A nationwide cohort study with propensity score matching. *Gut, 70*(1), 76–84. doi:10.1136/gutjnl-2020-322248.

Le Goaziou, M. F., Kellou, N., Flori, M., Perdrix, C., Dupraz, C., Bodier, E., & Souweine, G. (2013). Vitamin D supplementation for diffuse musculoskeletal pain: Results of a before-and-after study. *European Journal of General Practice, 20*(1), 3–9. doi:10.3109/13814788.2013.825769

Liddle, S. D., & Pennick V. (2015). Interventions for preventing and treating low-back and pelvic pain during pregnancy. *Cochrane Database of Systematic Reviews, 2015*(9), CD001139. doi:10.1002/14651858.CD001139.pub4

Madjunkova, S., Maltepe, C., & Koren, G. (2013). The leading concerns of American women with nausea and vomiting of pregnancy calling Motherisk NVP Helpline. *Obstetrics and Gynecology International*, 752980. doi:10.1155/2013/752980

Mahadevan, U., & Kane, S. (2006). American Gastroenterological Association Institute technical review on the use of gastrointestinal medications in pregnancy. *Gastroenterology, 131*(1), 283–311. doi:10.1053/j.gastro.2006.04.049

Marton, L. T., Barbalho, S. M., Sloan, K. P., Sloan, L. A., Goulart, R. A., Araújo, A. C., & Bechara, M. D. (2020). Curcumin, autoimmune and inflammatory diseases: going beyond conventional therapy—a systematic review. *Critical Reviews in Food Science and Nutrition, 62*(8):2140–2157. doi:10.1080/10408398.2020.1850417

Matok, I., Gorodischer, R., Koren, G., Sheiner, E., Wiznitzer, A., & Levy, A. (2009). The safety of metoclopramide use in the first trimester of pregnancy. *New England Journal of Medicine*, *360*(24), 2528–2535. doi: 10.1056/NEJMoa0807154

Matok, I., Levy, A., Wiznitzer, A., Uziel, E., Koren, G., & Gorodischer, R. (2012). The safety of fetal exposure to proton-pump inhibitors during pregnancy. *Digestive Diseases and Sciences*, *57*(3), 699–705. doi: 10.1007/s10620-011-1940-3

McDaid, F., Underwood, L., Fa Alili-Fidow, J., Waldie, K. E., Peterson, E. R., Bird, A., D Souza, S., & Morton, S. (2019). Antenatal depression symptoms in Pacific women: evidence from Growing Up in New Zealand. *Journal of Primary Health Care*, *11*(2), 96–108.

Mellman, T. A., Bell, K. A., Abu-Bader, S. H., & Kobayashi, I. (2018). Neighborhood stress and autonomic nervous system activity during sleep. *Sleep*, *41*(6), zsy059. doi:10.1093/sleep/zsy059

Mills, E., Duguoa, J., Perri, D., & Koren, G. (2006). *Herbal medicines in pregnancy and lactation: An evidence-based approach.* Taylor & Francis.

Mitchell, M. D., Gehrman, P., Perlis, M., & Umscheid, C. A. (2012). Comparative effectiveness of cognitive behavioral therapy for insomnia: A systematic review. *BMC Family Practice*, *13*, 40. doi:10.1186/1471-2296-13-40

Mottola, M. F., Davenport, M. H., Ruchat, S.-M., Davies, G. A., Poitras, V. J., Gray, C. E., … Zehr, L. (2018). 2019 Canadian guideline for physical activity throughout pregnancy. *British Journal of Sports Medicine*, *52*(21), 1339–1346. doi:10.1136/bjsports-2018-100056

Mulder, B., Schuiling-Veninga, C. C., Bos, H. J., De Vries, T. W., Jick, S. S., & Hak, E. (2014). Prenatal exposure to acid-suppressive drugs and the risk of allergic diseases in the offspring: A cohort study. *Clinical and Experimental Allergy*, *44*(2), 261–269. doi: 10.1111/cea.12227

Muscogiuri, G., Barrea, L., Scannapieco, M., Di Somma, C., Scacchi, M., Aimaretti, G., Savastano, S., Colao, A., & Marzullo, P. (2018). The lullaby of the sun: The role of vitamin D in sleep disturbance. *Sleep Medicine*, *54*, 262–265. doi:10.1016/j.sleep.2018.10.033

Ndumbe-Eyoh, S., Muzumdar, P., Betker, C., & Oickle, D. (2021). "Back to better": Amplifying health equity, and determinants of health perspectives during the COVID-19 pandemic. *Global health promotion*, *28*(2), 7–16. doi:10.1177/17579759211000975

Nuangchamnong, N., & Niebyl, J. (2014). Doxylamine succinate-pyridoxine hydrochloride (Diclegis) for the management of nausea and vomiting in pregnancy: An overview. *International Journal of Women's Health*, *6*, 401–409. doi: 10.2147/IJWH.S46653

Nunn, C. L., Samson, D. R., & Krystal, A. D. (2016). Shining evolutionary light on human sleep and sleep disorders. *Evolution, Medicine, and Public Health*, *2016*(1), 227–243. doi:10.1093/emph/eow018

Office of Dietary Supplements. (2021). *Vitamin D.* U.S. Department of Health and Human Services. https://ods.od.nih.gov/factsheets/VitaminD-HealthProfessional/.

Parker, S. E., Van Bennekom, C., Anderka, M., Mitchell, A. A., & National Birth Defects Prevention Study. (2018). Ondansetron for treatment of nausea and vomiting of pregnancy and the risk of specific birth defects. *Obstetrics and Gynecology*, *132*(2), 385–394. DOI: 10.1097/AOG.0000000000002679

Poskus, T., Buzinskien, D., Drasutiene, G., Samalavicius, N. E., Barkus, A., Barisauskiene, A., Tutkuviene, J., Sakalauskaite, I., Drasutis, J., Jasulaitis, A., & Jakaitiene, A. (2014). Haemorrhoids and anal fissures during pregnancy and after childbirth: A prospective cohort study. *BJOG*, *121*(13), 1666–1672. doi:10.1111/1471-0528.12838

Quach, D. T., Le, Y. T., Mai, L. H., Hoang, A. T., & Nguyen, T. T. (2021). Short meal-to-bed time is a predominant risk factor of gastroesophageal reflux disease in pregnancy. *Journal of Clinical Gastroenterology*, *55*(4), 316–320. doi:10.1097/MCG.0000000000001399

Quartarone, G. (2013). Gastroesophageal reflux in pregnancy: A systematic review on the benefit of raft forming agents. *Minerva Ginecologica*, *65*(5), 541–549.

Querejeta Roca, G., Anyaso, J., Redline, S., & Bello, N. A. (2020). Associations between sleep disorders and hypertensive disorders of pregnancy and materno-fetal consequences. *Current Hypertension Reports*, *22*(8), 53. doi: 10.1007/s11906-020-01066-w

Rezende, E., Lima, G. C., & Naves, M. (2021). Dietary fibers as beneficial microbiota modulators: A proposed classification by prebiotic categories. *Nutrition*, *89*, 111217. doi:10.1016/j.nut.2021.111217

Rivera, A. M., & Huberman, A. D. (2020). Neuroscience: A chromatic retinal circuit encodes sunrise and sunset for the brain. *Current Biology*, *30*(7), R316–R318. doi:10.1016/j.cub.2020.02.090

Romm, A. (2010). *Botanical medicine for women's health.* Churchill Livingstone Elsevier.

Salfi, F., Amicucci, G., Corigliano, D., D'Atri, A., Viselli, L., Tempesta, D., & Ferrara, M. (2021). Changes of evening exposure to electronic devices during the COVID-19 lockdown affect the time course of sleep disturbances. *Sleep*, *44*(9), zsab080. doi:10.1093/sleep/zsab080

Sharifzadeh, F., Kashanian, M., Koohpayehzadeh, J., Rezaian, F., Sheikhansari, N., & Eshraghi, N. (2018). A comparison between the effects of ginger, pyridoxine (vitamin B6) and placebo for the treatment of the first trimester nausea and vomiting of pregnancy (NVP). *Journal of Maternal-Fetal & Neonatal Medicine*, *31*(19), 2509–2514. doi:10.1080/14767058.2017.1344965

Shechter, A., Kim, E. W., St-Onge, M. P., & Westwood, A. J. (2018). Blocking nocturnal blue light for insomnia: A randomized controlled trial. *Journal of Psychiatric Research*, *96*, 196–202. doi:10.1016/j.jpsychires.2017.10.015

Sherman, P. W., & Flaxman, S. M. (2002). Nausea and vomiting of pregnancy in an evolutionary perspective. *American Journal of Obstetrics and Gynecology*, *186*(Suppl. 5), S190–S197. doi: 10.1067/mob.2002.122593

Shiri, R., Coggon, D., & Falah-Hassani, K. (2018). Exercise for the prevention of low back and pelvic girdle pain in pregnancy: A meta-analysis of randomized controlled trials. *European Journal of Pain*, *22*(1), 19–27. doi: 10.1002/ejp.1096

Sipponen, P., & Härkönen, M. (2010). Hypochlorhydric stomach: A risk condition for calcium malabsorption and osteoporosis. *Scandinavian Journal of Gastroenterology*, *45*(2), 133–138. doi: 10.3109/00365520903434117

Skokovic-Sunjic, Dragana. (2022). Clinical guide to probiotic products available in USA. http://www.usprobioticguide.com/PBCIntroduction.html?utm_source=intro_pg&utm_medium=civ&utm_campaign=USA_CHART

Sroykham, W., & Wongsawat, Y. (2013). Effects of LED-backlit computer screen and emotional self-regulation on human melatonin production. *IEEE Engineering in Medicine and Biology Society Conference Proceedings*, *2013*, 1704–1707. doi:10.1109/EMBC.2013.6609847

Stanisiere, J., Mousset, P. Y., & Lafay, S. (2018). How safe is ginger rhizome for decreasing nausea and vomiting in women during early pregnancy? *Foods*, *7*(4), 50. doi: 10.3390/foods7040050

Suarez, E. A., Boggess, K., Engel, S. M., Stürmer, T., Lund, J. L., & Funk, M. J. (2021). Ondansetron use in early pregnancy and the risk of late pregnancy outcomes. *Pharmacoepidemiology and Drug Safety*, *30*(2), 114–125. doi: 10.1002/pds.5151

Tait, R. C., & Chibnall, J. T. (2014). Racial/ethnic disparities in the assessment and treatment of pain: psychosocial perspectives. *American Psychologist*, *69*(2), 131–141. doi:10.1037/a0035204

Tan, P. C., Khine, P. P., Vallikkannu, N., & Omar, S. Z. (2010). Promethazine compared with metoclopramide for hyperemesis gravidarum: A randomized controlled trial. *Obstetrics and Gynecology*, *115*(5), 975–981. doi: 10.1097/AOG.0b013e3181d99290.

Tossetta, G., Fantone, S., Giannubilo, S. R., & Marzioni, D. (2021). The multifaced actions of curcumin in pregnancy outcome. *Antioxidants*, *10*(1), 126. doi:10.3390/antiox10010126

Tran-Duy, A., Connell, N. J., Vanmolkot, F. H., Souverein, P. C., de Wit, N. J., Stehouwer, C., Hoes, A. W., de Vries, F., & de Boer, A. (2019). Use of proton pump inhibitors and risk of iron deficiency: a population-based case-control study. *Journal of Internal Medicine*, *285*(2), 205–214. doi:10.1111/joim.12826

Trifan, A., Stanciu, C., Girleanu, I., Stoica, O. C., Singeap, A. M., Maxim, R., Chiriac, S. A., Ciobica, A., & Boiculese, L. (2017). Proton pump inhibitors therapy and risk of *Clostridium difficile* infection: Systematic review and meta-analysis. *World Journal of Gastroenterology*, *23*(35), 6500–6515. doi:10.3748/wjg.v23.i35.6500

Twohig-Bennett, C., & Jones, A. (2018). The health benefits of the great outdoors: A systematic review and meta-analysis of greenspace exposure and health outcomes. *Environmental Research*, *166*, 628–637. doi:10.1016/j.envres.2018.06.030

Tytgat, G. N., Heading, R. C., Müller-Lissner, S., Kamm, M. A., Schölmerich, J., Berstad, A., Fried, M., Chaussade, S., Jewell, D., & Briggs, A. (2003). Contemporary understanding and management of reflux and constipation in the general population and pregnancy: A consensus meeting. *Alimentary Pharmacology & Therapeutics*, *18*(3), 291–301.

U.S. Food and Drug Administration. (2018). Notice to US Food and Drug Administration of the conclusion that the intended use of curcumin is generally recognized as safe. https://www.fda.gov/media/132575/download

U.S. Food and Drug Administration. (2021). Over-the-counter (OTC) heartburn treatment. https://www.fda.gov/drugs/information-consumers-and-patients-drugs/over-counter-otc-heartburn-treatment

Vermani, E., Mittal, R., & Weeks, A. (2009). Pelvic girdle pain and low back pain in pregnancy: A review. *Pain Practice*, *10*(1), 60–71. doi: 10.1111/j.1533-2500.2009.00327.x.

Veugelers, P. J., Pham, T.-M., & Ekwaru, J. P. (2015). Optimal vitamin D supplementation doses that minimize the risk for both low and high serum 25-hydroxyvitamin D concentrations in the general population. *Nutrients*, *7*(12), 10189–10208. doi: 10.3390/nu7125527

Vieth R., & Holick M. F. (2018). The IOM–Endocrine Society controversy on recommended vitamin D targets. In D. Feldman (Ed.), *Vitamin D* (4th ed., pp. 1091–1107).

Vleeming, A., Albert, H. B., Ostgaard, H. C., Sturesson, B., & Stuge, B. (2008). European guidelines for the diagnosis and treatment of pelvic girdle pain. *European Spine Journal*, *17*(6), 794–819. doi: 10.1007/s00586-008-0602-4.

Wang, S. M., Dezinno, P., Maranets, I., Berman, M. R., Caldwell-Andrews, A. A., & Kain, Z. N. (2004). Low back pain during pregnancy: Prevalence, risk factors, and outcomes. *Obstetrics and Gynecology*, *104*(1), 65–70. doi:10.1097/01.AOG.0000129403.54061.0e

West, K. E., Jablonski, M. R., Warfield, B., Cecil, K. S., James, M., Ayers, M. A., Maida, J., Bowen, C., Sliney, D. H., Rollag, M. D., Hanifin, J. P., & Brainard, G. C. (2011). Blue light from light-emitting diodes elicits a dose-dependent suppression of melatonin in humans. *Journal of Applied Physiology*, *110*(3), 619–626. doi:10.1152/japplphysiol.01413.2009

Wu, Z., Malihi, Z., Stewart, A. W., Lawes, C. M., & Scragg, R. (2018). The association between vitamin D concentration and pain: A systematic review and meta-analysis. *Public Health Nutrition*, *21*(11), 2022–2037. doi:10.1017/S1368980018000551

Yamamichi, N., Mochizuki, S., Asada-Hirayama, I., Mikami-Matsuda, R., Shimamoto, T., Konno-Shimizu, M., Takahashi, Y., Takeuchi, C., Niimi, K., Ono, S., Kodashima, S., Minatsuki, C., Fujishiro, M., Mitsushima, T., & Koike, K. (2012). Lifestyle factors affecting gastroesophageal reflux disease symptoms: A cross-sectional study of healthy 19864 adults using FSSG scores. *BMC Medicine*, *10*, 45. doi:10.1186/1741-7015-10-45.

Yang, Z., Zhu, Z., Wang, C., Zhang, F., & Zeng, H. (2020). Association between adverse perinatal outcomes and sleep disturbances during pregnancy: a systematic review and meta-analysis. The *Journal of Maternal-Fetal & Neonatal Medicine*, 1–261. doi:10.1080/14767058.2020.1711727

Yong, W. C., Sanguankeo, A., & Upala, S. (2017). Effect of vitamin D supplementation in chronic widespread pain: A systematic review and meta-analysis. *Clinical Rheumatology*, *36*(12), 2825–2833. doi:10.1007/s10067-017-3754-y

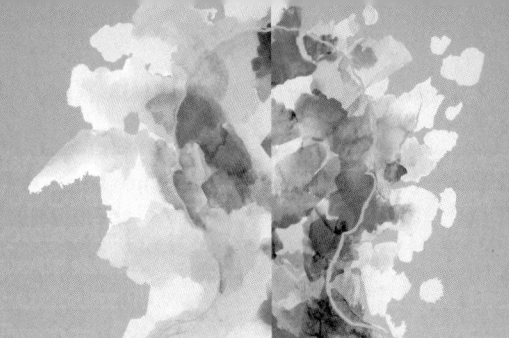

CHAPTER 33

Gestational Diabetes Mellitus: Early Detection and Management in Pregnancy

Kelly Wong McGrath, Maribeth Inturrisi, Julio Diaz-Abarca, and JoAnne M. Saxe

I. Introduction and general background

Normal pregnancy can be viewed as a progressive condition of insulin resistance, hyperinsulinemia, and mild postprandial hyperglycemia. The mild postprandial hyperglycemia serves to increase the amount of time that maternal glucose levels are elevated above the basal glucose levels after a meal, thereby increasing the flux of ingested nutrients from the pregnant person to the fetus and enhancing fetal growth.

During the fasting state (5 hours after food intake), the metabolic processes are relatively the same as in the non-pregnant state, except that they proceed at an accelerated rate (**Table 33-1**). By 10 weeks' gestation, placental hormones begin to alter the gestational parent's carbohydrate metabolism.

Early in pregnancy, estrogen and human chorionic somatomammotropin (hCS) tend to dominate such that during weeks 8–15, insulin resistance is low, resulting in lower glucose levels, especially in people with type 1 diabetes mellitus (DM). The fasting blood sugar in the normal pregnant person averages about 71 mg/dL (Hernandez et al., 2011). However, in the postprandial state, these same hormones cause a resistance to the cellular uptake of glucose by insulin-sensitive tissue, muscle, and fat. This pattern of insulin resistance tends to parallel the growth of the fetal–placental unit and the levels of hormones secreted by the placenta. In non-diabetic pregnant people, pancreatic β cells respond to insulin resistance by increasing their insulin secretion, resulting in normal circulating glucose levels (Barbour et al., 2007).

The fetus does most of its growing in the third trimester of pregnancy. During this time, the fetus is constantly "feeding," but the pregnant person is alternately fasting and feeding. Glucose is transported across the placenta from the pregnant person by facilitated diffusion. The concentration of glucose within the fetus is only slightly lower than that of the gestational parent.

Insulin does not cross the placenta. The fetus synthesizes their own insulin starting at about 9 weeks of gestation. The fetal β cells respond to both an increase in glucose and amino acids. Spikes in gestational parent glucose cause spikes in fetal insulin production.

A. Gestational diabetes mellitus: definition and overview

Gestational diabetes mellitus (GDM) is defined as glucose intolerance that is initially recognized during pregnancy and resolves after delivery of the placenta (World Health Organization [WHO], 2013). This suggests that pregnant people who develop gestational diabetes have some defect in carbohydrate metabolism that results in hyperglycemia when exacerbated by a greater demand for insulin production. Pregnant people with GDM cannot overcome the insulin resistance mediated by placental hormones. Pregnancy demands a doubling to tripling of insulin output. This requires β-cell adaptations, both functional and morphological, that begin before the onset of pregnancy-induced insulin resistance and are actually a response to pregnancy itself (Moyce & Dolinsky, 2018), changes that, for a variety of postulated factors, do not reliably occur in people with gestational diabetes.

The fetuses of pregnant people with GDM produce insulin in response to the circulating glucose levels. Fetal β cells, in turn, hypertrophy in utero, initiating a cascade of abnormal metabolic processes resulting in

Table 33-1 Major Placental Hormones and Their Impact on Maternal Carbohydrate Metabolism in All Pregnancies—Normal and With Diabetes

Placental Hormone	Effect on carbohydrate metabolism
Estrogen	Increases insulin binding to cells (insulin sensitivity) in early pregnancy, but this effect is canceled out by increases in progesterone and cortisol in the second half of pregnancy
Progesterone	Decreases insulin binding to cells, thus increasing insulin resistance
Human chorionic somatomammotropin (hCS)	Induces insulin release from the pancreas, but may also contribute to peripheral insulin resistance (in muscle and fat cells)
Human placental growth hormone (hPGH)	Causes severe peripheral insulin resistance
Tumor necrotizing factor alpha (TNFα)	Has the greatest effect of increasing insulin resistance. Changes in insulin sensitivity correlate specifically with increasing TNFα secretion from 22 to 35 weeks' gestation. TNFα is a cytokine, a proinflammatory agent, that impairs insulin's action of moving glucose from the bloodstream into cells (fat and muscle). In pregnant people with gestational diabetes mellitus, this downregulation of insulin action is increased.
Cortisol	Causes gluconeogenesis from the liver, increasing glucose in the bloodstream. Additionally, it diminishes insulin secretion from the pancreas.

Data from Barbour et al. (2007). Cellular mechanisms for insulin resistance in normal pregnancy and gestational diabetes. Diabetes Care, 30 Suppl 2.

fetal overgrowth and fetal hyperinsulinemia in the short term (Hillier et al., 2007). Some studies have suggested that GDM poses an increased risk for a variety of long-term metabolic and neurocognitive consequences for the fetus; however, these studies need to be regarded with caution because it has been difficult to control for important confounding factors (e.g., gestational parent total body weight, parental neurocognitive disorders) (Shou et al., 2019). Furthermore, to date, no studies have been able to demonstrate that treatment of GDM improves long-term fetal outcomes, suggesting the propensity for these outcomes is influenced more by parental genetics rather than in utero exposure (Shou et al., 2019).

Nevertheless, treatment of GDM does improve short-term fetal outcomes and thus is important in improving outcomes for both parent and child. Treatment of mild hyperglycemia during pregnancy has been shown to reduce serious perinatal morbidity (Horvath et al., 2010). In a meta-analysis by Horvath et al. (2010), the rate of macrosomia and birth trauma were found to be significantly reduced when comparing pregnant people who were treated for GDM versus not treated. Newborn intensive care admissions were decreased, as were shoulder dystocias. In one of the included studies (Crowther et al., 2005), pregnant people in the treatment group had a 50% decrease in weight gain during the treatment period and had less postpartum depression than those in the untreated group.

GDM is optimally managed by referral to a multidisciplinary health education team trained and skilled in the management of diabetes during pregnancy. Consultation with a registered dietitian or a practitioner skilled in nutritional counseling is recommended (American College of Obstetricians and Gynecologists [ACOG], 2018). Although studies on exercise and GDM outcomes are few and small, data show that exercise reduces the risk of GDM in pregnant people, and studies in individuals with type 2 DM, which shares mechanistic similarities with GDM, demonstrate improved insulin function with exercise (Golbidi & Laher, 2013).

B. *Prevalence and incidence*

Approximately 9% of all pregnancies in the United States are documented to be complicated by diabetes. It is estimated that 86% of these are GDM, whereas the remainder are preexisting diabetes (ACOG, 2018). The ongoing epidemic of obesity has led to more type 2 DM in individuals of childbearing age. The number of people entering pregnancy with undiagnosed type 2 DM has increased. In addition, it is estimated that 23% of individuals of childbearing age in the United States have prediabetes, also known as *glucose intolerance* (Centers for Disease Control and Prevention [CDC], 2014). Two out of three individuals with prediabetes do not know they have it (CDC, 2014). This translates to more individuals entering pregnancy with undiagnosed diabetes and prediabetes.

II. Database (may include but is not limited to)

In March 2010, the International Association of Diabetes and Pregnancy Study Groups (IADPSG) set forth global recommendations to change the way GDM is diagnosed (Metzger et al., 2010). These recommendations are based on data from the prospective double-blinded (patients and providers) epidemiologic study Hyperglycemia and Adverse Pregnancy Outcomes (HAPO; Metzger et al., 2008). The research subjects were 25,000 pregnant people from around the world who were given a 75-gm oral glucose tolerance test (OGTT) at 24–28 weeks' gestation to determine at what glucose level adverse outcomes for the fetus occurred. Removal from the study and treatment only occurred if glucose levels reached those consistent with overt diabetes. The Carpenter and Coustan (1982) 3-hour OGTT was designed to determine which pregnant people were at increased risk of developing type 2 DM in the future, not on outcomes for the fetus/newborn. The HAPO study showed that there was a continuous relationship between increasing maternal blood glucose levels and fetal fat deposition and fetal hyperinsulinemia. The proposed glucose values for a positive test were selected when the odds ratio reached 1.75. These blood glucose values conveyed a 75% increased risk for adverse fetal/neonatal outcomes such as macrosomia, hypoglycemia, and cesarean birth (Metzger et al., 2008, 2010).

The IADPSG translated the results into a one-step clinical practice guideline for the diagnosis of GDM at 24–28 weeks. Ideally, all pregnant people, and especially those with risk factors, should be screened for type 2 DM in the first trimester using one of the standard diagnostic criteria for diagnosing diabetes in the nonpregnant population (Metzger et al., 2010). If a pregnant person is found to have a fasting blood glucose (BG) of >125 mg/dL, an A1C of >6.4%, or a random BG of >199 mg/dL, a diagnosis of overt diabetes should be made (American Diabetes Association [ADA], 2015). According to the IADPSG recommendations, type 2 DM can be diagnosed during pregnancy, and management can be instituted early in order to limit the adverse effects of undiagnosed hyperglycemia.

The WHO, the ADA, and most countries outside the United States have adopted the IADPSG recommendations (ADA 2015; WHO, 2013). The ACOG, based on the 2015 Cochrane review that could not support either screening strategy as being optimal, has continued to endorse the two-step Carpenter and Coustan method (ACOG, 2018; Farrar et al., 2015). The National Institutes of Health (NIH) recommended further cost-effective studies and studies in which the improved outcomes could be related to the specific IADPSG testing recommendations (Mission et al., 2012). The NIH agreed that the adoption of a worldwide approach to the diagnosis of GDM is necessary to be able to study GDM for best-practice management guidelines (Van Dorsten et al., 2013).

Both the 2010 IADPSG method (using one step) and the 1982 Carpenter and Coustan method (using two steps) of diagnosing gestational diabetes are presented here and are used in current practice (ACOG, 2018; ADA, 2015).

A. Subjective

The ADA has identified a screening strategy for identifying pregnant people at risk for unidentified pregestational diabetes or early GDM (**Table 33-2**). All pregnant people should be asked about risk factors at the first prenatal visit.

Table 33-2 Screening Strategy for Detecting Pregestational Diabetes or Early Gestational Diabetes Mellitus

Consider testing in all pregnant people with a body mass index greater than 25 or greater than 23 for those of Asian descent and those who have one or more of the following additional risk factors:
- Physical inactivity
- First-degree relative with diabetes
- High-risk race or ethnicity (e.g., Black, Latinx, Native American, Asian, Pacific Islander)
- Have previously given birth to an infant weighing 4,000 g (approximately 9 lb) or more
- Previous gestational diabetes mellitus
- Hypertension (140/90 mm Hg or on therapy for hypertension)
- High-density lipoprotein cholesterol level less than 35 mg/dL (0.90 mmol/L); triglyceride level greater than 250 mg/dL (2.82 mmol/L)
- People with a history of polycystic ovarian syndrome
- A1C greater than or equal to 5.7%, impaired glucose tolerance, or impaired fasting glucose on previous testing
- Other clinical conditions associated with insulin resistance (e.g., greater prepregnancy total body weight, acanthosis nigricans)
- History of cardiovascular disease

Data from American Diabetes Association. Classification and Diagnosis of Diabetes. Diabetes Care 2017;40 (Suppl. 1):S11–S24. Copyright 2017 American Diabetes Association.

B. Objective/Assessment

For patients meeting the criteria listed earlier, ADA testing for undiagnosed type 2 DM or prediabetes is recommended at the first prenatal visit (ADA, 2015; Metzger et al., 2010). Some providers use the convenience of an A1C, which does not require fasting and can easily be added to the prenatal panel. However, any method to diagnose diabetes or prediabetes in nonpregnant people can be used (ADA, 2015). See **Table 33-3**.

The ACOG does not specify a preferred screening test for use in early pregnancy but does note that even if a patient screens negative early in pregnancy, screening should be repeated at 24–28 weeks' gestation because a substantial proportion of those with risk factors who screen negative early on will go on to develop GDM (ACOG, 2018). See **Table 33-4**. If any early screening is negative, the IADPSG, ADA, ACOG, and U.S. Preventive Services Task Force (USPSTF, 2014) recommend universal screening at 24–28 weeks' gestation by either a one-step method (ADA, 2015; WHO, 2013) or a two-step method (ACOG, 2018; Van Dorsten et al., 2013).

III. Goals of clinical management

A. *Identify pregnant people at risk; screen for and diagnose both type 2 DM and GDM.*
B. *Reduce adverse fetal and neonatal outcomes through treatment of pregnant people with GDM.*

Table 33-3 Criteria for the Diagnosis of Diabetes or Prediabetes in the Nonpregnant Population

Test	Overt Diabetes	Prediabetes
A1C The test should be performed in a laboratory using an NGSP-certified method that is standardized to the DCCT assay.*	≥6.5%	≥5.7% to ≤6.4%
FPG Fasting is defined as no caloric intake for at least 8 hours.*	≥126 mg/dL	≥100 mg/dL to ≤125 mg/dL
2-h plasma glucose during an OGTT The test should be performed as described by the WHO, using a glucose load containing the equivalent of 75 g of anhydrous glucose dissolved in water.*	≥200 mg/dL	≥140 mg/dL to ≤199 mg/dL
Random plasma glucose In a patient with classic symptoms of hyperglycemia or hyperglycemic crisis	≥200 mg/dL	

*In the absence of unequivocal hyperglycemia, result should be confirmed by repeat testing.
DCCT, Diabetes Control and Complications Trial; FPG, fasting plasma glucose;
NGSP, National Glycohemoglobin Standardization Program (now known only by the abbreviation); OGTT, oral glucose tolerance test; WHO, World Health Organization.
Data from American Diabetes Association. (2015). Classification and diagnosis of diabetes. Position statement: Gestational diabetes mellitus. Diabetes Care, 38 (Suppl. 1), S13–S14.

Table 33-4 Methods to Diagnose Gestational Diabetes

ONE-STEP INTERNATIONAL ASSOCIATION OF DIABETES AND PREGNANCY STUDY GROUPS (IADPSG) METHOD*:

- After an 8- to 12-hour fast, obtain fasting blood glucose (FBG)
- Administer a 2-hour 75-g oral glucose tolerance test (OGTT). The patient should remain seated.

If **any one** of the following values are reached or exceeded, the test may be terminated at that time and considered positive:

- FBG: 92 mg/dL; 1 hour—180 mg/dL; 2 hour—153 mg/dL

*Note: This method *does not* include a 50-g glucose challenge test (GCT)
(ADA, 2015; WHO, 2013)

TWO-STEP METHOD:
Step 1: Administer a 50-g non-fasting GCT.
If the result of the GCT is greater than the institutional threshold (institutional screening thresholds for the 1-hour glucose challenge range from 130 mg/dL to 140 mg/dL), proceed to step 2.
Step 2: Administer a fasting 3-hr 100-g OGTT.
If **any two** of the following values are reached or exceeded, the test may be terminated at that time and considered positive (ACOG, 2018):

- Carpenter and Coustan: FBG—95 mg/dL; 1 hour—180 mg/dL; 2 hours—155 mg/dL; 3 hours: 140 mg/dL
- National Diabetes Data Group: FBG—105 mg/dL; 1 hour—190 mg/dL; 2 hours—165 mg/dL; 3 hours—145 mg/dL

Data from American Diabetes Association. (2015). Classification and diagnosis of diabetes Position Statement: Gestational Diabetes Mellitus. Diabetes Care, 38 (Suppl.1), S13–S14.; World Health Organization. (2013). Diagnostic Criteria and Classification of Hyperglycaemia First Detected in Pregnancy. Geneva, World Health Org., (WHO/NMH/MND/13.2) and American College of Obstetricians and Gynecologists. (2018) ACOG Practice Bulletin No. 190. Obstetrics & Gynecology, 131(2), e49–e64.

C. Incorporate an interdisciplinary approach, including nutrition, psychosocial, and medical interventions, to help pregnant people with GDM successfully achieve normal BG levels and decrease perinatal morbidity.

D. Educate pregnant people with GDM regarding testing for overt diabetes every 1–3 years and about early testing in subsequent pregnancies.

E. Encourage people with a history of GDM in prior pregnancy to continue healthy eating and being active, as well as weight reduction if high total body weight, to prevent future GDM or overt diabetes.

IV. Plan
Educate all pregnant people with GDM about healthy lifestyle behaviors that can result in pregnancy outcomes that

closely match those of pregnant people without hyperglycemia in pregnancy.

A. *Healthy eating*

Lifestyle and nutrition adjustments can control GDM in approximately 70% of cases, which underscores the importance of evidence-based nutrition recommendations (ADA, 2017). In practice, three meals and two to three snacks are recommended to distribute carbohydrate intake and reduce postprandial glucose fluctuations (ACOG, 2018). Traditionally, carbohydrate restriction has been the cornerstone of GDM nutritional counseling, related to reductions in postprandial glucose levels. However, these recommendations typically result in poor adherence and the unintended consequence of replacing carbohydrates with unhealthy amounts of fat (Mahajan et al., 2019). Furthermore, a Cochrane review comparing trials of different GDM diets suggests that carbohydrate-restricted diets do not improve gestational parent or neonatal outcomes when compared to other GDM dietary counseling, including options that do not restrict carbohydrates (Han et al., 2017). Mahanjan et al. (2019) reviewed the evidence of specific approaches to GDM nutritional counseling and found that although no specific diet could be recommended at present, a diet that encouraged low-glycemic-index foods but was otherwise unrestricted was most consistently associated with improved glycemic control, reduced insulin use in the gestational parent, and decreased neonatal birth weights in systemic reviews. Regardless of specific dietary counseling, pregnant people with GDM should be cared for by clinicians who can provide well-rounded, culturally competent nutritional support at all prenatal encounters.

Recent research has shown a potential benefit of supplementing those at risk for developing GDM with myo-inositol, a dietary supplement known to modulate insulin. Although its use in preventing GDM is promising, there is also evidence of improvements in rates of macrosomia and preterm birth (Santamaria et al., 2018), which holds promise for its use in individuals already diagnosed with GDM. Larger trials are needed to confirm its efficacy as a mainstay in the treatment of GDM; however, given its low risk profile, it can be considered as a dietary supplement for those diagnosed with GDM.

Pregnancy weight-gain targets should be within those established by the Institute of Medicine (IOM, 2009), which have been associated with optimum outcomes for the birthing parent and baby (Cheng et al., 2008). Prepregnant body weight should be determined at the first visit. Weight-gain recommendations are determined according to prepregnant BMI (see **Figure 28-6** in Chapter 28, The Return Prenatal Visit). Weight gain should be followed closely and plotted on the appropriate IOM weight graphs (IOM, 2009).

B. *Physical activity*

Physical activity increases insulin sensitivity (ADA, 2015), and exercise after meals improves postprandial blood sugar more than exercise done at other times (Chang et al., 2019). It is recommended that all pregnant people work to achieve 20 to 30 minutes of moderate-intensity exercise on most or all days of the week (ACOG, 2020).

C. *Monitoring blood glucose*

Maintaining near-normal BG during pregnancy is associated with reduced macrosomia, preeclampsia, and neonatal hypoglycemia (Crowther et al., 2005; Landon et al., 2009). For this reason, a target fasting BG of <95 mg/dL and either a BG of <140 mg/dL 1 hour after the start of a meal or a BG of <120 mg/dL 2 hours after the start of a meal is recommended by both the ADA and the ACOG (ACOG, 2018; ADA, 2015).

Pregnant people who used daily self-monitoring of BG using home glucometers, test strips, and finger-sticking devices had less macrosomia than those who had their BG checked by weekly lab testing only (Hawkins et al., 2009). There is no evidence that blood sugar checks with finger sticks or with a continuous monitor are superior at improving outcomes; however, the latter may be more acceptable among users and therefore may improve adherence (Raman et al., 2017). Documenting food records and BG results that were reviewed by the providers at each visit was associated with improved BG levels (California Diabetes and Pregnancy Program [CDAPP], 2015; Parkin & Davidson, 2009).

D. *Healthy coping*

Approximately one-third of pregnant people with GDM will go on to have postpartum depression (Nicklas et al., 2012), which is higher than the background rate of 15%–20% in the general postpartum population (Davé et al., 2010). Nicklas et al. (2012) found that cesarean delivery and prenatal weight gain were associated with those postpartum individuals who went on to have depressive symptoms. Although it is recommended that all postpartum individuals be screened for postpartum depression, it is especially important that pregnant people with GDM be screened for depressive symptoms, both as recommended in pregnancy and in the postpartum, using a standardized depression screening tool for pregnant people (AAP, n.d.; ACOG, 2006). Comprehensive prenatal and postpartum care of the person with GDM should include regular review of their stress levels, tolerance for the lifestyle recommendations that have been made, and coping strategies. Referrals should be made to mental health providers as needed.

E. *Problem solving*

When working with patients who have GDM, it is important to help strategize around behaviors that will help them in achieving success around normal BG levels. Utilize the food log and corresponding BG levels to individualize recommendations that will support changes that will be achievable and meaningful (American Association of Diabetes Educators [AADE], 2010). Continuous monitoring may prove useful in patients who have BG patterns that deviate from those that are expected (CDAPP, 2015). Pregnant people should be taught the signs and symptoms of hyperglycemia and how to avoid it. When pregnant people are taking oral medication or insulin, it is important to teach them to recognize hypoglycemia, how to prevent it, and how to treat it (ADA, 2015; CDAPP, 2015).

F. *Reducing risks*

Habits such as smoking, alcohol use, and drug use should be reviewed and support provided to help with cessation when the patient is ready. As with all pregnant people, individuals with GDM should understand tests that evaluate fetal well-being, such as fetal movement awareness, and should understand recommendations for when additional evaluations are included in care (see later discussion), such as nonstress tests (NSTs) and amniotic fluid index (AFI; CDAPP, 2015). If clinically indicated (size greater than dates, poor BG control, refusal of medication), obtain ultrasound at 32–35 weeks for fetal growth (CDAPP, 2015).

For pregnant people with GDMA1 (achieves BG control with diet and exercise alone), NSTs are not indicated outside of the window otherwise recommended for those with late term pregnancy (>40w6d) in the absence of another clinical indication such as elevated blood pressure, macrosomia, history of intrauterine fetal demise, or decreased fetal movement. The GINEX-MAL trial, which examined induction of labor at 38 weeks versus expectant management in participants with GDM, found no difference in gestational parent or neonatal outcomes (Alberico et al., 2016). As such, pregnant people with well-controlled GDMA1 may continue pregnancy beyond 40 weeks with expectant management (ACOG, 2018).

For pregnant people with GDMA2 (requires the addition of medication to control BG), NST/AFI may be started weekly at 32 weeks and biweekly beginning at 36 weeks (CDAPP, 2015). Research has shown that those with GDMA2 that is well controlled with medication are at higher risk of shoulder dystocia when laboring beyond 40 weeks' gestation; induction of labor in this population in the 39th week of pregnancy did not result in a higher rate of cesarean section. As a result, the ACOG recommends that those with well-controlled GDMA2 time induction of labor between 39 0/7 and 39 6/7 (ACOG, 2018). When GDMA2 is not well controlled with medications, the care provider should weigh the risk of prematurity against the risk of stillbirth associated with poorly controlled GDM and consider in-hospital medication management of GDM before proceeding to preterm delivery (ACOG, 2018).

There is currently no evidence to suggest that an estimated fetal weight cutoff should be used to determine whether someone with GDM should have a trial of labor versus planned cesarean (ACOG, 2018). Ultrasound diagnosis of large-for-gestational age (LGA) infants correctly predicted LGA in only 22% of cases (Scifres et al., 2015).

G. *Taking medications*

Once diet and exercise have been optimized, if BG values exceed targets, consider adding medication (CDAPP, 2015). However, there is no evidence-based threshold at which the disadvantages of medication management are outweighed by the benefits of improved glucose control (ACOG, 2018). Providers should consult their institutional guidelines for the threshold at which patients are started on medications. When medication is added to treatment, the type of GDM is GDMA2.

Medical management is beyond the scope of this chapter; therefore, specific medication regimens will not be covered. Insulin is considered the first-line agent for medication management (ACOG, 2018; ADA, 2017). Although some research has shown a benefit of oral medications (metformin and glyburide) in reducing glucose levels in GDM, these medications are not considered first-line treatments because both agents cross the placental barrier, and long-term safety data for the neonate are unknown (ADA, 2019). The ACOG (2018) suggests reserving oral agents only for specific clinical scenarios (e.g., concern for poor adherence to insulin) and only after discussing the risks and benefits with the patient.

Insulin initiation should be done in consultation with a clinician who is experienced in medication management of GDM. For further discussion of considerations around insulin use, refer to the ACOG Practice Bulletin on Gestational Diabetes Mellitus (ACOG, 2018).

H. *Postpartum management of GDMA1 and GDMA2*

1. Encourage individuals to continue healthy eating and being active.
2. Nursing may be recommended because some data suggest this is a protective factor against high total body weight in childhood. However, these data remain disputed, and the exact mechanism for the association remains unknown (Ma et al., 2020). Early skin-to-skin contact should be recommended because there are benefits for the newborn and birthing patient, including reduced rates of neonatal hypoglycemia (Chertok et al., 2009).
3. Encourage individuals to reach a normal weight before their next pregnancy because high total body weight confers the same adverse outcomes as diabetes, and it increases the risk for GDM and overt diabetes (Roman et al., 2011).
4. Encourage avoidance of pregnancy for at least 18 months to allow the pancreas to "rest" from insulin resistance. Progesterone-only birth control methods, such as medroxyprogesterone (Depo Provera), etonogestrel, and progesterone-only pills, have been associated with an increase in the conversion rate of GDM to type 2 DM in Hispanic individuals who are breastfeeding (Xiang et al., 2006). Pregnancy will confer greater insulin resistance than progesterone; therefore, the risks must outweigh the benefits when considering birth control methods. The copper

or levonorgestrel interuterine devices may be good choices for their effectiveness and length of use. In spite of containing progesterone, the levonorgestrel intrauterine device has only a local effect on the uterus and has not been shown to increase insulin resistance (Damm et al., 2007). Barrier devices and nonhormonal options (Phexxi®) are also good options.

5. Reclassify glucose tolerance with 75-g OGTT (fasting plus 2 h postprandial) at 6–12 weeks (ACOG, 2018; ADA, 2020).
6. Educate individuals about screening for diabetes every 1–3 years using the baby's birthday as a reminder.
7. Obtain an early screen (first visit) for diabetes in future pregnancies (ACOG, 2018).
8. If prediabetes or overt diabetes has been identified in pregnancy, the person should be referred to a primary care provider and, when possible, to a diabetes program with educational classes for prediabetes and diabetes. Metformin was shown to reduce the rate of conversion to type 2 DM by 58% in individuals with previous GDM in the Diabetes Prevention Program Trial (Ratner et al., 2008).

I. Resources for professionals

The prenatal weight-gain charts are located at the California Department of Public Health website: http://www.publichealth.lacounty.gov/mch/cpsp/forms/Prenatal%20Weight%20Gain%20Grids.pdf
- CDPH 4472 B1 Prenatal Weight-Gain Grid: Prepregnancy Underweight Range
- CDPH 4472 B2 Prenatal Weight-Gain Grid: Prepregnancy Normal Weight Range
- CDPH 4472 B3 Prenatal Weight-Gain Grid: Prepregnancy Overweight Range
- CDPH 4472 B4 Prenatal Weight-Gain Grid: Prepregnancy Obese Weight Range

J. Resources for people with GDM

1. American Diabetes Association: (800)342-2383, http://www.diabetes.org
2. American Association of Diabetes Educators: (800)338-DMED, http://www.aadenet.org
3. Centers for Disease Control and Prevention, Division of Diabetes Translation: (877)232-3422, http://www.cdc.gov/diabetes
4. California Diabetes and Pregnancy Program: Sweet Success: http://www.cdappsweetsuccess.org/

References

Alberico, S., Erenbourg, A., Hod, M., Yogev, Y., Hadar, E., … Neri, F. (2016). Immediate delivery or expectant management in gestational diabetes at term: the GINEXMAL randomised controlled trial. *BJOG: An International Journal of Obstetrics & Gynaecology, 124*(4), 669–677. doi:10.1111/1471-0528.14389

American Academy of Pediatrics. (n.d.). *Edinburgh Postnatal Depression Scale*. https://www.aap.org/en/patient-care/screening-technical-assistance-and-resource-center/screening-tool-finder/edinburgh-postpartum-depression-scale-epds/

American Association of Diabetes Educators. (2010). *AADE 7 self-care behaviors*. http://www.diabeteseducator.org/ProfessionalResources/AADE7

American College of Obstetricians and Gynecologists. (2006). ACOG Committee Opinion No. 343: Psychosocial risk factors: Perinatal screening and intervention. *Obstetrics & Gynecology, 108*(2), 469–477. doi:10.1097/00006250-200608000-00046

American College of Obstetricians and Gynecologists. (2018). ACOG Practice Bulletin No. 190: Gestational diabetes mellitus. *Obstetrics & Gynecology, 131*(2), e49–e64. doi:10.1097/AOG.0000000000002501

American College of Obstetricians and Gynecologists. (2020). ACOG Committee Opinion No. 804: Physical activity and exercise during pregnancy and the postpartum period. *Obstetrics & Gynecology, 135*(4), e178–e188. doi:10.1097/AOG.0000000000004266

American Diabetes Association. (2015). Classification and diagnosis of diabetes. Position Statement: Gestational diabetes mellitus. *Diabetes Care, 38*(Suppl. 1), S13–S14.

American Diabetes Association. (2017). 13. Management of diabetes in pregnancy: Standards of medical care in diabetes—2018. *Diabetes Care, 41*(Suppl. 1), S137–S143. doi:10.2337/dc18-S013

Barbour, L. A., McCurdy, C. E., Hernandez, T. L., Kirwan, J. P., Catalano, P. M., & Friedman, J. E. (2007). Cellular mechanisms for insulin resistance in normal pregnancy and gestational diabetes. *Diabetes Care, 30*(Suppl. 2), S112–119. doi:10.2337/dc07-s202

California Diabetes and Pregnancy Program. (2015). *Guidelines for care*. https://www.cdappsweetsuccess.org/Portals/0/2015Guidelines/2015__CDAPPSweetSuccessGuidelinesforCare.pdf

Carpenter, M. W., & Coustan, D. R. (1982). Criteria for screening tests for gestational diabetes. *American Journal of Obstetrics and Gynecology, 144*, 768–773. doi:10.1016/0002-9378(82)90349-0

Centers for Disease Control and Prevention. (2014). *Prevalence of GDM in the US, Pregnancy Risk Assessment Monitoring System (PRAMS) 2007–2010*. http//www.cdc.gov/pcd/issues/2014/13_0415.htm

Chang, C. R., Francois, M. E., & Little, J. P. (2019). Restricting carbohydrates at breakfast is sufficient to reduce 24-hour exposure to postprandial hyperglycemia and improve glycemic variability. *American Journal of Clinical Nutrition, 109*(5), 1302–1130. doi:10.1093/ajcn/nqy261

Cheng, Y. W., Chung, J. H., Kurbisch-Block, I., Inturrisi, M., Shafer, S., & Caughey, A. B. (2008). Gestational weight gain and gestational diabetes mellitus: Perinatal outcomes. *Obstetrics and Gynecology, 112*(5), 1015–1022. doi:10.1097/AOG.0b013e31818b5dd9

Chertok, I. R. A., Raz, I., Shoham, I., Haddad, H., & Wiznitzer, A. (2009). Effects of early breastfeeding on neonatal glucose levels of term infants born to women with gestational diabetes. *Journal of Human Nutrition and Dietetics, 22*(2), 166–169. doi:10.1111/j.1365-277X.2008.00921.x

Crowther, C., Hiller, J., Moss, J., McPhee, A., Jeffries, W., & Robinson, J. (2005). Effect of treatment of gestational diabetes mellitus on pregnancy outcomes from the Australian Carbohydrate Intolerance Study in Pregnant Women (ACHOIS) trial. *New England Journal of Medicine, 352*(24), 2477–2486. doi:10.1056/NEJMoa042973

Damm, P., Mathiesen, E. R., Petersen, K. R., & Kjos, S. (2007). Contraception after gestational diabetes. *Diabetes Care, 30*(Suppl. 2), S236–241. doi:10.2337/dc07-s222

Davé, S., Petersen, I., Sherr, L., & Nazareth, I. (2010). Incidence of maternal and paternal depression in primary care. *Archives of Pediatrics & Adolescent Medicine, 164*(11), 1038–1044. doi:10.1001/archpediatrics.2010.184

Farrar, D., Duley, L., Medley, N., & Lawlor, D. A. (2015). Different strategies for diagnosing gestational diabetes to improve maternal and infant health. *Cochrane Database of Systematic Reviews, 2011*(10), CD007122. doi:10.1002/14651858.CD007122.pub2

Golbidi, S., & Laher, I. (2013). Potential mechanisms of exercise in gestational diabetes. *Journal of Nutrition and Metabolism*, 285948. doi:10.1155/2013/285948.

Han, S., Middleton, P., Shepherd, E., Van Ryswyk, E., & Crowther, C. A. (2017). Different types of dietary advice for women with gestational diabetes mellitus. *Cochrane Database of Systematic Reviews, 2017*(2), CD009275. doi:10.1002/14651858.CD009275.pub3

Hawkins, J. S., Casey, B. M., Lo, J. Y., Moss, K., McIntire, D. D., & Leveno, K. J. (2009). Weekly compared with daily blood glucose monitoring in women with diet-treated gestational diabetes. *Obstetrics & Gynecology, 113*(6), 1307–1312. doi:10.1097/AOG.0b013e3181a45a93

Hernandez, T. L., Friedman, J. E., Van Pelt, R. E., & Barbour, L. A. (2011). Patterns of glycemia in normal pregnancy: Should the current therapeutic targets be challenged? *Diabetes Care, 34*(7), 1660–1668. doi:10.2337/dc11-0241

Hillier, T. A., Pedula, K. L., Schmidt, M. M., Mullen, J. A., Charles, M. A., & Pettitt, D. J. (2007). Childhood obesity and metabolic imprinting: The ongoing effects of maternal hyperglycemia. *Diabetes Care, 30*(9), 2287–2292. doi:10.2337/dc06-2361

Horvath, K., Koch, K., Jeitler, K., Matyas, E., Bender, R., Bastian, H., Lange, S., & Siebenhofer, A. (2010). Effects of treatment in women with gestational diabetes mellitus: systematic review and meta-analysis. *BMJ, 340*, c1395–c1395. doi:10.1136/bmj.c1395

Institute of Medicine. (2009). *Weight gain during pregnancy: Re-examining the guidelines*. National Academies Press.

Landon, M. B., Spong, C. Y., Thom, E., Carpenter, M. W., Ramin, S. M., & Casey, B. (2009). A multicenter, randomized trial of treatment for mild gestational diabetes. *New England Journal of Medicine, 361*(14), 1339–1348. doi:10.1056/NEJMoa0902430

Ma, J., Qiao, Y., Zhao, P., Li, W., Katzmarzyk, P. T., Chaput, J. P., Fogelholm, M., Kuriyan, R., Lambert, E. V., Maher, C., Maia, J., Matsudo, V., Olds, T., Onywera, V., Sarmiento, O. L., Standage, M., Tremblay, M. S., Tudor-Locke, C., Hu, G., & ISCOLE Research Group. (2020). Breastfeeding and childhood obesity: A 12-country study. *Maternal & Child Nutrition, 16*(3), e12984. doi:10.1111/mcn.12984

Mahajan, A., Donovan, L. E., Vallee, R., & Yamamoto, J. M. (2019). Evidenced-based nutrition for gestational diabetes mellitus. *Current Diabetes Reports, 19*(10). doi:10.1007/s11892-019-1208-4

Metzger, B. E., Gabbe, S. G., Persson, B., Buchanan, T. A., Catalano, P. A., Damm, P., & Schmidt, M. I. (2010). International Association of Diabetes and Pregnancy Study Groups (IADPSG) recommendations on the diagnosis and classification of hyperglycemia in pregnancy. *Diabetes Care, 33*(3), 676–682. doi:10.2337/dc09-1848

Metzger, B. E., Lowe, L. P., Dyer, A. R., Trimble, E. R., Chaovarindr, U., Coustan, D. R., & Sacks, D. A. (2008). Hyperglycemia and Adverse Pregnancy Outcomes (HAPO). *New England Journal of Medicine, 358*(19), 1991–2002. doi:10.1056/NEJMoa0707943.

Mission, J. F., Ohno, M. S., Cheng, Y. W., & Caughey, A. B. (2012). Gestational diabetes screening with the new IADPSG guidelines: A cost-effectiveness analysis. *American Journal of Obstetrics and Gynecology, 207*(4), 326.e1-9. doi:10.1016/j.ajog.2012.06.048

Moyce, B., & Dolinsky, V. (2018). Maternal β-cell adaptations in pregnancy and placental signalling: Implications for gestational diabetes. *International Journal of Molecular Sciences, 19*(11), 3467. doi:10.3390/ijms19113467.

Nicklas, J. M., Miller, L. J., Zera, C. A., Davis, R. B., Levkoff, S. E., & Seely, E. W. (2012). Factors associated with depressive symptoms in the early postpartum period among women with recent gestational diabetes mellitus. *Maternal and Child Health Journal, 17*(9), 1665–1672. doi:10.1007/s10995-012-1180-y

Parkin, C. G., & Davidson, J. A. (2009). Value of self-monitoring blood glucose pattern analysis in improving diabetes outcomes. *Journal of Diabetes Science Technology, 3*(3), 500–508. oi:10.1177/193229680900300314

Raman, P., Shepherd, E., Dowswell, T., Middleton, P., & Crowther, C. A. (2017). Different methods and settings for glucose monitoring for gestational diabetes during pregnancy. *Cochrane Database of Systematic Reviews, 2017*(10), CD011069. doi:10.1002/14651858.CD011069.pub2

Ratner, R. E., Christophi, C. A., Metzger, B. E., Dabelea, D., Bennett, P. H., Pi-Sunyer, X., & Kahn, S. E. (2008). Prevention of diabetes in women with a history of gestational diabetes: Effects of metformin and lifestyle interventions. *Journal of Clinical Endocrinology and Metabolism, 93*(12), 4774–4779. doi:10.1210/jc.2008-0772

Roman, A. S., Rebarber, A., Fox, N. S., Klauser, C. K., Istwan, N., Rhea, D., & Saltzman D. (2011). The effect of maternal obesity on pregnancy outcomes in women with gestational diabetes. *Journal of Maternal, Fetal & Neonatal Medicine, 24*(5), 723–727. doi:10.3109/14767058.2010.521871

Santamaria, A., Alibrandi, A., Di Benedetto, A., Pintaudi, B., Corrado, F., Facchinetti, F., & D'Anna, R. (2018). Clinical and metabolic outcomes in pregnant women at risk for gestational diabetes mellitus supplemented with myo-inositol: A secondary analysis from 3 RCTs. *American Journal of Obstetrics and Gynecology, 219*(3), 300.e1–300.e6. doi:10.1016/j.ajog.2018.05.018

Scifres, C. M., Feghali, M., Dumont, T., Althouse, A. D., Speer, P., Caritis, S. N., & Catov, J. M. (2015). Large-for-gestational-age ultrasound diagnosis and risk for cesarean delivery in women with gestational diabetes mellitus. *Obstetrics & Gynecology, 126*(5), 978–986. doi:10.1097/AOG.0000000000000109

Shou, C., Wei, Y.-M., Wang, C., & Yang, H.-X. (2019). Updates in long-term maternal and fetal adverse effects of gestational diabetes mellitus. *Maternal-Fetal Medicine, 1*(2), 91–94. doi:10.1097/FM9.0000000000000019

U.S. Preventive Services Task Force. (2014). *Final recommendation statement gestational diabetes mellitus, screening.* http://www.uspreventiveservicestaskforce.org/Page/Document/RecommendationStatementFinal/gestational-diabetes-mellitus-screening

Van Dorsten, J. P., Dodson, W. C., Espeland, M. A., Grobman, W. A., Guise, J. M., Mercer, B. M., Minkoff, H. L., Poindexter, B., Prosser, L. A., Sawaya, G. F., Scott, J. R., Silver, R. M., Smith, L., Thomas, A., & Tita, A. T. N. (2013). NIH Consensus Development Conference: Diagnosing gestational diabetes mellitus. *NIH Consensus Statement Science Statements, 29*(1), 1–30.

World Health Organization. (2013). *Diagnostic criteria and classification of hyperglycaemia first detected in pregnancy*.

Xiang, A. H., Kawakubo, M., Kjos, S. L., & Buchanan, T. A. (2006). Long-acting injectable progestin contraception and risk of type 2 diabetes in Latino women with prior gestational diabetes mellitus. *Diabetes Care, 29*(3), 613–617. doi:10.2337/diacare.29.03.06.dc05-194

CHAPTER 34

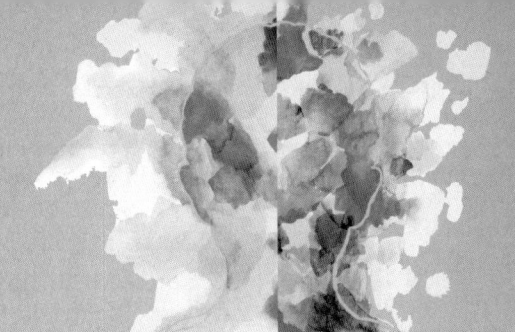

Hypertension Disorders in Pregnancy: Gestational Hypertension and Preeclampsia

Colleen Moreno and Jenna Shaw-Battista

I. Introduction and general background

Gestational hypertension and preeclampsia–eclampsia are hypertensive disease processes with unknown etiology that occur in pregnancy and the postpartum period and are characterized by new-onset hypertension occurring after 20 weeks of gestation that can affect multiple organ systems with disease progression over time (American College of Obstetricians and Gynecologists [ACOG], 2020; Druzin et al., 2021). Hypertensive disorders in pregnancy are outlined in **Table 34-1** and include chronic hypertension, gestational hypertension, preeclampsia without severe features, preeclampsia with severe features, chronic hypertension with superimposed preeclampsia and hemolysis, elevated liver enzymes, and low platelets (HELLP) syndrome. Chronic hypertension with superimposed preeclampsia and hemolysis, elevated liver enzymes, and low platelets (HELLP) syndrome, which are beyond the scope of this chapter, which is focused on the diagnosis and evidence-based management of gestational hypertension and preeclampsia–eclampsia.

Hypertensive disorders in pregnancy contribute as a leading cause of perinatal morbidity and mortality worldwide, affecting 8%–10% of pregnancies. Hypertensive disorders contribute to gestational parent death at varied rates worldwide: from 9% of gestational parent deaths in Africa and Asia to 16% of gestational parent deaths in high-income countries such as the United States, and 26% in Latin America and the Caribbean (ACOG, 2020).

It is important for clinicians to understand risk factors for hypertensive disorders. Early recognition and detection are critical in order to decrease adverse parental and fetal outcomes because any pregnant person is potentially affected. However, there are racial disparities in morbidity and mortality among pregnant persons of color, which requires all clinicians to be aware of the negative impacts of racism and discrimination on perinatal complications and outcomes, including hypertensive disorders (Druzin et al., 2021). African Americans have a two to three times higher risk for severe morbidity and mortality among gestational parents in the United States (Druzin et al., 2021) and experience a rate of preeclampsia that is 1.65 times greater than that of Caucasians in the United States (Henderson et al., 2014; Tanaka et al., 2007). Clinicians must be vigilant in detecting signs of preeclampsia while working to build rapport and trust with persons of color and decreasing stress experienced in healthcare environments that results from historic and contemporary bias and mistreatment (Druzin et al., 2021). This is one step toward personalized and equitable health care for all.

Preeclampsia typically includes both hypertension and proteinuria, but the presence of proteinuria is not required for diagnosis. As noted in Table 34-1, proteinuria is defined as at least 2+ on urine dipstick *or* ≥0.3 mg/dL on spot protein/creatinine ratio *or* ≥ 300 mg in 24-hour urine collection in a patient with new-onset hypertension results in the diagnosis of preeclampsia. The finding of 1+ protein on urine dipstick is not diagnostic of preeclampsia but prompts suspicion of preeclampsia and warrants further evaluation (Druzin et al., 2021). In the absence of proteinuria, preeclampsia can be diagnosed in the setting

Table 34-1 Hypertensive Disorders in Pregnancy

Diagnosis	Criteria
Chronic hypertension	Blood pressure ≥ 140/90 (two measurements at least 4 hours apart) with onset prior to 20 weeks of gestation; typically predates the pregnancy
Gestational hypertension	Systolic blood pressure ≥ 140 and/or diastolic ≥ 90 (two measurements at least 4 hours apart) with onset after 20 weeks of gestation; no proteinuria or other abnormal lab values; resolves by 6 weeks postpartum
Preeclampsia	1. Hypertension: Systolic blood pressure ≥ 140 and/or diastolic ≥ 90 with onset after 20 week gestation (two measurements at least 4 hours apart); *or* in severe range with systolic ≥ 160 and/or diastolic of 110 with onset after 20 weeks of gestation (can confirm diagnosis with elevated readings, 4 hours apart to expedite antihypertensive treatment in case of severe range blood pressure readings) 2. Proteinuria (at least 2+ on urine dipstick *or* ≥0.3 mg/dL on spot protein/creatinine ratio *or* ≥300 mg in 24-hour urine collection), **OR** in the absence of proteinuria, then new-onset of at least one of the following: • Pulmonary edema • Cerebral symptoms such as visual changes or new-onset headache unresponsive to medication not accounted for by alternative diagnosis • Thrombocytopenia (platelets < 100,000/mL) • Renal insufficiency: ≥1.1 mg/dL or a doubling of serum creatinine concentration. Impaired liver function: Twice the normal serum concentration of aspartate aminotransferase (AST) or alanine aminotransferase (ALT).
Preeclampsia with severe features	Presence of preeclampsia with any of the following: • Blood pressure ≥ 160/110 (two measurements at least 4 hours apart) • Pulmonary edema • Cerebral or visual symptoms • Thrombocytopenia (platelets < 100,000/mL) • ≥1.1 mg/dL or a doubling of serum creatinine concentration • Twice the normal concentration of AST or ALT
Chronic hypertension with superimposed preeclampsia	Chronic hypertension in the setting of: • Sudden increase in blood pressure • New onset of or increased proteinuria • Sudden manifestation or worsening of lab abnormalities • Onset of severe headaches, cerebral or visual symptoms, pulmonary edema, right upper quadrant pain
Hemolysis, elevated liver enzymes, and low platelets (HELLP) syndrome	Considered a severe subtype of preeclampsia; characterized by hemolysis, elevated liver enzymes, low platelets
Postpartum preeclampsia	Preeclampsia occurring in the postpartum period prior to 6 months postpartum
Eclampsia	New-onset grand mal seizures with preeclampsia in pregnancy or postpartum, in the absence of other causative conditions

Data from American College of Obstetricians and Gynecologists. (2020). Gestational Hypertension and Preeclampsia. Washington, DC: American College of Obstetricians and Gynecologists.

of hypertension plus end-organ involvement, indicating severe disease and evidenced by abnormal laboratory values (thrombocytopenia, elevated liver enzymes, or elevated serum creatinine), physical examination findings, or client symptomatology. During evaluation and diagnosis of hypertension, preeclampsia must be differentiated from gestational hypertension and white-coat hypertension, which do not include proteinuria or end-organ involvement. White-coat hypertension is recognized in pregnancy and defined as a systolic blood pressure of ≥140 mm Hg and/or diastolic of ≥90 mm Hg in the presence of healthcare providers but not on home monitoring. Continued surveillance of the patient presenting with white-coat hypertension is important. Approximately 40% will progress to gestational hypertension, and 8% will further progress to preeclampsia. Frequent self-monitoring with an automatic blood pressure cuff is recommended for confirmation of diagnosis and to assess for evolution of disease processes (Druzin et al., 2021).

The etiology of preeclampsia–eclampsia is largely unknown but multifactorial, with suspected genetic and immunologic pathways and several identified predisposing risk factors. The pathophysiology of preeclampsia involves abnormal development of placental vascularization and impaired implantation, which often contributes to reduced perfusion and uteroplacental insufficiency. Placental ischemia triggers the release of inflammatory and oxidative stress factors that cause endothelial dysfunction, resulting in the classic manifestations of preeclampsia, including hypertension. Preeclampsia typically progresses in severity as pregnancy advances, with a variable rate that cannot be reliably predicted. The disease can be resolved only through birth of the infant and placenta, but recovery does not occur immediately; symptoms may present or worsen in the first 24–48 hours postpartum, and new diagnoses have been reported up to 6 weeks later (ACOG, 2020; Ananth et al., 2013; Druzin et al., 2021, Henderson et al., 2014; Sibai, 2012).

There is no reliable predictive model for preeclampsia, and there are few preventive measures with demonstrable efficacy (ACOG, 2020). Daily low-dose aspirin therapy (81 mg) late in the first trimester reduces the risk of preeclampsia by 15% (Druzin et al., 2021) and is recommended for people with significant risk factors or a history of preeclampsia (**Table 34-2**). The best available research currently indicates daily low-dose aspirin should be started between 12 and 16 weeks and continued until birth; however, it may be beneficial to begin earlier or later, up to 28 weeks of gestation (ACOG, 2018; Druzin et al., 2021). Daily low-dose aspirin does not prevent the disease process of preeclampsia but rather delays the disease onset, often beyond 34 weeks gestation, thereby improving gestational parent and fetal morbidity and mortality, particularly when delivery is indicated for treatment (Druzin et al., 2021).

Evidence to support nutritional prevention of preeclampsia remains mixed and insufficient to support strong recommendations during pregnancy (ACOG, 2020). However, it may be beneficial to consider improved nutrition and exercise for health promotion and disease prevention, especially when caring for pregnant persons in low-income countries. People living in low-income countries are more likely to have a low dietary intake of calcium than those living in high-income countries (Hofmeyr et al., 2014). Oral calcium supplementation may reduce preeclampsia incidence among individuals with low dietary intake (<600 mg/day) and should be considered for clients with a history of diagnosis in prior pregnancies, keeping in mind that excessive calcium may be harmful (Hofmeyr et al., 2014; Rath & Fischer, 2009; Schoenaker et al., 2014; Sibai, 1998, 2005). Preeclampsia prevention with supplemental vitamins C, E, and D remains

Table 34-2 Clinical Risk Assessment for Preeclampsia and Use of Low-Dose Aspirin

Recommend low-dose aspirin if one or more risk factors are present:
- History of persistent high blood pressure either while pregnant or not (chronic hypertension, preeclampsia), especially if associated with an adverse outcome
- Pregnancies with more than one fetus
- Type 1 or 2 diabetes
- Renal disease
- Autoimmune disease (systemic lupus erythematosus, antiphospholipid syndrome)

Recommend low-dose aspirin if two of more risk factors are present:
- First pregnancy or greater than 10-year pregnancy interval
- Larger body habitus with excess adiposity
- Hypertensive disorder of pregnancy in a first-degree relative
- Individuals impacted by systemic racism and other sociodemographic characteristics known to be associated with greater life stress
- Birthing parent ≥ 35 years
- Personal history factors (e.g., low birth weight or small for gestational age, previous adverse pregnancy outcome)

Low-dose aspirin not recommended:
Previous uncomplicated full-term delivery

Adapted from U.S. Preventive Services Task Force. (2021). *Aspirin Use to Prevent Preeclampsia and Related Morbidity and Mortality: Preventive Medication* https://www.uspreventiveservicestaskforce.org/uspstf/recommendation/low-dose-aspirin-use-for-the-prevention-of-morbidity-and-mortality-from-preeclampsia-preventive-medication

controversial and lacks strong evidence to support routine or targeted recommendations, although low prepregnancy dietary intake of these vitamins may increase the risk of preeclampsia, and physical activity may be protective (ACOG, 2020; Dodd et al., 2014; Weinert & Silveiro, 2015). Thus, health education focused on nutrition and exercise may be particularly helpful before conception and in early pregnancy for persons with nutritional deficiencies as well as those of greater body weight and those with other risk factors for chronic hypertension.

Management of hypertensive disorders in pregnancy aims to prevent adverse gestational parent and fetal outcomes, which requires timely recognition and treatment to prevent progression of the disease process. Preeclampsia is one of the most common serious perinatal complications, affecting 1–2 out of every 10 pregnancies near term (Druzin et al., 2021). Almost half of pregnant persons diagnosed with gestational hypertension will develop preeclampsia, which confers greater risk for gestational parent and fetal morbidity and mortality (ACOG, 2020; Druzin et al., 2021). The risk of gestational parent and fetal morbidity is higher for preeclampsia with severe features versus without and for preeclampsia when diagnosed prior to 34 weeks of gestation (Druzin et al., 2021). Gestational parent morbidity is rare and includes placental abruption, stroke, pulmonary edema, myocardial infarction, and coagulopathy. Fetal and neonatal sequelae of severe disease may include fetal growth restriction and stillbirth. Preeclampsia also contributes to the iatrogenic preterm birth rate because management includes facilitating delivery with induction of labor or cesarean delivery prior to labor in the case of severe disease with rapid progression. When preeclampsia is unrecognized or untreated, it progresses to eclampsia, which is a clinical emergency associated with severe adverse outcomes, including gestational parent and fetal death. Eclampsia is new-onset grand mal seizures with preeclampsia in pregnancy or postpartum, in the absence of other etiologies (Druzin et al., 2021). Hypertensive disorders in pregnancy also confer an increased risk of cardiovascular disease and mental health diagnoses later in life. Early detection and management of hypertensive disorders in pregnancy reduce adverse perinatal outcomes and may improve long-term cardiovascular health among parents, although it remains unclear if preeclampsia causes cardiovascular changes or if preeclampsia is a manifestation of an underlying cardiovascular disease that also predisposes the person to subsequent cardiovascular disease (Druzin et al., 2021). Persons diagnosed with preeclampsia are also at greater risk for postpartum depression and posttraumatic stress disorder (PTSD) following childbirth, which may be limited with prevention efforts and prompt recognition and treatment of disease (Druzin et al., 2021; Senden et al., 2012). It is therefore critically important for persons diagnosed with a hypertensive disorder in pregnancy to receive follow-up physical and mental health care with a long-term focus on health maintenance and prevention, as well as preconception care planning if applicable.

II. Database (may include but is not limited to)

A. Subjective

Assess for the presence of risk factors and symptoms. Persons presenting with vague symptoms such as headache, visual disturbances, abdominal pain, shortness of breath, generalized swelling, and complaints of "I just don't feel right" should be evaluated for preeclampsia presentations and severe disease features because of the variable presentation of this serious complication of pregnancy (ACOG, 2020).

1. Past health history
   a. Medical history:
      Prepregnancy body mass index > 30; diabetes; chronic hypertension; renal, vascular, or autoimmune disease, such as systemic lupus erythematosus or antiphospholipid syndrome.
   b. Obstetric and gynecological history:
      First pregnancy, gestational parent age of >35 years; multiple gestation; in vitro fertilization; or history of preeclampsia, placental abruption, or fetal growth restriction
2. Family history:
   a. Mother or sister with hypertensive disorder in pregnancy
3. Review of systems:
   a. Constitutional signs and symptoms: decreased fetal movement, report of feeling unwell (e.g., fatigued, malaise, dizzy, lightheaded, anxious, or confused)
   b. Skin: Unexplained ecchymosis
   c. Eyes: visual disturbances including blurred vision, "spots," "stars," "flashing lights," or blindness (indicative of retinal detachment)
   d. Respiratory and cardiovascular: shortness of breath or dyspnea (may indicate concomitant pulmonary edema); increased swelling, particularly facial or periorbital.
   e. Gastrointestinal: epigastric pain or pain in the right upper quadrant of the abdomen, heartburn, nausea, or vomiting
   f. Genitourinary: decreased urinary output, vaginal bleeding (may indicate abruptio placentae resulting from severe hypertension)
   g. Neurologic: Paresthesia of hands, feet, or extremities (may accompany significant edema); report of seizure; change in mental status or loss of consciousness. Headaches, particularly with new onset or increased severity or frequency. Headaches associated with preeclampsia are often frontal or occipital and do not respond to conservative treatment (e.g., over-the-counter medication such as acetaminophen).

B. Objective

1. Vital signs
   a. Blood pressure greater than or equal to 140 mm Hg systolic and/or 90 mm Hg diastolic on at least two occasions more than 4 hours apart. If blood pressure is greater than or equal to 160 mm Hg

Table 34-3 Steps for Obtaining Accurate Blood Pressure Measurements

To ensure an accurate blood pressure measurement:
- Obtain correct-size cuff with width that encircles 80% of the arm.
- Assess for caffeine or nicotine consumption within 30 minutes.
- Be sure patient is sitting or semi-reclining with back supported and feet flat on floor (not dangling).
- Place cuff on bare upper arm without restrictive clothing, with arm supported at heart level.
- Auscultation is most accurate. If auscultating: Use first audible sound (Korotkoff I) as systolic pressure and use disappearance of sound (Korotkoff V) as diastolic pressure.
- For accuracy, a second reading should be taken within 15 minutes in the same position, with the highest reading recorded.
- If reading is greater than or equal to 140/90 on repeat, further evaluation for preeclampsia is warranted.
- Documentation should include the arm in which the blood pressure was taken.

---

systolic and/or 110 mm Hg diastolic, confirm with repeat measurement within minutes to ensure timely management of severe hypertension (**Table 34-3**).
  b. Rapid and excessive weight gain (>2 pounds per week)
2. Skin examination: petechiae, ecchymosis, or jaundice (may be present with hemolysis or thrombocytopenia)
3. Cardiovascular examination: generalized edema, particularly facial or periorbital, with or without pitting
4. Abdominal examination:
   a. Liver may be enlarged.
   b. Right upper quadrant abdominal pain on palpation or spontaneous
   c. Fundal height: If less than expected for gestational age, ultrasound imaging may be indicated to assess for oligohydramnios or fetal growth restriction, which may result from hypertension.
   d. Fetal heart tones
5. Genitourinary: Proteinuria of greater than or equal to 2+ protein on macrourinalysis with a clean, midstream sample. Refer to Table 34-1 for subsequent proteinuria measurement options and diagnostic criteria.
6. Neurologic examination: hyperreflexia, with or without clonus

III. Assessment
A. *Determine the diagnosis*
  1. Criteria for preeclampsia diagnosis: gestational hypertension and either proteinuria or evidence of severe features with end-organ involvement as described in Table 34-1
  2. Differential diagnosis: If criteria are not met, the differential diagnosis should include but is not limited to impending preeclampsia; chronic, white-coat, or gestational hypertension; liver or renal disease; or substance use (Sibai & Stella, 2009). Similarly, HELLP syndrome should be considered, especially when hemolysis, elevated liver enzyme levels, or low platelet counts are observed.

IV. Goals of clinical management
A. *Screening*
  Screen all pregnant people for risk factors at the first prenatal visit and with blood pressure checks at each prenatal visit.
B. *Prevention*
  Treat people at moderate to high risk with low-dose aspirin therapy.
C. *Identification*
  Order appropriate diagnostic laboratory tests when blood pressure is elevated, educate all pregnant people about preeclampsia symptoms, and screen for them during prenatal visits.
D. *Gestational parent and fetal well-being*
  Assure gestational parent and fetal well-being with blood pressure and symptom monitoring, and implement fetal surveillance and growth ultrasounds with the diagnosis of hypertensive disorders in pregnancy. Plan for induction of labor at the appropriate gestational age for each diagnosis, with reference to gestational age at onset and severity.

V. Plan
A. *Diagnostic tests*
  1. Blood pressure assessment: Repeat blood pressure assessment after a 10- to 30-minute rest period with the client in an upright or sitting position, using an appropriately sized sphygmomanometer cuff. Proper blood pressure assessment is essential and outlined in Table 34-3. Diagnosis of hypertensive disorders requires two or more elevated readings observed greater than 4 hours apart unless readings are in the severe range or abnormal lab results or severe symptoms are present. In the case of hypertensive emergency in pregnant or postpartum clients, it is not advisable to wait for at least two elevated blood pressure readings in 4 hours before initiating treatment. In the case of acute-onset or persistent (lasting 15 minutes or more) and severe systolic ($\geq$160 mm Hg) and/or diastolic ($\geq$110 mm Hg) hypertension, treat with antihypertensives within 30–60 minutes if blood pressures remain elevated 15 minutes after the initial severe finding (ACOG, 2020).
  2. Proteinuria assessment: Obtain a clean midstream urine sample to assess for protein on standardized laboratory macrourinalysis if not previously done. Inconsistencies in qualitative assessment of

macrourinalysis via dipstick suggest this method of diagnosis should be avoided, but in low-resource settings, a urine dipstick reading of 2+ is sufficient for diagnosis of proteinuria if found on two or more occasions at least 4 hours apart (ACOG, 2020). Consider urine culture and sensitivity to rule out urinary tract infection if proteinuria is present. Asymptomatic infection is common in pregnancy and could confound the diagnosis.

Initiate 24-hour urine collection or urine protein/creatinine ratio to assess for proteinuria if the pregnant person has gestational hypertension or 2+ protein on urine dipstick. A protein/creatinine ratio greater than or equal to 0.3 mg/dL *or* a 24-hour urine collection with protein levels equal to or greater than 300 mg is diagnostic of preeclampsia in a hypertensive pregnant person (ACOG, 2020).

3. Order serum testing: Complete blood count (CBC) with platelets and liver function panel that includes aspartate aminotransferase (AST), alanine aminotransferase (ALT), and creatinine. Note that alkaline phosphatase is typically elevated in pregnancy and is not indicative of preeclampsia. Although commonly ordered, uric acid has a 33% positive predictive value and is not a useful diagnostic tool (ACOG, 2020). Lactate dehydrogenase (LDH) and bilirubin levels are used to detect hemolysis associated with HELLP syndrome, in addition to thrombocytopenia assessment included in CBC results (ACOG, 2020; Druzin et al., 2021).

B. *Treatment and follow-up of gestational hypertension or preeclampsia without severe features*
   1. Delivery is recommended after 37 weeks of gestation after physician consultation; co-management may be appropriate.
   2. If less than 37 weeks of gestation, persons with the diagnosis of gestational hypertension and/or preeclampsia without severe features may receive outpatient care with gestational and fetal surveillance to identify disease progression and the development of severe features (ACOG, 2020; Druzin et al., 2021)
      a. Fetal surveillance and management (Druzin et al., 2021)
         i. Twice-weekly biophysical profile (BPP) or nonstress test (NST) plus amniotic fluid index (AFI) is recommended.
         ii. Ultrasound assessment of fetal growth is recommended upon diagnosis and continued at 3-week intervals until delivery.
      b. Gestational parent surveillance and management (ACOG, 2020; Druzin et al., 2021)
         i. Blood pressure and signs/symptom review (severe headache, visual changes, epigastric or right upper quadrant pain, shortness of breath) should be evaluated twice weekly to monitor for development of severe features. Once proteinuria is over the diagnostic threshold, 24-hour urine testing does not need to be repeated because this is no longer a diagnostic criterion for preeclampsia with severe features (Druzin et al., 2021).
         ii. Laboratory testing may be repeated weekly or sooner with worsening symptomatology: CBC, ALT/AST, serum creatinine, urine protein/creatinine ratio (ACOG, 2020; Druzin et al., 2021).
         iii. There is no compelling evidence that bed rest reduces disease progression or improves perinatal outcomes. However, lying down in the left lateral position may optimize uterine, placental, and fetal circulation and should be encouraged, particularly if significant edema is present. It is appropriate to encourage patients to engage in normal daily activities, yet caution against strenuous exercise (Druzin et al., 2021).
         iv. Home blood pressure monitoring and recording should be recommended at least twice daily for patients diagnosed with gestational hypertension who are being managed on an outpatient basis.
         v. During return prenatal visits, a complete a review of systems and physical exam should be performed as previously described. Discuss parameters for acute reevaluation, and ensure the person has appointments for subsequent fetal and gestational parent surveillance.
      c. Ongoing medical consultation about evolving conditions and collaborative management plan

C. *Treatment and follow-up of severe preeclampsia*
   1. Treatment and follow-up of preeclampsia with severe features require immediate physician consultation and probable referral to obstetrician or perinatology services. Treatment with magnesium sulfate will be recommended for seizure prophylaxis.
   2. If less than 34 weeks of gestation, admission to a tertiary facility should occur. Corticosteroids should be considered to enhance fetal lung development during expectant management, which is recommended in the absence of indications for immediate delivery. Severe cases at early gestational ages are more likely to progress rapidly and result in adverse outcomes compared to later-onset cases, necessitating ongoing surveillance and anticipatory guidance for the family.
   3. Delivery is recommended at 34 or more weeks of gestation.
   4. To minimize risk of gestational parent stroke, antihypertensives should be administered as soon as possible for those individuals with blood pressure greater than or equal to 160 mm Hg systolic or above 110 mm Hg diastolic (ACOG, 2020).

D. *Education and anticipatory guidance in the setting of suspected or confirmed preeclampsia*
   1. Advise the pregnant person to immediately report signs of preeclampsia: headache, visual changes,

epigastric or right upper quadrant pain, or shortness of breath.
2. Teach the pregnant person how to perform fetal kick counts twice daily after 28 weeks of gestation. Instruct them to notify providers if fewer than 10 fetal movements are felt in a 2-hour period, preferably when at rest following a meal.
3. If home blood pressure monitoring is initiated, teach how to use the machine and record values. Instruct the pregnant person to immediately report critical values ($\geq$160/110 mm Hg).
4. Discuss self-care, including nutrition, hydration, exercise, stress management, and relaxation.
5. Provide anticipatory guidance about disease progression and both immediate and long-term sequelae.
6. Clearly document the follow-up plan and shared decision-making process.
7. Provide anticipatory guidance regarding the recommendation of induction of labor in the setting of preeclampsia diagnosis (ACOG, 2020). Encourage individualized care planning, taking into consideration the pregnant person's own values and judgments (ACOG, 2020).

E. *Consultation and referral*

Refer to Chapter 30, Guidelines for Medical Consultation, Interprofessional Collaboration, and Transfer of Care During Pregnancy and Childbirth. Physician consultation is indicated for suspected or documented preeclampsia of any severity. Gestational hypertension and preeclampsia without severe features may be managed by nurse practitioners or nurse-midwives with physician consultation or may be collaboratively managed on either an inpatient or outpatient basis. Preeclampsia with severe features at any gestational age warrants evaluation by an obstetrician as soon as possible and may require referral and transfer of care to obstetrical care or a maternal–fetal medicine service, depending on the practice setting and standardized procedures used by nonphysician clinicians (ACOG, 2019).

F. *Postpartum and preconception considerations* (ACOG, 2020; Druzin et al., 2021)
1. It is important to rule out a diagnosis of preeclampsia in a postpartum patient who is presenting with new-onset hypertension (Druzin et al., 2021).
2. Signs and symptoms of preeclampsia can present more than 48 hours after delivery and up to 6 months postpartum, although they typically occur in the first 6 weeks (Druzin et al., 2021). Postpartum follow-up is recommended to monitor blood pressure. Persons who were diagnosed with hypertensive disease in pregnancy should be discharged home with a blood pressure cuff to monitor blood pressure and provided with parameters for when to seek medical care. They should also be scheduled for follow-up with a maternity care provider within 1 week after birth. If a postpartum person was treated with antihypertensive medications, follow-up should be scheduled within 3–7 days of discharge and within 7–14 days for those not treated with medication yet diagnosed with hypertension during hospital admission (Druzin et al., 2021).
3. Preeclampsia is associated with a greater risk of postpartum depression, PTSD, and lifelong cardiovascular disease. Psychological warning signs, support services, and healthy lifestyle changes to promote cardiovascular health should be included in postpartum education.
4. Any pregnant person with a history of preeclampsia should be advised of their increased risk of preeclampsia in subsequent pregnancy and the availability of low-dose aspirin therapy to lessen the recurrence rate.

In the preconception period, any persons at high risk for hypertensive disorders, such as those with high total body weight, chronic hypertension, renal disease, diabetes, or autoimmune disease, should be advised of their preeclampsia risk and provided support to improve health before conception.

References

American College of Obstetricians and Gynecologists. (2018). ACOG Committee Opinion No. 743: Low-dose aspirin use during pregnancy. *Obstetrics and Gynecology*, 132(1), e44–e52. doi:10.1097/AOG.0000000000002708

American College of Obstetricians and Gynecologists. (2019). ACOG Obstetric Care Consensus No. 9: Levels of maternal care. *Obstetrics and Gynecology*, 134(2), e41–e525. doi:10.1097/AOG.0000000000005128

American College of Obstetricians and Gynecologists. (2020). *ACOG Practice Bulletin No. 222: Gestational hypertension and preeclampsia*.

Ananth, C. V., Keyes, K. M., & Wapner, R. J. (2013). Pre-eclampsia rates in the United States, 1980–2010: Age-period-cohort analysis. *British Medical Journal*, 347(15), f6564. doi:10.1136/bmj.f6564

Dodd, J. M., O'Brien, C., & Grivell, R. M. (2014). Preventing preeclampsia: Are dietary factors the key? *BMC Medicine*, 12, 176. doi:10.1186/s12916-014-0176-4

Druzin, M., Shields, L., Peterson, N., Sakowski, C., Cape, V., & Morton, C. (2021). *Improving health care response to hypertensive disorders of pregnancy, a California Maternal Quality Care Collaborative quality improvement toolkit*. California Maternal Quality Care Collaborative.

Henderson, J. T., Whitlock, E. P., O'Connor, E., Senger, C. A., Thompson, J. H., & Rowland, M. G. (2014). Low-dose aspirin for prevention of morbidity and mortality from preeclampsia: A systematic evidence review for the U.S. Preventive Services Task Force. *Annals of Internal Medicine*, 10, 695–703. doi:10.7326/M13-2844

Hofmeyr, G. J., Belizan, J. M., von Dadelszen, P., & Calcium and Pre-eclampsia Study Group. (2014). Low-dose calcium supplementation for preventing pre-eclampsia: A systematic review and commentary. *British Journal of Obstetrics and Gynaecology, 8*, 951–957. doi:10.1111/1471-0528.12613

Rath, W., & Fischer, T. (2009). The diagnosis and treatment of hypertensive disorders of pregnancy: New findings for antenatal and inpatient care. *Deutsches Ärzteblatt International, 106*(45), 733–738. doi:10.3238/artebl.2009.0733

Schoenaker, D., Soedamah-Muthu, S. S., & Mishra, G. D. (2014). The association between dietary factors and gestational hypertension and pre-eclampsia: A systematic review and meta-analysis of observational studies. *BMC Medicine, 1*, 157. doi:10.1186/s12916-014-0157-7

Senden, I. P., Duivenvoorden, H. J., Filius, A., DeGroot, C. J., Steegers, E. A., & Passchier, J. (2012). Maternal psychosocial outcome after early onset preeclampsia and preterm birth. *Journal of Maternal-Fetal Neonatal Medicine, 25*, 272–276. doi:10.3109/14767058.2011.573829

Sibai, B. M. (1998). Prevention of preeclampsia: A big disappointment. *American Journal of Obstetrics & Gynecology, 179*, 1275–1278. doi:10.1016/s0002-9378(98)70146-2

Sibai, B. M. (2005). Diagnosis, prevention, and management of eclampsia. *Obstetrics & Gynecology, 105*(2), 402–410. doi:10.1097/01.AOG.0000152351.13671.99

Sibai, B. M. (2012). Etiology and management of postpartum hypertension-preeclampsia. *American Journal of Obstetrics and Gynecology, 203*(6), 470–475. doi:10.1016/j.ajog.2011.09.00

Sibai, B. M., & Stella, C. L. (2009). Diagnosis and management of atypical preeclampsia-eclampsia. *American Journal of Obstetrics and Gynecology, 200*(5), e481–e487. doi:10.1016/j.ajog.2008.07.048

Tanaka, M., Jaamaa, G., Kaiser, M., Hills, E., Soim, A., Zhu, M., Shcherbatykh, I. Y., Samelson, R., Bell, E., Zdeb, M., & McNutt, L.-A. (2007). Racial disparity in hypertensive disorders of pregnancy in New York State: A 10-Year longitudinal population-based study. *American Journal of Public Health, 97*(1), 163–170. doi:10.2105/AJPH.2005.068577

Weinert, L. S., & Silveiro, S. P. (2015). Maternal-fetal impact of vitamin D deficiency: A critical review. *Maternal and Child Health Journal, 19*(1), 94–101. doi:10.1007/s10995-014-1499-7

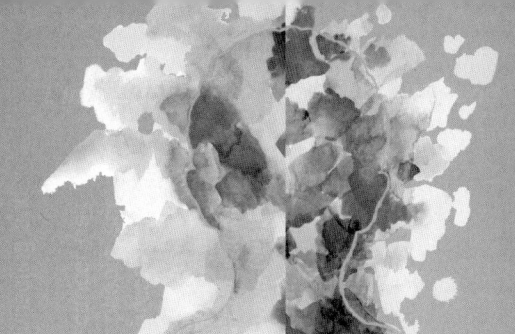

CHAPTER 35

Preterm Labor Management

Lisa Jensen

I. Introduction and general background

Preterm birth (PTB) has broad implications not only for its impact on maternal and child health but also for its economic and political significance, making it a major health index of a nation. Both the World Health Organization (WHO) and the United Nations (UN) consider the prevention of PTB to be a major focus and opportunity for improving health outcomes in pregnant people and newborn babies across the globe (Medley et al., 2018). In the United States, despite having access to advanced medical training and technology, the rates of PTB remain some of the highest in the world. This is exacerbated by the structural inequalities and racism that contribute to the disproportionately high rates of PTB among resource-poor individuals and people of color in this country. This chapter will define PTB, risk factors, signs and symptoms, treatments, and potential consequences.

A. *Definition*
1. PTB is defined as the birth of a live baby after 20 weeks and before 37 completed weeks of gestation (36 weeks, 6 days). The classification of PTB can be further subdivided into several categories of prematurity:
   a. Late preterm (>34 weeks and <37 weeks)
   b. Moderate preterm (>32 weeks and <34 weeks)
   c. Very preterm (>28 weeks and <32 weeks)
   d. Extremely preterm (<28 weeks)
2. PTB can be further classified according to its clinical presentation as either spontaneous or indicated (iatrogenic) (Feghali et al., 2015):
   a. Spontaneous labor precedes signs in 50% of PTBs and occurs when signs and symptoms of preterm labor (PTL) occur before 37 completed weeks of pregnancy.
   b. The remainder of PTBs occurs when a clinical determination is made to induce labor in the interest of the well-being of the pregnant person and/or the fetus. Indications for a preterm induction beyond 31 weeks most commonly include hypertensive disorders (preeclampsia, followed by chronic hypertension).

B. *Prevalence/incidence*
The global burden of PTB is significant, and across the globe, 15 million babies are born prematurely, a rate that has been increasing in almost all countries globally over the last two decades; PTBs account for roughly 11% of all births (da Fonseca et al., 2020). In the United States, after decades on the rise, PTB rates may be leveling out and may possibly be on the decline; however, the incidence remains high, with an estimated 10% of babies in the United States born prematurely in 2020 (Frey & Klebanoff, 2016; March of Dimes, 2022; Osterman et al., 2021). Of these premature babies, roughly 70% fall into the category of late PTB. This classification is consequential because potential consequences for the baby decline and chances of survival increase with each subsequent week of gestation (Manuck et al., 2016).

C. *Etiology*
PTB is a complex health issue with multiple etiologies. Millions of dollars a year are spent in research and clinical trials to better understand PTB, and yet we still have an incomplete understanding of its causes. In fact, two-thirds of PTBs occur among pregnant people with no discernable risk factors (American College of Obstetricians and Gynecologists [ACOG] Committee on Practice Bulletins—Obstetrics, 2021). Although PTB is discussed as a single outcome, there are many drivers, including social, environmental, hormonal, genetic, and other factors (DeFranco et al., 2008; Frey & Klebanoff, 2016). Our limited understanding of the complex interactions among these factors contributes to the lack of effective intervention strategies available to reduce the rate of PTB.

D. *Burden of PTB*
The health impacts associated with PTB are manifold. Seen as one of the leading health indicators of a nation, PTB is the highest cause of death in neonates and the second-most-common cause for all children under 5 years of age. Beyond mortality, the impacts of PTB

extend into both the neonatal and infant periods. Impacts can manifest as learning and developmental challenges in childhood, an increased risk of cardiovascular disease and diabetes in adulthood, and anxiety and depression later in life.

E. *Economic impact*

Financially, a seminal 2007 Institute of Medicine (IOM) study estimated the costs associated with prematurity in the United States alone as $26.2 billion annually (in 2005 dollars), or roughly $51,600 per preterm infant (Beam et al., 2020). However, the economic burdens of prematurity have most often been measured from a health insurance perspective and therefore have not adequately accounted for costs beyond the initial hospital interactions. Indeed, this number is likely much higher when set to include rehospitalization, subsequent outpatient and specialist services, medication over the life course, and/or nonmedical costs such as special education or lost productivity among families (Hodek et al., 2011). Summarized by Kelly and Li (2019) as an issue with multifactorial causes and a "global epidemic with psychosocial, economic, and physical ramifications affecting the child, family, and community at large (p.275)."

F. *Racial disparities*

Prematurity has societal implications and causality. Disparities in PTB rates reflect social and structural inequities: rates of PTB are highest in the United States for Black infants (14.2%), followed by American Indian and Alaska Natives (11.6%,) Whites (9.2%), and Asian/Pacific Islanders (8.8%) (Osterman et al., 2021). Black infants are 50% more likely to be born preterm and twice as likely to be born very preterm (Janevic et al., 2021). However, Black birthing people are not a monolith, and within this population, rates vary significantly by ancestry, country of origin, and ethnicity (Frey & Klebanoff, 2016; Medley et al., 2018). Being born outside the USA was also independently associated with a reduction in PTB risk, illustrating that the experience of being born Black in the United States—and the forces of systematic racism that influence economic opportunities and health status—negatively affect reproductive health.

The drivers of these racial disparities in PTB are not fully understood, but many researchers have hypothesized that socioeconomic inequities play a role. Among these, individual as well as neighborhood poverty, parental education, and stress are each associated with an increased risk (Behrman et al., 2007; Giurgescu et al., 2012; Jansen et al., 2009; Lu & Halfon, 2003). These indicators also interact with and modify each other in many ways, with race remaining as one of the defining factors. Indeed, studies have shown that racial disparities in PTB persist, with Black gestational parents facing higher rates even when all other factors have been adjusted for.

II. Database

A. *Subjective*

This section lists many of the factors that are screened for to identify individuals at risk for spontaneous PTB that have a reasonable evidence base. However, as noted earlier, there are many complex intertwining drivers that still do not fully explain the overall rates seen in the United States or elsewhere. Further, it is critical to note that approaches to create scores to classify pregnant people into risk categories have been shown to be problematic, with both low overall detection rates and high false-positive rates (da Fonseca et al., 2020).

1. Past reproductive history
    a. Other than having a twin pregnancy, the single greatest risk factor is a history of prior spontaneous birth, either (a) singleton live birth between 16 and 37 weeks' gestation or (b) a stillbirth before 24 weeks presenting as labor, ruptured membranes, or advanced cervical dilation.
    b. The risk of PTB increases multifold with each prior number of pregnancies resulting in a PTB.
    c. Pregnant people who deliver a twin pregnancy have a 5.8% greater risk of having a subsequent premature birth in a singleton pregnancy.
    d. Independent associations between nulliparity and spontaneous PTB have also been recorded.
    e. A matrilineal history of PTB within three generations, especially biological sisters, has been shown to correlate with PTB, with the heritability of PTB estimated at between 13% and 35%.
    f. Preeclampsia, placental abruption, stillbirth, neonatal death, or small for gestational age
2. Gynecological history
    a. Presence of a uterine anomaly, including didelphys, septate, bicornuate, and unicornuate uterus
    b. Previous cervical cone biopsy or excision with loop electrosurgical excision procedure (LEEP)
3. Medical history
    a. Chronic hypertension
    b. Types 1 and 2 diabetes and/or poorly controlled gestational diabetes, with higher rates among insulin-treated gestational diabetes mellitus (GDM) than those whose GDM is controlled with lifestyle changes
    c. The presence of an autoimmune disease, including but not limited to systemic lupus erythematosus, antiphospholipid syndrome, and scleroderma
    d. Indicators or diagnosis of thyroid dysfunction, both overt hypothyroidism and hyperthyroidism
    e. Chronic kidney disease
    f. Asthma
    g. Periodontal disease (periodontitis)
4. Pregnancy history and modifiable risk factors in the current pregnancy
    a. Accurate pregnancy dating by regular last menstrual period (LMP) or as confirmed by first trimester dating sonogram. Research suggests avoiding elective early-term deliveries before 39 weeks due to the possibility of incorrect estimations of gestational age and thus potential for preterm delivery.
    b. Multiple gestation

c. Vaginal bleeding caused by placental abnormalities (placenta previa or abruption)
d. Polyhydramnios or oligohydramnios
e. A history of spontaneous abortion (SAB), with the risk of PTB increasing following one or multiple SABs
f. Any abdominal or cervical surgery after 18 weeks' gestation. Treatment of cervical intraepithelial neoplasia (CIN) with surgery during pregnancy is associated with PTB and a high rate of recurrence or persistence.
g. Genital tract infections (chlamydia, gonorrhea, bacterial vaginosis, trichomoniasis). Although gonorrhea and chlamydia are associated with preterm and early PTB regardless of time of treatment, it is unclear whether treatment of trichomoniasis can reduce PTB.
h. Uterine infections
i. Singleton births conceived after fertility treatment, with both artificial reproductive technology (ART) and non-ART approaches are shown to have a higher risk of PTB, and rates are dependent on the mode of transfer, type of sperm used (fresh vs. frozen), number of embryos transferred, and the number of interuterine-insemination (IUI) cycles.
j. Presence of a fetus with a congenital anomaly
k. Short interpregnancy interval of less than 18 months
l. Body mass index (BMI): Both low and high BMI, as well as insufficient weight gain and gestational weight loss, regardless of the initial BMI. It should be noted that literature is now exploring the limits of BMI as an indicator in health due to the measurement approach but it is still noted as an important risk factor in the literature.
m. Smoking is strongly associated with PTB, with increased rates correlated to the number of cigarettes per day. However, some evidence has shown that smoking cessation early in pregnancy reduces the risk of PTB.
n. Cocaine use
o. Heroin use
p. Febrile illness/systemic infection during pregnancy
q. Inadequate prenatal care
r. Physically strenuous work as part of one's occupation
s. Environmental exposures, including:
   i. Environmental tobacco smoke
   ii. Lead
   iii. Air pollution
   iv. Endocrine-disrupting chemicals, such as phthalates and parabens
   v. Agrochemicals
t. Lower socioeconomic status (SES)
u. High social stress
v. Cervical length less than 25 mm

5. Presence of signs or symptoms of PTL
   a. Regular or frequent uterine contractions that are often painless
   b. Back pain, either constant or intermittent
   c. Menstrual-type cramping, with or without diarrhea
   d. Pelvic pressure
   e. Change in vaginal discharge (watery, mucous, or bloody)
   f. Vaginal spotting/bleeding (bloody show)
   g. Preterm premature rupture of membranes (PPROM)

B. *Objective*
   1. Assess abdomen/uterus tenderness identified through palpation.
   2. Continuous fetal monitoring: Although continuous fetal monitoring is indicated for an individual suspected of having PTL, it is important to note that no threshold of contraction frequency successfully identifies those who still progress to true labor.
   3. Sterile speculum exam for fetal fibronectin (fFN) specimen: Done when PTL is suspected between 22 and 34 weeks. Note that this must be done before a digital exam of the cervix and/or before taking other vaginal/cervical cultures or performing a transvaginal ultrasound (TVUS) to avoid a false positive.
   4. Evaluate fetal membrane status
   5. Check the cervix for dilation and effacement (length), consistency, position, and station of the baby's presenting part. If membranes have ruptured, avoid unnecessary digital examinations. TVUS may be useful for supporting the diagnosis or exclusion of PTL based on cervical length. PTB is associated with the following:
      a. Cervical dilation of ≥3 cm
      b. Cervical length of <20 mm on TVUS
      c. Cervical length of 20–30 mm and positive fetal fibronectin

III. Assessment

A. *At risk for preterm labor*

The factors listed previously can be used to help identify pregnant parents who may be at risk for PTL. In doing so, it is important to remember that there is no one single clear risk factor—or set groupings of risk factors—that place individuals into a definitive "high-risk" category. However, the presence of multiple factors across individual categories or within one category does indicate a potential higher likelihood of PTB. Because many of these risk factors are also indicators for other potential issues that may occur during pregnancy, it is always best to take a comprehensive, detailed, and patient-centered approach to screening.

B. *Threatened PTL*

If a pregnant parent shows signs and symptoms of PTL prior to 37 weeks of pregnancy, they should be assessed through the objective measurements listed earlier and be referred to more advanced care for further assessment.

IV. Goals of clinical management

A. *Identification*

The first step is to determine, through screening and a detailed history, pregnant people at a heightened risk for PTL.

B. *Prevention*

Given our lack of knowledge as to all the drivers of PTB and the myriad of fixed factors, PTB cannot be fully prevented. However, providers can reduce PTL and PTB rates by using interventions aimed at addressing individual identified risk factors. Careful monitoring of those at risk for PTB can also allow for interventions that help increase the gestational age of the baby at birth and those that can help mitigate the immediate and long-term consequences.

C. *Treatment*

Although the ACOG affirmed its recommendation to offer vaginal progesterone supplementation for individuals with a history of spontaneous PTB in 2021, a recent meta-analysis of high-quality studies could not confirm a reduction of recurrent PTB with treatment (Conde-Agudelo & Romero, 2022). Many practices still offer this treatment, and both ACOG and the Society for Maternal Fetal Medicine emphasize shared decision making that considers individual factors when offering treatment.

Refer those who have a prior history of PTB for serial cervical length assessments. Screen for those at risk for PTB and identify PTL early for referral to hospital birth units for assessment and possible medical management with antenatal corticosteroid therapy, group B streptococcal infection prophylaxis, magnesium sulfate for neuroprotection, and/or transfer to a facility with a higher level of neonatal care (as appropriate).

V. Plan

A. *Pregnant people at risk for PTL*

The following list contains suggestions for all pregnant people as well as those who have identified risk factors because there are unknown and significant drivers of PTB that remain unclear. The ones listed here are those with the most accepted evidence base. As the field of research rapidly develops, providers should continually reassess the evidence available.

1. Environmental:
    a. Consider supporting pregnant people in moving toward a midwife-led model of care, which has been shown in systematic reviews to be associated with lower rates of PTB (Medley et al., 2018)
    b. Evaluate personal/family resources and potential barriers to accessing care.
    c. Group antenatal care for pregnant persons may help reduce the likelihood of PTB (Medley et al., 2018).
2. Nutrition:
    a. Ensure adequate nutrition for all pregnant people:
        i. If BMI < 19, discuss recommended weight gain in pregnancy and refer to a nutritionist if needed.
        ii. Identify those with a history of disordered eating and refer to a nutritionist and/or social worker as needed.
        iii. Assess for food security/access and refer to social work or other institutional resources.
    b. Recommend zinc supplementation for pregnant people without systemic illness or contraindications for its use (Medley et al., 2018).
    c. Vitamin D supplementation alone for individuals without preexisting conditions (e.g., diabetes) may help reduce PTB.
    d. Assess for adequate levels of calcium. Low levels of calcium have been linked with hypertensive disorders, which are strongly associated with PTB.
3. Behavioral:
    a. Reduce, or preferably eliminate, exposure to smoking. Refer pregnant people with a history of smoking to cessation support programs. Educate all pregnant people on the dangers of second- and third-hand smoke. Pharmacological interventions for smoking cessation may be beneficial as well (Medley et al., 2018).
    b. Reduce, or preferably eliminate, the use of cannabis products, whether smoked, vaporized, or ingested, because recent evidence suggests all forms increase the risk for PTB (Frey & Klebanoff, 2016; Marchand et al., 2022; Wang et al., 2020).
    c. Utilize a harm-reduction model with respect to controlled substances. Pregnant people with a history of substance use disorders should be referred to cessation, support, and treatment programs.
4. Medical:
    a. Screen all pregnant people for lower genital tract infections such as asymptomatic bacteriuria and treat positive cases with antibiotics to reduce the risk of pyelonephritis and other complications associated with PTB (Smaill & Vazquez, 2019).
    b. Recommend low-dose aspirin for those with moderate to severe risk factors for preeclampsia/eclampsia, which is strongly associated with PTB.
    c. For those with a prior spontaneous PTB in a singleton pregnancy, progesterone supplementation, starting at 16–24 weeks and continued weekly until 36 weeks of pregnancy, may be beneficial.
        i. However, although intramuscular progesterone shots (17-OHP-C, or Makena) have been the standard for these patients, as of writing, the Center for Drug Evaluation and Research at the U.S. Food and Drug Administration (FDA) has called for its withdrawal from clinical use after findings showed that it failed to demonstrate a clinical benefit to newborns (Center for Drug Evaluation

and Research, 2021; Chang et al., 2020; da Fonseca et al., 2020)
   ii. Vaginal progesterone administered before 25 weeks for pregnant people with a prior history of PTB and short cervical length (≤25 mm) may be offered to help reduce spontaneous PTB and associated complications in the neonate (da Fonseca et al., 2020), although recent evidence is mixed. See the earlier Goals of Clinical Management section for further discussion of recent evidence regarding vaginal progesterone.
  d. For patients with a history of poor prior outcomes (e.g., multiple second-trimester losses subsequent to cervical dilation), consult after the first prenatal visit for possible cerclage placement between 12 and 25 weeks' gestation. For those who may have a shortened cervix on TVUS (<20 mm) or 1 cm or greater cervical dilation on vaginal exam, the period of placement is adjusted to 16–23 weeks' gestation (Eleje et al., 2020)
  e. Consider assessing cervical length at midpregnancy in pregnant people without a history of PTB. Although a shortened cervix is related to preterm delivery in individuals with PTL, it is not universally recommended because of its low accuracy as a single measure of PTB, general low prevalence in the population, and misidentification among clinicians (Melamed et al., 2013; Reicher et al., 2021).
  f. Please note that prior clinical practice has included both vaginal pessary and bed rest as interventions to aid in the prevention of PTB; there is no evidence to support the use of either approach (Conde-Agudelo et al., 2020; Medley et al., 2018).
B. *Pregnant people with signs and symptoms of PTL*
   The assessment and treatment of PTL and PTB significantly depend on the level of care available at your practice site. Sites that are remote from a hospital, or where transportation is an issue, may choose to monitor over a period of time, whereas more urban sites may refer directly for advanced care. When considering management options, in those presenting with signs or symptoms of PTL, less than 10% will actually give birth within 7 days of diagnosis. Further, approximately 30% of PTL spontaneously resolves, and 50% of those hospitalized for the presentation of PTL actually give birth at term (ACOG, 2016). For providers who have a patient presenting with suspected PTL, consider the following:
  1. Assess whether the patient meets diagnostic criteria for PTL:
     a. Gestational age between 20 weeks and 36 weeks 7 days, AND
     b. Documented regular contractions, AND
     c. Cervical dilation of ≥3 cm OR cervical length of <20 mm on transvaginal ultrasound OR cervical length of 20–30 mm on TVUS and positive fetal fibronectin
  2. If the pregnant person's obstetric history is unknown or no medical records indicating placental placement are available, do an ultrasound to rule out placenta previa.
  3. Perform a digital cervical exam if fetal membranes are intact, there is no bleeding, and there is no placenta previa on ultrasound.
  4. Obtain a clean-catch urine and dipstick and send for urinalysis to rule out urinary tract infection (asymptomatic bacteriuria).
  5. If not previously obtained, test for group B *Streptococcus* (GBS) and sexually transmitted infections.
  6. Assess fetal position with Leopold's maneuvers or transabdominal sonogram, and assess abdomen for contractions and tenderness. Place a tocometer to detect the presence of contractions.
  7. Evaluate fetal well-being with assessment of fetal heart-rate pattern.
  8. Depending on your clinical setting, refer to a birthing unit for further evaluation or continue observation in the ambulatory setting. If the latter:
     a. Assess cervical length and obtain a posterior fornix sample for fFN. Both alone have a poor positive predictive value and should be done in concert for best results (Lee et al., 2009; Reicher et al., 2021).
  9. Assess the status of placental membranes and for the presence of vaginal bleeding. If membranes are ruptured or bleeding is present, the pregnant person should be referred immediately to the hospital and/or advanced care support.
 10. Observe the pregnant person for 1–2 hours and have the same provider, whenever possible, recheck their cervix to limit individual-based measurement differences.
     If the birthing parent meets the criteria for PTL, refer them to a birthing unit for further evaluation, along with the fFN swab that was obtained. If no cervical change and no uterine contractions are appreciated after a 4- to 6-hour period of observation and fetal well-being is confirmed (e.g., by a reactive nonstress test), provide education regarding signs and symptoms of PTL, review recommendations for calling the healthcare provider, and arrange for follow-up in 1–2 weeks.
C. *Pregnant people with a diagnosis of PTL*
   When given a diagnosis of PTL at less than 34 weeks of gestation, pregnant people are recommended to be hospitalized, and the following treatments may be initiated:
  1. The administration of antenatal corticosteroids has been shown to be the most beneficial intervention for improvement in neonatal outcomes by promoting fetal lung maturity, regardless of membrane status, and is recommended as the standard of care for all impending preterm deliveries. This may be given

as a single dose or as a single course for pregnant people between 24 and 34 weeks of gestation who are at risk of delivery within a week. Corticosteroids are also indicated for those people at less than 34 weeks of gestation who are at risk for PTB in the next 7 days AND have had a course of antenatal steroids at least 14 days previously and at <28 weeks of gestation (ACOG, 2016; Medley et al., 2018). Note: Current evidence shows no benefits of corticosteroids after 34 weeks, and data show evidence of harm (Arimi et al., 2021; Groom, 2019); corticosteroids should thus be avoided.
2. Tocolytic drugs (beta-adrenergic agonist therapy, calcium channel blockers, or nonsteroidal anti-inflammatory drugs [NSAIDs]) may be given for up to 48 hours to delay birth so that betamethasone can be given with its maximum fetal effect (da Fonseca et al., 2020; van Winden et al., 2020).
3. Antibiotics may be given for a documented infection or for identified GBS but show no efficacy on their own, absent these conditions, in the treatment of PTL.
4. Magnesium sulfate for pregnancies at or between 24 and 32 weeks' gestation may be given for fetal neuroprotection against cerebral palsy (ACOG Committee on Practice Bulletins, 2010).

Critically, despite the many clinical options for the identification and attempted prevention of PTB, there is no one "magic bullet" for solving this epidemic. Therefore, it is critical for providers to be diligent in taking thorough histories, provide ample time to discuss and identify risk factors during prenatal visits, and both document and track potential signs and symptoms. Indeed, addressing PTB will likely require comprehensive, integrated approaches at both the clinical and societal levels to address the many socioenvironmental drivers of PTB.

References

American College of Obstetricians and Gynecologists. (2016). Practice Bulletin No. 171: Management of preterm labor. *Obstetrics & Gynecology*, 128(4), e155. doi:10.1097/AOG.0000000000001711

American College of Obstetricians and Gynecologists, Committee on Practice Bulletins. (2010). Opinion No. 455: Magnesium sulfate before anticipated preterm birth for neuroprotection. *Obstetrics & Gynecology*, 115(3), 669–671. doi:10.1097/AOG.0b013e3181d4ffa5

American College of Obstetricians and Gynecologists, Committee on Practice Bulletins—Obstetrics. (2021). ACOG Practice Bulletin No. 234: Prediction and prevention of spontaneous preterm birth. *Obstetrics & Gynecology*, 138(2), e65–e90. doi:10.1097/AOG.0000000000004479

Arimi, Y., Zamani, N., Shariat, M., & Dalili, H. (2021). The effects of betamethasone on clinical outcome of the late preterm neonates born between 34 and 36 weeks of gestation. *BMC Pregnancy and Childbirth*, 21(1), 774. doi:10.1186/s12884-021-04246-x

Beam, A. L., Fried, I., Palmer, N., Agniel, D., Brat, G., Fox, K., Kohane, I., Sinaiko, A., Zupancic, J. A. F., & Armstrong, J. (2020). Estimates of healthcare spending for preterm and low-birthweight infants in a commercially insured population: 2008–2016. *Journal of Perinatology*, 40(7), 1091–1099. doi:10.1038/s41372-020-0635-z

Behrman, R. E., Butler, A. S., & Institute of Medicine Committee on Understanding Premature Birth and Assuring Healthy Outcome. (2007). The role of environmental toxicants in preterm birth. In *Preterm Birth: Causes, Consequences, and Prevention*. National Academies Press. https://www.ncbi.nlm.nih.gov/books/NBK11368/

Center for Drug Evaluation and Research. (2021). *Makena (hydroxyprogesterone caproate injection) information*. https://www.fda.gov/drugs/postmarket-drug-safety-information-patients-and-providers/makena-hydroxyprogesterone-caproate-injection-information

Chang, C. Y., Nguyen, C. P., Wesley, B., Guo, J., Johnson, L. L., & Joffe, H. V. (2020). Withdrawing approval of Makena—a proposal from the FDA Center for Drug Evaluation and Research. *New England Journal of Medicine*, 383(24), e131. doi:10.1056/NEJMp2031055

Conde-Agudelo, A., & Romero, R. (2022). Does vaginal progesterone prevent recurrent preterm birth in women with a singleton gestation and a history of spontaneous preterm birth? Evidence from a systematic review and meta-analysis. *American Journal of Obstetrics and Gynecology*, 227(3), 440–461.e2.10.1016/j.ajog.2022.04.023

Conde-Agudelo, A., Romero, R., & Nicolaides, K. H. (2020). Cervical pessary to prevent preterm birth in asymptomatic high-risk women: A systematic review and meta-analysis. *American Journal of Obstetrics and Gynecology*, 223(1), 42–65.e2. doi:10.1016/j.ajog.2019.12.266

da Fonseca, E. B., Damião, R., & Moreira, D. A. (2020). Preterm birth prevention. *Best Practice & Research Clinical Obstetrics & Gynaecology*, 69, 40–49. doi:10.1016/j.bpobgyn.2020.09.003

DeFranco, E. A., Lian, M., Muglia, L. A., & Schootman, M. (2008). Area-level poverty and preterm birth risk: A population-based multilevel analysis. *BMC Public Health*, 8, 316. doi:10.1186/1471-2458-8-316

Eleje, G. U., Eke, A. C., Ikechebelu, J. I., Ezebialu, I. U., Okam, P. C., & Ilika, C. P. (2020). Cervical stitch (cerclage) in combination with other treatments for preventing spontaneous preterm birth in singleton pregnancies. *Cochrane Database of Systematic Reviews*, 2020(9), CD012871. doi:10.1002/14651858.CD012871.pub2

Feghali, M., Timofeev, J., Huang, C.-C., Driggers, R., Miodovnik, M., Landy, H. J., & Umans, J. G. (2015). Preterm induction of labor: Predictors of vaginal delivery and labor curves. *American Journal of Obstetrics and Gynecology*, 212(1), 91.e1–91.e7. doi:10.1016/j.ajog.2014.07.035

Frey, H. A., & Klebanoff, M. A. (2016). The epidemiology, etiology, and costs of preterm birth. *Seminars in Fetal and Neonatal Medicine*, 21(2), 68–73. doi:10.1016/j.siny.2015.12.011

Giurgescu, C., Zenk, S. N., Dancy, B. L., Park, C. G., Dieber, W., & Block, R. (2012). Relationships among neighborhood environment, racial discrimination, psychological distress, and preterm birth in African American women. *Journal of Obstetric, Gynecologic & Neonatal Nursing*, 41(6), E51–E61. doi:10.1111/j.1552-6909.2012.01409.x

Groom, K. M. (2019). Antenatal corticosteroids after 34 weeks' gestation: Do we have the evidence? *Seminars in Fetal and Neonatal Medicine*, 24(3), 189–196. doi:10.1016/j.siny.2019.03.001

Hodek, J.-M., von der Schulenburg, J.-M., & Mittendorf, T. (2011). Measuring economic consequences of preterm birth—Methodological recommendations for the evaluation of personal burden on children and their caregivers. *Health Economics Review, 1*(1), 6. doi:10.1186/2191-1991-1-6

Janevic, T., Glazer, K. B., Vieira, L., Weber, E., Stone, J., Stern, T., Bianco, A., Wagner, B., Dolan, S. M., & Howell, E. A. (2021). Racial/ethnic disparities in very preterm birth and preterm birth before and during the COVID-19 pandemic. *JAMA Network Open, 4*(3), e211816. doi:10.1001/jamanetworkopen.2021.1816

Jansen, P. W., Tiemeier, H., Jaddoe, V. W. V., Hofman, A., Steegers, E. A. P., Verhulst, F. C., Mackenbach, J. P., & Raat, H. (2009). Explaining educational inequalities in preterm birth: The generation r study. *Archives of Disease in Childhood. Fetal and Neonatal Edition, 94*(1), F28–34. doi:10.1136/adc.2007.136945

Kelly, M. M., & Li, K. (2019). Poverty, toxic stress, and education in children born preterm. *Nursing Research, 68*(4), 275–284. doi:10.1097/nnr.0000000000000360

Lee, H. J., Park, T. C., & Norwitz, E. R. (2009). Management of pregnancies with cervical shortening: A very short cervix is a very big problem. *Reviews in Obstetrics and Gynecology, 2*(2), 107–115. doi: 10.1023/a:1022537516969

Lu, M. C., & Halfon, N. (2003). Racial and ethnic disparities in birth outcomes: A life-course perspective. *Maternal and Child Health Journal, 7*(1), 13–30. doi:10.1023/a:1022537516969

Manuck, T. A., Rice, M. M., Bailit, J. L., Grobman, W. A., Reddy, U. M., Wapner, R. J., Thorp, J. M., Caritis, S. N., Prasad, M., Tita, A. T. N., Saade, G. R., Sorokin, Y., Rouse, D. J., Blackwell, S. C., Tolosa, J. E., & Eunice Kennedy Shriver National Institute of Child Health and Human Development Maternal-Fetal Medicine Units Network. (2016). Preterm neonatal morbidity and mortality by gestational age: A contemporary cohort. *American Journal of Obstetrics and Gynecology, 215*(1), 103.e1–103.e14. doi:10.1016/j.ajog.2016.01.004

March of Dimes. (2022). *Premature babies*. https://www.marchofdimes.org/complications/premature-babies.aspx

Marchand, G., Masoud, A. T., Govindan, M., Ware, K., King, A., Ruther, S., Brazil, G., Ulibarri, H., Parise, J., Arroyo, A., Coriell, C., Goetz, S., Karrys, A., & Sainz, K. (2022). Birth outcomes of neonates exposed to marijuana in utero: A systematic review and meta-analysis. *JAMA Network Open, 5*(1), e2145653. doi:10.1001/jamanetworkopen.2021.45653

Medley, N., Vogel, J. P., Care, A., & Alfirevic, Z. (2018). Interventions during pregnancy to prevent preterm birth: An overview of Cochrane systematic reviews. *Cochrane Database of Systematic Reviews, 2018*(11). doi:10.1002/14651858.CD012505.pub2

Melamed, N., Hiersch, L., Domniz, N., Maresky, A., Bardin, R., & Yogev, Y. (2013). Predictive value of cervical length in women with threatened preterm labor. *Obstetrics & Gynecology, 122*(6), 1279–1287. doi:10.1097/AOG.0000000000000022

Osterman, M., Hamilton, B., Martin, J., Driscoll, A., & Valenzuela, C. (2021). Births: Final data for 2020. *National Vital Statistics Reports, 70*(17). doi:10.15620/cdc:112078

Reicher, L., Fouks, Y., & Yogev, Y. (2021). Cervical assessment for predicting preterm birth—cervical length and beyond. *Journal of Clinical Medicine, 10*(4), 627. doi:10.3390/jcm10040627

Smaill, F. M., & Vazquez, J. C. (2019). Antibiotics for asymptomatic bacteriuria in pregnancy. *Cochrane Database of Systematic Reviews, 2019*(11), CD000490. doi:10.1002/14651858.CD000490.pub4

van Winden, T. M. S., Roos, C., Nijman, T. a. J., Kleinrouweler, C. E., Olaru, A., Mol, B. W., McAuliffe, F. M., Pajkrt, E., & Oudijk, M. A. (2020). Tocolysis compared with no tocolysis in women with threatened preterm birth and ruptured membranes: A propensity score analysis. *European Journal of Obstetrics, Gynecology, and Reproductive Biology, 255*, 67–73. doi:10.1016/j.ejogrb.2020.10.015

Wang, X., Lee, N. L., & Burstyn, I. (2020). Smoking and use of electronic cigarettes (vaping) in relation to preterm birth and small-for-gestational-age in a 2016 U.S. national sample. *Preventive Medicine, 134*, 106041. doi:10.1016/j.ypmed.2020.106041

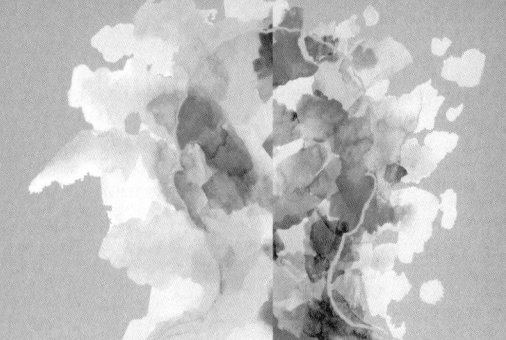

CHAPTER 36

Perinatal Mood and Anxiety Disorders (PMADs)

Laura Todaro

I. Introduction and general background

Perinatal mood and anxiety disorders (PMADs) are a group of mental health disorders that can occur during the period from pregnancy through 6–12 months of postpartum (sometimes called the *perinatal* or *peripartum period*). These can affect both birthing and nongestational individuals. They make up a significant portion of maternal morbidity and mortality in the United States (Gavin et al., 2005) and are therefore an important component of obstetric, pediatric, and primary care (Gavin et al., 2005). Previously, postpartum depression was used as a catchall term for any mental health problem in the perinatal period. More recently, the term *PMADs* has been adopted to reflect a more accurate and thorough description of the types of mental health problems new parents may experience, which can include depression, anxiety, obsessive–compulsive disorder (OCD), bipolar disorder, and psychosis (O'Hara & Wisner, 2014). In addition, some new parents experience post-traumatic stress disorder (PTSD) either from past trauma that is triggered during childbirth or trauma caused by the birth itself. Any new parent can experience symptoms of perinatal depression or mood disorders. However, there is increased risk if individuals have a personal or family history of depression, anxiety, or other mood disorders or if they are experiencing particularly stressful life events or inadequate support from family or friends (Robertson et al., 2004). Rapid changes in sex and stress hormones during pregnancy and after delivery, changes in relationships and at work, lack of sleep, situational life stressors, and physical discomfort may affect mood and contribute to depression.

II. Prevalence

PMADs are more prevalent than any other pregnancy and postpartum complication, with the rates in the United States ranging from 15% to 20%. This is higher than the rates for gestational hypertension (6%–8%), gestational diabetes (6%), and preeclampsia (6%–8%) (Oates, 2003). In addition, PMADs contribute to the high rate of death by suicide among pregnant and postpartum people. According to Lindahl et al. (2005), death by suicides account for up to 20% of postpartum deaths. Self-harm ideation is more common than suicide attempts or deaths, with thoughts of self-harm during pregnancy and the postpartum ranging from 5% to 14%. The risk for suicidality is significantly elevated among depressed individuals during the perinatal period, and death by suicide has been found to be the second-leading cause of death in this depressed population. New studies suggest that suicide rates among pregnant and postpartum people have dramatically increased. According to Admon et al. (2021), who studied 595,237 postpartum individuals from 2006 to 2017, the prevalence of suicidal ideation increased from 0.1% to 0.5% over that period. Intentional self-harm also doubled from 0.1% to 0.2%. Suicidality prevalence increased from 0.2% per 100 individuals in 2006 to 0.6% per 100 individuals in 2017. In California, from 2002 to 2007, 4% of non–obstetric-related deaths were from suicide, just below drug abuse and homicide (California Department of Public Health, 2018). Therefore, knowledge of the symptoms, screening, diagnosis, and treatment of PMADs is necessary for advanced practice nurses who may see new parents in OB/GYN, primary care, pediatrics, psychiatry, or other specialties.

III. Screening recommendations

Screening for PMADs increases the rate of detection from 6.3% to 35.4%. Therefore, it is important to include this as part of routine OB/GYN or pediatric care. PMADs are treatable, so screening is critical to improving outcomes. Currently, many advanced practice providers report feeling hesitant about asking postpartum parents about their emotional well-being; reasons may be due to (1) lack of time, (2) lack of understanding of the types of disorders, and (3) lack of knowledge or resources for treatment. When screening for perinatal mental health disorders, use a compassionate, nonjudgmental communication style that emphasizes patients' own agency. Questions such as "What are you already doing to manage your depression and anxiety?"; "Whom can you rely on for support?"; and "Do you think you need to be on medication?" are helpful interviewing tools. Many patients will use the phrase "I just don't feel like myself," which is a reliable indicator of illness.

In January 2016, the U.S. Preventive Services Task Force (USPTSF) updated its recommendation for depression screening in adults to include screening pregnant and postpartum people. In February 2019, the USPSTF recommended that clinicians provide or refer pregnant and postpartum people at increased risk of perinatal depression to counseling interventions (Siu et al., 2016). The recommendations for screening times are at entrance to prenatal care, at least once each in the second and third trimesters, at the 6-week (or sooner) postpartum visit, and at 6 and 12 months postpartum (American College of Obstetricians and Gynecologists [ACOG], 2016). In addition, pediatric visits should include PMAD screening at the 3-, 9-, and 12-month well-visits (Earls & Committee on Psychosocial Aspects of Child and Family Health American Academy of Pediatrics, 2010).

A. *Screening tools*
1. Edinburgh Postnatal Depression Screening (EPDS) (http://www.perinatalservicesbc.ca/Documents/Resources/HealthPromotion/EPDS/EPDSScoringGuide_March2015.pdf)
   a. Assesses anxiety with questions 4, 5, and 6
   b. 86% sensitivity, 76% specificity
2. Mood Disorders Questionnaire (MDQ) (https://www.sadag.org/images/pdf/mdq.pdf)
3. Patient Health Questionnaire—two-item version (PHQ-2) and Patient Health Questionnaire—nine-item version (PHQ-9)
4. SIGECAPS—mnemonic for symptoms of depression
   a. Sleep, Interest (pleasure/sex), Guilt, Energy (lack of), Cognition/Concentration, Appetite, Psychomotor (agitation or lethargy), Suicidal/Preoccupation with death)

It is important to note that these are screening tools and not diagnostic for PMADs. Upon a patient screening positive, the advanced practice nurse must either refer the patient to a qualified mental health professional or have the experience and skill to diagnose and treat the disorder, such as psychiatric nurse practitioners (NPs) or other NPs/certified nurse–midwives (CNMs) who have completed additional training, such as the Perinatal Mental Health certification through Postpartum Support International (PSI). Additional support may include the aid of a social worker, who can assist patients in finding appropriate mental health referrals and/or support groups, and preprinted information available for patients who are struggling.

IV. Diagnosis

Depression with peripartum onset, otherwise known as *postpartum depression* (PPD), is defined by the American Psychiatric Association (APA, 2013) as a depressive episode occurring during the third trimester of pregnancy or in the 4 weeks after delivery. The ACOG provides a more expansive definition, considering PPD to be a major or minor depressive episode that occurs during pregnancy or in the first 12 months after delivery (ACOG, 2023). Although depression during the postpartum period is frequently referred to as "postpartum depression," according to the *Diagnostic and Statistical Manual of Mental Disorders*, 5th edition (*DSM-5*; APA, 2013), depression during the postpartum period is classified as Major Depressive Disorder, with postpartum onset. The postpartum onset specifier can be applied to the current major depressive episode of major depressive disorder (MDD), bipolar I disorder, or bipolar II disorder. Some individuals have a recurrence of depression after childbirth, while others experience their first onset of depression in the postpartum period (APA, 2013). A diagnosis of a major depressive episode requires that at least five of the symptoms listed in **Table 36-1** must be present, one of which must be depressed mood or diminished pleasure or interest in activities. The symptoms must be present most of the day, nearly every day for 2 weeks, and there must be an associated decline in social and/or occupational functioning.

V. Types of disorders

A. *Postpartum depression*

Up to 70% of postpartum parents who have given birth can experience the "baby blues" in the first weeks after

Table 36-1 Symptoms of Postpartum Depression

1. Feeling sad or having a depressed mood
2. Loss of interest or pleasure in activities once enjoyed
3. Changes in appetite
4. Trouble sleeping or sleeping too much
5. Loss of energy or increased fatigue
6. Increase in purposeless physical activity (e.g., inability to sit still, pacing, handwringing) or slowed movements or speech (these changes must be severe enough to be observable by others)
7. Feeling worthless or guilty
8. Difficulty thinking, concentrating, or making decisions
9. Thoughts of death or suicide
10. Crying for "no reason"
11. Lack of interest in baby, not feeling bonded to baby, or feeling very anxious about/around baby
12. Feelings of being a bad parent
13. Fear of harming the baby or oneself

giving birth. This is characterized by short-lasting episodes of crying, restlessness, irritability, and anxiety. These changes do not interfere with the functions of daily living and resolve on their own within a few weeks without treatment. Conversely, postpartum depression is defined as an episode of depression with an onset of symptoms during the first 4 weeks after delivery; however, individuals remain at risk for developing depression for several months after delivery. These symptoms (**Table 36-1**) worsen over time without treatment and interfere with the postpartum parent's ability to care for themselves and their baby.

1. Consequences of untreated postpartum depression
   Untreated depression during the perinatal period not only affects the gestational parent's health but can also affect their babies—babies born prematurely (before 37 weeks' gestation) or with low birth weight (2500 g or less) have been correlated with untreated depression. Postpartum depression can also cause difficulty with bonding, as well as feeding and sleeping problems, and over time, they can negatively affect children's cognitive, emotional, developmental, verbal, and social skills (Field, 2010). Additional consequences of nontreatment for the family can include relationship problems, intimate partner violence (IPV), divorce, disability, unemployment, poor adherence to medical care, exacerbation of medical conditions, loss of financial resources, and increased tobacco and alcohol use (Field, 2010).

   Many parents are hesitant to consider antidepressants while nursing because of perceived risks to the baby, and healthcare providers may also perpetuate this myth as a result of outdated information. Therefore, when counseling patients, it is important to consider the risks associated with some antidepressants and the risks of untreated mental illness to the individual, baby, and extended family, which can include child abuse and neglect (Hoffman et al., 2017). One phrase many providers find helpful is "exposure always occurs," whether it is the exposure to medication or to the adverse effects of the illness itself.

2. Treatment options
   Treating PMADs is an evolving science that includes psychotherapy, pharmacological, and complementary medicine. It is valuable to have a shared decision-making conversation with patients to determine which methods are most appropriate based on the patient's beliefs and values. Psychotherapy is the first-line treatment option for individuals with mild to moderate perinatal depression. Cognitive–behavioral therapy (CBT) has been shown to be incredibly effective, as has acceptance and commitment therapy (ACT). CBT helps regulate thoughts, dialectical behavior therapy (DBT) helps build distress tolerance, and ACT helps with self-acceptance and directing energy into useful actions. It is critical to offer this information to patients because energy, time, and financial resources vary in this period, and sometimes a single unsatisfactory experience with dialectic therapy can cause treatment to be abandoned altogether. Antidepressant medication in combination with therapy is recommended for individuals with moderate to severe depression (Guille et al., 2013). In pregnancy, individuals who are stable on their current psychiatric medication should remain on it throughout pregnancy, with the exception of any that have clear documented risks to the fetus. There is also evidence that for individuals who have a prior history of depression or postpartum depression, starting antidepressants during pregnancy or at the time of delivery is effective at preventing recurrence (Wisner et al., 2004). Some individuals will require an increase in their current antidepressant medication because of physiological changes in pregnancy (Tosata et al., 2017).

3. Postpartum depression treatment considerations
   When considering treatment options for postpartum depression, it is wise to start with some basic lab work to rule out any underlying conditions and establish a baseline. These include a complete blood count (CBC), thyroid-stimulating hormone (TSH), T_4, thyroid peroxidase (TPO) antibody, vitamin D, ferritin, A1C, folate, and B_{12}, as well as a urine toxicology screen if substance use is suspected. Selective serotonin reuptake inhibitors (SSRIs) and serotonin and norepinephrine reuptake inhibitors (SNRIs) are the most commonly used antidepressants in the treatment of postpartum depression and/or anxiety. Citalopram, nortriptyline, sertraline, and paroxetine are first-line antidepressants because these medications, in therapeutic doses, are associated with low to undetectable serum concentrations in breastfed/chestfed babies (Davanzo et al., 2011). Sertraline is the most prescribed antidepressant during pregnancy and lactation because it is well tolerated and effective for many individuals, including those with anxiety. However, it can cause gastrointestinal (GI) disturbance, especially at initiation of therapy, so it is essential to warn patients of this. When initiating treatment, begin with a low dose and increase slowly to minimize side effects. For example, with Zoloft, start at 25 mg for 4 days, then 50 mg for 2 weeks, then increase as needed until symptoms are gone. It is important to consider that the maintenance dose necessary varies by individual; a higher dose is not an indicator of more severe illness. The goal is to treat to remission. Fortunately, 70% of patients respond to the first medication prescribed (Guille et al., 2013). It is ideal to wait at least 2–4 weeks without symptom improvement before changing medications. Set realistic expectations for patients by reminding them that it often takes 6–9 months for neurotransmitters to normalize. The goal is for patients to feel like themselves again, not to feel

numb or unable to have strong emotions. Patients should expect to remain on medication for 1 year from the time of remission and then slowly taper down over 1–2 months. If patients are not responding to several medication trials, consider gene testing for methylenetetrahydrofolate (MTHFR), which can affect the metabolism of some medications.

Recently, the U.S. Food and Drug Administration (FDA) approved the only medication for the treatment of postpartum depression, brexanolone. It is reserved for the treatment of severe depression only and is given in an inpatient setting through an intravenous (IV) line. Brexanolone is a proprietary version of allopregnanolone, a metabolite of progesterone, which rises throughout pregnancy, then falls quickly after childbirth. It is posited that this fall can lead to depressive symptoms in some postpartum patients. It has a rapid onset of action and can be administered intravenously, thus potentially mitigating the precipitous decline that occurs after childbirth. It may be superior to traditional antidepressants for some individuals because it is designed to treat perinatal depression rather than MDD that occurs during the perinatal period. The efficacy of brexanolone has been established in a total of three phase II/III studies. In each study, based on the change from baseline on the Hamilton Depression Rating Scale (HAM-D), brexanolone was found to be more efficacious than placebo at 60 hours (Faden & Citrome, 2020).

4. Risks of treatment

All medications come with side effects and risks. This is truer in the prenatal period when there are potentially two patients (or more in the case of multiple pregnancies) who may be affected. It is essential to know the basic physiology of pregnancy, including how medications can cross the placenta. The advanced practice nurse should be prepared to have a nuanced discussion weighing the risks and benefits of treatment. It can be helpful to utilize a chart showing stages of fetal development, which can help pregnant patients identify times in pregnancy that are more vulnerable than others. In 2015, the FDA retired its use of pregnancy letter categories A, B, C, D, and X because of the system's simplicity and frequent misinterpretation as a grading system and replaced it with the Pregnancy and Lactation Labeling Rule (PLLR). This new system includes information on pregnancy exposure registries, risk summaries, clinical considerations, and current data (Namazy et al., 2020). Healthcare providers and their patients can also access up-to-date information on drugs in pregnancy and lactation on the MotherToBaby website (https://mothertobaby.org/) and at the Infant Risk Center (https://www.infantrisk.com/), which collects information on medication in human milk.

In terms of nursing, it is generally accepted that levels of medication in human milk of less than 10% are acceptable. Although many medications are safe to use during lactation, it is always a consideration for patients to decide not to breastfeed if they feel it is not conducive to their recovery, especially if it has been challenging (FDA, 2015). Additionally, patients can enroll in registries to assist with collecting evidence on medication use in pregnancy and lactation.

As of 2021, there are no consistent studies showing fetal malformations or miscarriage rates associated with SSRI use, although it is hard to remove confounding factors, such as depression itself. The most common risk associated with antidepressant use among pregnant people is increased incidence of prematurity (averaging 5–7 days early) or low birth weight (averaging 97 g less). However, similar outcomes are associated with depressed gestational parents, so the benefits of treatment likely outweigh the potential risks. Approximately one-third of newborns exposed to SSRIs/SNRIs in utero will experience neonatal adaptation syndrome (NAS), which generally presents within a few hours after birth and may include a combination of respiratory distress, feeding difficulty, jitteriness, irritability, temperature instability, sleep problems, tremors, shivering, restlessness, jaundice, rigidity, and hypoglycemia. Typically, NAS symptoms are mild and transient, generally resolving within 2–3 weeks of delivery.

Persistent pulmonary hypertension of the newborn (PPHN) is defined as a failure of the normal relaxation in the fetal pulmonary vascular bed during the circulatory transition that occurs shortly after birth. PPHN is very rare and occurs with differing severity. There is a slightly increased risk of PPHN (from 1%–2% up to 2%–3%) in newborns exposed to SSRIs in utero; however, the absolute risk is very small. The pediatric team should be notified of the maternal use of SSRIs or SNRIs at the time of delivery in order to increase observation of the neonate (Forsberg et al., 2014). Another important aspect of prescribing SSRIs or SNRIs is the risk of serotonin syndrome, which can cause mild symptoms, such as shivering and diarrhea, to severe symptoms, such as muscle rigidity, fever, and seizures. Severe serotonin syndrome can cause death if not treated. Therefore, providers should review the list of serotonergic agents the patient may be taking, such as St. John's Wort.

5. Therapeutic and complementary approaches

Patients experiencing postpartum depression will benefit from increasing their social support system while undergoing treatment. This can include family members and friends, home visiting nurses, or postpartum doulas (Corrigan et al., 2015). Increased visits from their healthcare provider during the postpartum period will be essential for monitoring treatment success. Patients will benefit from an extended postpartum medical leave from work or utilizing their disability benefits, if they qualify. Interpersonal psychotherapy and/or group therapy facilitated by a perinatal mental health professional have been shown to be effective at treating individuals with postpartum depression alone or in combination with pharmacological therapy (Stuart, 2012). In some areas of the United States and Canada, there are inpatient treatment centers for patients with postpartum depression that allow them to get the rest and assistance with infant care they need (Guille et al., 2013). Additionally, self-care, such as exercise, yoga, and massage, have been found to be helpful adjuncts in treating postpartum depression (Deligiannidis & Freeman, 2014). There is also some evidence that vitamin D and omega-3 fatty acid supplementation can help reduce the occurrence of postpartum depression, although more studies need to be done (Abedi et al., 2018).

B. Postpartum anxiety

As many as two-thirds of individuals with postpartum depression also experience symptoms of anxiety; alternatively, anxiety can present on its own (Munk-Olsen et al., 2009). Although estimates vary, a 2016 study found that about 16% of people experience an anxiety disorder during pregnancy, and about 17% experience it during the postpartum period (Fairbrother et al., 2016). The symptoms may include rapid heart rate, a sense of impending doom, irrational fears and obsessions, feeling guilty and blaming oneself when things go wrong, worrying, and feeling panicky for no reason. One helpful definition of anxiety is perceived danger that is greater than coping skills; therefore, improving coping skills can help to alleviate the symptoms.

1. Treatment for postpartum anxiety

There are both therapeutic and pharmacological methods for treating postpartum anxiety that can be very effective. Treating anxiety is often more successful than treating depression, which tends to increase in severity with recurrences. Medications such as SSRIs are often effective, especially if the patient is also experiencing depression. It is important to note, however, that treatment for anxiety in the perinatal period will not be successful if patients are not getting adequate sleep. Therefore, short-term sleep aids, such as Unisom and trazadone, are often used in treatment plans. Other short-term benzodiazepines, such as Klonopin or lorazepam, can be used as a bridge until an SSRI reaches a therapeutic dose. Alprazolam is typically a last choice because it can cause lethargy in nursing infants. CBT is an effective treatment for anxiety and has been shown to reduce symptoms. CBT involves education about the nature and treatment of anxiety, identification of physical responses to anxiety and maladaptive thoughts and behaviors, followed by restructuring of these responses through exposure therapy. There are also group therapy and support group options for patients experiencing postpartum anxiety. It is important to note that symptoms of anxiety inherently make self-management of those symptoms difficult while those symptoms are active.

C. Postpartum OCD

Postpartum OCD is characterized by fears of deliberate or accidental harm or contamination; recurrent ordering or arranging; and constant checking of potentially hazardous conditions, such as leaving a stovetop on. These thoughts are highly distressing to the patient and may prevent them from discussing them with their family or healthcare provider. Therefore, it is important to ask questions that elicit specific responses, such as "Are you having any obsessive or intrusive thoughts about harming the baby?" About 11% of patients screen positive at 2 weeks postpartum and 5.5% at 6 months (Hudak & Wisner, 2012). It is important to note that there is a difference between intrusive thoughts and psychosis. Thoughts do not equal action for many patients who experience disturbing thoughts. In general, if the thoughts are alarming to the patient, there is very little risk of hurting the baby, and this is not a reason for notifying child protective services. Nonetheless, these thoughts can be terrifying for new parents and their families and therefore need immediate attention, which should include an immediate referral to a psychiatric professional. Treatment includes serotonergic drugs; education to help the patient understand that they are highly unlikely to harm their infant; and exposure with response prevention therapy, which involves exposure of the patient to the feared situations while simultaneously preventing the compulsive rituals (Forray et al., 2010).

D. Perinatal bipolar disorder

Bipolar illness can emerge during pregnancy or the postpartum period and is therefore an important consideration when screening for perinatal mental health disorders. Risk factors include a personal or family history of mood disorders; however, 50% of individuals with bipolar disorder are diagnosed for the first time in the postpartum period. Sixty percent of individuals with bipolar disorder present as clinically depressed, often leading to providers starting them on antidepressants, which then increases symptoms of mania (Sharma et al., 2008). It is often called the postpartum depression "imposter" for this reason. Bipolar I is defined as at least one lifetime episode of mania, that is, euphoria, agitation, decreased need for sleep, racing thoughts, increased productivity, pressured speech, and increased energy (up to 4 days in length). Bipolar disorder has two phases: the depression phase and the manic phase (**Table 36-2**). When these happen at the same time, it is considered a "mixed episode" (Azorin et al. 2012).

Patients who screen positive for a bipolar symptom should be referred to a mental health professional with experience treating bipolar disorder in the perinatal period. Treatment can include mood stabilizers and antipsychotic medications, along with therapy. Individuals with bipolar disorder who stop mood stabilizers in pregnancy have a twofold increased risk of recurrence, so it is essential for these individuals to see a psychiatric professional who can help manage their treatment options (Yonkers et al., 2004).

Table 36-2 Symptoms of Depression and Mania

- Severe sadness and irritability
- Elevated mood
- Rapid speech and racing thoughts
- Little or no sleep and high energy
- Impulsive decisions and poor judgment
- Delusions that can be grandiose or paranoid
- Hallucinations—seeing or hearing things that are not present

E. *Postpartum psychosis*

Postpartum psychosis is an extremely rare but often lethal condition that occurs in 1–2 of every 1,000 deliveries. The symptoms include insomnia, excessive energy, agitation, auditory or visual hallucinations, delusions, and extreme paranoia. Many individuals with postpartum psychosis have a personal or family history of bipolar disorder, but it can occur in anyone. Fifty percent of parents who experience postpartum psychosis had no previous psychiatric hospitalization. About 5% of parents with postpartum psychosis die by suicide, and 4.5% commit infanticide, so it is imperative to screen for this disorder and stress the importance of immediate treatment, most often through the emergency department at the nearest hospital. The typical onset is within 2 weeks of giving birth. Postpartum psychosis has a high incidence of recurrence, so patients with a prior history of psychosis should be started on antipsychotics immediately postpartum and have close psychiatric follow-up (Gabally et al., 2014).

1. Treatment of postpartum psychosis

    Upon identifying postpartum psychosis, advanced practice nurses should send patients to the nearest emergency room or call 911. This is a medical emergency with dire consequences if ignored, and because patients cannot distinguish normal thoughts and behavior from psychosis, they should be accompanied wherever they are going for treatment.

F. *Posttraumatic stress disorder*

Many pregnant and birthing people have a history of trauma that can manifest as PTSD during the perinatal period. High-risk factors include those who have experienced interpersonal violence (Mahenge et al., 2013) and/or sexual or physical abuse (Loveland Cook et al., 2004). Other factors that increase PTSD in pregnancy include hyperemesis gravidarum (Seng et al., 2013), pregnancy complications (Annagür et al., 2013), and fetal anomalies (Horsch et al., 2015). According to Yildiz et al. (2017), the prevalence of PTSD in pregnancy in community samples is 3.3%, and after birth, it is 4.0%. The increase in postpartum rates may be from traumatic events during childbirth that trigger a new episode of PTSD or exacerbate existing PTSD in pregnancy. PTSD rates increase in high-risk samples to 18.9% and 18.5% before and after birth, respectively.

Patients with PTSD are also more likely to exhibit avoidance and may be less forthcoming with their concerns or symptoms. Patients who experience birth trauma or obstetric violence during their delivery are also more likely to miss postpartum visits and, consequently, an important time for screening for mental health disorders (Alcorn et al., 2010). It is therefore essential to provide adequate follow-up for patients who had difficult or traumatic birth experiences. Advanced practice nurses would do well to establish a therapeutic rapport with medically vulnerable patient populations, especially those with a history of trauma. Trauma-informed care that includes assessment of adverse childhood events (ACEs) is essential because a higher ACE score may increase the risk of antenatal IPV and psychological distress, both of which may contribute to PPD (Mersky & Janczewski, 2018).

1. Treatment for PTSD

    Treatment options for patients with PTSD include group therapy, including confidential online groups (Vesel & Nickash, 2015). Giving patients time to share their experiences in a safe and nonjudgmental environment is essential. Fostering resilience is key in recovering from a traumatic birth. It is critical to mention that trauma is the result of a dislocation from safe connections; someone experiencing PMAD may feel a lack of trust of self as a parent resulting from their symptoms; may have experienced a rupture with a provider after violations of physical autonomy during birth or loss of agency in the process; or may be experiencing ongoing foundational lack of trust in their own original providers (usually parents), resulting in a dysregulated attachment style. Healing focuses on repairing that sense of safety with self and others.

VI. Health disparities and special populations

Due to the history of racism in both obstetrics and mental health care in the United States, many Black women report feeling distrustful of their healthcare providers and are less likely to attend their postpartum visits, therefore missing an important time to screen for perinatal mood disorders (Wouk et al., 2021). Having racial or ethnic concordance with their providers has been shown to improve outcomes among Black and Latinx patients, so it is important to support programs that recruit and retain providers of color (Dahlem et al., 2015). There are also specific programs for Black individuals through the Northwestern Family Institute (https://counseling.northwestern.edu/blog/mental-health-counseling-black-women-pregnancy/) and evidence that group prenatal care (i.e., Centering ™) with and by Black participants and providers can reduce these disparities (Kemet et al., 2021).

Many non–English-speaking patients have risk factors that increase the incidence of PMADs, such as undocumented immigration status, social isolation, and a greater likelihood of having experienced violence and/or sexual trauma in their home country or during their migration to the United States. The EPDS has been translated into many languages, so efforts should be made to have these available for non–English-speaking patients (https://medlineplus.gov/languages/postpartumdepression.html).

Adoptive parents can also experience perinatal mood disorders. According to Mott et al. (2011), when studying adoptive versus birthing parents, they had comparable levels of depressive symptoms, but adoptive parents reported greater well-being and less anxiety than postpartum parents. However, stressors (e.g., sleep deprivation, history of infertility, past psychological disorders, and less marital satisfaction) were all significantly associated with depressive symptoms among adoptive parents. It is important for healthcare providers interacting with adoptive parents to perform depression screenings (Mott et al., 2011).

Families who experience perinatal or neonatal death, including termination as a result of fetal anomalies, have higher levels of postpartum depression and PTSD but are less likely to receive treatment for it compared to those who did not experience a loss. According to Gold et al. (2016), bereaved individuals had nearly fourfold-higher odds of having a positive screen for depression and sevenfold-higher odds of a positive screen for PTSD after controlling for demographic and personal risk variables. Only a minority of screen-positive individuals were receiving any type of psychiatric treatment.

The EPDS has been found to be highly accurate in teens, who are at higher risk of experiencing PMADs because of situational circumstances, stigma, or lack of financial or family support. Nonbirthing and nongestational parents can also experience PMADs (Davé, 2010); the EPDS and PHQ-9 are both validated for nongestational parents, although they will require a 2-point-lower cutoff when screening for depression or anxiety than gestational parents (Matthey et al., 2001). Several studies have confirmed a higher prevalence of depression among lesbian, gay, bisexual, transgender, queer, and other (LGBTQ+) birthing parents (Ross et al., 2007). This may be the result of minority stress (e.g., stress created by anti-gay discrimination), which has been found to be related to depression and other psychiatric disorders in LGBTQ+ individuals (Frisell et al., 2010). Additionally, there are an increasing number of transgender men experiencing pregnancy and childbirth. The background risk of attempted suicide among transgender individuals, according to the U.S. Transgender Survey, is nearly nine times the national average. That already increased risk can be increased further in transgender men with the unwanted physical changes that come with pregnancy. One researcher stated, "The process of transitioning is long and arduous, and pregnancy, which is regarded as a feminine condition, forces these men to almost fully transition back to their sex assigned at birth, which can worsen gender dysphoria" (Brandt et al., 2019, p. 19). Special efforts should be made to use LGBTQ+-friendly intake forms when screening patients for PMADs.

VII. Summary

Perinatal mental health is an important aspect of caring for pregnant, birthing, and postpartum patients because it affects pregnancy and childbirth outcomes and child development over time. Postpartum depression, anxiety, and other mood disorders are more common than gestational diabetes or gestational hypertension during the peripartum period and therefore require the same level of knowledge of screening, diagnosis, appropriate treatment or referral, and follow-up. There are many forms of effective pharmacological and therapeutic approaches to treating PMADs, so it is essential to have systems in place that support access to these in all healthcare environments that care for pregnant and new parents. This is especially true for communities that have been historically underserved or discriminated against in health care, such as Black individuals and other people of color, non–English-speaking individuals, and LGBTQ+ individuals.

VIII. Resources

National Maternal Mental Health Hotline: :https://mchb.hrsa.gov/national-maternal-mental-health; hotline 1-833-943-5476 (1-833-9-HELP4MOMS)

MotherToBaby Medication Information and Fact Sheets: https://mothertobaby.org

PSI Helpline: https://www.postpartum.net/get-help/psi-helpline-english-and-spanish/

PSI online support groups: https://www.postpartum.net/get-help/psi-online-support-meetings/

Ayuda en Espanol: https://www.postpartum.net/get-help/psi-ayuda-en-espanol/

Columbia Suicide Severity Rating Scale: https://www.integration.samhsa.gov/clinical-practice/Columbia_Suicide_Severity_Rating_Scale.pdf

Massachusetts General Hospital Center for Women's Mental Health: https://womensmentalhealth.org

ACOG Maternal Mental Health Safety Bundle: https://www.acog.org/Womens-Health/Depression-and-Postpartum-Depression

PSI video *Healthy Mom, Happy Family* in English and Spanish (order for Centering)

on YouTube, "What postpartum depression feels like": https://youtu.be/U8ZSUzJ0KqU

Near Miss Closed Facebook group: https://www.facebook.com/groups/maternalnearmiss/

Internet-based CBT (iCBT) for perinatal anxiety: https://thiswayup.org.au/clinician-hub/

Postpartum OCD: https://iocdf.org/wp-content/uploads/2014/10/Postpartum-OCD-Fact-Sheet.pdf

National Pregnancy Registry for Psychiatric Medications: https://womensmentalhealth.org/research/pregnancyregistry/

Trauma and Birth Stress: http://tabs.org.nz

Solace for Mothers, including online support group: https://www.solaceformothers.org

Prevention and Treatment of Traumatic Childbirth: http://pattch.org

Action on Postpartum Psychosis: https://www.app-network.org

Resources for Non-Birthing Parents

https://www.padrecadre.com

https://www.postpartum.net/get-help/resources-for-fathers/

References

Abedi, P., Bovayri, M., Fakhri, A., & Jahanfar, S. (2018). The relationship between vitamin D and postpartum depression in reproductive-aged Iranian women. *Journal of Medicine and Life*, *11*(4), 286–292. doi:10.25122/jml-2018-0038

Admon, L. K., Dalton, V. K., Kolenic, G. E., Ettner, S. L., Tilea, A., Haffajee, R. L., Brownlee, R. M., Zochowski, M. K., Tabb, K. M., Muzik, M., & Zivin, K. (2021). Trends in suicidality 1 year before and after birth among commercially insured childbearing individuals in the United States, 2006–2017. *JAMA Psychiatry*, *78*(2), 171–176. doi:10.1001/jamapsychiatry.2020.3550

Alcorn, K. L., O'Donovan, A., Patrick, J. C., Creedy, D., & Devilly, G. J. (2010). A prospective longitudinal study of the prevalence of post-traumatic stress disorder resulting from childbirth events. *Psychological Medicine*, *40*(11), 1849–1859. doi:10.1017/S0033291709992224

American College of Obstetricians and Gynecologists. (2016, October 29). *Screening for perinatal depression*. https://www.acog.org/Resources-And-Publications/Committee-Opinions/Committee-on-Obstetric-Practice/Screening-for-Perinatal-Depression

American College of Obstetricians and Gynecologists. (2023, October 2). Summary of Perinatal Mental Health Conditions. https://www.acog.org/programs/perinatal-mental-health/summary-of-perinatal-mental-health-conditions

American Psychiatric Association. (2013). *Diagnostic and statistical manual of mental disorders* (5th ed.). doi:10.1176/appi.books.9780890425596

Annagür, B. B., Tazegül, A., & Gündüz, S. (2013). Do psychiatric disorders continue during pregnancy in women with hyperemesis gravidarum? A prospective study. *General Hospital Psychiatry*, *35*(5), 492–496. doi:10.1016/j.genhosppsych.2013.05.008

Azorin, J. M., Angst, J., Gamma, A., Bowden, C. L., Perugi, G., Vieta, E., & Young, A. (2012). Identifying features of bipolarity in patients with first-episode postpartum depression: findings from the international BRIDGE study. *Journal of Affective Disorders*, *136*(3), 710–715. doi:10.1016/j.jad.2011.10.003

Brandt, J. S., Patel, A. J., Marshall, I., & Bachmann, G. A. (2019). Transgender men, pregnancy, and the "new" advanced paternal age: A review of the literature. *Maturitas*, *128*, 17–21. doi:10.1016/j.maturitas.2019.07.004

California Department of Public Health. (2018). *The California Pregnancy-Associated Mortality Review. Report from 2002–2007. Maternal Death Reviews*. https://www.cdph.ca.gov/Programs/CFH/DMCAH/CDPH%20Document%20Library/PAMR/CA-PAMR-Report-1.pdf

Corrigan, C. P., Kwasky, A. N., & Groh, C. J. (2015). Social support, postpartum depression, and professional assistance: A survey of mothers in the midwestern United States. *Journal of Perinatal Education*, *24*(1), 48–60. doi:10.1891/1058-1243.24.1.48

Dahlem, C. H., Villarruel, A. M., & Ronis, D. L. (2015). African American women and prenatal care: perceptions of patient-provider interaction. *Western Journal of Nursing Research*, *37*(2), 217–235.

Davanzo, R., Copertino, M., De Cunto, A., Minen, F., & Amaddeo, A. (2011). Antidepressant drugs and breastfeeding: A review of the literature. *Breastfeeding Medicine*, *6*(2), 89–98. doi:10.1089/bfm.2010.0019

Davé, S., Petersen, I., Sherr, L., & Nazareth, I. (2010). Incidence of maternal and paternal depression in primary care: A cohort study using a primary care database. *Archives of Pediatrics & Adolescent Medicine*, *164*(11), 1038–1044. doi:10.1001/archpediatrics.2010.184

Deligiannidis, K. M., & Freeman, M. P. (2014). Complementary and alternative medicine therapies for perinatal depression. *Best Practice & Research: Clinical Obstetrics & Gynaecology*, *28*(1), 85–95. doi:10.1016/j.bpobgyn.2013.08.007

Earls, M. F., & Committee on Psychosocial Aspects of Child and Family Health American Academy of Pediatrics (2010). Incorporating recognition and management of perinatal and postpartum depression into pediatric practice. *Pediatrics*, *126*(5), 1032–1039. doi:10.1542/peds.2010-2348

Faden, J., & Citrome, L. (2020). Intravenous brexanolone for postpartum depression: What it is, how well does it work, and will it be used? *Therapeutic Advances in Psychopharmacology*, *10*, 2045125320968658. doi:10.1177/2045125320968658

Fairbrother, N., Janssen, P., Antony, M. M., Tucker, E., & Young, A. H. (2016). Perinatal anxiety disorder prevalence and incidence. *Journal of Affective Disorders*, *200*, 148–155. doi:10.1016/j.jad.2015.12.082

Field, T. (2010). Postpartum depression effects on early interactions, parenting, and safety practices: A review. *Infant Behavior & Development*, *33*(1), 1–6. doi:10.1016/j.infbeh.2009.10.005

Forray, A., Focseneanu, M., Pittman, B., McDougle, C. J., & Epperson, C. N. (2010). Onset and exacerbation of obsessive-compulsive disorder in pregnancy and the postpartum period. *Journal of Clinical Psychiatry*, *71*(8), 1061–1068. doi:10.4088/JCP.09m05381blu

Forsberg, L., Navér, L., Gustafsson, L. L., & Wide, K. (2014). Neonatal adaptation in infants prenatally exposed to antidepressants—clinical monitoring using Neonatal Abstinence Score. *PloS One*, *9*(11), e111327. doi:10.1371/journal.pone.0111327

Frisell, T., Lichtenstein, P., Rahman, Q., & Långström, N. (2010). Psychiatric morbidity associated with same-sex sexual behaviour: Influence of minority stress and familial factors. *Psychological Medicine*, *40*(02), 315–324. doi:10.1017/s0033291709005996

Galbally, M., Snellen, M., & Power, J. (2014). Antipsychotic drugs in pregnancy: A review of their maternal and fetal effects. *Therapeutic Advances in Drug Safety*, *5*(2), 100–109. doi:10.1177/2042098614522682

Gavin, N. I., Gaynes, B. N., Lohr, K. N., Meltzer-Brody, S., Gartlehner, G., & Swinson, T. (2005). Perinatal depression: A systematic review of prevalence and incidence. *Obstetrics & Gynecology*, *106*(5, Pt. 1), 1071–1083. doi:10.1097/01.AOG.0000183597.31630.db83

Gold, K. J., Leon, I., Boggs, M. E., & Sen, A. (2016). Depression and posttraumatic stress symptoms after perinatal loss in a population-based sample. *Journal of Women's Health*, *25*(3), 263–269. doi:10.1089/jwh.2015.5284

Guille, C., Newman, R., Fryml, L. D., Lifton, C. K., & Epperson, C. N. (2013). Management of postpartum depression. *Journal of Midwifery & Women's Health*, *58*(6), 643–653. doi:10.1111/jmwh.12104

Hoffman, C., Dunn, D. M., & Njoroge, W. (2017). Impact of postpartum mental illness upon infant development. *Current Psychiatry Reports*, *19*(12), 100. doi:10.1007/s11920-017-0857-8

Horsch, A., Jacobs, I., & McKenzie-McHarg, K. (2015). Cognitive predictors and risk factors of PTSD following stillbirth: A short-term longitudinal study. *Journal of Traumatic Stress*, *28*(2), 110–117. doi:10.1002/jts.21997

Hudak, R., & Wisner, K. L. (2012). Diagnosis and treatment of postpartum obsessions and compulsions that involve infant harm. *American Journal of Psychiatry*, *169*(4), 360–363. doi:10.1176/appi.ajp.2011.11050667

Kemet, S., Yang, Y., Nseyo, O., Bell, F., Yinpa-Ala Gordon, A., Mays, M., Fowler, M., & Jackson, M. (2021). "When I think of mental healthcare, I think of no care." Mental health services as a vital component of prenatal care for Black women. *Maternal and Child Health Journal*, 26(4), 778–787. doi:10.1007/s10995-021-03226-z

Lindahl, V., Pearson, J. L., & Colpe, L. (2005). Prevalence of suicidality during pregnancy and the postpartum. *Archives of Women's Mental Health*, 8(2), 77–87. doi:10.1007/s00737-005-0080-1

Loveland Cook, C. A., Flick, L. H., Homan, S. M., Campbell, C., McSweeney, M., & Gallagher, M. E. (2004). Posttraumatic stress disorder in pregnancy: Prevalence, risk factors, and treatment. *Obstetrics & Gynecology*, 103(4), 710–717. doi:10.1097/01.AOG.0000119222.40241.fb

Mahenge, B., Likindikoki, S., Stöckl, H., & Mbwambo, J. (2013). Intimate partner violence during pregnancy and associated mental health symptoms among pregnant women in Tanzania: a cross-sectional study. BJOG: An International Journal of Obstetrics & Gynaecology, 120(8), 940–947. doi:10.1111/1471-0528.12185

Matthey, S., Barnett, B., Kavanagh, D. J., & Howie, P. (2001). Validation of the Edinburgh Postnatal Depression Scale for men, and comparison of item endorsement with their partners. *Journal of Affective Disorders*, 64(2), 175–184. doi:10.1016/s0165-032

Mersky, J. P., & Janczewski, C. E. (2018). Adverse childhood experiences and postpartum depression in home visiting programs: Prevalence, association, and mediating mechanisms. *Maternal and Child Health Journal*, 22(7), 1051–1058. doi:10.1007/s10995-018-2488z

Mott, S. L., Schiller, C. E., Richards, J. G., O'Hara, M. W., & Stuart, S. (2011). Depression and anxiety among postpartum and adoptive mothers. *Archives of Women's Mental Health*, 14(4), 335–343. doi:10.1007/s00737-011-0227-1

Munk-Olsen, T., Laursen, T. M., Mendelson, T., Pedersen, C. B., Mors, O., & Mortensen, P. B. (2009). Risks and predictors of readmission for a mental disorder during the postpartum period. *Archives of General Psychiatry*, 66(2), 189–195. doi:10.1001/archgenpsychiatry.2008.528

Namazy, J., Chambers, C., Sahin, L., Johnson, T., Dinatale, M., Lappin, B., & Schatz, M. (2020). Clinicians' perspective of the New Pregnancy and Lactation Labeling Rule (PLLR): Results from an AAAAI/FDA survey. *Journal of Allergy and Clinical Immunology: In Practice*, 8(6), 1947–1952. doi:10.1016/j.jaip.2020.01.056

Oates, M. (2003). Perinatal psychiatric disorders: A leading cause of maternal morbidity and mortality. British Medical Bulletin, 67, 219–229. doi:10.1093/bmb/ldg011

O'Hara, M. W., & Wisner, K. L. (2014). Perinatal mental illness: Definition, description and aetiology. *Best Practice & Research: Clinical Obstetrics & Gynaecology*, 28(1), 3–12. doi:10.1016/j.bpobgyn.2013.09.002

Robertson, E., Grace, S., Wallington, T., & Stewart, D. E. (2004). Antenatal risk factors for postpartum depression: A synthesis of recent literature. *General Hospital Psychiatry*, 26(4), 289–295. doi:10.1016/j.genhosppsych.2004.02.006

Ross, L. E., Steele, L., Goldfinger, C., & Strike, C. (2007). Perinatal depressive symptomatology among lesbian and bisexual women. Archives of Women's Mental Health, 10(2), 53–59. doi:10.1007/s00737-007-0168-x

Seng, J. S., Sperlich, M., Low, L. K., Ronis, D. L., Muzik, M., & Liberzon, I. (2013). Childhood abuse history, posttraumatic stress disorder, postpartum mental health, and bonding: A prospective cohort study. *Journal of Midwifery & Women's Health*, 58(1), 57–68. doi:10.1111/j.1542-2011.2012.00237.x

Sharma, V., Khan, M., Corpse, C., & Sharma, P. (2008). Missed bipolarity and psychiatric comorbidity in women with postpartum depression. *Bipolar Disorders*, 10(6), 742–747. doi:10.1111/j.1399-5618.2008.00606.x

Siu, A. L., U.S. Preventive Services Task Force (USPSTF), Bibbins-Domingo, K., Grossman, D. C., Baumann, L. C., Davidson, K. W., Ebell, M., García, F. A. R., Gillman, M., Herzstein, J., Kemper, A. R., Krist, A. H., Kurth, A. E., Owens, D. K., Phillips, W. R., Phipps, M. G., & Pignone, M. P. (2016). Screening for depression in adults: US Preventive Services Task Force recommendation statement. *JAMA*, 315(4), 380–387.

Stuart, S. (2012). Interpersonal psychotherapy for postpartum depression. *Clinical Psychology & Psychotherapy*, 19(2), 134–140. doi:10.1002/cpp.1778

U.S. Food and Drug Administration. (2015). Drugs in pregnancy and lactation: Improved benefit-risk information. *FDA/CDER SBIA Chronicles.* https://www.fda.gov/files/drugs/published/%22Drugs-in-Pregnancy-and-Lactation--Improved-Benefit-Risk-Information%22-January-22--2015-Issue.pdf

Vesel, J., & Nickasch, B. (2015). An evidence review and model for prevention and treatment of postpartum posttraumatic stress disorder. *Nursing for Women's Health*, 19(6), 504–525. doi:10.1111/1751-486X.12234

Wisner, K. L., Perel, J. M., Peindl, K. S., Hanusa, B. H., Piontek, C. M., & Findling, R. L. (2004). Prevention of postpartum depression: A pilot randomized clinical trial. *American Journal of Psychiatry*, 161(7), 1290–1292. doi:10.1176/appi.ajp.161.7.1290

Wouk, K., Morgan, I., Johnson, J., Tucker, C., Carlson, R., Berry, D. C., & Stuebe, A. M. A Systematic review of patient-, provider-, and health system-level predictors of postpartum health care use by people of color and low-income and/or uninsured populations in the United States. *Journal of Women's*, 30(8), 1127–1159. doi:10.1089/jwh.2020.8738

Yildiz, P. D., Ayers, S., & Phillips, L. (2017). The prevalence of posttraumatic stress disorder in pregnancy and after birth: A systematic review and meta-analysis. *Journal of Affective Disorders*, 208, 634–645. doi:10.1016/j.jad.2016.10.009

Yonkers, K. A., Wisner, K. L., Stowe, Z., Leibenluft, E., Cohen, L., Miller, L., Manber, R., Viguera, A., Suppes, T., & Altshuler, L. (2004). Management of bipolar disorder during pregnancy and the postpartum period. *American Journal of Psychiatry*, 161(4), 608–620. doi:10.1176/appi.ajp.161.4.608

CHAPTER 37

Human Lactation

Serena Saeed-Winn

I. Introduction and background

The mammary gland and surrounding structures are made up of a complex matrix of epithelial, myoepithelial, adipose, fibroblast, immune, lymphatic, and vascular cells. Unlike any other organ in the human body, the mammary gland continues to grow, differentiate, and change in function throughout life.

The study of the structure and function of this gland has been primarily conducted in non-human animals. Mice have been used as a proxy for human tissue for decades because of the limited number of available human tissue samples, the short reproductive cycle of mice, and the ease of study of mice tissue. The similarities between mice and human cells are remarkable; however, fundamental differences in structure, hormonal influence, development, and cellular differentiation make comparisons acceptable but not perfect (Fu et al., 2020; Gusterson & Stein, 2012). In addition, much of the research on milk supply and mastitis comes from data on lactation from the dairy animal community. It is important to remember that there are differences between species, and it is important to note study subjects when analyzing results. Although non-human data may pose limitations, human studies also have their challenges. Many older studies are underpowered, and very few report the individual backgrounds (e.g., ethnicity, education levels, incomes, social support, knowledge of nursing, familial experiences, community views of nursing) of their subjects. Of the studies that do report subject demographics, a large portion of these U.S. and Australian studies focus on subjects who are White, educated (>14 years of schooling), and have mid- to high income, with much of the research being done in high-resourced countries and settings. Very little research is available that focuses on traditional practices, low-resourced communities, non-White people living in the United States and Australia, nonbinary people, community birth practitioners, and people not giving birth in a hospital. Prior to generalizing study findings to the population they are serving, it is important that providers investigate the study population and characteristics, methods, and possible biases in the research they are using.

II. Stages of lactation

The stages of lactation are marked by distinctly different physiological changes and characterized by different hormonal factors.

A. *Secretory differentiation (lactogenesis I)*

The maturation of the secretory cells occurs in pregnancy as a result of influences from hormones from the placenta (Fu et al., 2020). During pregnancy, the epithelial cells of the mammary gland experience rapid growth, cell differentiation, and proliferation. Under the influence of high levels of estrogen and progesterone from the placenta, the epithelial cells expand to create a highly branched ductal system terminating in lobules capable of producing milk. Histological studies of mammary cells have noted differential maturation of cells, leading to the theory that alveoli may be at different stages of development throughout lactation (Hassiotou & Geddes, 2013). This, along with the cellular plasticity noted in mammary cells, shows that the growth and development of the mammary gland is a dynamic series of events resulting in an ever-changing gland throughout lactation and a person's lifetime.

The amount of milk produced at this time is limited by the incomplete differentiation of the mammary epithelial cells into secretory cells, leading to only small amounts of colostrum being produced. If colostrum is not expressed, it is reabsorbed into the blood (Truchet & Honvo-Houéto, 2017).

By gestational week 16, lactation will occur, regardless of whether the pregnancy progresses. During pregnancy, milk production is suppressed by high levels of circulating estrogen, progesterone, and human placental lactogen from the placenta. These hormones work to prevent prolactin (the hormone responsible for milk production) from binding to receptor sites, as well as decreasing prolactin production.

B. *Secretory activation (lactogenesis II)*
The birth of the placenta marks the beginning of the next stage in mammary gland development. The secretory activation stage, or lactogenesis II, is marked by the production of colostrum followed by copious amounts of milk over the first 38–98 hours postpartum (Truchet & Honvo-Houéto, 2017). As the placenta is birthed, the levels of estrogen, progesterone, and placental lactogen drop significantly in the birthing person's circulation, thus ceasing the inhibition of prolactin. Prolactin, along with growth hormone and insulin, are now able to act directly on the mammary epithelial cells to initiate the differentiation of cells to secretory cells that enable mature milk production (Geddes & Sakalidis, 2016; Pandya, 2011; Wambach & Spencer, 2019). Although milk production at this stage is mainly endocrine mediated, changes at the cellular level contribute as well. Colostrum is produced in the first 4 days after birth. With the closure of the tight junctions of the mammary epithelial cells, the sodium and chloride levels fall as lactose, immunoglobulin A (IgA), lactoferrin (LTF), and other milk proteins rise (Truchet & Honvo-Houéto, 2017). These changes in the components of milk are noted to precede copious milk onset by close to 24 hours and usually takes roughly 72 hours to make this change (Nevelle, 1991).

The first few days after birth are essential for milk production. Timing of the first feed within 60 minutes of birth and feeding frequency on day 2 were correlated with milk volume on day 5 postpartum (Kent et al., 2012; Truchet & Honvo-Houéto, 2017). During the first feed, infants will take 0–5 mL of colostrum (Kent et al., 2016). The objective of this first latch is thought to be nipple stimulation and promotion of skin-to-skin contact, not delivery of nutrients. Over the next 2 days, intake of colostrum is 37–169 mL/day until transitional milk appears (Kent et al., 2016). Feeding frequency ranges from 8 to 12 times/day or every 2–3 hours. Parents are encouraged to maintain this frequency until milk supply has been established, at which time on-demand feeding is the preferred method of timing. A sign that milk supply has been established to adequate levels in an exclusively nursed infant is surpassing their birth weight after the initial newborn weight loss. On-demand feeding denotes a pattern of feeding in which infant hunger cues guide the timing, duration, and volumes of feeds.

C. *Galactopoiesis (lactogenesis III)*
Galactopoiesis refers to the time of sustained lactation and marks the shift from endocrine to autocrine regulation of milk supply. For this reason, this stage of lactation is often referred to as the "supply-and-demand" stage. Milk production varies in the first month after birth. After this time, quantities of milk remain relatively constant until 6 months or once the infant begins complementary foods. On average, milk production between 1 and 6 months is 750–800 mL/day, with a range of 440–1,220 mL/day (Kent et al., 2012). Frequency and demand for milk depend on the following factors: (1) storage capacity of the mammary gland (amount of milk available when the gland is full), (2) infant's stomach capacity, and (3) infant's gastric emptying time (Kent et al., 2012). It is important to note that the frequency and duration of feedings can vary greatly among infants based on these factors. Studies have found that the frequency of feeding can range from 5 to >18 times/day, with feeding session durations of 12 to 67 minutes (Hörnell et al., 1999; Ghosh, 2006; Saki et al., 2012; Shealy, 2008), indicating that there is a wide range of "normal" feeding patterns. This knowledge can help providers to alleviate parental anxieties as they compare their experiences with other parents around them.

Regulation of milk supply comes mainly from autocrine control related to the demand of the infant. Milk stasis leads to the release of autocrine proteins whose action is to decrease supply and downregulate the expression of prolactin receptors. Increase volumes of milk in the ducts cause mechanical stress, thus initiating inflammatory processes that affect lactocytes (Hilton et al., 2018; Kent et al., 2012; Saleem et al., 2018; Truchet & Honvo-Houéto, 2017). If milk is not expressed, permanent apoptosis can occur, and the process of involution begins.

Endocrine-mediated processes contribute to milk supply as well, as the nipple is stimulated and milk removed from the gland. The primary hormones involved in lactation are prolactin and oxytocin. Prolactin is responsible for milk production. Oxytocin is released to initiate the milk-ejection reflex, pushing milk out of the nipple.

D. *Involution*
While hormones influence the production and delivery of milk, local mediators control the amount of milk produced. During the interfeeding interval, milk produced by the lactocytes fill the ducts. If this milk is not expressed, a cascade of events takes place to stop production in the moment. If the breast/chest is not drained and milk stasis is sustained, cell death can occur, leading to the involution of the gland.

Involution is the regression of ducts and cells to a nonsecretory state. Involution occurs in two stages. Stage one is known as the *reversible* stage. During this time, milk production can be stimulated to continue by the process of milk removal. If milk is not removed, the *irreversible* phase begins, and milk production cannot restart without the hormonal cues of pregnancy (Truchet & Honvo-Houéto, 2017). Although the cellular and structural regressions that occur during involution return the gland to a nonsecretory state, the tissues, structural components, and external appearance of the gland will remain permanently changed, never regressing back to a prelactation state.

III. Common issues with lactation

Working with lactating people and families invites providers to have a wide view that includes attention to the individual and the community while remaining aware of the foundational anatomy and physiology of lactation. Ensuring that care plans are family centered, realistic, and tailored to the individual needs and desires of the client will help to create recommendations that families can sustain. The most common issues with nursing are discussed in this section.

A. *Low supply*

When assessing an infant–parent dyad, it is essential that signs of inadequate milk intake are noted and evaluated immediately. Low milk supply can place infants at risk for hypoglycemia, dehydration/hypernatremia, lethargy, poor feeding, weight loss or slow gain, hyperbilirubinemia (jaundice), and delayed stools (Kellams et al., 2017). One of the most common reasons people report for stopping nursing is "not having enough milk." The reasons for inadequate milk supply are varied. When triaging a patient, it is important to use the knowledge of lactational anatomy and physiology to guide your treatment plan.

The key physiologic components of milk extraction are (1) nipple stimulation to elicit the milk-ejection reflex, or neuroendocrine-mediated milk production, and cause erection of the nipple; (2) movement of the nipple into the soft palate–hard palate junction by the infant's tongue; (3) creation of a pressure differential in the infant's mouth by the sealing of the lips around the areola and movement of the infant's mandible and tongue; (4) coordination of the suck–swallow–breath pattern by the infant; and (5) sufficient draining of the ducts to prevent milk stasis, which can lead to inflammation, decreased production, and involution. Using this simplistic framework, providers can identify what part of the nursing dynamic is working and what is not.

1. Database

    Primary causes for low milk supply (e.g., hormonal, insufficient glandular tissue) are not nearly as common as secondary, modifiable causes. Careful history and examination are necessary to elicit the cause of low milk supply.

    a. Subjective
        i. Timing since birth
        ii. Mode of delivery and any notable complications
        iii. Frequency and duration of feedings
        iv. Number of infant voids and stools in last 24 h
        v. Coloring and characteristics of stool
        vi. Infant behavior and response to feedings
        vii. Parental report of breast/chest changes in pregnancy and history of breast/chest surgery or abnormal development of the breast/chest is a key indicator of the ability to produce milk.
        viii. Parental report of breast/chest changes that represent secretory activation: feelings of fullness or "hard spots" in the breast/chest, increase in amount of milk secreted, change in milk color (yellow to white) and texture (sticky and thick to thin and milky)
        ix. Secretory activation (SA) is considered delayed if there are no signs of SA at >72 hours after birth.
        x. Volume of expressed milk if expressing

    b. Objective
        i. Exam of breast/chest to assess for fullness, nipple damage, and type of milk present
        ii. Infant weight: Excessive weight loss (EWL) in infants is defined by >10% weight loss after birth, with most infants losing <8% of their birth weight (DiTomasso & Cloud, 2019; Flaherman et al., 2017; Thulier, 2017).

            Obtaining regular weights on the newborn can offer important insights into how feeding is going and allow early recognition of issues. Using the appropriate validated assessment tools is essential for accurate diagnosis and monitoring. The American Academy of Pediatrics (AAP) and the Centers for Disease Control (CDC) support the use of the World Health Organization (WHO) growth charts for children under the age of 2. In contrast to many of the growth charts that existed at the time of this study, an important aim was to "establish the breastfed infant as the normative model for growth and development" (de Onis et al., 2004, p. S15). Resources for evaluating infant growth can be found in the Resources section of this chapter.

            It is important to remember that infants lose on average 5% to 8% of their birth weight in the first 4 days of life, with a return to their birth weight by 7–14 days of life (DiTomasso & Cloud, 2019; Flaherman et al., 2017; Thulier, 2017). A loss of greater than 8%–10% of their birth weight may indicate an infant experiencing inadequate nutritional intake. The majority of the studies in the field define excess weight loss as the loss of >10% of the infant's birth weight. However, there is evidence that labor events can influence infant weight loss after birth. Fluid overload during labor can lead to findings of EWL in the postpartum. Intravenous (IV) fluid rates of >200 mL/hour, 100–200 mL/hour, and total IV fluids of >1,200 have been associated with increased weight loss in the first 24 hours of life, leading to the idea that diuresis by the infant to correct fluid balance after birth can be falsely interpreted as EWL (Chantry et al., 2011; Noel-Weiss et al., 2011).

Timely and accurate evaluations of the nursing dyad are essential. There is not professional consensus on the optimal timing of obtaining infant weights. One proposed schedule is as follows: after birth, every 8–12 hours if admitted to the hospital, within 8–12 hours before discharge, 24–48 hours after discharge if risk factors for inadequate weight gain are present, or within 48–72 hours for low-risk dyads (Feldman-Winter et al., 2020). Many community midwives evaluate weight loss for low-risk dyads at birth and at 24 hours, 72 hours, and 7 days postpartum. The frequency of weight evaluations should be tailored to the individual based on clinical findings and risk factors.
2. Differential diagnosis
   a. Hormonal imbalance
   b. Inadequate milk removal
   c. Insufficient glandular tissue
3. Goals for clinical management
   a. Clinical management of low supply requires a good understanding of the underlying concern. **Table 37-1** outlines common issues and proposed treatment strategies. **Box 37-1** outlines galactagogues, or medications and supplements, used to treat the underlying cause of low supply.
   b. Shared decision making should be used when discussing when and how to begin supplementary feeding (**Box 37-2**). Families and caregivers can work as a team to create a plan that meets the needs and desires of the family and the needs of the infant. The plan should be flexible and families are supported in their decisions.
4. Referral
   A vital part of providing patient-centered care is the creation of a list of professional providers and services that clinicians can refer their patients to. Examples of possible referrals include lactation consultant or International Board Certified Lactation Consultant (IBCLC), pediatric provider, social worker, milk banks, educational resources and videos, nutritional services, patient rights advocates, traditional Chinese medicine/ayurvedic practitioner, herbalist, chiropractor/cranial-sacral practitioner, naturopath, mental health professional, spiritual guide, trauma counselor, and support groups.
B. *Tongue-tie*
Ankyloglossia, also known as *tongue-tie*, is defined by the tethering of the tongue to the floor of the mouth by a short and/or tight frenulum, which restricts the movement of the tongue. The presence of a short frenulum can lead to suboptimal latching, decreased milk intake, pain with feeding for the parent, difficulty with speech later in life, and maxillofacial malformation in the infant (Geddes et al., 2008; Shekher et al., 2021). The prevalence of tongue-tie in infants ranges from 4% to 10% and up to 16% in some studies, depending on the timing of evaluation (Shekher et al., 2021), geographic location, and evaluation technique.
1. Database
   a. Subjective
      i. Weight-gain trend of infant since birth
      ii. Frequency and duration of feedings
      iii. Quality and comfort of latch
      iv. Infant behavior during nursing session

Table 37-1 Treating Low Supply

Issue	Possible Causes	Physiological Impact on Milk Supply	Treatment
Low prolactin levels or decreased receptor expression	■ Genetic predisposition to low levels ■ Milk stasis ■ Inadequate nipple stimulation ■ Retained placental fragments secreting hormones ■ Medications (especially dopamine agonists) ■ Increased dopamine levels	Prolactin stimulates milk production; low levels of this hormone will reduce milk production.	Pharmacological (used off-label): Dopamine antagonists: domperidone (not available in the United States), metoclopramide 1. Nonpharmacological: • Increase nipple stimulation through increased frequency of feedings and hand expression. • Decrease milk stasis (see next row in table). • Removal of retained placental fragments, if identified

III. Common issues with lactation

Issue	Possible Causes	Physiological Impact on Milk Supply	Treatment
Milk stasis or inadequate milk removal	<ul><li>Poor latch</li><li>Poor suck</li><li>Nipple damage</li><li>Ill-fitting pump flange</li><li>Infrequent feedings</li><li>Moving to other breast/chest too quickly</li><li>Oversupply</li></ul>	Milk stasis occurs if milk is not removed from the gland regularly and completely. This leads to a decrease in milk production through autocrine and inflammatory processes that can lead to cell death and permanent effects on supply.	<ul><li>Evaluate infant latch, tongue-tie, and nursing session (see Resources for tools).</li><li>Nursing and expression of milk should not cause damage to the epidermis or underlying tissue and must result in adequate draining of the mammary gland. A correctly fit flange is comfortable and pulls the nipple halfway into the flange. The nipple should not touch the end of the flange during pumping but should be elongated so that the curve of the flange is stimulating the areola during the pumping session. A blanched or erythematous ring visible around the nipple or areola after pumping is an indicator of a flange that is too small. Difficulty in achieving a good seal and "popping off" may be a sign the flange is too big.</li><li>Allow the infant to lick, touch, and nuzzle the breast/chest and nipple before they latch on to stimulate the smooth muscle around the nipple and areola to cause nipple erection to aid in attachment.</li><li>Evaluate for engorgement.</li><li>Evaluate the feeling of the breast/chest after feeding (should feel soft and nontender); if breast/chest still feels full, encourage draining one side completely before switching to the other side.</li><li>Consider breast/chest massage and changing feeding positions during the day to ensure all ducts are being drained equally.</li><li>Increase feeding frequency (every 2–3 hours until supply is well established).</li><li>Consider triple feeding: 1. Nurse infant. 2. Pump after feeds to fully drain mammary gland. 3. Give pumped milk to infant as a supplement.</li></ul>
Decreased oxytocin levels or expression of receptor	<ul><li>A stressful environment can interfere with release of oxytocin.</li><li>Postpartum depression has been noted in parents with lower serum oxytocin levels.</li><li>Labor events (long labor, use of synthetic oxytocin)</li><li>Separation of infant and birthing parent after birth</li><li>Genetic predisposition</li></ul>	Oxytocin is needed for the milk-ejection reflex (MER). The MER contracts the myocytes of the alveoli to push milk into the ducts and out of the nipple. This is an essential step in the nursing process.	<ul><li>Allow the infant to lick, touch, and nuzzle the breast/chest and nipple before they latch on. Breast/chest massage and nipple stimulation increase oxytocin to elicit the MER.</li><li>Oxytocin nasal spray 10–40 units/mL 1–2 sprays per nostril before feeds</li><li>Create relaxed and comfortable environment when feeding or expressing milk.</li><li>Increase skin-to-skin time for parent and infant.</li><li>Minimize separation of infant and birthing parent.</li></ul>

(continues)

Table 37-1 Treating Low Supply (continued)

Issue	Possible Causes	Physiological Impact on Milk Supply	Treatment
Delayed lactogenesis or decreased production due to parental causes	■ Hypoplasia due to inadequate ductal-lobular development ■ History of breast/chest surgery ■ Diabetes mellitus ■ Higher body weight ■ Excessive blood loss in labor ■ Thyroid disorder ■ History of polycystic ovary syndrome (PCOS)	■ Hypoplasia due to inadequate development: insufficient number of alveoli needed to create milk ■ History of breast/chest surgery: injury to nerves innervating the nipple–areola complex, which can reduce afferent signals to stimulate endogenous response; reduction of ductal tissue; preexisting signs of hypoplasia masked by augmentation ■ Diabetes: Insulin is needed for initial lactation onset. ■ Higher total body weight: Increased rates of early nursing cessation and low supply have been noted in patients with higher total body weight; the etiology is yet unknown. ■ Excessive blood loss in labor: risk of damage to the pituitary gland (Sheehan syndrome) ■ PCOS: effect of abnormal hormonal environment during puberty affecting breast/chest development, hyperinsulinemia ■ Thyroid disorders: impact endocrine-mediated milk production and expression	Hypoplasia: ■ Routine prenatal breast/chest exams to increase early identification of people at risk for hypoplasia ■ Create a plan to support parents with signs of hypoplasia in the postpartum. Breast/chest surgery: ■ Identification prenatally: Create plan for adequate support in the postpartum. Diabetes: ■ Prenatal focus on stable blood sugar levels and focus on postpartum support Higher total body weight: ■ Support with feeding positions and comfort with nursing ■ Nonjudgmental care ■ Identification and treatment of comorbidities such as diabetes, hypertension, or thyroid disorder Excessive blood loss in labor: ■ Note in history. ■ Nutritional and supplemental iron as needed Thyroid disorder: ■ Screen all patients prenatally. ■ Referral to endocrinology as needed History of PCOS: ■ Prenatal breast/chest exam to look for abnormal development ■ Screen for comorbidities.
Idiopathic	Low supply is often a combination of various factors, a direct case is not always clear	The human body is a complex structure with processes and interconnections still not well understood by science	■ Galactagogues (see Box 37-1) ■ Adequate nutrition ■ Increase skin-to-skin time with infant. ■ Offer social support to allow parent time to bond with baby during feeds. ■ Patient education on techniques to support nursing

       v. Report of pain with nursing at the nipple–areolar complex
  b. Objective
       i. Evaluate infant tongue using a validated diagnostic tool: Hazelbaker Assessment Tool for Lingual Frenulum Function (ATLFF; Hazelbaker Lactation Institute, 2021) or Bristol Tongue Assessment Tool (BTAT) (see Resources).
      ii. Evaluate nursing session using validated tools (**Box 37-3**): LATCH score or B-R-E-A-S-T F EED Observation Form.
      iii. Evaluate appearance of the nipple after nursing session (a good, deep latch will result in a round, symmetrical nipple that is intact, with no bruising or cracking).
2. Differential diagnosis
  a. Tongue-tie

Box 37-1 Galactagogues

Herbal

The use of herbs in practice differs greatly from allopathic uses of medications. Herbs often work slowly, some needing weeks to show changes in the human body. Herbal medicine is also very individualized. There are professional herbalists that practice in many communities as well as a wealth of resources online and in text. Providers may find it helpful to learn more about the herbs they are suggesting through study and discussions with herbalists.

Most Commonly Used in Practice

- Goat's rue (*Galegae officinalis herba*): 1–2 mL of tincture, 2–3 times a day
  - Makeup similar to metformin, can influence blood sugar levels
  - Reports of hypotonia, lethargy, emesis, weak cry, poor sucking in infants from parents drinking "herbal tea" have been reported in a few sources, including the LactMed database; however, it is important to evaluate the source of this information. The original article was a letter to the editor warning against the use of herbs in nursing parents. The author recounts two cases of infants (15 and 22 days old) admitted for slow weight gain and difficulty feeding. Examination revealed hypotonia, lethargy, emesis, weak cry, and poor sucking. Both nursing parents were drinking >2 L/day of an herbal tea mixture containing licorice, fennel, anise, and *G. officinalis*. The infants were worked up for infection or central nervous system (CNS) involvement, and no cause was found. Nursing was stopped, and the symptoms improved over 24–36 hours. Nursing resumed after 2 days (the nursing parents had stopped drinking the teas), and no other issues were reported. The author's theory was that the effects were caused by the chemical anethole, found in anise and fennel. Studies on goat's rue proving toxic effects have not been found by this author.
- Fenugreek (*Foenugraeci semen*): 6 g, in capsule form, daily
  - May cause diarrhea in parent or baby, evaluation of infant stools important
  - May increase asthma symptoms
  - Cross-reactivity with peanut allergy
  - May affect blood sugar levels of parent
  - Fenugreek may have hypothyroid effects; use with caution in patients with thyroid disorders (Majumdar et al., 2017).
- Milk thistle (*Cardui mariae herba*): 12 to 15 g daily as brewed tea (equal to 200–400 mg of silibinin)
  - Laxative effect
  - Some people are allergic to milk thistle.
  - Often works synergistically with fenugreek and/or goat's rue
- Fennel (*Foeniculi fructus*): 0.1 to 0.6 mL of oil (equal to 100–600 mg) daily

Dietary Galactagogues

For information on specific dietary galactagogues please see https://journals.sagepub.com/doi/10.1177/1941406415579718

Off-Label Pharmacological Drugs

- Domperidone*: 10 to 20 mg 4 times a day or 30 mg 3 times a day, 3 to 8 weeks or as long as needed to maintain supply
  * Note: Not approved by the U.S. Food and Drug Administration for use in breast/chest feeding people in the United States.

- Metformin 500 to 2500 mg per day taken in 2 divided doses for 3 to 10 weeks

Data from Nice FJ. Selection and Use of Galactogogues. ICAN: Infant, Child, & Adolescent Nutrition. 2015;7(4):192-194. doi:10.1177/1941406415579718

---

   b. Buccal tie
   c. Lip tip
   d. Latching issues unrelated to oral structures: nipple shape, nursing position, gastroesophageal reflux disease (GERD) (see Resources for infant feeding positions)
3. Goals of clinical management
   a. Improved quality and comfort of latch
   b. Thriving infant

4. Referral
Referral for treatment of tongue-tie should be individualized to the patient and family. Research and clinical practice have been mixed on the impact of tongue-tie on nursing effectiveness and the appropriate treatment for ankyloglossia (Geddes et al., 2008; Muldoon et al., 2017; O'Shea et al., 2017; Shekher et al., 2021). Considerations for recommendation of frenotomy or frenectomy include the

Box 37-2 Supplementary Feeding

Informed Consent and Patient Education:

- Anticipatory guidance on milk production, nursing frequency, and expectations
- Benefits of nursing for parent and child: These include but are not limited to the ability of the content of human milk to change based on the needs of the infant the parent is feeding (Ballard & Marrow, 2013; Breakey, 2015; Feist, 2000; Hassiotou & Geddes, 2013), the presence of immunological factors and beneficial bacteria specific to the environment the infant is living in (Witkowska-Zimny, 2017), the presence of growth factors and essential fatty acids (e.g., docosahexaenoic acid [DHA]), and hormonally influenced infant–parent bonding.
- Cost is a factor when determining the optimal feeding modality for one's infant. Nursing costs to consider: time away from work to either nurse or pump, storage ability for pumped milk, pumping supplies and psychological, familial and social impacts of nursing. Formula or donor milk feeding costs are cost of the formula, cost of storage, cost of bottles and psychological, familial and social impacts of formula or donor milk feeding.
- Strategies to increase milk production and maintain nursing practices desired by the client (Table 37-1)
- Supplementation methods: cup, spoon, supplemental nursing system, finger feeds, bottle
- Choice of supplement: donor human milk, expressed milk, or formula
- Availability of supplies and support: pumps, lactation consultants, feeding supplies

Initiation:

- Create a clear plan with the family and the care team. Supplementation plans must include the following: type and method of supplement (see Resources), timing and volume of supplement (see Resources), activities to increase/maintain supply (if desired), activities to maintain parent–infant bonding, activities to involve family support people, referral for support or supplies, and criteria for discontinuation of supplementation.

Follow-Up Evaluation:

- Regular follow-up and evaluation: Schedule timely evaluations to ensure that the plan is adjusted to the changing needs of the infant, parent, and family.
- Criteria for discontinuation of supplementation: Indications include but are not limited to meeting targeted weight-gain goals, improvement of lab values (e.g., bilirubin, glucose), adequate parental milk production, and improved infant latch and/or coordination of suck–swallow–breath pattern.

Box 37-3 Tools for Evaluation of a Nursing Session

Evaluation of a nursing session may include the following elements:

1. Comfort of parent
2. Comfort of infant
3. Ability to latch on and stay on breast/chest
4. Parent's response to the nursing session
5. Evaluation of the latch quality (use validated tools such as LATCH or B-R-E-A-S-T—see Resources)
6. Evaluation of quantity of milk expressed
7. Evaluation of infant response to nursing

following: availability of a qualified provider to do the procedure, cost, impact of tongue-tie on milk intake and infant weight gain, parental pain, and implications for future infant development. In addition, complementary therapies can include tongue massage and exercise, body work (cranial-sacral, chiropractic, etc.), and lactation consultation.

C. *Pain with nursing*

The body of literature specifically related to pain and nursing is sparse. The experience of pain in the body is a subject that is not well understood; nursing-related pain is no different. Often, the approach to nursing pain is one of trial and error, using reported response to treatment and mammary gland anatomy

and physiology as a guide. Pain is often multifaceted and will almost always include a multilayer treatment approach.
1. Database
    a. Subjective
        i. Nursing history
        ii. Reported stress levels
        iii. Nutrition status
        iv. Sleeping patterns
        v. Pain history
        vi. Past medical history
        vii. Mental health history and current mental health status
        viii. Infant history
        ix. Support systems available to parent
    b. Objective
        i. Appearance
        ii. Sensitivity
        iii. Pain triggers of the patient
        iv. Observation of a nursing session or expressing session
2. Differential diagnosis
    a. Nipple damage
    b. Dermatosis
    c. Infection/inflammation
    d. Vasospasm/Raynaud
    e. Allodynia/functional pain
3. Goals for clinical management
    a. Identification of underlying cause of pain resulting in adequate treatment: Clinical management steps for the potential causes of nipple pain are outlined in **Table 37-2**.
4. Referral
Because of the complex nature of pain, referrals for nipple/breast/chest discomfort are guided by the etiology of the pain. Referrals may include lactation consultants, dermatology, pediatric dentistry, functional medicine, naturopaths, psychology, psychiatry, Chinese medicine, and more.

D. *Mastitis*
Mastitis can occur at any time in a person's life. The most common type of mastitis and the focus of this chapter is lactational mastitis, herein referred to as *mastitis*. Mastitis is most common in the first 6 weeks after birth (Sun et al., 2017). The risk factors for the development of mastitis can be separated into four categories: (1) nipple damage, (2) milk stasis/constriction of milk flow, (3) infection/illness, and (4) personal and family history.

Table 37-2 Possible Causes of Nipple or Breast/Chest Pain

Abnormal Latch/Suck Dynamics

Infant Factors

- Gestational age/prematurity: Suck–swallow–breath coordination improves with maturity (Kellams et al., 2017).
- Oral/mandibular anatomy or congenital abnormalities: effect of anatomy on creating adequate pressure in mouth, ability to move nipple into the hard palate–soft palate junction (Elad et al., 2014; Geddes et al., 2016)
- Muscle tone/low oral tone: inability to sustain suck–swallow–breath coordination and create adequate pressure (Lau, 2006)
- Neurological maturity: effects on suck–swallow–breath coordination and tone
- Reflux/aspiration: can cause infant to come off nipple during feeds (Kellems, 2016)
- Ankyloglossia (tongue-tie): Restricted tongue movement can affect the ability to create a good latch and increase nipple pain.
- Biting or jaw clenching: Underlying conditions that may elicit this behavior include clavicle fracture, torticollis, head/neck/facial trauma, mandibular asymmetry, oral defensiveness as a result of aggressive feeding or hard oral suctioning at birth, tonic bite reflex, nasal congestion, teething, and response to overactive milk-ejection reflex (Kellams et al., 2017).

Parental Factors

- Nipple shape, size, elasticity, and level of eversion: Anatomy can affect latch and milk-extraction volumes (e.g., more elastic nipples are shown to have lower extracted milk volumes; inverted or flat nipples adversely affect nursing) (Hill, 2019; Lau, 2006).
- Engorgement: May be physiologic in the first few days of lactogenesis or may occur because of oversupply. Engorgement can flatten the nipple and make latching more difficult.
- Fluid overload: Third spacing of extra fluid can cause edema in the area and flatten the nipple, leading to a poor latch.
- Positioning: Poor positioning while nursing can lead to suboptimal latch (defined as a LATCH score of <8) (Dewey et al., 2003).

(continues)

Table 37-2 Possible Causes of Nipple or Breast/Chest Pain (continued)

Management

- Counseling and support to improve latch
- Treatment of tongue-tie if needed
- Use of nipple shield during feeding to improve latch and allow nipple to heal if damaged
- Nipple creams: Although the subject is understudied, traditional practices suggest the application of the parent's own milk on the affected part. In cases where cream is needed, ensure it is compatible with infant consumption.
- Nipple protectors or cups worn in the bra between feeds prevent the raw tissue from sticking to the material.
- Nutrition and rest to aid in healing and strengthening of the immune system to avoid infection
- Use of nipple everter, inverted syringe, or areolar massage to aid in latching on to an inverted or flat nipple
- Reverse-pressure softening to reduce edema in the areola and nipple—especially useful for cases of third spacing or edema in areola

Dermatoses

Underlying Factors (Coexisting Infection May Also Be Present)

- Atopic dermatitis and eczema: Affects 2%–3% of adults. Symptoms include pruritus, history of or current flexural lesions, sparing of groin and axillary, xerosis (dry skin), atopy (personal/family history, immunoglobulin E [IgE] reactivity) (Eichenfield et al., 2014).
- Contact dermatitis (irritant or allergic): Inflammatory skin disorder caused by irritant effects of reactive chemicals or metal ions that induce an immune response. Symptoms include erythema and scaling with visible borders, itching, and discomfort. Acute symptoms include erythema, vesicles, and bullae; chronic cases may involve lichen with cracks and fissures (Novak-Bilić et al., 2018).
- Psoriasis: An immune-mediated skin disorder. Symptoms include inflammation that appears as raised plaques and scales. Often occurs 4–6 weeks postpartum (Mervic, 2014).
- Paget disease: Rare form of carcinoma often associated with ductal cancer. Symptoms present much like eczema, with thickened, sometimes pigmented, eczematoid, erythematous weeping, or crusted lesions with irregular borders, with the lesion being limited to the nipple or extended to the areola. Defining features differing from eczema include unilateral presentation, association with palpable mass, advancing lesion resulting in ulceration, and destruction of the nipple (Karakas, 2011).

Treatment

Dermatitis/eczematous (based on Kellams et al., 2017):

- Identify and reduce triggers.
- Apply emollient to affected area.
- Apply low-/medium-strength steroid ointment to affected area twice a day for 2 weeks immediately after feed to reduce infant contact.
- Second-generation antihistamines for pruritus
- For resistant cases: oral prednisolone or prednisone (<3-week course recommended)

Psoriasis

- Phototherapy (ultraviolet B [UVB]) to affected area
- Apply emollient to affected area.
- Apply low-/medium-strength steroid ointment to affected area twice a day for 2 weeks immediately after feed to reduce infant contact.
- Apply topical vitamin D creams or gels.
- Avoid immunomodulating agents on nipple to reduce risk of infant oral absorption.

Paget Disease

- Immediate referral to oncology for evaluation and treatment

Bacterial Infection

Superficial infections: including impetigo, cellulitis, and underlying dermatitis

- Symptoms: weeping lesions; yellow crusted lesions; erythema; deep, dull aching breast pain during and/or after feedings; breast tenderness, especially with deep touch; bilateral pain and burning quality to the pain (Barrett et al., 2013)
- Treatment: Topical mupirocin or bacitracin ointment; oral antibiotics such as cephalosporin or penicillinase-resistant penicillin (Kellams et al., 2017)

Bacterial Infection

Infection of the lactiferous ducts or dysbiosis of the gland: Bacterial overgrowth, presence of biofilm, and coexisting *Candida* infections can lead to inflammation and narrowing of the ducts.
- Symptoms: constant, dull, aching pain felt deep in the mammary gland; tenderness with palpation (Eglash et al., 2006)
- Treatment: Oral antibiotics have been shown to be superior to topical treatments (Barrett et al., 2013).
- Probiotics to support beneficial bacterial growth (conflicting results on efficacy)

Candida: The presence of *Candida* infections is still a source of controversy; if symptoms do not improve with antifungal treatment, explore other causes (Jiménez et al., 2017; Kellams et al., 2016).
- Symptoms: shooting or burning pain with nursing, erythema of nipple and areola, oral thrush or *Candida* diaper rash in infant
- Treatment: topical antifungals, treatment of infant with oral antifungals if indicated, consideration of oral antifungals for parent if systemic infection is noted

Viral Infection

Herpes Simplex
- Symptoms: Painful blister on nipple–areola complex
- Treatment: Antivirals. Do not feed on infected side, and discard milk from that side while lesion is present (CDC, 2023).

Herpes Zoster
- Symptoms: Lesions erupt along dermatome from spine to chest.
- Treatment: Antivirals. Do not feed on infected side, and discard milk from that side while lesion is present.

Vasospasm/Raynaud Syndrome

- Symptoms: Spasm of the arterioles in the nipple–areola complex leads to a triphasic color change (white to blue to red) in response to stimuli such as cold temperature or nursing. Vasospasms are associated with intense pain.
- Treatment: Warming nipple/whole person, nifedipine 30–60 mg sustained release daily or immediate release 10–20 mg three times a day for 2 weeks initially; if pain persists, a longer course or repeat treatment can be offered (Kellams et al., 2017).

Engorgement

- Symptoms: swelling of the breast/chest; feeling of tight, tender, and sore breast/chest
- Treatment: Massage of the area with attention to the direction of lymph drainage (Bolman et al., 2013; Witt et al., 2016), cabbage leaf application to affected area (place a cold leaf on the breast/chest until withered; Boi et al., 2012; Zakarija-Grkovic & Stewart, 2020). Cactus and aloe compresses and cold gel packs may be helpful (Zakarija-Grkovic & Stewart, 2020).

Blocked Ducts

- Symptoms: hard, possibly rubbery area in breast/chest that is tender to touch; duct may be swollen and tender in a wedge-shaped area; may be associated with engorgement on affected side; pain increased before feed and with letdown; supply on affected side may temporarily decrease; thick, fatty milk may be noted, being expressed once plug is cleared.
- Treatment: adequate hydration, immune support, and rest (prevention of mastitis), frequent and thorough nursing to empty breast/chest, heat (hot compress or warm shower) before feeds, massage of affected side before and during feed toward nipple to dislodge plug, "dangle feeding" or use of gravity to aid in removal of plug, analgesia, cold compress after feeds for symptom relief, lecithin dietary supplement (Bonyata, 2021; U.S. National Library of Medicine, 2021)

Oversupply

- Symptoms: recurrent engorgement and/or milk stasis; hard, tight appearance and feel of the mammary gland; feeling of fullness after feed; reflux in infant after feeds

- Treatment: stimulation of nipple/surrounding tissues only with feeds, herbal medicines to reduce milk supply (e.g., sage, peppermint), cold packs

(continues)

Table 37-2 Possible Causes of Nipple or Breast/Chest Pain (continued)

Blocked Nipple Pore (Milk Bleb or Milk Blister)

- Symptoms: painful area on nipple that appears as a white, clear, or yellow dot on nipple
- Treatment: Epsom salt or saline soaks of nipple, removal of overlying skin through rubbing or sterile needle, good hygiene after removal to prevent infection, warm compress before feeds (Bonyata, 2021)

Allodynia/Functional Pain

Sensation of pain in response to a stimulus that would not normally elicit pain
- Symptoms: pain with light touch, history of other pain disorders
- Treatment: nonsteroidal anti-inflammatory drugs (NSAIDs), propranolol, antidepressants, trigger point evaluation massage, psychotherapy

---

There are varied definitions of mastitis found in practice and in the literature. In this chapter, *mastitis* is defined as the inflammation of the mammary gland tissue (Amir, 2014; Ingman et al., 2014; WHO, 2000). This inflammation results in the presence of clinical symptoms that often present quickly and are associated with parental discomfort. Mastitis was once thought to be solely caused by bacterial infections, however newer research has led to the discovery of inflammatory mediators and processes that may contribute to the symptoms of mastitis even in the absence of pathogenic bacteria.

1. Database
    a. Subjective
        i. Clinical symptoms: tender, hot, swollen, wedge-shaped area of breast/chest associated with a temperature of 38.5°C (101.3°F) or greater; chills; flu-like aching; and systemic illness (AMB, 2014; Barbosa-Cesnik et al., 2003; Wambach & Spenser, 2019)
        ii. Stress and sleep levels: The connection between mood disorders and mastitis has been hypothesized to relate to the inflammatory nature of depression and neuroendocrine effects on the body, including mammary tissue (Ingman et al., 2014; Kvist, 2010; Leonard, 2010; Schiller et al., 2015; Stuebe et al., 2012).
        iii. Latch quality and comfort/pump flange fit: See Resources for tools to evaluate latch. See Table 37-1.
    b. Objective
        i. A clinical exam will reveal unilateral edema with a hot, erythematous, wedge-shaped area that is tender to touch. If an abscess is present, this area may feel hard and fluctuant, depending on the amount of fluid within the abscess (Barbosa-Cesnik, 2003; Wambach & Spencer, 2019). Bilateral presentation can occur in some cases, and evaluation of both glands is required.
        ii. Evaluation of temperature >38.5°C (101.3°F)
2. Differential diagnosis
    a. Bacterially mediated mastitis
    b. Non–bacterially mediated mastitis
3. Goals for clinical management
    a. Choose appropriate nonpharmacological or pharmacological treatment modalities based on etiology: Contrary to previous beliefs, mastitis is not always related to increased bacterial counts (Ingman et al., 2014). The presence of common pathogens has been noted in the milk and on the nipple of people without symptoms (Arroyo et al., 2011; Ingman et al., 2014; Patel et al., 2017). As noted, connections between mood disorders and mastitis have also been hypothesized to relate to the inflammatory nature of depression and neuroendocrine effects on the body, including mammary tissue (Ingman et al., 2014; Kvist, 2010; Leonard, 2010; Schiller et al., 2015; Stuebe et al., 2012). The WHO and the ABM agree that other treatment modalities should be attempted for 24 hours before starting antibiotics (ABM, 2014; WHO, 2000). This recommendation, in addition to the growing attention to antibiotic overuse and resulting bacterial resistance, should encourage providers to explore alternative treatments for mastitis before prescribing antibiotics. Underlying causes and prevention strategies are outlined in **Table 37-3**.
4. Referral

An understanding the connection between parental mood, inflammation, and mastitis can help the provider to create treatment plans that are holistic in nature. Creating a plan for a patient with mastitis should include attention to mental health,

Table 37-3 Mastitis Causes, Treatment, and Prevention

Category	Possible Causes	Prevention/Patient Education/Treatment
Milk stasis	<ul><li>Poor latch</li><li>Plugged duct</li><li>Milk blister</li><li>Infrequent feedings</li><li>Infant immaturity, causing inability to suck adequately</li><li>Oversupply</li><li>Rapid weaning</li><li>Use of pumped or expressed milk with bottle (due to inadequate draining)</li><li>Tight bra</li><li>Wrapping chest before complete involution</li></ul>	<ul><li>Frequent feedings (<4 hours between feedings)</li><li>Breast/chest should feel soft to touch after feeding/pumping (unless oversupply is suspected).</li><li>Early recognition and treatment of oversupply</li><li>Teach hand expression.</li><li>Breast/chest lymphatic massage before and during feed</li><li>Well-fitted bra</li></ul>
Infection/illness/ genetic component	<ul><li>Presence of infection in parent</li><li>Increase levels of parental stress</li><li>Decreased immunity</li><li>Pathological bacteria on skin of nipple that can enter if nipple is damaged</li><li>Antibiotic or antifungal treatments</li></ul>	<ul><li>Antibiotic can be started after 24 hours of conservative treatment.</li><li>Dicloxacillin or flucloxacillin 500 mg by mouth four times per day for 10–14 days</li><li>Cephalexin is usually safe in women with suspected penicillin allergy, but clindamycin is suggested for cases of severe penicillin hypersensitivity.</li><li>Offer immune support through nutrition, rest, and hydration; increased vitamin C, vitamin D, and zinc supplementation; probiotic foods or supplements; and herbal support.</li><li>Decrease parental stress levels.</li><li>Offer increased immune support to parents with family or personal history of mastitis.</li></ul>
Damaged nipple	<ul><li>Poor latch</li><li>Ill-fitting pump</li><li>Dermatitis</li><li>Use of pumped or expressed milk with bottle (Inadequate draining, ill-fitting pump parts, damage from high level suction)</li></ul>	<ul><li>Evaluation, support, and patient education to improve latch</li><li>Evaluation of infant's oral cavity to rule out tongue or lip restriction</li><li>Ensure well-fitting flange.</li><li>Patient education on pumping techniques</li><li>Offer treatments for dermatitis.</li></ul>

Data from Amir, L. H., & Academy of Breastfeeding Medicine Protocol Committee. (2014). ABM clinical protocol# 4: Mastitis, revised March 2014. Breastfeeding Medicine, 9(5), 239-243, Berens, P., Eglash, A., Malloy, M., Steube, A. M., & Academy of Breastfeeding Medicine. (2016). ABM clinical protocol# 26: persistent pain with breastfeeding. Breastfeeding Medicine, 11(2), 46-53, Sun, K., Chen, M., Yin, Y., Wu, L., & Gao, L. (2017). Why Chinese mothers stop breastfeeding: Mothers' self-reported reasons for stopping during the first six months. Journal of Child Health Care, 21(3), 353-363, Zarshenas, M., Zhao, Y., Poorarian, S., Binns, C. W., & Scott, J. A. (2017). Incidence and risk factors of mastitis in shiraz, Iran: results of a cohort study. Breastfeeding Medicine, 12(5), 290-296, Fernandez, L., Mediano, P., García, R., Rodríguez, J. M., & Marín, M. (2016). Risk factors predicting infectious lactational mastitis: decision tree approach versus logistic regression analysis. Maternal and child health journal, 20(9), 1895-1903, Wilson, E., Woodd, S. L., & Benova, L. (2020). Incidence of and risk factors for lactational mastitis: A systematic review. Journal of Human Lactation, 36(4), 673-686, Ingman, W. V., Glynn, D. J., & Hutchinson, M. R. (2014). Inflammatory mediators in mastitis and lactation insufficiency. Journal of mammary gland biology and neoplasia, 19(2), 161-167.

support, and overall wellness. Referral options may include mental health providers and practical support (childcare, postpartum doula, housecleaner, and more). In cases that this is outside of the financial or practical realities of the families practitioner should get to know resources in their area that can help support families on a practical level.

IV. Contraindications to nursing

Before recommending cessation of nursing, ensure that the provider is aware of the most up-to-date, current research on the impact of various factors. For situations necessitating temporary cessation, parents should be encouraged to pump and/or hand express according to their baby's feeding schedule to maintain their milk supply.

According to the CDC (2022), the following conditions are contraindicated with nursing:

- Infant diagnosed with classic galactosemia, a rare genetic metabolic disorder
- Nursing parent infected with HIV (Note: Recommendations about nursing and HIV differ in different countries. The Global Breastfeeding Collective published an advocacy brief in January 2019; this information can be found at http://www.who.int/publications/i/item/WHO-NMH-NHD-18.14.)
- Nursing parent infected with human T-cell lymphotropic virus type I or II
- Nursing parent using an illicit street drug, such as phencyclidine (PCP) or cocaine (exception: narcotic-dependent parents who are enrolled in a supervised methadone program and have a negative screening for other illicit drugs)
- Nursing parent has suspected or confirmed Ebola virus disease.

Temporary cessation of feeding should recommended in the following cases:

- Nursing parent infected with untreated brucellosis
- Nursing parent taking certain medications (see Resources)
- Nursing parent undergoing diagnostic imaging with radiopharmaceuticals. Consult with provider to review medications that will used.
- Nursing parent has active herpes simplex virus (HSV) infection, with lesions present on the breast/chest. (Note: Nursing parent can breastfeed directly from the unaffected breast if lesions on the affected breast are covered completely to avoid transmission.)

Expressed milk may be given in the following scenarios if the infant is not directly nursing:

- Nursing parent has untreated, active tuberculosis (may resume breastfeeding once treated appropriately for 2 weeks and is documented to no longer be contagious).
- Nursing parent has active varicella (chickenpox) infection that developed around the time of birth (within the 5 days prior to delivery to the 2 days following delivery).

V. Medications and nursing

Prescribing medications to the nursing parent involves a risk–benefit calculation that requires adequate resources and information for the clinician to use. **Box 37-4** outlines factors to consider before prescribing medications. One metric the clinician can use to calculate risk is the relative infant dose (RID). This number is calculated by dividing the dose in the infant (from milk) by the dose in the parent. An RID of <10% is considered relatively safe to use. Calculated RIDs can be found in medication texts and databases such as LactMed (see Resources). Impacts of the medication on the milk supply should also be considered. Encourage nursing parents to discuss all medications, supplements, and herbs that they are taking in order to ensure safety for the infant and lessen impact on milk supply.

Box 37-4 Medication Considerations While Nursing

- Avoid unnecessary medications, herbs, or supplements.
- Choose lowest therapeutic dose for shortest duration possible.
- Relative infant dose (RID) of <10% is considered safe.
- Drugs may transfer at a higher rate into milk if they:
  - Attain high concentrations in parental plasma
  - Are low in molecular weight (<800)
  - Are low in protein binding
  - Cross blood–brain barrier easily
- Choose drugs with published data, in contrast to newer drugs.
- Medications used in the first 3–4 days (before onset of SA) usually produce subclinical levels in the infant because of the low volume of milk.
- Most medications are safe in nursing, and consideration for the cessation of nursing should weigh the desires or the client, the health benefits of human milk and length of treatment.
- Consider the health, age, and weight of the infant, with the understanding that larger, healthier, and older infants will tolerate medications better. Exercise more caution with premature or ill infants.
- Medications that are also pediatric-approved drugs are generally safer choices. Review U.S. Food and Drug Administration (FDA) and American Academy of Pediatrics (AAP) updates as a guide.
- Evaluation of the medication's impact on milk supply should be considered.

Data from Hale, T.; Rowe, H. (2017). Medications and Mother's Milk, 17th Edition, Springer Publishing Company.

VI. Resources

Nursing patient resources:
- Global Health Media: http://www.globalhealthmedia.org
- Penn State Health. (2023). *Newborn weight loss tool. Newt.* https://www.newbornweight.org/
- KellyMom: https://www.kellymom.com
- UNICEF Baby Friendly Initiative: http://www.unicef.org.uk/babyfriendly/baby-friendly-resources/breastfeeding-resources/off-to-the-best-start
- La Leche League International http://www.llli.org/breastfeeding-info/

Milk-storage guidelines:
- Proper storage and preparation of breast milk (CDC): https://www.cdc.gov/breastfeeding/recommendations/handling_breastmilk.htm
- Infant formula preparation and storage (CDC): https://www.cdc.gov/nutrition/InfantandToddlerNutrition/formula-feeding/infant-formula-preparation-and-storage.html

Medication safety:
- LactMed database: https://www.ncbi.nlm.nih.gov/books/NBK501922/
- Thomas Hale and Hillary Rowe's book *Medications and Mother's Milk*

Nursing session observation tools:
- The LATCH score: Jensen, D., Wallace, S., & Kelsay, P. (1994). LATCH: A breastfeeding charting system and documentation tool. *Journal of Obstetric, Gynecologic, & Neonatal Nursing, 23*(1), 27–32. doi:10.1111/j.1552-6909.1994.tb01847.x
- B-R-E-A-S-T Feeing Observation Form: https://www.who.int/nutrition/publications/infantfeeding/bf_counselling_participants_manual1.pdf

Supplementary feeding:
- Techniques:
  - Kellams, A., Harrel, C., Omage, S., Gregory, C., Rosen-Carole, C., & Academy of Breastfeeding Medicine. (2017). ABM Clinical Protocol #3: Supplementary feedings in the healthy term breastfed neonate, revised 2017. *Breastfeeding Medicine, 12*(4), 188–198. doi:10.1089/bfm.2017.29038.ajk
  - La Leche League International: https://www.llli.org/breastfeeding-info/
- Target volumes: https://abm.memberclicks.net/assets/DOCUMENTS/PROTOCOLS/3-supplementation-protocol-english.pdf.

Tongue-tie assessment tools:
- Hazelbaker Assessment Tool for Lingual Frenulum Function (HATLFF): https://hazelbakerinstitute.com/course/using-the-assessment-tool-for-lingual-frenulum-function/
- Bristol Tongue Assessment Tool (BTAT): Ingram, J., Johnson, D., Copeland, M., Churchill, C., Taylor, H., & Emond, A. (2015). The development of a tongue assessment tool to assist with tongue-tie identification. *Archives of Disease in Childhood. Fetal and Neonatal Edition, 100*(4), F344–F348. doi:10.1136/archdischild-2014-307503

Supporting nursing:
- 10 Steps to Successful Breastfeeding from the Baby-Friendly Hospital Initiative (BFHI), WHO, and UNICEF: https://www.who.int/teams/nutrition-and-food-safety/food-and-nutrition-actions-in-health-systems/ten-steps-to-successful-breastfeeding
- Baby-Friendly USA, Inc. (BFUSA)—accrediting body and national authority for the BFHI in the United States: https://www.babyfriendlyusa.org
- Baby Friendly Initiative. (2022, February 11). *Breastfeeding assessment tools.* https://www.unicef.org.uk/babyfriendly/baby-friendly-resources/implementing-standards-resources/breastfeeding-assessment-tools/
- International Code of Marketing of Breast-Milk Substitutes: https://www.babyfriendlyusa.org/for-facilities/practice-guidelines/10-steps-and-international-code/
- International Board of Lactation Consultant Examiners: https://iblce.org/
- Coverage of breast pumps through insurance: https://www.healthcare.gov/coverage/breast-feeding-benefits/
- State laws protecting nursing parents: https://www.ncsl.org/research/health/breastfeeding-state-laws.aspx
- Federal laws supporting nursing parents: https://www.womenshealth.gov/supporting-nursing-moms-work/what-law-says-about-breastfeeding-and-work

References

Amir, L. H. (2014). ABM clinical protocol #4: Mastitis, revised March 2014. *Breastfeeding Medicine, 9*(5), 239–243. doi:10.1089/bfm.2014.9984

Arroyo, P., Mediano, P., Martin, V., Jimenez, E., Delgado, S., Fernandez, L., Marin, M., & Rodriguez, J. M. (2011). Etiological diagnosis of infectious mastitis: proposal of a protocol for the culture of human milk samples. *Acta Pediátrica Española, 69*(6), 276–281.

Barbosa-Cesnik, C., Schwartz, K., & Foxman, B. (2003). Lactation mastitis. *JAMA, 289*(13), 1609–1612. doi:10.1001/jama.289.13.1609

Barrett, M. E., Heller, M. M., Fullerton Stone, H., & Murase, J. E. (2013). Dermatoses of the breast in lactation. *Dermatologic therapy, 26*(4), 331–336. doi:10.1111/dth.12071

Ballard, O., & Morrow, A. L. (2013). Human milk composition: Nutrients and bioactive factors. *Pediatric clinics of North America, 60*(1), 49–74. doi:10.1016/j.pcl.2012.10.002

Boi, B., Koh, S., & Gail, D. (2012). The effectiveness of cabbage leaf application (treatment) on pain and hardness in breast engorgement and its effect on the duration of breastfeeding. *JBI library of systematic reviews, 10*(20), 1185–1213. doi:10.11124/01938924-201210200-00001

Bolman, M., Saju, L., Oganesyan, K., Kondrashova, T., & Witt, A. M. (2013). Recapturing the art of therapeutic breast massage during breastfeeding. *Journal of human lactation: Official journal of International Lactation Consultant Association, 29*(3), 328–331. doi:10.1177/0890334413475527

Bonyata, K. (2021). Plugged ducts and mastitis. https://kellymom.com/bf/concerns/mother/mastitis/

Breakey, A. A., Hinde, K., Valeggia, C. R., Sinofsky, A., & Ellison, P. T. (2015). Illness in breastfeeding infants relates to concentration of lactoferrin and secretory Immunoglobulin A in mother's milk. *Evolution, Medicine, and Public Health, 2015*(1), 21–31. doi:10.1093/emph/eov002

Chantry, C. J., Nommsen-Rivers, L. A., Peerson, J. M., Cohen, R. J., & Dewey, K. G. (2011). Excess weight loss in first-born breastfed newborns relates to maternal intrapartum fluid balance. *Pediatrics, 127*(1), e171–e179. doi:10.1542/peds.2009-2663

Centers for Disease Control and Prevention. (2023). Herpes Simplex Virus (HSV). https://www.cdc.gov/breastfeeding/breastfeeding-special-circumstances/maternal-or-infant-illnesses/herpes.html#:~:text=A%20mother%20may%20breastfeed%20her,of%20herpes%20to%20her%20infant

de Onis, M., Garza, C., Victora, C. G., Onyango, A. W., Frongillo, E. A., & Martines, J. (2004). The WHO Multicentre Growth Reference Study: planning, study design, and methodology. *Food and nutrition bulletin, 25*(1), S15–S26. doi:10.1177/15648265040251S103

Dewey, K. G., Nommsen-Rivers, L. A., Heinig, M. J., & Cohen, R. J. (2003). Risk factors for suboptimal infant breastfeeding behavior, delayed onset of lactation, and excess neonatal weight loss. *Pediatrics, 112*(3), 607–619 doi:10.1542/peds.112.3.607

DiTomasso, D., & Cloud, M. (2019). Systematic review of expected weight changes after birth for full-term, breastfed newborns. *Journal of obstetric, gynecologic, and neonatal nursing: JOGNN, 48*(6), 593–603. doi:10.1016/j.jogn.2019.09.004

Eglash, A., Plane, M. B., & Mundt, M. (2006). History, physical and laboratory findings, and clinical outcomes of lactating women treated with antibiotics for chronic breast and/or nipple pain. *Journal of human lactation: Official journal of International Lactation Consultant Association, 22*(4), 429–433. doi:10.1177/0890334406293431

Eichenfield, L. F., Tom, W. L., Chamlin, S. L., Feldman, S. R., Hanifin, J. M., Simpson, E. L., Berger, T. G., Bergman, J. N., Cohen, D. E., Cooper, K. D., Cordoro, K. M., Davis, D. M., Krol, A., Margolis, D. J., Paller, A. S., Schwarzenberger, K., Silverman, R. A., Williams, H. C., Elmets, C. A., ... & Sidbury, R. (2014). Guidelines of care for the management of atopic dermatitis: Section 1. Diagnosis and assessment of atopic dermatitis. *Journal of the American Academy of Dermatology, 70*(2), 338–351. doi:10.1016/j.jaad.2013.10.010

Elad, D., Kozlovsky, P., Blum, O., Laine, A. F., Po, M. J., Botzer, E., Dollberg, S., Zelicovich, M., & Sira, L. B. (2014). Biomechanics of milk extraction during breast-feeding. *Proceedings of the National Academy of Sciences, 111*(14), 5230–5235. doi:10.1073/pnas.1319798111

Feist, N., Berger, D., & Speer, C. (2000). Anti-endotoxin antibodies in human milk: Correlation with infection of the newborn. *Acta Pædiatrica, 89*, 1087–1092. doi:10.1111/j.1651-2227.2000.tb03356.x

Feldman-Winter, L., Kellams, A., Peter-Wohl, S., Taylor, J. S., Lee, K. G., Terrell, M. J., Noble, L., Maynor, A. R., Younger Meek, J., & Stuebe, A. M. (2020). Evidence-based updates on the first week of exclusive breastfeeding among infants ≥ 35 weeks. *Pediatrics, 145*(4), e2018369. doi:10.1542/peds.2018-3696

Fernández, L., Mediano, P., & García, R. et al. (2016). Risk factors predicting infectious lactational mastitis: Decision tree approach *versus* logistic regression analysis. *Maternal and child health journal, 20*, 1895–1903. doi:10.1007/s10995-016-2000-6

Flaherman, V. J., Schaefer, E. W., Kuzniewicz, M. K., Li, S., Walsh, E., & Paul, I. M. (2017). Newborn weight loss during birth hospitalization and breastfeeding outcomes through age 1 month. *Journal of human lactation: Official journal of International Lactation Consultant Association, 33*(1), 225–230. doi:10.1177/0890334416680181

Flavahan, N. (2015). A vascular mechanistic approach to understanding Raynaud phenomenon. *Nat rev rheumatol, 11*, 146–158. doi:10.1038/nrrheum.2014.195

Fu, N. Y., Nolan, E., Lindeman, G. J., & Visvader, J. E. (2020). Stem cells and the differentiation hierarchy in mammary gland development. *Physiological Reviews, 100*(2), 489–523. doi:10.1152/physrev.00040.2018

Geddes, D. T., Langton, D. B., Gollow, I., Jacobs, L. A., Hartmann, P. E., & Simmer, K. (2008). Frenulotomy for breastfeeding infants with ankyloglossia: Effect on milk removal and sucking mechanism as imaged by ultrasound. *Pediatrics, 122*(1), e188-194. doi:10.1542/peds.2007-2553

Geddes, D. T., & Sakalidis, V. S. (2016). Ultrasound imaging of breastfeeding--A window to the inside: Methodology, normal appearances, and application. *Journal of human lactation: Official journal of International Lactation Consultant Association, 32*(2), 340–349. doi:10.1177/0890334415626152

Gusterson, B. A., & Stein, T. (2012, July). Human breast development. *Seminars in Cell and Developmental Biology, 23*(5), 567–573. doi:10.1016/j.semcdb.2012.03.013

Ghosh, R., Mascie-Taylor, C. N., & Rosetta, L. (2006). Longitudinal study of the frequency and duration of breastfeeding in rural Bangladeshi women. *American journal of human biology: The official journal of the Human Biology Council, 18*(5), 630–638. doi:10.1002/ajhb.20533

Hassiotou, F., & Geddes, D. (2013). Anatomy of the human mammary gland: Current status of knowledge. *Clinical anatomy (New York, N.Y.), 26*(1), 29–48. doi:10.1002/ca.22165

Hazelbaker Lactation Institute. (2021). Using the Assessment Tool for Lingual Frenulum Function. https://hazelbakerinstitute.com/course/using-the-assessment-tool-for-lingual-frenulum-function/

Hill, R. (2019). Implications of Ankyloglossia on breastfeeding. *MCN. The American journal of maternal child nursing, 44*(2), 73–79. doi:10.1097/NMC.0000000000000501

Hilton, H. N., Clarke, C. L., & Graham, J. D. (2018). Estrogen and progesterone signalling in the normal breast and its implications for cancer development. *Molecular and cellular endocrinology, 466*, 2–14. doi:10.1016/j.mce.2017.08.011

Hörnell, A., Aarts, C., Kylberg, E., Hofvander, Y., & Gebre-Medhin, M. (1999). Breastfeeding patterns in exclusively breastfed infants: a longitudinal prospective study in Uppsala, Sweden. *Acta paediatrica, 88*(2), 203–211. doi:10.1080/08035259950170402

Ingman, W. V., Glynn, D. J., & Hutchinson, M. R. (2014). Inflammatory mediators in mastitis and lactation insufficiency. *Journal of mammary gland biology and neoplasia, 19*(2), 161–167. doi:10.1007/s10911-014-9325-9

Jiménez, E., Arroyo, R., Cárdenas, N., Marín, M., Serrano, P., Fernández, L., & Rodríguez, J. M. (2017). Mammary candidiasis: A medical condition without scientific evidence?. *PloS one*, *12*(7), e0181071. doi:10.1371/journal.pone.0181071

Jonas, W., & Woodside, B. (2016). Physiological mechanisms, behavioral and psychological factors influencing the transfer of milk from mothers to their young. *Hormones and behavior*, *77*, 167–181. doi:10.1016/j.yhbeh.2015.07.018

Karakas, C. (2011). Paget's disease of the breast. *Journal of Carcinogenesis*, *10*, 31. doi:10.4103/1477-3163.90676

Kellams, A., Harrel, C., Omage, S., Gregory, C., Rosen-Carole, C., & Academy of Breastfeeding Medicine. (2017). ABM Clinical protocol #3: Supplementary feedings in the healthy term breastfed neonate, revised 2017. *Breastfeeding Medicine*, *12*(4), 188–198. doi:10.1089/bfm.2017.29038.ajk

Kent, J. C., Gardner, H., & Geddes, D. T. (2016). Breastmilk production in the first 4 weeks after birth of term infants. *Nutrients*, *8*(12), 756. doi:10.3390/nu8120756

Kent, J. C., Prime, D. K., & Garbin, C. P. (2012). Principles for maintaining or increasing breast milk production. *Journal of obstetric, gynecologic, and neonatal nursing: JOGNN*, *41*(1), 114–121. doi:10.1111/j.1552-6909.2011.01313.x

Kvist L. J. (2010). Toward a clarification of the concept of mastitis as used in empirical studies of breast inflammation during lactation. *Journal of human lactation: Official journal of International Lactation Consultant Association*, *26*(1), 53–59. doi:10.1177/0890334409349806

Lau, C. (2006). Oral feeding in the preterm infant. *NeoReviews*, *7*(1), e19–e27. doi:10.1542/neo.7-1-e19

Majumdar, J., Chakraborty, P., Mitra, A., Sarkar, N. K., & Sarkar, S. (2017). Fenugreek, A potent hypoglycaemic herb can cause central hypothyroidism via leptin - a threat to diabetes phytotherapy. *Experimental and clinical endocrinology & diabetes: Official journal, German Society of Endocrinology [and] German Diabetes Association*, *125*(7), 441–448. doi:10.1055/s-0043-103458

Leonard B. E. (2010). The concept of depression as a dysfunction of the immune system. *Current immunology reviews*, *6*(3), 205–212. doi:10.2174/157339510791823835

Mervic, L. (2014). Management of moderate to severe plaque psoriasis in pregnancy and lactation in the era of biologics. *Acta dermatovenerologica Alpina, Pannonica, et Adriatica*, *23*(2), 27–31. doi:10.15570/actaapa.2014.7

Muldoon, K., Gallagher, L., McGuinness, D., & Smith, V. (2017). Effect of frenotomy on breastfeeding variables in infants with ankyloglossia (tongue-tie): A prospective before and after cohort study. *BMC pregnancy and childbirth*, *17*(1), 373. doi:10.1186/s12884-017-1561-8

Neville, M. C., Allen, J. C., Archer, P. C., Casey, C. E., Seacat, J., Keller, R. P., Lutes, V., Rasbach, J., & Neifert, M. (1991). Studies in human lactation: milk volume and nutrient composition during weaning and lactogenesis. *The American journal of clinical nutrition*, *54*(1), 81–92. doi:10.1093/ajcn/54.1.81

Noel-Weiss, J., Woodend, A. K., Peterson, W. E., Gibb, W., & Groll, D. L. (2011). An observational study of associations among maternal fluids during parturition, neonatal output, and breastfed newborn weight loss. *International breastfeeding journal*, *6*, 9. doi:10.1186/1746-4358-6-9

Novak-Bilić, G., Vučić, M., Japundžić, I., Meštrović-Štefekov, J., Stanić-Duktaj, S., & Lugović-Mihić, L. (2018). Irritant and allergic contact dermatitis - skin lesion characteristics. *Acta clinica Croatica*, *57*(4), 713–720. doi:10.20471/acc.2018.57.04.13

O'Shea, J. E., Foster, J. P., O'Donnell, C. P., Breathnach, D., Jacobs, S. E., Todd, D. A., & Davis, P. G. (2017). Frenotomy for tongue-tie in newborn infants. *Cochrane Database of Systematic Reviews*, *2017*(3), CD011065. doi:10.1002/14651858.CD011065.pub2

Patel, S. H., Vaidya, Y. H., Patel, R. J., Pandit, R. J., Joshi, C. G., & Kunjadiya, A. P. (2017). Culture independent assessment of human milk microbial community in lactational mastitis. *Scientific Reports*, *7*(1), 1–11. doi:10.1038/s41598-017-08451-7

Saki, A., Eshraghian, M. R., & Tabesh, H. Patterns of daily duration and frequency of breastfeeding among exclusively breastfed infants in Shiraz, Iran, a 6-month follow-up study using Bayesian generalized linear mixed models. *Global Journal of Health Science*, 5(2):123-133. doi:10.5539/gjhs.v5n2p123

Saleem, M., Martin, H., & Coates, P. (2018). Prolactin biology and laboratory measurement: an update on physiology and current analytical issues. *The Clinical biochemist. Reviews*, *39*(1), 3–16. PMID: 30072818; PMCID: PMC6069739.

Shealy, K. R., Scanlon, K. S., Labiner-Wolfe, J., Fein, S. B., & Grummer-Strawn, L. M. (2008). Characteristics of breastfeeding practices among US mothers. *Pediatrics*, *122*(Suppl 2), S50–S55. doi:10.1542/peds.2008-1315f

Shekher, R., Lin, L., Zhang, R., Hoppe, I. C., Taylor, J. A., Bartlett, S. P., & Swanson, J. W. (2021). How to treat a tongue-tie: An evidence-based algorithm of care. *Plastic and Reconstructive Surgery Global Open*, *9*(1), e3336. doi:10.1097/GOX.0000000000003336

Stuebe, A. M., Grewen, K., Pedersen, C. A., Propper, C., & Meltzer-Brody, S. (2012). Failed lactation and perinatal depression: Common problems with shared neuroendocrine mechanisms? *Journal of women's health (2002)*, *21*(3), 264–272. doi:10.1089/jwh.2011.3083

Sun, K., Chen, M., Yin, Y., Wu, L., & Gao, L. (2017). Why Chinese mothers stop breastfeeding: Mothers' self-reported reasons for stopping during the first six months. *Journal of Child Health Care*, *21*(3), 353–363. doi:10.1177/1367493517719160

Thulier, D. (2017). Challenging expected patterns of weight loss in full-term breastfeeding neonates born by cesarean. *Journal of obstetric, gynecologic, and neonatal nursing: JOGNN*, *46*(1), 18–28. doi:10.1016/j.jogn.2016.11.006

Truchet, S., & Honvo-Houéto, E. (2017). Physiology of milk secretion. Best practice & research. *Clinical endocrinology & metabolism*, *31*(4), 367–384. doi:10.1016/j.beem.2017.10.008

Wambach, K., & Spencer, B. (2019). *Breastfeeding and human lactation*. Jones & Bartlett Learning.

Wilson, E., Woodd, S. L., & Benova, L. (2020). Incidence of and risk factors for lactational mastitis: A systematic review. *Journal of human lactation: Official journal of International Lactation Consultant Association*, *36*(4), 673–686. doi:10.1177/0890334420907898

Witkowska-Zimny, M., & Kaminska-El-Hassan, E. (2017). Cells of human breast milk. *Cellular & molecular biology letters*, *22*, 11. doi:10.1186/s11658-017-0042-4

Witt, A. M., Bolman, M., Kredit, S., & Vanic, A. (2016). Therapeutic Breast massage in lactation for the management of engorgement, plugged ducts, and mastitis. *Journal of human lactation: Official journal of International Lactation Consultant Association*, *32*(1), 123–131. doi:10.1177/0890334415619439

Zakarija-Grkovic, I., & Stewart, F. (2020). Treatments for breast engorgement during lactation. *Cochrane Database of Systematic Reviews*, *2020*(9), CD006946. doi:10.1002/14651858.CD006946.pub4

Zarshenas, M., Zhao, Y., Poorarian, S., Binns, C. W., & Scott, J. A. (2017). Incidence and risk factors of mastitis in Shiraz, Iran: Results of a cohort study. *Breastfeeding Medicine*, *12*(5), 290–296.

SECTION VI

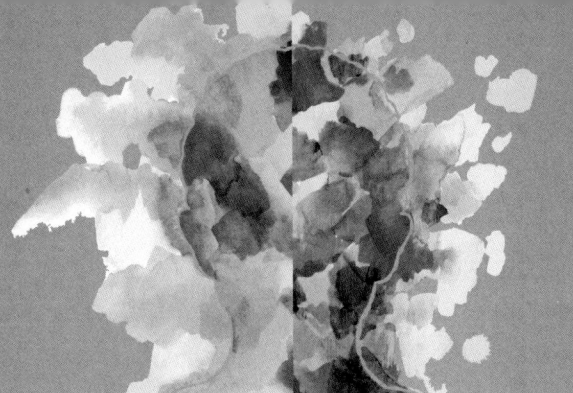

Adult Gerontology Health Maintenance and Promotion

CHAPTER 38	Adult Health Maintenance and Promotion	443
CHAPTER 39	Healthcare Maintenance for Adults with Developmental Disabilities	479
CHAPTER 40	Healthcare Maintenance for Transgender and Gender Expansive (TGE) Adults	495

CHAPTER 38

Adult Health Maintenance and Promotion

Helen R. Horvath

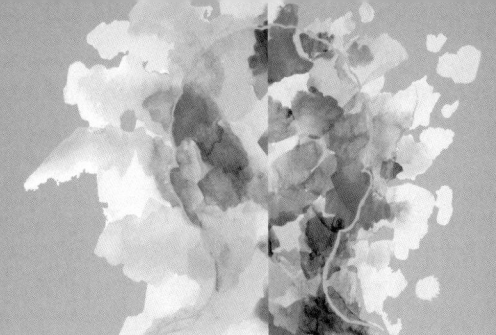

I. Introduction and general background

Health maintenance and promotion, also called *preventive health care* and *healthcare maintenance*, comprise interventions that aim to prevent and minimize disease and promote health. Preventive healthcare interventions include counseling, immunizations, preventive medications (chemoprophylaxis), and screening. This chapter focuses on evidence-based interventions to prevent disease (primary prevention) and detect asymptomatic conditions (secondary prevention) in adults.

Populations vary and have different needs in health maintenance and promotion. This chapter will include guidance for the care of older adults in addition to adults more generally. Additional guidelines which address the unique needs of adolescents, people who are pregnant, people with developmental disabilities, and people who are transgender can be found in the chapters of this book that focus on those populations.

The U.S. Preventive Services Task Force (USPSTF), an independent group of experts in primary care, prevention, and evidence-based medicine, evaluates peer-reviewed evidence regarding clinical preventive services. The USPTF then grades the quality of the evidence and makes recommendations regarding which interventions have a high likelihood of benefitting patients, are unlikely to benefit patients, or have insufficient evidence to make a recommendation one way or the other. The USPSTF's strongest recommendations in favor of interventions are given a grade A or B. Per the USPSTF, grade A is given if "(t)here is high certainty that the net benefit is substantial" (USPTF, 2018, table row 1). When an intervention is given a grade of B, "(t)here is high certainty that the net benefit is moderate or there is moderate certainty that the net benefit is moderate to substantial" (USPTF, 2018, table row 2).

Tables 38-1–38-3 provide an overview of USPSTF grade A and B recommendations. The first column of each table may be used as a guide for clinicians determining which interventions may be appropriate for their individual patient. USPSTF recommendations, along with supporting resources for providers and patients, can be found at the website of the USPSTF (https://www.uspreventiveservicestaskforce.org). Medicare and most private insurers in the United States are required to cover these services without copay.

Many professional associations, such as the American Heart Association, the American Cancer Society, and the American Geriatrics Society, also make recommendations for preventive healthcare interventions specific to their areas of focus. These guidelines may conflict with each other and with the USPSTF recommendations. Each USPSTF recommendation contains a section titled "Recommendations of Others" that can help the clinician understand the landscape of varying guidance. The provider must use clinical judgment in conjunction with evidence-based guidelines to assess which interventions are most appropriate for the patient for whom they are providing care.

The Centers for Disease Control and Prevention (CDC) publishes immunization schedules annually. These schedules are based on the recommendations of the Advisory Committee on Immunization Practices and are approved by a variety of national professional medical organizations. The latest schedule is available in many formats from the CDC website (https://www.cdc.gov/vaccines/). The 2022 schedule is included here as **Figure 38-1**.

Despite strong evidence for effective and cost-effective preventive healthcare interventions, many of these measures remain underused among the U.S. population—in

Table 38-1 U.S. Preventive Services Task Force (USPSTF) Grade A and B Age-Based Recommendations for Screening and Interventions

Target Population	USPSTF Topic and Date of Latest Recommendation	Intervention	Comments
Adults	Tobacco Smoking Cessation in Adults, Including Pregnant Persons: Interventions Grade A January 2021 https://www.uspreventiveservicestaskforce.org/uspstf/recommendation/tobacco-use-in-adults-and-pregnant-women-counseling-and-interventions	Ask all adults about tobacco use. If they use tobacco, advise them to stop. Provide behavioral interventions for cessation. Provide nonpregnant adults who use tobacco U.S. Food and Drug Administration (FDA)-approved medication for cessation. Interval: The USPSTF provides no guidance on appropriate interval for screening for tobacco use.	See USPSTF Recommendation section "Practice Considerations" on USPSTF website for common approaches to assessing tobacco use. See USPSTF Recommendation on USPSTF website for a discussion of the use of e-cigarettes for cessation. The evidence is insufficient to assess the balance of benefits and harms of e-cigarettes for cessation.
Adults	Weight Loss to Prevent Obesity-Related Morbidity and Mortality in Adults: Behavioral Interventions Grade B September 2018 https://www.uspreventiveservicestaskforce.org/uspstf/recommendation/obesity-in-adults-interventions	Assess body mass index (BMI), calculated as weight in kilograms divided by height in meters squared. Those with a BMI of 30 or higher should be referred to intensive, multicomponent behavioral interventions. Interval: Not specified	Potentially effective intervention types reviewed by the USPSTF include: ■ Behavioral counseling ■ Behavior-based weight loss and weight-loss maintenance ■ Pharmacotherapy-based weight loss and weight-loss maintenance See USPSTF Recommendation section "Clinical Considerations" on USPSTF website for more information.

Adults without known hypertension	Hypertension in Adults: Screening
	Grade A
	April 2021
	https://www.uspreventiveservicestaskforce.org/uspstf/recommendation/hypertension-in-adults-screening
		Office blood pressure measurement
		Interval:
		■ Age 18–39 and at increased risk for hypertension: screen annually
		Increased risk for hypertension:
		  • Black persons
		  • Persons with high-normal blood pressure
		  • Persons who are overweight or obese (body mass index [BMI] ≥25 [calculated as weight in kilograms divided by height in meters squared])
		■ Age 18 to 39 years not at increased risk for hypertension and with a prior normal blood pressure reading: screen every 3–5 years
		■ Age 40 or older: screen annually
			The USPSTF recommends obtaining blood pressure measurements outside of the clinical setting for diagnostic confirmation before starting treatment.

Population	Recommendation	Screening tools/intervals
Adults, including pregnant and postpartum persons, and older adults (65 years or older)	Depression and Suicide Risk in Adults: Screening Grade B June 2023 https://www.uspreventiveservicestaskforce.org/uspstf/recommendation/screening-depression-suicide-risk-adults	Screening tool options: ■ Patient Health Questionnaire (PHQ) ■ Geriatric Depression Scale ■ Edinburgh Postnatal Depression Scale (EPDS) ■ Center for Epidemiologic Studies Depression Scale (CES-D) Interval: Optimal interval unknown
Adults when services for accurate diagnosis, effective treatment, and appropriate care can be offered or referred to	Unhealthy Drug Use: Screening Grade B June 2020 https://www.uspreventiveservicestaskforce.org/uspstf/recommendation/drug-use-illicit-screening	Screening tools: ■ National Institute on Drug Abuse (NIDA) Quick Screen (4 questions about use of alcohol, tobacco, nonmedical use of prescription drugs, and illegal drugs in the past year) ■ Alcohol, Smoking and Substance Involvement Screening Test (ASSIST) (8-item screen) ■ Tobacco, Alcohol, Prescription Medication, and Other Substance Use (TAPS) Note: A positive screen does not diagnose drug dependence, abuse, addiction, or drug use disorders. A positive screen should be followed up with more in-depth assessment and treatment if needed. Interval: Optimal interval unknown Per the USPSTF, "For the purposes of this recommendation, 'unhealthy drug use' is defined as the use of substances (not including alcohol or tobacco products) that are illegally obtained or the nonmedical use of prescription psychoactive medications; that is, use of medications for reasons, for duration, in amounts, or with frequency other than prescribed or by persons other than the prescribed individual. These substances are ingested, inhaled, injected, or administered using other methods to affect cognition, affect, or other mental processes; to 'get high'; or for other nonmedical reasons."

(continues)

Table 38-1 U.S. Preventive Services Task Force (USPSTF) Grade A and B Age-Based Recommendations for Screening and Interventions *(continued)*

Target Population	USPSTF Topic and Date of Latest Recommendation	Intervention	Comments
Adults when services for accurate diagnosis, effective treatment, and appropriate care can be offered or referred to	Unhealthy Alcohol Use in Adolescents and Adults: Screening Grade B November 2018 https://www.uspreventiveservicestaskforce.org/uspstf/recommendation/unhealthy-alcohol-use-in-adolescents-and-adults-screening-and-behavioral-counseling-interventions	Brief screening tools: ■ Alcohol Use Disorders Identification Test-Consumption (AUDIT-C)—3 questions ■ Single Alcohol Screening Question (SASQ—"How many times in the past year have you had five (four for cis-gender women) or more drinks in a day?" A response of greater than zero is a positive screen. In gender-minority people, five or more drinks in a day is an effective number for identifying possible unhealthy alcohol use (Flentje et al., 2020). A positive result on a brief screening instrument (e.g., SASQ or AUDIT-C) does not diagnose substance use disorder. It should trigger follow-up with a more in-depth assessment to confirm unhealthy alcohol use and determine the next steps. Interval: Optimal interval unknown	There are other screening tools that target particular populations, including pregnant people and older people. Persons diagnosed as engaging in unhealthy alcohol use should be provided with brief behavioral counseling interventions to reduce unhealthy alcohol use. The Cut down, Annoyed, Guilty, Eye-opener (CAGE) tool only detects alcohol dependence rather than the full range of unhealthy alcohol use. The American Society of Addiction Medicine defines unhealthy alcohol use as follows: "Unhealthy alcohol … use is any use that increases the risk or likelihood for health consequences (hazardous use) or has already led to health consequences (harmful use). Unhealthy use is an umbrella term that encompasses all levels of use relevant to health, from at-risk use through addiction" (Saitz et al., 2021, p3).
Adults aged 15 to 65 years	Human Immunodeficiency Virus (HIV) Infection: Screening Grade A June 2019 https://www.uspreventiveservicestaskforce.org/uspstf/recommendation/human-immunodeficiency-virus-hiv-infection-screening	HIV-1/2 antigen/antibody immunoassay Reactive tests should be followed by HIV-1/HIV-2 antibody differentiation immunoassay. For more information, see the Centers for Disease Control and Prevention (CDC) 2018 Quick reference guide: "Recommended Laboratory HIV Testing Algorithm for Serum or Plasma Specimens" (https://stacks.cdc.gov/view/cdc/50872). Interval: Optimal interval unknown. Consider risk. The CDC recommends annual screening in persons at increased risk (DiNenno, 2017).	Younger adolescents and older adults who are at increased risk of infection, especially those with new sex partners, should also be screened.

Adults aged 18–79 years	Hepatitis C Virus (HCV) Infection in Adolescents and Adults: Screening Grade B March 2020 https://www.uspreventiveservicestaskforce.org/uspstf/recommendation/hepatitis-c-screening	Anti–HCV antibody test Reactive tests should be followed by a confirmatory polymerase chain reaction (PCR) test for HCV RNA. Interval: Screen one time for most people. For those at ongoing increased risk of HCV, such as persons who inject drugs, consider periodic screening.	The USPSTF also suggests that clinicians consider screening persons younger than 18 years and older than 79 years who are at high risk for infection (e.g., those with past or current injection drug use).
Women of reproductive age Transgender people: See Comments	Intimate Partner Violence: Screening Grade B October 2018 https://www.uspreventiveservicestaskforce.org/uspstf/recommendation/intimate-partner-violence-and-abuse-of-elderly-and-vulnerable-adults-screening	Screening tool options: ■ Humiliation, Afraid, Rape, Kick (HARK) ■ Hurt/Insult/Threaten/Scream (HITS) ■ Extended Hurt/Insult/Threaten/Scream (E-HITS) ■ Partner Violence Screen (PVS) ■ Woman Abuse Screening Tool (WAST) Provide or refer those who screen positive to ongoing support services. Interval: Optimal interval unknown	For older and vulnerable adults, women not of reproductive age, and men, the USPSTF found that current evidence is insufficient to assess the balance of benefits and harms of screening. A 2021 study completed after the latest USPSTF evidence review found universal intimate partner violence (IPV) screening among transgender clients in a trans-competent primary care clinic to be effective in facilitating referral and engagement in IPV-related services (Das et al., 2021).
Adults with a cervix aged 21 to 65 years	Cervical Cancer: Screening Grade A August 2018 Update in Progress https://www.uspreventiveservicestaskforce.org/uspstf/recommendation/cervical-cancer-screening	21–29 years: cervical cytology every 3 years 30–65 years: choose one of the following options: ■ Cervical cytology (Pap) every 3 years ■ High-risk human papillomavirus (hrHPV) every 5 years ■ hrHPV testing in combination with cytology (cotesting) every 5 years	See the "Clinical Considerations" section for the relative benefits and harms of alternative screening strategies for people 21 years or older. For guidance on cervical cancer screening with transgender people, see sections titled "General approach to cancer screening in transgender people" and "Screening for cervical cancer in transgender men" by in *Guidelines for the Primary and Gender Affirming Care of Transgender and Gender Nonbinary People* (Deutsch, 2016).

(continues)

Table 38-1 U.S. Preventive Services Task Force (USPSTF) Grade A and B Age-Based Recommendations for Screening and Interventions *(continued)*

Target Population	USPSTF Topic and Date of Latest Recommendation	Intervention	Comments
Women aged 50–74 years Transgender people: See Comments	Breast Cancer: Screening Grade B January 2016 Update in progress* https://www.uspreventiveservicestaskforce.org/uspstf/recommendation/breast-cancer-screening	Screening mammography Interval: Every 2 years	For guidance on breast cancer screening for transgender people, see sections titled "General approach to cancer screening in transgender people," "Screening for breast cancer in transgender women," and "Breast cancer screening in transgender men" in the *Guidelines for the Primary and Gender Affirming Care of Transgender and Gender Nonbinary People* (Deutsch, 2016). For those over age 75 who have a life expectancy of 10 years or more, it is reasonable to consider breast cancer screening while incorporating the patient's values and preferences, along with overall health and function (Kotwal & Walter, 2020). There are many different professional guidelines for breast cancer screening. See the CDC table "Breast Cancer Screening Guidelines for Women" (https://www.cdc.gov/cancer/breast/pdf/breast-cancer-screening-guidelines-508.pdf).

*Update in progress as of November 14, 2023
Data from Source of information is USPSTF Recommendations unless otherwise noted.

Das, K. J. H., Peitzmeier, S., Berrahou, I. K., & Potter, J. (2021). Intimate Partner Violence (IPV) Screening and Referral Outcomes among Transgender Patients in a Primary Care Setting. *Journal of Interpersonal Violence*, 08862605211997460. https://doi.org/10.1177/08862605211997460
Deutsch, M. B. [Ed.]. (2016). Guidelines for the primary and gender affirming care of transgender and gender nonbinary people. UCSF Center of Excellence for Transgender Health. https://transcare.ucsf.edu/guidelines.
DiNenno, E. A. (2017). Recommendations for HIV Screening of Gay, Bisexual, and Other Men Who Have Sex with Men—United States, 2017. *Morbidity and Mortality Weekly Report*, 66. https://doi.org/10.15585/mmwr.mm6631a3

Table 38-2 U.S. Preventive Services Task Force (USPSTF) Grade A and B Characteristic-Based Recommendations for Screening and Interventions

Target Population	USPSTF Topic and Date of Latest Recommendation	Intervention	Comments
Adolescents and adults at increased risk for hepatitis B virus (HBV) infection Groups with an HBV prevalence of ≥2% that should be screened include: ■ Persons born in countries and regions with a high prevalence of HBV infection (≥2%), such as Asia, Africa, the Pacific Islands, and parts of South America ■ U.S.-born persons not vaccinated as infants whose parents were born in regions with a very high prevalence of HBV infection (≥8%) ■ HIV-positive persons ■ Persons with injection drug use ■ Men who have sex with men ■ Household contacts or sexual partners of persons with HBV infection For more information on countries and regions with a high prevalence of HBV infection, visit https://wwwnc.cdc.gov/travel/yellowbook/2020/travel-related-infectious-diseases/hepatitis-b#5182.	Hepatitis B Virus (HBV) Infection in Adolescents and Adults: Screening Grade B December 2020 https://www.uspreventiveservicestaskforce.org/uspstf/recommendation/hepatitis-b-virus-infection-screening	Hepatitis B surface antigen (HbsAg) test Reactive tests should be followed by confirmatory test (usually automatically done by the lab). Interval: Use clinical judgment	For more detailed guidance on HBV screening and follow-up in specific circumstances, see the Centers for Disease Control and Prevention (CDC) web page titled "Recommendations for Routine Testing and Follow-up for Chronic Hepatitis B Virus (HBV) Infection" (https://www.cdc.gov/hepatitis/hbv/HBV-RoutineTesting-Followup.htm). In many circumstances, it makes sense to simultaneously test for hepatitis B surface antigen (HBsAg) and total hepatitis B core antibody (anti-HBc) or hepatitis B surface antibody (anti-HBs). Confirmatory testing following a positive HbsAg is often done automatically by the lab as a "reflex."
Adults at increased risk for latent tuberculosis infection (LTBI) Risk assessment—groups with increased risk for tuberculosis (TB) infection: ■ Persons who live in, or have lived in, high-risk congregate settings (e.g., homeless shelters and correctional facilities) ■ Persons who were born in, or are former residents of, countries with increased TB prevalence. Per the CDC (2016), this includes most countries in Latin America, the Caribbean, Africa, Asia, Eastern Europe, and Russia. Local demographic patterns may vary across the United States. Consult local or state health departments for more information about local populations at risk.	LTBI: Screening Grade B May 2023 https://www.uspreventiveservicestaskforce.org/uspstf/recommendation/latent-tuberculosis-infection-screening	Screening tests: ■ Tuberculin skin test (Mantoux test) ■ Interferon-gamma release assay (IGRA) blood test Choose based on setting, cost, availability Interval: Optimal interval unknown	

(continues)

Table 38-2 U.S. Preventive Services Task Force (USPSTF) Grade A and B Characteristic-Based Recommendations for Screening and Interventions *(continued)*

Target Population	USPSTF Topic and Date of Latest Recommendation	Intervention	Comments
Adults with cardiovascular disease (CVD) risk factors: ■ Hypertension ■ Dyslipidemia ■ Combination of risk factors, such as metabolic syndrome or an estimated 10-year CVD risk of 7.5% or greater (calculate with fasting or nonfasting total cholesterol and high-density lipoprotein [HDL] lab tests and American College of Cardiology [ACC]/American Heart Association [AHA] pooled cohort equations: https://tools.acc.org/ascvd-risk-estimator-plus/)	Healthy Diet and Physical Activity for CVD Prevention: Behavioral Counseling Interventions Grade B November 2020 https://www.uspreventiveservicestaskforce.org/uspstf/recommendation/healthy-diet-and-physical-activity-counseling-adults-with-high-risk-of-cvd	Behavioral counseling interventions reviewed by the USPSTF combine counseling on a healthy diet with counseling on physical activity and are intensive, with multiple individual and/or group counseling sessions over 6–18 months. Interval: Not specified	Most interventions reviewed by the USPSTF were performed in the primary care setting but were delivered by nonclinicians, including nurses, registered dietitians, nutritionists, exercise specialists, physical therapists, masters- and doctoral-level counselors trained in behavioral methods, and lifestyle coaches. See the USPSTF Recommendation section "Practice Considerations" and Table 2 for more info. For guidance in calculating CVD risk with transgender people, see the section titled "Cardiovascular disease" in *Guidelines for the Primary and Gender Affirming Care of Transgender and Gender Nonbinary People* (Deutsch, 2016). There are other CVD risk calculators better suited to non-U.S. populations. For a discussion about the use of race in pooled cohort equations and over- and underprediction in some communities, see the USPSTF 2022 draft recommendation "Statin Use for the Primary Prevention of Cardiovascular Disease in Adults" (https://www.uspreventiveservicestaskforce.org/uspstf/draft-recommendation/statin-use-primary-prevention-cardiovascular-disease-adults).

Adults, including pregnant people, who have screened positive for unhealthy alcohol use	Unhealthy Alcohol Use in Adolescents and Adults: Behavioral Counseling Interventions Grade B November 2018 https://www.uspreventiveservicestaskforce.org/uspstf/recommendation/unhealthy-alcohol-use-in-adolescents-and-adults-screening-and-behavioral-counseling-interventions	Various interventions were evaluated by the USPSTF. See USPSTF Recommendation section "Clinical Considerations" on USPSTF website for more information. The Screening, Brief Intervention, and Referral to Treatment (SBIRT) approach may be used in primary care settings.	For more information on SBIRT, see the U.S. Department of Health and Human Services Substance Abuse and Mental Health Services Administration web page at https://www.samhsa.gov/sbirt.
Women 24 years or younger who are sexually active Women 25 years or older who are at increased risk for infection Transgender people: See Comments Circumstances that may increase risk include but are not limited to: - New sex partner - More than 1 sex partner - Sex partner with concurrent partners - Sex partner who has an sexually transmitted infection (STI) - Inconsistent condom use when not in a mutually monogamous relationship - Previous or coexisting STI - Exchanging sex for money or drugs - History of incarceration. There is local variation in risk. Consider contacting local public health authorities for information about local epidemiology.	Chlamydia and Gonorrhea: Screening Grade B September 2021 https://www.uspreventiveservicestaskforce.org/uspstf/recommendation/chlamydia-and-gonorrhea-screening	Nucleic acid amplification tests (NAATs) for *Chlamydia trachomatis* and *Neisseria gonorrhoeae* (CT/GC) Urine, pharyngeal, or rectal sample depending on reported sexual behaviors and exposure Interval: Optimal interval unknown. A reasonable approach is to screen patients whose sexual history reveals new or persistent risk factors since the last negative test result.	For guidance on STI screening, including chlamydia and gonorrhea, for transgender people, see section titled "Transgender people and STIs" in *Guidelines for the Primary and Gender Affirming Care of Transgender and Gender Nonbinary People* (Deutsch, 2016). See the CDC's "Sexually Transmitted Infections Treatment Guidelines, 2021" (https://www.cdc.gov/std/treatment-guidelines/toc.html) for more detail and other guidance on STI screening strategies. The CDC recommends routine chlamydia and gonorrhea screening for men who have sex with men (see https://www.cdc.gov/std/treatment-guidelines/screening-recommendations.html).

(continues)

Table 38-2 U.S. Preventive Services Task Force (USPSTF) Grade A and B Characteristic-Based Recommendations for Screening and Interventions *(continued)*

Target Population	USPSTF Topic and Date of Latest Recommendation	Intervention	Comments
Asymptomatic, nonpregnant adolescents and adults who are at increased risk for syphilis infection. When deciding which persons to screen for syphilis, consider the prevalence of syphilis infection in the local community. Other factors associated with increased prevalence of syphilis infection: ■ Male sex ■ Men who have sex with men ■ Living with HIV ■ Young adults ■ History of incarceration ■ History of sex work ■ History of military service Per the 2022 USPSTF recommendation, "Higher infection rates in persons of some racial and ethnic groups have been reported, but more likely reflect a combination of factors, including social determinants of health (e.g., disparities of income, low educational achievement, and unstable housing)" (see https://uspreventiveservicestaskforce.org/uspstf/recommendation/syphilis-infection-nonpregnant-adults-adolescents-screening.	Syphilis Infection in Nonpregnant Adolescents and Adults: Screening Grade A September 2022 https://uspreventive servicestaskforce.org/uspstf/recommendation/syphilis-infection-nonpregnant-adults-adolescents-screening	Traditional two-step screening algorithm: 1. Nontreponemal test (Venereal Disease Research Laboratory [VDRL] or rapid plasma reagin [RPR] test) 2. If the initial test is reactive, follow with a confirmatory treponemal antibody detection test *Treponema pallidum* particle agglutination [TPPA] test) (likely will be a reflex test at the lab). Use of a newer reverse-sequence algorithm may be dictated by local lab. This consists of an initial treponemal test followed by one or more confirmatory tests. Interval: Optimal screening frequency is not well established. Men who have sex with men or persons living with HIV may benefit from screening every 3–6 months.	Per the September 2022 USPSTF recommendation, sensitivity may be low for rapid point-of-care testing for antibodies to *T. pallidum*.

I. Introduction and general background   453

Sexually active adolescents and adults at increased risk Circumstances that increase an individual's risk of STI include but are not limited to: ■ Diagnosed with an STI within the past year ■ Not consistently using condoms ■ Multiple sex partners ■ Partner or partners at high risk for STIs ■ Sexual and gender minorities ■ Living with HIV ■ Injection drug use ■ Transactional sex (exchange sex for money, drugs, housing, etc.) ■ Recently having been in a correctional facility	STI: Behavioral Counseling Grade B August 2020 https://www.uspreventiveservicestaskforce.org/uspstf/recommendation/sexually-transmitted-infections-behavioral-counseling	Behavioral counseling intervention approaches include in-person counseling, videos, websites, written materials, telephone support, and text messages. See USPSTF Recommendation section "Clinical Considerations" on USPSTF website for many related resources.	Some interventions reviewed by the USPSTF were group and/or individual counseling delivered by researchers, facilitators, nursing professionals, counselors, health educators, trained peer counselors, or physicians. Others were media-based interventions without in-person counseling.
Women who have family members with or personal history of these types of cancer: ■ Breast ■ Ovarian ■ Tubal ■ Peritoneal Transgender people: Follow sex assigned at birth.	Breast cancer gene (BRCA)-Related Cancer: Risk Assessment, Genetic Counseling, and Genetic Testing Grade B August 2019 https://www.uspreventiveservicestaskforce.org/uspstf/recommendation/brca-related-cancer-risk-assessment-genetic-counseling-and-genetic-testing	Brief familial risk assessment tool, such as International Breast Cancer Intervention Study instrument (https://ibis.ikonopedia.com/). See USPSTF Recommendation section "Clinical Considerations" on USPSTF website for other validated tools. Positive result on the risk assessment tool should trigger referral to genetic counseling and, if indicated after counseling, genetic testing. Interval: Repeat if personal or family history of cancer changes.	Per the USPSTF, "the net benefit estimates are driven by biological sex (i.e., male/female) rather than gender identity. Persons should consider their sex at birth to determine which recommendation best applies to them" (see https://www.uspreventiveservicestaskforce.org/uspstf/recommendation/brca-related-cancer-risk-assessment-genetic-counseling-and-genetic-testing). For guidance on BRCA-related cancer risk assessment for transgender people, see section titled "Screening for breast cancer in transgender women" and "Breast cancer screening in transgender men" in *Guidelines for the Primary and Gender Affirming Care of Transgender and Gender Nonbinary People* (Deutsch, 2016).

(continues)

Table 38-2 U.S. Preventive Services Task Force (USPSTF) Grade A and B Characteristic-Based Recommendations for Screening and Interventions *(continued)*

Target Population	USPSTF Topic and Date of Latest Recommendation	Intervention	Comments
Young adults, adolescents, children, and parents of young children with fair skin types Because most trials of skin cancer counseling predominantly include persons with fair skin types, the USPSTF limited its recommendation to this population.	Skin Cancer Prevention: Behavioral Counseling Grade B March 2018 https://www.uspreventiveservicestaskforce.org/uspstf/recommendation/skin-cancer-counseling	Counseling about minimizing exposure to ultraviolet (UV) radiation for persons aged 6 months to 24 years with fair skin types to reduce their risk of skin cancer. Interventions reviewed by the USPSTF included tailored mailings, print materials, and in-person counseling by health professionals. See USPSTF Recommendation section "Clinical Considerations" on USPSTF website for more information.	Patient-oriented skin cancer prevention information from the CDC can be found at https://www.cdc.gov/cancer/skin/.
Adults aged 35 to 70 years who have a body mass index (BMI) ≥ 25 (calculated as weight in kilograms divided by height in meters squared) For Asian American people, consider screening at BMI ≥23 Consider screening at an earlier age for people with these circumstances: ■ From groups with disproportionately high incidence and prevalence of diabetes (American Indian/Alaska Native, Asian American, Black, Hispanic/Latino, or Native Hawaiian/Pacific Islander persons) ■ Family history of diabetes ■ Personal history of gestational diabetes or polycystic ovarian syndrome	Prediabetes and Type 2 Diabetes: Screening Grade B August 2021 https://www.uspreventiveservicestaskforce.org/uspstf/recommendation/screening-for-prediabetes-and-type-2-diabetes	Calculate BMI to establish need for further screening. Serum fasting plasma glucose, hemoglobin A1c level, or an oral glucose tolerance test Interval: Optimal interval unknown, but data suggests every 3 years is reasonable	Those with test results indicating prediabetes should be referred to or offered effective preventive interventions.

I. Introduction and general background 455

Adults aged 45–75 years who are at average risk of colon cancer Average risk: ■ No personal or family history of known genetic disorders that predispose one to a high lifetime risk of colorectal cancer, such as Lynch syndrome or familial adenomatous polyposis ■ No prior diagnosis of: • Colorectal cancer • Adenomatous polyps • Inflammatory bowel disease	Colorectal Cancer: Screening Grade A (50–75 years) Grade B (45–49 years) May 2021 https://www.uspreventiveservicestaskforce.org/uspstf/recommendation/colorectal-cancer-screening	Recommended screening strategies include: ■ High-sensitivity guaiac fecal occult blood test (HSgFOBT) or fecal immunochemical test (FIT) every year ■ Stool DNA-FIT every 1–3 years ■ Computed tomography colonography every 5 years ■ Flexible sigmoidoscopy every 5 years ■ Flexible sigmoidoscopy every 10 years + annual FIT ■ Colonoscopy screening every 10 years	For those over age 75 who have a life expectancy of 10 years or more, it is reasonable to consider colorectal cancer screening while incorporating the patient's values and preferences along with overall health and function (Kotwal & Walter, 2020).
Adults aged 50–80 years with: ■ 20 pack-year smoking history and ■ Currently smoke or have quit within the past 15 years	Lung Cancer Grade B March 2021 https://www.uspreventiveservicestaskforce.org/uspstf/recommendation/lung-cancer-screening	Low-dose computed tomography (LDCT) Interval: USPSTF recommends annual screening.	Screening should be discontinued once a person has not smoked for 15 years or develops a health problem that substantially limits life expectancy or the ability or aim to have curative lung surgery.

(continues)

Table 38-2 U.S. Preventive Services Task Force (USPSTF) Grade A and B Characteristic-Based Recommendations for Screening and Interventions *(continued)*

Target Population	USPSTF Topic and Date of Latest Recommendation	Intervention	Comments
- Women age 65 and older - Women younger than 65 who are postmenopausal and at increased risk of osteoporosis as determined by a formal clinical risk assessment tool, such as the Fracture Risk Assessment (FRAX) tool Risk factors include: - History of fracture - History of hip fracture in a parent - Smoking - Excessive alcohol consumption - Glucocorticoid use - Low body weight Transgender people: See Comments. The FRAX tool has been validated in more cohorts than other tools (Marques et al., 2015). A FRAX result of greater than 8.4% risk of major osteoporotic fracture over the next 10 years indicates increased risk (see https://www.sheffield.ac.uk/FRAX/).	Osteoporosis: Screening June 2018 Update in progress* https://www.uspreventiveservicestaskforce.org/uspstf/recommendation/osteoporosis-screening	Bone mineral density (BMD) testing (also called dual-energy x-ray absorptiometry [DEXA or DXA]) Interval: Optimal interval unknown	There are many different professional guidelines for osteoporosis screening. See USPSTF Recommendation section "Recommendations of Others" for more information (available at https://www.uspreventiveservicestaskforce.org/uspstf/recommendation/osteoporosis-screening). For guidance on osteoporosis screening for transgender people, see section titled "Bone health and osteoporosis" in Guidelines for the Primary and Gender Affirming Care of Transgender and Gender Nonbinary People (Deutsch, 2016). For a discussion of the use of race in the FRAX tool, see Vyas et al. (2020) and Lewiecki et al. (2020).
Adults 65 years or older who are at increased risk for falls Risk assessment: - History of falls - Limited mobility and impaired physical function - Standardized tools such as Timed Up and Go test	Falls Prevention in Community-Dwelling Older Adults: Interventions April 2018 https://www.uspreventiveservicestaskforce.org/uspstf/recommendation/falls-prevention-in-older-adults-interventions	Exercise interventions: Multiple options, including supervised individual and group classes, tai chi, physical therapy. Interval: Not specified	

	Abdominal Aortic Aneurysm: Screening December 2019 https://www.uspreventiveservicestaskforce.org/uspstf/recommendation/abdominal-aortic-aneurysm-screening	Abdominal duplex ultrasonography Interval: One time only	Per USPSTF, "the net benefit estimates are driven by biologic sex (i.e., male/female) rather than gender identity. Persons should consider their sex at birth to determine which recommendation best applies to them" (see https://www.uspreventiveservicestaskforce.org/uspstf/recommendation/abdominal-aortic-aneurysm-screening). Insufficient evidence to assess the balance of benefits and harms of screening for abdominal aortic aneurysm (AAA) in women aged 65–75 years who have ever smoked or have a family history of AAA.
Men aged 65 to 75 years who have ever smoked (100 or more cigarettes) Transgender people: Follow sex assigned at birth.			

*Update in progress as of November 14, 2023.

Data from Source of information is USPSTF Recommendations unless otherwise noted.

Deutsch, M. B. (Ed.). (2016). Guidelines for the primary and gender affirming care of transgender and gender nonbinary people. UCSF Center of Excellence for Transgender Health. https://transcare.ucsf.edu/guidelines.

Kotwal, A. A., & Walter, L. C. (2020). Cancer Screening Among Older Adults: A Geriatrician's Perspective on Breast, Cervical, Colon, Prostate, and Lung Cancer Screening. Current Oncology Reports, 22(11), 108. https://doi.org/10.1007/s11912-020-00968-x.

Lewiecki, E. M., Wright, N. C., & Singer, A. J. (2020). Racial disparities, FRAX, and the care of patients with osteoporosis. Osteoporosis International: A Journal Established as Result of Cooperation between the European Foundation for Osteoporosis and the National Osteoporosis Foundation of the USA, 31(11), 2069–2071. https://doi.org/10.1007/s00198-020-05655-y

Marques, A., Ferreira, R. J. O., Santos, E., Loza, E., Carmona, L., & da Silva, J. A. P. (2015). The accuracy of osteoporotic fracture risk prediction tools: A systematic review and meta-analysis. Annals of the Rheumatic Diseases, 74(11), 1958–1967. https://doi.org/10.1136/annrheumdis-2015-207907

Vyas, D. A., Eisenstein, L. G., & Jones, D. S. (2020). Hidden in Plain Sight—Reconsidering the Use of Race Correction in Clinical Algorithms. New England Journal of Medicine, 0(0), null. https://doi.org/10.1056/NEJMms2004740

Table 38-3 U.S. Preventive Services Task Force (USPSTF) Grade A and B Recommendations for Preventive Medications

Target Population	USPSTF Topic and Date of Latest Recommendation	Intervention	Comments
Women who are at increased risk for breast cancer and at low risk for adverse medication effects. Transgender people: See comments. Sample tool for risk assessment: National Cancer Institute (NCI) Breast Cancer Risk Assessment Tool (https://bcrisktool.cancer.gov/) Includes these characteristics: ■ Age ■ Age at the start of menstruation ■ Age at first live birth of a child ■ Number of first-degree relatives (mother, sisters, daughters) with breast cancer ■ Number of previous breast biopsies (whether positive or negative) ■ Presence of atypical hyperplasia in a biopsy	Breast Cancer Risk-Reducing Medication Grade B September 2019 https://www.uspreventiveservicestaskforce.org/uspstf/recommendation/breast-cancer-medications-for-risk-reduction	Offer to prescribe risk-reducing medications, such as tamoxifen, raloxifene, or aromatase inhibitors. See USPSTF Recommendation section "Clinical Considerations" on USPSTF website for information about assessing risk and balancing harms and benefits.	This recommendation does not apply to people who have a current or previous diagnosis of breast cancer or ductal carcinoma in situ (DCIS). In trials reviewed by the USPSTF, participants typically used risk-reducing medications for 3–5 years. For guidance on breast cancer screening for transgender people, see sections titled "General approach to cancer screening in transgender people," "Screening for breast cancer in transgender women," and "Breast cancer screening in transgender men" in *Guidelines for the Primary and Gender Affirming Care of Transgender and Gender Nonbinary people* (Deutsch, 2016).
People who are planning or capable of pregnancy who are at average risk of pregnancy affected by neural tube defects Characteristics indicating average risk: ■ Not affected previously by neural tube defects ■ No family history of neural tube defects ■ Not on high-risk medication, including antiseizure medications and some others	Folic Acid for the Prevention of Neural Tube Defects Grade A January 2017 Update in progress* https://www.uspreventiveservicestaskforce.org/uspstf/recommendation/folic-acid-for-the-prevention-of-neural-tube-defects-preventive-medication	Recommend daily supplement containing 0.4–0.8 mg (400–800 μg) of folic acid	This guideline does not apply to those at high risk of a pregnancy affected by neural tube defects (affected previously; family history; high-risk medication use, including antiseizure medications and some others). Those at high risk should be taking significantly higher doses of folic acid than those at average risk. This dose of folic acid can be found in commonly available multivitamins.

I. Introduction and general background

Population	Recommendation	Details	Notes
People at high risk of HIV acquisition Circumstances that increase an individual's risk of HIV include but are not limited to: - Having a partner or partners with HIV - Not consistently using condoms - Shared injection drug equipment - Transactional sex (exchange sex for money, drugs, housing, etc.) See USPSTF Recommendation section "Clinical Considerations" on USPSTF website for more detailed risk information.	Preexposure Prophylaxis (PrEP) for Prevention of HIV Infection Grade A June 2019 Update in progress* https://www.uspreventiveservicestaskforce.org/uspstf/recommendation/prevention-of-human-immunodeficiency-virus-hiv-infection-pre-exposure-prophylaxis	Centers for Disease Control and Prevention (CDC) 2021 PrEP Guidelines: - Emtricitabine (F) 200 mg in combination with tenofovir disoproxil fumarate (TDF) 300 mg (F/TDF; brand name, Truvada®) - For sexually active men and transgender women, consider emtricitabine (F) 200 mg in combination with tenofovir alafenamide (TAF) 25 mg (F/TAF; brand name, Descovy®). For details on how to assess for and prescribe PrEP, see CDC (2021) guidelines.	The CDC's 2021 PrEP Guidelines recommend clinicians inform all sexually active adults and adolescents that PrEP can protect them from getting HIV and that providers should offer PrEP to anyone who asks for it.
Adults aged 40–75 years adults without a history of cardiovascular disease (CVD) who meet both of the following criteria: - At least one CVD risk factor (i.e., dyslipidemia, diabetes, hypertension, or smoking) - 10-year risk of a cardiovascular event of 10% or greater [calculate with the American College of Cardiology (ACC)/American Heart Association (AHA) pooled cohort equations (available at https://tools.acc.org/ascvd-risk-estimator-plus/)], which require fasting or nonfasting total cholesterol and high-density lipoprotein (HDL) lab tests.	Statin for Primary Prevention of CVD Grade B November 2016 Update in progress* Draft available in 2022 reaffirms 2016 recommendation. https://www.uspreventiveservicestaskforce.org/uspstf/recommendation/statin-use-in-adults-preventive-medication	For primary prevention, use a low- to moderate-dose statin. Example: simvastatin 10 mg, low dose; 20–40 mg, moderate dose	There are other CVD risk calculators better suited to non-U.S. populations For those over age 75, randomized controlled trial data are limited. Consider patient values and preferences as well as prognosis and time to benefit. For guidance in calculating CVD risk with transgender people, see the section titled "Cardiovascular disease" in Deutsch (2016). See USPSTF Recommendation section "Practice Considerations" on USPSTF website for a discussion of race in pooled cohort equations and over- and underprediction in some communities.

*Update in progress as of November 14, 2023.

Data from Source of information is USPSTF Recommendations unless otherwise noted.

Centers for Disease Control and Prevention. (2021). Preexposure Prophylaxis for the Prevention of HIV Infection in the United States – 2021 Update Clinical Practice Guideline. https://www.cdc.gov/hiv/pdf/risk/prep/cdc-hiv-prep-guidelines-2021.pdf

Recommended Adult Immunization Schedule for ages 19 years or older

UNITED STATES 2022

How to use the adult immunization schedule

1. Determine recommended vaccinations by age **(Table 1)**
2. Assess need for additional recommended vaccinations by medical condition or other indication **(Table 2)**
3. Review vaccine types, frequencies, intervals, and considerations for special situations **(Notes)**
4. Review contraindications and precautions for vaccine types **(Appendix)**

Vaccines in the Adult Immunization Schedule*

Vaccine	Abbreviation(s)	Trade name(s)
Haemophilus influenzae type b vaccine	Hib	ActHIB® Hiberix® PedvaxHIB®
Hepatitis A vaccine	HepA	Havrix® Vaqta®
Hepatitis A and hepatitis B vaccine	HepA-HepB	Twinrix®
Hepatitis B vaccine	HepB	Engerix-B® Recombivax HB® Heplisav-B®
Human papillomavirus vaccine	HPV	Gardasil 9®
Influenza vaccine (inactivated)	IIV4	Many brands
Influenza vaccine (live, attenuated)	LAIV4	FluMist® Quadrivalent
Influenza vaccine (recombinant)	RIV4	Flublok® Quadrivalent
Measles, mumps, and rubella vaccine	MMR	M-M-R II®
Meningococcal serogroups A, C, W, Y vaccine	MenACWY-D MenACWY-CRM MenACWY-TT	Menactra® Menveo® MenQuadfi®
Meningococcal serogroup B vaccine	MenB-4C MenB-FHbp	Bexsero® Trumenba®
Pneumococcal 15-valent conjugate vaccine	PCV15	Vaxneuvance™
Pneumococcal 20-valent conjugate vaccine	PCV20	Prevnar 20™
Pneumococcal 23-valent polysaccharide vaccine	PPSV23	Pneumovax 23®
Tetanus and diphtheria toxoids	Td	Tenivac® Tdvax™
Tetanus and diphtheria toxoids and acellular pertussis vaccine	Tdap	Adacel® Boostrix®
Varicella vaccine	VAR	Varivax®
Zoster vaccine, recombinant	RZV	Shingrix

*Administer recommended vaccines if vaccination history is incomplete or unknown. Do not restart or add doses to vaccine series if there are extended intervals between doses. The use of trade names is for identification purposes only and does not imply endorsement by the ACIP or CDC.

Recommended by the Advisory Committee on Immunization Practices (www.cdc.gov/vaccines/acip) and approved by the Centers for Disease Control and Prevention (www.cdc.gov), American College of Physicians (www.acponline.org), American Academy of Family Physicians (www.aafp.org), American College of Obstetricians and Gynecologists (www.acog.org), American College of Nurse-Midwives (www.midwife.org), and American Academy of Physician Associates (www.aapa.org), and Society for Healthcare Epidemiology of America (www.shea-online.org).

Report
- Suspected cases of reportable vaccine-preventable diseases or outbreaks to the local or state health department
- Clinically significant postvaccination reactions to the Vaccine Adverse Event Reporting System at www.vaers.hhs.gov or 800-822-7967

Injury claims
All vaccines included in the adult immunization schedule except pneumococcal 23-valent polysaccharide (PPSV23) and zoster (RZV) vaccines are covered by the Vaccine Injury Compensation Program. Information on how to file a vaccine injury claim is available at www.hrsa.gov/vaccinecompensation.

Questions or comments
Contact www.cdc.gov/cdc-info or 800-CDC-INFO (800-232-4636), in English or Spanish, 8 a.m.–8 p.m. ET, Monday through Friday, excluding holidays.

Download the CDC Vaccine Schedules app for providers at www.cdc.gov/vaccines/schedules/hcp/schedule-app.html.

Helpful information
- Complete Advisory Committee on Immunization Practices (ACIP) recommendations: www.cdc.gov/vaccines/hcp/acip-recs/index.html
- General Best Practice Guidelines for Immunization (including contraindications and precautions): www.cdc.gov/vaccines/hcp/acip-recs/general-recs/index.html
- Vaccine information statements: www.cdc.gov/vaccines/hcp/vis/index.html
- Manual for the Surveillance of Vaccine-Preventable Diseases (including case identification and outbreak response): www.cdc.gov/vaccines/pubs/surv-manual
- Travel vaccine recommendations: www.cdc.gov/travel
- Recommended Child and Adolescent Immunization Schedule, United States, 2022: www.cdc.gov/vaccines/schedules/hcp/child-adolescent.html
- ACIP Shared Clinical Decision-Making Recommendations: www.cdc.gov/vaccines/acip/acip-scdm-faqs.html

Scan QR code for access to online schedule

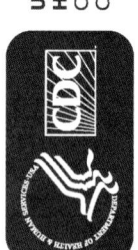

U.S. Department of
Health and Human Services
Centers for Disease
Control and Prevention

Figure 38-1 Centers for Disease Control and Prevention (CDC) Vaccine Schedule 2022

Table 1 Recommended Adult Immunization Schedule by Age Group, United States, 2022

Vaccine	19–26 years	27–49 years	50–64 years	≥65 years
Influenza inactivated (IIV4) or **Influenza recombinant** (RIV4)	1 dose annually	1 dose annually	1 dose annually	1 dose annually
Influenza live, attenuated (LAIV4)	1 dose annually	1 dose annually		
Tetanus, diphtheria, pertussis (Tdap or Td)	1 dose Tdap each pregnancy; 1 dose Td/Tdap for wound management (see notes) then Td or Tdap booster every 10 years			
Measles, mumps, rubella (MMR)	1 or 2 doses depending on indication (if born in 1957 or later)			
Varicella (VAR)	2 doses (if born in 1980 or later)		2 doses	2 doses
Zoster recombinant (RZV)	2 doses for immunocompromising conditions (see notes)		2 doses	2 doses
Human papillomavirus (HPV)	2 or 3 doses depending on age at initial vaccination or condition	27 through 45 years		
Pneumococcal (PCV15, PCV20, PPSV23)		1 dose PCV15 followed by PPSV23 OR 1 dose PCV20 (see notes)	1 dose PCV15 followed by PPSV23 OR 1 dose PCV20	1 dose PCV15 followed by PPSV23 OR 1 dose PCV20
Hepatitis A (HepA)	2 or 3 doses depending on vaccine			
Hepatitis B (HepB)	2, 3, or 4 doses depending on vaccine or condition			
Meningococcal A, C, W, Y (MenACWY)	1 or 2 doses depending on indication, see notes for booster recommendations			
Meningococcal B (MenB)	19 through 23 years	2 or 3 doses depending on vaccine and indication, see notes for booster recommendations		
Haemophilus influenzae type b (Hib)	1 or 3 doses depending on indication			

Legend:
- Recommended vaccination for adults who meet age requirement, lack documentation of vaccination, or lack evidence of past infection
- Recommended vaccination for adults with an additional risk factor or another indication
- Recommended vaccination based on shared clinical decision-making
- No recommendation/Not applicable

Figure 38-1 (Continued)

Table 2 Recommended Adult Immunization Schedule by Medical Condition or Other Indication, United States, 2022

Vaccine	Pregnancy	Immunocompromised (excluding HIV infection)	HIV infection CD4 percentage and count <15% or <200 mm³	HIV infection CD4 percentage and count ≥15% and ≥200 mm³	Asplenia, complement deficiencies	End-stage renal disease, or on hemodialysis¹	Heart or lung disease; alcoholism¹	Chronic liver disease	Diabetes	Health care personnel²	Men who have sex with men
IIV4 or RIV4	1 dose annually										
LAIV4	Contraindicated	Contraindicated	Contraindicated				Precaution			1 dose annually	
Tdap or Td	1 dose Tdap each pregnancy	1 dose Tdap, then Td or Tdap booster every 10 years									
MMR	Contraindicated*	Contraindicated	Contraindicated		1 or 2 doses depending on indication						
VAR	Contraindicated*	Contraindicated	Contraindicated		2 doses						
RZV			2 doses at age ≥19 years					2 doses at age ≥50 years			
HPV	Not Recommended*	3 doses through age 26 years			2 or 3 doses through age 26 years depending on age at initial vaccination or condition						
Pneumococcal (PCV15, PCV20, PPSV23)					1 dose PCV15 followed by PPSV23 OR 1 dose PCV20 (see notes)						
HepA					2 or 3 doses depending on vaccine or condition						
HepB	3 doses (see notes)				2, 3, or 4 doses depending on vaccine or condition						
MenACWY		1 or 2 doses depending on indication, see notes for booster recommendations									
MenB	Precaution				2 or 3 doses depending on vaccine and indication, see notes for booster recommendations						
Hib		3 doses HSCT³ recipients only			1 dose						

Legend:
- Recommended vaccination for adults who meet age requirement, lack documentation of vaccination, or lack evidence of past infection
- Recommended vaccination for adults with an additional risk factor or another indication
- Recommended vaccination based on shared clinical decision-making
- Precaution—vaccination might be indicated if benefit of protection outweighs risk of adverse reaction
- Contraindicated or not recommended—vaccine should not be administered. *Vaccinate after pregnancy.
- No recommendation/Not applicable

1. Precaution for LAIV4 does not apply to alcoholism. 2. See notes for influenza; hepatitis B; measles, mumps, and rubella; and varicella vaccinations. 3. Hematopoietic stem cell transplant.

Figure 38-1 (*Continued*)

Recommended Adult Immunization Schedule for ages 19 years or older, United States, 2022

Notes

For vaccine recommendations for persons 18 years of age or younger, see the Recommended Child and Adolescent Immunization Schedule.

COVID-19 Vaccination

COVID-19 vaccines are recommended within the scope of the Emergency Use Authorization or Biologics License Application for the particular vaccine. ACIP recommendations for the use of COVID-19 vaccines can be found at www.cdc.gov/vaccines/hcp/acip-recs/vacc-specific/covid-19.html.

CDC's interim clinical considerations for use of COVID-19 vaccines can be found at www.cdc.gov/vaccines/covid-19/clinical-considerations/covid-19-vaccines-us.html.

Haemophilus influenzae type b vaccination

Special situations

- **Anatomical or functional asplenia (including sickle cell disease):** 1 dose if previously did not receive Hib; if elective splenectomy, 1 dose, preferably at least 14 days before splenectomy
- **Hematopoietic stem cell transplant (HSCT):** 3-dose series 4 weeks apart starting 6–12 months after successful transplant, regardless of Hib vaccination history

Hepatitis A vaccination

Routine vaccination

- **Not at risk but want protection from hepatitis A** (identification of risk factor not required): 2-dose series HepA (Havrix 6–12 months apart or Vaqta 6–18 months apart [minimum interval: 6 months]) or 3-dose series HepA-HepB (Twinrix) at 0, 1, 6 months (minimum intervals: dose 1 to dose 2: 4 weeks / dose 2 to dose 3: 5 months)

Special situations

- **At risk for hepatitis A virus infection:** 2-dose series HepA or 3-dose series HepA-HepB as above
- **Chronic liver disease** (e.g., persons with hepatitis B, hepatitis C, cirrhosis, fatty liver disease, alcoholic liver disease, autoimmune hepatitis, alanine aminotransferase [ALT] or aspartate aminotransferase [AST] level greater than twice the upper limit of normal)
- **HIV infection**
- **Men who have sex with men**
- **Injection or noninjection drug use**
- **Persons experiencing homelessness**
- **Work with hepatitis A virus** in research laboratory or with nonhuman primates with hepatitis A virus infection
- **Travel in countries with high or intermediate endemic hepatitis A** (HepA-HepB [Twinrix] may be administered on an accelerated schedule of 3 doses at 0, 7, and 21–30 days, followed by a booster dose at 12 months)
- **Close, personal contact with international adoptee** (e.g., household or regular babysitting) in first 60 days after arrival from country with high or intermediate endemic hepatitis A (administer dose 1 as soon as adoption is planned, at least 2 weeks before adoptee's arrival)
- **Pregnancy** if at risk for infection or severe outcome from infection during pregnancy
- **Settings for exposure, including** health care settings targeting services to injection or noninjection drug users or group homes and nonresidential day care facilities for developmentally disabled persons (individual risk factor screening not required)

Hepatitis B vaccination

Routine vaccination

- **Age 19 through 59 years:** complete a 2- or 3-, or 4-dose series
- 2-dose series only applies when 2 doses of Heplisav-B* are used at least 4 weeks apart
- 3-dose series Engerix-B or Recombivax HB at 0, 1, 6 months [minimum intervals: dose 1 to dose 2: 4 weeks / dose 2 to dose 3: 8 weeks / dose 1 to dose 3: 16 weeks])
- 3-dose series HepA-HepB (Twinrix at 0, 1, 6 months [minimum intervals: dose 1 to dose 2: 4 weeks / dose 2 to dose 3: 5 months])
- 4-dose series HepA-HepB (Twinrix) accelerated schedule of 3 doses at 0, 7, and 21–30 days, followed by a booster dose at 12 months
- 4-dose series Engerix-B at 0, 1, 2, and 6 months for persons on adult hemodialysis (note: each dosage is double that of normal adult dose, i.e., 2 mL instead of 1 mL)

*Note: Heplisav-B not recommended in pregnancy due to lack of safety data in pregnant women

Special situations

- **Age 60 years or older* and at risk for hepatitis B virus infection:** 2-dose (Heplisav-B) or 3-dose (Engerix-B, Recombivax HB) series or 3-dose series HepA-HepB (Twinrix) as above
- **Chronic liver disease** (e.g., persons with hepatitis C, cirrhosis, fatty liver disease, alcoholic liver disease, autoimmune hepatitis, alanine aminotransferase [ALT] or aspartate aminotransferase [AST] level greater than twice upper limit of normal)
- **HIV infection**
- **Sexual exposure risk** (e.g., sex partners of hepatitis B surface antigen [HBsAg]-positive persons; sexually active persons not in mutually monogamous relationships; persons seeking evaluation or treatment for a sexually transmitted infection; men who have sex with men)
- **Current or recent injection drug use**
- **Percutaneous or mucosal risk for exposure to blood** (e.g., household contacts of HBsAg-positive persons; residents and staff of facilities for developmentally disabled persons; health care and public safety personnel with reasonably anticipated risk for exposure to blood or blood-contaminated body fluids; hemodialysis, peritoneal dialysis, home dialysis, and predialysis patients; patients with diabetes)
- **Incarcerated persons**
- **Travel in countries with high or intermediate endemic hepatitis B**

*Note: Anyone age 60 years or older who does not meet risk-based recommendations may still receive Hepatitis B vaccination.

Human papillomavirus vaccination

Routine vaccination

- HPV vaccination recommended for all persons through age 26 years: 2- or 3-dose series depending on age at initial vaccination or condition:
- **Age 15 years or older at initial vaccination:** 3-dose series at 0, 1–2 months, 6 months (minimum intervals: dose 1 to dose 2: 4 weeks / dose 2 to dose 3: 12 weeks / dose 1 to dose 3: 5 months; repeat dose if administered too soon)
- **Age 9–14 years at initial vaccination and received 1 dose or 2 doses less than 5 months apart:** 1 additional dose
- **Age 9–14 years at initial vaccination and received 2 doses at least 5 months apart:** HPV vaccination series complete, no additional dose needed

Figure 38-1 (Continued)

Notes

- **Interrupted schedules:** If vaccination schedule is interrupted, the series does not need to be restarted
- **No additional dose recommended when any HPV vaccine series has been completed using the recommended dosing intervals.**

Shared clinical decision-making
- Some adults age 27–45 years: Based on shared clinical decision-making, 2- or 3-dose series as above

Special situations
- Age ranges recommended above for routine and catch-up vaccination or shared clinical decision-making also apply in special situations
  - Immunocompromising conditions, including HIV infection: 3-dose series, even for those who initiate vaccination at age 9 through 14 years.
  - Pregnancy: Pregnancy testing is not needed before vaccination; HPV vaccination is not recommended until after pregnancy; no intervention needed if inadvertently vaccinated while pregnant

Influenza vaccination

Routine vaccination
- Age 19 years or older: 1 dose any influenza vaccine appropriate for age and health status annually
- For the 2021–2022 season, see www.cdc.gov/mmwr/volumes/70/rr/rr7005a1.htm
- For the 2022–23 season, see the 2022–23 ACIP influenza vaccine recommendations.

Special situations
- **Egg allergy, hives only:** any influenza vaccine appropriate for age and health status annually
- **Egg allergy–any symptom other than hives** (e.g., angioedema, respiratory distress) or required epinephrine or another emergency medical intervention: see Appendix listing contraindications and precautions
- **Severe allergic reaction (e.g., anaphylaxis) to a vaccine component or a previous dose of any influenza vaccine:** see Appendix listing contraindications and precautions
- **History of Guillain-Barré syndrome within 6 weeks after previous dose of influenza vaccine:** Generally, should not be vaccinated unless vaccination benefits outweigh risks for those at higher risk for severe complications from influenza

Recommended Adult Immunization Schedule, United States, 2022

Measles, mumps, and rubella vaccination

Routine vaccination
- No evidence of immunity to measles, mumps, or rubella: 1 dose
  - **Evidence of immunity:** Born before 1957 (health care personnel, see below), documentation of receipt of MMR vaccine, laboratory evidence of immunity or disease (diagnosis of disease without laboratory confirmation is not evidence of immunity)

Special situations
- **Pregnancy with no evidence of immunity to rubella:** MMR contraindicated during pregnancy; after pregnancy (before discharge from health care facility), 1 dose
- **Nonpregnant women of childbearing age with no evidence of immunity to rubella:** 1 dose
- **HIV infection with CD4 percentages ≥15% and CD4 count ≥200 cells/mm³ for at least 6 months and no evidence of immunity to measles, mumps, or rubella:** 2-dose series at least 4 weeks apart; MMR contraindicated for HIV infection with CD4 percentage <15% or CD4 count <200 cells/mm³
- **Severe immunocompromising conditions:** MMR contraindicated
- **Students in postsecondary educational institutions, international travelers, and household or close, personal contacts of immunocompromised persons with no evidence of immunity to measles, mumps, or rubella:** 2-dose series at least 4 weeks apart if previously did not receive any doses of MMR or 1 dose if previously received 1 dose MMR
- **Health care personnel:**
  - **Born before 1957 with no evidence of immunity to measles, mumps, or rubella:** Consider 2-dose series at least 4 weeks apart for measles or mumps or 1 dose for rubella
  - **Born in 1957 or later with no evidence of immunity to measles, mumps, or rubella:** 2-dose series at least 4 weeks apart for measles or mumps or at least 1 dose for rubella

Meningococcal vaccination

Special situations for MenACWY
- **Anatomical or functional asplenia (including sickle cell disease), HIV infection, persistent complement component deficiency, complement inhibitor (e.g., eculizumab, ravulizumab) use:** 2-dose series MenACWY-D (Menactra, Menveo, or MenQuadfi) at least 8 weeks apart and revaccinate every 5 years if risk remains
- **Travel in countries with hyperendemic or epidemic meningococcal disease, or microbiologists routinely exposed to Neisseria meningitidis:** 1 dose MenACWY (Menactra, Menveo, or MenQuadfi) and revaccinate every 5 years if risk remains
- **First-year college students who live in residential housing (if not previously vaccinated at age 16 years or older) or military recruits:** 1 dose MenACWY (Menactra, Menveo, or MenQuadfi)
- For MenACWY booster dose recommendations for groups listed under "special situations" and in an outbreak setting (e.g., in community or organizational settings and among men who have sex with men) and additional meningococcal vaccination information, see www.cdc.gov/mmwr/volumes/69/rr/rr6909a1.htm

Shared clinical decision-making for MenB
- **Adolescents and young adults age 16–23 years (age 16–18 years preferred) not at increased risk for meningococcal disease:** Based on shared clinical decision-making, 2-dose series MenB-4C (Bexsero) at least 1 month apart or 2-dose series MenB-FHbp (Trumenba) at 0, 6 months (if dose 2 was administered less than 6 months after dose 1, administer dose 3 at least 4 months after dose 2); MenB-4C and MenB-FHbp are not interchangeable (use same product for all doses in series)

Special situations for MenB
- **Anatomical or functional asplenia (including sickle cell disease), persistent complement component deficiency, complement inhibitor (e.g., eculizumab, ravulizumab) use, or microbiologists routinely exposed to Neisseria meningitidis:**
  2-dose primary series MenB-4C (Bexsero) at least 1 month apart or 3-dose primary series MenB-FHbp (Trumenba) at 0, 1–2, 6 months (if dose 2 was administered at least 6 months after dose 1, dose 3 not needed); MenB-4C and MenB-FHbp are not interchangeable (use same product for all doses in series); 1 dose MenB booster 1 year after primary series and revaccinate every 2–3 years if risk remains

Figure 38-1 (Continued)

Notes — Recommended Adult Immunization Schedule, United States, 2022

- **Pregnancy:** Delay MenB until after pregnancy unless at increased risk and vaccination benefits outweigh potential risks
- **For MenB booster dose recommendations** for groups listed under "Special situations" and in an outbreak setting (e.g., in community or organizational settings and among men who have sex with men) and additional meningococcal vaccination information, see www.cdc.gov/mmwr/volumes/69/rr/rr6909a1.htm

Note: MenB vaccines may be administered simultaneously with MenACWY vaccines if indicated, but at a different anatomic site, if feasible.

Pneumococcal vaccination

Routine vaccination

- **Age 65 years or older** who have not previously received a pneumococcal conjugate vaccine or whose previous vaccination history is unknown: 1 dose PCV15 or 1 dose PCV20. If PCV15 is used, this should be followed by a dose of PPSV23 given at least 1 year after the PCV15 dose. A minimum interval of 8 weeks between PCV15 and PPSV23 can be considered for adults with an immunocompromising condition,* cochlear implant, or cerebrospinal fluid leak to minimize the risk of invasive pneumococcal disease caused by serotypes unique to PPSV23 in these vulnerable groups.
- For guidance for patients who have already received a previous dose of PCV13 and/or PPSV23, see www.cdc.gov/mmwr/volumes/71/wr/mm7104a1.htm.

Special situations

- **Age 19–64 years** with certain underlying medical conditions or other risk factors** who have not previously received a pneumococcal conjugate vaccine or whose previous vaccination history is unknown: 1 dose PCV15 or 1 dose PCV20. If PCV15 is used, this should be followed by a dose of PPSV23 given at least 1 year after the PCV15 dose. A minimum interval of 8 weeks between PCV15 and PPSV23 can be considered for adults with an immunocompromising condition,* cochlear implant, or cerebrospinal fluid leak to minimize the risk of invasive pneumococcal disease caused by serotypes unique to PPSV23 in these vulnerable groups.
- For guidance for patients who have already received a previous dose of PCV13 and/or PPSV23, see www.cdc.gov/mmwr/volumes/71/wr/mm7104a1.htm.

*__Note:__ Immunocompromising conditions include chronic renal failure, nephrotic syndrome, immunodeficiency, iatrogenic immunosuppression, generalized malignancy, human immunodeficiency virus, Hodgkin disease, leukemia, lymphoma, multiple myeloma, solid organ transplants, congenital or acquired asplenia, sickle cell disease, or other hemoglobinopathies.

**__Note:__ Underlying medical conditions or other risk factors include alcoholism, chronic heart/liver/lung disease, chronic renal failure, cigarette smoking, cochlear implant, congenital or acquired asplenia, CSF leak, diabetes mellitus, generalized malignancy, HIV, Hodgkin disease, immunodeficiency, iatrogenic immunosuppression, leukemia, lymphoma, multiple myeloma, nephrotic syndrome, solid organ transplants, or sickle cell disease or other hemoglobinopathies.

Tetanus, diphtheria, and pertussis vaccination

Routine vaccination

- **Previously did not receive Tdap at or after age 11 years:** 1 dose Tdap, then Td or Tdap every 10 years

Special situations

- **Previously did not receive primary vaccination series for tetanus, diphtheria, or pertussis:** 1 dose Tdap followed by 1 dose Td or Tdap at least 4 weeks after Tdap and another dose Td or Tdap 6–12 months after last Td or Tdap (Tdap can be substituted for any Td dose, but preferred as first dose), Td or Tdap every 10 years thereafter
- **Pregnancy:** 1 dose Tdap during each pregnancy, preferably in early part of gestational weeks 27–36
- **Wound management:** Persons with 3 or more doses of tetanus-toxoid-containing vaccine: For clean and minor wounds, administer Tdap or Td if more than 10 years since last dose of tetanus-toxoid-containing vaccine; for all other wounds, administer Tdap or Td if more than 5 years since last dose of tetanus-toxoid-containing vaccine. Tdap is preferred for persons who have not previously received Tdap or whose Tdap history is unknown. If a tetanus-toxoid-containing vaccine is indicated for a pregnant woman, use Tdap. For detailed information, see www.cdc.gov/mmwr/volumes/69/wr/mm6903a5.htm

Varicella vaccination

Routine vaccination

- **No evidence of immunity to varicella:** 2-dose series 4–8 weeks apart if previously did not receive varicella-containing vaccine (VAR or MMRV [measles-mumps-rubella-varicella vaccine] for children); if previously received 1 dose varicella-containing vaccine, 1 dose at least 4 weeks after first dose
- Evidence of immunity: U.S.-born before 1980 (except for pregnant women and health care personnel [see below]), documentation of 2 doses varicella-containing vaccine at least 4 weeks apart, diagnosis or verification of history of varicella or herpes zoster by a health care provider, laboratory evidence of immunity or disease

Special situations

- **Pregnancy with no evidence of immunity to varicella:** VAR contraindicated during pregnancy; after pregnancy (before discharge from health care facility), 1 dose if previously received 1 dose varicella-containing vaccine or dose 1 of 2-dose series (dose 2: 4–8 weeks later) if previously did not receive any varicella-containing vaccine, regardless of whether U.S.-born before 1980
- **Health care personnel with no evidence of immunity to varicella:** 1 dose if previously received 1 dose varicella-containing vaccine; 2-dose series 4–8 weeks apart if previously did not receive any varicella-containing vaccine, regardless of whether U.S.-born before 1980
- **HIV infection with CD4 percentages ≥15% and CD4 count ≥200 cells/mm^3 with no evidence of immunity:** Vaccination may be considered (2 doses 3 months apart); VAR contraindicated for HIV infection with CD4 percentage <15% or CD4 count <200 cells/mm^3
- **Severe immunocompromising conditions:** VAR contraindicated

Zoster vaccination

Routine vaccination

- **Age 50 years or older:** 2-dose series RZV (Shingrix) 2–6 months apart (minimum interval: 4 weeks; repeat dose if administered too soon), regardless of previous herpes zoster or history of zoster vaccine live (ZVL, Zostavax) vaccination (administer RZV at least 2 months after ZVL)

Special situations

- **Pregnancy:** There is currently no ACIP recommendation for RZV use in pregnancy. Consider delaying RZV until after pregnancy.
- **Immunocompromising conditions (including HIV):** RZV recommended for use in persons age 19 years or older who are or will be immunodeficient or immunosuppressed because of disease or therapy. For detailed information, see www.cdc.gov/mmwr/volumes/71/wr/mm7103a2.htm.

Figure 38-1 (*Continued*)

Appendix: Recommended Adult Immunization Schedule, United States, 2022

Guide to Contraindications and Precautions to Commonly Used Vaccines

Adapted from Table 4-1 in Advisory Committee on Immunization Practices (ACIP) General Best Practice Guidelines for Immunization: Contraindication and Precautions available at www.cdc.gov/vaccines/hcp/acip-recs/general-recs/contraindications.html and ACIP's Recommendations for the Prevention and Control of 2021-22 Seasonal Influenza with Vaccines available at www.cdc.gov/mmwr/volumes/70/rr/rr7005a1.htm

Interim clinical considerations for use of COVID-19 vaccines including contraindications and precautions can be found at www.cdc.gov/vaccines/covid-19/clinical-considerations/covid-19-vaccines-us.html

Vaccine	Contraindications[1]	Precautions[2]
Influenza, egg-based, inactivated injectable (IIV4)	• Severe allergic reaction (e.g., anaphylaxis) after previous dose of any influenza vaccine (i.e., any egg-based IIV, ccIIV, RIV, or LAIV of any valency) • Severe allergic reaction (e.g., anaphylaxis) to any vaccine component[3] (excluding egg)	• Guillain-Barré syndrome (GBS) within 6 weeks after a previous dose of any type of influenza vaccine • Persons with egg allergy with symptoms other than hives (e.g., angioedema, respiratory distress) or required epinephrine or another emergency medical intervention: Any influenza vaccine appropriate for age and health status may be administered. If using egg-based IIV4, administer in medical setting under supervision of health care provider who can recognize and manage severe allergic reactions. May consult an allergist. • Moderate or severe acute illness with or without fever
Influenza, cell culture-based inactivated injectable [(ccIIV4), Flucelvax® Quadrivalent]	• Severe allergic reaction (e.g., anaphylaxis) to any ccIIV of any valency, or to any component[3] of ccIIV4	• Guillain-Barré syndrome (GBS) within 6 weeks after a previous dose of any type of influenza vaccine • Persons with a history of severe allergic reaction (e.g., anaphylaxis) after a previous dose of any egg-based IIV, RIV, or LAIV of any valency. If using ccIIV4, administer in medical setting under supervision of health care provider who can recognize and manage severe allergic reactions. May consult an allergist. • Moderate or severe acute illness with or without fever
Influenza, recombinant injectable [(RIV4), Flublok® Quadrivalent]	• Severe allergic reaction (e.g., anaphylaxis) to any RIV of any valency, or to any component[3] of RIV4	• Guillain-Barré syndrome (GBS) within 6 weeks after a previous dose of any type of influenza vaccine • Persons with a history of severe allergic reaction (e.g., anaphylaxis) after a previous dose of any egg-based IIV, ccIIV, or LAIV of any valency. If using RIV4, administer in medical setting under supervision of health care provider who can recognize and manage severe allergic reactions. May consult an allergist. • Moderate or severe acute illness with or without fever
Influenza, live attenuated [LAIV4, Flumist® Quadrivalent]	• Severe allergic reaction (e.g., anaphylaxis) after previous dose of any influenza vaccine (i.e., any egg-based IIV, ccIIV, RIV, or LAIV of any valency) • Severe allergic reaction (e.g., anaphylaxis) to any vaccine component[3] (excluding egg) • Adults age 50 years or older • Anatomic or functional asplenia • Immunocompromised due to any cause including, but not limited to, medications and HIV infection • Close contacts or caregivers of severely immunosuppressed persons who require a protected environment • Pregnancy • Cochlear implant • Active communication between the cerebrospinal fluid (CSF) and the oropharynx, nasopharynx, nose, ear, or any other cranial CSF leak • Received influenza antiviral medications oseltamivir or zanamivir within the previous 48 hours, peramivir within the previous 5 days, or baloxavir within the previous 17 days.	• Guillain-Barré syndrome (GBS) within 6 weeks after a previous dose of any type of influenza vaccine • Asthma in persons aged 5 years old or older • Persons with egg allergy with symptoms other than hives (e.g., angioedema, respiratory distress) or required epinephrine or another emergency medical intervention: Any Influenza vaccine appropriate for age and health status may be administered. If using LAIV4 (which is egg based), administer in medical setting under supervision of health care provider who can recognize and manage severe allergic reactions. May consult an allergist. • Persons with underlying medical conditions (other than those listed under contraindications) that might predispose to complications after wild-type influenza virus infection (e.g., chronic pulmonary, cardiovascular (except isolated hypertension), renal, hepatic, neurologic, hematologic, or metabolic disorders (including diabetes mellitus)] • Moderate or severe acute illness with or without fever

1. When a contraindication is present, a vaccine should NOT be administered. Kroger A, Bahta L, Hunter P. ACIP General Best Practice Guidelines for Immunization. www.cdc.gov/vaccines/hcp/acip-recs/general-recs/contraindications.html
2. When a precaution is present, vaccination should generally be deferred but might be indicated if the benefit of protection from the vaccine outweighs the risk for an adverse reaction. Kroger A, Bahta L, Hunter P. ACIP General Best Practice Guidelines for Immunization. www.cdc.gov/vaccines/hcp/acip-recs/general-recs/contraindications.html
3. Vaccination providers should check FDA-approved prescribing information for the most complete and updated information, including contraindications, warnings, and precautions. Package inserts for U.S.-licensed vaccines are available at www.fda.gov/vaccines-blood-biologics/approved-products/vaccines-licensed-use-united-states.

Figure 38-1 (Continued)

Appendix

Recommended Adult Immunization Schedule, United States, 2022

Vaccine	Contraindications[1]	Precautions[2]
Haemophilus influenzae type b (Hib)	• Severe allergic reaction (e.g., anaphylaxis) after a previous dose or to a vaccine component[3] • For Hiberix, ActHIB, and PedvaxHIB only: History of severe allergic reaction to dry natural latex	• Moderate or severe acute illness with or without fever
Hepatitis A (HepA)	• Severe allergic reaction (e.g., anaphylaxis) after a previous dose or to a vaccine component[3] including neomycin	• Moderate or severe acute illness with or without fever
Hepatitis B (HepB)	• Severe allergic reaction (e.g., anaphylaxis) after a previous dose or to a vaccine component[3] including yeast • For Heplisav-B only: Pregnancy	• Moderate or severe acute illness with or without fever
Hepatitis A–Hepatitis B vaccine [HepA-HepB, (Twinrix®)]	• Severe allergic reaction (e.g., anaphylaxis) after a previous dose or to a vaccine component[3] including neomycin and yeast	• Moderate or severe acute illness with or without fever
Human papillomavirus (HPV)	• Severe allergic reaction (e.g., anaphylaxis) after a previous dose or to a vaccine component[3]	• Moderate or severe acute illness with or without fever
Measles, mumps rubella (MMR)	• Severe allergic reaction (e.g., anaphylaxis) after a previous dose or to a vaccine component[3] • Severe immunodeficiency (e.g., hematologic and solid tumors, receipt of chemotherapy, congenital immunodeficiency, long-term immunosuppressive therapy or patients with HIV infection who are severely immunocompromised) • Pregnancy • Family history of altered immunocompetence, unless verified clinically or by laboratory testing as immunocompetent	• Recent (≤11 months) receipt of antibody-containing blood product (specific interval depends on product) • History of thrombocytopenia or thrombocytopenic purpura • Need for tuberculin skin testing or interferon-gamma release assay (IGRA) testing • Moderate or severe acute illness with or without fever
Meningococcal ACWY (MenACWY), [MenACWY-CRM (Menveo®); MenACWY-D (Menactra®); MenACWY-TT (MenQuadfi®)]	• Severe allergic reaction (e.g., anaphylaxis) after a previous dose or to a vaccine component[3] • For MenACWY-D and Men ACWY-CRM only: severe allergic reaction to any diphtheria toxoid– or CRM197-containing vaccine • For MenACWY-TT only: severe allergic reaction to a tetanus toxoid-containing vaccine	• Moderate or severe acute illness with or without fever
Meningococcal B (MenB) [MenB-4C (Bexsero); MenB-FHbp (Trumenba)]	• Severe allergic reaction (e.g., anaphylaxis) after a previous dose or to a vaccine component[3]	• Pregnancy • For MenB-4C only: Latex sensitivity • Moderate or severe acute illness with or without fever
Pneumococcal conjugate (PCV15)	• Severe allergic reaction (e.g., anaphylaxis) after a previous dose or to a vaccine component[3] • Severe allergic reaction (e.g., anaphylaxis) to any diphtheria-toxoid–containing vaccine or to its vaccine component[3]	• Moderate or severe acute illness with or without fever
Pneumococcal conjugate (PCV20)	• Severe allergic reaction (e.g., anaphylaxis) after a previous dose or to a vaccine component[3] • Severe allergic reaction (e.g., anaphylaxis) to any diphtheria-toxoid–containing vaccine or to its vaccine component[3]	• Moderate or severe acute illness with or without fever
Pneumococcal polysaccharide (PPSV23)	• Severe allergic reaction (e.g., anaphylaxis) after a previous dose or to a vaccine component[3]	• Moderate or severe acute illness with or without fever
Tetanus, diphtheria, and acellular pertussis (Tdap); Tetanus, diphtheria (Td)	• Severe allergic reaction (e.g., anaphylaxis) after a previous dose or to a vaccine component[3] • For Tdap only: Encephalopathy (e.g., coma, decreased level of consciousness, prolonged seizures), not attributable to another identifiable cause, within 7 days of administration of previous dose of DTP, DTaP, or Tdap	• Guillain-Barré syndrome (GBS) within 6 weeks after a previous dose of tetanus-toxoid–containing vaccine • History of Arthus-type hypersensitivity reactions after a previous dose of diphtheria-toxoid–containing or tetanus-toxoid–containing vaccine; defer vaccination until at least 10 years have elapsed since the last tetanus-toxoid-containing vaccine • Moderate or severe acute illness with or without fever • For Tdap only: Progressive or unstable neurological disorder, uncontrolled seizures, or progressive encephalopathy until a treatment regimen has been established and the condition has stabilized
Varicella (VAR)	• Severe allergic reaction (e.g., anaphylaxis) after a previous dose or to a vaccine component[3] • Severe immunodeficiency (e.g., hematologic and solid tumors, receipt of chemotherapy, congenital immunodeficiency, long-term immunosuppressive therapy or patients with HIV infection who are severely immunocompromised) • Pregnancy • Family history of altered immunocompetence, unless verified clinically or by laboratory testing as immunocompetent	• Recent (≤11 months) receipt of antibody-containing blood product (specific interval depends on product) • Receipt of specific antiviral drugs (acyclovir, famciclovir, or valacyclovir) 24 hours before vaccination (avoid use of these antiviral drugs for 14 days after vaccination) • Use of aspirin or aspirin-containing products • Moderate or severe acute illness with or without fever
Zoster recombinant vaccine (RZV)	• Severe allergic reaction (e.g., anaphylaxis) after a previous dose or to a vaccine component[3]	• Moderate or severe acute illness with or without fever • Current herpes zoster infection

1. When a contraindication is present, a vaccine should NOT be administered. Kroger A, Bahta L, Hunter P. ACIP General Best Practice Guidelines for Immunization. www.cdc.gov/vaccines/hcp/acip-recs/general-recs/contraindications.html
2. When a precaution is present, vaccination should generally be deferred but might be indicated if the benefit of protection from the vaccine outweighs the risk for an adverse reaction. Kroger A, Bahta L, Hunter P. ACIP General Best Practice Guidelines for Immunization. www.cdc.gov/vaccines/hcp/acip-recs/general-recs/contraindications.html
3. Vaccination providers should check FDA-approved prescribing information for the most complete and updated information, including contraindications, warnings, and precautions. Package inserts for U.S.-licensed vaccines are available at www.fda.gov/vaccines-blood-biologics/approved-products/vaccines-licensed-use-united-states.

Figure 38-1 *(Continued)*

Centers for Disease Control and Prevention, Recommended Adult Immunization Schedule, United States, 2023

particular, where the burden of the respective preventable chronic conditions is high (Levine, 2019). In 2015, only 8% of American adults aged 35 and older had received all high-priority preventive healthcare interventions that were appropriate and recommended for them (Borsky et al., 2018).

Furthermore, disadvantaged groups, such as those affected by systemic racism, people with disabilities, people living with mental illness, people with low socioeconomic status, and people living in rural areas, experience additional barriers in accessing preventive healthcare interventions. These barriers contribute to disproportionately poorer health for disadvantaged groups (Aggarwal et al., 2013; Cole et al., 2013; Ramjan et al., 2016; Rivera et al., 2020; Tung et al., 2017; Xu et al., 2017).

In 2021, the USPSTF developed new strategies for its recommendation process that will support the Task Force in its efforts to eliminate health inequities for people affected by systemic racism (USPTF, 2021). Among many challenges in this mission are the gaps in clinical evidence due to the exclusion of Black, Indigenous, and Hispanic/Latino populations in prevention-related research. Information gaps and bias itself can lead to unfair and inaccurate assessment of risk via algorithms that include race or proxies of racism. The USPSTF aims to assess for bias in the evidence it uses and present information about such deficiencies in a transparent way.

Another avenue to advance health equity is to employ evidence-based preventive healthcare implementation plans as identified by the Community Preventive Services Task Force (CPSTF). The CPSTF, in collaboration with the CDC and the Agency for Healthcare Research and Quality, conducts systematic reviews and makes evidence-based recommendations for implementing programs and systems to improve the delivery of preventive health care. Examples of interventions that have been evaluated by the CPSTF and found to be effective are text messaging programs for tobacco cessation, patient reminders for breast and colon cancer screening, and workplace-based digital and telephone interventions to improve healthy eating and physical activity. Additionally, the CPSTF recommends tenant-based housing voucher programs and "housing first" programs to advance health and health equity. CPSTF findings and recommendations can be found at the CPSTF website (https://www.thecommunityguide.org).

II. Individualizing screening decisions in the geriatric population (**Figure 38-2**)

A key concept in the care of older adults is the notion that decisions about screening for preventable illnesses need to be individualized rather than based solely on age. The large heterogeneity of comorbidities, life expectancy, and goals of treatment in this population mean that decisions based simply on age can lead to both over- and undertreatment and potential harm. Screening adults whose life expectancy is shorter than the time it would take them to benefit from a screening intervention subjects them to the potential harms of screening without the potential benefits. Conversely, not screening an individual, based on their age, who would be expected to live long enough to benefit from the intervention would deny them the potential benefit of screening (Lee, Leipzig, et al., 2013). The difficulty for the clinician arises when the time to benefit and the estimated life expectancy are similar, and it is not clear whether potential harms or potential benefits are greater. In these cases, what can guide the clinician is the individual's values and preferences regarding healthcare interventions (Walter & Covinsky, 2001; Yourman et al., 2012). The following section provides the clinician with a framework for making clinical decisions about offering screening to older adults.

Decision making about individualized screening requires three elements: (1) estimating the patient's life expectancy, (2) estimating the time to benefit of the proposed intervention or screening procedure, and (3) evaluating the patient's preferences around the potential harms and benefits of the intervention (Lee, Leipzig, et al., 2013).

Incorporating a person's comorbidities and functional status with their age can provide a more accurate picture of life expectancy than age alone (Walter & Covinsky, 2001; Yourman et al., 2012). Those with fewer comorbidities and higher functional ability can be expected to live longer than the average, whereas those with more comorbidities and lower functional ability will have a shorter-than-average life expectancy. **Figure 38-3** shows life expectancy by age and quartile and can be used to make prognosis estimates based on whether one has more or fewer comorbidities and functional impairments than the average person.

Prognostic indices have been developed based on single dominant terminal conditions, such as dementia, cancer, heart failure, or coronary artery disease (Levy et al., 2006; McClelland et al., 2015; Mitchell et al., 2010; Xie et al., 2008; Ziepert et al., 2010). Other indices have been developed to address prognosis among older adults who do not have a dominant terminal illness. A systematic review of the literature for this population has led to a repository of indices on the internet called ePrognosis (https://ePrognosis.ucsf.edu). The ePrognosis website includes a user interface to easily access the most relevant index in order to help estimate life expectancy (Yourman et al., 2012). Along with age, this calculator incorporates such factors as the location of the patient (community, skilled nursing facility, hospital), functional ability, and comorbidities to pair the clinical question with the appropriate index. As with other clinical decisions, one must assess whether the population studied to develop an index is comparable to the patient one is addressing.

When considering an intervention such as screening, the provider should evaluate how long it would take the patient to benefit from the intervention that would likely be triggered by a positive screen. How soon will the intervention help the patient? Are they likely to live long enough

II. Individualizing screening decisions in the geriatric population (Figure 38-2)

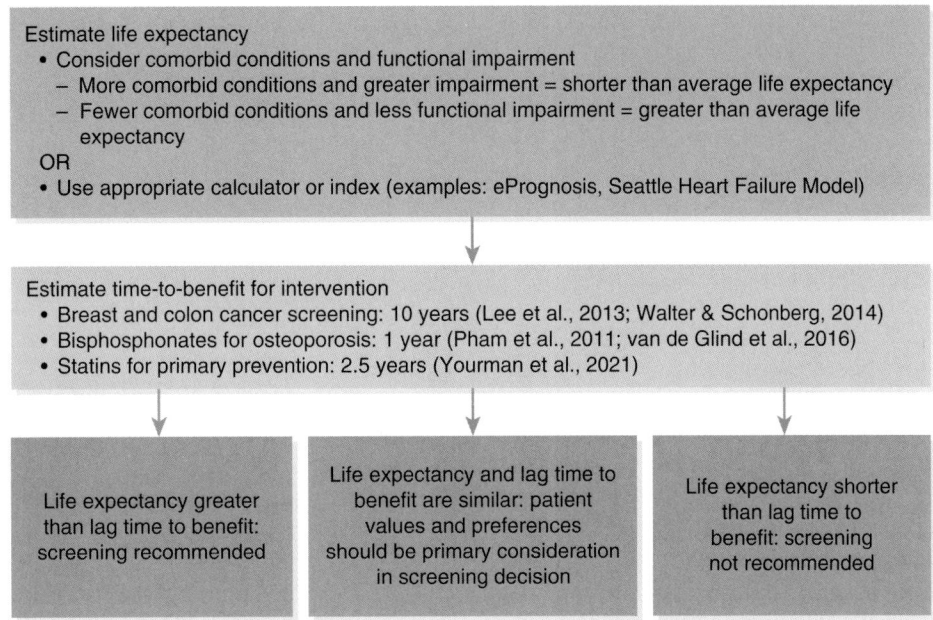

Figure 38-2 Individualizing Screening Decision-Making for Older Adults

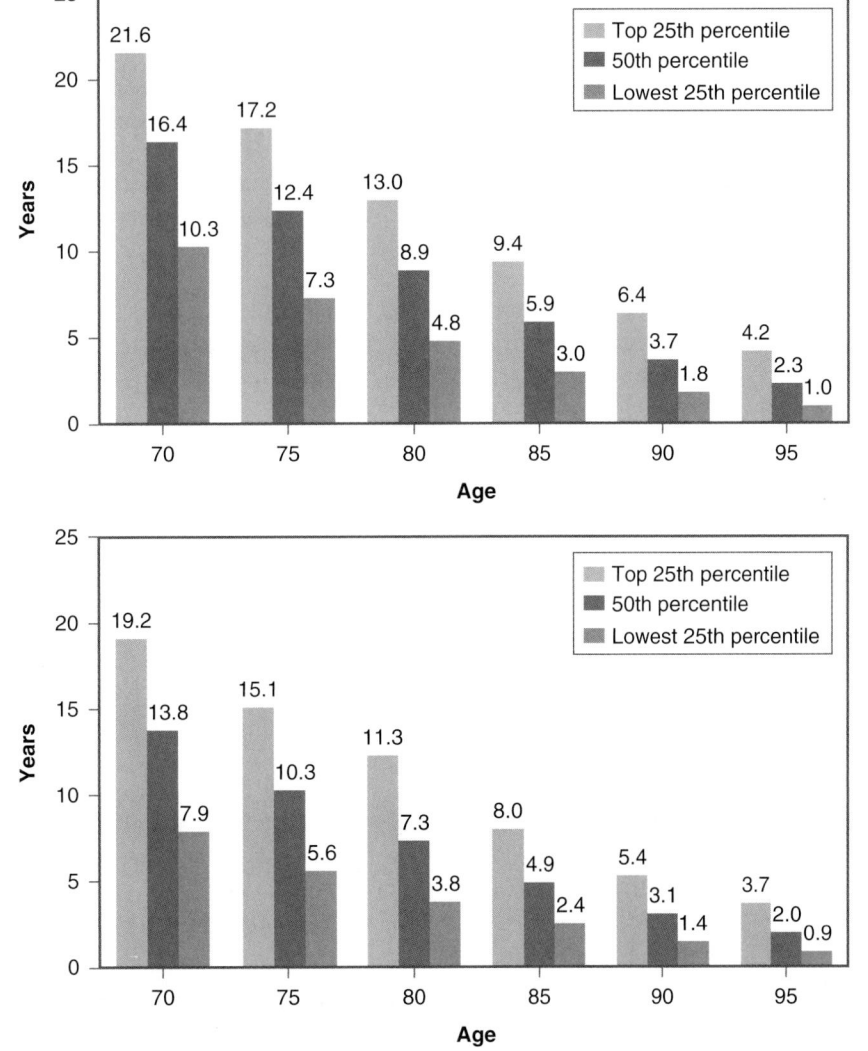

Figure 38-3 Upper, middle, and lower quartiles of life expectancy for women and men at selected ages.

for this benefit? If not, they are susceptible to harms only. Time-to-benefit estimation seeks to answer the question, "When will it help?" Unfortunately, these data are rarely reported directly in clinical trials (Holmes et al., 2013). Some current research is attempting to fill this gap. A 2013 meta-analysis found that the time to benefit for breast and colorectal cancer screening is 10 years (Lee, Boscardin, et al., 2013). Treatment for osteoporosis can be clinically significant at 1 year (Pham et al., 2011; van de Glind et al., 2016), and statin use for primary prevention of myocardial infarction is significant at 2.5 years (Yourman et al., 2021). In older adults with diabetes, microvascular complications of diabetes are reduced only after 8 years of glycemic control, whereas treatment of hypertension shows benefits in 2–3 years (Brown et al., 2003). This information allows the clinician to consider whether the patient's life expectancy is great enough to benefit from treatment for screened-for conditions. The ePrognosis website (https://eprognosis.ucsf.edu/time_to_benefit.php) described above includes an evidence-based time-to-benefit figure that can assist clinicians with these decisions.

In addition to the potential benefits of screening interventions, it is necessary to evaluate how a particular intervention fits with an individual's values, preferences, and goals of treatment. Harms to be considered include overdiagnosis—the identification and subsequent treatment of disease that would not have become clinically significant during the patient's lifetime, false positives leading to additional diagnostic procedures with potential complications, and physical and psychologic discomfort from screening (Pham et al., 2011). Discussions of screening should include information on treatments that would be expected to follow a positive screening result. General treatment goals for a particular patient may include longevity, preserving function, comfort, or some combination of the three. Clarifying how a particular screening intervention fits within the patient's goals can help facilitate decision making.

III. Database
A. Subjective
1. Symptoms that would trigger diagnosis/management rather than screening
2. Risk factors for diseases that can be appropriately screened for (Tables 38-1, 38-2, and 38-3)
   a. Behavioral characteristics
   b. Past medical history
   c. Family history
   d. Occupational history
   e. Personal-social history
3. Functional status (as a contributor to life expectancy and ability to undergo screening/treatment)
4. Behavioral factors affecting the ability to make healthy lifestyle changes
5. Patient values/preferences related to illness prevention and health care

B. Objective
1. Demographics (e.g., age, place of birth, sex)
2. Initial common screening physical exam assessments to consider:
   a. Blood pressure
   b. Total body weight
   c. Timed Up-and-Go or other balance/mobility exam for older adults

IV. Assessment
A. Establish what currently undiagnosed conditions the patient is at risk for based on subjective and objective characteristics.
B. Select appropriate screening, immunizations, chemoprophylaxis, and counseling based on risk.
   1. Use evidence-based recommendations from USPSTF, CDC, or other appropriate source (Figure 38-1 and **Tables** 38-1–**38-4**).
   2. Consider life expectancy and time to benefit of intervention (**Figures 38-2** and **38-3**).
C. Consider health maintenance interventions related to previously diagnosed conditions following evidence-based guidelines.
D. Consider patient's values and preferences related to recommended measures, particularly if life expectancy and time to benefit are similar.
E. Evaluate patient's ability and desire to engage in recommended measures to prevent illness (**Box 38-1**).

V. Plan
A. Order screening tests, immunizations, and chemoprophylaxis as appropriate.
B. Provide education and counseling as appropriate.

VI. Goals of clinical management
A. Primary prevention—prevent injury and disease by minimizing risk factors.
   1. Counseling (e.g., behavioral counseling for those at risk for sexually transmitted infections)
   2. Immunizations (e.g., influenza, pneumococcal, human papillomavirus)
   3. Chemoprophylaxis (e.g., statin for prevention of cardiovascular disease)
   4. Screening for modifiable risk factors for disease (e.g., screening for hypertension, higher body weight, and hyperlipidemia as risk factors for cardiovascular disease)
B. Secondary prevention—identify asymptomatic disease when treatment can prevent it from progressing. Be sure to weigh risks and benefits of secondary prevention screening and anticipated management of positive screens before initiating screening.

Table 38-4 Screening Recommendations and Considerations Referenced in Centers for Disease Control and Prevention (CDC) 2021 Sexually Transmitted Infection (STI) Treatment Guidelines and Original Sources

Transgender and Gender Diverse Persons	
Chlamydia	■ Screening recommendations should be adapted based on anatomy (i.e., annual, routine screening in cis-gender women <25 years old should be extended to all transgender men and gender-diverse people with a cervix; if over 25 years old, persons with a cervix should be screened if at increased risk).[2] ■ Consider screening at the rectal site based on reported sexual behaviors and exposure.[2]
Gonorrhea	■ Screening recommendations should be adapted based on anatomy (i.e., annual, routine screening for gonorrhea in cisgender women <25 years old should be extended to all transgender men and gender-diverse people with a cervix; if over 25 years old, screen if at increased risk).[2] ■ Consider screening at the pharyngeal and rectal sites based on reported sexual behaviors and exposure.[2]
Syphilis	■ Consider screening at least annually based on reported sexual behaviors and exposure.[2]
HIV	■ HIV screening should be discussed and offered to all transgender persons. Frequency of repeat screenings should be based on level of risk.[2,15]
HPV, Cervical Cancer, Anal Cancer	■ Screening for people with a cervix should follow current screening guidelines for cervical cancer.[2]
Women	
Chlamydia	■ Sexually active women under 25 years of age[1] ■ Sexually active women 25 years of age and older if at increased risk (those who have a new sex partner, more than one sex partner, a sex partner with concurrent partners, or a sex partner who has an STI)[1] ■ Retest approximately 3 months after treatment.[2] ■ Rectal chlamydial testing can be considered in females based on reported sexual behaviors and exposure, through shared clinical decision between the patient and the provider.[3,4]
Gonorrhea	■ Sexually active women under 25 years of age[1] ■ Sexually active women 25 years of age and older if at increased risk (those who have a new sex partner, more than one sex partner, a sex partner with concurrent partners, or a sex partner who has an STI or transactional sex)[1] ■ Retest 3 months after treatment.[2] ■ Pharyngeal and rectal gonorrhea screening can be considered in females based on reported sexual behaviors and exposure, through shared clinical decision between the patient and the provider.[3,4]
Syphilis	■ Screen asymptomatic adults at increased risk (history of incarceration or transactional sex work, geography, race/ethnicity, and being a male younger than 29 years) for syphilis infection.[2,5]
Herpes	■ Type-specific HSV serologic testing can be considered for women presenting for an STI evaluation (especially for women with multiple sex partners).[2,6]
Trichomonas	■ Consider screening for women receiving care in high-prevalence settings (e.g., STI clinics and correctional facilities) and for asymptomatic women at high risk for infection (e.g., women with multiple sex partners, transactional sex, drug misuse, or a history of STI or incarceration).[2]
HIV	■ All women aged 13–64 years (unless they opt out)*[7,8] ■ All women who seek evaluation and treatment for STIs[2,8]
HPV, Cervical Cancer, Anal Cancer	■ Women 18–29 years of age every 3 years with cytology ■ Women 30–65 years of age every 3 years with cytology, or every 5 years with a combination of cytology and HPV testing[9-11]
Hepatitis B Screening	■ Women at increased risk (having had more than one sex partner in the previous 6 months, evaluation or treatment for an STI, past or current injection-drug use, and an HBsAg-positive sex partner)[12]
Hepatitis C Screening	■ All adults over age 15 years should be screened for hepatitis C except in settings where the hepatitis C infection (HCV) positivity is <0.1%.[13]

(continues)

Table 38-4 Screening Recommendations and Considerations Referenced in Centers for Disease Control and Prevention (CDC) 2021 Sexually Transmitted Infection (STI) Treatment Guidelines and Original Sources *(continued)*

Men Who Have Sex with Women	
Chlamydia	■ There is insufficient evidence for screening among heterosexual men who are at low risk for infection; however, screening of young men can be considered in high-prevalence clinical settings (adolescent clinics, correctional facilities, STI/sexual health clinic).[1,14]
Gonorrhea	■ There is insufficient evidence for screening among heterosexual men who are at low risk for infection.[1,14]
Syphilis	■ Screen asymptomatic adults at increased risk (history of incarceration or commercial sex work, geography, race/ethnicity, and being a male younger than 29 years) for syphilis infection.[2,5]
Herpes	■ Type-specific HSV serologic testing can be considered for men presenting for an STI evaluation (especially for men with multiple sex partners).[2,6]
HIV	■ All men aged 13-64 years (unless they opt out)*[7] ■ All men who seek evaluation and treatment for STIs[2]
Hepatitis B Screening	■ Men at increased risk (i.e., by sexual or percutaneous exposure)[12]
Hepatitis C Screening	■ All adults over age 15 years should be screened for hepatitis C except in settings where the hepatitis C infection (HCV) positivity is <0.1%.[13]
Men Who Have Sex with Men (MSM)	
Chlamydia	■ At least annually for sexually active MSM at sites of contact (urethra, rectum), regardless of condom use[2] ■ Every 3-6 months if at increased risk (i.e., MSM on PrEP, with HIV infection, or if they or their sex partners have multiple partners)[2]
Gonorrhea	■ At least annually for sexually active MSM at sites of contact (urethra, rectum, pharynx), regardless of condom use[2] ■ Every 3-6 months if at increased risk[2]
Syphilis	■ At least annually for sexually active MSM[2] ■ Every 3-6 months if at increased risk[2]
Herpes	■ Type-specific serologic tests can be considered if infection status is unknown in MSM with previously undiagnosed genital tract infection.[2,6]
HIV	■ At least annually for sexually active MSM if HIV status is unknown or negative and the patient or their sex partner(s) have had more than one sex partner since most recent HIV test[2,8,15] ■ Consider the benefits of offering more frequent HIV screening (e.g., every 3-6 months) to MSM at increased risk for acquiring HIV infection.
HPV, Cervical Cancer, Anal Cancer	■ Digital anorectal exam[2] ■ Data are insufficient to recommend routine anal cancer screening with anal cytology.[2]
Hepatitis B Screening	■ All MSM should be tested for HBsAg, HBV core antibody, and HBV surface antibody[12]
Hepatitis C Screening	■ All adults over age 15 years should be screened for hepatitis C except in settings where the hepatitis C infection (HCV) positivity is <0.1%.[13]
Persons with HIV	
Chlamydia	■ For sexually active individuals, screen at first HIV evaluation and at least annually thereafter.[2,17] ■ More frequent screening might be appropriate depending on individual risk behaviors and the local epidemiology.[2]
Gonorrhea	■ For sexually active individuals, screen at first HIV evaluation and at least annually thereafter.[2,17] ■ More frequent screening might be appropriate depending on individual risk behaviors and the local epidemiology.[2]
Syphilis	■ For sexually active individuals, screen at first HIV evaluation and at least annually thereafter.[6,18] ■ More frequent screening might be appropriate depending on individual risk behaviors and the local epidemiology.[2]
Herpes	■ Type-specific HSV serologic testing should be considered for persons presenting for an STI evaluation (especially for those persons with multiple sex partners).[2]

Persons with HIV	
Trichomonas	■ Recommended for sexually active women at entry to care and at least annually thereafter[2,18]
HPV, Cervical Cancer, Anal Cancer	■ Women with HIV should be screened within 1 year of sexual activity using conventional or liquid-based cytology; testing should be repeated 6 months later. With 3 normal and consecutive Pap tests, screening should be every 3 years.[16,19]
Hepatitis B Screening	■ Test for HBsAg and anti-HBc and/or anti-HBs[12]
Hepatitis C Screening	■ Serologic testing at initial evaluation[2,13] ■ Annual HCV testing in MSM with HIV infection[2,13]

anti-HBc, hepatitis B core antibody; *anti-HBs*, hepatitis B surface antibody; *HBsAg*, hepatitis B surface antigen; *HBV*, hepatitis B virus; *HCV*, hepatitis C virus; *HPV*, human papillomavirus; *HSV*, herpes simplex virus; *PrEP*, pre-exposure prophylaxis.

* USPSTF recommends screening in adults and adolescents ages 15–65.

[1] LeFevre, M. L. (2014). Screening for chlamydia and gonorrhea: U.S. Preventive Services Task Force recommendation statement. *Annals of Internal Medicine, 161*(12), 902–910. doi:10.7326/M14-1981

[2] Workowski, K. A., Bachmann, L., Chan, P., Johnston, C., Muzny, C., Park, I., Reno, H., Zenilman, J., & Bolan, G. (2021). Sexually transmitted infections, 2021. *MMWR Recommendations and Reports, 70*(RR-04), 1–187. doi:10.15585/mmwr.rr7004a1

[3] Bamberger, D. M., Graham, G., Dennis, L., & Gerkovich, M. M. (2019). Extragenital gonorrhea and chlamydia among men and women according to type of sexual exposure. *Sexually Transmitted Diseases, 46*(5), 329–334. doi:10.1097/OLQ.0000000000000967

[4] Chan, P. A., Robinette, A., Montgomery, M., Almonte, A., Cu-Uvin, S., Lonks, J. R., Chapin, K. C., Kojic, E. M., & Hardy, E. J. (2016). Extragenital infections caused by *Chlamydia trachomatis* and *Neisseria gonorrhoeae*: A review of the literature. *Infectious Diseases in Obstetrics and Gynecology*, 5758387. doi:10.1155/2016/5758387

[5] Bibbins-Domingo, K. (2016). Screening for syphilis infection in nonpregnant adults and adolescents. U.S. Preventive Services Task Force recommendation statement. *JAMA, 315*(21), 2321–2327. doi:10.1001/jama.2016.5824

[6] Type-specific HSV-2 serologic assays for diagnosing HSV-2 are useful in the following scenarios: recurrent or atypical genital symptoms or lesions with a negative HSV polymerase chain reaction (PCR) or culture result, clinical diagnosis of genital herpes without laboratory confirmation, and a patient's partner has genital herpes. HSV-2 serologic screening among the general population is not recommended. Patients who are at higher risk for infection (e.g., those presenting for an STI evaluation, especially for persons with ≥10 lifetime sex partners, and persons with HIV infection) might need to be assessed for a history of genital herpes symptoms, followed by type-specific HSV serologic assays to diagnose genital herpes for those with genital symptoms.

[7] Branson, B. M., Handsfield, H. H., Lampe, M. A., Janssen, R. S., Taylor, A. W., Lyss, S. B., Clark, J. E., & Centers for Disease Control and Prevention (CDC). (2006). Revised recommendations for HIV testing of adults, adolescents, and pregnant women in healthcare settings. *Morbidity and Mortality Weekly Report, 55*(RR-14), 1–17.

[8] Owens, D. K. (2019). Screening for HIV infection: U.S. Preventive Services Task Force recommendation statement. *JAMA, 321*(23), 2326–2336. doi:10.1001/jama.2019.658

[9] Committee on Practice Bulletins—Gynecology. (2016). Practice Bulletin No. 157: Cervical cancer screening and prevention. *Obstetrics and Gynecology, 127*(1), e1–20. doi:10.1097/AOG.0000000000001263

[10] Fontham, E. T. H., Wolf, A. M. D., Church, T. R., Etzioni, R., Flowers, C. R., Herzig, A., Guerra, C. E., Oeffinger, K. C., Shih, Y. T., Walter, L. C., Kim, J. J., Andrews, K. S., DeSantis, C. E., Fedewa, S. A., Manassaram-Baptiste, D., Saslow, D., Wender, R. C., & Smith, R. A. (2020). Cervical cancer screening for individuals at average risk: 2020 guideline update from the American Cancer Society. *CA: A Cancer Journal for Clinicians, 70*(5), 321–346. doi:10.3322/caac.21628

[11] US Preventive Services Task Force, Curry, S. J., Krist, A. H., Owens, D. K., Barry, M. J., Caughey, A. B., Davidson, K. W., Doubeni, C. A., Epling, J. W., Jr, Kemper, A. R., Kubik, M., Landefeld, C. S., Mangione, C. M., Phipps, M. G., Silverstein, M., Simon, M. A., Tseng, C. W., & Wong, J. B. (2018). Screening for cervical cancer: U.S. Preventive Services Task Force Recommendation Statement. *JAMA, 320*(7), 674–686. doi:10.1001/jama.2018.10897

[12] Schillie, S., Vellozzi, C., Reingold, A., Harris, A., Haber, P., Ward, J. W., & Nelson, N. P. (2018). Prevention of hepatitis B virus infection in the United States: Recommendations of the Advisory Committee on Immunization Practices. *MMWR Recommendations and Reports, 67*(RR-1), 1–31. doi:10.15585/mmwr.rr6701a1

[13] US Preventive Services Task Force, Owens, D. K., Davidson, K. W., Krist, A. H., Barry, M. J., Cabana, M., Caughey, A. B., Donahue, K., Doubeni, C. A., Epling, J. W., Jr, Kubik, M., Ogedegbe, G., Pbert, L., Silverstein, M., Simon, M. A., Tseng, C. W., & Wong, J. B. (2020). Screening for hepatitis C virus infection in adolescents and adults: U.S. Preventive Services Task Force recommendation statement. *JAMA, 323*(10), 970–975. doi:10.1001/jama.2020.1123

[14] Rietmeijer, C. A., Hopkins, E., Geisler, W. M., Orr, D. P., & Kent, C. K. (2008). *Chlamydia trachomatis* positivity rates among men tested in selected venues in the United States: A review of the recent literature. *Sexually Transmitted Diseases, 35*(11), S8–18. doi:10.1097/OLQ.0b013e31816938ba

[15] DiNenno, E. A., Prejean, J., Irwin, K., Delaney, K. P., Bowles, K., Martin, T., Tailor, A., Dumitru, G., Mullins, M. M., Hutchinson, A. B., & Lansky, A. (2017). Recommendations for HIV screening of gay, bisexual, and other men who have sex with men—United States, 2017. *Morbidity and Mortality Weekly Report, 66*(31), 830–832.

[16] Data are insufficient to recommend routine anal cancer screening with anal cytology among populations at risk for anal cancer. Certain clinical centers perform anal cytology to screen for anal cancer among populations at high risk (e.g., persons with HIV infection, MSM, and those having receptive anal intercourse), followed by high-resolution anoscopy (HRA) for those with abnormal cytologic results (e.g., ACS-US, LSIL, or HSIL).

[17] Thompson, M. A., Horberg, M. A., Agwu, A. L., Colasanti, J. A., Jain, M. K., Short, W. R., Singh, T., & Aberg, J. A. (2020). Primary care guidelines for persons with HIV: 2020 update by the HIV Medicine Association of the Infectious Diseases Society of America. *Clinical Infectious Disease, 73*(11), e3572–e3605. doi:10.1093/cid/ciaa1391

[18] Centers for Disease Control and Prevention, Health Resources and Services Administration, National Institutes of Health, American Academy of HIV Medicine, Association of Nurses in AIDS Care, International Association of Providers of AIDS Care, the National Minority AIDS Council, and Urban Coalition for HIV/AIDS Prevention Services. (2014, December 11). *Recommendations for HIV prevention with adults and adolescents with HIV in the United States, 2014.* http://stacks.cdc.gov/view/cdc/26062

[19] Panel on Opportunistic Infections in Adults and Adolescents with HIV. (n.d.). *Guidelines for the prevention and treatment of opportunistic infections in adults and adolescents with HIV.* https://clinicalinfo.hiv.gov/sites/default/files/guidelines/documents/adult-adolescent-oi/guidelines-adult-adolescent-oi.pdf

CDC Sexually Transmitted Infections Treatment Guidelines, 2021, Screening Recommendations and Considerations Referenced in Treatment Guidelines and Original Sources by Population. Retrieved from https://www.cdc.gov/std/treatment-guidelines/screening-recommendations.htm on 3/22/22.

Box 38-1 Assessing a Client's Readiness for Behavior Change

Counseling interventions regarding lifestyle and healthy behaviors begins with an assessment of the client's recognition of unhealthy behavior and an assessment of the client's readiness to make health-directed changes. Readiness to change is one of many frameworks designed to help the primary care provider choose an interviewing approach that will be most meaningful to the patient. The Transtheoretical Model defines behavior change as a process that occurs in stages (Huddleston, 2009). These stages, often referred to as "stages of change," help the clinician tailor motivational interviewing strategies to help the client move closer to changing unhealthy behaviors (Walley, 2016).

Stage of Change	Definition	Patient Approach
Precontemplation	The client has not recognized the behavior as unhealthy or they are not ready to change the behavior	<ul><li>Inform and educate the client about the unhealthy behavior and health consequences</li><li>Convey support for the client and their life ambitions and encouragement to continue seeking care</li></ul>
Contemplation	The client understands his or her behavior is unhealthy but is ambivalent about making a change	<ul><li>Elicit reasons for ambivalence</li><li>Support and reinforce positive behavior change</li><li>Acknowledge negative effects of the unhealthy behavior</li></ul>
Preparation or Determination	The client makes a decision to change	<ul><li>Commend the decision to change the behavior</li><li>Assist in choosing treatment path</li></ul>
Action	The client is active in some change of the behavior	<ul><li>Support the changes made and provide encouragement to sustain the changes</li><li>Provide support for co-occurring vulnerabilities such as pain or depression</li></ul>
Maintenance	The client has made behavior change and is stable	<ul><li>Recognize the client's commitment and continued struggle to maintain the healthy behavior</li><li>Anticipate difficulties that may challenge maintenance</li><li>Address relapse without judgment</li></ul>

Data from Huddleston, J. S. (2009). Health Promotion and Behavior Change. In A. J. Lowenstein, L. Foord-May, & J. Romano (Eds.), Teaching strategies for health education and health promotion: Working with patients, families, and communities. Jones and Bartlett Publishers

Prochaska, J. O., Norcross, J. C., & DiClemente, C. C. (2006). Changing for good (First Collins paperback edition). William Morrow, an imprint of HarperCollins Publishers.

Walley, A. Y. (2016). Principles of Caring for People Who Use Alcohol and Other Drugs. In T. E. King & M. B. Wheeler (Eds.), Medical Management of Vulnerable and Underserved Patients: Principles, Practice, and Populations (2nd ed.). McGraw-Hill. "

---

1. Screening for cancer (e.g., mammogram for breast cancer, colonoscopy for colorectal cancer)
2. Screening for other conditions (e.g., depression, abdominal aortic aneurysm, sexually transmitted infections)

C. *Tertiary prevention—interventions to minimize complications of disease once it is diagnosed. Not addressed in this chapter—see chapters dedicated to particular conditions for prevention of disease-specific complications.*

VII. Resources for health professionals and consumers

See the section titled "Clinical Considerations" or "Practice Considerations" in each USPSTF recommendation for suggested tools and resources. For additional recommendations, see **Table 38-5**.

Table 38-5 Resources for Consumers and Health Professionals

Multilingual printable consumer information on many preventive health topics	National Institutes of Health (NIH), National Library of Medicine: MedlinePlus, Health https://medlineplus.gov/languages/all_healthtopics.html#A *Information available in over 50 languages*
Alcohol and substance use disorders prevention	NIH, National Institute on Alcohol Abuse and Alcoholism https://niaaa.nih.gov/publications/clinical-guides-and-manuals Centers for Disease Control and Prevention (CDC) Fact Sheets: Preventing Excessive Alcohol Use https://cdc.gov/alcohol/fact-sheets/prevention.htm Substance Abuse and Mental Health Services Administration (SAMHSA): Prevention of Substance Abuse and Mental Illness https://samhsa.gov/prevention NIH, National Institute on Drug Abuse: DrugFacts: Lessons From Prevention Research https://drugabuse.gov/publications/drugfacts/lessons-prevention-research SAMHSA: Screening, Brief Intervention, and Referral to Treatment (SBIRT) https://samhsa.gov/sbirt Massachusetts Department of Public Health Bureau of Substance Abuse Services: SBIRT: A Step-By-Step Guide for Screening and Intervening for Unhealthy Alcohol and Other Drug Use http://files.hria.org/files/SA3522.pdf
Cancer screening	NIH, National Cancer Institute: Cancer Screening https://www.cancer.gov/about-cancer/screening
Diabetes	CDC: National Diabetes Prevention Program https://www.cdc.gov/diabetes/prevention/index.html CDC: Diabetes and Asian Americans https://www.cdc.gov/diabetes/library/spotlights/diabetes-asian-americans.html
Falls	NIH, National Institute on Aging: Prevent Falls and Fractures https://www.nia.nih.gov/health/prevent-falls-and-fractures International Osteoporosis Foundation: Falls Prevention https://www.osteoporosis.foundation/patients/prevention/falls-prevention
HIV prevention (including pre-exposure prophylaxis [PrEP])	CDC: HIV https://www.cdc.gov/hiv U.S. Department of Health and Human Services (supported by the Minority HIV/AIDS Fund) https://www.hiv.gov/ Health Resources and Services Administration (HRSA), AIDS Education and Training Center (AETC): Prescribing PrEP: A Guide for Healthcare Providers https://aidsetc.org/prep
Nutrition	U.S. Department of Agriculture (USDA) and other government agencies https://www.nutrition.gov/ *Some Spanish*
Occupational health	CDC, National Institute for Occupational Safety and Health (NIOSH): Stress at Work https://cdc.gov/niosh/topics/stress CDC, NIOSH: Occupational Violence https://cdc.gov/niosh/topics/violence CDC, NIOSH: Total Worker Health® Program https://www.cdc.gov/niosh/twh/default.html CDC, NIOSH: Workplace Safety and Health Topics: Safety & Prevention https://www.cdc.gov/niosh/topics/safety.html
Osteoporosis	Bone Health & Osteoporosis Foundation (BHOF) https://www.bonehealthandosteoporosis.org/ International Osteoporosis Foundation https://www.osteoporosis.foundation/

(continues)

Table 38-5 Resources for Consumers and Health Professionals (continued)

Physical activity	CDC: Physical Activity Basics https://cdc.gov/physicalactivity/everyone/guidelines/adults.html
Sexually transmitted infection prevention	CDC: Sexually Transmitted Diseases (STDs): Prevention https://cdc.gov/std/prevention *Includes Fact Sheets on individual STIs in multiple languages*
Skin cancer prevention	National Council on Skin Cancer Prevention https://skincancerprevention.org CDC: Skin Cancer https://cdc.gov/cancer/skin *Materials in English and Spanish*
Tuberculosis	World Health Organization: Tuberculosis https://www.who.int/health-topics/tuberculosis#tab=tab_1
Tobacco use and cessation	U.S. Department of Health and Human Services, NIH, National Cancer Institute, and USA.gov: https://smokefree.gov/ https://espanol.smokefree.gov/ (Spanish) Agency for Health Research and Quality: Five Major Steps to Intervention (the "5 A's") https://ahrq.gov/professionals/clinicians-providers/guidelines-recommendations/tobacco/5steps.html
Violence prevention	CDC: Injury Prevention & Control: Division of Violence Prevention https://cdc.gov/violenceprevention

References

Aggarwal, A., Pandurangi, A., & Smith, W. (2013). Disparities in breast and cervical cancer screening in women with mental illness. *American Journal of Preventive Medicine, 44*(4), 392–398. doi:10.1016/j.amepre.2012.12.006

Borsky, A., Zhan, C., Miller, T., Ngo-Metzger, Q., Bierman, A. S., & Meyers, D. (2018). Few Americans receive all high-priority, appropriate clinical preventive services. *Health Affairs, 37*(6), 925–928. doi:10.1377/hlthaff.2017.1248

Brown, A. F., Mangione, C. M., Saliba, D., & Sarkisian, C. a. (2003). Guidelines for improving the care of the older person with diabetes mellitus. *Journal of the American Geriatrics Society, 51*(5 Suppl Guidelines), S265–S280. https://doi.org/10.1046/j.1532-5415.51.5s.1.x

Cole, A. M., Jackson, J. E., & Doescher, M. (2013). Colorectal cancer screening disparities for rural minorities in the United States. *Journal of Primary Care & Community Health, 4*(2), 106–111. doi:10.1177/2150131912463244

Holmes, H. M., Min, L. C., Yee, M., Varadhan, R., Basran, J., Dale, W., & Boyd, C. M. (2013). Rationalizing prescribing for older patients with multimorbidity: Considering time to benefit. *Drugs & Aging, 30*(9), 655–666. doi:10.1007/s40266-013-0095-7

Lee, S. J., Boscardin, W. J., Stijacic-Cenzer, I., Conell-Price, J., O'Brien, S., & Walter, L. C. (2013). Time lag to benefit after screening for breast and colorectal cancer: Meta-analysis of survival data from the United States, Sweden, United Kingdom, and Denmark. *BMJ (Clinical Research Ed.), 346*, e8441. doi:10.1136/bmj.e8441

Lee, S. J., Leipzig, R. M., & Walter, L. C. (2013). Incorporating lag time to benefit into prevention decisions for older adults. *JAMA: The Journal of the American Medical Association, 310*(24), 2609–2610. doi:10.1001/jama.2013.282612

Levine, S. (2019). Health care industry insights: Why the use of preventive services is still low. *Preventing Chronic Disease, 16*, e30. doi:10.5888/pcd16.180625

Levy, W. C., Mozaffarian, D., Linker, D. T., Sutradhar, S. C., Anker, S. D., Cropp, A. B., Anand, I., Maggioni, A., Burton, P., Sullivan, M. D., Pitt, B., Poole-Wilson, P. A., Mann, D. L., & Packer, M. (2006). The Seattle Heart Failure Model: Prediction of survival in heart failure. *Circulation, 113*(11), 1424–1433. doi:10.1161/CIRCULATIONAHA.105.584102

McClelland, R. L., Jorgensen, N. W., Budoff, M., Blaha, M. J., Post, W. S., Kronmal, R. A., Bild, D. E., Shea, S., Liu, K., Watson, K. E., Folsom, A. R., Khera, A., Ayers, C., Mahabadi, A.-A., Lehmann, N., Jöckel, K.-H., Moebus, S., Carr, J. J., Erbel, R., & Burke, G. L. (2015). 10-year coronary heart disease risk prediction using coronary artery calcium and traditional risk factors: Derivation in the MESA (Multi-Ethnic Study of Atherosclerosis) with validation in the HNR (Heinz Nixdorf Recall) study and the DHS (Dallas Heart Study). *Journal of the American College of Cardiology, 66*(15), 1643–1653. doi:10.1016/j.jacc.2015.08.035

Mitchell, S. L., Miller, S. C., Teno, J. M., Davis, R. B., & Shaffer, M. L. (2010). The advanced dementia prognostic tool: A risk score to estimate survival in nursing home residents with advanced dementia. *Journal of Pain and Symptom Management, 40*(5), 639–651. doi:10.1016/j.jpainsymman.2010.02.014

Pham, A. N., Datta, S. K., Weber, T. J., Walter, L. C., & Colón-Emeric, C. S. (2011). Cost-effectiveness of oral bisphosphonates for osteoporosis at different ages and levels of life expectancy.

Journal of the American Geriatrics Society, 59(9), 1642–1649. doi:10.1111/j.1532-5415.2011.03571.x

Ramjan, L., Cotton, A., Algoso, M., & Peters, K. (2016). Barriers to breast and cervical cancer screening for women with physical disability: A review. *Women & Health, 56*(2), 141–156. doi:10.1080/03630242.2015.1086463

Rivera, M. P., Katki, H. A., Tanner, N. T., Triplette, M., Sakoda, L. C., Wiener, R. S., Cardarelli, R., Carter-Harris, L., Crothers, K., Fathi, J. T., Ford, M. E., Smith, R., Winn, R. A., Wisnivesky, J. P., Henderson, L. M., & Aldrich, M. C. (2020). Addressing disparities in lung cancer screening eligibility and healthcare access. An Official American Thoracic Society Statement. *American Journal of Respiratory and Critical Care Medicine, 202*(7), e95–e112. doi:10.1164/rccm.202008-3053ST

Saitz, R., Miller, S. C., Fiellin, D. A., & Rosenthal, R. N. (2021). Recommended Use of Terminology in Addiction Medicine. *Journal of Addiction Medicine, 15*(1), 3. https://doi.org/10.1097/ADM.0000000000000673

Tung, E. L., Baig, A. A., Huang, E. S., Laiteerapong, N., & Chua, K.-P. (2017). Racial and ethnic disparities in diabetes screening between Asian Americans and other adults: BRFSS 2012–2014. *Journal of General Internal Medicine, 32*(4), 423–429. doi:10.1007/s11606-016-3913-x

U.S. Preventive Services Task Force. (2018). *Grade definitions*. https://www.uspreventiveservicestaskforce.org/uspstf/about-uspstf/methods-and-processes/grade-definitions

U.S. Preventive Services Task Force. (2021). Actions to transform US Preventive Services Task Force methods to mitigate systemic racism in clinical preventive services. *JAMA, 326*(23), 2405–2411. doi:10.1001/jama.2021.17594

van de Glind, E. M. M., Willems, H. C., Eslami, S., Abu-Hanna, A., Lems, W. F., Hooft, L., de Rooij, S. E., Black, D. M., & van Munster, B. C. (2016). Estimating the time to benefit for preventive drugs with the statistical process control method: An Example with alendronate. *Drugs & Aging, 33*(5), 347–353. doi:10.1007/s40266-016-0344-7

Walter, L. C., & Covinsky, K. E. (2001). Cancer screening in elderly patients: A framework for individualized decision making. *JAMA, 285*(21), 2750–2756. doi:10.1001/jama.285.21.2750

Xie, J., Brayne, C., & Matthews, F. E. (2008). Survival times in people with dementia: Analysis from population based cohort study with 14 year follow-up. *BMJ (Clinical Research Ed.), 336*(7638), 258–262. doi:10.1136/bmj.39433.616678.25

Xu, X., Mann, J. R., Hardin, J. W., Gustafson, E., McDermott, S. W., & Deroche, C. B. (2017). Adherence to US Preventive Services Task Force recommendations for breast and cervical cancer screening for women who have a spinal cord injury. *Journal of Spinal Cord Medicine, 40*(1), 76–84. doi:10.1080/10790268.2016.1153293

Yourman, L. C., Cenzer, I. S., Boscardin, W. J., Nguyen, B. T., Smith, A. K., Schonberg, M. A., Schoenborn, N. L., Widera, E. W., Orkaby, A., Rodriguez, A., & Lee, S. J. (2021). Evaluation of time to benefit of statins for the primary prevention of cardiovascular events in adults aged 50 to 75 years: A meta-analysis. *JAMA Internal Medicine, 181*(2), 179–185. doi:10.1001/jamainternmed.2020.6084

Yourman, L. C., Lee, S. J., Schonberg, M. A., Widera, E. W., & Smith, A. K. (2012). Prognostic indices for older adults: A systematic review. *JAMA, 307*(2), 182–192. doi:10.1001/jama.2011.1966

Ziepert, M., Hasenclever, D., Kuhnt, E., Glass, B., Schmitz, N., Pfreundschuh, M., & Loeffler, M. (2010). Standard international prognostic index remains a valid predictor of outcome for patients with aggressive CD20+ B-cell lymphoma in the rituximab era. *Journal of Clinical Oncology: Official Journal of the American Society of Clinical Oncology, 28*(14), 2373–2380. doi:10.1200/JCO.2009.26.2493

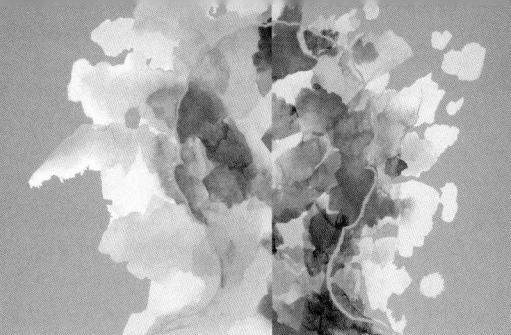

CHAPTER 39

Healthcare Maintenance for Adults With Developmental Disabilities

Geraldine Collins-Bride and Clarissa Kripke

I. Introduction and general background

Individuals with developmental disabilities (DD) experience health disparities across a number of domains. In the context of disability, a healthcare disparity is a population with a difference in health status not directly attributable to the condition leading to or associated with the disability. Disparities are caused in part by inadequate access to appropriate medical care, accommodations, services, and supports. They are compounded by intersectional issues with social determinants of health, such as poverty, social exclusion, and implicit racial bias (Andresen et al., 2013; Engleman et al., 2019; Horner-Johnson et al., 2013; Vanderbaum et al., 2018).

The current healthcare system presents an array of structural deficits that severely limit its ability to provide appropriate care for this population. These deficits include:
- Lack of clinicians who are knowledgeable and skilled in the treatment of adults with DD
- Lack of regular health assessment and care
- Lack of coordination among provider teams
- Limited availability of services in places where patients with DD live and reside
- Lack of access to health-related, long-term care services and supports
- Exclusion from research and proven care guidelines (Bear et al., 2020; Autistic Self Advocacy Network, Office of Developmental Primary Care, 2014)

Life expectancy and quality of life have improved significantly over the past several decades as people with DD moved from institutional settings to community-based care. The life expectancy of younger adults with DD approaches that of the general population (Patja et al., 2000).

With the rise in life expectancy comes the increased risk for chronic diseases. Many of the chronic illnesses acquired by elders with DD are similar to those seen in the general population, such as cardiovascular disease, cancers, pulmonary disease, diabetes, and renal diseases. Although individuals with DD do have an increased incidence of respiratory, gastrointestinal, and musculoskeletal problems, it is imperative that the clinician not focus solely on these conditions and perform routine screening for other chronic diseases, as well as for secondary conditions that some patients with disabilities may be at increased risk of developing, such as hearing loss, dental caries, osteoporosis, and contractures.

People with DD have a higher prevalence of chronic medical conditions such as epilepsy and neurologic disorders, dermatologic problems, fractures and orthopedic problems, gastrointestinal disorders, cardiovascular disorders, and mental health concerns. They are at risk for secondary conditions such as pressure sores, constipation, medication side effects, and injuries. To access healthcare services and manage their health, they may need support or accommodations for communication, decision making, mobility, sensory processing, personal care, or behavior (Folch et al., 2019; van Timmeren et al., 2016).

Currently, most adults with DD live in the community in their own homes, with their families, or in group homes. Some lead very independent lives, and others require a variety of services. Supports can include, but are not limited to, healthcare advocates, independent living coaches, vocational coaches, and case managers. They can also include personal assistants, including direct support professionals, paid or unpaid family members, home health workers, and board and care home staff.

Transition of care from the child-oriented to an adult healthcare system is a particularly challenging and vulnerable time for patients, families, and clinicians. Clinicians who serve children have accumulated a wealth of information about the individual and often have a well-established, trusting relationship with the patient and the family or caregivers. Clinicians who serve adults are rarely trained in this field and often do not have the resources to provide the range of services required for comprehensive care. It is not uncommon for pediatric healthcare providers to continue to provide care for individuals with DD well beyond the age of 21 (Levy et al., 2020; Kripke, 2014).

A. *Definition of developmental disabilities*

The Developmental Disabilities Assistance and Civil Rights Act of 2000 defines DD as a severe, chronic disability caused by physical or mental impairments manifesting before the age of 22 that is expected to continue indefinitely. These impairments cause limitations in three or more of the following categories: self-care, learning, receptive and expressive language, mobility, self-direction, capacity for independent living, and economic self-sufficiency (Developmental Disabilities Assistance and Bill of Rights Act, 2000; American Association on Intellectual and Developmental Disabilities, 2010). Many states define DD according to specific diagnoses or functions and have different age cutoffs. To receive Medicaid funding, states must have a mechanism of delivering supports and services to individuals meeting the state eligibility requirements for DD, although the structure of each system varies by state. Both federal and state statutes have been established to determine when an individual is eligible for services and supports. Some states use diagnostic labels such as intellectual disability, autism, or cerebral palsy in their eligibility criteria. Nobody's cognition should be summarized by a two- or three-digit number on a standardized test, and the cognition of people who do not have a robust form of fluent expressive communication cannot be accurately assessed. Neuropsychological or neuroeducational assessments use a variety of assessment tools and methods to characterize cognitive strengths and challenges and are more useful for selecting services and interventions than standardized intelligence tests.

Clinicians can refer individuals to the local or regional developmental resource center for an eligibility consultation or determination of changes to their services and supports as their needs evolve.

There is a strong self-advocacy movement, and the disability rights community has fought hard to dispel the old notion that individuals with disabilities are limited in their capacity to contribute meaningfully and be fully included in society. People with disabilities have the same rights to lead productive, independent lives as other citizens, and communities benefit from diversity, including having people with DDs integrated into school, work, religious, and social organizations. The Americans With Disabilities Act guarantees people with disabilities the right to access healthcare services, although many physical, financial, and programmatic barriers still exist. The *Olmstead v. LC* Supreme Court decision holds that people with disabilities have a right to receive state-funded supports and services in the community rather than in institutions.

B. *Overview of common syndromes seen in primary care*
1. Intellectual disability

Intellectual disability (ID) is a disability characterized by significant limitations in both intellectual functioning (reasoning, learning, problem solving) and adaptive behavior, which covers a range of everyday social and practical skills. The environment and expectations of a community affect adaptive behavior. This disability originates before the age of 22 (Schalock et al., 2021). Etiologies of ID include genetic conditions; intrauterine factors (asphyxia, maternal infections, trauma, and substance use); perinatal factors (hypoxic-ischemic encephalopathy, sepsis, and prematurity); and postnatal causes, such as childhood infections, environmental toxins, trauma, and severe malnutrition. Alcohol exposure during pregnancy is the toxin most clearly linked to ID. IDs are complex neurodevelopmental conditions that typically affect many areas of life function. The prevalence of ID is approximately 2% and covers a wide range of cognitive traits and characteristics. The majority of adults with ID (80%) have mild ID. Regardless of functional ability, people with IDs benefit from exposure to rich life experiences. Clinicians should presume competence, which means to assume that all people communicate and all people have the capacity to learn, grow, and improve skills. It is important not to make assumptions about people's intellect when it cannot be accurately assessed because of limitations in expressive communication. People with profound expressive communication problems can have normal receptive language. Individuals with more severe functional limitations and communication challenges are at particular risk for not receiving regular preventive health screening and lifestyle counseling. Counseling, health education, and information should be delivered directly to patients and their supporters using plain language, pictures, or other visual supports and demonstrations, regardless of whether the patient's understanding of the messages can be confirmed. Patients with ID often understand far more than is apparent from their facial expressions, body movements, or other responses. Also, cognitive challenges with understanding health information; with the executive function or skills to follow through on healthcare recommendations; or with memory, concentration, and focus can be missed if patients do not have obvious speech difficulties. It is helpful to ask how your patient learns best and if they have any supporters who help them with their medical care.

2. Cerebral palsy

Cerebral palsy (CP) is a term used to describe a group of chronic conditions affecting body movement and muscle coordination. It is caused by differences in one or more specific areas of the brain, usually occurring during fetal development; before, during, or shortly after birth; or during infancy. Thus, these conditions are not caused by problems in the muscles or nerves. Instead, damage to motor areas in the brain affect the brain's ability to control movement and posture. The diagnosis of CP is not appropriate for individuals with motor impairments caused by spinal cord injuries, peripheral nerve injuries, myopathies, or any other etiology that is not brain based. Historically, individuals with a physical exam consistent with CP were given the diagnosis only if the brain abnormalities or injuries occurred within the first 1–2 years of life—the period associated with the greatest amount of brain development. The time frame for applying the CP diagnosis has expanded over the last several years because of the recognition that the brain continues to develop throughout childhood. Children with brain damage secondary to central nervous system infections, tumors, or nonaccidental or accidental trauma that causes motor impairments meet the criteria for a CP diagnosis, even if the injury occurs after 2 years of age. Co-occurring sensory, perceptual, cognitive, and behavioral differences are common. There is no longer an exact age cutoff for applying the diagnosis; clinical judgment is used to identify children with clear brain-related motor limitations.

Cerebral refers to the brain, and *palsy* refers to muscle weakness and difficulty with control. Because people may not be able to voluntarily control muscles, this can have an impact on the ability to speak, gesture, or type. CP itself is not progressive (i.e., brain changes do not evolve); however, secondary conditions such as muscle spasticity can develop, which may get better over time, get worse, or remain the same. CP is not communicable. It is not a disease and should not be referred to as such. Although CP is not "curable" in the accepted sense, training, therapy, adaptive equipment, and an accommodating physical and social environment and access to education, employment, and services can greatly improve function and quality of life (Vitrikas et al., 2020; Wimalasundera & Stevenson, 2016).

The prevalence of CP is 2.1–3.3 per 1,000 live births, with higher rates seen in males and African Americans (Durkin et al., 2016). The greatest risk factor for CP is prematurity. An estimated one in three very low-birth-weight children (<1,500 g) are eventually diagnosed with CP. CP occurs as a consequence of the perinatal course. Spastic diplegia (greater involvement in the legs than the arms) is the type of CP most commonly associated with prematurity, with hallmark findings of periventricular leukomalacia commonly seen on computed tomography (CT). Hemiplegic (one side of the body) CP is almost always caused by an in utero or perinatal stroke, which should raise concerns about possible familial hypercoagulable disorders. Other etiologies for CP include chromosomal and brain anomalies, genetic and metabolic conditions, infection, and trauma.

Individuals with CP frequently have problems with spasticity, seizures, mobility, dystonia, dysarthria, swallowing, constipation, and gastroesophageal reflux (Fortuna et al., 2018). People with CP have a wide range of intellect, so it is important not to make assumptions about people's intellect based on their appearance or method of expressive communication. Many people with CP have normal intelligence, even if they have difficulty producing clear speech and controlling their bodies (Stadskleiv, 2020). Performing clinical interviews with nonverbal patients requires special techniques or adaptive equipment. For video models of appropriate interview techniques, visit https://www.youtube.com/watch?v=YGOm7NKGGWM. Symptoms of fatigue, depression, impaired mobility, and musculoskeletal problems frequently worsen with aging. Individuals with CP have high rates of cardiovascular and respiratory disease, with aspiration pneumonia as the leading cause of death across all age groups (Jonsson et al., 2021).

3. Autism spectrum disorders

Autism spectrum disorders (ASDs) are heterogeneous neurodevelopmental conditions of unclear etiology that are classified according to the *Diagnostic and Statistical Manual of Mental Disorders*, 5th edition (*DSM-5*; American Psychiatric Association, 2013) criteria, which include atypical development in two major areas: (1) communication used for social purposes and (2) restricted, repetitive patterns of interests, behaviors, or activities. The hallmark of ASD is atypical social interaction. This can result from sensory-motor or movement differences or problems with language or social understanding. In addition, current *DSM-5* criteria require deficits in the use of nonverbal communication (e.g., quality of eye contact, use of gestures, odd facial expressions, misreading other people's facial expressions, tone of voice) and difficulties with establishing meaningful relationships with peers. Other criteria include a series of highly focused interests over their lifetime that are either unusual or highly focused, a need for routines and rituals and distress with change, and repetitive motor mannerisms (hand-flapping, finger flicking, or shuddering, occurring most often when the individual is happy or distressed). Although it has long been recognized that people with ASD react in atypical ways to various sensory inputs, ranging from extreme negative reactions to sounds, smells, or touch to fascination or soothing related to sounds, visual stimuli, or movement, it was not until the publication of the *DSM-5* that sensory issues were included in the diagnostic criteria for ASD. It is extremely important for the clinician to understand the particular sensory issues that the individual with ASD experiences in order to deliver good care.

People on the autism spectrum have a wide range of strengths and challenges, which is one of the reasons that the condition is considered to be a spectrum. Language skills range from nonverbal to normal or advanced language skills. Problems with motor planning and coordination, sometimes affecting speech, are increasingly being recognized in persons with ASD. Speech is a motor function. Language is processed in other parts of the brain. Therefore, nonspeaking autistic people can have normal receptive language and can benefit from high- or low-technology augmentative and alternative communication. A toolkit for accessing communication assessments, funding, and accommodations can be found at https://odpc.ucsf.edu/communications-paper. Like people with CP, people with autism can benefit from voice output devices, keyboards, or letterboards (United for Communication Choice, n.d.). They may need extensive training to develop the motor skills to use the technology or a communication regulation partner to assist. Individuals with average to advanced expressive and receptive language skills may demonstrate deficits in how to use language for social purposes (referred to as *pragmatic* language).

Some people on the autism spectrum are highly verbal or skilled in writing and mechanical skills. Some have challenges with communication and motor skills, including difficulty with articulation and controlling and coordinating movements. Sensory processing differences combined with communication and motor planning problems and lack of accommodation and understanding can lead to difficulties with social interaction, misinterpreted behavior, and difficulty developing friendships and peer relationships. They can also lead to the behaviors seen in ASD, as described previously, or regulating "stims" (self-stimulating behaviors); a narrow focus on specific interests or activities; and difficulties with changes to routine, environments, or transitions.

The prevalence of people diagnosed with ASD continues to rise, but how much of the increase can be attributed to changes in diagnostic criteria, access to services, and reclassification of individuals with other DDs continues to be a subject of debate.

ASDs are diagnosed in boys four times more frequently than girls. The incidence of intellectual impairment is much lower than previously estimated once testing using appropriate methods is done. Standardized tests that require speech or normal sensory and motor control should not be administered to people with speech, sensory, and motor deficits because they lead to misleading results. Many individuals with ASD experience sensory integration problems and may be extremely sensitive to sounds or stimuli in the environment. Sensory processing differences should be explored to learn how to increase the comfort of people with autism in medical environments and during the physical examination. Many people with ASD also have seizure disorders and associated mental health conditions. Anxiety almost always accompanies ASD, with depression being quite common as the individual approaches the teenage and adult years. Although individuals with ASD may experience the same range of health problems as the general population, the communication and behavioral features of this condition often require accommodations to deliver high-quality care in primary care settings. These accommodations should be individualized but might include preparation for the visit or examination ahead of time and the use of a timer to indicate the start and stop of the examination (Nicolaidis et al., 2014).

4. Genetic disorders

There are many genetic disorders associated with ID and DD. The completion of the Human Genome Project in 2003 sparked the discovery of new genetic testing examining the whole genome for duplications and deletions associated with ID and DD. One of the most common and well characterized of these genetic conditions is Down syndrome, a chromosomal disorder with an estimated incidence of 1 in 700 babies born (Centers for Disease Control [CDC], 2020). The risk for Down syndrome rises with increasing maternal age, although prenatal diagnosis has reduced the incidence of Down syndrome. This demographic change may change with increasing restrictions on pregnancy terminations. The distinguishing characteristics of Down syndrome include facial dysmorphology (the term *dysmorphic* indicates an abnormal appearance), muscle hypotonia, and ID of varying degrees. Numerous medical problems are seen with Down syndrome, including visual and hearing impairments, higher body weight, sleep apnea, hypothyroidism, cardiac and respiratory diseases, celiac disease and other gastrointestinal disorders, autoimmune disorders, and early-onset Alzheimer (Bull, 2020). There are healthcare guidelines for following individuals with Down syndrome from the American Academy of Pediatrics Council on Genetics Health Supervision for Children and Adolescents With Down Syndrome (Bull et al., 2022; Tsou, 2020).

When genetic syndromes are suspected or the etiology of a DD is unclear, referral to genetics can be helpful. Given the advances in today's genetic testing, it may be helpful to refer adults with

unidentified ID for a genetics evaluation for further diagnostic testing.
5. Epilepsy
Epilepsy refers to a group of conditions that are characterized by the recurrent disturbance of cerebral function (seizures) caused by excessive neuronal discharges in the brain occurring in a paroxysmal manner. An epileptic seizure occurs when the cerebral cortex is rendered hyperexcitable (because of an increase in excitatory neurotransmission, a decrease in inhibitory neurotransmission, or a disturbance in brain circuitry) by any of a number of causes, including metabolic disturbances, injuries, strokes, tumors, and developmental abnormalities. For further discussion of epilepsy, see Chapter 51, Epilepsy.

II. Database

A. *Subjective*

It can be challenging to obtain an accurate and comprehensive history in individuals with DD, especially when the individual has communication or cognitive impairments. Ask how best to support a patient's communication and what accommodations they need. In order to gather a comprehensive and accurate understanding of the patient, start by collecting information directly from the patient. Historical data can be obtained from a variety of sources, including supporters, family, case managers, ID and DD nurses, school or developmental services records, and medical record review.

Supported healthcare decision making is a process where people with disabilities can name trusted supporters to assist them with communicating, accessing healthcare services, making decisions, and implementing their healthcare plan. People with disabilities should have the same right to make healthcare choices as everyone else. Supported healthcare decision-making recognizes that people can manage their own health care even if they cannot do so independently. The person with the disability retains the right to choose whom they trust to provide support, the type of support they want, and the right to make all final healthcare decisions.

Supported healthcare decision making recognizes that people learn to make decisions by making decisions and that they can develop skills to direct their lives and health care when given opportunities and support. In guardianships or conservatorships, a judge denies those rights not just for the current decision but for all future decisions. In guardianship or conservatorship, the right to make decisions is assigned by a judge to someone else. Judges may name family members as conservators, or they may choose to name a stranger.

Sometimes a person lacks the capacity to make a specific decision at a specific moment in time. *Capacity* means a person understands the options, understands the risks and benefits of each option, can weigh them against each other, and can communicate a choice. If a person is unable to complete this process, they can name a healthcare proxy or power of attorney. If they are unable to name a proxy, the medical center or hospital protocols should be followed. To support your patient's abilities to make decisions, ask your patient:

- How do we communicate best?
- What can I do to accommodate you?
- Do you use any services or supports?
- What information would you like shared with others?
- Would you like more information about supported healthcare decision making or a referral to social, legal, or disability services?
- Presume competence and start with your usual shared decision-making process.
- Move to supported and, finally, substituted decision-making processes as needed.

Some respectful ways to ask about supports include the following:

- Do you have any legal documents, such as a supported healthcare decision-making agreement, power of attorney, or advance directive?
- Do you have a trusted supporter who helps you make decisions?
- How do you make decisions? Is there someone who assists you with that?
- Is there someone you would like to consult to help you make your decision?
- Do you need more time to make a decision?
- Do you want to think about it at home and tell me later?

Do you have a health passport, accommodation letter, or medical summary that describes how I can best support yous (National Resource Center for Supported Decision-Making, n.d.; Office of Developmental Primary Care, 2021)?

In some systems, a structured health interview and examination tool is used to collect and document important past and current health issues. An example of such a tool can be found at https://inclusivehealth.specialolympics.org/resources/tools/idd-toolkit-for-primary-care-providers. This yearly health assessment form is a component of many healthcare delivery models for adults with DDs throughout the world, although it is not consistently in use in the United States. These health assessment forms have been well studied and capture key information on functional, behavioral, developmental, and psychosocial issues pertinent to adults with DD (Byrne et al., 2015; Carey et al., 2017; Robertson et al., 2014). Regardless of the type of data collection tool used for the history and physical examination, when possible, the clinician should allow extra time for appointments when seeing individuals with DD. It can also be helpful to schedule visits at regular or more frequent intervals to address the complexities of the patient's healthcare issues. Periodic telehealth or video visits can be a nice compliment to in person visits and allow the clinician to provide care when transportation or behavioral factors limit the feasibility of an office visit. Flexibility and creativity are often required to ensure a successful office visit. Home visits or visits in community settings can be very effective ways to provide care. Such strategies as desensitization, telephone conferences with supporters, and obtaining assistance from health advocates or case managers can allow the visit to proceed more smoothly. Always attempt to prepare the individual for the appointment and enlist support from a trusted supporter. For severely agitated patients, sedation with a low dose of benzodiazepines, such as lorazepam, 0.5–1 mg, may be indicated. A test dose of the medication can be tried at home first to determine the timing of peak effect and dose and because some patients have been known to experience a paradoxical reaction where agitation actually increases rather than decreases. Multidisciplinary telemedicine consultation has been shown to be an effective option for addressing difficult behavioral, medical, and psychiatric issues in some patients with complex DDs (Krysta et al., 2021; Lankamp et al., 2015).

1. Pertinent past medical history, as outlined in Chapter 38 (Adult Health Maintenance and Promotion), with a focus on the following additional data:
   a. Etiology of DD, with review of pediatric records and medical summary when possible. Note previous developmental and genetic evaluations. Note any history of institutionalizations.
   b. Previous medical illnesses, noting history of:
      i. Epilepsy: frequency of seizures, medications, use of seizure tracking logs, and emergency management plan
      ii. Gastroesophageal reflux disease: previous workup, treatment, and *Helicobacter pylori* testing
      iii. Constipation: Unrecognized or untreated constipation can be a significant cause of morbidity and mortality. Note previous workup and treatment.
      iv. Visual impairment: use of eyeglasses or contact lenses and date of last ophthalmology examination
      v. Hearing impairment: use of hearing devices and date of last audiology examination
      vi. Sensory perceptual differences: Note processing of sounds, touch, taste, and sensation, which may affect the physical examination or interpretation of pain behavior. Document recommendations from patients, supporters, family, and others about accommodations, strategies, and the best methods of approaching individuals with sensory integration differences.
   c. Communication: Document the patient's usual method of communication (verbal, written, sign language, behaviors, or gestures) and use of augmentative or alternative communication methods or technology.
   d. Mobility and neuromotor function: Note if the patient is ambulatory or nonambulatory, use of adaptive equipment, and how much time per day is spent using the equipment. Note how the person transfers if non–weight bearing and what assistance is needed for transfers (equipment, such as a Hoyer lift; staff or family and how many are needed). Note fine and gross motor skills, spasticity, and changes in motor tone, either increased or decreased.
   e. Swallowing and feeding: episodes of choking or coughing with eating, history of aspiration, pneumonia, last swallowing study, and speech therapy treatments
   f. Bowel and bladder function: constipation, urinary incontinence or retention, and use of diapers or other incontinence supplies
   g. Dental health issues: Caries, periodontal disease, and gingival hyperplasia. Identification of risk factors for dental disease is important to avoid the effects of premature demineralization. Often, patients have undiagnosed conditions of gastric reflux, resulting in dental erosion, or medication-induced xerostomia, which leaves the oral cavity hyperacidic and prone to premature demineralization. Checking for adequate and healthy saliva can help minimize the effects of dental disease. Prevention strategies of neutralizing the acids in the mouth through sodium bicarbonate rinses, increasing hydration, and possible fluoride varnishes or sealants can prevent dental caries (American Academy of Pediatric Dentistry, 2021). Inquire about ongoing dental care, cleanings, and need for sedation before dental visits.
   h. Mental health issues: Depression, posttraumatic stress disorder, and anxiety are the most common disorders, with rates similar to those in the general population. There is a much lower incidence of psychotic disorders, although antipsychotic medication is often overprescribed to control behavior that is considered to be "difficult." Ask specifically how symptoms manifest themselves. Some patients may be capable of verbally expressing mood symptoms, and others may express symptoms as a change in behavior. Behavior needs to be interpreted developmentally. For example, a person with an ID may have imaginary friends and may have tantrums when frustrated. This behavior may be appropriate to the person's intellectual development and not an indication of a mental illness. Document the patient's baseline behavior and review annually for changes (Fletcher, 2018).
   i. Medications: Polypharmacy is a significant issue, with multiple medications often used to treat the same health problem. This is an especially

common, ineffective, and harmful practice used in the treatment of aggressive or other problem behaviors. It is important to note the indications and duration of use for all medications, with attention to any side effects, drug interactions, and medication efficacy.
  j. Immunization status: In addition to the primary vaccination series and scheduled boosters, note if the patient has received vaccines for hepatitis A and B, pneumococcal disease, COVID, RSV and seasonal flu.
  k. History of injuries or falls
  l. History of abuse, victimization, or human trafficking: This is especially prevalent in those individuals with ID, but it is also seen with high frequency in all individuals with disabilities. The majority of abusers are family members, relatives, caregivers, neighbors, classmates, educators, or staff members assigned to support the person with disabilities (Collins & Murphy, 2021; Tomsa et al., 2021).
  m. History of resistive or challenging behavior: Behavior is often a form of communication but can easily be misinterpreted, especially in disabilities that affect sensory processing and movement. Difficult behaviors that are new or a change from the individual's usual level of functioning may signify an undiagnosed medical or psychiatric problem or may be a sign of a mismatch between a person's needs and the services and supports they are receiving or the environments in which they live and work. Behaviors can also be the result of difficulties with motor initiation, impulsivity, or compulsions and are not purposeful or under the person's control. New behaviors always warrant a medical evaluation. Additionally, new behaviors or a significant change in behaviors can indicate that the individual has experienced abuse or neglect; therefore, assessment specific to this is also important. Note previous medical and psychiatric evaluations of behavior change. Document behavioral, environmental, and pharmacologic therapies used for treatment.
2. Family history, with emphasis on developmental and genetic disorders
3. Occupational history: People with DD work in a variety of settings. Inquire about a job coach or other personnel support present at work. Obtain specific details about job tasks to screen for repetitive-motion injuries. Ask about job satisfaction and relationships with coworkers.
4. Personal and social history
   a. Housing status and supports: Note if the patient lives independently and what support is required for independent living, such as in-home support services, independent living coaches, or case management support. Include type of housing (apartment, family, or residential group home), noting how many individuals live in the home and the ratio of staff/caregivers needed to provide a safe environment.
   b. Relationships and social support network: Note significant relationships with family, friends, and sexual and life partners. Inquire about the quantity and quality of social contact and relationships (Office of Developmental Primary Care, n.d.).
   c. Future goals: Note desired future personal, educational, and occupational goals.
5. Habits
   a. Nutrition
   b. Exercise and activity
   c. Tobacco, alcohol, and substance use
   d. Sleep
   e. Sexual activity
6. Interdisciplinary healthcare team members: Note each team member's name and contact information, which may include a case manager, nurse, dentist, psychologist, behavior specialist, pharmacist, physical therapist, occupational therapist, speech and language therapist, psychotherapist, and medical specialists (**Figure 39-1**).

B. Objective
1. Perform an annual physical examination, with blood pressure, height, weight, and total body weight. The physical examination is particularly important for patients with cognitive and communication impairments, where subjective symptoms may be difficult to elicit (**Figure 39-2**).
2. Pay particular attention to a careful oral examination, given the frequency of dental disease (National Institute of Dental and Craniofacial Research, 2009; Sullivan et al., 2018).
3. Perform annual office-based vision and hearing screening examinations (Sullivan et al., 2018).
4. Document the patient's baseline, typical behavior, and method of communication.
5. Schedule a separate appointment dedicated solely to the gynecologic examination. Extra time is needed for the pelvic examination because these examinations can be challenging for providers and for women with disabilities (**Figure 39-3**).

III. Assessment

A. *Identify the patient's general and specific health risk profile. If the cause of the DD is unknown or unclear, consider a referral to genetics for an evaluation (Sullivan et al., 2018). According to the 2021 American College of Medical Genetics and Genomics (ACMG) practice guideline, whole-exome and whole-genome sequencing have a much higher diagnostic yield than previous standard genetic testing (Manickam et al., 2021). Many adults with neurodevelopmental disorders have not had a comprehensive diagnostic evaluation and may benefit from further testing, although insurance companies often deny payment for these evaluations.*

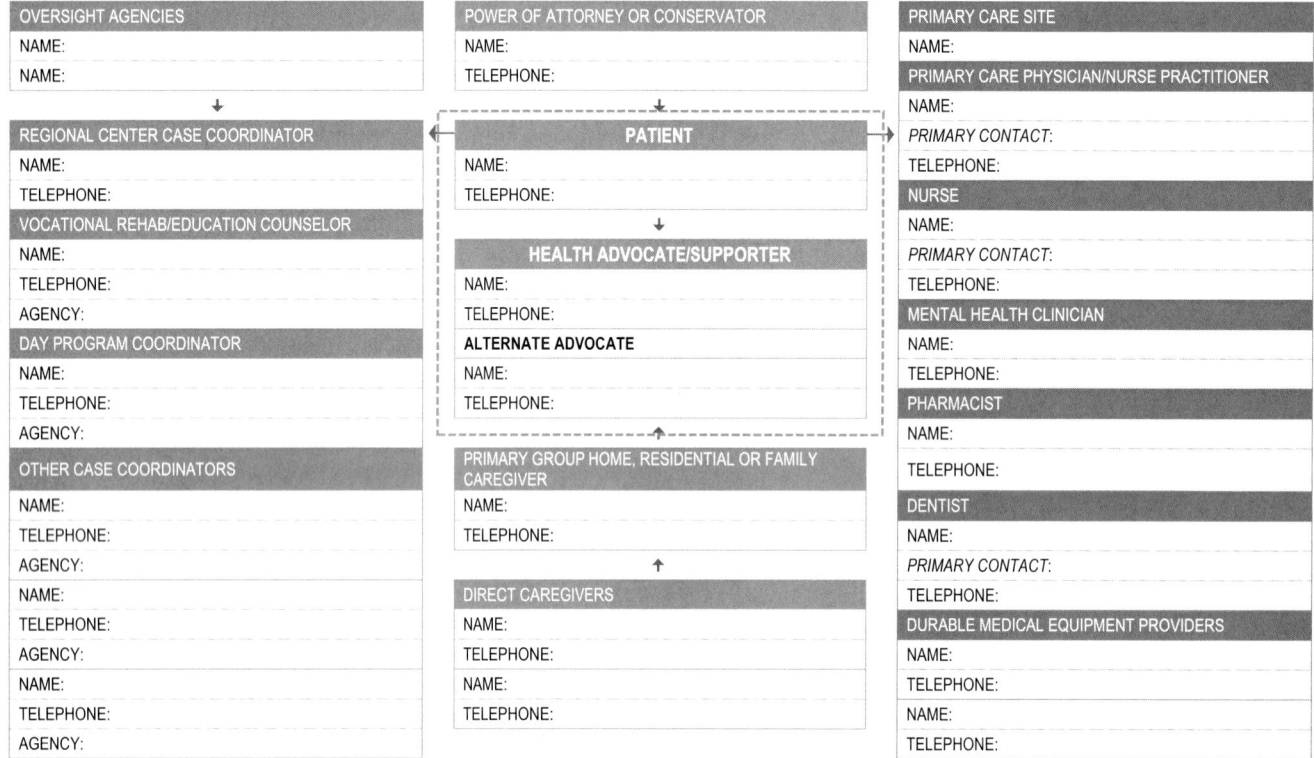

Figure 39-1 Interdisciplinary Healthcare Team Chart
Reproduced from Office of Developmental Primary Care, University of California, San Francisco. http://odpc.ucsf.edu

B. Recognize health habits that benefit from lifestyle modification.
C. Ascertain additional members of the interdisciplinary health team who would be beneficial to improve the healthcare plan (Figure 39-1).
D. Determine the support needed for medical decision making and informed consent for diagnostic testing and procedures. Document whether the individual has a power of attorney or a legal decision maker for healthcare decisions. Although many individuals with ID and DD require the support of families and supporters for decision making, it is important to remember that people with ID and DD have the right to make decisions about their lives and their health care. For individuals who lack the capacity for decision making even with support, and have no identified power of attorney for health care, the state developmental disability service can be contacted for procedures to support medical decision making for diagnostic, treatment, or emergency decisions.
E. Assess the patient and supporter's assets, barriers, and resources needed for implementing recommendations.

IV. Plan
A. Diagnostics (screening and secondary prevention tests)
Follow screening guidelines recommended for the general population, as outlined in Chapter 38, Adult Healthcare Maintenance and Promotion. Disparities in preventive screening tests for people with disabilities as compared to the general population have been well documented for years. These disparities can be improved significantly with some understanding of the support and accommodations needed to be successful. Examples of these accommodations can be seen with breast and colon cancer screening. Mammography screening for breast cancer for women with mobility problems may require that radiology technicians have additional training. Colonoscopy screening for colorectal cancer may require that the individual have extra support to complete the bowel prep. Some individuals may need to be admitted to the hospital the day prior to the exam for the prep to be successfully completed. Although these strategies require extra thought and time, individuals with DD deserve the same quality of

You may need to provide support to communicate with a patient with a developmental disability. Communication may take more thought and planning. Assess whether your patient uses spoken language; if not, he or she may use other forms of language, such as sign language, written language, or augmentative and alternative communication. Even people who do not use language can communicate through behavior, facial expressions, and sounds. Listening to your patient may require using more of your senses. The following are some ideas, but ask your patient and caregivers what works best for them.

- Order an interpreter if spoken English is not the patient's primary language.
- Use person-first or identity-first language for the autistic, deaf, and blind communities (unless your patient prefers something else).
- Talk directly to your patient in an adult voice and listen attentively for your patient to respond and to finish. If your patient appears to be thinking, wait quietly.
- A patient may have better receptive than expressive language. Use plain language without jargon.
- If your patient is not using words to communicate, then try nonverbal communication strategies, such as demonstrations, pictures, touch, gestures, and facial expressions.
- Get your patient's attention before speaking to him or her.
- Check for understanding by repeating and asking your patient to repeat.
- If necessary, use short, concrete questions that require yes or no answers.
- If necessary, ask questions that can be answered nonverbally. For example, "Show me how you say yes."
- Sit at eye level and treat wheelchairs as personal space. Don't touch a wheelchair without permission.
- Before helping, offer assistance, and wait for a response and instructions.
- Offer to shake hands even if your patient has limited use of hands or an artificial limb.
- Identify yourself and others to people with visual disabilities and indicate to whom you are speaking.
- It is okay to use common idioms that refer to vision or hearing such as, "Have you heard about …" or "See the light …"

Figure 39-2 Exam Room Etiquette
Used with permission from the Office of Developmental Primary Care, Department of Family & Community Medicine, University of California, San Francisco.

For some women with disabilities, pelvic exams can be frightening and potentially uncomfortable. If the situation permits, focus the first visit on history and relationship building alone. The following may be helpful to reduce both the patient's and the provider's anxiety about the pelvic examination:

- Get to know your patient before attempting a pelvic exam.
- Educate the patient and caregivers about the exam.
- Don't assume that a pelvic exam will be any more difficult or uncomfortable for a person with a disability than for anyone else. You don't know until you try.
- Women with disabilities, including those with intellectual disabilities, can and do have sex.
- Use anatomy models with visual demonstration before the visit.
- Allow extra time (this is a must!).
- Encourage your patient to bring a supportive person to the appointment.
- If needed, locate the cervix manually.
- The anatomy of women with disabilities is often normal. However, it may be helpful to have several different pediatric and adult-sized speculums available.
- Pelvic exams can be done in a variety of positions. You may need assistants to hold a flashlight or help the patient maintain a comfortable position.
- Use a soothing voice, deep breathing, visualization, and praise.
- Consider pelvic ultrasound if bimanual exam is not possible.
- Consider using a short-acting benzodiazepine for sedation before a pelvic exam for women who have anxiety, spasticity, or agitation. Obtain consent from the patient or decision maker. Consider a test dose at home prior to the visit. Ask the caregiver to carefully document the patient's reaction, as well as the peak action of the medication.
- Consider doing the exam under conscious sedation or general anesthesia especially if the patient has a scheduled surgical or dental procedure under anesthesia. Other exams, such as echocardiograms, labs, EKG, hearing tests, etc., can be coordinated at the same time.

Figure 39-3 Tips for a Successful Pelvic Exam
Used with permission from the Office of Developmental Primary Care, Department of Family & Community Medicine, University of California, San Francisco.

health care as others in our communities. Depending on the patient's comorbidities, anesthesia risk may outweigh the benefits of colonoscopy.

1. Patients with mobility disorders, spasticity, and/or cognitive impairment may require hospital admission the day prior to testing with colonoscopy and sigmoidoscopy for professional assistance with bowel preparation.
2. Screen for diseases and conditions specific to the patient's underlying DD or known specific developmental syndrome. For specific screening and diagnostic test recommendations, see **Table 39-1**.

Table 39-1 Healthcare Maintenance Guidelines for Adults with Developmental Disabilities

Health Problem	Who to Screen	Test & Frequency	Special Considerations
Abuse & Neglect	All adults	■ Screen yearly with history & physical exam looking for unexplained physical, mental and/or behavioral signs and symptoms such as unexplained bruising, falls, injuries, oral trauma, weight loss, depression, and behavior changes	■ Risk factors include caregiver stress, residential living ■ Signs of neglect can be seen with missed appointments, nonadherence and nonengagement (Sullivan, et al., 2018).
Alcohol & Substance Use	■ All adults	■ Screen yearly with history (although best screening interval is unknown).	■ Traditional screening tools such as the CAGE & AUDIT have not been well tested in this population (Pezzoni & Kouimtsidis, 2015). ■ Substance use disorders are often under-recognized in DD. Alcohol and cannabis misuse can be seen more commonly in mild ID & those living independently (Sullivan, et al., 2018).
Cervical Spine Atlanto-Axial Instability	Adults with Down syndrome	■ Perform an annual neurologic examination for signs and symptoms of cervical myelopathy for patients with Down syndrome. ■ Order cervical spine x-ray with lateral flexion and extension if symptoms develop, such as changes in behavior or activity, changes in hand preference or urinary incontinence. If this is the first C-spine film, also order an anteroposterior view.	Routine screening cervical spine films for asymptomatic individuals with Down syndrome is not recommended (Tsou, et al., 2020), although some organizations continue to require this prior to participation in athletics and other activities.
Dental Disease	■ All adults	■ Perform an annual oral exam. ■ Refer to dentist for regular dental care including cleaning every 6 months or as recommended by the dentist ■ **Check for adequate saliva flow and amount (should be watery and abundant, not bubbly, stringy, or thick)**	■ Pay special attention to dental and gum health in persons with certain syndromes, such as Cornelia de Lange, cerebral palsy, Down, Prader-Willi, Turner, Rett, Williams, and tuberous sclerosis. ■ USPSTF recommends application of fluoride varnish on individuals with high caries risk.
		Comments *Patients with developmental disabilities are at high risk for periodontal disease and dental caries for numerous reasons, including: difficulty maintaining hygiene, lack of access to regular dental care, syndrome-specific susceptibilities, and medication side effects (xerostomia).* *In some patients unable to tolerate office exams and treatment, hospital dentistry under anesthesia may be indicated. Other necessary diagnostic testing should be considered while patient is sedated.*	

Health Problem	Who to Screen	Test & Frequency	Special Considerations
Depression	■ All adults	■ Screen annually or sooner for behaviors or emotions that may indicate depression.	*Patients with developmental disabilities may have difficulty recognizing and communicating symptoms such as depressed mood, anxiety, and sadness. Mental health symptoms are often expressed in physical or behavioral changes. It is critical that healthcare providers obtain information about the patient's usual level of functioning, skills, and behavior in order to assess the potential for mental health disorders.* ■ *See Diagnostic Manual-Intellectual Disabilities for more in-depth discussion on assessment.* (Fletcher, 2018).
Fall Risk	■ All adults	■ Evaluate as part of the annual physical examination including an evaluation of the medication profile for drugs that may affect balance and/or gait. Screen more frequently if there is a change in gait/balance or for individuals at high risk, such as those who have a history of two or more falls in the previous year. ■ For patients with no previous mobility impairments who report one or more falls, consider performing the Get-Up and Go Test: www.ncbi.nlm.nih.gov/pubmed/3487300. Patients having difficulty with this test should be referred to a physical/occupational therapist for a full fall evaluation.	■ If the patient has had an increase in falls or a decline in function, a medical evaluation of the cause is warranted.
Hearing	■ All adults	■ Screen annually subjectively or objectively with office-based testing (Whisper Test). ■ Refer to audiology at regular intervals. ■ Refer to audiology for hearing assessment every 5 years after age 45 (every 3 years throughout life for patients with Down syndrome).	■ Reevaluate hearing if problems are reported or changes in behavior are noted.

Comments
Other syndromes associated with hearing impairments include Cornelia de Lange, Noonan, Usher, and Smith-Magenis.
Methods for testing may include the following:

Method	Applicable for Developmental Age (years)
OtoAcoustic Emissions (OAE)	> 0
Auditory Brainstem Responses (ABR)	> 0
Behavioral observation audiometry	> 0
Pure tone audiometry with visual reinforcement	> 1
Whispered speech	> 3
Pure tone (play) audiometry	> 3–4

(continues)

Table 39-1 Healthcare Maintenance Guidelines for Adults with Developmental Disabilities *(continued)*

Health Problem	Who to Screen	Test & Frequency	Special Considerations
Obesity	■ All adults	■ Measure height and weight annually.	■ Consider weight on home scale in more familiar setting. ■ Accommodations for patients unable to stand include using a Lift Team, a wheelchair scale, Hoyer Lift, and/or hospital bed that includes a scale.
Osteoporosis	■ Women ≥ age 65 & younger women whose 10-year fracture risk is ≥ 9.3% ■ All adults with ID/DD at high risk.	■ Bone mineral density (BMD) screening with dual-energy x-ray absorptiometry (DEXA) testing at the spine and hip earlier and at regular intervals for high-risk patients ■ Recommended screening interval is unknown.	■ The typical sites for DEXA scans (lumbar spine & hip) may be very difficult for some individuals with mobility impairments &/or spasticity. Alternate testing methods are needed.
	–	■ Although the age to begin screening is unclear, some authors suggest age 40 for patients residing in institutions and age 45 for patients residing in the community. ■ Check serum vitamin D 25 OH levels at regular intervals	

Comments
High-risk factors in patients with developmental disabilities include mobility impairments, long-term use of antiepileptic drugs or antipsychotics, nutritional issues, and oral-motor problems. Patients with Down syndrome, cerebral palsy, and Prader-Willi syndrome are also at greater risk.
High-risk factors in the general population include osteopenia on plain films, history of vertebral fractures, early menopause, chronic steroid use, low body weight, cigarette use, and positive family history of osteoporosis.
See FRAX: WHO Fracture Risk Assessment Tool: www.shef.ac.uk/FRAX/. Note that mobility is not calculated in this assessment tool.

Thyroid Disease	■ Adults with Down syndrome	■ Monitor thyroid-stimulating hormone (TSH) every 1-2 years beginning at age 21 (Tsou, et al., 2020).	

Comments
Symptoms of thyroid disease are often not elicited due to cognitive impairment and/or communication differences in patients with developmental disabilities.
Consider TSH testing if unexplained change in behavior or level of functioning.
Increased risk for thyroid disease seen in patients with Down syndrome and the elderly.

Tuberculosis	All adults with DD	Screen routinely with tuberculin skin test (TST) or serum Quantiferon-TB Gold test based on likelihood of exposure	Serum Quantiferon-TB Gold test if the individual is unlikely to return to have TST read or those who have had previous Bacillus Calmette–Guérin (BCG) vaccination.

Comments
Consider tuberculin skin testing every 1 to 2 years for patients who live or work in aggregate settings (board and care homes, intermediate care facilities, day programs).

Health Problem	Who to Screen	Test & Frequency	Special Considerations
Vision	■ All adults with DD	■ Screen annually subjectively or objectively with office-based tests (Snellen test). ■ Refer to ophthalmology for exam and glaucoma screening at least once before age 40 ■ Refer for ophthalmologic exam and glaucoma screening every 5 years after age 45 or as recommended by ophthalmologist	
	■ Adults with Down syndrome	■ Refer to ophthalmology for exam and glaucoma screening by age 30 for patients with Down syndrome.	
	Comments *Screen more frequently for persons with diabetes, those on long-term psychiatric medication, and those with syndromes associated with vision deficits/ocular abnormalities, such as Cornelia de Lange, Fragile X, Down, Smith-Magenis, tuberous sclerosis, and Velocardiofacial.*		
Counseling			
Lifestyle Modification/ Healthy Quality of Life	**Discuss:** ■ Adequate calcium and vitamin D supplementation ■ Dental hygiene ■ Fall risk assessment and prevention ■ Nutrition—Excellent resource is the Montana Disability & Health Program: Nutrition for Individuals with Intellectual or Developmental Disabilities, http://mtdh.ruralinstitute.umt.edu/?page_id=813 ■ Physical activity (regular schedule with structured staff training to support & reinforce) ■ Tobacco and substance abuse cessation ■ Sexual health, including: contraception, sexually transmitted infection prevention, and healthy relationships		
	Comments *Critical to include supporters, health advocates, and parents/family members to help reinforce teaching concepts.*		
Advanced directives & end-of-life planning	■ Schedule dedicated time for discussion with the individual and support team ■ Excellent resource: Thinking Ahead Matters (End-of-Life Planning for People with DD, http://coalitionccc.org/tools-resources/people-with-developmental-disabilities/		
Medication Review	■ Review medications at regular intervals with patients and caregivers to ensure adherence with regimen and evaluate for side effects and drug interactions.		
	Comments *High rates of polypharmacy exist. See medication watch list*: http://odpc.ucsf.edu/sites/odpc.ucsf.edu/files/pdf_docs/MedFest-Medical-Watch-List.pdf		
Safety	■ Review safety practices per individual circumstance, such as stranger and street safety for patients who live independently; prevention of head trauma in patients with frequent seizures; and street safety for patients with unpredictable behavior.		

©2022 Geraldine Collins-Bride, MS, ANP-BC, FAAN. Non-commercial use with attribution is permitted.

B. *Treatment/Plan*
1. For general health guidelines, see Chapter 38, Adult Healthcare Maintenance and Promotion.
2. For recommendations targeted toward individuals with DDs, see Table 39-1.
3. For immunizations: See the CDC Recommended Adult Immunization Schedule at http://www.cdc.gov/vaccines/schedules/index.html.
4. For bone health: Advise adequate calcium (1,500 mg per day) and vitamin D (400–800 IU per day)

> Person-first language was developed by disability advocates to educate the community at large. It emphasizes the individual before the disability. For example, "Tom has Down syndrome." Some people, especially those in the autistic, blind, and deaf communities, view their disability as an integral part of who they are. They may use identity-firstlanguage such as "autistic man" or "blind person." Language evolves and the disability community is diverse. It is always appropriate to inquire about and use the language your patient prefers.
>
> Avoid describing people with disabilities as overly courageous, brave, or special merely for having a disability. It is not unusual for people with disabilities to accomplish significant things and participate in and manage activities of daily living despite functional limitations. It is always appropriate to celebrate the achievement of personal goals and milestones.
>
> Also, avoid describing people with disabilities as overly pitiful and unfortunate. Most people with disabilities do not consider their lives tragic. They rate their quality of life far higher than many nondisabled people estimate.
>
> Likewise, don't assume that people are unhappy or heroic simply because they are caring for a relative or friend who has a disability. It is helpful to inquire what challenges they face and assistance they need. Most caregivers appreciate empathy and assistance if they struggle with discrimination or lack of respite and accommodation.
>
> | Instead of... | Use ... |
> |---|---|
> | Afflicted with... suffers from... | She has Down syndrome |
> | Confined to a wheelchair/wheelchair-bound | Uses a wheelchair |
> | Caretaker | Caregiver, or person who cares for, advocates for, or serves people... |
> | Handicapped parking | Accessible parking |
> | Mentally retarded | Person with an intellectual disability |
> | "Normal" or "healthy" | Nondisabled/typical/neurotypical |

Figure 39-4 Communicating with Patients with Developmental Disabilities
Used with permission from the Office of Developmental Primary Care, Department of Family & Community Medicine, University of California, San Francisco.

supplementation for those patients with a high-risk profile for osteoporosis (mobility impairments, long-term use of antiepileptic or antipsychotic medications, Down syndrome, CP, Prader–Willi syndrome, history of fractures, history of amenorrhea, and cigarette smoking).

5. For mental health: Consult with other members of the interprofessional team to help identify potential environmental and social issues contributing to symptoms. Review common stress management strategies with patients and supporters (Hwang & Kearney, 2013). Emphasize the importance of healthy nutrition, physical activity, and good sleep (Kapsal et al., 2019). Provide prompt referral to mental health professionals knowledgeable in providing care of people with DD (Tsou et al., 2020; Sullivan et al., 2018).

6. For oral health: To reduce dental caries and gingival disease, an expert dental panel recommends:
   a. Brushing teeth twice daily for 2 minutes with a fluoridated toothpaste containing triclosan.
   b. Using xylitol for 5 minutes, three times per day. If the patient tolerates chewing, use chewing gum. If chewing is not possible, use a dissolved lozenge, spray, mint, or lollipop.
   c. Referral for regular dental cleanings and care to a dentist with experience providing care for people with special needs. Consult with a dentist regarding fluoride varnishes, rinses, and chlorhexidine rinses (National Institute of Dental and Craniofacial Research, 2009).

C. Patient education
   1. Primary focus should be on developing a trusting relationship with the patient and supporters (**Figure 39-4**).
   2. Provide lifestyle modification counseling to promote a healthy and happy quality of life (Table 39-1, **counseling section**).
   3. Provide information on community resources to support patients, supporters, and families.
   4. Review safety practices for prevention of accidents and victimization.
   5. Always presume competence. This means assume that all people deserve dignity, privacy, autonomy, access, and respect. Assume all people have the potential to learn. Do not assume that someone who does not speak cannot understand. Assume all people communicate; all lives are meaningful and valuable; and all people can learn, grow, and benefit from inclusion and opportunity. Speak directly to patients in a normal, adult tone of voice. Offer accommodations to help, but ask before assisting.

   Not all disabilities are visible, and many people develop skills or find ways to accommodate their disabilities that make them less apparent to others. However, this does not mean that those individuals do not have significant challenges.

V. Self-management resources and tools
   A. Healthcare provider resources
      1. Office of Developmental Primary Care, University of California, Department of Family & Community Medicine, https://odpc.ucsf.edu
      2. Health care for adults with intellectual and developmental disabilities: Toolkit for Primary Care Providers, https://iddtoolkit.vkcsites.org/
      3. Health assessment forms, yearly health checks, and other information, https://cddh.monashhealth.org/index.php/health-professionals/resources-and-links-health-practitioners/
      4. Health Watch Tables: information on select developmental disability syndromes, https://ddprimarycare.surreyplace.ca/tools-2/health-watch-tables/
      5. AASPIRE Healthcare Toolkit: Primary Care Resources for Adults on the Autism Spectrum and Their Primary Care Providers (Academic Autistic Spectrum Partnership in Research and Education, 2015) http://autismandhealth.org/
      6. American Academy of Developmental Medicine and Dentistry: resources for clinicians and students on neurodevelopmental disorders and health care for adults with DDs, https://www.aadmd.org
      7. Developmental Disability Nurses Association (resources for healthcare providers and families), https://www.ddna.org
      8. Coalition for Compassionate Care of California: Thinking Ahead Matters: Addressing the needs of the intellectual and developmentally disabled community when preparing for the end of life, https://coalitionccc.org/CCCC/Resources/People-With-Developmental-Disabilities-Resources.aspx
      9. National Institute of Dental and Craniofacial research: information and resources on oral health, https://www.nidcr.nih.gov/health-info/developmental-disabilities
   B. Patient and caregiver resources
      1. State of California Department of Developmental Services, https://www.dds.ca.gov
      2. Support for Families, https://www.supportforfamilies.org
      3. Family Voices, https://www.familyvoices.org

References

Academic Autistic Spectrum Partnership in Research and Education. (2015). *AASPIRE healthcare toolkit: Primary care resources for adults on the autism spectrum and their primary care providers.* http://www.autismandhealth.org/

American Academy of Pediatric Dentistry. (2021). *Management of dental patients with special health care needs.* https://www.aapd.org/media/Policies_Guidelines/BP_SHCN.pdf

American Association on Intellectual and Developmental Disabilities. (2010). *Definition of intellectual disability.* https://www.aamr.org/content_100.cfm?navID=21.

American Psychiatric Association. (2013). *Diagnostic and statistical manual of mental disorders* (5th ed.).

Andresen, E. M., Peterson-Besse, J. J., Krahn, G. L., Walsh, E. S., Horner-Johnson, W., & Iezzoni, L. I. (2013). Pap, mammography, and clinical breast examination screening among women with disabilities: A systematic review. *Women's Health Issues, 23*(4), e205–e214. doi:10.1016/j.whi.2013.04.002

Autistic Self Advocacy Network, Office of Developmental Primary Care. (2014). *Our lives, our health care: Self-advocates speaking out about our experiences with the medical system.* http://odpc.ucsf.edu/sites/odpc.ucsf.edu/files/pdf_docs/Our%20Lives%20Our%20Health%20Care%20Final_0.pdf.

Bear, A., Drew, C., Zuckerman, K. E., & Phelps, R. A. (2020). Understanding barriers to access and utilization of developmental disability services facilitating transition. *Journal of Developmental Behavioral Pediatrics, 41*(9), 680–689. doi:10.1097/DBP.0000000000000840

Bull, M. J. (2020). Down syndrome. *New England Journal of Medicine, 382*(24), 2344–2352. doi:10.1056/NEJMra1706537

Bull, M. J., Trotter, T., Santoro, S., Christensen, C., & Grout, R. W. (2022). Health supervision for children and adolescents with Down syndrome. *Pediatrics, 149*(5), e2022057010. doi:10.542/peds.2022-057010

Byrne, J. H., Ware, R. S., & Lennox, N. G. (2015). Health actions prompted by health assessments for people with intellectual disability exceed actions recorded in general practitioners' records. *Australian Journal of Primary Health, 21*(3), 317–320. doi:10.1071/PY14007

Carey, I. M., Hosking, F. J., Harris, T., DeWilde, S., Beighton, C., & Cook, D. G. (2017). *An evaluation of the effectiveness of annual health checks and quality of health care for adults with intellectual disability: An observational study using a primary care database.* NIHR Journals Library.

Centers for Disease Control and Prevention, National Center on Birth Defects and Developmental Disabilities. (2020). *Data and statistics on Down syndrome.* https://www.cdc.gov/ncbddd/birthdefects/downsyndrome/data.html

Collins, J., & Murphy, G. H. (2021). Detection and prevention of abuse of adults with intellectual and other developmental disabilities in care services: A systematic review. *Journal of Applied Research in Intellectual Disabilities, 35*(2), 338–373. doi:10.1111/jar.12954

Developmental Disabilities Assistance and Bill of Rights Act of 2000. P. L. 106-402 (2000). https://www.acl.gov/Programs/AIDD/DDA_BOR_ACT_2000/Index.aspx

Durkin, M. S., Benedict, R. E., Christensen, D., Dubois, L. A., Fitzgerald, R. T., Kirby, R. S., Maenner, M. J., Van Naarden Braun, K., Wingate, M. S., & Yeargin-Allsopp, M. (2016). Prevalence of cerebral palsy among 8-year-old children in 2010 and preliminary evidence of trends in its relationship to low birthweight. *Pediatric Perinatal Epidemiology, 30*(5), 496–510. doi:10.1111/ppe.12299

Engelman, A., Valderama-Wallace, C., Nouredini, S. (2019). State of the profession: The landscape of disability justice, health inequities, and access for patients with disabilities. *Advances in Nursing Science, 42*(3), 231–242. doi:10.1097/ANS.0000000000000261

Fletcher, R. (2018). *Diagnostic manual—intellectual disability: A clinical guide for diagnosis of mental disorders in persons with intellectual disability* (2nd ed.). NADD Press.

Folch, A., Salvador-Carulla, L., Vicens, P., Cortés, M. J., Irazábal, M., Muñoz, S., Rovira, L., Orejuela, C., González, J. A., & Martínez-Leal, R. (2019). Health indicators in intellectual developmental disorders: The key findings of the POMONA-ESP project. *Journal of Applied Research in Intellectual Disabilities, 32*(1), 23–34. doi:10.1111/jar.12498

Fortuna, R. J., Holub, A., Turk, M. A., Meccarello, J., & Davidson, P. W. (2018). Health conditions, functional status and health care utilization in adults with cerebral palsy. *Family Practice, 35*(6), 661–670. doi:10.1093/fampra/cmy027.

Horner-Johnson, W., Dobbertin, K., & Lee, J. (2013). Disparities in chronic conditions and health status by type of disability. *Disability and Health Journal, 6*(4), 280–286.

Hwang, Y. S., & Kearney, P. (2013). A systematic review of mindfulness intervention for individuals with developmental disabilities: Long-term practice and long-lasting effects. *Research in Developmental Disabilities, 34*(1), 314–326. doi:10.1016/j.ridd.2012.08.008

Jonsson, U., Eek, M.N., Sunnerhagen, K.S., & Himmelmann, K. (2021). Changes in walking ability, intellectual disability, and epilepsy in adults with cerebral palsy over 50 years: a population-based follow-up study. *Developmental Medicine & Child Neurology, 63*(7), 839–845. doi: 10.1111/dmcn.14871. Epub 2021 Mar 27.

Kapsal, N. J., Dicke, T., Morin, A. J. S., Vasconcellos, D., Maïano, C., Lee, J., & Lonsdale, C. (2019). Effects of physical activity on the physical and psychosocial health of youth with intellectual disabilities: A systematic review and meta-analysis. *Journal of Physical Activity and Health, 16*(12), 1187–1195. doi: 10.1123/jpah.2018-0675.

Kripke, C. C. (2014). Primary care for adolescents with developmental disabilities. *Primary Care, 41*(3), 507–518.

Krysta, K., Romanczyk, M., Diefenbacher, A., & Krzystanek, M. (2021). Telemedicine treatment and care for patients with intellectual disability. *International Journal of Environmental Research and Public Health, 18*(4), 1746. doi:10.3390/ijerph18041746

Lankamp, D. L., McManus, M. D., & Blakemore, S. D. (2015). Telemedicine for children with developmental disabilities: A more effective clinical process than office-based care. *Telemedicine Journal and E-Health, 21*(2), 110–114. doi:10.1089/tmj.2013.0379

Levy, B., Song, J., Luong, D., Perrier L, Bayley MT, Andrew G, Arbour-Nicitopoulos K, Chan B, Curran CJ, Dimitropoulos G, Hartman L, Huang L, Kastner M, Kingsnorth S, McCormick A, Nelson M, Nicholas D, Penner M, Thompson L, ... Munce, J. (2020). Transitional care interventions for youth with disabilities: A systematic review. *Pediatrics, 146*(5), e20200187. doi:10.1542/peds.2020-0187

Manickam, K., McClain, M., Demmer, L., Biswas, S., Kearney, H., Malinowski, J., Massingham, L. J., Miller, D., Yu, T. W., Hisama, F. M., & ACMG Board of Directors. (2021). Exome and genome sequencing for pediatric patients with congenital anomalies or intellectual disability: An evidence-based clinical guideline of the American College of Medical Genetics and Genomics (ACMG). *Genetics in Medicine, 23*(11), 2029–2037. doi:10.1038/s41436-021-01242-6

National Institute of Dental and Craniofacial Research. (2009). *Practical oral care for people with intellectual disability.* http://www.nidcr.nih.gov/oralhealth/Topics/DevelopmentalDisabilities/PracticalOralCarePeopleIntellectualDisability.htm

National Resource Center for Supported Decision-Making. (n.d.). *Home page.* http://supporteddecisionmaking.org

Nicolaidis, C., Kripke, C., & Raymaker, D. (2014). Primary care for adults on the autism spectrum. *Medical Clinics of North America, 98*(5), 1169–1191. doi:10.1016/j.mcna.2014.06.011

Office of Developmental Primary Care. (n.d.). *Interdisciplinary healthcare team chart.* http://odpc.ucsf.edu/odpc/html/for_clinicians/charts_forms_c.htm.

Office of Developmental Primary Care. (2021). *Partners in health: Implementing supported healthcare decision-making for users of augmentative and alternative communication in California.* https://odpc.ucsf.edu/advocacy/supported-health-care-decision-making

Patja, K., Iivanainen, M., Vesala, H., Oksanen, H., & Ruoppila, I. (2000). Life expectancy of people with intellectual disability: A 35-year follow-up study. *Journal of Intellectual Disability Research, 44*(Pt. 5), 591–599. doi:10.1046/j.1365-2788.2000.00280.x

Pezzoni, V., & Kouimtsidis, C. (2015). Screening for alcohol misuse within people attending intellectual disability community service. *Journal of Intellectual Disability Research, 59*(4), 353–359. doi:10.1111/jir.12168

Robertson, J., Hatton, C., Emerson, E., & Baines, S. (2014). The impact of health checks for people with intellectual disabilities: An updated systematic review of evidence. *Research in Developmental Disabilities, 35*(10), 2450–2462. doi:10.1016/j.ridd.2014.06.007

Schalock, R. L., Luckasson, R., & Tassé, M. J. (2021). *Intellectual disability: Definition, diagnosis, classification, and systems of supports* (12th ed.). American Association on Intellectual and Developmental Disabilities.

Stadskleiv, K. (2020). Cognitive functioning in children with cerebral palsy. *Developmental Medicine & Child Neurology, 62*(3), 283–289. doi:10.1111/dmcn.14463

Sullivan, W. F., Diepstra, H., Heng, J., Ally, S., Bradley, E., Casson, I., Hennen, B., Kelly, M., Korossy, M., McNeil, K., Abells, D., Amaria, K., Boyd, K., Gemmill, M., Grier, E., Kennie-Kaulbach, N., Ketchell, M., Ladouceur, J., Lepp, A., ... Witherbee, S. (2018). Primary care of adults with intellectual and developmental disabilities: 2018 Canadian consensus guidelines. *Canadian Family Physician, 64*(4), 254–279.

Tomsa, R., Gutu, S., Cojocaru, D., Gutiérrez-Bermejo, B., Flores, N., & Jenaro, C. (2021). Prevalence of sexual abuse in adults with intellectual disability: Systematic review and meta-analysis. *International Journal of Environmental Research and Public Health, 18*(4), 1980. doi:10.3390/ijerph18041980

Tsou, A. Y., Bulova, P., Capone, G., Chicoine, B., Gelaro, B., Harville, T. O., Martin, B. A., McGuire, D. E., McKelvey, K. D., Peterson, M., Tyler, C., Wells, M., Whitten, M. S., & Global Down Syndrome Foundation Medical Care Guidelines for Adults with Down Syndrome Workgroup. (2020). Medical care of adults with Down syndrome: A clinical guideline. *Journal of the American Medical Association, 324*(15), 1543–1556. doi:10.1001/jama.2020.17024

United for Communication Choice. (n.d.). *Home page.* https://unitedforcommunicationchoice.org/

van Timmeren, E. A., van der Putten, A. A., van Schrojenstein Lantman-de Valk, H. M., van der Schans, C. P., & Waninge, A. (2016). A. Prevalence of reported physical health problems in people with severe or profound intellectual and motor disabilities: A cross-sectional study of medical records and care plans. *Journal of Intellectual Disability Research, 60*(11), 1109–1118. doi:10.1111/jir.12298

Vanderbom, K. A., Eisenberg, Y., Tubbs, A. H., Washington, T., Martínez, A. X., & Rauworth, A. (2018). Changing the paradigm in public health and disability through a knowledge translation center. *International Journal of Environmental Research and Public Health, 15*(2), 328. doi:10.3390/ijerph15020328

Vitrikas, K., Dalton, H., & Breish, D. (2020). Cerebral palsy: An overview. *American Family Physician, 101*(4), 213–220. PMID: 32053326.

Wimalasundera, N., & Stevenson, V. L. (2016). Cerebral palsy. *Practical Neurology, 16*(3), 184–94. doi:10.1136/practneurol-2015-001184

CHAPTER 40

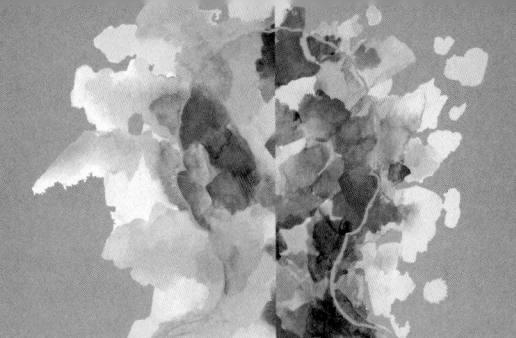

Healthcare Maintenance for Transgender and Gender Expansive (TGE) Adults

Bennett Lareau-Meredith and Isabella Ventura

I. Introduction and general background

Transgender and gender expansive (TGE) people living in the United States are a marginalized and medically underserved population. Although the term *transgender* or *trans* is an acceptable encompassing adjective commonly used to describe individuals of trans experience, not all trans people self-identify as such. Historically, healthcare services for transgender populations have been relatively scarce or nonexistent. Oftentimes, providing transition-related health services was used as a tool for HIV prevention and care, such as was the case for Transgender Tuesday at Tom Waddell Health Center's model of care in San Francisco, California. In recent years, a growing body of literature has been published on providing effective gender-affirming care to TGE populations, but these guidelines are mostly based on expert opinion. There is a need for more research and data to support these clinical recommendations.

Understanding transgender populations' diverse healthcare needs, barriers, and facilitators to care are important first steps in providing gender-affirming care. Some of the barriers to care faced by many people in trans communities are as follows.

First, transgender populations are vulnerable to stigma and discrimination, which stems primarily from transphobia (White Hughto et al., 2015). Transphobia is the irrational fear, discrimination against, and hatred of TGE populations. Providers and health systems need to prioritize eliminating transphobia in the healthcare setting. The 2015 United States Transgender Survey (USTS) survey conducted by the National Center for Transgender Equality (NCTE), with 27,715 respondents in the United States and territories, shows that 1 in 3 trans people has had at least one negative experience in a healthcare setting in the past year (James et al., 2016). The most common complaints include verbal, physical, and sexual abuse; treatment refusal; deadnaming (use of a trans person's birth name when they no longer use that name, regardless of whether it is still the person's legal name); misgendering by using the wrong pronouns; and having to educate their healthcare provider on how to provide appropriate care.

Access to affordable health insurance that covers transition-related health benefits is another barrier to care. Nearly one-third of the respondents in the NCTE's USTS reported living in poverty, and the unemployment rate is three times higher (15%) than that of the general U.S. population (12%) (James et al., 2016). Addressing other basic necessities, such as housing, food, and clothing, might be on the top of most transgender people's priorities before health care. Access to affordable health care for trans populations also depends on local, state, and federal laws and regulations. As of September 2023, 22 U.S. states have banned or restricted gender affirming care for minors, with a few states extending restrictions to adults (Davis, 2023). Understanding the provisions of health services to transgender populations and advocating for and with trans people on health coverage and expansion of transition-related health benefits will help address inequities in access to quality and cost-effective health care.

Lastly, there is a greater need to address clinicians' competency in providing adequate gender-affirming care to transgender patients. The lack of knowledge, skills, and willingness to care for this population due to transphobia is a barrier to providing effective TGE care (Chisolm-Straker et al., 2018; Shires et al., 2018). Research indicates that providers, particularly nurse practitioners, have strong intentions to provide care to TGE adults, but they lack knowledge, training, and experience in providing care to these populations (Paradiso & Lally, 2018). Education and training of existing and future healthcare providers on gender-affirming care must be addressed at every level of education and our healthcare system.

As a result of these barriers to care, the rates of preventable illnesses such as HIV are higher in the transgender community than in any other population (Centers for Disease Control and Prevention, 2015). However, it has been demonstrated that routine medical care focusing on healthcare maintenance for transgender individuals can be delivered in the primary care setting safely and compassionately, without the need for specialty or psychiatric referrals (Davidson et al., 2013). Creating a trans-inclusive clinical environment is essential to increasing patient engagement in care. A safe and welcoming environment should include continuous training of all clinical and administrative staff on trans issues and common language used in the communities, using patients' preferred names and pronouns, providing "all gender" bathrooms and safe waiting spaces, and hiring staff from within trans communities. Increasing the capacity for comprehensive gender-affirming care utilizing intersectional gender-affirming, trauma-informed, and trans-centered principles across all aspects of care by providers is crucial in supporting some of the basic needs of these populations. There are numerous online resources available to support medical clinics in improving access to care, including those offered by the National LGBTQIA+ Education Center.

It should be noted that all healthcare providers will likely care for transgender patients in the course of their careers, regardless of whether these patients are seeking transgender-specific care from a particular clinical setting. Therefore, it is imperative that all clinics take action to create an inclusive and welcoming environment and develop culturally congruent gender-affirming care.

Gender-affirming care, derived from a gender-affirmation framework (Sevelius, 2013), is a scope of medical, behavioral, social, and psychological practices and interventions that affirms and centers one's current gender identity and expression. The lack of gender affirmation in clinical and social settings can lead to psychological distress, such as depression, anxiety, low self-esteem, and internalized transphobia, resulting in TGE adults engaging in high-risk behaviors such as heavy substance use, unprotected sexual encounters, and even self-harm (Glynn et al., 2016; Sevelius, 2013). On the other end of the spectrum, providing gender-affirming medical, social, and mental health services, including gender-affirming surgical interventions, promotes a reduction in psychological distress (44%), a reduction in suicidal ideation (44%), and overall improved health and well-being among transgender and gender diverse people (James et al., 2016; Sevelius et al., 2021).

A. *Transgender identity*
  1. Definition and overview
    Data collection and epidemiologic estimates concerning the transgender community in the United States have been challenging because of the lack of inclusive survey or data collection forms, lack of reliability due to fear of stigma or discrimination from self-identification, and overgeneralization of the term *transgender*. In 2016, the Williams Institutes at the University of California, Los Angeles, estimated that 0.6% of adults, or 1.4 million adults, in the United States identify as transgender (Flores et al., 2016). These numbers, however, are likely underestimated, both because the US Census does not include data on gender identity and current surveys on TGE population statistics contain methodological flaws (Lett & Everhart, 2022; Meerwijk & Sevelius, 2017).

    The terms *transgender* and *trans* are broadly used to describe people whose gender identity is different from their assigned sex at birth. Included in the *Diagnostic and Statistical Manual of Mental Disorders* (*DSM*) as of 1980, the term *gender identity disorder* has been reclassified as *gender dysphoria* in the current 5th edition (*DSM-5*; American Psychiatric Association, 2013) guidelines. Labeling transgender patients with a mental disorder is controversial and offensive to most transgender people, although a corresponding diagnosis code is often needed for billing purposes and insurance coverage. For transgender patients who have concerns with the gender dysphoria diagnosis, an alternative diagnosis of *endocrine disorder, nonspecified* may be used. It is important to recognize that gender is seen by many as more than a binary concept.

  2. Definitions (Note that language specific to gender identity is continually evolving and is culturally and regionally dependent.)
    Sex: sex assigned at birth; based on an assessment of external genitalia, chromosomes, and gonads
    Gender identity: a person's internal sense of gender (i.e., being a man, a woman, masculine, feminine, nonbinary, etc.)
    Gender expression: describes a person's gender presentation or communication of gender to the world via clothing, behavior, speech, and so forth
    Sexual orientation: describes a person's identity based on pattern of sexual and/or emotional attraction
    Transgender: Describes an individual whose gender identity is not congruent with their sex assigned at birth. Note that the term *transgendered* is outdated and should not be used, and *transgender* should not be used as a noun.
    Cisgender: describes a person whose gender identity is congruent with their sex assigned at birth
    Transmasculine: Describes someone assigned female at birth (AFAB) whose identity is on the masculine spectrum. Includes people who may identify within either a binary gender (e.g., a trans man) or nonbinary gender.
    Transfeminine: Describes someone assigned male at birth (AMAB) whose identity is on the feminine spectrum. Includes people who may identify within either a binary gender (e.g., a trans woman) or nonbinary gender.

Nonbinary, gender-variant, bigendered, genderqueer, gender nonconforming, agender, genderfluid, Two Spirit: Individuals who may choose to identify as both or neither male or female or along a nonbinary gender spectrum. Some people may use multiple terms to describe their gender identity and may include terms not written in this document.

II. Database

A. *Subjective*

When taking a history from a transgender patient, it is important to use the principles of trauma-informed care. Trauma-informed care takes into consideration various points of trauma that a person may have experienced throughout their life and informs opportunities for greater patient empowerment in the healthcare context. For transgender patients specifically, it is critical to account for the multiple barriers to care, stressors, and social oppression that have been outlined earlier in this chapter when approaching care of these populations. First and foremost, rapport should be established, and questions that may be perceived as invasive or "othering" should be given context by the provider or medical staff taking the history. Given the historical context of marginalization in both medical settings and wider society, trans patients may rightly be wary of discrimination within the clinical context. Not all of the following information is necessary to gather for every patient; keep the following data points in mind as potentially relevant for transgender patients, particularly if they embody multiple marginalized identities that increase risk factors for issues such as housing instability, unemployment, sexually transmitted infection risk, violence, deportation, or mental health issues caused or exacerbated by stress due to both institutional and interpersonal oppression and trauma.

1. Pertinent past medical history, as outlined in Chapter 38, Adult Healthcare Maintenance and Promotion, with a focus on the following additional data:
   a. Previous medical illnesses, with emphasis on a history of coronary disease and/or thromboembolic events
   b. Risk for sexually transmitted infection and HIV status, including assessment of sexual activities (oral, anal, vaginal, insertive, receptive, etc.), number of sex partners, preferred sex partners (cis male, cis female, trans woman, trans man, nonbinary, etc.), date and results of last screening tests
   c. Surgical history, with emphasis on any gender-affirming procedures (feminizing procedures include mammoplasty, facial feminization surgery [commonly referred to as FFS], orchiectomy, vaginoplasty, and body contouring; masculinizing procedures include mastectomy with male chest reconstruction, facial masculinization surgery, metoidioplasty, phalloplasty, and body contouring)
   d. Nonsurgical procedures, including those done by nonlicensed laypersons, such as facial fillers and silicone injections.
   e. Previous psychiatric hospitalizations and/or any suicide attempts
   f. Medications, with emphasis on hormone therapy, including names of medications, dosage, route, and source (i.e., previous providers, nonmedical sources such as online, friends, etc.)
   g. Immunization status, with emphasis on hepatitis A, B, and human papillomavirus (HPV) vaccines
   h. Hepatitis C risk factors and antibody status
   i. Screening for abuse and intimate partner violence
2. Family history, with emphasis on cardiovascular disease and cardiac risk factors
3. Occupational history
4. Personal and social history including:
   a. History of alcohol, tobacco, and drug use
   b. History of depression, anxiety, other mental health/psychiatric diagnosis, trauma, suicidal ideation or attempts
   c. Relationships and social support
   d. Housing status

B. *Objective*

Physical examination may be deferred until a strong clinician–patient relationship is established, unless review of symptoms warrants immediate examination. Furthermore, as with any patient, physical exams should be limited to what is necessary for a patient's presenting health concern or for specific cancer-related screening. The patient should be prepared for the need for a physical examination in advance and given an opportunity to discuss feelings about being examined. Guidelines suggest implementing physical exams, screening, and healthcare maintenance needs based on the anatomy that is present, regardless of patient's self-identification (Deutsch, 2016). Efforts should be made to provide a medical chaperone for the patient if they wish, regardless of the gender of the provider. Keep in mind that a lack of transgender providers and/or staff in a clinical setting may create more barriers in trust-building and patient comfort.

1. Genital, rectal, and breast/chest examinations deserve particular sensitivity because they may cause particular distress for patients if they experience dysphoria related to these physical attributes. Discuss with the patient in advance the rationale for the examination and ascertain how the patient would like one to refer to their anatomy (i.e., *genitals* instead of *penis* or *vagina*, *chest* instead of *breasts*). For transmasculine patients needing a speculum or bimanual exam, consider providing a prescription for a benzodiazepine 1 hour prior to a scheduled visit for those anticipating a distressing experience.
2. For patients who have had silicone injections, the clinician should carefully examine the patient for signs of cellulitis, granulomas, or more serious systemic complications (Zevin & Deutsch, 2016).

III. Assessment

A. The current risk factors and health status of the patient should be identified, and the patient's motivation to change potentially risky behaviors should be assessed. A harm-reduction approach should be utilized in supporting a patient's goals.

B. Identify the patient's medical and/or surgical gender-affirmation goals and barriers to the goals.

Assess for benefits of hormonal therapy and potential for reversible and irreversible effects, including but not limited to weight gain or fat redistribution, increased cardiovascular risk, increased breast mass, hair growth and/or loss, mood changes, and changes in libido or sexual function. Some effects of hormonal therapy may be more desired by some patients, whereas others may perceive certain physical changes to be drawbacks.

C. Identify psychosocial needs of the patient.

IV. Plan

A. Diagnostics (screening and secondary prevention tests)
   1. Screen for diseases and conditions based on the patient's risk profile. Note that normal laboratory values are often gender specific. Although there are no established guidelines for determining normal laboratory values for transgender patients, physiologic hormone levels in cisgender people are used as reference ranges. In many cases, sex-specific non-hormone labs, such as hemoglobin, hematocrit, and creatinine, should be interpreted using the reference range of the non-natal sex of the patient. (Center of Excellence for Transgender Health, 2014).
   2. Similar healthcare maintenance and screening needs as general populations: **Table 40-1** outlines healthcare maintenance guidelines and special considerations for transgender patients (Center of Excellence for Transgender Health, 2014).

B. Treatment
   1. Immunization recommendations are not sex specific, follow general guidelines.
   2. For prescribing guidelines for transition-related medical therapy, see the Resources list at the end of this chapter. Consensus on the practice of hormone therapy is ever-evolving; there are numerous free resources available on the internet that

Table 40-1 Healthcare Maintenance Guidelines for the Transgender Patient

Patients Who Are Transfeminine/Assigned Male at Birth (AMAB)	Patients Who Are Transmasculine /Assigned Female at Birth (AFAB)
Prostate cancer (CA) screening per general population (prostate-specific antigen can be low; use digital rectal exam if necessary to evaluate based on review of systems)	Cervical CA screening per general population with the following considerations:
Breast CA screening by mammography in presence of other risk factors (estrogen/progestin use > 5 years, family history, increased adiposity ≥ 35) (It is recommended that screening mammography be performed every 2 years, once the age of 50 and 5–10 years of feminizing hormone use criteria have been met. Providers and patients should engage in discussions that include the risks of overscreening and an assessment of individual risk factors [Feldman & Deutsch, 2021]).	*If patient has had total hysterectomy and has prior history of high-grade cervical dysplasia → do pap cotest of vaginal cuff until 3 consecutive normal, then every 3 years for a total of 25 years thereafter per American Society for Colposcopy and Cervical Pathology (ASCCP) guidelines.*
Pap smears are not required if a patient has neovagina, but consider periodic visual inspection to assess for lesions or granulation tissue. If available, examination of the neovagina may be done with an anoscope; otherwise, a small speculum can be used if necessary (consider a pediatric-sized speculum as needed; neovagina width and depth vary significantly, and the tissue does not readily stretch).	*If patient has had ovaries removed but uterus/cervix is intact, follow the standard cervical cancer screening guidelines.* *Note that atrophy from testosterone use can mimic dysplasia, and providers should note on the cytology requisition if the patient uses testosterone.
Blood pressure (BP) screening routinely	Uterine CA: *Evaluate all spontaneous vaginal bleeding that cannot be explained by missed testosterone doses or changes in dosing.*
Lipid screening based on U.S. Preventive Services Task Force (USPSTF) guidelines	Chest/breast exams, depending on age, follow current evidence-based guidelines.
Consider liver function tests (LFTs) if on hormones AND higher risk (increased alcohol use, weight gain, or at risk for hepatitis C)	BP screening routinely
Periodic mental health screenings with the Patient Health Questionnaire, 9-item version (PHQ-9) and the Generalized Anxiety Disorder 7-item (GAD-7) scale	Lipid screening based on USPSTF guidelines
Sexual health screening as appropriate, based on sexual practices; may include HIV and sexually transmitted infection testing, hepatitis B and C screening, and prevention	Consider LFTs based on specific risk factors. Periodic mental health screenings with PHQ-9 and GAD-7 Sexual health screening as appropriate, based on sexual practices; may include HIV and sexually transmitted infection testing, hepatitis B and C screening, and prevention

Table 40-2 Feminizing Therapy

Anti-Androgens	Estrogen
Decreased facial/body hair, male-pattern baldness	Breast development
Decreased libido	Redistribution of body fat
Decreased erections	Softening of skin
Mild breast growth	Suppression of testosterone production
Decreased benign prostatic hyperplasia (BPH)	Atrophy of testes
	Decreased/altered libido mood changes
Therapies: Spironolactone, finasteride, gonadotropin-releasing hormone (GnRH) agonists	*Therapies: Estradiol (transdermal, oral, injection, pellet)*

Table 40-3 Masculinizing Therapy

Androgens
Changes/deepening of voice pitch
Increased libido
Increased muscle mass and strength
Hair growth on face, chest, extremities
Cessation of menses
Redistribution of body fat
Clitoral enlargement Male-pattern hair loss Mood changes
Therapies: Testosterone (injection, transdermal, pellet)

Table 40-4 Considerations/Contraindications (Individualize Risk Versus Benefit) of Estrogen Use

History of or current thrombophlebitis or venous thromboembolic disorders—pulmonary embolism, deep vein thrombosis
History of or active arterial thromboembolic disease—myocardial infarction, cerebrovascular accident
Estrogen-dependent tumor
End stage chronic liver disease

Data from Lexicomp. (2015); Center for Excellence for Transgender Health. (2016). Feminizing medications for transgender clients. Retrieved from http://transhealth.ucsf.edu/pdf/protocols/Sample_3_Feminizing%20Medications.pdf; Vancouver Coastal Health Transgender Health Information Program. (2016). Feminizing hormones. Retrieved from http://transhealth.vch.ca/medical-options/hormones/feminizing-hormones.

are updated periodically regarding the provision of gender-affirming hormone therapy. Use the appropriate drug interaction database when prescribing hormone therapy to avoid adverse drug interactions.

3. Discuss fertility goals with all patients initiating or taking hormones because treatment may interfere with fertility (Amato, 2016). Some patients may consider oocyte or sperm banking.

   Table 40-2 outlines the effects of feminizing therapies. **Table 40-3** outlines the effects of masculinizing therapies. Note that the use of hormones for gender affirmation is off-label, and the provider should obtain informed consent before initiating therapy.

4. **Transfeminine patients:** Most patients seeking feminizing hormone therapy can transition with the use of estrogen and spironolactone alone. Progesterone can also be used; however, it may not be as effective as spironolactone in suppressing testosterone and likely carries excess cardiovascular risks (Tangpricha & Safer, 2021). Some providers prescribe progesterone to enhance the development of natural breast contour; this practice has strong anecdotal reports but has not been well studied. **Table 40-4** outlines clinical considerations with estrogen use. Always limit estrogen to one type and use the lowest effective dose. There are differing recommendations regarding baseline and monitoring labs; therefore, it is recommended to review the available resources and check periodically for updates in evidence and literature informing these recommendations.

5. **Transmasculine patients:** Discuss contraceptive use with patients having receptive genital sex with partners who have sperm because testosterone is not a contraceptive. Advise patients that it may take up to 6 months for menses to cease once on testosterone therapy. Any contraceptive option can be used by transgender patients using testosterone; however, provider sensitivity is advised because some patients may have dysphoria associated with hormonal options, estradiol in particular. Testosterone dose should not necessarily be reduced after hysterectomy or gender-affirming surgery. Hormone

therapy should be continued in patients who have had an oophorectomy for osteoporosis protection until around the average age of menopause (51 years old).
6. Particular emphasis should be placed on smoking cessation strategies for patients receiving estrogen therapy because of the increased risk of thromboembolism. Consider patch versus oral or intramuscular (IM) estrogen. Aspirin 81 mg may be added for cardiovascular protection.
7. Consider referring HIV-positive patients for care at a specialty clinic, unless the provider is trained in HIV/AIDS.
8. Consider a psychiatric or mental health referral for patients who have mental health concerns outside of the provider's scope of practice. Routine referral for psychiatric care is not otherwise warranted and may alienate patients, but note that one or more letters written by mental health professionals assessing a patient's surgical readiness are often a prerequisite for patients considering gender transition surgery. This particular requirement is usually insurance-driven and based on prior World Professional Association for Transgender Health (WPATH) recommendations. (Deutsch, 2016)

C. Surgical options
1. If a patient is interested in surgical intervention, assess patient readiness for surgery, including support before and after surgery, and provide the patient with surgical options and education, as well as referrals to applicable surgeon(s). See **Table 40-5** for a list of common surgical options.

Table 40-5 Surgical Options for the Transgender Patient

Feminizing	Masculinizing
Breast augmentation/mammoplasty: Saline or silicone implants	**Mastectomy with male chest reconstruction:** Also called "top surgery," this is the removal of breast tissue with alteration and reconstruction of surrounding area to create a male-appearing contoured chest.
Facial feminization: A broad range of surgical procedures. May include forehead contouring, brow lift, hairline adjustment, jaw restructuring, rhinoplasty, cheek implants, and lip augmentation.	**Hysterectomy:** Removal of uterus and/or total removal of uterus and cervix
Thyroid chondroplasty (chondrolaryngoplasty): Sometimes referred to as "tracheal shave," this is the surgical reduction of the thyroid cartilage to reduce appearance of an "Adam's apple."	**Salpingo-Oophorectomy:** Removal of fallopian tubes and ovaries. This procedure results in irreversible infertility unless oocyte banking has been done prior to surgery.
Orchiectomy: Surgical removal of testicles, which results in reduced levels of testosterone in the body. Results in irreversible infertility unless sperm banking is done prior to surgery.	**Vaginectomy:** Removal of the vagina
Penectomy: Surgical removal of penis with relocation of urethral opening to allow for urination in sitting position	**Colpocleisis:** Surgical closure of the vagina, often performed when patients choose metoidioplasty or phalloplasty procedures
Vaginoplasty: Surgical creation of vaginal canal, commonly using penile inversion technique; peritoneal pull-through technique increasingly accessible. Goal of surgery is to create a neovagina that has sensation and sufficient depth and width for penetration.	**Metoidioplasty:** Surgical creation of a phallus using existing genital tissue. Expected phallus size is smaller than average male penis, but testosterone use for 2+ years prior to surgery may help add length to new phallus. Successful metoidioplasty results in retained sensation and erectile capability.
Labiaplasty: Surgical creation of labia minora and majora using skin from existing penis and scrotum	**Scrotoplasty:** Surgical creation of scrotum using existing tissue from genital area and testicular implants
Clitoroplasty: Surgical creation of clitoris	**Phalloplasty:** Highly complex surgical construction of a penis using skin from abdomen, forearm, or inner thigh. Differs from metoidioplasty in that new phallus length is closer to average male penis, and erections are possible only through permanently implanted rod or use of implanted pump.

Reproduced from San Francisco Department of Public Health Transgender Health Services Resources.

D. Patient education
   1. Primary focus should be on developing a trusting relationship with the patient and assisting the patient to overcome previous negative experiences with healthcare providers.
   2. Provide health counseling, with particular attention to sexually transmitted infection, HIV, alcohol use, cigarette use, nutrition, and physical activities.
   3. Harm reduction as needed based on findings of subjective and objective assessments
   4. Provide information on community resources, such as legal advice, housing assistance, and mental health counseling.
   5. Periodic health counseling as outlined in Chapter 38, Adult Healthcare Maintenance and Promotion
E. Resources and tools
   1. The Center of Excellence for Transgender Health at the University of California, San Francisco, provides education, advocacy, and current research around transgender health needs for both trans individuals and providers (http://transhealth.ucsf.edu/).
   2. Transcare BC (formerly Vancouver Coastal Health) has excellent resources for both providers and patients on a variety of topics related to transgender health promotion, mental health, and other topics (http://www.phsa.ca/transcarebc/health-professionals).
   3. The WPATH conducts academic research and promotes the development of evidence-based medicine for transsexual, transgender, and gender-nonconforming individuals (http://www.wpath.org/). Updated Standards of Care (SOC) were released in 2022.
   4. Project Health focuses on advocacy, education, and leadership for transgender health. Project Health hosts a national online trans medical consultation service for healthcare providers (http://project-health.org).
   5. Fenway Health/National LGBTQIA+ Health Education Center: https://www.lgbtqiahealtheducation.org/
   6. Cedar Rivers Transgender Health Care Toolkit: http://www.cedarriverclinics.org/transtoolkit/
   7. Endocrine Society Guidelines: https://www.endocrine.org/clinical-practice-guidelines/gender-dysphoria-gender-incongruence
   8. The Transgender Law Center advocates for individuals who have faced discrimination based on their gender identity or expression (http://transgenderlawcenter.org/).
   9. The NCTE is an advocacy organization working to advance the equality of transgender individuals (http://transequality.org/).
   10. Trauma-informed care for trans and gender-diverse individuals: https://www.lgbtqiahealtheducation.org/wp-content/uploads/2020/06/9e.-Trauma-Informed-Care.pptx.min_.pdf
   11. San Francisco Department of Public Health's Gender Health SF provider resources: https://www.0sfdph.org/dph/comupg/oprograms/THS/ClinicalResources.asp

References

American Psychiatric Association. (2013). *Diagnostic and statistical manual of mental disorders* (5th ed.).

Amato, P. (2016) *Fertility options for transgender persons.* UCSF Transgender Care and Treatment Guidelines. https://transcare.ucsf.edu/guidelines/fertility

Centers for Disease Control and Prevention. (2015). *HIV among transgender people.* http://www.cdc.gov/hiv/risk/transgender/index.html

Chisolm-Straker, M., Willging, C., Daul, A. D., McNamara, S., Sante, S. C., Shattuck, D. G., & Crandall, C. S. (2018). Transgender and gender-nonconforming patients in the emergency department: What physicians know, think, and do. *Annals of Emergency Medicine, 71*(2), 183–188. doi:10.1016/j.annemergmed.2017.09.042

Coleman, E., Radix, A. E., Bouman, W. P., Brown, G. R., de Vries, A. L., Deutsch, M. B., Ettner, R., Fraser, L., Goodman, M., Green, J., Hancock, A. B., Johnson, T. W., Karasic, D. H., Knudson, G. A., Leibowitz, S. F., Meyer-Bahlburg, H. F., Monstrey, S. J., Motmans, J., Nahata, L., ... Arcelus, J. (2022). Standards of care for the health of transgender and gender diverse people, version 8. *International Journal of Transgender Health, 23*(sup1). https://doi.org/10.1080/26895269.2022.2100644

Davidson, A., Francivich, J., Freeman, M., Lin, R., Martinez, L., Monihan, M., Porch, M., Samuel, L., Stukalin, R., Vormohr, J., & Zevin, B. (2013). *Tom Waddell Health Center protocols for hormonal reassignment of gender.* https://www.sfdph.org/dph/comupg/oservices/medSvs/hlthCtrs/TransGendprotocols122006.pdf

Davis, E. (2023, September 13). States that have restricted gender-affirming care for trans youth in 2023. *US News and World Report.* Retrieved September 26, 2023, from https://www.usnews.com/news/best-states/articles/2023-03-30/what-is-gender-affirming-care-and-which-states-have-restricted-it-in-2023.

Deutsch, M. B. (2016). UCSF Transgender Care and Treatment Guidelines. https://transcare.ucsf.edu/guidelines/

Feldman, J., & Deutsch, M. (2021). Primary care of transgender individuals. *UpToDate.* http://www.uptodate.com/contents/primary-care-transgender-individuals

Flores, A. R., Herman, J. L., Gates, G. J., & Brown, T. N. T. (2016). *How many adults identify as transgender in the United States?* The Williams Institute.

Gynn, T. R., Gamarel, K., Kahler, C., Iwamoto, M., Operario, D., & Nemoto, T. (2016). The role of gender affirmation in psychological well-being among transgender women. *Psychology of Sexual Orientation and Gender Diversity, 3*(3), 336–344. doi/10.1037/sgd0000171

James, S. E., Herman, J. L., Rankin, S., Keisling, M., Mottet, L., & Anafi, M. (2016). *The report of the 2015 U.S. Transgender Survey.* National Center for Transgender Equality.

Lett, E., & Everhart, A. (2022). Considerations for Transgender Population Health Research based on US National Surveys.

Annals of Epidemiology, 65, 65–71. https://doi.org/10.1016/j.annepidem.2021.10.009

Meerwijk, E. L., & Sevelius, J. M. (2017). Transgender population size in the United States: A meta-regression of population-based probability samples. *American Journal of Public Health*, 107(2). https://doi.org/10.2105/ajph.2016.303578

Paradiso, C., & Lally, R. M. (2018). Nurse practitioner knowledge, attitudes, and beliefs when caring for transgender people. *Transgender Health*, 3(1), 48–56. doi:10.1089/trgh.2017.0048

San Francisco Department of Public Health. (n.d.). *Gender Health SF.* https://www.sfdph.org/dph/comupg/oprograms/THS/procedures.asp

Sevelius, J. M. (2013). Gender affirmation: A framework for conceptualizing risk behavior among transgender women of color. *Sex Roles*, 68(11–12), 675–689. doi:10.1007/s11199-012-0216-5

Sevelius, J. M., Xavier, J., Chakravarty, D., Keatley, J., Shade, S., & Rebchook, G. (2021). Correlates of engagement in HIV care among transgender women of color in the United States of America. *AIDS and Behavior*, 25(Suppl. 1), 3–12. doi:10.1007/s10461-021-03306-9

Shires, D. A., Stroumsa, D., Jaffee, K. D., & Woodford, M. R. (2018). Primary care clinicians' willingness to care for transgender patients. *Annals of Family Medicine*, 16(6), 555–558. doi:10.1370/afm.2298

Tangpricha, V., & Safer, J. (2021). Transgender women: Evaluation and management. *UpToDate.* http://www.uptodate.com/contents/transgender-women-evaluation-and-management

Transcare BC. (2023, March). *Gender-affirming care for trans, two-spirit, and gender diverse patients in BC: A primary care toolkit.* http://www.phsa.ca/transcarebc/Documents/HealthProf/Primary-Care-Toolkit.pdf

White Hughto, J. M., Reisner, S. L., & Pachankis, J. E. (2015). Transgender stigma and health: A critical review of stigma determinants, mechanisms, and interventions. *Social Science & Medicine*, 147, 222–231. doi:10.1016/j.socscimed.2015.11.010

Zevin, B., & Deutsch, M. B. (2016, June 17). *Free silicone and other filler use.* UCSF Transgender Care and Treatment Guidelines. https://transcare.ucsf.edu/guidelines/silicone-filler

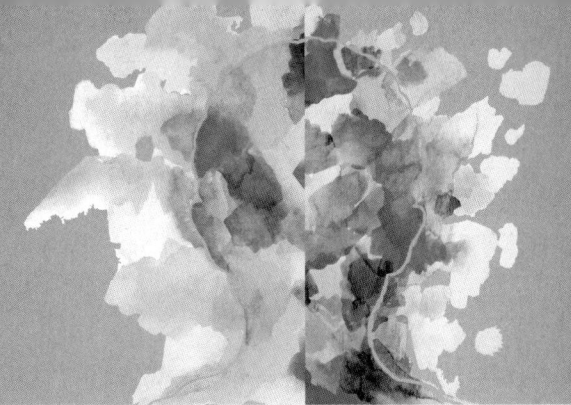

SECTION VII

Common Complex Adult Gerontology Presentations

CHAPTER 41	Anemia	505
CHAPTER 42	Anxiety	521
CHAPTER 43	Asthma in Adolescents and Adults	529
CHAPTER 44	Cancer Survivorship	545
CHAPTER 45	Chronic Obstructive Pulmonary Disease	553
CHAPTER 46	Chronic Nonmalignant Pain Management	569
CHAPTER 47	Chronic Wound Care	579
CHAPTER 48	Dementia	587
CHAPTER 49	Depression	599
CHAPTER 50	Diabetes Mellitus	615
CHAPTER 51	Epilepsy	627
CHAPTER 52	Gastroesophageal Reflux Disease	637
CHAPTER 53	Geriatric Syndromes	645
CHAPTER 54	Heart Failure	655
CHAPTER 55	Herpes Simplex Virus	665

CHAPTER 56	HIV Infection in Adolescents and Adults	675
CHAPTER 57	Hypertension	701
CHAPTER 58	Intimate Partner Violence (Domestic Violence)	711
CHAPTER 59	Irritable Bowel Syndrome	721
CHAPTER 60	Lipid Disorders	729
CHAPTER 61	Low Back Pain	743
CHAPTER 62	Nonalcoholic Fatty Liver Disease (NAFLD)	757
CHAPTER 63	Weight	765
CHAPTER 64	Substance Use and Substance Use Disorders	775
CHAPTER 65	Thyroid Disorders	805
CHAPTER 66	Upper Back and Neck Pain Syndromes	817
CHAPTER 67	Upper Extremity Tendinopathy: Shoulder (Bicipital and Rotator Cuff), Elbow, and De Quervain Tendinopathy	833

CHAPTER 41

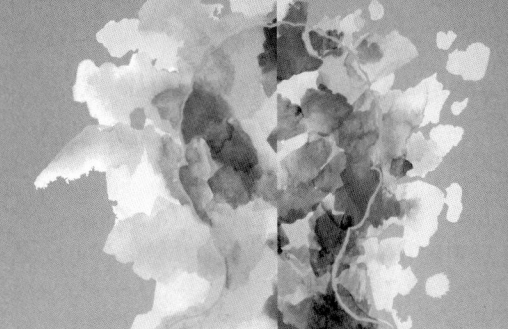

Anemia

Michelle M. Marin

I. Introduction and general background

Anemia is defined as a decrease in the red blood cell (RBC) number with hemoglobin (Hgb) concentration inadequate to carry oxygen to meet physiological demands (Newhall et al., 2020). The World Health Organization (WHO) defines anemia by laboratory definition as Hgb of less than 12.0 g/dL for premenopausal women and 13 g/dL for adults. The American Society of Hematology defines anemia differently using levels of 13.5 g/dL for men and 12 g/dL for women. Anemia affects 1/3 of the world population (Chaparro & Suchdev, 2019). Globally, most anemias are caused by iron deficiency, hemoglobinopathies, and hemolytic anemias (Safiri et al., 2021). Anemia is not a diagnosis but a collection of symptoms presenting from a potentially multifactorial condition creating the decreased red blood cells. The degree of symptoms depends on the type of anemia; how quickly the anemia develops and its severity; and the presence of comorbidities, especially cardiovascular disease. Gradual onset of anemia is better tolerated because of compensatory mechanisms. Symptoms can be subtle until anemia becomes severe, defined as 10 g/dL (Cascio & DeLourery, 2017). Certain races and ethnic groups are at increased risk for anemia because of genetic factors, and socioeconomic disadvantage, especially with untreated chronic illness, also increases risk (Maakaron, 2023). In older adults, anemia prevalence is 10%–24% and increasing, because of both better diagnostics and changing demographics (Stauder et al., 2018). Although more than one cause of anemia may coexist, creating a complex picture, correct identification of the underlying disease is essential for appropriately managed care.

Erythropoiesis is the regulated process of RBC production through a series of steps (Satish, K., et al. 2016). In adults, this process occurs in the bone marrow of the sternum, ribs, vertebrae, and pelvis. The process begins when pluripotent stem cells are dedicated and the hematopoietic precursor cells mature with growth factors and hormones. Stem cells become reticulocytes for 3 days before becoming a mature RBC, typically surviving in the circulation for 120 days. The key to erythropoietin production is the availability of oxygen, which is carried to the tissues bound to the Hgb. When oxygen is low, then erythropoietin (90% from the kidney) triggers the RBC production to meet tissue demand. This production feedback system can occur only when all the needed substrates are in place: normal renal production of erythropoietin, functioning bone marrow, and adequate support of substrates of Hgb synthesis.

Anemia is often seen during pregnancy, when the blood volume increases by about 50% to meet the demands of increased circulation of the placenta and maternal-fetal tissue. This increase in intravascular volume starts at 6 weeks, peaks at about 28–34 weeks, and levels off during the last 6 weeks of pregnancy. Because plasma volume expansion is faster and greater than RBC production, there is a lowering of the Hgb and hematocrit, referred to as *physiologic anemia*. Hgb below 10.5 dL is a true anemia regardless of gestational age (Breyman C, 2015). Nutritional anemias do occur, with iron deficiency being the most common because pregnancy results in increased iron demand. Folate and cobalamin, necessary for fetal growth and maternal tissue development, add to deficiencies, contributing to anemia in pregnancy (Patel & Balanchivadze, 2021). If there is no significant blood loss during the intrapartum period, the Hgb and hematocrit typically return to normal at about 6 weeks postpartum. Severe anemia in pregnancy is associated with an increased risk of spontaneous abortion, low birth weight, preterm birth, and fetal death (Brabin et al., 2001). Persistent severe anemia increases the risk of maternal mortality (Sifakis & Pharmakides, 2000).

Anemia classifications are based on causative mechanisms, including (1) excessive RBC loss, (2) inadequate or ineffective RBC production, (3) abnormal RBC destruction, or (4) morphologic characteristics. Morphological appearance helps provide insight using cell characteristics to point toward a diagnosis. (**Table 41-1**). Evaluation of anemia should begin with assessing the mean corpuscular volume (MCV), allowing for a stepwise approach to diagnosis (**Table 41-2**). Common microcytic anemias (MCV < 80 fL) include iron deficiency, thalassemia, lead poisoning, and sideroblastic anemia. The most common causes of normocytic anemias (MCV 80–110 fL) include anemia of chronic disease, hemolytic anemia, bone marrow failure or infiltration, endocrine disorders, and renal disease. Common macrocytic anemias (MCV > 100 fL) include vitamin B_{12} and folate deficiencies. Outside the usual categories of anemia lies a unique group of poorly diagnosed anemias that occurs in the geriatric population, accounting for 43% of hypoproliferative anemias with reduced oral intake, poor absorption and excessive blood loss as contributors. (Makipour et al., 2008; Kumar et al, 2022) (**Table 41-3**). Multiple etiologies of anemia can coexist together, requiring a stepwise diagnostic approach that is critical to not missing a treatable cause.

A. Microcytic anemias
   1. Iron-deficiency anemia (IDA)
      a. Definition and overview: Iron deficiency is a microcytic and hypochromic (decrease in Hgb concentration) anemia. It occurs when the bone marrow iron stores are less than what is needed to produce RBCs. Hgb definitions can vary by

Table 41-1 Red Blood Cell (RBC) Morphology

Description of RBC		Associated With Disease
Anisocytosis	Excessive number of RBCs of various sizes	Larger size = vitamin B_{12} or folate deficiency, drug effect Smaller size = iron deficiency
Hypochromia (decreased hemoglobin [Hgb] content in the RBC)	Central pallor	Iron deficiency (Hgb < 10 g/dL)
Macro-ovalocytes	Oval red blood cell	Vitamin B_{12} or folate deficiency, liver disease, myelodysplastic syndrome
Polychromasia	Wright's stain: large grayish blue with pink	Reticulocytes Increased levels in a peripheral smear may result from a variety of anemias or from damage to the bone marrow.
Poikilocytosis	Abnormal red blood cell shapes, such as:	(The following is not inclusive list.)
	Acanthocytes (spur cells)	Severe liver disease
	Echinocytes (burr cells)	Uremia, hyperlipidemia, artifact
	Schistocytes Helmet cells	Microangiopathic or intravascular damage to red cell Hemolytic anemia
	Spherocytes	Autoimmune hemolytic anemia, glucose-6-phosphate dehydrogenase (G6PD) deficiency, hereditary spherocytosis
	Target cells	Thalassemia, liver disease, hemoglobin C, sickle cell disease
	Teardrop cells	Myelofibrosis, infiltrative processes of marrow
	Rouleaux formation	Paraproteinemia, such as multiple myeloma, inflammatory states
RBC inclusions		(The following is not inclusive list.)
	Basophilic stippling	Lead poisoning, thalassemia, myelofibrosis
	Pappenheimer (iron) bodies	Sideroblastic anemia, lead poisoning
	Parasites	Malaria, babesiosis
Hypersegmentation	Neutrophil nuclei with more than seven lobes	Vitamin B_{12} or folate deficiency, drug effects

Table 41-2 Separating Anemia by Mean Corpuscular Volume (MCV)

Hypochromic Microcytic MCV < 80 μm³	Iron deficiency	Thalassemia	Sideroblastic	Hemoglobinopathies	Lead poisoning
Normochromic/ Normocytic MCV 80–100 fL	Acute hemorrhage	Acute hemolysis	Early iron deficiency, folate, and vitamin B_{12} deficiency	Anemia of chronic disease Chronic inflammation Acute and chronic infections Cancer Kidney disease	Myelodysplastic syndromes: bone marrow failure, pregnancy
Macrocytic MCV > 100 fL	Megaloblastic: vitamin B_{12} and folate deficiencies and drug induced	Reticulocytosis: intense red blood cell stimulation caused by acute hemolysis or hemorrhage (reticulocytes are large and young red blood cells)	Chronic liver disease	Myelodysplastic syndromes: bone marrow failure or infiltration	Endocrinopathies Postsplenectomy

Reproduced from Collins-Bride, G., & Saxe, J. (Eds.). (1998). *Nurse practitioner/physician collaborative practice: Clinical guidelines for ambulatory care.* UCSF Nursing Press. Used with permission from the UCSF Nursing Press.

Table 41-3 Differentiating Microcytic Anemias

	MCV	RDW	Retics	Iron	TIBC	% Sat	Ferritin
Iron deficiency	D	I	D	D	I	D	D
Iron depletion	N	N	N	N	I	D	D
β-Thalassemia	DQ	D	I	N	N	N	N
Sideroblastic	D	H	I	NII	NID	NII	N
Chronic disease	D or N	N	NID	D	N/D	N/I/D	N
Lead poisoning	D	N	I	N	N	N	N

D, decreased; *DQ*, decreased greater than expected in iron deficiency; *I*, increased; *II*, increased significantly; *MCV*, mean corpuscular volume; *N*, normal; *RDW*, red blood cell distribution width; *TIBC*, total iron-binding capacity.

age, sex, elevation above sea level, and smoking status (Garcia-Casal et al., 2019). According to WHO, those living at higher altitudes and smokers will have higher Hgb. Estimates are that 15% to 35% of female endurance athletes are at risk, whereas their male counterparts have a 5% to 11% risk for IDA (Sims et al., 2019). Risk factors for IDA include age, sex, lactation, and pregnancy. Common causes of iron deficiency are:

  i. Increased demand for RBC: Pregnancy accounts for about 75% of non physiologic anemia in the pregnant population (American College of Obstetricians and Gynecologists [ACOG], 2008). This is due to an increased demand for iron during pregnancy for Hgb synthesis, as well as for fetal liver storage, which is necessary to meet the needs of the infant in the first 6 months of life. The demand for iron increases in the second half of pregnancy as red cell mass increases along with the demands of the growing fetus.

  ii. Malnutrition: diets with inadequate iron intake

  iii. Malabsorption: Individuals with gastric atrophy, achlorhydria, erythropoiesis-stimulating agents, and proton pump inhibitors (Cappellini et al., 2020; Kryssia et al, 2018) may experience anemia as a result of not appropriately absorbing iron that is present in the diet.

  iv. Increased blood loss: blood loss caused by menstrual bleeding, malignancy, gastrointestinal blood loss, urinary loss, bleeding disorders and other coagulative factors, trauma, and surgery

 b. Prevalence and incidence: IDA is the most common nutritional deficiency (Umbreit, 2005). Estimates are that 5.6% of the U.S. population and 17% of older adults had anemia in 2012 (Lanier et al., 2018; Le, 2016). Iron deficiency results in increased maternal and child mortality, reduced work productivity, and delayed childhood development. Individuals with mild to moderate deficiency experience an increased risk for developing infectious diseases, sleep disturbances, and heart failure (Leung et al., 2020). In older adults, anemia is associated with a significant increase in morbidity and mortality, including functional decline affecting mobility and balance (Lanier et al., 2019).

2. Thalassemia
 a. Definition and overview: Thalassemia syndromes are a group of inherited autosomal-recessive anemias classified by defects in the synthesis of one or more of the Hgb globin-chain subunits. These defects can occur either in the α or β globin chains of Hgb. The combined imbalances of globin and inadequate Hgb production result in a variety of clinical manifestations, and both cause hemolysis. The former causes hypochromia and microcytosis; the latter leads to ineffective erythropoiesis. However, new thinking about thalassemia syndromes expands beyond genotypes to include clinical severity, specifically transfusion dependent or non–transfusion dependent (Viprakasit & Ekwattanakit, 2018).
 b. Prevalence and incidence: Thalassemia is the most common genetic disorder. It is encountered in every ethnic group and geographic location. Alpha thalassemia is seen most often in persons of Southeast Asian and African descent (Muncie & Campbell, 2009). Beta thalassemia is more common in persons descended from Southeast Asia, Africa, and the Mediterranean. Thalassemia prevalence in these regions ranges from 1% to 40% (Merkeley & Bolster, 2020). In a world of immigration and intermarriage, new patterns of thalassemia have emerged. In some European countries, β-thalassemia and other hemoglobinopathies are the most common genetic anemia (Kattamis et al., 2020). Even in the United States, this once-rare disease is being seen more frequently (Sayani & Kwiatkowski, 2015).

3. Sideroblastic anemia
 a. Definition and overview: Sideroblastic anemias are a group of acquired and congenital disorders with ringed iron-laden sideroblasts in the bone marrow, accompanied by moderate to severe microcytic anemia. Despite having normal iron levels, the iron inside the red cell is inadequate for function. X-linked inherited forms are the most common and typically present in early adulthood; other rare forms are recognized earlier in life. Acquired types are caused by exposures to toxins such as alcohol, lead, or zinc, as well as deficiencies of copper and vitamin B_6. Exposures to drugs such as isonicotinic acid hydrazide (INH), hormones, and antibiotics may also lead to acquired sideroblastic anemia. Once the offending toxin is removed, supportive therapy usually sustains normal survival (Bottomley & Fleming, 2014). Other acquired anemias include those of the myelodysplastic syndrome as a refractory anemia.
 b. Prevalence and incidence: The incidence of sideroblastic anemia is low. Acquired types are more prevalent in older adults, whereas hereditary types usually are seen in the young. Many individuals are stable for years, but a subset of patients who belong to the myelodysplastic syndrome category go on to develop leukemia.

B. Normocytic anemias
1. Definition and overview: In a normocytic anemia, the MCV is within normal limits, but Hgb and hematocrit are decreased mildly to moderately. Individuals are generally not symptomatic but may have symptoms due to underlying disease. Nearly all anemias are normocytic in their initial stages (Brill & Baumgardner, 2000). Most normocytic anemias appear to be a result of impaired RBC production (Yilmaz & Shaikh, 2021). The reticulocyte count differentiates hypoproliferative (<2%) from hyperproliferative (>2%) anemias. Hyperproliferative anemias include hematological malignancies and aplastic anemias, which are associated with pancytopenia.
2. Anemia of chronic disease (ACD) and anemia of chronic inflammation (AI)
 a. Definitions and overview: ACD is a chronic, normocytic, normochromic, mildly microcystic anemia with a low reticulocyte count (hypoproliferative). This anemia is caused by the underproduction of RBCs as a result of one or more of three major pathways: iron restriction, inflammatory suppression of erythropoietic activity, and decreased RBC lifespan. Hepcidin, an iron-regulatory peptide produced by the liver, is thought be the central regulator of the uptake and release of iron. This is regulated by iron supply, the state of inflammation, and erythrocytosis (Agarwal & Yee, 2019). ACD or AI is a diagnosis of exclusion and has characteristics of iron

homeostasis, hypoferremia, and hyperferritinemia (Weiss et al., 2019). Common causes include:
   i. Chronic systemic diseases, such as congestive heart failure and chronic obstructive pulmonary disease
   ii. Chronic autoimmune inflammation disorders, such as rheumatoid arthritis and inflammatory bowel disease
   iii. Neoplasm
   iv. Chronic liver and kidney disease
   v. Chronic infection, such as HIV
   vi. Endocrine deficiencies, such as hypothyroidism, diabetes, adrenal or pituitary insufficiencies, and hypogonadism
   vii. Uncompensated blood loss
   viii. Hypersplenism
   ix. Infections
   x. Higher body weight
   b. Prevalence and incidence: With rising numbers of chronic illnesses and older individuals in the population, ACD is increasingly common. It is the most common anemia in hospitalized and chronically ill patients (Weiss et al., 2019). ACD and other anemias can coexist, creating a normocytic pattern.
3. Hemolytic anemia
   a. Definition and overview: Hemolytic anemia is a normocytic or macrocytic, normochromic anemia or where there is a premature destruction of RBCs through cold and warm antibodies for which the bone marrow cannot compensate (Jager et al., 2020). This tends to be a hyperproliferative anemia because the bone marrow attempts to produce more reticulocytes. RBC shape is crucial in making this diagnosis. Depending on the cause, symptoms can be on a spectrum from chronic to life-threatening, with the etiology and management dictating survival. The numerous causes of this anemia include exposure to various drugs, infections, spider and snake bites, pregnancy, blood transfusions, and immune disorders or inheritance (Barcellini et al., 2018; Phillips & Henderson, 2018). Congenital types occur with recognition early in life, as in sickle cell disease, or later in life when exposed to a stressor such as fava beans or aspirin, as in glucose-6-phosphate dehydrogenase (G6PD) deficiency. The acquired type usually occurs in adulthood and in those persons older than 40 years of age and with mechanical hemolysis, paroxysmal nocturnal hemolysis, and those with reactive antibodies. Individuals with autoimmune hemolytic anemia with severe anemia at diagnosis are at increased risk of relapse.
   b. Prevalence and incidence: Hemolytic anemia represents 5% of all anemias (Schick, 2010). The incidence of autoimmune hemolytic anemia is 1 case per 100,000 years (Hill et al., 2017).

C. *Macrocytic anemias*

Macrocytic anemia is classified as megaloblastic or nonmegaloblastic anemia. Macrocytosis can be seen without megaloblastic changes in liver disease, hypothyroidism, and myelodysplastic syndromes (Nagao & Hirokawa, 2017). Megaloblastic anemias are a group of diverse anemias that share the feature of failure in the synthesis and assembly of DNA, resulting in ineffective erythropoiesis and hemolysis. The most common causes of megaloblastic anemia are folate and vitamin B_{12} deficiencies, with pernicious anemia being a primary cause especially in persons of European or African descent (Socha et al., 2020, Stabler & Allen 2004). Vitamin B_{12} is highly prevalent in those consuming a vegan diet (no diary or eggs) (Woo et al., 2014). However, medications that are folate agonists (e.g., methotrexate), other drugs (e.g., anticonvulsants, oral contraceptives), and inborn errors of metabolism can interfere with folate levels. Findings of MCV greater than 100 suggest megaloblastic anemia, but with MCV greater than 110, it is much more likely to be present. Deficiencies of one of these vitamins can cause malabsorption of the other vitamins. Megaloblastic disease, especially when combined with microcytic anemia, can present as normocytic.

1. Vitamin B_{12} deficiency
   a. Definitions and overview: Vitamin B_{12} (cobalamin) deficiency is a problem of either inadequate intake over several years or inadequate absorption. Lifelong subclinical vitamin B_{12} deficiency, 50% with normal vitamin B_{12} levels, when challenged with abnormal absorption or altered metabolism, can tip individuals into symptomatic deficiency. Initially, microcystic anemia precedes the megaloblastosis. Consider screening high-risk individuals for megaloblastic anemia. Common causes are:
      i. Pernicious anemia associated with autoimmune disorders and atrophic gastritis
      ii. Gastrectomy, bariatric surgery, and intestinal surgeries
      iii. Small-bowel disorders, such as inflammatory bowel disease, bacterial overgrowth, tapeworms, enteritis, sprue, and celiac disease, all affecting the terminal ileum
      iv. Malnutrition and long-term vegan diets without dairy products or eggs
      v. Medications inhibiting absorption, such as metformin, proton pump inhibitors, and histamine 2 blockers
      vi. Food: cobalamin malabsorption syndrome when nutritional intake is adequate and there is no evidence of other causes of malabsorption or pernicious anemia
   b. Prevalence and incidence: It is estimated that vitamin B_{12} deficiency occurs in 6% of those older than 60 years. In the elderly, rates increase from 5% to 20%. Those 31–51 years old have a 4%

incidence and have a subclinical presentation (Shipton & Thachil, 2015). Although usually seen in adults older than 40 of Scandinavian or northern European ancestry, it can also be seen in any population. Nutritional deficiency is seen worldwide; however, in affluent countries, inadequate absorption is most common.
2. Folic acid deficiency
   a. Definitions and overview: Folic acid is present in fruits, nuts, meat, eggs, and leafy vegetables. A typical diet of 50 mg/d should be adequate. Common causes of folic acid deficiency include:
      i. Inadequate intake
      ii. Decreased absorption in small bowel, as in inflammatory bowel disease, sprue, and celiac disease
      iii. Cultural or ethnic cooking destroying folate, as in prolonged stewing
      iv. Medications interfering with absorption, such as methotrexate, phenytoin, acyclovir, oral contraceptives, colchicine, and trimethoprim
      v. Increased demand in pregnancy, hemolytic anemia, puberty, eczematous conditions, and malignancy infiltration in the bone marrow
   b. Prevalence and incidence: The U.S. Food and Drug Administration (FDA) mandated that folic acid be added to enriched grain products in 1998, which resulted in a significant decrease in folate deficiency (Hildebrand et al., 2021). In the United States, folate deficiency is most common in those with alcohol use disorder, those who are homeless, and those born elsewhere. Tropical sprue, which is endemic near the equator, results in malabsorption of this critical vitamin.

II. Database
A. *Subjective: microcytic*
1. IDA, thalassemia, and sideroblastic anemia
   a. Past health history
      i. Medical illnesses: recurrent IDA, anorexia, chronic kidney disease, gastrointestinal or genitourinary malignancy, celiac disease, atrophic gastritis, helminthic infections, and chronic inflammatory conditions
      ii. Surgical history: partial or total gastroenterostomy, gastric resection, splenectomy, or recent surgery
      iii. Obstetric and gynecological history: heavy menses, multiparty, recent pregnancy, and parturition
      iv. Medication history: nonsteroidal anti-inflammatory drugs, steroids, chemotherapy, iron or multivitamins, salicylates, antacids that block iron absorption, and health food products
      v. Exposure history: toxic exposures, such as lead poisoning (exposure to lead-based paint, lead-contaminated dust, and lead-contaminated residential soil), potent marrow-toxic agents, and radiation
   b. Family history
      i. Anemia
      ii. Chronic inflammatory diseases
      iii. Malignancy
      iv. Lead poisoning
   c. Personal and social history
      i. Diet inadequate in iron, dairy, or animal products
      ii. Heavy alcohol use
      iii. Travel to sub-Sahara Africa, exposing the person to *Schistosoma*, such as *Trichuris* infections, and malarial zones
      iv. Regular blood donations
2. Thalassemia
   a. Past health history
      i. Medical illnesses: chronic microcytic anemia and iron overload.
      ii. Surgical history: splenectomy or hematopoietic stem cell transplant.
      iii. Obstetric history: pregnancy or stillborn fetus caused by hydrops fetalis
      iv. Medication history: chelation therapy, iron intake, and RBC transfusions
   b. Family history
      i. Thalassemia and hemoglobinopathies or bleeding disorders
      ii. Ethnicity: Mediterranean, Southeast Asian, Chinese, and African American descent
3. Sideroblastic anemia
   a. Past health history
      i. Medical illness: copper deficiency, vitamin B_6 deficiency, and myelodysplastic syndrome
      ii. Medication history: excessive use of zinc supplements, antibiotics, copper chelating agents, antituberculosis agents, and chemotherapy
      iii. Exposure history: lead poisoning and prolonged exposure to cold
   b. Family history
      i. Sideroblastic anemia
      ii. Mitochondrial disease
   c. Personal and social history
      i. Chronic excessive alcohol intake
      ii. Tobacco use
4. Review of systems for microcytic anemias
   a. Constitutional: The degree of symptoms depends on the degree and rate of anemia development. Marked fatigue with weakness and decreased exercise tolerance may be the earliest symptoms, along with postural faintness, headache, and weight loss. Easy bruising, night sweats, and weight loss suggest a hematological

malignancy (Mehta, 2022). Pica, especially eating of ice, is commonly seen in children.
   b. Skin and nails: pallor, bruising, koilonychia (spoon nails), brittle nails, bronze-colored skin, and hair thinning
   c. Ears, nose, and throat: bleeding, fissures at corners of mouth, painful mouth
   d. Neck: swollen neck glands
   e. Pulmonary: cough, shortness of breath, and hemoptysis
   f. Cardiac: chest pain, palpitations, and tachycardia
   g. Abdomen: tenderness; masses; changes in bowel habits; fatty, bulky stools with foul odor; bleeding hemorrhoids; hematemesis; melena or bright-red blood per rectum; distention; and difficulty swallowing
   h. Genitourinary: bloody urine
   i. Gynecological: heavy and or irregular menses, pregnancy, and multiple pregnancies
   j. Skeletal: bone tenderness
B. *Subjective: normocytic anemias*
   1. Anemia of chronic disease
      a. Past health history
         i. Medical illness: anemia; chronic diseases, such as renal disease; inflammatory bowel disease; autoimmune disorders; malignancies; sickle cell disease; and liver disease
         ii. Surgical history: cholecystectomy, prosthetic cardiac valves, and stem cell transplant
         iii. Medications
         iv. Exposure history: parvovirus B19
      b. Family history
         i. G6PD deficiency
         ii. Sickle cell disease
         iii. Hereditary anemia disorders
         iv. Autoimmune disorders
         v. Renal or liver disease
      c. Personal and social history
         i. Diet including fava beans
   2. Hemolytic anemia
      a. Past medical history
         i. Medical illnesses: previous hemolysis, chronic hemolytic anemia, systemic lupus erythematosus, rheumatoid arthritis, chronic lymphocytic leukemia, non-Hodgkin lymphoma, various carcinomas, idiopathic thrombocytopenic purpura and thrombotic thrombocytopenic purpura, G6PD deficiency, malaria, and cold agglutinin disease
         ii. Surgical: prosthetic heart valves, patches, and vascular grafts
         iii. Medications: antimalarials, sulfonamides, nitrofurantoin, sulfonylureas, rifampin, quinidine, interferon, metronidazole, penicillin, and blood transfusions
         iv. Exposures: infectious agents, such as parasites; viruses, such as Epstein–Barr or cytomegalovirus; measles; syphilis; enteric bacteria; spider bites and snake venom; copper; and organic compounds
      b. Family history
         i. G6PD deficiency
         ii. Autoimmune hemolytic anemia and sideroblastic anemia
         iii. RBC membrane disorders
      c. Personal and social history
         i. Aggressive exercise causing microvascular trauma
   3. Review of symptoms for normocytic anemia and ACD and hemolysis
      a. Constitutional: fatigue, weakness, postural faintness, poor exercise tolerance, and abrupt or gradual onset
      b. Skin: rash, yellowing color, bruising, petechiae, pale skin, and nails
      c. Neck: swollen lymph nodes
      d. Pulmonary: shortness of breath
      e. Cardiac: palpitations, tachycardia, and chest pain
      f. Abdominal: right upper quadrant pain, abdominal fullness, and decreased appetite
      g. Extremities: leg ulcers and edema
      h. Joints: swollen, painful joints
      i. Bladder: dark or bloody urine
C. *Subjective: macrocytic and megaloblastic*
   1. Vitamin B_{12} deficiency
      a. Past health history
         i. Medical history: autoimmune thyroid disease, type I diabetes mellitus, Addison disease, idiopathic hypoparathyroidism, autoimmune hemolytic diseases, tropical sprue, atrophic gastritis, regional enteritis, or gastric cancer
         ii. Surgical: gastrectomy, bariatric surgery, or intestinal surgery
         iii. Medications: metformin, thyroid replacement, colchicine, allopurinol, histamine 2 blockers, proton pump inhibitors
         iv. Exposures: intestinal tapeworm infestation and repeated and prolonged (>6 hour) nitrous oxide inhalation, especially in the elderly (Longo, 2009)
      b. Family history
         i. Pernicious anemia
         ii. Autoimmune disorders, such as diabetes mellitus type 1 and thyroid disorders, vitiligo, hypoparathyroidism, and Addison disease
      c. Personal and social history
         i. Vegan diet, high folate intake
         ii. Alcohol use
   2. Folate deficiency
      a. Past health history
         i. Medical history: vitamin B_{12} deficiency, chronic hemolytic anemia, sprue, atrophic gastritis, small bowel disease, psoriasis, epilepsy, and chronic hemodialysis

ii. Obstetric and gynecological history: pregnancy
iii. Medications: methotrexate, pentamidine, trimethoprim, cancer chemotherapy, triamterene, phenytoin, primidone, phenobarbital, and sulfasalazine
b. Family history
i. Hereditary disorders
ii. Gluten sensitivities
c. Personal and social history
i. Alcohol abuse
ii. Inadequate diet
3. Review of systems: macrocytic or megaloblastic anemia, vitamin B_{12} or folic acid deficiency
a. Constitutional: fatigue, decreased exercise tolerance, weakness, and weight loss
b. Skin: yellow skin, pallor, vitiligo, and rashes
c. Mouth: cheilosis, stomatitis, sore red smooth tongue, and atrophic glossitis
d. Neck: sense of fullness in the thyroid region
e. Pulmonary: shortness of breath
f. Cardiac: tachycardia, chest pain, palpitations.
g. Abdominal: diarrhea, pain, anorexia, nausea, constipation, bowel incontinence, and sense of fullness
h. Bladder: incontinence
i. Neurologic: paresthesia, balance problems, and difficulty walking
j. Extremities: edema
k. Neuropsychiatric: depression, irritability, dementia, and insomnia
D. Physical examination
1. Evaluate weight and height.
2. Complete vital signs: postural blood pressure and pulse, respiratory rate, oxygen saturation and temperature
3. See **Table 41-4** for physical examination findings seen in anemia.

III. Assessment
A. *Determine the diagnosis*
After the health history and physical examination, guide the workup based on the clues found. Review previous complete blood cell count (CBC) to evaluate the individual's trend of RBC counts. Those individuals with active or severe bleeding, severe anemia, or pancytopenias require referrals for rapid evaluation and stabilization.
B. *Differentiate the anemia and assess the severity of the disease.*
1. Microcytic anemias
a. Iron-deficiency anemia
i. CBC: White blood cell and platelet abnormalities give clues about bone marrow malfunction, such as myelodysplastic or myeloproliferative disorder.
ii. Assess anemia based on the MCV (Table 41-2).
iii. Order iron studies: Ferritin, iron, total iron-binding capacity (TIBC), transferrin serum iron saturation (TSAT), and reticulocyte count with a peripheral blood smear (Table 41-1). Ferritin <30 ug/L and TSAT <20% are most suggestive of IDA. Additionally, IDA is associated with reactive thrombocytosis.
iv. Determine the type of microcytic anemia. If iron deficiency, order fecal occult blood testing and urinalysis to rule out blood loss from the gastrointestinal and genitourinary tracts, respectively. It is critical not to miss an occult gastrointestinal lesion, frequently a malignancy. Refer postmenopausal women and men with IDA to gastroenterology for bidirectional endoscopy and colonoscopy (Bouri & Martin, 2018). For asymptomatic premenopausal women with IDA, the American Gastroenterological Association recommends bidirectional endoscopy (Ko et al, 2020). Older premenopausal woman can be referred depending on the clinical picture particularly if she has prior GI screening. Usually, younger patients with IDA have non-gastrointestinal etiologies and do not need referral unless they are GI symptoms or have a strong family history of colon disease. Celiac disease can be evaluated by a serum tissue transglutaminase immunoglobulin A (tTG-IgA) test.
v. Consider other causes of IDA, especially in older adults, such as myeloma and combined anemias.
vi. Pregnant women and young menstruating women who are asymptomatic and otherwise healthy likely have IDA caused by menses or increased iron demands from a growing fetus in the context of dietary iron intake (ACOG, 2008).
vii. A limited therapeutic trial of iron reevaluating the results can be helpful because only an iron-deficient state will improve with iron supplementation (see the treatment section). A 1.0-g/dL increase on day 14 predicts the overall response to oral iron (Okam et al., 2017).
b. Thalassemia anemia
i. If iron studies are normal and an abnormal peripheral smear is reported, consider thalassemia based on the individual's history. Milder forms of thalassemia need to be distinguished from iron deficiency, and more severe forms need to be distinguished from other hemoglobinopathies. The diagnosis of thalassemia is made by an Hgb electrophoresis test (**Table 41-5**). Most individuals

Table 41-4 Physical Examination Findings Seen With Anemia

Location	Finding	Implication
Skin and nails	Pallor	Decreased number of red blood cells
	Petechiae	Thrombocytopenia, leukemia, disseminated intravascular coagulation
	Telangiectasia and spider angiomas	Liver disease
	Jaundice, icterus Bronze-tinged skin	Hemolytic and megaloblastic anemia, liver disease Sideroblastic anemia
	Decreased elasticity of skin, brittle nails	Long-standing anemia
	Koilonychia (spoon nails) Hair loss	Long-standing iron-deficiency anemia
	Rash	Systemic lupus erythematosus
Neck	Thyromegaly or masses	Endocrinopathies
Mucous membranes	Pallor, cheilosis, and stomatitis	Leukemia, pernicious anemia, or severe iron deficiency
	Smooth red tongue, atrophic glossitis	Vitamin B_{12} deficiency
Lymph nodes	Lymphadenopathy	Leukemia, lymphoma, HIV
Heart	Tachycardia, loud murmurs, decreased point of maximal impulse (PMI), congestive heart failure, functional murmurs	Severe anemia, pregnancy, renal disease
Pulmonary	Tachypnea	Severe anemia
Abdomen	Splenomegaly, hepatomegaly, or hepatic tenderness Scars of prior surgeries	Leukemia, hemolytic anemia Liver disease, autoimmune disorder
Central nervous system	Decreased vibratory and position sense/ataxia and decreased vibration of 256-degree tuning fork	Pernicious anemia Lead poisoning causing ringed sideroblasts
Skeletal	Bone tenderness, swollen joints Back pain	Hematologic disease, rheumatoid arthritis, autoimmune disorders, myeloma
Rectal	Guaiac-positive stool or bright-red blood per rectum	Gastrointestinal bleeding
Extremities	Edema	Heart failure, renal failure, cirrhosis, hepatitis
	Leg ulcers	Chronic hemolytic anemia, iron deficiency

with thalassemia can be monitored and should not be given iron unless they have documented iron deficiency.
ii. Thalassemias are congenital. Compare current CBC to previous CBCs. Microcytosis is usually significant, whereas the RBC count is normal or elevated.
iii. If a birthing parent is thought to be a carrier, the nonbirthing parent of the baby should be tested. A CBC and Hgb electrophoresis should be done.

c. Sideroblastic anemia
   i. Review the CBC, peripheral smear, and iron studies with reticulocytes; iron overload is suggestive of clonal sideroblastic anemia.
   ii. A bone marrow biopsy with appropriate staining ultimately is the gold standard for this diagnosis.

d. Lead poisoning
   i. Review the CBC and iron studies.
   ii. Consider getting a zinc protoporphyrin or free erythrocyte protoporphyrin (an elevated

Table 41-5 Thalassemia Percentage of Abnormal Hemoglobin (Hgb) and Degrees of Anemia

	HgbA	HgbA2	HgbF	Comments
Normal	97%–99%	1%–3%	<1%	
β-Thalassemia (minor)	80%–95%	4%–8%	1%–5%	Mean corpuscular volume (MCV) 55–75 fL, hematocrit (Hct) 28%–40%, peripheral smear mildly abnormal, heterozygous trait
β-Thalassemia (intermediate)	0%–30%	0%–10%	6%–100%	Moderate anemia
β-Thalassemia (major)	0%	4%–10%	90%–96%	Homozygous trait, marked microcytosis with severe anemia
α-Thalassemia trait	Normal	Normal	Normal	Heterozygous trait, 2/4 genes normal, MCV 60–70 fL, Hct 28–40%, diagnosis of exclusion

Data from Collins-Bride, G., & Saxe, J. (Eds.). (1998). *Nurse practitioner/physician collaborative practice: Clinical guidelines for ambulatory care*. UCSF Nursing Press. Used with permission from the UCSF Nursing Press.

level suggests lead poisoning or IDA) because either test can be used as an indication of lead exposure over the past 3 months.
iii. Obtain a serum lead level.
2. Normocytic anemia
   a. ACD: This is a diagnosis of exclusion when CBC, reticulocyte, and iron stores are normal. Ferritin of <30 ug/L is associated with iron deficiency with transferrin saturation below 20% (Cappellini et al., 2020). Ferritin of <100 ug/L with inflammatory conditions suggests iron deficiency, whereas ferritin of 100–300 ug/L and transferrin saturation of <20% is still suggestive of iron deficiency. ACD without inflammatory conditions is suggested by ferritin of >100 ug/L. A C-reactive protein can distinguish the two conditions. Identify potential causes of this anemia.
      i. Consider ordering an erythrocyte sedimentation rate and a C-reactive protein to look for chronic inflammatory states, both of which are elevated in infection and inflammation.
      ii. Rule out liver disease with liver functions tests and hepatitis screen; thyroid disease with thyroid function tests; and renal disease with a serum creatinine with blood urea nitrogen (BUN), creatinine clearance, and urinalysis. Consider an erythropoietin level for Hgb < 10 g/dL and chronic renal failure (Colbert, 2020). Based on history and physical findings, rheumatoid factor, antinuclear antibodies, and serum creatine kinase can be considered.
   b. Hemolytic anemia
      i. With a careful health and medication history and physical examination, look at the normocytic anemia MCV with reticulocytosis.
      ii. Order an indirect bilirubin, haptoglobin, and lactate dehydrogenase (LDH) blood test. Elevated LDH and bilirubin with low haptoglobin in suggestive of hemolytic anemia. A urine dipstick may show blood, but a urine microscopy will be negative for RBCs if hemolysis is intravascular, leading to hemoglobinuria (Hill et al., 2017).
      iii. Consider ordering a direct antiglobulin test (DAT) with monospecific anti-immunoglobulin G (anti-IgG) anti-c3d (Barcellini et al., 2018). This suggests an immune cause, but it is not specific. If autoimmune hemolytic anemia is suspected, those positive on DAT should be screened for a cold antibody test.
3. Macrocytic and megaloblastic anemias
   a. Vitamin B_{12} deficiency
      i. CBC with elevated MCV and a peripheral smear with macro-ovalocytes and hypersegmented polymorphonuclear cells are seen with vitamin B_{12} and folate deficiency.
      ii. Order a vitamin B_{12} and a folate level to differentiate the common causes of megaloblastic anemia. They can co-occur and can occur separately. Consider screening high-risk individuals, especially those with health conditions resulting in a high cell turnover, such as after a prolonged or critical illness, and normal MCV, as well as those who have taken proton pump inhibitors for more than 12 months or metformin for more than 4 months and those with strict vegan diets of longer than 3 years (Langan & Goodbred, 2017; Langan & Zawistoski, 2011).
      iii. Order a serum methylmalonic acid (MMA) level, which has increased sensitivity and

specificity for confirming vitamin B_{12} deficiency and homocysteine. Serum vitamin B_{12} of <200 pg/mL is diagnostic of deficiency (Langan & Goodbred, 2017). When levels are between 200 and 300 pg/mL, checking MMA and homocysteine is helpful to distinguish folate and vitamin B_{12} deficiencies. Additional serologic testing for parietal cell antibodies and anti–intrinsic factor (IF) is used to diagnose pernicious anemia (Mehta, 2022).

iv. Low cobalamin distinguishes vitamin B_{12} deficiency from myelodysplastic syndrome Folate deficiency: with normal vitamin B_{12} level, low serum folate level, normal methylmalonic level, and elevated homocysteine, folate deficiency is the probable diagnosis.

IV. Goals of clinical management
A. *Choose a cost-effective approach for diagnosing anemia.*
B. *Choose a treatment plan that normalizes serum RBC level and minimizes the risk of anemia relapse (Table 41-6).*
C. *Select an approach that maximizes the patient's short- and long-term adherence to treatment.*

V. Plan
A. **Microcytic anemias**
   1. Iron-deficiency anemia
      a. Encourage intake of iron-rich foods: lean red meat, poultry, seafood, egg yolks, beans, nuts, dried fruit, and dark leafy greens.
      b. Review foods (e.g., coffee, tea, soda, dairy) and medications (e.g., antacids, proton pump inhibitors, calcium supplements) that interfere with iron absorption.
      c. Ferrous sulfate therapy, 325 mg (65 mg elemental iron) daily to three times daily, depending on severity of anemia treatment. In pregnancy, this should be given in addition to prenatal vitamins (Graves & Barger, 2001). A 4-week trial of iron supplementation for mild anemia before a definitive diagnosis of IDA with iron studies is an acceptable initial intervention. If the follow-up CBC is normal, it is reasonable to assume the anemia was caused by a deficiency in iron. Plan to give iron for 1–2 months for anemia correction, then for an additional 4–5 months to replenish iron stores (ferritin level to 50 mcg/mL).
      d. *Keep iron out of the hands of children; ingesting only 10–20 pills can be fatal.*
      e. Discuss ways to increase iron intake and absorption: take with juice with vitamin C and in between meals on an empty stomach.
      f. Review side effects of supplementation: constipation; nausea; bloating; very dark, charcoal-colored stool; and abdominal cramps.
      g. If iron is poorly tolerated because of side effects, encourage increasing fluid intake and fiber and adding a stool softener. Switching to ferrous fumarate, ferrous gluconate, or a different preparation may help tolerance. Starting iron supplements slowly, then increasing the dose also may help individuals with side effects.
      h. If the patient has mild anemia, consider intermittent dosing (120 mg elemental iron one to two times weekly).
      i. Elemental iron interferes with zinc absorption, so zinc supplementation (25 mg, which is the amount found in prenatal vitamins) is recommended in pregnant patients (Graves & Barger, 2001).
      j. Repeat CBC and reticulocyte count in 2–4 weeks after initiation of treatment. An increased reticulocyte count after 7–10 days confirms that the bone marrow is responding.
      k. Although medication nonadherence is the most common cause of response failure, having the incorrect diagnosis has to be considered.
      l. Plan for patient follow-up with laboratory values at 1, 2, 4, and 6 months to ensure full recovery.
      m. Intravenous iron should be considered when oral iron is ineffective, particularly in those persons with gastrointestinal impairment (duodenal resection, celiac disease), high blood loss (menorrhagia), or intolerance of oral preparations (Jimenez et al., 2015).
      n. Medically stable individuals with Hgb <7 to 8 g/dL should be considered for blood transfusion, depending on patient characteristics (Szczepiorkowski & Dunbar, 2013).
      o. In pregnancy, obtain medical consultation if severe anemia (Hgb is less than 9 g/dL) despite initiation of therapy or if anemia is chronic.
      p. Patients who are hemodynamically unstable or do not respond to treatments should be referred to a physician.
   2. Thalassemia
      a. Individuals with mild disease should be identified to prevent repeated unnecessary diagnostic anemia evaluations and to prevent patients from taking iron unnecessarily.
      b. Individuals who have severe anemia and need to be treated with RBC transfusions and chelation therapy should be referred to a hematologist.
      c. Pregnant women who are found to be carriers and whose partners are also a carrier of either a thalassemia or sickle cell trait should have genetic counseling because of the risk of fetal hemoglobinopathy. Women who either have a thalassemia or sickle cell disease may have profound anemia with considerable neonatal morbidity and therefore should be cared for by a specialist in obstetrics and hematology (ACOG, 2008).
   3. Sideroblastic anemia
      a. If medically stable, no treatment is needed. Patients often do not respond to erythropoietin therapy.

Table 41-6 Laboratory Tests With Normal Values

*Note that each lab has its own result standards.

Test	Normal	Comment
Complete blood count Hemoglobin (Hgb) Hematocrit (Hct)	Hemoglobin: F: 12–15.5 g/dL M: 13.6–17.5 g/dL Hematocrit: F: 35%–49% M: 39%–49%	Physiologic variation because of age, smoking, exercise, and altitude. Hemoglobin reflects amount of oxygen-carrying protein. Hematocrit measures percentage of Hgb in blood.
Red blood cell count (RBC)	F: 3.5–5.2 × 10^6/mcL M: 4.3–6 × 10^6/mcL	Elevated in dehydration, lung disease, smoking, polycythemia vera
Mean cell volume (MCV)	80–100 fL	Reflects size of red cell
Mean cell hemoglobin concentration (MCHC)	31–36 g/dL	Increased with spherocytosis, hemolysis; decreased in other anemias
Mean cell Hgb (MCH)	26–34 pg	Calculation of average amount of Hgb in RBC
Red blood cell distribution width (RDW)	11.5%–14.5%	Calculation of variation of RBC size; increased in iron deficiency; normal in thalassemia
White blood cell count	4.5–11 × 10^3/mcL	
Platelets	15,000–450,000 µL	
Reticulocyte count	33–137 × 10^3/mcL >400 reflects RBC loss or destruction <200 reflects low production, macrocytosis, anemia of chronic disease (ACD), or myelodysplastic disease	Expect increase of 2 to 3 times in 10 days after anemia starts if normal erythropoietin and bone marrow.
Iron supply studies	50–175 mcg/dL	
Serum iron, total iron-binding capacity	250–460 mcg/dL	Decreased in iron-deficiency anemia
Transferrin saturation	25%–50%	Low in iron deficiency (<16%)
Ferritin	M: 10–200 µg/mL F: 10–200 µg/mL	Most useful in separating iron deficiency from ACD, thalassemia; lowest levels correlate with depleted bone marrow
Haptoglobin	4–316	High levels helpful in ruling out significant intravascular hemolysis
Folate	165–760 ng/mL	
Vitamin B_{12}	140–820 pg/mL	

Data from Gomella, L., & Haist, S. (2007). *The famous scut monkey handbook: Clinician's pocket reference* (11th ed.). McGraw-Hill; Nicoll, D., McPhee, S., Pignone, M., & Lu, C. (2007). *Pocket guide to diagnostic tests* (5th ed.). McGraw-Hill Medical.

b. Occasionally, these patients need RBC transfusions. A hematologist should be managing their anemia because of problems with iron overload.
  4. Lead poisoning
     a. Further investigate the patient's possible lead exposures: exposure to lead-based paint, lead-contaminated dust, lead-contaminated residential soil (U.S. Environmental Protection Agency, 2023).
     b. Refer patient to the public health department to help with investigation of lead exposure.
     c. Consult with a hematologist to evaluate for a plan of treatment (e.g., need for therapeutic administration of a chelating agent).
B. Normocytic anemias
  1. Anemia of chronic disease
     a. Treat underlying conditions.
     b. In most cases, correction of anemia is not indicated unless coexisting with iron deficiency. However, erythropoietin can be effective for those individuals with renal failure (Hgb < 10), cancer, and ACD. Refer to a specialist for guidance on erythropoietin use.
  2. Hemolytic anemias
     a. Treat illness and discontinue drugs that may have triggered this anemia.
     b. Prednisone is the standard initial treatment in autoimmune hemolytic anemia. Symptomatic individuals may receive transfusions. In those who fail remission or cannot sustain remission, a splenectomy is recommended. Immunosuppressive and modulating agents are used in those persons who fail to respond to splenectomy.
     c. In those individuals with G6PD deficiency, avoid giving oxidant medications. Classically, fava beans, sulfa drugs, and primaquine are triggers; the medication list to avoid is extensive (Phillips & Henderson, 2018).
     d. In those susceptible to hemolysis, avoid giving medications known to trigger hemolytic anemia.
     e. Hematology evaluation and management are indicated.
     f. For pregnant patients with sickle cell trait, the nonbirthing parent of the baby should be tested (CBC and Hgb electrophoresis). If the nonbirthing is found to be a sickle cell trait carrier, refer to genetics for counseling.
     g. For pregnant patients with a child with sickle disease, refer to genetics for counseling.
C. Macrocytic and megaloblastic anemias
  1. Vitamin B_{12} deficiency anemia
     a. Vitamin B_{12} is available in the form of pills, intramuscular injections, sublingual lozenges, and nasal spray. The decision for treatment depends on the etiology. Individuals with intrinsic factor deficiency, such as those with pernicious anemia or extensive bowel or gastric resection, require parenteral dosing. Individuals with neurological symptoms should be started on parenteral dosing as well. Expect lifetime treatment.
     b. Administer cobalamin 1,000 mg, parenterally daily for 1 week, then weekly for 1 month, then monthly lifelong. In severe anemia, serum potassium and hematocrit may drop with initial treatment with cobalamin. Hematologic changes improve after 8 weeks and neurological symptoms, improve in 8 weeks to 3 months (Shipton &Thachil, 2015).
     c. Oral cobalamin, 1,000–2,000 mcg daily, is commonly used effectively in those with vegan diets.
     d. Follow-up labs include CBC and reticulocytes, which peak at 5–7 days. Check a CBC and reticulocyte count 4 weeks after starting treatment. Expect Hgb to normalize in 4–8 weeks. In those with pernicious anemia, checking MMA 4 weeks after therapy initiation and every 6 months to a year ensures response to vitamin B_{12} (Socha et al., 2020).
     e. Those individuals who do not respond to vitamin B_{12} treatment, who are medically unstable, or whose vitamin B_{12} and folic acid levels are normal should be referred to a hematologist.
  2. Folate-deficiency anemia
     a. Avoid treating patients with potential cobalamin deficiency with folate alone unless vitamin B_{12}–deficiency anemia has been ruled out and treated because this may lead to progressively severe neuropsychiatric disease caused by untreated vitamin B_{12} deficiency.
     b. Administer folate, 1–5 mg daily. In 1 week, the patient should begin to have a sense of improvement, along with an increase in reticulocytes. CBC corrects in 2 months. Continue folate as long as needed.
D. Patient education
  1. Provide verbal and written information regarding the following:
     a. The disease process, including signs and symptoms and underlying etiologies
     b. Diagnostic tests that include a discussion about preparation, actual procedures, and follow-up care
     c. Management plan: rationale, action, use, side effects, and cost of therapeutic interventions; the need for adhering to the long-term treatment plans

VI. **Self-management resources and tools**
A. The American Society of Hematology's website is http://www.bloodthevitalconnection.org. This website provides both an overview of anemia and other links for additional information for patients.
B. The National Institutes of Health has a collection of patient information sites that discuss anemia, as well as handouts: http://www.nhi.gov.
C. University of California, San Francisco (UCSF): Anemia and Pregnancy: http://www.ucsfhealth.org/education/annemia and pregnancy

References

Agarwal, A., & Yee, J. (2019). Hepcidin. *Advances in Chronic Kidney Disease. 26*(4), 298–305. doi:10.10.53/jack.2019.04.005

American College of Obstetricians and Gynecologists. (2008). ACOG Practice Bulletin No. 95: Anemia in pregnancy. *Obstetrics & Gynecology, 112*(1), 201–207. doi:10.97/aog06013e3181809.cod

Barcellini, W., Fattizzo, B., & Zaninoni, A. (2018). Current and emerging treatment options for autoimmune hemolytic anemia. *Expert Review of Clinical Immunology, 14*(10), 857–872. doi:10.1080/1744666x,2018.1521722

Bottomley, S., & Fleming, M. (2014). Sideroblastic anemia: Diagnosis and management. *Hematolgy-Oncology Clinics of North America, 28*(4), 653–670. doi:10.1016/j.hoc2014.04.008epub2014June22

Bouri, S., & Martin, J. (2018). Investigation of iron deficiency anemia. *Clinical Medicine, 18*(3), 242–244. doi:10.7861/clinmedicine.18-3-242

Brabin, B. J., Hakimi, M., & Pelletier, D. (2001). An analysis of anemia and pregnancy-related maternal mortality. *Journal of Nutrition, 131*(2S-2), 604S–614S. doi:10.1093/jn/131.2.604S

Breymann C. (2015). Iron deficiency anemia in pregnancy. *Seminars in Hematology, 52*(4), 339–347. doi:10.1053/j.seminhematol.2015.07.003

Brill, J., & Baumgardner, D. (2000). Normocytic anemia. *American Family Physician, 62*(10), 2255. PMID111126852.

Cappellini, M., Musallam, K., & Taher, A. (2020). Iron deficiency anemia revisited. *Journal of Internal, 287*, 153–170. doi:10.1111joim.13004

Cascio, M., & DeLzourghery, T. (2017). Anemia: Evaluation and diagnostic tests. *Medical Clinics of North America, 101*(2), 263–284. doi:10.1016/j.mcna.2016.09.003

Chaparro, C., & Suchdev, P. (2019). Anemia epidemiology, pathophysiology and etiology in low- and middle-income countries. *Annals New York Academy of Science, 1450*(1), 15–31. doi:10.1111/nyas.14092

Colbert, G. (2020). Anemia of chronic disease and kidney failure. *Medscape*. https://emedicine.medscape.com/article/1389854-overview

Garcia-Casal, M., Pasricha, S., Sharma, A., & Peña-Rosa, J. P. (2019). Use and interpretation of hemoglobin concentrations for assessing anemia status in individuals and populations: results from a WHO technical meeting. *Annals New York Academy of Science, 1450*(1), 5–14. doi:10.1111/nyas.14090

Graves, B. W., & Barger, M. K. (2001). A "conservative" approach to iron supplementation during pregnancy. *Journal of Midwifery & Women's Health, 46*(3), 159–160. PMID: 11480748.

Hildebrand, L., Duma, B., Milirod, C., & Hudspeth, C. (2021). Folate deficiency in an urban safety next population. *American Journal of Medicine, 134*(10), 1065–1269. doi:10.1016/j.amjmed 2021.04.028

Hill, Q., Stamps, R., Massey, E., Grainger, J., Provan, D., & Hill, A. (2017). The diagnosis and management of primary autoimmune haemolytic anemia. *British Journal of Haemotology, 176*(3), 395–411. doi:10.1111/bjh14478

Jäger, U., Barcellini, W., Broome, C. M., Gertz, M. A., Hill, A., Hill, Q. A., Jilma, B., Kuter, D. J., Michel, M., Montillo, M., Röth, A., Zeerleder, S. S., & Berentsen, S. (2020). Diagnosis and treatment of autoimmune hemolytic anemia in adults: Recommendations from the first international consensus meeting. *Blood Review, 41*, 100648. doi:10.1016/j.blre.2019.100648

Jimenez, K., Kulnigg-Dabsch, S., & Gashe, C. (2015). Management of iron deficiency anemia. *Gastroenterology & Hepatology, 11*(4), 241–249. PMID: 27099596; PMCID: PMC4836595.

Kattamis, A., Fornia, G., Aydinok, Y., & Viprakasit, V. (2020). Changing patterns in the epidemiology of B-thalassemia. *European Journal of Haematology, 105*(6), 692–703. doi:10.1111/ejh.13512

Ko, C., Siddique, S., Patel, A., Harris, A., Sultan, S., Altayar, O., & Falck-Ytter, Y. (2020). AGA clinical practice guideline on the gastrointestinal evaluation of iron deficiency anemia. *Gastroenterology, 159*(3), 1085–1094. doi:10.1053/jgastro.2020.6.046

Kryssia, I., Marilisa, F., Antonio, N., Chiara, M., Antonio, N., Gioacchinio, L., Tiziana, M., Gian, L., & Francesco, D. (2018). Clinical manifestations of chronic atrophic gastritis. *Acta Biomedica, 89*(8), 88–92. doi:10.23750/abm.v8918S.7919

Kumar, A., et al. (2022). Iron deficiency anaemia: pathophysiogy, assessment and practical management. *BMJ Open Gastroenterology, 9*(1). doi:10.1136/bmjgast-2021-0000759

Langan, R., & Goodbred, A. (2017). Vitamin B_{12} deficiency: Recognition and management. *American Family Physician, 96*(6), 384–389. PMID: 28925645.

Lanier, J., Park, J., & Callahan, R. (2018). Anemia in older adults. *American Family Physician. 98*(7), 437–442. PMID: 302252420.

Le, C. (2016). The prevalence of anemia and moderate severe anemia in the US population (NHANES 2003–2012). *PlosONE, 11*(11), 1–14. doi: 10.1371/journal pone.0166635

Leung, W., Singh, I., McWilliams, S., Stockler, S., & Ipsiroglu, O. (2020). Iron deficiency and sleep—a scoping review. *Sleep Medicine Review, 51*, 101274. doi:10.1016/j.smrv,2020.12174

Longo, D. (2009). Examination of blood smears and bone marrow and red blood cell disorders. In A. Fauci, E. Braunwald, D. Kasper, S. Hauser, D. Longo, J. Jameson, & J. Loscalzo (Eds.), *Harrison's manual of medicine, 17*, 321–328. McGraw-Hill.

Maakaron, J. (2023). Anemia. *Medscape*. https://emedicine.medscape.com/article/198475-overview

Makipour, S., Kanapuru, B., & Ershler, W. B. (2008). Unexplained anemia in the elderly. *Seminars in Hematology, 45*(4), 250–254. doi:10.1053/j.seminhematol.2008.06.003

Mehta, A. (2022). Best practice: assessment of anemia. *British Medical Journal BMJ Best Practices online*. BMJ.com>topics

Merkeley, H., & Bolster, L. (2020). Thalassemia. *Canadian Medical Association Journal, 192*(41), 192. doi:10.1053/cmaj.191613

Muncie, H., & Campbell, J. (2009). Alpha and beta thalassemia. *American Family Physician, 80*(4), 339–344. PMID: 19678601.

Nagao, T., & Hirokawa, M. (2017). Diagnosis and treatment of macrocytic anemias in adults. *Journal of General and Family Medicine, 18*(5), 200–204. doi:10.1002/jgf2.31

Newhall, D., Oliver, R., & Lugthart, S. (2020). Anemia: A disease or symptom? *The Netherlands Journal of Medicine, 78*(3), 104–110. PMID: 32332184.

Okam, M., Koch, T., & Tran, M. (2017). Iron supplementations, response in iron-deficiency anemia: Analysis of 5 trials. *The American Journal of Medicine, 130*(8), 991. doi:10.1016/j.amjmed.2017.03.045

Patel, P., & Balanchivadze, N. (2021). Hematologic findings in pregnancy: A guide for the internist. *Cureus, 13*(5), 1–14. doi:10.7759/cureus.15149

Phillips, J., & Henderson, A. (2018). Hemolytic anemia: Evaluation and differential diagnosis. *American Family Physician, 98*(6), 354–361. PMID: 30215915.

Safiri, S., Kolahi, A., Noori, M., Nejadghaderi, S., Karamzad, N., Bragazzi, N., Sullman, M., Abdollahi, M., Collins, G., Kaufman, J., & Grieger, J. (2021). Burden of anemia and its underlying causes in 2014 countries and territories, 1990–2019: Results from the

Global Burden of Disease Study 2019. *Journal of Hematology & Oncology, 14*, 185. doi:10.1186/s51304-021-01202-2

Nandakumar, S. K., Ulirsch, J. C., & Sankaran, V. G. (2016). Advances in understanding erythropoiesis: evolving perspectives. *British journal of haematology, 173*(2), 206–218. https://doi.org/10.1111/bjh.13938

Sayani, F., & Kwiatkowski, J. (2015). Increasing prevalence of thalassemia in America: Implications for primary care. *Annals of Medicine, 47*(7), 592–604. doi:10.3109/07853890.2015.1691942

Schick, P. (2010). Hemolytic anemia. *Medscape.* http://emedicine.medscape.com/article/201066-overview

Szczepiorkowski, Z. M., & Dunbar, N. M. (2013). Transfusion guidelines: when to transfuse. *Hematology. American Society of Hematology. Education Program, 2013*, 638–644. doi:10.1182/asheducation-2013.1.638

Sifakis, S., & Pharmakides, G. (2000). Anemia in pregnancy. *Annals of the New York Academy of Sciences, 900*, 125–126. doi:1111/j.1749-6632.20000.tb06223.x.uj

Sim, M., Garvican-Lewis, L., Cox, G., Govus, A., McKay, A., Stellingwerff, T., & Peeling, P. (2019). Iron considerations for the athlete: A narrative review. *European Journal of Applied Physiology, 119*(7), 1463–1478. PMID: 31055680.

Shipton, M., & Thachil, J (2105). Vitamin B12 deficiency-A 21st perspective. *Clinical Medicine, 15*(2), 145–150. doi:10.7861/clinmedicine.15-2-145

Socha, D., DeSouza, S., Flagg, A., Sekeres, M., & Rogers, H. (2020). Severe megaloblastic anemia: Vitamin deficiency and other causes. *Cleveland Clinic Journal of Medicine Cleveland, 87*(3), 153–163. PMID: 32127439.

Stabler, S. P., & Allen, R. H. (2004). Vitamin B12 deficiency as a worldwide problem. *Annual review of nutrition, 24*, 299–326. https://doi.org/10.1146/annurev.nutr.24.012003.132440

Stauder, R., Valent., P., & Theurl, I. (2018). Anemia at older age: Etiologies, clinical implications and management. *Blood, 131*(5), 505–513. doi:10.1182/blood-2017-07-746446

Umbreit, J. (2005). Iron deficiency: A concise review. *American Journal of Medicine, 78*(3), 225–231. doi:10.1002/ajh.20249

U.S. Environmental Protection Agency. (2023). *Hazard standards and clearance l levels in lead in paint, dust and soil.* http://www.epa.gov/lead

Viprakasit, V., & Ekwattanakit, S. (2018). Clinical classification, screening and diagnosis of thalassemia. *Hematology-Oncology Clinics, 32*(2), 193–221. doi:10.1016/j.hoc,2017.11.006

Weiss, G., Ganz, T., & Goodnough, L. T. (2019). Anemia of inflammation. *Blood, 133*(1), 40–50. https://doi.org/10.1182/blood-2018-06-856500

Yilmaz, G., & Shaikh, H. (2021). Normochromic normocytic anemia. *StatPearls.* https://www.ncbi.nlm.nih.gov/books/NBK565880/

Woo, K, Kwok, T, & Celermajer, D. (2014). Vegan diet, subnormal vitamin B-12 status and cardiovascular health. *Nutrients, 6*(8), 3259-3273. doi:10.3390/nu6083259

CHAPTER 42

Anxiety

Amanda Ling and Esker-D Ligon

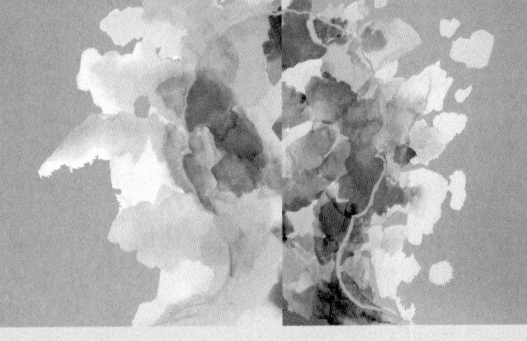

I. Introduction and general background

Anxiety disorders are among the most common mental health conditions in the United States, with about 8% of adults reporting symptoms of an anxiety disorder in a given month and 31% of adults and adolescents experiencing an anxiety disorder in their lifetime (Kessler et al., 2012; Terlizzi & Schiller, 2021). Despite increased awareness, less than half of patients identified as having an anxiety disorder receive adequate treatment in primary care (Chapdelaine et al., 2018; Lamoureux-Lamarche et al., 2021). These disorders contribute to functional impairments, disability, decreased health outcomes, comorbidity, and high use of health services. Given the impact and cost of anxiety disorders at the individual and societal levels, primary care providers should be equipped to properly screen and treat patients presenting with these conditions.

Anxiety disorders can be differentiated from typical stress or worry by the persistence of symptoms and disruption to daily function. People with anxiety may overestimate the level of threat in a situation and respond in a manner that seems disproportional to others. Accompanying activation of the sympathetic nervous system response can cause physical symptoms.

The etiology of anxiety disorders is multifactorial, involving environmental, biochemical, psychosocial, and genetic factors. These guidelines focus on the identification and treatment of the most common anxiety disorders: generalized anxiety disorder, social anxiety disorder, and panic disorder, as well as posttraumatic stress disorder (PTSD). PTSD has many symptoms in common with anxiety disorders, although it is differentiated in the *Diagnostic and Statistical Manual of Mental Disorders*, 5th edition (*DSM-5*) as a trauma- and stressor-related disorder (American Psychiatric Association [APA], 2013).

Screening and assessment for anxiety disorders in the primary care setting are guided by a number of factors. Patients may clearly describe panic, worry, or fear or may present with less obvious somatic complaints or sleep issues. Consistent use of a screening questionnaire is a straightforward way to elicit anxiety symptoms and determine the need for further evaluation. The Generalized Anxiety Disorder 7-item (GAD-7) scale is brief and patient administered, although some patients may need assistance because of limited language or health literacy. Patients who describe anxiety symptoms or score positive on a screening tool should be assessed clinically to determine whether they meet the criteria for diagnosis and treatment.

Many anxiety symptoms overlap with those of other psychiatric, medical, or substance use disorders. Healthcare providers should maintain a broad differential and rule out medical conditions that require treatment, such as cardiac or endocrine disorders (Locke, Kirst, & Schultz, 2015). Comorbidities such as mood and substance use disorders are common, with substances often used to cope with anxiety symptoms (Grant et al., 2015). Substances, including caffeine, can also precipitate or exacerbate anxiety. Determining whether a temporal relationship exists between consumption and peak anxiety symptoms or a trial off the substance can help narrow the differential.

Social context shapes the presentation of anxiety disorders, and communication techniques that enhance provider–patient rapport and elicit patient perspectives and background may improve patient experience and outcomes (Jarvis et al., 2020; Kirmayer & Ryder, 2016). Healthcare providers should cultivate awareness of personal biases or lack of knowledge pertaining to particular issues or cultural standards. Providers should maintain a nonjudgmental tone and ensure privacy when discussing anxiety and other topics that patients may find difficult. Patients may feel embarrassed and guarded, and the interviewer should phrase questions creatively and in different ways if needed. Rather than asking, "What do you do to manage your anxiety?", a provider could ask, "Are there things you do or anything you're using that helps you relax?". The second question is framed in a gentler and more curious tone while normalizing the experience of seeking relief and relaxation as something that everyone might do, avoiding clinical language. The re-framing allows for the possibility that patient may not have any methods of relaxation, while encouraging broad responses of positive or negative coping mechanisms, such as gardening or drinking alcohol, that patients may not recognize as anxiety management.

Situationally appropriate anxiety should not be pathologized as a psychiatric condition. For example, patients may feel nervous during their appointment as they meet a new healthcare provider or try to remember information from their history. Other factors that may cause a patient to present as anxious or distressed include difficulty navigating to the clinic, concern for their health, fear of bias or judgment, and actual or perceived sociocultural differences between provider and patient. Additionally, traditional office settings can be noisy and congested, often requiring patients to wait well beyond scheduled visit times. Verbal acknowledgment of the stress that can accompany healthcare appointments and a sincere apology for delays can go a long way toward improving patients' situational anxiety.

II. Database (may include but is not limited to)
A. *Subjective*
　1. Symptomatology and relevant supporting data
　　Patients may present with a variety of complaints related to anxiety disorders. Providers should inquire about the duration of symptoms, effect of symptoms on patient functioning, and relationships between symptoms and contributory factors. Providers should assess for the following:
　　a. Feelings of nervousness, anxiety, panic, excessive worry, or feeling generally stressed and overwhelmed
　　b. Negative thoughts, ruminative or obsessive thinking, unrelenting pessimism, feelings of foreboding, and excessive guilt
　　c. Adrenergic effects: irregular heartbeat, tachycardia, palpitations, shortness of breath, diaphoresis, lightheadedness, paresthesias, and tremor
　　d. Sleep disturbances, including insomnia, hypersomnia, nightmares, and restless sleep
　　e. Marked avoidance of specific situations and social withdrawal
　　f. Restlessness, irritability, agitation, and excessive anger
　　g. Appetite disturbance
　　h. Difficulty with memory or concentration
　　i. Persistent sense of fear, foreboding, apprehension, and hypervigilance
　　j. Suicidality: ideation, thoughts of being better off dead or that life is not worth living, and planned or attempted suicidal acts
　　k. Somatic complaints: headaches, gastrointestinal complaints, back and neck pain, chest pain, and excessive concern with physical health
　　l. Precipitating stressors, events, and losses (including community violence and vicarious trauma)
　　m. Substance use: changes in types, frequency, and quantity of alcohol or drugs, including caffeine, nicotine, street drugs, and prescribed medications
　　n. Past health history: history of other mental health disorders and medical illnesses causing or exacerbating signs and symptoms of anxiety (e.g., hyperthyroidism, attention-deficit/hyperactivity disorder [ADHD], major depression, bipolar disorder, and schizophrenia)
B. *Objective*
　1. Appearance and kinetic behavior: restlessness, wringing hands, biting nails, shaking legs or feet, rocking, sitting unusually still, appearing tense, and altered grooming and hygiene
　2. Mental status examination, which includes appearance, mood, affect, speech, thought content, thought process, memory and concentration, and assessment of insight and judgment
　3. Evidence-based screening tools: Consistent use of screening tools in primary care practice settings allows for systematic identification of anxiety disorders:
　　a. The GAD-7 scale (**Figure 42-1**) is a useful screening tool for common anxiety disorders in primary care (Spitzer et al., 2006). Although the GAD-7 is designed for generalized anxiety disorder, a positive result may also be indicative of social anxiety disorder, panic disorder, or PTSD, and clinical assessment is needed to clarify and confirm a diagnosis. Higher GAD-7 scores correlate with more severe symptoms and more functional impairment. Screening should be repeated periodically to objectively track changes, especially after behavioral or psychotherapeutic intervention.
　4. Diagnostic studies: Include laboratory testing for thyroid disorders, hormonal imbalances, substance use or withdrawal, electrolyte imbalances, vitamin B_{12} deficiency, and hypo- or hyperglycemia.
　5. Collateral data: Include information from members of a multidisciplinary treatment team when possible. With the permission of the patient, a brief discussion with family members or friends may yield corroborating or missing information about manifestations of the patient's anxiety or provide perspective on the cause, duration, intensity, and possible remedies of the patient's condition. Collateral contacts may also yield helpful information regarding suicidal statements, failure to eat or function normally, or substance use.

III. Assessment
A. *Determining a diagnosis*
　The following are summarized criteria for anxiety and trauma-related disorders common to primary care settings. As in all areas of physical and mental health, these diagnostic criteria are guidelines to be informed by further assessment and clinical judgment. Symptoms attributable to the effects of a substance or another medical or psychiatric condition should be treated at the root cause. Providers

GAD-7

Over the last 2 weeks, how often have you been bothered by the following problems? (Use "✓" to indicate your answer)	Not at all	Several days	More than half the days	Nearly every day
1. Feeling nervous, anxious or on edge	0	1	2	3
2. Not being able to stop or control worrying	0	1	2	3
3. Worrying too much about different things	0	1	2	3
4. Trouble relaxing	0	1	2	3
5. Being so restless that it is hard to sit still	0	1	2	3
6. Becoming easily annoyed or irritable	0	1	2	3
7. Feeling afraid as if something awful might happen	0	1	2	3

Total Score ____ = ____ + ____ + ____

Scoring and Interpretation:

GAD-2 Score	GAD-7 Score
Provisional Diagnosis	Provisional Diagnosis
0–2 None	0–7 None
3–6 Probable anxiety disorder	8+ Probable anxiety disorder
*GAD-2 is the first 2 questions of the GAD-7	

Figure 42-1 Generalized Anxiety Disorder 7-Item (GAD-7) Scale

Pfizer. (n.d.). GAD-7. Retrieved from www.phqscreeners.com. Developed by Drs. Robert L. Spitzer, Janet B.W. Williams, Kurt Kroenke, and colleagues, with an educational grant from Pfizer Inc. No permission required to reproduce, translate, display, or distribute. Scoring and interpretation table modified from www.lifesolutionsforyou.com

who are confident after an initial assessment that a patient suffers from an anxiety disorder can suggest treatment even if further visits may be needed to differentiate between specific disorders: serotonin reuptake inhibitors or individual psychotherapy are effective treatments for all anxiety and trauma-related disorders and are contraindicated for none. However, a clear diagnosis will improve the specificity of treatment, monitoring, patient education, and self-management tools.

1. Panic attack: A feature of many anxiety disorders (not only panic disorder) characterized by an abrupt surge of fear or intense discomfort that reaches a peak within minutes. Panic attacks may occur in response to known triggers or unexpectedly.
   a. Physical symptoms during panic may include palpitations, sweating, trembling, shortness of breath or feelings of choking, chest pain or pressure, nausea, dizziness, and sensations of numbness, tingling, chills, or heat.
   b. Thoughts during panic may include feeling detached from reality or from one's self, fear of losing control or "going crazy," or fear of dying.
2. Panic disorder: recurrent unexpected panic attacks with at least one of the attacks being followed by at least 1 month of either of the following:
   a. Persistent worry about additional attacks or their consequences
   b. Significant, maladaptive change in behavior related to attacks

Panic disorder may include both unexpected attacks and attacks that are expected or triggered by a known stressor. However, a patient who experiences only panic attacks triggered by a known stressor likely has a different disorder, such as a specific phobia or PTSD.
3. Generalized anxiety disorder: Excessive anxiety and worry about a variety of situations. Patients often seek help in primary care for somatic symptoms related to autonomic hyperactivity.
   a. Patients report difficulty controlling the anxiety and that symptoms interfere with daily function.
   b. Anxiety is associated with at least three of the following: restlessness, fatigue, difficulty concentrating, irritability, muscle tension, and sleep disturbance.
4. Social anxiety disorder: fear or anxiety about one or more social situations when exposed to possible scrutiny by others
   a. Feared situations may include but are not limited to having a conversation, meeting unfamiliar people, being observed eating or drinking, or performing in front of others.
   b. Exposure to the feared situation provokes anxiety out of proportion to the actual threat of the situation.
   c. The feared situation is avoided or endured with intense anxiety.
5. Agoraphobia: Fear or anxiety about being in situations in which escape might be difficult or help may not be available. Often but not always comorbid with panic disorder.
   a. Feared situations may include but are not limited to public transportation, open spaces, enclosed spaces like shops or theaters, standing in line or a crowd, or being outside the home alone.
   b. Feared situations are avoided or endured with intense anxiety, or a companion is required to function.
6. PTSD: Response after exposure to actual or threatened death, serious injury, or sexual violence through direct experience, witnessing the event occur to others, learning that the event occurred to close family or friend, or experiencing repeated or extreme exposure of details of traumatic events (e.g., by first responders, healthcare providers). Onset may be shortly after the event or months to years later. The disorder is characterized by the following:
   a. The presence of intrusive symptoms associated with the event, including recurrent involuntary memories, recurrent distressing dreams or nightmares, dissociative reactions or flashbacks, or psychological distress to internal or external cues related to the event
   b. Persistent avoidance of stimuli associated with the trauma, which may include avoidance of internal memories, thoughts, or feelings associated with the trauma or avoidance of external reminders, places, activities, or situations associated with the trauma
   c. Negative alterations in cognitions and mood associated with the traumatic event, which may include inability to remember an important aspect of the event, diminished interest or participation in activities, feeling detached, feeling unable to experience positive emotions, or experiencing persistent negative emotions or beliefs
   d. Alterations in arousal and reactivity, which may include sleep disturbance, irritability, poor concentration, hypervigilance, exaggerated startle response, or reckless or self-destructive behavior

B. *Functional assessment and severity of illness*
   1. Consider the patient's current clinical status, psychosocial factors affecting the clinical situation, the patient's highest level of past functioning, and the patient's quality of life.
   2. A functional assessment may be useful for assessing strengths and disease severity and should focus on the patient's ability to perform essential activities of daily living. Information gathered may facilitate monitoring of treatment efficacy by allowing comparison of function before and after treatment.

IV. Plan

Anxiety disorders and PTSD are common and can affect many aspects of daily life. Treatment is indicated when symptoms of the disorder cause significant distress or interfere with functioning. Provider and patient should work together to clearly define the areas of function affected by anxiety and develop goals and priorities for treatment. Effective treatment for anxiety disorders should reduce the intensity of symptoms, with the goal of enabling effective self-care and returning to premorbid levels of function. Treatment should optimally yield full remission of disproportionate and maladaptive anxiety responses. However, aiming to suppress or remove anxiety entirely is unrealistic.

A range of evidence-based psychosocial and pharmacological interventions can be effective in treating anxiety disorders. Either medication or psychotherapy can be used as first-line treatment, and a comprehensive plan may combine multiple approaches (Locke, Kirst, & Schultz, 2015). Considerations that guide initial treatment planning include patient preference, the risks and benefits of treatment, past treatment history and efficacy, presence of co-occurring conditions, cost, and treatment availability.

Patients should be engaged as active and equal participants in treatment planning alongside the healthcare provider and other members of the treatment team. Not only is this good general practice, but most anxiety treatments are effective only after a commitment of time and effort. First-line medications take time to reach efficacy, and several trials may be necessary. Psychotherapy and relaxation training require consistency and willingness to practice techniques outside of sessions. Establishing patient buy-in early on through collaborative planning and education is key.

A. *Medication selection*

Selective serotonin reuptake inhibitors (SSRIs) and serotonin–norepinephrine reuptake inhibitors (SNRIs) are first-line agents for the treatment of anxiety disorders and PTSD. Escitalopram (Lexapro) and sertraline (Zoloft) are common first picks, but any SSRI or SNRI is a reasonable choice, depending on the side-effect profile, drug interactions, and patient history or preference. If a patient has found an SSRI effective previously, restart it. If barriers prevent consistent adherence, choose fluoxetine (Prozac) for its long half-life. Before starting any antidepressant–anxiolytic, providers should assess for history of mania associated with bipolar disorder. Any patients with a history of mania should be referred to psychotherapy as the first-line anxiety treatment and to specialty psychiatry for management of bipolar disorder because antidepressants can precipitate manic episodes.

Another medication option for generalized anxiety disorder is the serotonin partial agonist buspirone (Buspar). This can be used to augment a first-line SSRI or SNRI or as monotherapy for patients who cannot tolerate the first-line agents. Buspirone has not shown clear efficacy for other anxiety disorders or PTSD.

Serotonergic medications may have some effect within 4–6 weeks, but they take 6–8 weeks to reach full efficacy. For patients with severe anxiety, short-acting medications can augment initial treatment or be continued longer term if the serotonergic medication only partially relieves symptoms. These medications have more severe side-effect profiles and have not been found effective as monotherapy. Options include hydroxyzine (Vistaril), gabapentin (Neurontin), or propranolol (Inderal), and these can be dosed scheduled or as needed for acute symptoms. Benzodiazepines and hypnotic sleep medications are highly effective but have long-term risks, including physical dependence and withdrawal. Benzodiazepines with a longer half-life, such as clonazepam (Klonopin), provide better coverage and are easier to taper and discontinue. In primary care, benzodiazepines should only be prescribed for patients without a substance abuse history who are able to commit to a specific time frame and plan for discontinuation. Benzodiazepines are not recommended, especially for prolonged use, for patients with PTSD or depression (Bandelow et al., 2012).

PTSD may manifest with a variety of physical and psychiatric symptoms, and treatment should target symptoms that are most distressing or cause the most functional impairment. Symptoms of anxiety and sleep disturbance may need to be addressed separately, and several medications are helpful in PTSD but not anxiety disorders. Prazosin (Minipress) is an antihypertensive alpha-blocker that can reduce or relieve PTSD-related nightmares and improve sleep quality (Lipinska, Baldwin, & Thomas, 2016). Providers should reference the dosing and titration protocol for prazosin because the therapeutic dose varies between patients, and underdosing is common. The second-generation antipsychotic quetiapine (Seroquel) may also be helpful as monotherapy or augmentation, but it is not considered a first-line treatment because it has less evidence and carries a significant risk of metabolic side effects. Antidepressants other than SSRIs and SNRIs have not shown clear benefit for PTSD without comorbid depression. Patients with severe symptoms and inadequate response to a first-line medication should be referred to psychotherapy and specialty psychiatric care. Refer to **Table 42-1** for possible pharmacotherapeutic options to treat PTSD.

B. *Medication management*

1. Educate patients about the likely course of treatment associated with a particular medication, particularly how long a medication will take to reach efficacy and the possible need for dose titration. Effective medications should be continued for 12 months after stabilization of symptoms to limit relapse. In case of chronic or recurrent symptoms, SSRIs or SNRIs can be safely continued long term.

2. Patients with anxiety disorders can be sensitive to medication side effects; thus, low starting doses of medications are recommended, with a gradual increase to therapeutic dose over several days and as tolerated by the patient. Side effects are most common after beginning or increasing the dose of anxiolytic medications but will spontaneously remit after 1–2 weeks of treatment.

3. Medication monitoring involves assessment of side effects and changes in symptoms, such as frequency and intensity of panic attacks, level of anticipatory anxiety, degree of avoidance, quality of sleep, persistence of somatic symptoms, and severity of distress and impaired function related to anxiety.
   a. Patients benefit from monitoring every 2 weeks when starting a new medication.
   b. Appointment frequency can then be reduced to every 3–4 weeks while titrating and assessing and less frequently once symptoms are stable.
   c. If there is no response or only partial response after 4–8 weeks at the initial therapeutic dose, higher doses should be trialed as tolerated.

4. Discontinuing medication should be done in a gradual and collaborative manner. This allows for assessment of recurring anxiety symptoms and symptoms related to discontinuation. If required, treatment may be quickly reinitiated at a previously effective dose. Medications can be discontinued abruptly in situations such as drug interaction, pregnancy, or significant adverse effects. Provider and patient should collaboratively discuss the risks and benefits of discontinuation, taking into account the patient's history of mood or anxiety episodes, current or impending psychosocial stressors, and patient motivation to discontinue the medication.

Table 42-1 Pharmacotherapeutic Options for Treating Anxiety and Posttraumatic Stress Disorder (PTSD)

Medication	Mechanism of Action	Therapeutic dose (mg/day)
First-line selective serotonin reuptake inhibitors (SSRIs)		
Fluoxetine (Prozac®)	Selective serotonin 5-HT reuptake inhibitor	20-60 mg/day
Paroxetine (Paxil®)		50-200 mg/day
Sertraline (Zoloft®)		20-40 mg/day
Citalopram (Celexa®)		10-20 mg/day
Escitalopram (Lexapro®)		20-60 mg/day
Fluvoxamine (Luvox®)		100-300 mg/day
First-line serotonin–norepinephrine reuptake inhibitors (SNRIs)		
Desvenlafaxine (Pristiq®)	5-HT, norepinephrine and dopamine reuptake inhibitor	50-100 mg/day
Venlafaxine ER (Effexor®) is commonly used for ease of once-daily dosing		75-300 mg/day
Duloxetine (Cymbalta®)		30-60 mg/day
Augmenting agents		
Antiadrenergic agents		
Prazosin	Alpha-1 adrenergic antagonist	1-7 mg QHS
Propranolol* (Inderal®)	Beta-1, beta-2 adrenergic antagonist	60-120 mg/day
Mood stabilizers/anticonvulsants		
Gabapentin* (Neurontin®)	May modulate calcium channels	600-2400 mg/day
Atypical antipsychotics		
Consider referral to a psychiatric specialist if atypical antipsychotics are required for treatment.		
Quetiapine (Seroquel®)	Dopamine D_2, serotonin $5-HT_2$, histamine H_1 antagonist	800 mg/day
Miscellaneous agents		
Hydroxyzine* (Vistaril®)	Histamine H_1 antagonist	25-100 mg/day
Buspirone (Buspar)	Serotonin $5-HT_{1A}$ partial agonist	15-60 mg/day

*Hydroxyzine, gabapentin, and propranolol are often dosed as needed for short-acting treatment of anxiety but can also be scheduled in split dosing.

Garakani, A., Murrough, J.W., Freire, R.C., Thom, R.P., Larkin, K., Buono, F.D., & Iosifescu, D.V. (2020). Pharmacotherapy of anxiety disorders: Current and emerging treatment options. *Frontiers in Psychiatry*, 11, e595584. doi: 10.3389/fpsyt.2020.595584

C. Psychosocial interventions

Psychotherapy is considered a first-line treatment for anxiety disorders and PTSD, alongside serotonergic medications, and may be preferred for patients who are pregnant or hesitant about pharmacologic treatment. Barriers to therapy can include access to qualified clinicians and scheduling availability. However, options such as group, online or telephone live sessions, or self-guided modules can still be effective for patients willing to engage consistently. (Olthuis, Watt, Bailey, Hayden, & Stewart, (2016).

1. Cognitive–behavioral therapy (CBT): CBT has been found effective for anxiety disorders across a range of populations (Locke, Kirst, & Schultz, 2015). The treatment course is time-limited, generally 10–15 weekly sessions, and yields durable effects. CBT for anxiety disorders often includes self-monitoring of worry and thinking patterns, guided exposure to triggers and fear cues, and relaxation training.

2. Relaxation training: Specific techniques for relaxation have also been found effective for anxiety. These typically focus on reducing physical stress responses related to autonomic hyperarousal (Kim & Kim, 2018). Examples include applied relaxation (AR), which teaches patients to recognize early anxiety and respond by rapidly reducing muscle

tension, and mindfulness-based stress reduction (MSBR), which encourages awareness of the present moment, including conscious observation of thoughts and feelings. Full treatment courses can last 8 weeks or more, but basic techniques can be taught in even a single session and practiced without further supervision.

3. Switching between or combining psychosocial and pharmacological treatment should be considered for patients who have failed to respond to initial treatment. Combined treatment may enhance long-term outcomes and reduce the likelihood of relapse if pharmacologic treatment is discontinued.

D. *Referral to specialty care*

Complex cases or significant comorbid diagnoses may require consultation or referral to a psychiatric provider. If the primary care provider and patient are confident in the diagnosis of anxiety, but initial treatment with either psychotherapy or serotonin reuptake inhibitor at the maximum tolerated dose does not provide adequate relief, the next steps are either augmenting the initial treatment modality with another, switching the treatment modality, or switching the serotonergic medication. After first-line treatments and augmentation strategies have been exhausted, providers are encouraged to consult with experienced colleagues or refer the patient to dedicated psychiatric services.

V. Special populations

A. *Dually diagnosed patients*

Comorbidity of anxiety disorders and substance use disorders is common. Evidence suggests multiple pathways leading to co-occurrence: shared vulnerabilities may predispose patients to both types of disorder, patients with anxiety may self-medicate their symptoms by using substances, and substance use may precipitate anxiety (Vorspan et al., 2015). Integrated treatment of both conditions through psychotherapy and a serotonin reuptake inhibitor can improve outcomes; however, more research is needed on medications for comorbid anxiety and substance use. When prescribing medications, providers should be aware of potential interactions and screen for moderate to severe hepatic impairment, which may require reduced dosing. Benzodiazepines should be used infrequently outside of structured withdrawal and tapering protocols, and patients should be educated about the additive effects of benzodiazepines, alcohol, and opiates.

B. *Pregnant persons*

Psychotherapy is the preferred treatment for anxiety disorders occurring during pregnancy, nursing, or pregnancy planning. However, SSRIs are considered relatively safe, and initiation or continuation of an SSRI may be indicated for moderate to severe symptoms (Dragioti et al., 2019). Collaborative treatment planning should include both the patient and the obstetrician or midwife and should consider the risks of medication alongside the risks of untreated psychiatric illness for the parent and child.

C. *Older adults*

Generalized anxiety disorder is the most common anxiety disorder in older adults and may be precipitated by chronic illness or psychosocial stressors. Assessment and treatment recommendations are consistent for adults of any age; however, providers treating older adults should be aware of medication safety concerns. Many SSRIs affect the metabolism of other drugs through inhibition of liver enzymes. Fluoxetine and paroxetine are the most potent inhibitors, whereas escitalopram is the weakest and least likely to interact with other drugs through this pathway. Short-acting anxiety medications often contribute to an increased risk of falls in older adults because of their sedating effects. Providers should start medications at a low dose, titrate slowly, and discuss safety and side-effect monitoring with patients. Check the American Geriatrics Society Beers Criteria Medication List at http://www.dcri.org for potentially harmful medications for older adults.

D. *Children and adolescents*

Children and adolescents may present with different symptoms than adults and benefit from specialized assessment and treatment. Psychotherapy, specifically CBT, is the first-line approach for all pediatric anxiety, but concurrent treatment with an SSRI may be indicated for severe symptoms. Evidence suggesting a higher risk of suicidal thoughts and behaviors associated with SSRIs in children and adolescents remains controversial, and studies at the population level suggest that higher rates of these prescriptions are associated with lower rates of suicide in adolescents (Dragioti et al., 2019; Dwyer & Bloch, 2019). Providers should collaborate closely with pediatric patients and their families in treatment planning, discuss potential adverse effects of SSRIs as compared to risks of undertreated anxiety, and monitor for suicidal thoughts or changes in behavior.

VI. Self-management resources and tools

A. *Patient education and resources*

Encouraging patients to take an active role in monitoring symptoms and making lifestyle adjustments is an important part of collaborative care. Providers should also provide education about physiological causes of anxiety. Understanding how the sympathetic nervous system fuels the cycle of anxiety empowers patients to learn about and track routine aspects of their daily life that increase or decrease sympathetic activation. Caffeine is a common and overlooked contributor to sympathetic activation and anxiety, whereas improved sleep hygiene and physical exercise have been shown to decrease anxiety.

Advice websites and online forums may contain misleading or outdated information. The following resources are evidence-based and maintained by trustworthy organizations.

1. The Anxiety and Depression Association of America (ADAA) shares patient-centered information about anxiety, co-occurring disorders, treatment, and self-management techniques. The website is easy to navigate and includes helpful tips on accessing different types of treatment and support. (https://adaa.org/)
2. The National Institute for Mental Health (NIMH) website has a variety of educational handouts for patients and families, which can be downloaded and printed for distribution. Handouts are available in multiple languages and updated periodically. (https://www.nimh.nih.gov/health/topics/anxiety-disorders)
3. The National Alliance on Mental Illness (NAMI) shares resources and directions to access local or online support groups for mental health conditions, including anxiety disorders and PTSD. (https://www.nami.org)
4. The National Center for PTSD website has information on diagnosis and types of treatment. Much of the information is broadly applicable, although some resources are specifically for veterans. (https://www.ptsd.va.gov)
5. A wide variety of mobile phone apps aim to help users reduce stress and improve mental well-being. Individual patients may find benefit in easily accessible apps that teach skills or encourage consistency, although research suggests these are not as helpful as more structured interventions, such as psychotherapy (Goldberg et al., 2022). One Mind PsyberGuide is a nonprofit website with expert reviews of mental health apps. (https://onemindpsyberguide.org/)

References

American Psychiatric Association. (2013). *Diagnostic and statistical manual of mental disorders* (5th ed.).

Bandelow, B., Sher, L., Bunevicius, R., Hollander, E., Kasper, S., Zohar, J., & Möller, H-J. (2012). Guidelines for the pharmacological treatment of anxiety disorders, obsessive-compulsive disorder, and posttraumatic stress disorder in primary care. *International Journal of Psychiatry in Clinical Practice*, 16(2), 77–84. doi:10.3109/13651501.2012.667114

Chapdelaine, A., Carrier, J. D., Fournier, L., Duhoux, A., & Roberge, P. (2018). Treatment adequacy for social anxiety disorder in primary care patients. *PLOS One*, 13(11), e0206357. doi:10.1371/journal.pone.0206357

Dragioti, E., Solmi, M., Favaro, A., Fusar-Poli, P., Dazzan, P., Thompson, T., Stubbs, B., Firth, J., Fornaro, M., Tsartsalis, D., Carvalho, A. F., Vieta, E., McGuire, P., Young, A. H., Il Shin, J., Correll, C. U., & Evangelou, E. (2019). Association of antidepressant use with adverse health outcomes: a systematic umbrella review. *JAMA Psychiatry*, 76(12), 1241–1255. doi:10.1001/jamapsychiatry.2019.2859

Dwyer, J. B., & Bloch, M. H. (2019). Antidepressants for pediatric patients. *Current Psychiatry*, 18(9), 26.

Goldberg, S. B., Lam, S. U., Simonsson, O., Torous, J., & Sun, S. (2022). Mobile phone-based interventions for mental health: A systematic meta-review of 14 meta-analyses of randomized controlled trials. *PLOS Digital Health*, 1(1), e0000002. doi:10.1371/journal.pdig.0000002

Grant, B. F., Goldstein, R. B., Saha, T. D., Chou, S. P., Jung, J., Zhang, H., Pickering, R. P., Ruan, W. J., Smith, S. M., Huang, B., & Hasin, D. S. (2015). Epidemiology of DSM-5 alcohol use disorder: Results from the National Epidemiologic Survey on Alcohol and Related Conditions III. *JAMA Psychiatry*, 72(8), 757–766. doi: 10.1001/jamapsychiatry.2015.0584

Jarvis, G. E., Kirmayer, L. J., Gómez-Carrillo, A., Aggarwal, N. K., & Lewis-Fernández, R. (2020). Update on the cultural formulation interview. *Focus*, 18(1), 40–46. doi:10.1176/appi.focus.20190037

Kessler, R. C., Petukhova, M., Sampson, N. A., Zaslavsky, A. M., & Wittchen, H. (2012). Twelve-month and lifetime prevalence and lifetime morbid risk of anxiety and mood disorders in the United States. *International Journal of Methods in Psychiatric Research*, 21(3), 169–184. doi:10.1002/mpr.1359

Kim, H. S., & Kim, E. J. (2018). Effects of relaxation therapy on anxiety disorders: A systematic review and meta-analysis. *Archives of Psychiatric Nursing*, 32(2), 278–284. doi:10.1016/j.apnu.2017.11.015

Kirmayer, L. J., & Ryder, A. G. (2016). Culture and psychopathology. *Current Opinion in Psychology*, 8, 143–148.

Lamoureux-Lamarche, C., Berbiche, D., & Vasiliadis, H. M. (2021). Treatment adequacy and remission of depression and anxiety disorders and quality of life in primary care older adults. *Health and Quality of Life Outcomes*, 19(1), 1–12.

Lipinska, G., Baldwin, D. S., & Thomas, K. G. (2016). Pharmacology for sleep disturbance in PTSD. *Human Psychopharmacology: Clinical and Experimental*, 31(2), 156–163. doi:10.1002/hup.2522

Locke, A., Kirst, N., & Schultz, C. G. (2015). Diagnosis and management of generalized anxiety disorder and panic disorder in adults. *American Family Physician*, 91(9), 617–624.

Olthuis, J. V., Watt, M. C., Bailey, K., Hayden, J. A., & Stewart, S. H. (2016). Therapist-supported Internet cognitive behavioural therapy for anxiety disorders in adults. *Cochrane Database of Systematic Reviews*, 2016(3), CD011565. doi:10.1002/14651858.CD011565

Spitzer, R. L., Kroenke, K., Williams, J. B. W., & Lowe, B. (2006). A brief measure for assessing generalized anxiety disorder: The GAD-7. *Archives of Internal Medicine*, 166(10), 1092–1097. doi:10.1001/archinte.166.10.1092

Terlizzi, E. P., & Schiller, J. S. (2021). *Estimates of mental health symptomatology, by month of interview: United States, 2019*. National Center for Health Statistics. https://www.cdc.gov/nchs/data/nhis/mental-health-monthly-508.pdf

Vorspan, F., Mehtelli, W., Dupuy, G., Bloch, V., & Lépine, J. P. (2015). Anxiety and substance use disorders: Co-occurrence and clinical issues. *Current Psychiatry Reports*, 17(2), 1–7. doi:10.1007/s11920-014-0544-y

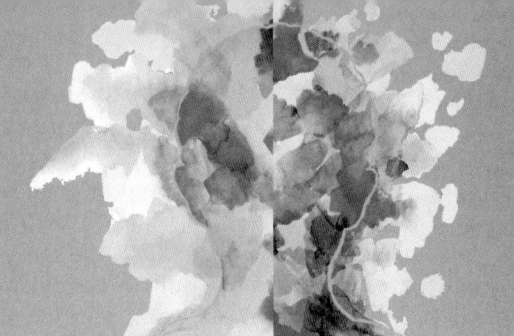

CHAPTER 43

Asthma in Adolescents and Adults

Susan L. Janson and Shaadi Settecase

I. Introduction and general background

Asthma is a chronic inflammatory disorder of the lower airways characterized by intermittent airway inflammation and bronchial hyperresponsiveness, resulting in airway narrowing and airflow obstruction that is reversible, either spontaneously or with treatment. The role of inflammation is a critical feature of asthma and contributes to bronchoconstriction of the airway smooth muscle, airway edema, and plugging of the airways with mucus, causing variable reductions in airflow. The heterogeneity of airway inflammation is explained by mechanistic biologic pathways (endotypes). Clinical manifestations (phenotypes) include recurrent episodes of wheezing, coughing, and breathlessness and a sensation of chest tightness that occurs particularly at night or early in the morning. In some patients, persistent changes in airway structure occur, resulting in airway remodeling and loss of lung function that are not fully reversible (National Asthma Education and Prevention Program [NAEPP], 2007).

A. Pathogenesis

The etiology of asthma is unknown, but the strongest predictor for developing asthma is atopy, the genetic predisposition for the development of an immunoglobulin (Ig) E–mediated response to common environmental aeroallergens. Viral respiratory infections may also contribute and are the most important cause of asthma exacerbations. The onset of asthma for most people begins early in life with recurrent wheezing, atopic disease, and a history of parental asthma.

Asthma is a complex immunologic syndrome with considerable variability in the underlying mechanisms of the disease and patterns of airway inflammation. There are multiple cellular elements and inflammatory mediators involved in its pathophysiology, in particular, neutrophils, eosinophils, lymphocytes, mast cells, macrophages, and epithelial cells. Asthma endotypes are type 2 high and type 2 low. Identification of the endotype is central to asthma management. There has been remarkable progress in our understanding of the pathogenesis of asthma as endotype variations are identified. As our understanding of the distinct genetic variations evolves, asthma therapeutics will become more precise, and future management will eventually be determined by asthma endotype.

Initial understandings of asthma pathogenesis focused on lymphocytes and, in particular, the imbalance of Th1 and Th2 in allergic IgE-mediated asthma, with an overexpression of Th2 cells resulting in eosinophilic inflammation and the development of the airway hyperresponsiveness that is characteristic of asthma (Harper & Zeki, 2015). However, only about 50% of people with asthma show an overexpression of type 2 cytokines (interleukin 4, 5, and 13), which trigger airway eosinophils, mucus production, and bronchial hyperresponsiveness, as well as IgE synthesis. People with high type 2 respond to anti-inflammatory corticosteroids. The other 50% have low type 2 expression and different immune responses, with more airway neutrophils, systemic inflammation related to obesity, and little other immune response (Lambrecht et al., 2019; Lazarus et al., 2019). These people are more likely not to respond to corticosteroid therapy and may require a different therapeutic approach that targets bronchoconstriction, such as long-acting beta$_2$-agonists (LABAs) and long-acting muscarinic agonists (LAMAs) (Lambrecht et al., 2019). LABAs are preferred over LAMAs because they seem to be more effective (NAEPP, 2020).

The type 2 high and type 2 low paradigm has provided a framework for understanding the pathogenesis of the disease, with recent research looking to more fully characterize the multiple pathways that lead to the clinical manifestations of asthma. As the understanding of these biological differences evolves, there will be an impetus for improved targeted therapies and a precision-medicine approach to treatment.

B. *Prevalence*

Asthma affects more than 25 million people in the United States (Centers for Disease Control and Prevention [CDC], 2021) and more than 262 million worldwide (World Health Organization, 2023). Early in life, the prevalence of asthma is higher in boys, but at puberty, the gender ratio shifts toward girls, and asthma is seen predominantly in women after puberty. Racial and ethnic disparities result in higher prevalence, morbidity, and mortality among Black, Hispanic, and American Indians/Alaska Native groups compared to White non-Hispanic populations. Thus, the burden of asthma falls hardest on these groups. Black Americans are 1.5 times more likely to have asthma and are 5 times more likely to visit the emergency department for exacerbations. Black women have the highest death rates from asthma (Asthma & Allergy Foundation of America, 2020). Asthma exacerbations are responsible for many emergency department visits and hospitalizations each year. Among those with current asthma, the prevalence of asthma exacerbations/attacks within the previous 12 months is 8,007,395 (39.6%) (CDC, 2021). Overall, among people with current asthma, 35% have intermittent worsening, and 65% have persistent symptoms. Exacerbations and hospitalizations cost more than $50 billion in direct costs and nearly $12 billion in indirect costs (missed work or school, low productivity) annually in the United States (Barnett & Numagambetov, 2011). Severe, difficult-to-control asthma affects approximately 10% of the population with asthma and accounts for 50% of asthma-related health costs (Sullivan et al., 2007).

C. *Factors that precipitate or aggravate asthma*
  1. Allergens: Exposure to aerosolized environmental allergens (aeroallergens) for people who are sensitized to them is an important precipitant of asthma. Outdoor allergens are primarily pollens from trees and plants that occur in seasonal waves. Patients with these sensitivities have more frequent exacerbations during the time of heavy pollination. Even more problematic for sensitized patients are the perennial indoor allergens (molds, house dust mites, cockroaches, and animal dander) because of the length of time people stay indoors.
  2. Irritants: The most significant airway irritant exposure is environmental tobacco smoke. Other irritants include bleach, sprays like perfume, strong odors (paint fumes, cooking gas, and wood smoke), and air pollution, with increased exposure in closed, poorly ventilated areas.
  3. In adults and adolescents who have asthma, respiratory viruses, predominantly rhinoviruses, are a significant cause of asthma exacerbations.
  4. Medication and drugs: Some medications are known to trigger airway constriction through neural or metabolic pathways. These include β-blockers, aspirin, and nonsteroidal anti-inflammatory drugs (NSAIDs).
  5. Other factors that can worsen asthma: Sulfites found in beer, wine, and food; strong emotions; cold air; weather changes; and exercise are common triggers for asthma symptoms.
  6. Comorbid conditions that exacerbate asthma: Among the chronic conditions that can increase nocturnal respiratory symptoms and make asthma harder to control are gastroesophageal reflux disease (GERD), rhinitis and sinusitis, high total body weight, untreated obstructive sleep apnea (OSA), and chronic stress and depression. Efforts should be made to treat and control all of these conditions when present, especially when asthma symptoms are resistant to treatment.

II. Database

A. *Subjective*
  1. Symptom description: The most common signs and symptoms of asthma are intermittent dyspnea, cough, and wheezing. These symptoms occur together, creating a well-recognized syndrome.
     a. Presenting symptoms: recurrent wheezing, shortness of breath, chest tightness, cough that is worse at night, and sputum production
     b. Pattern of symptoms
        i. Perennial, seasonal, or both
        ii. Continual, episodic, or both
        iii. Onset, duration, and frequency (number of days or nights per week or month)
        iv. Diurnal variations, especially nocturnal and on awakening in early morning
     c. Precipitating or aggravating factors
        i. Viral respiratory infections
        ii. Environmental allergens, indoor (e.g., mold, house dust mites, cockroaches, and animal dander or secretions) and outdoor (e.g., pollens)
        iii. Home characteristics (age, location, heating and cooling system, wood-burning stove, humidifier, carpeting over concrete, molds or mildew, floor coverings, and stuffed or upholstered furniture)
        iv. Smoking and/or exposure to secondhand smoke: tobacco products, including cigarettes, cigars, pipes, hookah, and vaping; inhaling or vaping cannabis
        v. Exercise, especially when breathing cold air
        vi. Occupational chemicals or allergens
        vii. Environmental change (relocation or remodeling)
        viii. Irritants (secondhand tobacco smoke, strong odors, air pollutants, dusts, particulates, vapors, gases, and aerosols)
        ix. Emotions (e.g., fear, anger, frustration, hard crying or laughing) or stress

x. Medications (e.g., aspirin, other NSAIDs, β-blockers)
xi. Food, food additives, and preservatives (e.g., sulfites)
xii. Changes in weather and exposure to cold air
xiii. Endocrine factors (e.g., menses, pregnancy, and thyroid disease)
xiv. Comorbid conditions (e.g., sinusitis, allergic rhinitis, GERD, OSA, and allergic responses to specific foods or alcohol)
2. Past health history
   a. Age of onset of disease
   b. History of emergency department visits, hospitalizations, need for intubation, and mechanical ventilation
   c. Need for systemic or oral corticosteroids and frequency of use
   d. History of exacerbations
      i. Prodromal signs and symptoms
      ii. Rapidity of onset, duration, and frequency
      iii. Severity (need for urgent care, hospitalization, or intensive care unit care)
      iv. Impact (number of days missed from work or school, limitation of activities, nocturnal awakening, and economic impact)
3. Family history: allergies, atopy, or asthma
4. Occupational and environmental history: work-related exposures, such as vapors, gas, dusts, fumes, isocyanates, or cedar
5. Personal and social history: tobacco smoking and secondhand tobacco exposure
6. Review of systems
   a. Constitutional signs and symptoms: fatigue caused by sleep disruption
   b. Ear, nose, and throat: congestion, sneezing, runny nose, sinus headache, and postnasal drip
   c. Respiratory: recurrent wheezing, cough, breathlessness, chest tightness, and increased mucus production
   d. Cardiac: palpitations during times of severe breathlessness
   e. Gastrointestinal: heartburn or dyspepsia
   f. Psychiatric: anxiety or depression

B. *Objective*
1. Physical findings
   a. General appearance: anxious, labored breathing; hyperexpansion of the chest (especially in children); use of accessory muscles; hunched shoulders; and deformed chest
   b. Ear, nose, and throat: pale and boggy nasal mucosa, thin and watery nasal secretions, red or streaked posterior pharynx, and thrush (associated with inhaled corticosteroid use)
   c. Lungs: diffuse or scattered expiratory wheezes, prolonged expiration, wheezing with forced exhalation, and decrease in air entry and movement
   d. Cardiac: tachycardia (if hypoxic or recent beta-agonist use)
   e. Skin: atopic dermatitis or eczema; pallor or cyanosis (if hypoxic)
2. Supporting data from relevant diagnostic tests, such as bronchoprovocation and, especially, spirometry

III. Assessment
A. *Differential diagnosis*
1. Asthma
2. Chronic obstructive pulmonary disease (COPD) (e.g., emphysema and/or chronic bronchitis)
3. Upper airway disease: allergic rhinitis and sinusitis
4. Vocal cord dysfunction
5. Obstruction of large airways (foreign body, tumor, and lymph nodes)
6. Obstruction of small airways (cystic fibrosis, bronchiolitis, and bronchopulmonary dysplasia)
7. Recurrent cough secondary to medications
8. Aspiration
9. Congestive heart failure

B. *Asthma severity, control, and response to treatment*
1. Classify asthma severity (**Table 43-1**) as intermittent, mild persistent, moderate persistent, or severe persistent. Asthma severity is the intrinsic intensity of the disease and is most easily determined when the patient is not on long-term treatment. Severity is measured in two domains: impairment and risk of future exacerbations. Impairment is assessed by history of symptoms, nocturnal awakenings, short-acting beta$_2$-agonist (SABA) use for relief of symptoms, activity limitation, and spirometry to assess airway caliber. It is important to assess the quantity and quality of sleep, limits to desired activity, and need for medication to gain a full picture of impairment. If these components are missed during history taking, asthma severity may be misclassified. Risk is assessed by the patient or caregiver's recall of events during the previous 2–4 weeks, the likelihood of frequent exacerbations, and forced expiratory volume in 1 second (FEV_1). Predictors of asthma exacerbation include severe airflow obstruction, two or more emergency department visits or hospitalizations in the last year, intubation or intensive care unit admission for asthma in the last 5 years, patient report of feeling in danger from asthma, depression, and certain demographic characteristics (female, non-White, not using corticosteroid medication, and current smoking). Asthma severity may be assessed retrospectively, after 2–3 months of treatment, based on the level of therapy needed to control asthma symptoms and prevent exacerbations (Global Initiative for Asthma [GINA], 2021).
2. Classify asthma control (**Table 43-2**): Asthma can be classified as well controlled, not well controlled, or very poorly controlled. Asthma control is classified when the patient is currently on a controller medication, considering domains of impairment

Table 43-1 Classifying Asthma Severity and Initiating Treatment in Adolescents ≥ 12 Years of Age and Adults (*in patients who are not currently taking long-term control medications*)

Components of Severity		Classification of Asthma Severity			
		Intermittent	Persistent Mild	Persistent Moderate	Persistent Severe
Impairment	Symptoms	≤2 days/week	≥ 2 days/week but not daily	Daily	Throughout the day
	Nighttime awakenings	≤ 2 times per month	3-4 times per month	> 1 per week but not nightly	Often 7 times/week
	SABA use for symptom control (not prevention of EIB)	≤2 days/week	> 2 days/week but not daily, and not more than once on any day	Daily	Several times per day
	Interference with normal activity	None	Minor limitation	Some limitation	Extremely limited
	Lung function Normal FEV_1/FVC: 8-19 yr 85% 20-39 yr 80% 40-59 yr 75% 60-80 yr 70%	■ Normal FEV_1 between exacerbations ■ FEV_1 > 80% predicted ■ FEV_1/FVC normal	■ FEV_1 > 80% predicted ■ FEV_1/FVC normal	■ FEV_1 60-80% ■ FEV_1/FVC reduced 5%	■ FEV_1 < 60% ■ FEV_1/FVC reduced > 5%
Risk	Asthama exacerbations requiring oral systemic corticosteroids	0-1/year	≥ 2/year *Generally, more frequent and intense events indicate greater severity**		
			Consider severity and interval since last asthma exacerbation. Frequency and severity may flucuate over time for patients in any severity category. Relative annual risk of exacerbations may be related to FEV_1.		
Recommended Step for Initiating Therapy *The stepwise approach is meant to assist, not replace, the clinical decision making required to meet individual patient needs.*		Step 1	Step 2	Step 3 *Consider short course of oral systemic corticosteroids*	Step 4 or 5 *Consider short course of oral systemic corticosteroids*
			In 2–6 weeks, depending on severity, assess level of asthma control achieved and adjust therapy as needed.		

Abbreviations: EIB, exercise-induced bronchospasm; FEV_1, forced expiratory volume in 1 second; FVC, forced vital capacity.

* Data are insufficient to link frequencies of exacerbation with different levels of asthma control. Generally, more frequent and intense exacerbations (e.g. requiring urgent care, hospital or intensive care admission, and/or oral corticosteroids) indicate greater underlying disease severity. For treatment purposes, patients with ≥2 exacerbations in a year may be considered to have persistent asthma, even in the absence of impairment levels consistent with persistent asthma.

Notes:

Level of severity is determined by assessment of impairment and risk. Assess impairment by patient or caregiver's recall of events during the previous 2-4 weeks; assess risk over the last year. Assign severity to the most severe category in which any feature occurs.

National Heart, Lung and Blood Institute, National Asthma Education and Prevention Program, & National Institutes of Health. (2007). *Expert panel report 3: Guidelines for the Diagnosis and Management of Asthma* (publication No. 97-4051). Bethesda, MD: Author.

and risk. Control is the degree to which the symptoms, impairments, and risk are minimized and the goals of therapy are met. Control is assessed by symptoms, nighttime awakenings, the need for SABA use for relief of symptoms, the ability to engage in usual activities, and the frequency of exacerbations requiring treatment with oral corticosteroids. Several standardized questionnaires have been developed for the assessment of asthma control as reported by patients, as shown in **Table 43-2**.

3. Assess responsiveness to therapy: Responsiveness is the ease with which asthma control is achieved by therapy.

Table 43-2 Assessing Asthma Control and Adjusting Therapy in Adolescents ≥ 12 years of Age and Adults

Components of Control		Levels of Asthma Control		
		Well Controlled	**Not Well Controlled**	**Very Poorly Controlled**
Impairment	Symptoms	≤2 days/week	>2 days/week	Throughout the day
	Nightime awakenings	≤2 times/month	1-3 times/week	≥4 times/week
	Interference with normal activity	None	Some limitation	Extremely limited
	SABA use for symptom control (not to prevent EIB)	≤2 days/week	>2 days/week	Several times/day
	Lung Function FEV_1 (% predicted) or peak flow (% personal best)	> 80%	60-80%	<60%
	Validated questionnaires♦ ■ ATAQ ■ ACQ ■ ACT	0 ≤0.75* ≥20	1-2 ≥1.5 16-19	3-4 Not applicable ≤15
Risk	Asthma exacerbations requiring oral systemic corticosteroids §	0-1/year	≥2/year	
		Consider severity and interval since last asthma exacerbation		
	Progressive loss of lung function	*Evaluation requires long-term follow-up care*		
	Treatment-related adverse effects	*Medication side effects can vary in intesity from none to very troublesome and worrisome. The leve of intensity does not correlate to specific levels of control but should be considered in the overall assessment of risk.*		
Recommended Action for Treatment *The stepwise approach is meant to help, not replace, the clinical decision making needed to meet individual patient needs.*		Maintain current step. Regular follow-up every 1-6 months. Consider step down if well controlled for at least 3 months.	Step up 1 step Reevalate in 2-6 weeks. *Before step up in treatment: Review adherence to medication, inhaler technique, and environmental control. If alternative treatment was used, discontinue and use preferred treatment for that step. For side effects, consider alternative treatment options.*	Consider short course of oral systemic corticosteroids. Step up 1-2 steps. Reevaluate in 2 weeks.

Abbreviations: ACQ, Asthma Control Questionnaire©; ACT, Asthma Control Test™; ATAQ, Asthma Therapy Assessment Questionnaire©; EIB, exercise induced bronchospasm; FEV_1, forced expiratory volume in 1 second; SABA, short-acting beta$_2$-agonist

♦Validated questionnaires for the impairment domain (the questionnaires do not assess lung function or the risk domain). Minimal important difference: 1.0 for the ATAQ; 0.5 for the ACQ; not determined for the ACT.

* ACQ values of 0.76-1.4 are indeterminate regarding well-controlled asthma.

Validated questionnaires for the impairment domain (questionnaires do not assess lung function or the risk domain)

ATAQ = Asthma Therapy Assessment Questionnaire © (user package may be obtained from https://eprovide.mapi-trust.org/instruments/asthma-therapy-assessment-questionnaire-adult)

ACQ = Asthma Control Questionnaire© (user package may be obtained from http://www.qoltech.co.uk/index.htm)

ACT = Asthma Control Test™ (https://www.asthma.com/understanding-asthma/severe-asthma/asthma-control-test/)

§ Data are insufficient to link frequencies of exacerbation with different levels of asthma control. Generally, more frequent and intense exacerbations (e.g. requiring urgent care, hospital or intensive care admission, and/or oral corticosteroids) indicate poorer asthma control.

Notes:

The level of control is based on the most severe component of impairment (symptoms and functional limitations) or risk (exacerbations). Assess impairment by patient's or caregiver's recall of previous 2-4 weeks and by spirometry and/or peak flow measures. Symptom assessment for longer periods should reflect a global assessment, such as inquiring whether the patient's ashtma is better or worse since the last visit. Assess risk by recall of exacerbations during the previous year and since the last visit.

National Heart, Lung and Blood Institute, National Asthma Education and Prevention Program, & National Institutes of Health. (2007). *Expert panel report 3: Guidelines for the Diagnosis and Management of Asthma* (publication No. 97-4051). Bethesda, MD: Author.

C. *Significance and motivation*

Assess the significance of asthma to the patient and family, including how much asthma interferes with quality of life, work, and play. Determine willingness and ability to follow the treatment plan and properly inhale medications. Identifying the patient's personal treatment goals and incorporating shared decision making into the asthma management plan have been shown to be important components of optimizing asthma control (GINA, 2021).

IV. Goals of clinical management to control asthma

A. *Reduce impairment*
   1. Prevent chronic symptoms and nighttime awakenings.
   2. Require only infrequent use of SABA (≤2 days/week) for quick relief of symptoms
   3. Maintain normal (or near normal) lung function.
   4. Maintain normal activity levels: exercise and attendance at work and school.

B. *Reduce risk*
   1. Prevent recurrent exacerbations and minimize need for urgent care.
   2. Prevent progressive loss of lung function; for youth, prevent reduced growth.
   3. Provide optimal pharmacotherapy with minimal or no adverse effects.

V. Plan

A. *Diagnostic tests*
   1. Pulmonary function testing (spirometry) (**Figure 43-1**): Spirometry, which measures airflow obstruction, is needed to diagnose asthma because medical history and physical examination are not reliable ways to exclude other causes of respiratory impairment. The key measures are FEV_1, forced vital capacity (FVC), and FEV_1/FVC ratio. For those who cannot sustain expiration for the length of time necessary to measure FVC, FEV in 6 seconds is used as a substitute for FVC. Significant reversibility is demonstrated by an increase in FEV_1 or FVC of 200 mL and ≥12% change from baseline after inhaling two puffs of albuterol at 90 mcg/puff (Pellegrino et al., 2005). Some patients with severe symptoms of asthma do not demonstrate reversibility until treatment is maximized according to level of severity; thus, follow-up spirometry measures are indicated as asthma control improves (NAEPP, 2007).
   2. Chest radiograph to exclude other causes of airway obstruction
   3. Allergy testing by skin tests or in vitro tests
   4. Exhaled nitric oxide (FeNO) testing should not be used in isolation to assess asthma control or predict risk of exacerbation or severity, but it may be used in conjunction with other clinical data as part of an ongoing monitoring and management strategy that includes frequent assessments (NAEPP, 2020).

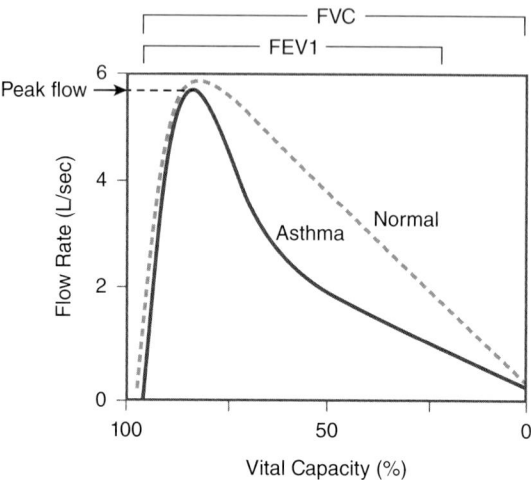

Figure 43-1 Spirometry in asthma versus normal results.

Data from Pellegrino, R., Viegi, G., Brusasco,V., Crapo, R. O., Burgos, F., Casaburi, R., et al. (2005). Interpretive strategies for lung function tests. European Respiratory Journal, 26, 948–968.

   5. Additional pulmonary function tests that are not routinely necessary but can be useful when considering alternative diagnoses:
      a. Flow–volume loops to assess the presence of inspiratory airflow obstruction (see **Figure 43-1** for normal versus asthmatic flow–volume loops)
      b. Bronchoprovocation challenge testing with methacholine or cold air may be helpful when asthma is suspected but spirometry is normal or near normal.
      c. Diffusing capacity to assess for emphysema
      d. Total lung volumes to assess for restrictive ventilatory defects

B. *Management*

The NAEPP of the National Heart, Lung, and Blood Institute (NHLBI) released a focused update to its asthma guidelines in 2020 using data through 2016. GINA releases ongoing twice-yearly updates to its asthma management recommendations. There are some recommendation differences between the 2020 NAEPP guidelines and the 2020 GINA report. In patients with intermittent asthma, using a SABA for as-needed symptom relief has been the traditional approach. GINA no longer recommends treating adults and adolescents with a SABA alone. Instead, the GINA report recommends the use of inhaled corticosteroids (ICSs) for *all* patients in any treatment step; specifically, the combination of low-dose ICS-formoterol is the preferred treatment for controller and reliever therapy. The second-track alternative treatment option GINA recommends is the use of a low-dose ICS whenever a SABA is used for symptom relief, administered consecutively one after the other. With this new approach, GINA seeks to highlight that patients classified as having mild intermittent symptoms are still at risk of severe exacerbations, and this risk is reduced with the use of a low-dose glucocorticoid inhaler compared with SABA use alone because lung function improves with ICSs containing treatment by reducing chronic airway inflammation (GINA, 2021). This recommendation differs from the NAEPP 2020 update, but it is an important facet of asthma management that is being utilized in primary and specialty care.

1. Medications: A stepwise approach to pharmacologic therapy is recommended (**Table 43-3**) using preferred therapy or alternative therapy based on the NAEPP (2020) *Focused Updates to the Asthma Management Guidelines*. GINA recommendations are inserted where different from the NAEPP guidelines. When initiating therapy, monitor at 2- to 4-week intervals to ensure that asthma control is achieved. Preferred options are the best choices supported by the evidence and reviewed by the NAEPP 2020 expert panel. Alternative therapies listed have limited availability in the United States, have an increased risk of adverse effects, or require monitoring. If patients continue to have poorly controlled symptoms after 2–3 months of treatment, assess adherence, inhaler technique, allergen exposure, and comorbidities before stepping up therapy. Poor inhaler technique is common and often contributes to uncontrolled asthma. Patients with severe uncontrolled asthma should be referred to specialist care.
    a. Quick relief "rescue" medication regimens:
        i. SABAs: These include albuterol-hydrofluoroalkane (HFA) and levalbuterol-HFA, which are prescribed for any severity of asthma. Patients should be instructed to inhale two puffs every 4–6 hours as needed for symptoms of asthma. They may also be used 20–30 minutes before exercise to prevent exercise-induced bronchospasm.
        ii. As-needed ICS and SABA used concomitantly one after the other: The NAEPP 2020 recommendations include "intermittent" ICS dosing as a treatment option in step 2 therapy for mild persistent asthma. "Intermittent" is defined as the temporary use of an ICS in response to worsening asthma on an as-needed basis in individuals not taking ICS controller therapy regularly. This may not be a good option in patients with a low or high perception of symptoms; in these patients, it is preferable to use a daily low-dose ICS with an as-needed SABA to avoid under- or overtreatment. Currently, these medications need to be administered sequentially in two separate inhalers. Combination inhalers with albuterol and ICS are currently undergoing clinical trials and may be available in the United States in the future.
        iii. ICS-formoterol used as both daily controller and reliever therapy: The NAEPP 2020 guidelines suggest ICS-formoterol in a single inhaler used as both daily maintenance to treat airway inflammation and as needed for acute symptoms (referred to as *single maintenance and reliever therapy*, or SMART) for moderate to severe persistent asthma in steps 3–4. SMART is preferred compared to either a higher-dose ICS as daily controller therapy and PRN SABA or same-dose daily ICS-LABA and PRN SABA for worsening asthma symptoms. Only formulary combinations with formoterol can be used in this way because formoterol has a rapid onset of action (providing symptom relief within 5 minutes) and a maximum daily dose that allows it to be used more than twice daily. The two ICS-formoterol inhalers that can be used for SMART are low to medium strengths of Symbicort® and Dulera®, 2 puffs BID and 1–2 puffs PRN for asthma symptoms, for a maximum of 10 puffs per day. Patients on the SMART plan must stop all other inhalers, including albuterol. If the patient needs more than 2 rescue doses per week, increase the strength of the dose to gain control. There is no need to change a daily ICS-LABA with a PRN SABA if it is providing adequate control. However, if asthma control is inadequate with this regimen, administer SMART before advancing to a higher step of therapy. Patients and providers should be aware that a 1-month supply of ICS-formoterol may not last a month if the inhaler is used for maintenance and reliever therapy, and this may affect insurance coverage. When prescribing a new inhaler, always check inhaler technique.
    b. Long-acting "controller" medication regimens:
        i. ICSs are the most effective therapy to reduce airway inflammation and control persistent asthma (A comparison of asthma medications can be found at Clinical Resource, Comparison of Asthma Meds. Pharmacist's Letter/Prescriber's Letter. December 2022 [381217]). For patients who have had well-controlled asthma for at least 3 months, it is essential to step down therapy to identify the minimum medication necessary to maintain control. For individuals with mild to moderate persistent asthma who are taking a daily controller ICS, increasing the regular daily ICS dose for short periods in response to worsening asthma symptoms is not recommended. This is especially important for young adolescents when there is the potential for growth suppression secondary to prolonged high-dose ICS exposure (NAEPP, 2020).
        ii. In individuals with moderate to severe persistent asthma, if asthma control is not achieved with ICS therapy, step up therapy with an ICS plus a LABA (steps 3–4), preferably in one inhaler. Consider SMART before moving to a higher step of therapy.

Table 43-3 Stepwise Approach for Managing Asthma in Adolescents 12+ Years and Adults

Intermittent Asthma	Persistent Asthma: Daily Medication Consult with asthma specialist if step 4 care or higher is required. Consider consultation at step 3					
Step 1 Preferred: PRN SABA (GINA preferred treatment: PRN low dose ICS-formoterol; Alternative: SABA and low-dose ICS taken right after the SABA)	**Step 2** Preferred: Daily low-dose ICS and PRN SABA♦ or PRN concomitant ICS and SABA (see notes) Alternative: Daily LTRA and PRN SABA or Cromolyn*, or Nedocromil*, or Zileuton*, or Theophylline*, and PRN SABA (GINA preferred treatment: PRN low dose ICS formoterol)	**Step 3** Preferred: Daily and PRN combination low-dose ICS-formoterol♦ Alternative: Daily medium-dose ICS and PRN SABA or Daily low-dose ICS-LABA, or daily low-dose ICS + LAMA♦, or daily low-dose ICS + LTRA*, and PRN SABA or Daily low-dose ICS + Theophylline* or Zileuton*, and PRN SABA	**Step 4** Preferred: Daily and PRN combination medium-dose ICS-formoterol♦ Alternative: Daily medium dose ICS-LABA or daily medium-dose ICS+ LAMA, and PRN SABA♦ or Daily medium-dose ICS + LTRA*, or daily medium dose ICS + Theophylline*, or daily medium-dose ICS + Zileuton*, and PRN SABA	**Step 5** Preferred: Daily medium-high dose ICS-LABA + LAMA, and PRN SABA♦ Alternative: Daily medium-high dose ICS-LABA or daily high-dose ICS + LTRA*, and PRN SABA	**Step 6** Preferred: Daily high-dose ICS-LABA + oral systemic corticosteroids + PRN SABA	**Step up if needed:** First, check adherence, inhaler technique, environmental control, and comorbid conditions 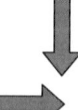 ASSESS CONTROL **Step down if possible:** if asthma is well controlled for at least 3 months

Steps 2–4: Consider subcutaneous immunotherapy as an adjunct treatment to standard pharmacotherapy for patients who have allergic asthma♦ (see notes)	Steps 5 & 6: consider adding Asthma Biologics (e.g. anti-IgE, anti-IL5, anti-IL5R, anti-IL4/IL13)

 Each step: patient education, environmental control, and management of comorbidities.

Quick_relief medication for all patients
- Use SABA as needed for symptoms. Intensity of treatment depends on the severity of symptoms: up to 3 treatments at 20-minute intervals as needed.
- Based on the 2020 guidelines, in steps 3 & 4, the preferred options include the use of ICS-formoterol 1–2 puffs as needed up to a maximum total daily maintenance and rescue dose of 12 puffs (54 mcg).
- Use of SABA > 2 days a week for symptom relief (not prevention of EIB) generally indicates inadequate control and the need to step up treatment.

Abbreviations: EIB, exercise-induced bronchospasm; ICS, inhaled corticosteroid; LABA, long-acting beta2-agonist; LAMA, long acting muscarinic antagonist; LTRA, leukotriene receptor antagonist; SABA, inhaled short-acting beta2-agonist

♦ New recommendations based on the NHLBI 2020 Focused Updates. GINA recommendations added where different from NHLBI guidelines.

⁺ Since 2020 The Global Initiative for Asthma (GINA) recommends the use of low dose ICS for all patients, specifically ICS-formoterol is preferred as maintenance and and reliever therapy in any treatment step. GINA does not recommend the use of SABA alone. This differs from the NHLBI 2020 guidelines.

*Cromolyn, Nedocromil, LTRAs including Zileuton and montelukast, and Theophylline are less desirable alternatives due to limited studies as adjunctive therapy, an increased risk of adverse effects, and the need for monitoring. Zileuton requires monitoring of liver function. Theophylline requires monitoring of serum concentration levels. The FDA issued a Boxed Warning for montelukast in March 2020.

Notes:

The stepwise approach is meant to assist, not replace, the clinical decision making required to meet individual patient needs.

If alternative treatment is used and response is inadequate, discontinue it and use the preferred treatment before stepping up.

Step 2: For mild persistent asthma, either daily low-dose ICS and PRN SABA for symptom relief, or intermittent PRN SABA and ICS administered sequentially for worsening asthma. For intermittent therapy, consider 2-4 puffs of albuterol followed by 80-250 mcg of beclomethasone equivalent every 4 hours as needed for symptom relief. Therapy can be initiated at home with regular follow up to ensure intermittent therapy is still appropriate.

Steps 2-4: subcutaneous immunotherapy (SCIT) conditionally recommended as adjunct treatment for individuals with allergic sensitization and evidence of worsening asthma symptoms after exposure to specific antigens. Do not initiate, increase or administer SCIT while individual is having asthma symptoms. Not recommended in individuals with severe asthma.

Steps 3 & 4: for individuals with moderate to severe persistent asthma already on daily ICS controller therapy, the preferred treatment is ICS-formoterol in a single inhaler used both daily and as needed for worsening symptoms (SMART). The terms ICS-LABA and ICS-formoterol refer to combination therapy with both an ICS and a LABA, preferably in a single inhaler. Where formoterol is specified, it is because the evidence is based on studies specific to formoterol. Maximum daily dose of formoterol not to exceed 12 puffs (54 µg) for ages 12 years and above.

ICS-formoterol should not be used as quick relief therapy in patients taking ICS-salmeterol as maintenance therapy.

National Heart, Lung and Blood Institute, National Asthma Education and Prevention Program, & National Institutes of Health. (2020). Expert panel report: The 2020 Focused Updates to the Asthma Management Guidelines (Publication No. 91-6749). Bethesda, MD: Author.

Global Initiative for Asthma. (2021). Global Strategy for Asthma Management and Prevention. Retrieved from www.ginasthma.org

---

iii. If asthma is not controlled with SMART, adding a LAMA in a second inhaler is recommended to achieve control. Individuals at risk for urinary retention or who have glaucoma should not use a LAMA.

iv. Consider adding a leukotriene receptor antagonist (e.g., montelukast [sold as Singulair®]) if allergies are a strong component of the asthma. The role of allergy in asthma is greater in children than in adults.

c. Asthma biologics: Anti-IgE therapy—for example, omalizumab (Xolair®), benralizumab (Fasenra®), dupilumab (Dupixent®), and mepolizumab (Nucala®)

i. Consider for adolescents older than 12 years and adults with severe uncontrolled asthma, skin or in vitro test positive to perennial allergens, and elevated IgE, as add-on treatment for patients with the eosinophilic phenotype.

Omalizumab is given subcutaneously under direct observation. Benralizumab, dupilumab, and mepolizumab come in prefilled pens and autoinjectors to facilitate ease of administration. Dupilumab and mepolizumab have additional indications for treatment, including atopic dermatitis (dupilumab) and chronic rhinosinusitis with nasal polyposis (dupilumab and mepolizumab). Be aware that biologics may cause hypersensitivity reactions (anaphylaxis, angioedema, etc.). Patients should be referred to a specialist for consideration of these medications.

2. Bronchial thermoplasty (BT): This is a procedure that uses heat to remove muscle tissue from the airways of adults with moderate to severe asthma.

a. BT may reduce severe asthma exacerbations, but there is limited evidence that this treatment improves long-term asthma outcomes. Risks and benefits should be reviewed with experienced specialists with training in BT (NAEPP, 2020).

3. Environmental control

a. Reduce exposure to allergens to which the patient is sensitized (dust mites, animal dander, mold, cockroaches, and pollens).

b. Effective allergen mitigation requires a multifaceted, comprehensive approach (e.g., carpets harbor dust mites, so remove or vacuum often; use allergen-proof mattress and pillow covers to protect against dust mites; wash all bed linens in hot water at least every 2 weeks; eliminate any cockroach infestations, and do not leave food or garbage out or exposed; remove mold and mildew; and repair leaks). Because these mitigations can be costly and burdensome to patients, the recent recommendations suggest only tailored allergen-specific intervention strategies for individuals with asthma whose asthma symptoms are related to exposure to identified aeroallergen, confirmed by allergy testing or clinical history.

c. Avoid exposure to environmental tobacco smoke and other respiratory irritants (woodsmoke, perfume, strong odors and fumes, bleach, and cleaning products).

d. Avoid exertion outside when air pollution levels are high.

e. Avoid use of nonselective β-blockers.

f. Avoid sulfite-containing food and foods to which the patient is sensitive.

4. Treat and control comorbid diseases that aggravate asthma.

a. Allergic rhinitis or sinusitis (consider leukotriene receptor antagonist, antihistamine, nasal corticosteroid spray, and nasal saline washes)

b. GERD: Consider use of a proton pump inhibitor; elevate head of bed at night; no food at bedtime; and decrease use of alcohol and caffeine. See Chapter 52, Gastroesophageal Reflux Disease, for further suggestions.

c. Other conditions that make asthma harder to control include higher total body weight, depression, OSA, vocal cord dysfunction, and psychosocial barriers to self-management.

5. Consider specialty consultation for uncontrolled asthma that has not responded to maximal therapy, when allergy immunotherapy or asthma biologics are being considered, or when exacerbations require hospitalizations.
6. Follow-ups should be at frequent intervals until control is achieved and then at 3- to 6-month intervals to maintain control. More frequent follow-up is determined by individual characteristics, past history, and psychosocial factors that increase risk.

C. Patient education and training in self-management of asthma
1. Shared decision making will help individuals with asthma to make choices compatible with their risks, values, and preferences. Elicit the patient's concerns and questions regarding asthma.
2. Describe airway inflammation and bronchospasm (Asthma & Allergy Foundation, 2021).
3. Teach the patient how to recognize and avoid individual triggers: explain the cumulative effect of precipitating factors. Use the teach-back technique to ensure understanding.
4. Instruct the patient not to smoke and to avoid secondhand smoke.
5. Review all asthma medications with the patient, including the purpose, actions, dosage, side effects, and interactions. Explain how each medication works to relieve, control, or prevent asthma signs and symptoms.
6. Demonstrate the proper use of the metered-dose inhaler or dry-powder inhaler and also the spacer device for metered-dose inhalers containing corticosteroid medication (**Box 43-1**). Have the patient demonstrate proper use periodically or at each follow-up visit.
7. For patients who meet the criteria for moderate-persistent or severe-persistent asthma, demonstrate the use of and rationale for peak flow meters (for use at home or in the office) before the initiation of therapy. See the Patient Education Supplement: Peak Flow Meter Use and Peak Expiratory Flow Rate Monitoring (**Box 43-2**). Recommend daily morning measurements on awakening before inhaling medications. Teach the patient how to

Box 43-1 Patient Instructions for Various Asthma Inhalers

Instructions for Using a Metered-Dose Inhaler (MDI) With or Without a Spacer

1. To begin, shake the inhaler five or six times.
2. Remove the mouthpiece cover. If using a spacer, place the spacer over the mouthpiece at the end of the inhaler.
3a. Use of an MDI without a spacer: Bring the inhaler to your lips and close your lips tightly over the inhaler mouthpiece. Breathe in slowly. As you do so, squeeze the top of the canister once to dispense medication. Continue to inhale slowly and deeply.
3b. Use of the MDI with a spacer: Put your lips over the mouthpiece. Squeeze the top of the canister once to dispense medication, and then breathe in slowly. Keep inhaling even after you finish the squeeze. Continue inhaling slowly and deeply.
4. After inhaling, remove the inhaler or spacer from your mouth and hold your breath for up to 10 seconds.
5. Rinse your mouth with water and gargle after using the inhaler.
6. If you need another dose of medication, repeat the previous steps.

Patient Instructions for Dry-Powder Inhalers (DPIs)

Diskus (Advair® Diskus®; Wixela® Inhub®)

1a. Advair®: Hold the disk horizontally in one hand. With the other hand, place your thumb in the thumb grip and slide the cover away from you as far as it will go to reveal the mouthpiece. Keeping the inhaler in a horizontal position, use your thumb to push the lever away from you until it clicks. The medication is now loaded. Do not shake the inhaler.
1b. Inhub®: Hold the inhaler vertically and pull the cover down to reveal the mouthpiece. Keeping the inhaler in a vertical position, push the yellow lever down toward the purple arrows as far as it will go—you may or may not hear a click. The medication is now loaded. Do not shake the inhaler.
2. Exhale as much air as you can from your lungs away from the mouthpiece.
3. Put your lips around the mouthpiece. Breathe in quickly and deeply through your mouth.
4. After inhaling, remove the disk from your mouth and hold your breath for up to 10 seconds.
5a. Advair®: To close the disk, put your thumb in the thumb grip of the cover and slide it over the mouthpiece as far as it will go. The disk will click shut, and the lever will automatically return to its original position. The disk is now ready for your next dose.
5b. Inhub®: Push the mouthpiece cover back up to the closed position and make sure the cover is completely closed. The lever will automatically return to its original position. The disk is now ready for your next dose.
6. Rinse your mouth with water and gargle after using the inhaler.

Ellipta Inhaler

1. Open the cover by placing your thumb on the groove of the cover and pressing down until you hear a click. The medication is now loaded and ready to use. Do not shake the inhaler.
2. Exhale as much air as you can from your lungs away from the mouthpiece.
3. Hold the inhaler in a horizontal position and bring to your mouth. Place lips around the mouthpiece to create a seal. Take a long, steady, deep breath in.
4. Remove the mouthpiece from your mouth and hold your breath for up to 10 seconds.
5. To close the inhaler, slide the cover up over the mouthpiece as far as it will go.
6. Rinse your mouth with water and gargle after using the inhaler.

Flexhaler®

1. To begin, hold the inhaler in the upright position, twist the cover off, and set it down.
2. The inhaler has to be primed when using for the very first time: turn the bottom base to the left as far as it will go and then twist to the right until you hear a click. Repeat this process a second time. You do not have to prime the Flexhaler after the first use.
3. Next, load the dose of medication. Keeping the inhaler upright, twist the bottom base to the left as far as it will go and then twist to the right until you hear a click. The medication is now loaded. Do not shake the inhaler.
4. Exhale as much air from your lungs away from the mouthpiece of the inhaler.
5. Bring the inhaler to your lips, close your lips tightly over the mouthpiece, and take a fast and deep breath through your mouth.
6. Hold your breath for up to 10 seconds.
7. If you need another dose of medication, repeat the previous steps. The Flexhaler is designed to deliver one dose at a time.
8. When you are finished, place the cover back on the inhaler and twist shut.
9. Rinse your mouth with water and gargle after using the inhaler.

Handihaler Device

1. Open the inhaler by pressing the piercing button and pull dust cap up to expose the mouthpiece.
2. Pull the mouthpiece up away from the base to access the center chamber.
3. Remove 1 capsule from the blister pack. Insert the capsule into the center chamber. Only remove the capsules from the sealed foil packs immediately before use.
4. Close the mouthpiece over the center chamber until you hear a click, leaving the dust cap open.
5. Holding the device upright, press the piercing button completely 1 time. Do not shake the device.
6. Exhale as much air as you can from your lungs away from the mouthpiece.
7. Bring mouthpiece to your mouth horizontally. Close your lips around the mouthpiece to create a tight seal. Take a rapid, deep breath through your mouth. You should hear/feel the capsule vibrate.
8. Remove Handihaler from your mouth and hold your breath for up to 10 seconds. Exhale and repeat inhalation a second time for the same capsule to ensure you get the full dose.
9. To remove the used capsule, pull the mouthpiece up and tip out the used capsule into the trash, trying not to touch it. Close the mouthpiece and dust cap for storage.

RespiClick®, Redihaler®

1. Hold the inhaler upright with the mouthpiece cover at the bottom.
2. Open the cap all the way until you hear a click. The medication is now loaded. Do not shake the device.
3. Exhale as much air as you can from your lungs away from the mouthpiece. Do not block the air vent with your mouth or fingers.
4. Bring the inhaler to your lips, close your lips tightly over the mouthpiece, and take a deep breath in through your mouth.
5. Take the inhaler out of your mouth and hold your breath for 10 seconds.
6. Close the cap all the way. Repeat previous steps if more than 1 puff prescribed.

Twisthaler®

1. To begin, hold the inhaler in the upright position and grip the colored base on the bottom.
2. Twist the cap counterclockwise while keeping the inhaler in an upright position. You will hear and feel a click as the dose counter counts down. The medication is now loaded in the inhaler and ready to use. Do not shake the inhaler. Lift the cap off. Make sure the arrow is lined up with the dose counter.
3. Exhale as much air from your lungs as possible away from the mouthpiece of the inhaler.

(continues)

Box 43-1 Patient Instructions for Various Asthma Inhalers (continued)

4. Hold the inhaler horizontally; bring the inhaler to your lips; put your lips over the mouthpiece to create a seal; and take a fast and deep, powerful breath through your mouth.
5. Remove the inhaler from your mouth and hold your breath for about 10 seconds.
6. Wipe the mouthpiece dry and put the cap back on. Turn the cap in a clockwise direction as you gently press down. You will hear a click to let you know the cap is fully closed. The cap must be closed to load the next dose.
7. Rinse your mouth with water and gargle after using the inhaler.

Soft Mist Inhaler (SMI)
Respimat®

1. When using the Respimat for the first time, prepare and prime the inhaler: press the safety release and pull off the clear base. Push the narrow part of the cartridge into the inhaler until it clicks. Put the plastic base back onto the inhaler. Holding the inhaler upright, turn the clear base in the direction of the white arrows until it clicks. Open the cap and push the button to dispense medication. Repeat twisting of the base, opening the cap and pressing the button 3 times until a visible mist of medication can be seen. Close the cap. The inhaler is now primed and ready for use. There is no need to shake the inhaler.
2. Exhale as much air from your lungs as possible away from the mouthpiece of the inhaler.
3. Twist the clear base until it clicks. Open the cap, put the inhaler in your mouth, and create a tight seal with your lips. Press the button and take a slow, deep breath. Once the button is pressed, the inhaler will release a slow mist of medication.
4. Remove inhaler from your mouth and hold your breath for 10 seconds.
5. Repeat if your dose is more than 1 puff. Close the cap after use.

Box 43-2 Patient Education Supplement: Peak Flow Meter Use and Peak Expiratory Flow Rate Monitoring

- What is a peak flow meter?

A peak flow meter is a portable, inexpensive device for home use to measure peak expiratory flow rates.

- What is a peak expiratory flow rate?

Peak expiratory flow rate is a measurement of the highest speed at which you can blow out air when you exhale as hard and as fast as you can. This measurement tells us how much impediment, or obstruction, there is in your airways. Flow rates decrease when asthma obstructs or narrows your airways. Flow rates are normal when there is no or minimal obstruction of your airways. Monitoring this measurement will help you to manage your asthma.

- When and how often should you measure and record peak flow rates?

You and your provider will plan this during your visits.

- What are the steps to measuring a peak expiratory flow rate using a peak flow meter?

1. Ask your clinician about where to set the color-coded indicators on the peak flow meter. They can help determine the status of your airflow.
2. To begin, hold the meter by the handgrip. Slide the measurement arrow to the bottom of the scale, next to the mouthpiece. (One device requires you to shake the arrow to the bottom of the device).
3. Stand up or sit up straight with head erect.
4. Take a deep breath.
5. Place the meter in your mouth and close your lips around the mouthpiece. Make sure your lips act as a seal over the mouthpiece so that no air escapes. Make sure your tongue is not in the mouthpiece.
6. Blow out as hard and as fast as possible.
7. The measurement arrow will slide up the scale. The number that it stops on is your peak flow reading. Write down this number.
8. Repeat this process two more times. Each time, remember to slide the measurement arrow back to its start position near the mouthpiece.
9. Record the highest of the three measurements with the date and time. Your clinician will help determine a personalized scale to use with your meter, dependent on your age, height, and gender.

Data from National Asthma Education and Prevention Program. (1997). *Expert panel report 2: Guidelines for the diagnosis and management of asthma* (NIH Publication No. 97-4051). National Heart, Lung, and Blood Institute; National Asthma Education and Prevention Program. (2007). *Expert panel report 3: Guidelines for the diagnosis and management of asthma* (NIH Publication 07-4051). National Heart, Lung, and Blood Institute.

measure and interpret the peak flow rate readings (**Box 43-2**). Provide written guidelines for what the patient should do when the readings fall below a specified level.
8. Have a written asthma action plan directing the patient what to do during an exacerbation (**Figure 43-2**). Include when the patient should call the provider, increase or add medications, or go to the emergency department.
9. Encourage adequate hydration, proper nutrition, and adequate rest.
10. Encourage the patient to keep regular appointments for follow-up and evaluation, even if the symptoms of asthma are not present.

D. *Asthma education resources*
1. American Academy of Allergy, Asthma, and Immunology: http://www.aaaai.org
2. American Lung Association: http://www.lung.org
3. Association of Asthma Educators: http://www.asthmaeducators.org
4. Centers for Disease Control and Prevention National Asthma Control Program: https://www.cdc.gov/asthma/nacp.htm
5. NHLBI Information Center: http://www.nhlbi.nih.gov
6. U.S. Environmental Protection Agency: http://www.airnow.gov

VI. Future update topics in asthma

The NAEPP (2020) *Focused Updates to the Asthma Management Guidelines* have suggested the following areas for future research opportunities:

1. Update asthma severity by incorporating asthma phenotypes and endotypes.
2. Further clarify the role of FeNO measurements as a diagnostic tool and for monitoring therapy for asthma management.
3. Undertake further research into the effectiveness of allergen mitigation interventions.
4. Determine differences by race and ethnicity of the risks and benefits of the ICS recommendations.
5. Undertake further studies examining LAMA therapy and comparing ICS-LAMA versus ICS-LABA in ethnically diverse populations.
6. Undertake studies of more diverse populations to examine whether race or ethnicity affects the efficacy and safety of immunotherapy.
7. Undertake longitudinal studies looking at the risks and benefits of BT.

Additional areas of future research:
- Biomarkers as predictors of response to medication and for monitoring response to therapy are an important area of developing research. There is a lot of potential for future research in this area as we move toward delivering targeted therapeutics. For example, specific biologics are now being developed to target type 2 high endotypes.
- The differences between the NAEPP 2020 updated recommendations and the latest GINA reports highlight the need for further studies on the use of as-needed ICS-formoterol versus a SABA alone in patients with mild persistent asthma.
- The role of technology in enhancing patient engagement in self-management

ASTHMA ACTION PLAN

For: _____ Doctor: _____ Date: _____

Doctor's Phone Number: _____ Hospital/Emergency Department Phone Number: _____

GREEN ZONE — DOING WELL

- No cough, wheeze, chest tightness, or shortness of breath during the day or night
- Can do usual activities

And, if a peak flow meter is used,
Peak flow: more than _____
(80 percent or more of my best peak flow)
My best peak flow is: _____

Daily Medications

Medicine	How much to take	When to take it

Before exercise   ☐ 2 or ☐ 4 puffs   5 minutes before exercise

YELLOW ZONE — ASTHMA IS GETTING WORSE

- Cough, wheeze, chest tightness, or shortness of breath, or
- Waking at night due to asthma, or
- Can do some, but not all, usual activities

-Or-

Peak flow: _____ to _____
(50 to 79 percent of my best peak flow)

1st Add: quick-relief medicine—and keep taking your GREEN ZONE medicine.

☐ _____ (quick-relief medicine)   _____ Number of puffs or ☐ Nebulizer, once

2nd If your symptoms (and peak flow, if used) return to GREEN ZONE after 1 hour of above treatment:
☐ Continue monitoring to be sure you stay in the green zone.

-Or-

If your symptoms (and peak flow, if used) do not return to GREEN ZONE after 1 hour of above treatment:

☐ Take: _____ (quick-relief medicine)   _____ Number of puffs or ☐ Nebulizer   Can repeat every _____ minutes up to maximum of _____ doses

☐ Add: _____ (oral steroid)   _____ mg per day   For _____ (3–10) days

☐ Call the doctor ☐ before / ☐ within _____ hours after taking the oral steroid.

RED ZONE — MEDICAL ALERT!

- Very short of breath, or
- Quick-relief medicines have not helped, or
- Cannot do usual activities, or
- Symptoms are same or get worse after 24 hours in Yellow Zone

-Or-

Peak flow: less than _____
(50 percent of my best peak flow)

Take this medicine:

☐ _____ (quick-relief medicine)   _____ Number of puffs or ☐ Nebulizer

☐ _____ (oral steroid)   _____ mg

Then call your doctor NOW. Go to the hospital or call an ambulance if:
- You are still in the red zone after 15 minutes AND
- You have not reached your doctor.

DANGER SIGNS
- Trouble walking and talking due to shortness of breath
- Lips or fingernails are blue

- Take _____ puffs of _____ (quick-relief medicine) AND
- Go to the hospital or call for an ambulance _____ NOW!
  (phone)

See the reverse side for things you can do to avoid your asthma triggers.

Figure 43-2 NIH Asthma Action Plan

National Heart, Lung, and Blood Institute. (2020). *Asthma action plan.* https://www.nhlbi.nih.gov/health-topics/all-publications-and-resources/asthma-action-plan-2020

HOW TO CONTROL THINGS THAT MAKE YOUR ASTHMA WORSE

This guide suggests things you can do to avoid your asthma triggers. Put a check next to the triggers that you know make your asthma worse and ask your doctor to help you find out if you have other triggers as well. Keep in mind that controlling any allergen usually requires a combination of approaches, and reducing allergens is just one part of a comprehensive asthma management plan. Here are some tips to get started. These tips tend to work better when you use several of them together. Your health care provider can help you decide which ones may be right for you.

ALLERGENS

☐ **Dust Mites**

These tiny bugs, too small to see, can be found in every home—in dust, mattresses, pillows, carpets, cloth furniture, sheets and blankets, clothes, stuffed toys, and other cloth-covered items. If you are sensitive:

- Mattress and pillow covers that prevent dust mites from going through them should be used along with high efficiency particulate air (HEPA) filtration vacuum cleaners.
- Consider reducing indoor humidity to below 60 percent. Dehumidifiers or central air conditioning systems can do this.

☐ **Cockroaches and Rodents**

Pests like these leave droppings that may trigger your asthma. If you are sensitive:

- Consider an integrated pest management plan.
- Keep food and garbage in closed containers to decrease the chances for attracting roaches and rodents.
- Use poison baits, powders, gels, or paste (for example, boric acid) or traps to catch and kill the pests.
- If you use a spray to kill roaches, stay out of the room until the odor goes away.

☐ **Animal Dander**

Some people are allergic to the flakes of skin or dried saliva from animals with fur or hair. If you are sensitive and have a pet:

- Consider keeping the pet outdoors.
- Try limiting to your pet to commonly used areas indoors.

☐ **Indoor Mold**

If mold is a trigger for you, you may want to:

- Explore professional mold removal or cleaning to support complete removal.
- Wear gloves to avoid touching mold with your bare hands if you must remove it yourself.
- Always ventilate the area if you use a cleaner with bleach or a strong smell.

☐ **Pollen and Outdoor Mold**

When pollen or mold spore counts are high you should try to:

- Keep your windows closed.
- If you can, stay indoors with windows closed from late morning to afternoon, when pollen and some mold spore counts are at their highest.
- If you do go outside, change your clothes as soon as you get inside, and put dirty clothes in a covered hamper or container to avoid spreading allergens inside your home.
- Ask your health care provider if you need to take or increase your anti-inflammatory medicine before the allergy season starts.

IRRITANTS

☐ **Tobacco Smoke**

- If you smoke, visit smokefree.gov or ask your health care provider for ways to help you quit.
- Ask family members to quit smoking.
- Do not allow smoking in your home or car.

☐ **Smoke, Strong Odors, and Sprays**

- If possible, avoid using a wood-burning stove, kerosene heater, or fireplace. Vent gas stoves to outside the house.
- Try to stay away from strong odors and sprays, such as perfume, talcum powder, hair spray, and paints.

☐ **Vacuum Cleaning**

- Try to get someone else to vacuum for you once or twice a week, if you can. Stay out of rooms while they are being vacuumed and for a short while afterward.
- If you must vacuum yourself, using HEPA filtration vacuum cleaners may be helpful.

☐ **Other Things That Can Make Asthma Worse**

- Sulfites in foods and beverages: Do not drink beer or wine or eat dried fruit, processed potatoes, or shrimp if they cause asthma symptoms.
- Cold air: Cover your nose and mouth with a scarf on cold or windy days.
- Other medicines: Tell your doctor about all the medicines you take. Include cold medicines, aspirin, vitamins and other supplements, and nonselective beta-blockers (including those in eye drops).

For more information and resources on asthma, visit *nhlbi.nih.gov/BreatheBetter*.

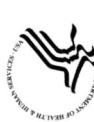

U.S. Department of Health and Human Services
National Institutes of Health
National Heart, Lung, and Blood Institute

NIH Publication No. 20-HL-5251
February 2021

Figure 43-2 (*Continued*)

References

Asthma & Allergy Foundation of America. (2020). *Asthma disparities in America: A roadmap to reducing burden on racial & ethnic minorities.* https://aafa.org/asthmadisparities

Asthma & Allergy Foundation of America. (2021). *Asthma medicines and treatments.* https://www.aafa.org/asthma-treatment/

Barnett, S. B., & Nurmagambetov, T. A. (2011). Costs of asthma in the United States: 2002–2007. *The Journal of allergy and clinical immunology, 127*(1), 145–152. doi:10.1016/j.jaci.2010.10.020

Centers for Disease Control and Prevention. (2021). *Most Recent National Asthma Data.* https://www.cdc.gov/asthma/most_recent_national_asthma_data.htm#print

Clinical Resource. (2022). *Comparison of Asthma Meds: Pharmacist's Letter/Prescriber's Letter.* December 2022 [381217].

Global Initiative for Asthma. (2021). *Global strategy for asthma management and prevention.* http://www.ginasthma.org.

Harper, R.W., & Zeki, A.A. (2015). Immunobiology of the critical asthma syndrome. *Clinical Reviews in Allergy & Immunology, 48,* 54–65.

Lambrecht, B. N., Hammad, H., & Fahy, J. V. (2019). The Cytokines of Asthma. *Immunity, 50*(4), 975–991. doi:10.1016/j.immuni.2019.03.018

Lazarus, S. C., Krishnan, J. A., King, T. S., Lang, J. E., Blake, K. V., Covar, R., Lugogo, N., Wenzel, S., Chinchilli, V. M., Mauger, D. T., Dyer, A., Boushey, H. A., Fahy, J. V., Woodruff, P. G., Bacharier, L. B., Cabana, M. D., Cardet, J. C., Castro, M., Chmiel, J., Denlinger, L., . . . Sorkness, C. A. (2019). Mometasone or tiotropium in mild asthma with a low sputum eosinophil level. *New England Journal of Medicine, 380,* 2009–2019.

National Asthma Education and Prevention Program. (1997). *Expert panel report 2: Guidelines for the diagnosis and management of asthma* (Publication No. 97-4051). National Heart, Lung, and Blood Institute.

National Asthma Education and Prevention Program. (2007). *Expert panel report 3: Guidelines for the diagnosis and management of asthma* (Publication No. 07-4051). National Heart, Lung, and Blood Institute.

National Asthma Education and Prevention Program. (2020). *Expert panel report: The 2020 focused updates to the asthma management guidelines* (Publication No. 91-6749). National Heart, Lung, and Blood Institute.

Pellegrino, R., Viegi, G., Brusasco, V., Crapo, R. O., Burgos, F., Casaburi, R., Coates, A., van der Grinten, C. P., Gustafsson, P., Hankinson, J., Jensen, R., Johnson, D. C., MacIntyre, N., McKay, R., Miller, M. R., Navajas, D., Pedersen, O. F., & Wanger, J. (2005). Interpretative strategies for lung function tests. *The European Respiratory Journal, 26*(5), 948–968. doi:10.1183/09031936.05.00035205

Sullivan, S. D., Rasouliyan, L., Russo, P. A., Kamath, T., Chipps, B. E., & TENOR Study Group. (2007). Extent, patterns, and burden of uncontrolled disease in severe or difficult-to-treat asthma. *Allergy, 62*(2), 126–133.

CHAPTER 44

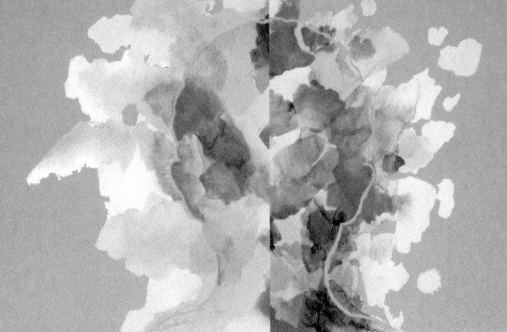

Cancer Survivorship

Tara D. Lacey and Sheila N. Lindsay

I. Introduction and background

There were an estimated 16.9 million cancer survivors living in the United States as of January 1, 2019. The estimated number of new cases of cancer in 2022 was over 1.9 million. Advances in early detection and treatment in some cancers resulted in a 32% decrease in cancer deaths between 1991 and 2019, leading to a substantial increase in the number of cancer survivors (American Cancer Society [ACS], 2022).

A. Definition and overview

The concept of cancer survivorship dates back to a 1985 *New England Journal of Medicine* article by Fitzhugh Mullan, a physician and cancer survivor, where he stated, "The challenge in overcoming cancer is not only to find therapies that will prevent or arrest the disease quickly, but also to map the middle ground of survivorship and minimize its medical and social hazards" (Mullan, 1985). The first definition of cancer survivorship was originated in 1986 by the National Coalition for Cancer Survivorship (NCCS) and was the foundation for the current definition developed by the National Cancer Institute (NCI) that defines a cancer survivor as "an individual from the time of diagnosis, through the balance of his or her life. Family members, friends, and caregivers are also impacted by the survivorship experience and are therefore included in this definition" (Hewitt et al., 2005). In 2005, a seminal report from the Institute of Medicine (IOM) called *From Cancer Patient to Cancer Survivor: Lost in Translation* highlighted the importance of cancer survivorship and the multifaceted aspects of caring for those with a history of cancer. The IOM report defined essential components of survivorship care, including the following : (1) prevention and detection of new and recurrent cancers; (2) surveillance for cancer spread, recurrence, or second cancers; (3) intervention for consequences of cancer and its treatment; and (4) coordination between specialists and primary care providers to ensure that all of a person's health needs are met (Hewitt et al., 2005). The American Society for Clinical Oncology (ASCO) further defined high-quality cancer survivorship care by recommending addressing psychosocial effects of cancer diagnosis; providing health education; promoting a healthy lifestyle, including diet and exercise guidance; providing resources for financial hardships; and empowering cancer survivors to be their own healthcare advocate (McCabe et al., 2013).

Oncology providers have historically been the coordinators of cancer survivorship care. The burden on oncology providers is daunting, given the increasing number of survivors requiring follow-up care. There is evidence to suggest that the increased lack of time and decreased workforce will not be able to manage the increasing number of cancer survivors. This, in combination with the increased access to care through the Affordable Care Act, has contributed to the burden of oncology providers (Chandak et al., 2014; Edwards et al., 2014). The need for a multidisciplinary approach that includes primary care providers is warranted to ensure continuity and complete cancer survivorship care.

Many models of care for survivorship have been identified, including disease specific, population specific, various provider-led programs, shared care, and transitional care between providers (Hewitt et al., 2007; Keesing et al., 2015; Nekhlyudov et al., 2017; Rowland et al., 2006). Across institutions, there is no consensus on the optimal model of healthcare delivery for cancer survivors at this time, but as a result of the demand for oncology specialists, it is evident that primary care providers will continue to be key members of the cancer survivor's care team (Gilbert et al., 2008).

Figure 44-1 shows the Cancer Care Trajectory taken from the IOM report *From Cancer Patient to Cancer Survivor: Lost in Translation* (Hewitt et al., 2005).

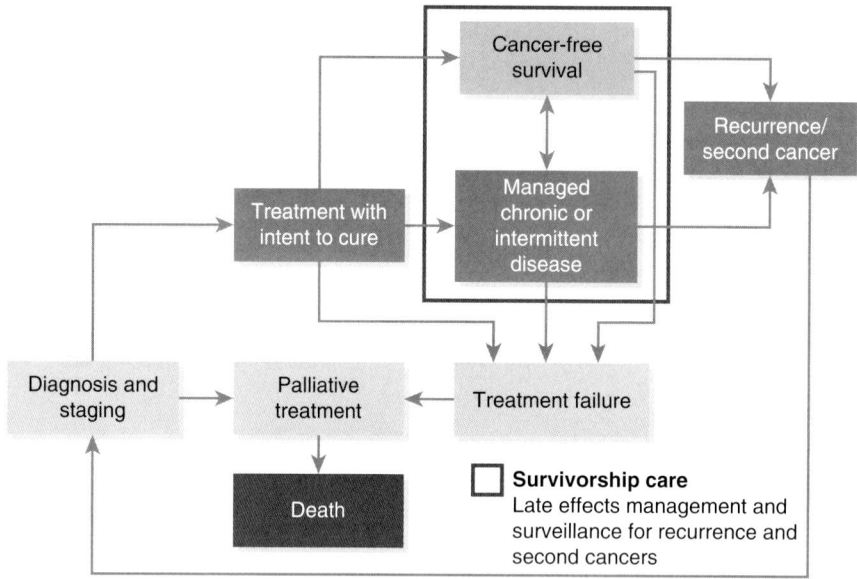

Figure 44-1 Cancer care trajectory.

Reproduced from Hewitt, M., Greenfield, S, & Stoval, E. (2005). *From Cancer Patient to Cancer Survivor - Lost in Transition* (T. N. A. Press Ed.). Washington, DC: The National Academies Press.

B. *Epidemiology*

In 2019, the Surveillance, Epidemiology, and End Results (SEER) database showed that 64% of survivors were 65 years or older, and this is expected to increase to 73% by 2040. The most common cancers among survivors are female breast cancer (31%), prostate cancer (27%), lung cancer (12%–13%), colorectal cancer (8%), and gynecologic cancer (8%) (Siegel et al., 2022). Survival rates and ages vary between cancer types. In all cancer sites, the relative 5-year cancer survival rate is estimated at 67.7%. The majority of those survivors, about 33%, are less than 5 years from diagnosis, 11% are 15 to 20 years from diagnosis, and only 6% are greater than 30-year cancer survivors (Howlader et al., 2018).

C. *Healthcare disparities and financial toxicity in cancer survivorship*

Disparities in health care in the United States are influenced by social determinants of health (SDOH), including race or ethnicity, sex or sexual identity, age, disability, economic burden, access and quality of education, access to and quality of health care, environment, and social and community context (Office of Disease Prevention and Health Promotion, n.d.). The community of cancer survivors is not immune to this, and there are subgroups of survivors that may be at higher risk for disparities. Black individuals have the highest mortality rate and lowest overall 5-year survival of any racial or ethnic group in the United States (ACS, 2019). Work is starting to address these disparities across racial, ethnic, and socioeconomic groups within cancer care and to understand more fully the differences in tumor biology and outcomes. SDOH are being recognized as key areas in understanding the different subpopulations of cancer survivors, particularly when developing cancer survivorship studies.

Healthcare equity is of great importance. As the number of cancer survivors continues to increase, the need for continued research and health initiatives to bridge the gaps in care for all cancer survivors is imperative and urgent. This work is critical to optimizing the health and quality of life for cancer survivors.

The financial burden experienced by patients and their families is often difficult to capture. The literature describes both the objective financial burden, including the monetary burden of paying for cancer treatment, and the subjective financial distress experienced by patients with a cancer diagnosis (Carrera & Kantarjian, 2018). The relationship is complex, with multiple intertwined layers. Financial toxicity (FT) has been associated with poorer outcomes, including an increase in mortality, decreased quality of life, and nonadherence to treatment (Arastu et al., 2020). Almost 50% of cancer survivors were found to experience financial hardship 1 year after diagnosis, and such hardship was more prevalent in Black and Hispanic populations (Pisu et al., 2015). Other contributing factors found by Gordon et al. (2017) include being female, low income at baseline, loss of income, younger age, adjuvant therapies, antineoplastic therapies, more recent diagnosis, advanced cancer, lack of health insurance, and living farther away from treatment centers.

Cancer survivors are at the highest risk for FT as a result of ongoing surveillance and treatment. Although there is an effort to mitigate the costs to cancer patients, as supported by the American Society of Oncologists, the American Society for Therapeutic Radiation and Oncology, and the Commission on Cancer, little movement in legislation has helped the direct effects on cancer patients. Discussing financial hardships is an important first step in assessing the burden in your patients. Understanding the coping mechanisms to treat these hardships and access to resources are important areas of possible intervention to assist in preventing poorer outcomes.

II. Database
A. *Subjective*
  1. Cancer history: specific type, stage at diagnosis, and histology; age at diagnosis
  2. Cancer treatment history:
     a. Chemotherapy: therapeutic agents used, including dose and date initiated and completed
     b. Immunotherapy/targeted therapy: therapeutic agents used, including dose and date initiated and completed
     c. Radiotherapy: region treated, radiation dose, date initiated and completed
     d. Surgery: surgical procedure, date of surgical procedure, pathology, and surgical complications
     e. Hereditary risk and genetic testing: Assess if genetic counseling was completed, including results. Follow screening guidelines for moderate- to high-risk cancer survivors (Wood et al., 2012).
     f. Complications from treatment course: hospitalizations, toxicities during treatment, ongoing toxicity at completion of treatment, and functional and performance status
  3. Medications: current medications for ongoing cancer therapy, current medications for cancer treatment sequelae, complementary and alternative medicine practices
  4. Past medical history: Comorbid conditions, both pre– and post–cancer diagnosis; gynecologic and obstetric history, including menstrual history, contraception, and sexually transmitted diseases
  5. Family history: Cancer history in family. Obtain a three-generation pedigree for hereditary cancer risk (Rowland et al., 2006).
  6. Personal and social history: past and current alcohol intake and tobacco use; history of higher body weight; sexual history, including fertility preservation, desire to have children, and current sexual practices; relationship and living situation; and ethnicity
  7. Occupational history: environmental exposures and cancer-related employment changes
  8. Review of systems
     A complete review of systems should be assessed at regular intervals.
     a. Constitutional: weight gain or loss, fatigue, fevers, sweats, pain, changes or limitations in exercise ability
     b. Skin and integument: treatment-related skin changes from radiotherapy, surgery, or chemotherapy; skin changes, including fibrosis, telangiectasia, or thinning of skin; hair loss
     c. Head, eyes, ear, nose, throat, and mouth: vision or hearing changes, dental problems, jaw pain or nonhealing sores, and xerostomia
     d. Pulmonary: cough, shortness of breath or dyspnea on exertion
     e. Cardiovascular: signs or symptoms of congestive heart failure, palpitations, coronary ischemia, pleuropericardial chest pain, claudication or vascular ischemic symptoms, Reynaud phenomenon, hypertension
     f. Breast: new lumps or bumps, nipple or skin changes, nipple discharge
     g. Gastrointestinal: diarrhea, constipation, nausea, emesis, abdominal pain, ostomy site problems, hepatitis, and cirrhosis
     h. Genitourinary: incontinence, dysuria, hematuria, urinary frequency or hesitancy, erectile dysfunction
     i. Gynecologic: premature menopause, vasomotor changes
     j. Endocrine, reproductive, and sexual functioning: symptoms of hypothyroidism, metabolic syndrome, vaginal dryness, dyspareunia, decreased libido, body image issues, decreased sexual functioning
     k. Hematologic and lymphatic: bleeding, easy bruising, recurrent or chronic infections, lymphedema
     l. Musculoskeletal: chronic pain, height changes, joint swelling, decreased range of motion, new lumps or bumps
     m. Neurologic: peripheral neuropathy, neuropathic pain, hearing loss, decreased cognitive function, mental acuity
     n. Psychiatric/Psychosocial: depression; posttraumatic stress disorder; cancer-related changes in health, relationships, and finance; fear of recurrence or new cancers
B. *Objective*
  1. Physical examination
     A problem-focused physical exam should occur at regular intervals. **Table 44-1** shows the late effects of both radiotherapy and chemotherapy on organ systems, including which chemotherapy drugs are used, as a reference for physical exam findings.
  2. Diagnostics
     a. Diagnostic testing should be based on the following: review of systems and physical exam findings, surveillance tests based on specific cancer history and hereditary risk factors, and standard of care cancer screening and prevention (Smith et al., 2014).
     b. Immunizations: Influenza vaccine (only inactive or recombinant) for all cancer survivors; pneumococcal vaccine; tetanus, diphtheria, and pertussis (Tdap); human papillomavirus (HPV) in survivors aged 26 or younger. Zoster vaccines in survivors aged 50 or older without active or ongoing immunodeficiency, no history of cellular immunodeficiency or hematopoietic stem cell transplant, or who have not received

Table 44-1 Late Effects for Cancer Treatment

Organ/System	Late Effects of Radiotherapy	Late Effects of Chemotherapy	Some of the Drugs Responsible
Cardiovascular	Pericardial effusion, pericarditis, coronary artery disease	Cardiomyopathy, congestive heart failure, hypertension	Anthracyclines (doxorubicin, daunorubicin, epirubicin, mitoxantrone), cyclophosphamide, monoclonal antibodies (trastuzumab and pertuzumab)
Central nervous system	Cognitive deficits, structural changes, hemorrhage, increased risk of stroke, hearing loss, psychiatric and psychosocial distress	Cognitive deficits, seizure, hemiplegia, hearing loss, psychiatric and psychosocial distress	Methotrexate, cisplatin
Gastrointestinal	Malabsorption, stricture, liver abnormalities	Abnormal liver function tests, hepatic fibrosis/failure, cirrhosis	Methotrexate, carmustine (BCNU®)
Genitourinary	Bladder fibrosis, contractures	Bladder fibrosis, hemorrhagic cystitis, urination dysfunction and malignancy	Cyclophosphamide, ifosfamide
Hematology/Lymph	Cytopenias, myelodysplasia	Myelodysplastic syndrome, acute myeloid leukemia	Alkylating agents, platinum agents (cisplatin, carboplatin, and oxaliplatin)
Musculoskeletal/ Soft tissue	Fibrosis, atrophy, osteonecrosis, secondary malignancies, cosmetic changes, lymphedema	Avascular necrosis, osteoporosis, pain	Steroids, methotrexate, aromatase inhibitors (letrozole, anastrozole, exemestane)
Ophthalmologic	Cataracts, retinopathy, double vision	Cataracts	Steroids, tamoxifen, busulfan
Oral health	Poor enamel and root formation, xerostomia	Xerostomia, increased incidence of caries	All chemotherapies
Peripheral nervous system	Peripheral neuropathy	Peripheral neuropathy, hearing loss	Cisplatin, taxanes (paclitaxel, docetaxel, and albumin-bound paclitaxel), vinca alkaloids (vincristine, vinorelbine), proteasome inhibitors (thalidomide)
Pulmonary	Pulmonary fibrosis, decreased lung volumes	Pulmonary fibrosis, interstitial pneumonitis	Bleomycin, BCNU, methotrexate, anthracyclines (doxorubicin, daunorubicin, epirubicin, mitoxantrone), *MTOR/PI3K* inhibitors (temsirolimus and everolimus)
Renal	Decreased creatinine clearance, hypertension	Decreased creatinine clearance, increased serum creatinine	Methotrexate, nitrosoureas, ifosfamides, Platinum agents (cisplatin, carboplatin, and oxaliplatin)

Organ/System	Late Effects of Radiotherapy	Late Effects of Chemotherapy	Some of the Drugs Responsible
Reproductive	Men: risk of sterility, Leydig cell dysfunction Women: ovarian failure, premature menopause	Men: sterility, deficient or insufficient testosterone Women: sterility, premature menopause	Alkylating agents (cyclophosphamide and ifosfamide), procarbazine, antiestrogen therapies (tamoxifen, anastrozole, letrozole, and exemestane), platinum agents
Endocrine	Hypothyroidism, nodules, growth hormone deficiencies, pituitary deficiencies		

Data from Ganz, P. A. (2001). Late effects of cancer and its treatment. *Seminars in Oncology Nursing, 17*(4), 241–248. doi: http://dx.doi.org/10.1053/sonu.2001.27914; Oeffinger, K. C., Hudson, M. M., & Landier, W. (2009). Survivorship: Childhood Cancer Survivors. *Primary Care, 36*(4), 743–780. doi: 10.1016/j.pop.2009.07.007

chemotherapy or radiotherapy in the past 3 months. COVID-19 vaccination is recommended for all patients receiving active therapy, understanding that there are limited safety and efficacy data in these patients. Currently, the COVID-19 vaccination guidelines for those patients who have had hematopoietic cell transplantation or engineered cellular therapy recommended a delay of at least 3 months for COVID-19 vaccination to maximize vaccine efficacy. This may change as more data become available; refer to the most recent Centers for Disease Control and Prevention (CDC) and National Comprehensive Cancer Network (NCCN, 2022a) guidelines.

III. Assessment

The NCI guidelines and clinical practice guidelines in oncology for survivorship recommend that a provider see an adult cancer survivor at regular intervals. These intervals are driven by individual cancer history and follow-up recommendations (NCCN, 2022b). At each visit, the differential diagnosis is based on the survivor's symptoms. The guidelines recommend addressing the following subjects at regular intervals to see if there are contributing and/or reversible factors affecting health: current disease status, functional/performance status, medications, comorbid conditions, cancer history, family history, psychosocial factors, and health behaviors that can modify cancer or comorbidity risk (NCCN, 2022b).

IV. Goals of clinical management

The IOM report created the foundation of survivorship care and its essential components (Hewitt et al., 2005). These principles of cancer survivorship care have been used as the backbone for subsequent discussions and are the overarching goals of management of the cancer survivor.

1. Prevention and detection of new cancers and recurrent cancer
2. Surveillance for cancer spread and secondary cancers
3. Intervention for the consequences of cancer and its treatment
4. Coordination between specialists and primary care providers to ensure health needs are met

The etiologies of secondary malignancies or recurrence in cancer survivors have many factors, including lifestyle, environment, hereditary risks, and late effects from treatment (Wood et al., 2012). The risk of subsequent primary cancers is increased in both incidence and mortality in cancers associated with smoking or higher body weight (Sung et al., 2020). It is important to identify those at higher risk and address health behaviors that are modifiable, including counseling on smoking cessation and alcohol usage, physical activity, nutrition, and sun exposure (NCCN, 2022b).

The timing and patterns of local regional recurrence and metastatic disease are disease-site specific, and surveillance is very individualized. The NCCN has created disease-specific guidelines that are useful for the primary care provider to help navigate the care of the cancer survivor (Morgan & Denlinger, 2014). In addition, prevention of new cancers, including age-appropriate cancer screening, should be considered (Smith et al., 2014).

The consequences of cancer and its treatment affect every individual and their family differently and can affect all aspects of their lives, including physical, psychosocial, financial, and employment aspects, as well as interpersonal relationships. The late effects of treatment can be long-lived and contribute to chronic physical and psychosocial changes such as fatigue, pain, anxiety, depression, and fear of recurrence. Assessments of these areas are essential and affect the quality of life of cancer survivors. Cancer survivorship requires a multidisciplinary team of specialists who, along with the primary care provider, can help navigate the transition from patient to survivor. A physical exam should be completed at every visit, and sites of previous cancers should be assessed (Wood et al., 2012).

The ASCO and the American College of Surgeons Commission on Cancer Program Standard for 2020 recommend treatment summaries and survivorship care plans for all cancer survivors (McCabe et al., 2013; American College of Surgeons Commission on Cancer, 2019). The survivorship care plan is designed to enhance communication between the oncology team and the primary care provider, in addition to patient–provider communication. It should consist of two components: the treatment summary and follow-up plan. Together, these two components help to facilitate continuity of care and promote high-quality survivorship care.

The treatment summary should consist of the specific diagnosis; stage at diagnosis, including histology; specific treatment modalities; ongoing toxicities of all treatments; and genetic or hereditary risk factors. The specific treatment modalities include surgical procedures; individually listed cancer therapies with names and dates of treatment; and radiotherapy, including anatomic location and end date (Mayer et al., 2014).

The follow-up plan should consist of oncology team members, including supportive care team members such as nutrition and physical therapy; contact information; ongoing need for adjuvant therapy, along with planned duration; schedule for follow-up visits; recommended surveillance tests for recurrence; cancer screening for new cancers; other periodic testing needed as applicable; symptoms of concern for recurrence; a list of clinically significant late or long-term effects of treatment; a general statement emphasizing modifiable risk factors; and a list of resources to address ongoing psychosocial, financial, employment, or parenting issues (Mayer et al., 2014).

V. Plan

A. *Diagnostic tests*

Diagnostic testing is based on the specific cancer history, symptoms at presentation, and subjective and objective findings. These diagnostic tests can include laboratory tests, including tumor markers, and/or imaging studies including computed tomography (CT) scan, bone scan, or positron emission tomography (PET) scan. The NCCN and ASCO guidelines outline specific follow-up recommendations based on cancer diagnosis, stage at presentation, and risk. These guidelines are widely available and useful when managing cancer survivors (NCCN 2022b; ASCO survivorship guidelines can be retrieved from http://www.asco.org/guidelines/survivorship).

There is also an indication for ongoing cancer screening and preventative imaging studies for cancer survivors. These include screening for breast, prostate, cervical, colorectal, and lung cancer (Ganz & Casillas, 2020; Smith et al., 2014).

B. *Patient education*

It is important for survivors to be educated that recovery takes time. They need to understand that their journey is not completed with the end of acute treatment but continues throughout their lifespan. Cancer survivors should be provided information about their individual care plan, symptoms to watch for, and lifestyle modifications that can aid in managing long-term effects and reduce risks.

1. Lifestyle interventions

    Cancer survivors often request information and advice from providers about what they can do to improve their quality of life and increase survival following cancer treatment. Healthcare providers have a marked opportunity to counsel and advise cancer survivors on lifestyle modifications that can decrease their risk of recurrence, manage cancer treatment effects, and improve quality of life. The lifestyle modifications that have been shown to make the greatest impact are physical activity, weight management, nutrition, and smoking cessation (Pekmezi & Demark-Wahnefried, 2011; Sung et al., 2020).

    There is no consensus on the optimal type of physical activity for cancer survivors. However, there is strong evidence that combined aerobic and resistance training may improve cancer-related health outcomes, including improved physical function, decreased pain, decreased anxiety and depression, improved cognitive function, and decreased cancer-related fatigue (Campbell et al., 2019). The current physical activity recommendations from both the ACS and NCCN are that cancer survivors should engage in regular physical exercise, with the goal of 150–300 minutes of moderate aerobic activity or 75 minutes of vigorous aerobic activity per week. Loss of muscle mass during cancer therapy was independently associated with decreased survival (Blauwhoff-Buskermolen et al., 2016). Therefore, in addition to aerobic activity, the ACS and NCCN recommend two to three sessions per week of resistance or strength training. Exercise programs should be tailored to individual needs (NCCN, 2022b; Rock et al., 2012).

    Nutrition and dietary choices have also been shown to play a role in cancer recurrence risk, improved quality of life after cancer treatment, and overall survival (Pekmezi & Demark-Wahnefried, 2011). Although more data are needed to further investigate the role nutrition and weight management play in cancer survivorship, the current recommendations follow those for the general population. There has been an increased risk of mortality associated with cancer survivors who eat a primarily Western type of diet (Schwedhelm et al., 2016). It is recommended that cancer survivors maintain a healthy weight, with a body mass index (BMI) of <25, and consume a plant-based diet high in vegetables, fruits, and whole grains (Kushi et al., 2012; Rock et al., 2012).

C. *Consultations and referrals*

The care of the adult cancer survivor is complex. Each survivor has their own specific cancer story and follow-up recommendations. It is imperative to consult with the oncology team for any questions or concerns regarding surveillance and possible recurrence. The open line of communication will ensure high-quality care.

In addition, the mental, psychosocial, and financial health of the cancer survivor should not be overlooked. Referrals to psycho-oncology, psychology, psychiatry, and social work should be used to address those needs.

VI. **Self-management resources**
A. *Educational resources*
American Cancer Society—information regarding tips on staying healthy and active during and after cancer treatments.
http://www.cancer.org/treatment/survivorshipduringandaftertreatment/index
National Coalition for Cancer Survivorship—survivorship checklist
https://canceradvocacy.org/resourcessurvivorship-checklist/#checklist-form
Journey Forward—health topics related to cancer survivorship
https://www.journeyforward.org/category/information/
Cancer.Net—survivorship information for both survivors and their family members and friends; available in English and Spanish
https://www.cancer.net/survivorship
Centers for Disease Control and Prevention—information on staying healthy after cancer treatment and survivorship care plans in Spanish and English
https://www.cdc.gov/cancer/survivors/index.htm
Livestrong—both direct services and community programs for living after cancer treatment brochures; available in multiple languages/cultures/lesbian, gay, bisexual, transgender, queer or questioning (LGBTQ+)
http://www.livestrong.org/we-can-help/healthy-living-after-treatment
National Cancer Institute—offers PDF/Kindle/ePub publication *Facing Forward: Life After Cancer Treatment*
https://www.cancer.gov/publications/patient-education/facing-forward
Memorial Sloan Kettering Cancer Center Integrative Medicine—a database for the public and healthcare professionals to determine the value of herbs and dietary supplements
https://www.mskcc.org/cancer-care/diagnosis-treatment/symptom-management/integrative-medicine/herbs

B. *Community support groups*
 1. The ACS provides a resource link where survivors can look up local support groups based on location: http://www.cancer.org/treatment/supportprogramsservices/app/resource-search
 2. Cancer Care is a national organization that provides free, professional support services and information to help survivors manage the emotional, practical, and financial challenges of cancer. The organization provides online, telephone, and face-to-face support groups: http://www.cancercare.org/support_group

References

American Cancer Society. (2019). *Cancer facts & figures for African Americans 2019–2021.*

American Cancer Society. (2022). *Cancer facts & figures 2022.*

American College of Surgeons Commission on Cancer. (2019). *National Cancer Database, 2016 data submission.*

Arastu, A., Patel, A., Mohile, S. G., Ciminelli, J., Kaushik, R., Wells, M., Culakova, E., Lei, L., Xu, H., Dougherty, D. W., Mohamed, M. R., Hill, E., Duberstein, P., Flannery, M. A., Kamen, C. S., Pandya, C., Berenberg, J. L., Aarne Grossman, V. G., Liu, Y., & Loh, K. P. (2020). Assessment of financial toxicity among older adults with advanced cancer. *Journal of the American Medical Association Network Open, 3*(12), e2025810. https://doi.org/10.1001/jamanetworkopen.2020.25810

Blauwhoff-Buskermolen, S., Versteeg, K. S., de van der Schueren, M. A., den Braver, N. R., Berkhof, J., Langius, J. A., & Verheul, H. M. (2016). Loss of muscle mass during chemotherapy is predictive for poor survival of patients with metastatic colorectal cancer. *Journal of Clinical Oncology, 34*(12), 1339–1344. https://doi.org/10.1200/JCO.2015.63.6043

Campbell, K. L., Winters-Stone, K. M., Wiskemann, J., May, A. M., Schwartz, A. L., Courneya, K. S., Zucker, D. S., Matthews, C. E., Ligibel, J. A., Gerber, L. H., Morris, G. S., Patel, A. V., Hue, T. F., Perna, F. M., & Schmitz, K. H. (2019). Exercise guidelines for cancer survivors: Consensus statement from international multidisciplinary roundtable. *Medicine & Science in Sports & Exercise, 51*(11), 2375–2390. https://doi.org/10.1249/MSS.0000000000002116

Carrera, P. M., & Kantarjian, H. M. (2018). Blinder VS. The financial burden and distress of patients with cancer: Understanding and stepping-up action on the financial toxicity of cancer treatment. *CA: A Cancer Journal for Clinicians, 68*(2), 153–165. https://doi.org/10.3322/caac.21443

Chandak, A. N., Loberiza, F. R., Deras, M., Armitage, J. O., Vose, J. M., & Stimpson, J. P. (2014). Estimating the state-level supply of cancer care providers: Preparing to meet workforce needs in the wake of health care reform. *Journal of Oncology Practice, 11*(1), 32–37. https://doi.org/10.1200/JOP.2014.001565

Edwards, B. K., Noone, A. M., Mariotto, A. B., Simard, E. P., Boscoe, F. P., Henley, S. J., Jemal, A., Cho, H., Anderson, R. N., Kohler, B. A., Eheman, C. R., & Ward, E. M. (2014). Annual report to the nation on the status of cancer, 1975–2010, featuring prevalence of comorbidity and impact on survival among persons with lung, colorectal, breast, or prostate cancer. *Cancer, 120*(9), 1290–1314. https://doi.org/10.1002/cncr.28509

Ganz, P. A., & Casillas, J. N. (2020). Incorporating the risk for subsequent primary cancers into the care of adult cancer survivors: Moving beyond 5-year survival. *Journal of the American Medical Association, 324*(24), 2493–2495. https://doi.org/10.1001/jama.2020.23410.

Gilbert, S. M., Miller, D. C., Hollenbeck, B. K., Montie, J. E., & Wei, J. T. (2008). Cancer survivorship: Challenges and changing paradigms. *Journal of Urology, 179*(2), 431–438. https://doi.org/10.1016/j.juro.2007.09.029

Gordon, L. G., Merollini, K. M. D., Lowe, A., & Chan, R. J. (2017). A systematic review of financial toxicity among cancer survivors: We can't pay the co-pay. *Patient, 10*(3), 295–309. https://doi.org/10.1007/s40271-016-0204-x

Hewitt, M., Greenfield, S., & Stoval, E. (Eds.). (2005). *From cancer patient to cancer survivor: Lost in transition* (T. N. A. Press ed.). National Academies Press.

Hewitt, M. E., Bamundo, A., Day, R., & Harvey, C. (2007). Perspectives on post-treatment cancer care: Qualitative research with survivors, nurses, and physicians. *Journal of Clinical Oncology, 25*(16), 2270–2273. https://doi.org/10.1200/jco.2006.10.0826

Howlader, N., Noone, A. M., Krapcho, M., Miller, D., Brest, A., Yu, M., Ruhl, J., Tatalovich, Z., Mariotto, A., Lewis, D. R., Chen, H. S., Feuer, E. J., & Cronin, K. A. (Eds.). (2018). *SEER cancer statistics review, 1975–2018*. National Cancer Institute. https://seer.cancer.gov/csr/1975_2018/

Keesing, S., McNamara, B., & Rosenwax, L. (2015). Cancer survivors' experiences of using survivorship care plans: A systematic review of qualitative studies. *Journal of Cancer Survivorship, 9*(2), 260–268. https://doi.org/10.1007/s11764-014-0407-x

Kushi, L. H., Doyle, C., McCullough, M., Rock, C. L., Demark-Wahnefried, W., Bandera, E. V., Gapstur, S., Patel, A. V., Andrews, K., & Gansler, T. (2012). American Cancer Society guidelines on nutrition and physical activity for cancer prevention: Reducing the risk of cancer with healthy food choices and physical activity. *CA: A Cancer Journal for Clinicians, 62*(1), 30–67. https://doi.org/10.3322/caac.20140

Mayer, D. K., Nekhlyudov, L., Snyder, C. F., Merrill, J. K., Wollins, D. S., & Shulman, L. N. (2014). American Society of Clinical Oncology clinical expert statement on cancer survivorship care planning. *Journal of Oncology Practice, 10*(6), 345–351. https://doi.org/10.1200/jop.2014.001321

McCabe, M. S., Bhatia, S., Oeffinger, K. C., Reaman, G. H., Tyne, C., Wollins, D. S., & Hudson, M. M. (2013). American Society of Clinical Oncology statement: Achieving high-quality cancer survivorship care. *Journal of Clinical Oncology, 31*(5), 631–640. https://doi.org/10.1200/jco.2012.46.6854

Morgan, M. A., & Denlinger, C. S. (2014). Survivorship: Tools for transitioning patients with cancer. *Journal of the National Comprehensive Cancer Network, 12*(12), 1681–1687. https://doi.org/10.6004/jnccn.2014.0170

Mullan, F. (1985). Seasons of survival-reflections of a physician with cancer. *New England Journal of Medicine, 313*(4), 270–273. https://doi.org/10.1056/nejm198507253130421

National Comprehensive Cancer Network. (2022a). *NCCN: Cancer and COVID-19 Vaccination* (v.6.0 4/27/2022). https://www.nccn.org/docs/default-source/covid-19/2021_covid-19_vaccination_guidance_v5-0.pdf?sfvrsn=b483da2b_114

National Comprehensive Cancer Network. (2022b). *NCCN clinical practice guidelines in oncology™: Survivorship* (v.1.2022). http://www.nccn.org/professionals/physician_gls/f_guidelines.asp#survivorship

Nekhlyudov, L., O'Malley, D. M., & Hudson, S. V. (2017). Integrating primary care providers in the care of cancer survivors: gaps in evidence and future opportunities. *Lancet Oncology, 18*(1), e30–e38. https://doi.org/10.1016/S1470-2045(16)30570-8

Office of Disease Prevention and Health Promotion. (n.d.). Social determinants of health. *Healthy People 2030*. U.S. Department of Health and Human Services. https://health.gov/healthypeople/objectives-and-data/social-determinants-health

Pekmezi, D. W., & Demark-Wahnefried, W. (2011). Updated evidence in support of diet and exercise interventions in cancer survivors. *Acta Oncologica, 50*(2), 167–178. https://doi.org/10.3109/0284186X.2010.529822

Pisu, M., Kenzik, K. M., Oster, R. A., Drentea, P., Ashing, K. T., Fouad, M., & Martin, M. Y. (2015). Economic hardship of minority and non-minority cancer survivors 1 year after diagnosis: Another long-term effect of cancer? *Cancer, 121*(8), 1257–1264. https://doi.org/10.1002/cncr.29206

Rock, C. L., Doyle, C., Demark-Wahnefried, W., Meyerhardt, J., Courneya, K. S., Schwartz, A. L., Bandera, E. V., Hamilton, K. K., Grant, B., McCullough, M., Byers, T., & Gansler, T. (2012). Nutrition and physical activity: Guidelines for cancer survivors. *CA: A Cancer Journal for Clinicians, 62*(4), 243–274. https://doi.org/10.3322/caac.21142

Rowland, J. H., Hewitt, M., & Ganz, P. A. (2006). Cancer survivorship: A new challenge in delivering quality cancer care. *Journal of Clinical Oncology, 24*(32), 5101–5104. https://doi.org/10.1200/jco.2006.09.2700

Schwedhelm, C., Boeing, H., Hoffmann, G., Aleksandrova, K., & Schwingshackl, L. (2016). Effect of diet on mortality and cancer recurrence among cancer survivors: A systematic review and meta-analysis of cohort studies. *Nutrition Reviews, 74*(12), 737–748. https://doi.org/10.1093/nutrit/nuw045

Siegel, R. L., Miller, K. D., Fuchs, H. E., & Jemal, A. (2022). Cancer statistics, 2022. *CA: A Cancer Journal for Clinicians, 72*(1), 7–33. https://doi.org/10.3322/caac.21708

Smith, R. A., Manassaram-Baptiste, D., Brooks, D., Cokkinides, V., Doroshenk, M., Saslow, D., & Brawley, O. W. (2014). Cancer screening in the United States, 2014: A review of current American Cancer Society guidelines and current issues in cancer screening. *CA: A Cancer Journal for Clinicians, 64*(1), 31–51. https://doi.org/10.3322/caac.21212

Sung, H., Hyun, N., Leach, C. R., Yabroff, K. R., & Jemal, A. (2020). Association of first primary cancer with risk of subsequent primary cancer among survivors of adult-onset cancers in the United States. *Journal of the American Medical Association, 324*(24), 2521–2535. https://doi.org/10.1001/jama.2020.23130.

Wood, M. E., Vogel, V., Ng, A., Foxhall, L., Goodwin, P., & Travis, L. B. (2012). Second malignant neoplasms: Assessment and strategies for risk reduction. *Journal of Clinical Oncology, 30*(30), 3734–3745. https://doi.org/10.1200/jco.2012.41.8681

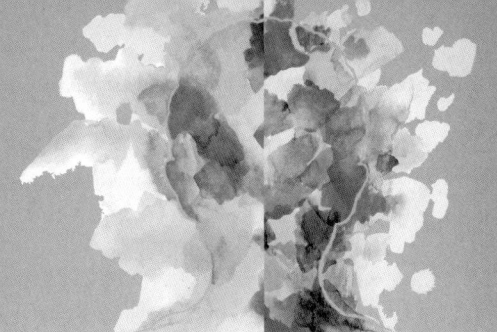

CHAPTER 45

Chronic Obstructive Pulmonary Disease

Emily Casabar

I. Introduction and background

Chronic obstructive pulmonary disease (COPD) is a chronic respiratory disorder involving both airway and lung parenchyma pathology that results in chronic airflow limitation. The Global Initiative for Chronic Obstructive Lung Disease (GOLD), a project of the National Heart, Lung, and Blood Institute (NHLBI) and the World Health Organization (WHO), organized pulmonary experts and multidisciplinary health professionals to bring awareness of the burden of COPD and develop guidelines for its early detection, prevention, and management (Rodriguez-Roisin, 2020).

A. Definition

Prior definitions of COPD included the terms *emphysema* and *chronic bronchitis* and related to smoking tobacco, which failed to identify early stages of the disorder and defined it as a single disease, limiting the role of the different causes of COPD (Celli et al., 2022). The new definition was updated in the 2023 GOLD report, which states that COPD is "a heterogeneous lung condition characterized by chronic respiratory symptoms (dyspnea, cough, sputum production and/or exacerbations) due to abnormalities of the airways (bronchitis, bronchiolitis) and/or alveoli (emphysema) that cause persistent, often progressive, airflow obstruction" (p. 15).

B. Pathophysiology

1. Inflammatory changes

   The pathological changes of COPD variably occur in four different areas of the lungs: central airways, peripheral airways, lung parenchyma, and pulmonary vasculature; the predominant changes occur in the small airways, which become narrow and reduce in number, leading to airway collapse (European Respiratory Society & American Thoracic Society [ERS/ATS], 2004). Inflammatory and structural changes increase the severity of airflow obstruction and can persist after smoking cessation. Both COPD and asthma are associated with chronic inflammation of the respiratory tract; however, there are differences in the inflammatory cells and mediators in the two diseases. COPD is characterized by an increased number of macrophages in peripheral airways, lung parenchyma, and pulmonary vessels, together with increased activated neutrophils and lymphocytes, whereas asthma is associated with inflammation due to eosinophils and group 2 innate lymphoid cells (ILC2), which are a subtype of lymphoid cells (GOLD, 2023).

2. Structural changes

   Chronic inflammation causes structural changes, including narrowing of small airways; exudates in the small airways; and the destruction of lung parenchyma, contributing to gas trapping and lung hyperinflation. Structural changes in the alveoli, airways, and pulmonary circulation alter the normal ventilation–perfusion distributions and can result in different degrees of arterial hypoxemia and hypercapnia in the patient with COPD (GOLD, 2023). Pulmonary vasculature changes, which may precede emphysema, are multifactorial and can be attributed to one or more of the following: pulmonary artery remodeling via tobacco smoke, endothelial dysfunction, structural and functional lung anomalies, inflammation, and genetic predisposition. The sequelae of these changes include pulmonary hypertension (PH), which is thought to be due to increased vascular resistance and left ventricular filling pressures or elevated intrathoracic pressure due to air trapping in the lungs (Kovacs et al., 2018).

C. *Epidemiology*

COPD is a leading cause of morbidity and mortality worldwide, with disease prevalence and burden projected to increase over the coming decades (GOLD, 2023). In 2018, approximately 15.7 million Americans reported a diagnosis of COPD, making it the fourth-leading cause of death that year (Centers for Disease Control and Prevention [CDC], 2021a). Morbidity due to COPD increases with age and in those with comorbidities at an earlier age. Currently annual deaths globally are estimated at 3 million, which is projected to increase to over 5.4 million by 2060, especially in high-income countries that have increased prevalence of smoking and aging populations (GOLD, 2023).

D. *Risk factors*

COPD results from lifetime cumulative and dynamic genetic and environmental interactions that can damage the lungs or alter the normal developmental or aging process (GOLD, 2023). Cigarette smoking is a key environmental risk factor for COPD. Those who smoke cigarettes have a higher prevalence of respiratory symptoms and lung function abnormalities compared to those who do not smoke. Other types of tobacco and marijuana smoking are also risk factors for developing COPD. Nonsmoking risk factors for COPD include the following (GOLD, 2023):
  a. Biomass exposure, including wood, animal dung, crop residues, and coal
  b. Occupational exposures, including organic and inorganic dusts and chemical agents and fumes
  c. Air pollution
  d. Genetic factors, including hereditary alpha-1 antitrypsin deficiency
  e. Lung growth and development: reduced peak lung function in early adulthood and/or accelerated lung function decline later in life
  f. Asthma and airway hyperreactivity
  g. Chronic bronchitis
  h. Respiratory infections, including history of severe childhood respiratory infections, chronic bronchial infection, and tuberculosis
  i. Passive smoke exposure
  j. Poverty and lower socioeconomic status
  k. Sex-based differences in immune pathways, although more research is needed in this area

E. *Taxonomy*

Traditionally, COPD was classified as a single disease caused by tobacco smoking. GOLD (2023) expanded the classification of COPD to include non–smoking-related COPD types, highlighting the need to explore current and future therapies related to the other etiologies. The proposed taxonomy for COPD is as follows:
- Genetically determined COPD (COPD-G)
- COPD due to abnormal lung development (COPD-D)
- Environmental COPD: cigarette smoking COPD (COPD-C) and biomass and pollution exposure COPD (COPD-P)
- COPD due to infections (COPD-I)
- COPD and asthma (COPD-A)
- COPD of unknown cause (COPD-U)

II. **Confirming COPD diagnosis**

A. *Subjective*
  1. History: The Diagnosis of COPD should be considered in any patient who reports symptoms of cough, sputum production, or dyspnea, particularly if the patient's exposure history reveals risk factors for the disease. The comprehensive medical history should include the following (GOLD, 2023):
     a. Patient's exposure to risk factors, including smoking and environmental exposures
     b. Past medical history, including early life events, asthma, allergy, sinusitis or nasal polyps, respiratory infections in childhood, HIV, and tuberculosis
     c. Family history of lung disease, including COPD
     d. Pattern of symptom development
     e. History of exacerbation and/or previous hospitalization for respiratory disorder
     f. Presence of comorbidities
     g. Impact of disease on the patient's life
     h. Social and family support available to patient
     i. Possibilities for reducing risk factors, especially smoking cessation
  2. Symptoms: The common symptoms of COPD are chronic cough with or without sputum and chronic dyspnea. Other symptoms may include wheezing, chest tightness, and fatigue. Weight loss and anorexia can indicate severe disease.

  Cough can be the first symptom of COPD and is often thought of as a consequence of smoking or other environmental exposure by patients. Chronic cough in patients with COPD can initially present as intermittent and be productive or nonproductive. In some patients with significant airflow limitation, cough may be absent. Sputum production is common in the patient with COPD and may occur with intermittent periods of flares and remissions. Chronic bronchitis is defined as regular sputum production for 3 or more months in 2 consecutive years in the absence of any other known etiology (GOLD, 2023).

  Dyspnea, especially during exertion or physical activity, is a cardinal symptom of COPD and is present across all stages of airflow obstruction. Patients with COPD may describe dyspnea as an increased effort to breathe, chest heaviness, air hunger, and/or gasping. Various dyspnea scales, including the Modified Medical Research Council (MMRC) scale and the COPD Assessment Test (CAT), are used to evaluate the patient's activity limitation due to dyspnea symptoms (**Figure 45-1** and **Figure 45-2**). The MMRC is integrated into the GOLD clinical classification scheme because patients with high dyspnea scores are associated with higher healthcare

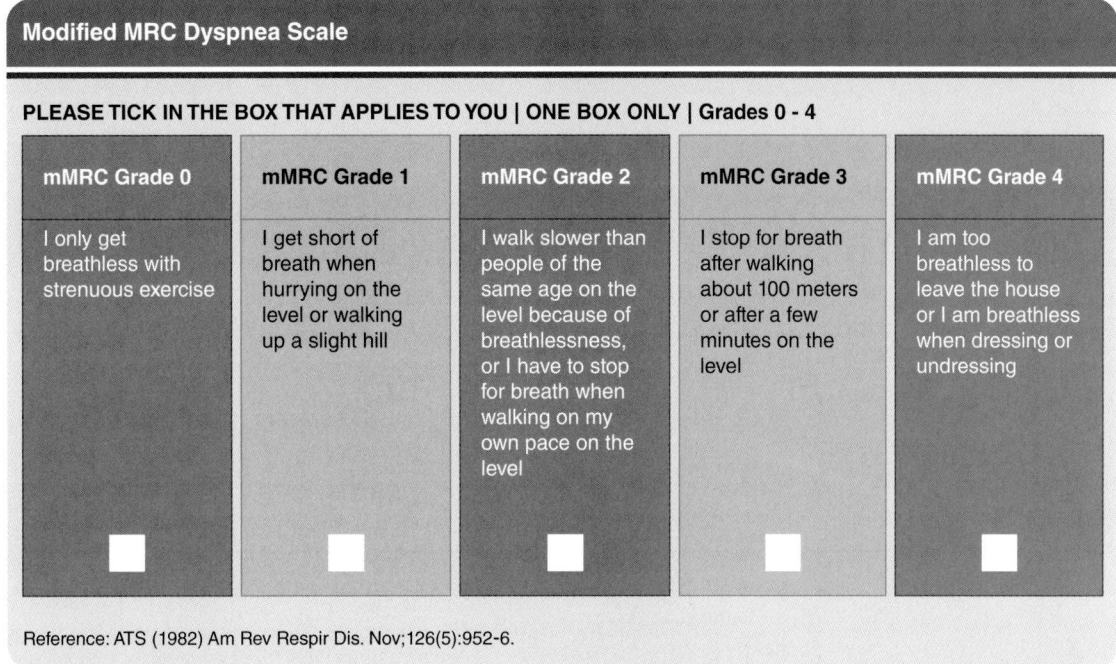

Figure 45-1 Modified Medical Research Council (MMRC) dyspnea scale.

Reproduced from "Global strategy for the diagnosis, management, and prevention of chronic obstructive pulmonary disease, 2022 report," by Global Initiative for Chronic Lung Disease, 2022, p. 30 (https://goldcopd.org/2022-gold-reports-2/). The mMRC is open access.

resource utilization and costs (GOLD, 2023). The CAT expands the patient's subjective assessment of impairment by including other factors in the score. The results of these scales contribute to creating a therapeutic plan for the patient with COPD.

B. *Objective*
1. Physical exam: The absence of physical signs does not exclude the diagnosis of COPD because a normal physical exam can be a common finding in early COPD (ERS/ATS, 2004). Physical signs of airflow limitation are usually not present until lung function is significantly impaired. Various physical exam findings in patients with COPD can include lung hyperinflation and cyanosis, but their absence does not exclude the diagnosis (GOLD, 2023).
2. Spirometry. Spirometry is the most reproducible objective measurement of airflow limitation and is cheap and readily available. It is a pulmonary function test that measures the presence and severity of airflow obstruction with reference values based on age, height, sex, and race, and it is helpful in discerning whether the symptoms are related to a respiratory disease or other conditions. Spirometry should be performed in adults who report symptoms concerning for COPD or other risk factors for COPD, including >20 pack-year smoking history, recurrent chest infections, and early life events. Results can be used to determine the presence and severity of airflow obstruction for prognostic value and can be used in follow-up assessments when choosing therapies and monitoring for disease progression. The most valuable spirometric measurements include the following (GOLD, 2023) (**Figure 45-3**):
   - Forced vital capacity (FVC): the volume of air forcibly exhaled from the point of maximal inspiration
   - Forced expiratory volume in 1 second (FEV_1): the volume of air exhaled during the first second of the FVC
   - The ratio of the two measurements (FEV_1/FVC): confirms the presence of non–fully reversible airflow obstruction.
3. The spirometric criteria for airflow obstruction is a post-bronchodilator ratio of $FEV_1/FVC < 0.7$ (GOLD, 2023). Further classification of post-bronchodilator FEV_1 is used to assess the severity of airflow limitation in COPD. Spirometry should be augmented with formal symptomatic assessment using the MMRC questionnaire described in the previous section.
4. Measuring lung volumes by body plethysmography or helium dilution can be useful in characterizing the severity of COPD. Gas trapping increases residual volume (RV) and is exhibited in the early stages of COPD; as airflow limitation worsens, static hyperinflation is demonstrated by increased total lung capacity (TLC) (GOLD, 2023).

Additionally, interpreting the diffusion capacity (DLCO) is a useful clinical tool to evaluate gas

COPD Assessment Test

Your name: _____

Today's date: _____

How is your COPD? Take the COPD Assessment Test™ (CAT)

This questionnaire will help you and your healthcare professional measure the impact COPD (Chronic Obstructive Pulmonary Disease) is having on your wellbeing and daily life. Your answers, and test score, can be used by you and your healthcare professional to help improve the management of your COPD and get the greatest benefit from treatment.

For each item below, place a mark (X) in the box that best describes you currently. Be sure to only select one response for each question.

Example: I am very happy [0] [X=1] [2] [3] [4] [5] I am very sad

Statement (Low)	Score (0–5)	Statement (High)	SCORE
I never cough	0 1 2 3 4 5	I cough all the time	☐
I have no phlegm (mucus) in my chest at all	0 1 2 3 4 5	My chest is completely full of phlegm (mucus)	☐
My chest does not feel tight at all	0 1 2 3 4 5	My chest feels very tight	☐
When I walk up a hill or one flight of stairs I am not breathless	0 1 2 3 4 5	When I walk up a hill or one flight of stairs I am very breathless	☐
I am not limited doing any activities at home	0 1 2 3 4 5	I am very limited doing activities at home	☐
I am confident leaving my home despite my lung condition	0 1 2 3 4 5	I am not at all confident leaving my home because of my lung condition	☐
I sleep soundly	0 1 2 3 4 5	I don't sleep soundly because of my lung condition	☐
I have lots of energy	0 1 2 3 4 5	I have no energy at all	☐

TOTAL SCORE ☐☐

COPD Assessment Test and the CAT logo are trademarks of the GlaxoSmithKline group of companies.
©2009 GlaxoSmithKline. All rights reserved.

Note. From "Development and first validation of the COPD assessment test," by P.W. Jones et al., 2009, *European Respiratory Journal* 34(3).

Figure 45-2 COPD Assessment Test™ (CAT).

Reproduced from "Development and first validation of the COPD assessment test," by P.W. Jones et al., 2009, European Respiratory Journal 34(3). (https://erj.ersjournals.com/content/erj/34/3/648.full.pdf). Copyright 2009 by GlaxoSmithKline group of companies. Adapted with permission.

GOLD Grades and Severity of Airflow Obstruction in COPD (based on post-bronchodilator FEV1)

In COPD patients (FEV1/FVC < 0.7):

GOLD 1:	Mild	FEV1 ≥ 80% predicted
GOLD 2:	Moderate	50% ≤ FEV1 < 80% predicted
GOLD 3:	Severe	30% ≤ FEV1 < 50% predicted
GOLD 4:	Very Severe	FEV1 < 30% predicted

Figure 45-3 GOLD grades and severity of airflow obstruction in chronic obstructive pulmonary disease (COPD).

Reproduced from Global strategy for the diagnosis, management, and prevention of chronic obstructive pulmonary disease, 2022 report, by Global Initiative for Chronic Lung Disease, 2022, p. 29 (https://goldcopd.org/2022-gold-reports-2/). Copyright 2021 by Global Initiative for Chronic Lung Disease, Inc. Adapted with permission.

transfer within the respiratory system. DLCO should be performed when the patient's dyspnea symptoms are disproportionate to the degree of airflow obstruction. In patients with COPD, decreased DLCO of less than 60% of predicted is associated with decreased exercise capacity, increased symptoms, worse health status, and increased risk of death (GOLD, 2023).

5. Oximetry and arterial blood gas. Pulse oximetry or oxygen saturation (SpO_2) is a useful and noninvasive tool to evaluate a patient's arterial oxygen saturation and assess the need for supplemental oxygen therapy (GOLD, 2023). It should be used to assess all patients with clinical signs of respiratory failure or right heart failure. If the SpO_2 is less than 92%, the arterial partial pressure of oxygen (PaO_2) should be assessed via an arterial blood gas measurement. The ATS definition of severe hypoxemia is SpO_2 ≤ 88% or PaO_2 ≤ 55 mm Hg, assessed by arterial blood gas; moderate hypoxemia is defined as SpO_2 of 89%–93% or PaO_2 of 56–60 mm Hg (ATS, 2020a). Arterial blood gas can also be used to evaluate for chronic hypercapnia, which is defined as a resting partial pressure of carbon dioxide ($PaCO_2$) of >45 mm Hg outside of an exacerbation episode (ATS, 2020b).

6. Exercise testing: The 6-minute walk test (6MWT) is a self-paced test of walking capacity in which patients are asked to walk as far as possible along a flat surface in 6 minutes (ERS/ATS, 2014). The distance walked is recorded in meters or feet while the patient's heart rate and SpO_2 are measured continuously. Subjective measurements include the patient's report of dyspnea and fatigue. Objectively measured exercise impairment is a powerful indicator of health status and prognostic tool (GOLD, 2023).

7. Laboratory. There are no specific laboratory tests to diagnose COPD. However, various laboratory values may help in the initial evaluation of the patient with dyspnea (ATS, 2012):
   a. Complete blood count to rule out anemia
   b. D-dimer to rapidly identify patients with a low probability of pulmonary embolism
   c. B-type natriuretic peptide (BNP) and N-terminal pro-BNP (NT-pro-BNP) to determine the possibility of heart failure, especially in the setting of acute dyspnea

   Alpha-1 antitrypsin deficiency (AATD) screening is recommended for all patients with a diagnosis of COPD, especially in areas with high AATD prevalence (GOLD, 2023). Low concentration, less than 20% of normal, is suggestive of homozygous deficiency, in which case the patient should be referred to specialist centers for advice and management and also be screened with family members (GOLD, 2023).

8. Chest imaging. Chest radiography is not a useful tool in the diagnosis of COPD but can rule out alternative diagnoses and assess for comorbidities, including respiratory (pulmonary fibrosis, bronchiectasis, and diseases of the pleura), skeletal (kyphoscoliosis), and cardiac illnesses (cardiomegaly or enlarged pulmonary artery diameter). Chest radiography signs associated with COPD include lung hyperlucency (an excess of air in the parenchyma or a decrease in mass of the parenchyma often associated with emphysema), lung hyperinflation (flattened diaphragm with retrosternal air space volume increase), and rapid tapering of the vascular markings (GOLD, 2023). Computed tomography (CT) should be considered for patients with COPD

who have persistent exacerbations, symptoms out of proportion to disease severity based on lung function testing, FEV_1 of less than 45% of predicted with significant hyperinflation and gas trapping, or for patients who meet the criteria for lung cancer screening (GOLD, 2023).

C. *Exacerbation and risk stratification*
1. Combined initial COPD assessment: In 2011, for the purpose of guiding initial pharmacological treatment, GOLD proposed to move from the simple spirometric grading system for disease severity assessment to a combined assessment strategy based on the level of symptoms, the severity of airflow limitation (FEV_1), and frequency of exacerbations. The result of this combined assessment created the four categories of A, B, C, and D. The 2023 GOLD report proposes a further evolution of the combined assessment tool that recognizes the clinical relevance of exacerbations independently of the level of symptoms of the patient. This change merges the prior C and D groups into a single group, E, to highlight the clinical relevance of exacerbations (GOLD, 2023). Groups A and B remain unchanged (**Figure 45-4**).
2. The BODE index: The BODE index, calculated from **b**ody mass index, degree of airflow **o**bstruction (FEV_1), level of **d**yspnea (MMRC scale), and **e**xercise capacity (6MWT), is another validated grading system that is simple to calculate and requires no special equipment (**Table 45-1**). The 4-year survival calculated from this combination of indices is a better predictor of survival from any cause, and *a composite score is a better predictor of subsequent survival than any single component,* such as FEV_1 alone. During prospective validation studies, lower scores were seen among survivors compared with those who died from any cause and in the cohort of those with a respiratory cause of death (Celli et al., 2004). In COPD, the BODE index can be used to assess the impact of exacerbations, interventions, and disease progression, especially in the setting of lung transplant evaluation (Cote et al. 2007).

III. Management

The aim of COPD therapy is to decrease symptoms, decrease exacerbations, and improve exercise tolerance and quality of life. Managing COPD consists of patient education and counseling, pharmacologic therapy, and nonpharmacologic therapy.

A. *General management for all patients*
1. Education and self-management: Patient knowledge is an important step toward behavior change. Personalized education and training that aim to enhance long-term functionality and appropriate health behaviors are likely to provide more benefit. Education topics, including smoking cessation, correct use of inhaler devices, early recognition of

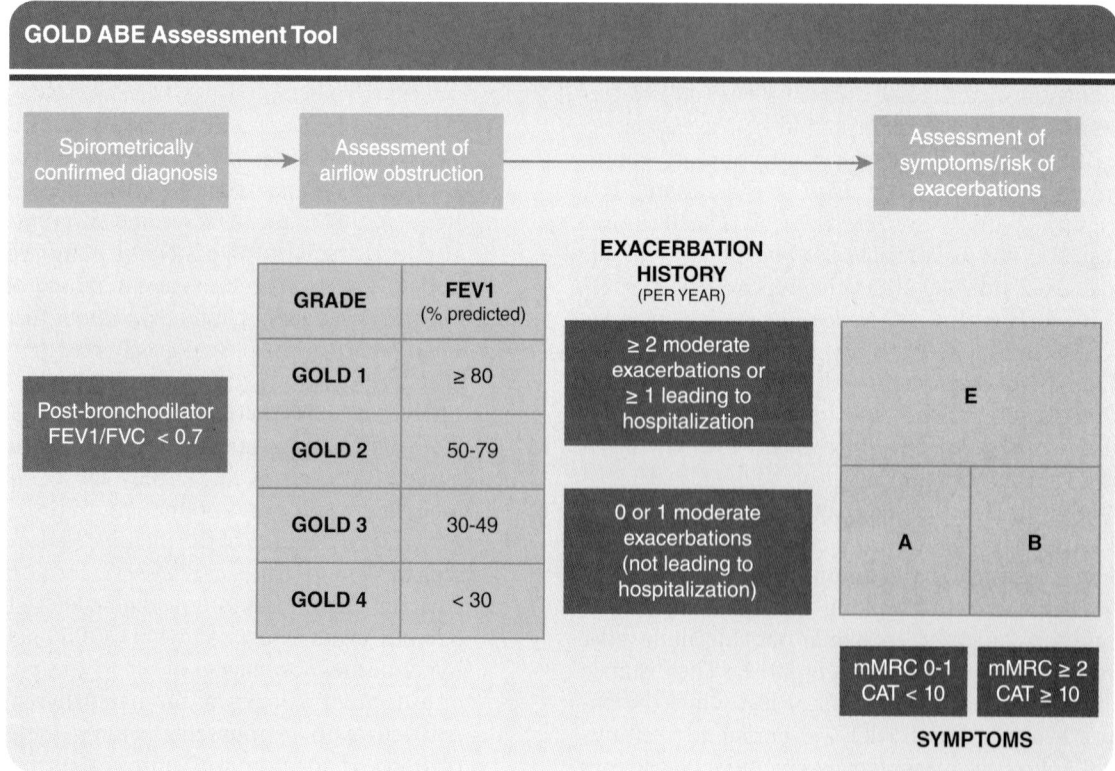

Figure 45-4 GOLD ABE assessment tool.

Reproduced from Global strategy for the diagnosis, management, and prevention of chronic obstructive pulmonary disease, 2022 report, by Global Initiative for Chronic Lung Disease, 2022, p. 33 (https://goldcopd.org/2022-gold-reports-2/). Copyright 2021 by Global Initiative for Chronic Lung Disease, Inc. Adapted with permission.

Table 45-1 Variables and Point Values Used for the Computation of the Body Mass Index, Degree of Airflow Obstruction and Dyspnea, and Exercise Capacity (BODE) Index*

Variable	Points on BODE Index			
	0	1	2	3
FEV$_1$ (% of predicted)[†]	≥65	50–64	36–49	≤35
Distance walked in 6 min (m)	≥350	250–349	150–249	≤149
MMRC dyspnea scale[‡]	0–1	2	3	4
Body mass index[§]	>21	>21		

FEV, forced expiratory volume in 1 second; *MMRC*, Modified Medical Research Council.

* The cutoff values for the assignment of points are shown for each variable. The total possible values range from 0 to 10.
[†] The FEV$_1$ categories are based on stages identified by the American Thoracic Society.
[‡] Scores on the modified MMRC dyspnea scale can range from 0 to 4, with a score of 4 indicating that the patient is too breathless to leave the house or becomes breathless when dressing or undressing.
[§] The values for body mass index were 0 or 1 because of the inflection point in the inverse relation between survival and body mass index at a value of 21.

Reproduced from The Body-Mass Index, airflow obstruction, dyspnea, and exercise capacity index in chronic obstructive pulmonary disease," by B.R. Celli et al., 2004, *The New England Journal of Medicine* 350(10), p. 1007 (https://www.nejm.org/doi/pdf/10.1056/NEJMoa021322?articleTools=true). Copyright 2004 by Massachusetts Medical Society. Adapted with permission.

exacerbation, and consideration of advance directives, can be approached using the self-management intervention model. A COPD self-management intervention is structured and personalized, with the goals of motivating, engaging, and supporting patients to positively adapt their health behaviors through repetitive coaching interactions with the patient (GOLD, 2023). COPD-specific patient education resources are available from various organizations, including the following:
- American Lung Association: https://www.lung.org/copd
- COPD Foundation: https://www.copdfoundation.org
- ATS COPD fact sheet: https://www.thoracic.org/patients/patient-resources/resources/copd-intro.pdf
- National Heart Lung & Blood Institute: https://www.nhlbi.nih.gov/health/copd

2. Risk reduction: Identifying risk factors and discussing their reduction is important when treating and preventing COPD. Smoking is the most common risk factor for COPD, and cessation should be encouraged at every available opportunity. Smoking cessation should be individualized for each patient and can include pharmacological products and behavioral counseling. Avoidance of other risk factors, such as indoor and outdoor pollution and occupational exposures, should also be encouraged.

3. Infection prevention: Lower respiratory tract infections can cause serious illness and death in patients with COPD. The Center for Disease Control and Prevention (CDC) recommends that adults with chronic lung disease, including COPD, receive various vaccines for infection prevention, including the following:

- Pneumococcal vaccine series (CDC, 2019)
- Annual influenza vaccine (CDC, 2021c)
- COVID-19 vaccine (CDC, 2021b)
- Recombinant zoster vaccine to protect against shingles in adults aged 50 years and older with COPD (CDC, 2018)
- Tetanus, diphtheria, and pertussis (Tdap) for those who were not vaccinated in adolescence (CDC, 2020)

B. *Pharmacologic therapy*
Pharmacological therapy for COPD is used to reduce symptoms, reduce frequency and severity of exacerbations, and improve exercise tolerance and health status. Each treatment regimen should be individualized because the relationship between the severity of symptoms, airflow obstruction, and severity of exacerbations can differ between patients. Drug classes commonly used as maintenance medications for COPD include methylxanthines, bronchodilators (beta-agonists and antimuscarinics), inhaled corticosteroids, and combination medication (e.g., triple-combination inhalers) (GOLD, 2023) (**Figure 45-5**). Inhaled therapy is a key component in the management of COPD. Because adherence to therapy can be challenging, prescribing strategies that improve medication adherence include selecting devices with a similar inhalation technique and a single combination inhaler therapy, which is more convenient and effective than multiple inhalers (GOLD, 2023).

1. Methylxanthines: Theophylline is the most used methylxanthine and may have a bronchodilator effect in the patient with COPD, although various studies showed no difference compared with placebo in the number of COPD exacerbations (GOLD, 2023). It is metabolized by the cytochrome P450 enzyme, with clearance of the drug declining with age. Adverse effects include toxicity which, is dose

COMMONLY USED MAINTENANCE MEDICATIONS IN COPD*

Generic Drug Name	Inhaler Type	Nebulizer	Oral	Injection	Duration Of Action
BETA$_2$-AGONISTS					
SHORT-ACTING (SABA)					
Fenoterol	MDI	√	pill, syrup		4-6 hours
Levalbuterol	MDI	√			6-8 hours
Salbutamol (albuterol)	MDI & DPI	√	pill, syrup, extended release tablet	√	4-6 hours 12 hours (ext. release)
Terbutaline	DPI		pill	√	4-6 hours
LONG-ACTING (LABA)					
Arformoterol		√			12 hours
Formoterol	DPI	√			12 hours
Indacaterol	DPI				24 hours
Olodaterol	SMI				24 hours
Salmeterol	MDI & DPI				12 hours
ANTICHOLINERGICS					
SHORT-ACTING (SAMA)					
Ipratropium bromide	MDI	√			6-8 hours
Oxitropium bromide	MDI				7-9 hours
LONG-ACTING (LAMA)					
Aclidinium bromide	DPI, MDI				12 hours
Glycopyrronium bromide	DPI		solution	√	12-24 hours
Tiotropium	DPI, SMI, MDI				24 hours
Umeclidinium	DPI				24 hours
Glycopyrrolate		√			12 hours
Revefenacin		√			24 hours
COMBINATION SHORT-ACTING BETA$_2$-AGONIST PLUS ANTICHOLINERGIC IN ONE DEVICE (SABA/SAMA)					
Fenoterol/ipratropium	SMI,	√			6-8 hours
Salbutamol/ipratropium	SMI, MDI	√			6-8 hours
COMBINATION LONG-ACTING BETA$_2$-AGONIST PLUS ANTICHOLINERGIC IN ONE DEVICE (LABA/LAMA)					
Formoterol/aclidinium	DPI				12 hours
Formoterol/glycopyrronium	MDI				12 hours
Indacaterol/glycopyrronium	DPI				12-24 hours
Vilanterol/umeclidinium	DPI				24 hours
Olodaterol/tiotropium	SMI				24 hours
METHYLXANTHINES					
Aminophylline			solution	√	Variable, up to 24 hours
Theophylline (SR)			pill	√	Variable, up to 24 hours
COMBINATION OF LONG-ACTING BETA$_2$-AGONIST PLUS CORTICOSTEROID IN ONE DEVICE (LABA/ICS)					
Formoterol/beclometasone	MDI, DPI				12 hours
Formoterol/budesonide	MDI, DPI				12 hours
Formoterol/mometasone	MDI				12 hours
Salmeterol/fluticasone propionate	MDI, DPI				12 hours
Vilanterol/fluticasone furoate	DPI				24 hours
TRIPLE COMBINATION IN ONE DEVICE (LABA/LAMA/ICS)					
Fluticasone/umeclidinium/vilanterol	DPI				24 hours
Beclometasone/formoterol/glycopyrronium	MDI				12 hours
Budesonide/formoterol/glycopyrrolate	MDI				12 hours
PHOSPHODIESTERASE-4 INHIBITORS					
Roflumilast			pill		24 hours
MUCOLYTIC AGENTS					
Erdosteine			pill		12 hours
Carbocysteine[†]			pill		
N-acetylcysteine[†]			pill		

*Not all formulation are available in all countries. In some countries other formulations and dosages may be available. [†]Dosing regimens are under discussion. MDI = metered dose inhaler; DPI = dry powder inhaler; SMI = soft mist inhaler. Note that glycopyrrolate & glycopyrronium are the same compound.

Figure 45-5 Commonly used maintenance medications in COPD*.

Reproduced from Global strategy for the diagnosis, management, and prevention of chronic obstructive pulmonary disease, 2022 report," by Global Initiative for Chronic Lung Disease, 2022, p. 49 (https://goldcopd.org/2022-gold-reports-2/). Copyright 2021 by Global Initiative for Chronic Lung Disease, Inc. Adapted with permission.

related and problematic given the narrow therapeutic index, with the most efficacy at near-toxic doses. Toxicity symptoms include palpitations due to atrial and ventricular arrhythmias and grand mal convulsions; other side effects that can occur within the therapeutic range of serum levels include headache, insomnia, nausea, and heartburn (ERS/ATS, 2004).

2. Bronchodilators: Bronchodilators used in COPD include beta$_2$-agonists, which act by altering airway smooth muscle tone and improving expiratory flow, resulting in improved FEV_1 and other spirometric values (ERS/ATS, 2004). Short-acting beta$_2$-agonists (SABAs) usually wear off within 4 to 6 hours. Long-acting beta$_2$-agonists (LABAs) have a duration of 12 hours or more. Adverse effects of beta$_2$-adrenergic therapy include resting sinus tachycardia and exaggerated somatic tremor; hypokalemia can occur, especially when beta$_2$-agonists are used in combination with thiazide diuretics (GOLD, 2023).

Antimuscarinics block the bronchoconstrictor effects of acetylcholine on muscarinic receptors expressed in airway smooth muscle. Short-acting antimuscarinics (SAMAs) block the M2 muscarinic receptor, whereas long-acting antimuscarinics (LAMAs) have prolonged binding to M3 muscarinic receptors, resulting in prolonged duration of bronchodilator effect. Adverse effects of antimuscarinic drugs include dryness of mouth and occasional reports of urinary symptoms. The use of solutions with a facemask can precipitate acute glaucoma, probably as a direct result of the contact between the solution and the eye (GOLD, 2023).

3. Corticosteroids: Corticosteroids act at multiple points within the inflammatory cascade, although their effects in COPD are more modest compared to use in asthma. Both current and former smokers with COPD benefit from the use of inhaled corticosteroids (ICSs) with regard to lung function and exacerbation rates, although ICSs alone do not curb the long-term decline of FEV_1 or the mortality risk in patients with COPD. An ICS combined with a LABA, however, is more effective than either component alone in improving lung function and health status and reducing exacerbations. Factors that favor adding an ICS to long-acting bronchodilators include one or more moderate COPD exacerbations per year and blood eosinophil values of 100 to 300 cells/µL (GOLD, 2023). Adverse effects of ICSs include a higher prevalence of oral candidiasis, hoarse voice, skin bruising, and pneumonia. Given the risk of adverse effects, adding an ICS may be appropriate in certain conditions (**Figure 45-6**).

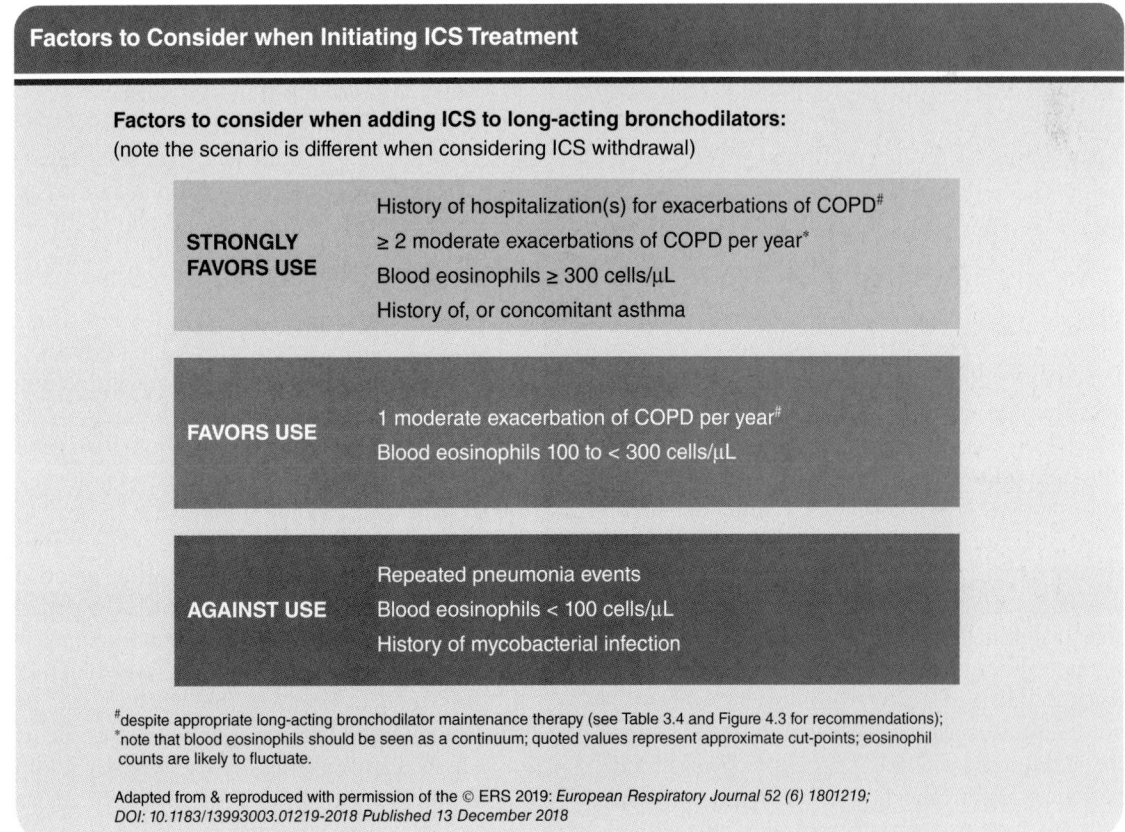

Figure 45-6 Factors to consider when initiating inhaled corticosteroid (ICS) treatment.

Reproduced from Global strategy for the diagnosis, management, and prevention of chronic obstructive pulmonary disease, 2022 report, by Global Initiative for Chronic Lung Disease, 2022, p. 55 (https://goldcopd.org/2022-gold-reports-2/). Copyright 2021 by Global Initiative for Chronic Lung Disease, Inc. Adapted with permission.

4. Combination therapy: Combining bronchodilators with different mechanisms and durations of action may increase the degree of bronchodilation, with a lower risk of side effects compared to increasing the dose of a single bronchodilator. Combinations of SABA + SAMA are superior compared to either medication alone in improving FEV_1 and symptoms; additionally, combination treatment with a LABA + LAMA increases FEV_1, reduces symptoms, and reduces exacerbations compared with monotherapy. Inhaled treatment with triple therapy, LABA + LAMA + ICS, has been shown to reduce exacerbations and improve lung function and patient-reported outcomes when compared to LAMA alone, LABA + LAMA, and LABA + ICS (GOLD, 2023).

C. Other pharmacologic therapy

For patients who experience refractory symptoms and/or recurrent exacerbation of COPD despite optimal inhaled pharmacotherapy, potential pharmacologic options include a trial of theophylline, roflumilast, or chronic azithromycin. The ATS recommends a personalized shared decision-making approach to consider opioid-based therapy for patients with COPD who experience advanced refractory dyspnea despite optimal therapy (ATS, 2020c). Oral glucocorticoids play a role in the management of acute COPD exacerbations; however, GOLD (2023) recommends against the use of oral glucocorticoids in the chronic daily treatment therapy of COPD, given the lack of benefit and high risk of systemic complications.

1. Roflumilast: Roflumilast is a once-daily oral phosphodiesterase-4 (PDE4) inhibitor with anti-inflammatory effects via the inhibition of intracellular cyclic adenosine monophosphate (cAMP) breakdown; it does not provide bronchodilation. It has been shown to reduce moderate and severe exacerbations and improve lung function in combination with a LABA. The effects were reported to be greater in patients with a prior history of hospitalization for acute exacerbation. Side effects of roflumilast include diarrhea, nausea, decreased appetite, weight loss, abdominal pain, sleep disturbance, and headache. Given the adverse side effects, it is recommended to monitor the weight trend during therapy and avoid roflumilast in underweight patients (GOLD, 2023).
2. Azithromycin: Azithromycin carries both antimicrobial and immunomodulatory effects and has been found to significantly decrease the COPD exacerbation rate, although there are no data showing the efficacy or safety of using chronic azithromycin to prevent COPD exacerbation beyond 1 year of treatment. Additional analysis suggests active smokers experience lesser benefit. Risks of azithromycin therapy include bacterial resistance, prolonged QTc interval, and impaired hearing (GOLD, 2023).
3. Mucolytics: Mucolytics reduce exacerbations and modestly improve health status in patients with COPD who are not receiving ICSs (GOLD, 2023). Mucolytics, such as carbocysteine and N-acetylcysteine, loosen sputum by changing the physical properties of the secretions, allowing for easier expectoration. The ATS and ERS recommend oral mucolytic treatment for patients with COPD who have moderate or severe airflow limitation and exacerbation despite optimal inhaled therapy (ERS/ATS, 2017).

D. Initial pharmacological management

In addition to prescribing rescue short-acting bronchodilators (SABDs) for immediate symptom relief for all patients with COPD, GOLD (2023) recommends pharmacological management as follows:
- Group A patients should be offered bronchodilator treatment, either short or long acting, which can be continued if benefit is documented.
- Group B patients should be initiated on a LABA + LAMA combination inhaler. It is also recommended to investigate and treat other possible etiologies of symptoms because group B patients are likely to have comorbidities.
- Group E patients should be initiated on a LABA + LAMA inhaler, with a strong recommendation to consider triple therapy (LABA + LAMA + ICS inhaler) in the presence of a history of hospitalization for exacerbation, eosinophils $\geq$ 300 cells/µL, and a history of or concomitant asthma. GOLD favors the addition of an ICS to long-acting bronchodilators in patients with COPD who have a history of one moderate exacerbation per year and blood eosinophils of 100 to <300 cells/µL.

E. Follow-up pharmacological management

Follow-up pharmacological treatment can be applied to any patient who is on maintenance treatments, irrespective of the GOLD group allocated at treatment initiation, and should integrate the following principles (GOLD, 2023):
1. Review symptoms and exacerbation risk.
2. Assess inhaler technique and adherence.
3. Adjust pharmacological treatment, including escalation and de-escalation and changing inhaler device. Any change in treatment requires a subsequent review of the clinical response.

F. Nonpharmacologic therapies
1. Pulmonary rehabilitation: Pulmonary rehabilitation is a "comprehensive intervention based on a thorough patient assessment followed by patient-tailored therapies, which include, but are not limited to, exercise training, education, and behavior change, designed to improve the physical and psychological condition of people with chronic respiratory disease and to promote the long-term adherence of health-enhancing behaviors" (ATS, 2013a, p. 16). It has been shown to be an effective therapeutic strategy to improve exercise tolerance and health-related quality of life across all grades of COPD severity. GOLD (2023) suggests optimum benefits are

achieved from programs lasting 6–8 weeks and recommends exercise training at least twice weekly. Exercise can include endurance and interval training, resistance and strength training, and walking.
2. Supplemental oxygen therapy: Progressive airflow limitation and emphysema causing ventilation–perfusion mismatch (V/Q) is the primary cause of hypoxemia in COPD patients. Other causes of V/Q mismatch in COPD include pulmonary exacerbations, high body weight, and reduced ventilatory drive. Chronic hypoxemia contributes to adverse consequences of COPD, such as PH, secondary polycythemia, skeletal muscle dysfunction, and systemic inflammation, all of which reduce quality of life and increase the risk of exacerbation and death (Kent et al., 2011). The ATS recommends prescribing long-term oxygen therapy for at least 15 hours per day in patients with COPD who have severe chronic resting room air hypoxemia, defined as (a) $Pa_{O_2} \leq 55$ mm Hg or $Sp_{O_2} \leq 88\%$ or (b) $Pa_{O_2} = 56–59$ mm Hg or $Sp_{O_2} = 89\%$, as well as edema, hematocrit $\geq 55\%$, or P pulmonale on an electrocardiogram; ambulatory oxygen is also recommended for adults with COPD who have severe exertional room air hypoxemia (ATS, 2020a).
3. Noninvasive ventilation: For patients with COPD with stable hypercapnic respiratory failure (resting $PaCO_2 > 45$), to target normalization of $PaCO_2$, ATS (2020b) suggests the use of nocturnal noninvasive ventilation (NIV) without the need for in-laboratory overnight polysomnography for titration or screening of obstructive sleep apnea. The initiation of long-term NIV use is not advised during hospitalization for acute-on-chronic hypercapnic respiratory failure; the recommendation is to reassess for its need 2–4 weeks after resolution of acute symptoms (ATS, 2020b).
4. Interventional therapy: In a select population of patients with COPD, procedural or surgical interventional therapy can be considered. Therapies include airway and emphysematous-predominant treatment (GOLD, 2023):
    a. Lung volume reduction surgery (LVRS) involves resecting portions of lungs containing the most emphysematous changes to reduce hyperinflation and increase lung elastic recoil pressure and density. LVRS can be performed unilaterally or bilaterally. Factors increasing mortality with LVRS include $FEV_1 \leq 20\%$ predicted, homogenous emphysema on high-resolution CT, DLCO $\leq 20\%$ predicted, and lower body weight. To achieve successful outcomes, a multidisciplinary team is imperative to the selection of potential LVRS patients and the coordination of their postoperative care.
    b. Bronchoscopy can also be used to perform lung volume reduction through interventions such as self-activating lung coils, sealants or one-way valves, and thermal ablative techniques. Endobronchial one-way valves (EBVs) are the most well-studied therapy and showed significant increases in FEV_1 and 6-minute walk distance, as well as improved health status.
    c. Surgical bullectomy is a rare but effective procedure for surgical resection of bullae, which are air-filled spaces of at least 1 centimeter in diameter resulting from emphysematous destruction of the parenchyma. Bullectomy is offered when a bulla occupies more than one-third of a hemithorax and compresses adjacent viable lung tissue.
    d. Lung transplantation can be considered in patients with progressive disease despite maximal medical treatment who are not candidates for LVRS or other interventional therapies and have a BODE index of 5–6, a $PaCO_2 > 50$ mm Hg, and/or a $PaO_2 < 60$ mm Hg and $FEV_1 < 25\%$, without relevant contraindications. The complications most seen in patients with COPD after lung transplantation include acute rejection, bronchiolitis obliterans, opportunistic infections, and lymphoproliferative disease.
    The BODE index is useful when considering interventional therapy for patients with COPD. When assessing 5-year survival following LVRS, the postoperative BODE index was found to correlate with survival. Decrease to a lower BODE score was associated with decreased mortality (Imfeld et al., 2006). A BODE index score of 5–6 is one of the indications when considering referral for lung transplantation evaluation, and a score of ≥ 7 is an indication for listing (International Society for Heart and Lung Transplantation, 2021).
5. Supportive, palliative, end-of-life, and hospice care: Patients who continue to experience distressing symptoms despite receiving optimal medical therapy can be improved by wider use of palliative therapies. The goals of palliative care are to prevent and relieve suffering and support the best possible quality of life for patients and their families regardless of the stage of disease (GOLD, 2023). Multiple therapeutic approaches can be considered, including palliative treatment of dyspnea; nutritional support for patients who are malnourished; and treatment of panic, anxiety, and depression associated with their disease. End-of-life care should include discussions with patients and their families regarding resuscitation, advance directives, and place-of-death preferences. Hospice services may provide additional benefits for patients with very advanced or terminal illness.

G. *COPD exacerbation*
1. Definition: *COPD exacerbation* is defined as "an event characterized by increased dyspnea and/or cough and sputum that worsens in < 14 days, which may be accompanied by tachypnea and/or tachycardia and is often associated with increased local and systemic inflammation caused by

infection, pollution, or other insult to the airways" (GOLD, 2023, p. 134).

Exacerbations negatively affect health status, rates of hospitalization and readmission, and disease progression. Patients with COPD are at increased risk for other acute events that may mimic or aggravate COPD exacerbation, such as heart failure, pneumonia, and pulmonary embolism. Currently, COPD exacerbation is classified after the event has occurred and is defined based on the treatment that was used: mild exacerbation treated with SABDs only; moderate exacerbation treated with SABDs and oral corticosteroids with or without antibiotics; or severe exacerbation requiring hospitalization or emergency room level of care, with or without associated acute respiratory failure. GOLD (2023) supports the Rome proposal, which proposes a new classification of COPD exacerbation using clinical variables obtained at the time of the patient encounter, which can help define the severity of exacerbations in clinical practice, research, and clinical trials (**Figure 45-7**). The five clinical variables discussed in the Rome proposal are dyspnea, respiratory rate, heart rate, oxygen saturation, and serum C-reactive protein (Celli et al., 2021).

2. COPD exacerbation treatment: Treatment goals are to minimize the negative impact of the current exacerbation and prevent subsequent events because they negatively affect health status, increase rates of hospitalization and readmission, and contribute to disease progression. The three classes of medications commonly used for COPD exacerbations are bronchodilators, corticosteroids, and antibiotics (GOLD, 2023).
    a. SABDs via nebulizer or metered dosed inhaler (MDI) are the initial bronchodilator treatment for acute COPD exacerbation, with recommendations for use via MDI in lieu of continuous nebulization; the recommended MDI dosing is one or two puffs every hour for two to three doses, then every 2–4 hours based on the patient's response.
    b. The use of oral glucocorticoids in COPD exacerbation can shorten recovery time, may improve lung function and oxygenation, and is associated with fewer hospitalizations. A course of prednisone at 40 mg daily for no longer than 5–7 days is recommended; longer courses are associated with an increased risk of pneumonia and mortality.
    c. Antibiotic therapy in exacerbations is controversial because viral or bacterial infections can cause COPD exacerbation. A course of antibiotics of 5 or less days for COPD exacerbation is recommended for patients who are (a) experiencing the three cardinal COPD exacerbation symptoms (increase in dyspnea, sputum volume, and sputum purulence), (b) experiencing increased sputum purulence and one additional cardinal symptom, or (c) require mechanical ventilation.

    Additional management of severe but non–life-threatening exacerbations includes blood gases, chest radiography, consideration for supplemental oxygen therapy and/or noninvasive mechanical ventilation, monitoring of fluid balance, consideration of thromboembolism prophylaxis, and treatment of associated conditions. Potential indications for hospitalization assessment include severe symptoms such as worsening of resting dyspnea, high respiratory rate, decreased oxygen saturation, drowsiness, acute respiratory failure, onset of new physical findings, failure of therapy with initial medical management, presence of serious comorbidities, and insufficient home support (GOLD, 2023).
3. Follow-up: Early follow-up (within 1 month), especially after hospital discharge, has been related to fewer exacerbation-related readmissions, with additional follow-up at 3–4 months to ensure the patient returns to a stable clinical state. Pulmonary rehabilitation initiated within 4 weeks after acute exacerbation of COPD requiring hospitalization reduces readmission and mortality. Strong encouragement of smoking cessation should be discussed at all patient encounters, especially in times of COPD exacerbation (GOLD, 2023).

IV. Specific population considerations

Several systematic reviews and meta-analyses support a higher prevalence of COPD in current and past smokers compared to nonsmokers and in those aged 40 years and older. Sex-related differences in immune pathways and patterns of airway damage may be clinically important; however, more work in this area is needed (GOLD, 2023). Poverty and lower socioeconomic status are associated with an increased risk of developing COPD, although it is not clear whether exposures to household and air pollutants, crowding, poor nutrition, infections, or other factors are related to low socioeconomic status (GOLD, 2023). The economic burden associated with COPD is expected to increase over the next 20 years in the United States. Both direct and indirect costs associated with COPD can be detrimental to the economy, especially in low- and middle-income countries.

A. *Smoking*

Smoking remains the main risk factor for developing COPD. Tobacco cessation is a key focus in preventing and treating COPD. The CDC recommends that comprehensive statewide tobacco control programs coordinate community-level interventions that counter tobacco industry marketing and focus on (a) preventing initiation among youth and young adults, (b) promoting quitting among young adults and youth, (c) eliminating exposure to second-hand smoke, and (d) identifying and eliminating tobacco-related disparities among population groups (CDC, 2014).

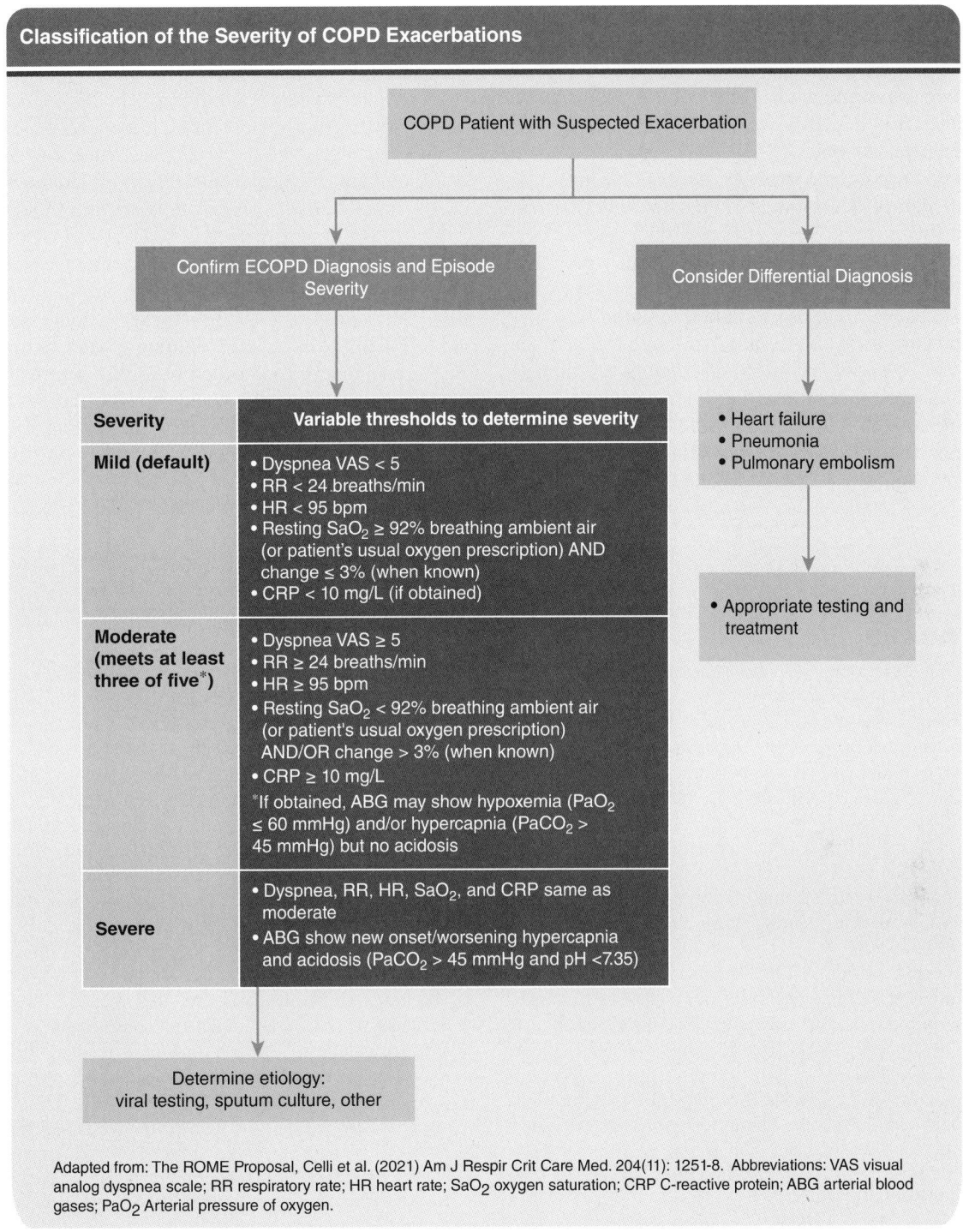

Figure 45-7 Classification of the severity of chronic obstructive pulmonary disease (COPD) exacerbations.

Reproduced from Global strategy for the diagnosis, management, and prevention of chronic obstructive pulmonary disease, 2022 report, by Global Initiative for Chronic Lung Disease, 2022, p. 116 (https://goldcopd.org/2022-gold-reports-2/). Copyright 2021 by Global Initiative for Chronic Lung Disease, Inc. Adapted with permission.

B. Lung development, age, and sex

GOLD (2023) reports that age is often listed as a risk factor for COPD; however, it is unclear if healthy aging leads to COPD or if age reflects the sum of cumulative exposures throughout life.

Factors occurring during gestation and birth and exposures during childhood and adolescence can affect lung function in adulthood. Smoking during pregnancy can affect lung growth and development in utero and may pose a risk for the fetus. Other childhood factors that can affect lung function in adult life include birth weight, early childhood lung infections, and exposure to air pollution (GOLD, 2023).

Past epidemiologic studies reported greater prevalence and mortality among men than women; however, later data from developed countries show that the prevalence of COPD is now almost equal in males and females, likely reflecting the changing patterns of tobacco smoking. Comorbidities such as bronchiectasis and sleep apnea might also be present in women with COPD (GOLD, 2023).

C. *Socioeconomic status*

Lower socioeconomic status is associated with an increased risk of developing COPD. However, it is not clear if this is due to exposures to indoor and outdoor pollutants, overpopulation, poor nutritional status, infections, or other influences of low socioeconomic rank (GOLD, 2023). Lower socioeconomic status poses significant barriers when treating COPD because treatment can be costly and treatment options are limited. These barriers affect health behaviors and adherence. The ERS and ATS support access of patients with respiratory disease to health care and specialists, as well as to other national programs designed to decrease healthcare disparities (ATS, 2013b).

D. *Action at the national level*

1. COPD National Action Plan: The NHLBI collaborated with the CDC and multiple stakeholders, including patients, providers, and policy makers, to address the growing incidence of COPD in the United States. The result of their collaboration was the COPD National Action Plan, launched in 2021 as the first multi-stakeholder model, with its primary objective being to raise awareness about COPD and reduce the impact of the disease. The COPD National Action Plan (NHLBI, 2020) goals include building awareness to recognize and reduce the burden of COPD, improving quality of care across the healthcare continuum, managing COPD-related public health data, increasing and supporting COPD research, and setting policy into action.

References

American Lung Association. (n.d.). *Chronic obstructive pulmonary disease.* https://www.lung.org/copd

American Thoracic Society. (2012). An official American Thoracic Society statement: Update on the mechanisms, assessment, and management of dyspnea. *American Journal of Respiratory and Critical Care Medicine, 185*(4), 435–452. https://doi.org/10.1164/rccm.201111-2042ST

American Thoracic Society. (2013a). An American Thoracic Society/European Respiratory Society statement: Key concepts and advances in pulmonary rehabilitation. *American Journal of Respiratory and Critical Care Medicine, 188*(8), 13–64. https://doi.org/10.1164/rccm.201309-1634ST

American Thoracic Society. (2013b). An official American Thoracic Society/European Respiratory Society policy statement: Disparities in respiratory health. *American Journal of Respiratory and Critical Care Medicine, 188*(7), 865–871. https://doi.org/10.1164/rccm.201308-1509ST

American Thoracic Society. (2020a). Home oxygen therapy for adults with chronic lung disease: An official American Thoracic Society clinical practice guideline. *American Journal of Respiratory and Critical Care Medicine, 202*(10), 121–141. https://doi.org/10.1164/rccm.202009-3608ST

American Thoracic Society. (2020b). Long-term noninvasive ventilation in chronic stable hypercapnic chronic obstructive pulmonary disease: An official American Thoracic Society clinical practice guideline. *American Journal of Respiratory and Critical Care Medicine, 202*(4), 74–87. https://doi.org/10.1164/rccm.202006-2382ST

American Thoracic Society. (2020c). Pharmacologic management of chronic obstructive pulmonary disease: An official American Thoracic Society clinical practice guideline. *American Journal of Respiratory and Critical Care Medicine, 201*(9), 56–69. https://doi.org/10.1164/rccm.202003-0625ST

American Thoracic Society. (2021). *Patient education information series: Chronic obstructive pulmonary disease (COPD).* https://www.thoracic.org/patients/patient-resources/resources/copd-intro.pdf

Celli, B. R., Cote, C. G., Marin, J. M., Casanova, C., Montes de Oca, M., Mendez, R. A., Plata, V. P., & Cabral, H. J. (2004). The body-mass index, airflow obstruction, dyspnea, and exercise capacity index in chronic obstructive pulmonary disease. *New England Journal of Medicine, 350*(10), 1005–1012. https://doi.org/10.1056/NEJMoa021322?articleTools=true

Celli, B. R., Fabbri, L. M., Aaron, S. D., Agusti, A., Brook, R., Criner, G. J., Franssen, F. M. E., Humbert, M., Hurst, J. R., O'Donnell, D., Pantoni, L., Papi, A., Rodriguez-Roisin, R., Sethi, S., Torres, A., Vogelmeier, C. F., & Wedzicha, J. A. (2021). An updated definition and severity classification of chronic obstructive pulmonary disease exacerbations: The Rome proposal. *American Journal of Respiratory and Critical Care Medicine, 204*(11), 1251–1258. https://doi.org/10.1164/rccm.202108-1819PP

Celli, B., Fabbri, L., Criner, G., Martinez, F. J., Mannino, D., Vogelmeier, C., Montes de Oca, M., Papi, A., Sin, D. D., Han, M. K., & Agusti, A. (2022). Definition and nomenclature of chronic obstructive pulmonary disease: Time for its revision. *American Journal of Respiratory and Critical Care Medicine, 206*(11), 1317–1325. https://doi.org/10.1164/rccm.202204-0671PP

Centers for Disease Control and Prevention. (2014). *Best practices for comprehensive tobacco control programs.* National Center for Chronic Disease Prevention and Health Promotion, Office on Smoking and Health. https://www.cdc.gov/tobacco/stateandcommunity/guides/pdfs/2014/comprehensive.pdf

Centers for Disease Control and Prevention. (2018). Recommendations of the advisory committee on the immunization practices for the use of herpes zoster vaccines. *Morbidity and Mortality Weekly Report, 67*(3), 103–108. https://doi.org/10.15585/mmwr.mm6703a5

Centers for Disease Control and Prevention. (2019). Use of 13-valent pneumococcal conjugate vaccine and 23-valent pneumococcal polysaccharide vaccine among adults aged ≥65 years: Updated recommendations of the advisory committee on immunization practices. *Morbidity and Mortality Weekly Report, 68*(46), 1069–1075. https://doi.org/10.15585/mmwr.mm6846a5

Centers for Disease Control and Prevention. (2020). Use of tetanus toxoid, reduced diphtheria toxoid, and acellular pertussis vaccines: Updated recommendations of the advisory committee on immunization practices—United States, 2019. *Morbidity and Mortality Weekly Report*, 69(3), 77–83. https://doi.org/10.15585/mmwr.mm6903a5

Centers for Disease Control and Prevention. (2021a). *Basics about COPD.* https://www.cdc.gov/copd/basics-about.html

Centers for Disease Control and Prevention. (2021b). *COVID-19: People with certain medical conditions.* https://www.cdc.gov/coronavirus/2019-ncov/need-extra-precautions/people-with-medical-conditions.html

Centers for Disease Control and Prevention. (2021c). Prevention and control of seasonal influenza with vaccines: Recommendations of the advisory committee on immunization practices, United States, 2021–22 influenza season. *Morbidity and Mortality Weekly Report*, 70(5), 1–28. https://doi.org/10.15585/mmwr.rr7005a1

COPD Foundation. (2022). *What is COPD?* https://www.copdfoundation.org

Cote, C. G., Dordelly, L. J., & Celli, B. R. (2007). Impact of COPD exacerbations on patient-centered outcomes. *CHEST Journal*, 131(3), 696–704. https://doi.org/10.1378/chest.06-1610

European Respiratory Society & American Thoracic Society. (2004). Standards for the diagnosis and treatment of patients with COPD: A summary of the ATS/ERS position paper. *European Respiratory Journal*, 23(6), 932–946. https://doi.org/10.1183/09031936.04.00014304

European Respiratory Society & American Thoracic Society. (2014). An official European Respiratory Society/American Thoracic Society technical standard: Field walking tests in chronic respiratory disease. *European Respiratory Journal* 44(6), 1428–1446. https://doi.org/10.1183/09031936.00150314

European Respiratory Society & American Thoracic Society. (2017). Prevention of COPD exacerbations: A European Respiratory Society/American Thoracic Society guideline. *European Respiratory Journal* 50(3), 1602265. https://doi.org/10.1183/13993003.02265-2016

Global Initiative for Chronic Lung Disease. (2023). *Global strategy for the diagnosis, management, and prevention of chronic obstructive pulmonary disease, 2023 report.* https://goldcopd.org/2023-gold-report-2/

Imfeld, S., Bloch, K. E., Weder, W., & Russi, E. W. (2006). The BODE index after lung volume reduction surgery correlates with survival. *CHEST Journal*, 129(4), 873–878. https://doi.org/10.1378/chest.129.4.873

International Society for Heart and Lung Transplantation. (2021). Consensus document for the selection of lung transplant candidates: An update from the International Society for Heart and Lung Transplantation. *Journal of Heart and Lung Transplantation*, 40(11), 1349–1379. https://doi.org/10.1016/j.healun.2021.07.005

Kent, B. D., Mitchell, P. D., & McNicholas, W. T. (2011). Hypoxemia in patients with COPD: Cause, effects, and disease progression. *International Journal of COPD*, 6, 199–208. https://doi.org/10.2147/COPD.S10611

Kovacs, G., Agusti, A., Barberà, J. A., Celli, B., Criner, G., Humbert, M., Sin, D. D., Voelkel, N., & Olschewski, H. (2018). Pulmonary vascular involvement in chronic obstructive pulmonary disease. Is there a pulmonary vascular phenotype? *American Journal of Respiratory and Critical Care Medicine*, 198(8), 1000–1011. https://doi.org/10.1164/rccm.201801-0095PP

National Heart, Lung, and Blood Institute. (2020). *COPD national action plan: Our goals.* U.S. Department of Health and Human Services. https://www.nhlbi.nih.gov/health-topics/education-and-awareness/COPD-national-action-plan/our-goals#health_professionals

National Heart, Lung, and Blood Institute. (2022). *COPD: What is COPD?* Department of Health and Human Services. https://www.nhlbi.nih.gov/health/copd

Rodriquez-Roisin, R. (2020). *Twenty years of GOLD (1997–2017). The origins.* https://goldcopd.org/wp-content/uploads/2019/03/GOLD-Origins-Final-Version-mar19.pdf

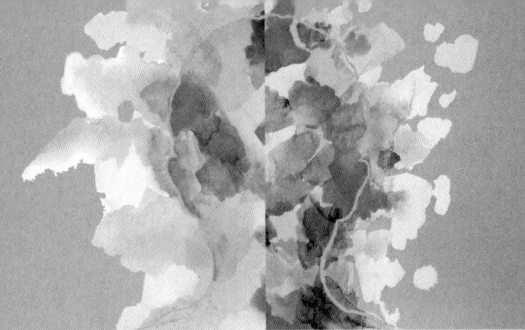

CHAPTER 46

Chronic Nonmalignant Pain Management

Caitlin Garvey and JoAnne M. Saxe

I. Introduction

This chapter examines multimodal treatments for chronic pain (CP), including pharmaceuticals. Inherent in this discussion is the use of opioids and long-term opioid therapy (LTOT) for the management of CP not associated with cancer, acute manifestations of chronic conditions (e.g., acute sickle cell crisis), or end-of-life care.

A. General background

Pain is one of the most common presenting complaints in primary care and affects over 100 million Americans (Institute of Medicine [IOM], 2011). It can be associated with a wide array of conditions encountered in primary care, including arthritis, diabetes, vascular disease, neuralgias, fibromyalgia, sickle cell disease, headache, gastrointestinal disease, and more. Pain is the number-one cause of disability in the United States (Centers for Disease Control and Prevention [CDC], 2009). Patients with CP report impacts on enjoyment of life, mood, concentration, energy, and sleep (American Pain Foundation, 2008). Anxiety and depression are common comorbidities, and the patient often has difficulty with work and personal life (Saxe et al., 2013; Yalcin & Barrot, 2014).

Opioid safety is an important responsibility of the primary care provider because about half of opioid prescriptions come from primary care settings (Daubresse et al., 2013). Opioid-related deaths, opioid use disorder (OUD), and the use of nonprescribed opioids have risen significantly over the past two decades (National Institute for Drug Abuse [NIDA], 2017), prompting the escalating phenomenon to be declared an opioid epidemic.

Additionally, there are concerns that both the opioid epidemic and CP may increase as the result of the COVID-19 pandemic, in response to the infection itself (e.g., musculoskeletal, nervous system and inflammatory implications that may result in prolonged symptoms) and in response to the psychological, social, and economic factors combined with disruptions to healthcare and safety-net systems.

The goal of therapy for the clinician is to provide adequate management of CP in a timely, safe, and effective manner for the patient while preserving or enhancing function. National guidelines (Veterans Affairs [VA]/Department of Defense [DoD], CDC) recommend biopsychosocial, multimodal, and interdisciplinary pain care. Therapy generally should incorporate multiple modalities (pharmacological, behavioral, physical, manual, interventional) and active self-management. Efficacy of therapy should be measured by reduction in pain interference scores (not simply pain severity scores), progress toward functional goals, and meaningful engagement in the things that matter most to the patient (return to social activities, hobbies, family responsibilities, work, etc.).

Bias, prejudice and discrimination exist in health care and in the treatment of chronic pain (Morales & Yang, 2021). Patients notice this. For example, in a 2005 survey, African American and Hispanic respondents perceived lower accessibility to pain care compared to white respondents and had lower confident that providers would understand or treat their pain (Nguyen et al., 2005). More research is required to understand disparities, underlying causes and solutions. Meghani et al. (2012) has recommended a framework that can used to guide macro level change at the structural/system, policy, workforce, provider and research levels.

B. Definition and context
C. Prevalence and costs

In 2023, a CDC analysis of data from the National Health Interview Survey estimated that one-fifth, or

51.6 million, adults in the United States had chronic pain and 17.1 million experienced symptoms severe enough to result in substantial reduction in daily activities (Rikard, Strahan, Schmit, & Guy, 2023). This survey also explored demographic data revealing higher prevalence of pain in adults with disabilities, adults with poor general health, older adults, women, American Indian or Alaska Native adults, individuals identifying as bisexual, unemployed adults, adults who are divorced or separated, Veterans and those living in poverty. There is substantial research demonstrating disparities in the treatment of pain, with race, socioeconomic status and other factors impacting assessment and treatment of chronic pain (Morales & Yang, 2021). Significant financial burden is attributed to this syndrome because of loss of productivity and disability and the direct cost of physician visits and medication treatment (Turk, 2006). Costs associated with CP have been estimated to be $635 billion each year in medical treatment and lost productivity (IOM, 2011).

II. Database
A. *Subjective*
1. History of the presenting complaint
   The history of the presenting symptom should include the identification of pain: its source onset, location, radiation, duration, characteristics, alleviating factors, aggravating factors, nonpharmacological and pharmacological treatments tried, and the response to treatments. The significance of pain (i.e., impact on work, relationships, and activities of daily living) should also be assessed. Pain and functional scales can be helpful in measuring the subjective report of pain. Note: Because pain and related functional assessments are challenging to assess in nonverbal individuals, such as persons affected by advanced dementia, behavioral pain assessment tools or surrogate pain reports may need to be used (Herr et al., 2006).
2. Past health history
   a. Medical and psychiatric illnesses, surgical history, hospitalizations, and physical and psychological trauma in relation to the pain syndrome
   b. Medications: current and history of medications
   c. Medication allergies and drug interactions: Pharmaceutical treatments for CP draw from multiple classes and mechanisms of action. Polypharmacy and the potential for interactions are particularly common in this setting. Be vigilant for potential serotoninergic overload, agents that can compound liver or renal injury, agents that may result in enzymatic inhibition or induction of another medication, and the compounding effects of central nervous system (CNS) depressants.
3. Family medical history, with emphasis on CP, musculoskeletal disorders, neurological disorders, mood disorders, and substance use disorders
4. Occupational history: If pain occurred as a result of a job injury, note any related litigation issues (including whether these are active or resolved), present ability to work, and goals for work in the future. Please note that not all work is paid, and a patient may be experiencing losses related to valuable unpaid work, such as parenting, caregiving, volunteering, or supporting a family business without pay.
5. Psychosocial history: This should include an assessment of aspects of biopsychosocial health, including housing, relationships, hobbies/personal interests, and health-related behaviors, including substance use history, diet, and physical activity.
6. Review of systems: Particular focus may be given to a system based on the location of pain and/or disease state; for example, if CP is related to abdominal pain, a more thorough gastrointestinal, urological, and reproductive system assessment would be indicated, whereas these systems are less valuable if CP is associated with isolated wrist pain due to carpal tunnel syndrome. Some symptomatic and medical histories may inform or preclude certain treatment initiations or titrations, regardless of the nature of the CP complaint.
   a. General: fatigue, weight change, fever/chills
   b. Head, eyes, ears, nose, throat: diplopia, photophobia, changes in hearing acuity, change in voice, loss of smell, xerostomia
   c. Skin: scar tissue, including trauma or surgical scars, rash, lesions, color change, ecchymosis
   d. Cardiovascular: chest pain, intermittent claudication, orthopnea, or arrhythmias
   e. Respiratory: shortness of breath, frequency and severity of asthma or chronic obstructive pulmonary disease (COPD) symptoms, signs of sleep apnea
   f. Gastrointestinal: nausea, vomiting, diarrhea, constipation, heartburn, symptoms of frank or occult bleeding, bowel incontinence
   g. Genitourinary: urinary incontinence or obstruction, dyspareunia, dysmenorrhea, erectile dysfunction
   h. Musculoskeletal: joint erythema, swelling and/or warmth, pain, decreased range of motion, arthralgias, myalgias, stiffness, and muscle wasting
   i. Neurologic: paresthesia, gait disturbance, weakness, muscle symmetry, dizziness, cognitive deficit
   j. Hematology: abnormal bleeding or clotting
   k. Endocrine/Metabolic: polyuria, polyphagia
   l. Psychological: mood change, depression, anxiety, sleep disruption, suicidality

B. *Objective*
1. The physical examination: Focus on the areas affected, which will typically include the completion of targeted musculoskeletal, orthopedic, and neurologic examinations but may also include an abdominal exam, skin exam, and so forth, based on presenting location or other characteristics of pain history. Even for a focused musculoskeletal exam, keep in mind to assess the area of complaint as part of the larger functioning body, and assess for

possible contributions from the areas above, deeper, and below the area of symptomatic presentation. The initial examination should also include a baseline cardiopulmonary examination, especially if opioids are currently prescribed or being considered.
   2. Screening and diagnostic tools
      a. Pain assessment should be multidimensional and include behavioral, functional, and mood sequelae and comorbidities alongside focal diagnostics relating to the differential diagnosis. Risk assessment tools are recommended for patients for whom you may be considering opioid treatment.
         i. Pain, function, and interference assessment: The PEG (pain intensity [P], interference with enjoyment of life [E], and interference with general activity [G]) Scale (Krebs et al., 2009) is valuable for repeated and brief pain assessments. All items are weighted on a scale of 0 (no pain or major interference) to 10 (severe to major interference). The PEG Scale can be accessed at https://health.gov/hcq/trainings/pathways/assets/pdfs/PEG_scale.pdf.
            For elderly individuals who are nonverbal, assessment tools have been developed to evaluate their pain (Herr et al., 2006). One such tool is the Pain Assessment Scale for Seniors With Severe Dementia, which includes an assessment of facial expressions, social/personality/mood indicators, activity/body movement, and physiological indicators/eating/sleeping changes/vocal behaviors (Fuchs-Lacelle & Hadjistavropoulos, 2004). Other tools are also available, such as the Pain Catastrophizing Scale (Sullivan et al., 1995).
         ii. Mood assessment: For depression screening, the Patient Health Questionnaire–9 (Kroenke, Spitzer, & Williams, 2001) or an equivalent resource may be used. (The Patient Health Questionnaire–9 can be accessed at https://www.ncbi.nlm.nih.gov/pmc/articles/PMC1495268/.) The Generalized Anxiety Disorder–2-item version (GAD-2) or Generalized Anxiety Disorder–7-item version (GAD-7) may be used to screen for anxiety (Spitzer et al., 2006).
         iii. Substance use and abuse risk: CAGE-AID (available at http://www.cqaimh.org/pdf/tool_cageaid.pdf) or another tool that is validated for substance and alcohol abuse
         iv. Opioid risk assessment (Cheatle et al., 2019)
         v. Document history of substance use.

III. Assessment
A. *Determine the diagnosis*
   Use the appropriate International Classification of Diseases–10 codes (available at http://www.icd10data.com/) (e.g., chronic primary osteoarthritis of the right hip: M16.11).
B. *Severity*
   Assess severity of symptoms (e.g., "moderate pain with frequent episodes of severe pain related to activity interfering with sleep and ability to work").
C. *Significance and motivation*
   Assess significance of diagnosis in relation to functional capacity, mood, and support systems. Determine the patient's strengths, ability to follow the treatment plan, and risk for nonadherence and/or substance misuse.

IV. Goals of clinical management
Focus on the patient's desired goals and expected outcomes, which may include but are not limited to the following:
A. *Improve and maximize functioning in relationships, at work, or at home.*
B. *Decrease related depression and anxiety.*
C. *Minimize pain and pain-related distress and disability.*
D. *Minimize adverse effects and/or associated risks from pain management strategies, medication transitions, and withdrawal/discontinuation syndromes (see following discussion).*

V. Plan
A. *Nonmedication strategies*
   Special considerations: As is the case in most chronic disease management, behavioral and lifestyle changes are some of the most potent interventions for CP management. They are also the most difficult part of the care plan to execute, for both the clinician and the patient. The guiding principles of effective CP care planning and goal setting should be to educate, align, empower, and remind—and repeat through *all* phases of treatment.
   1. Patient education and expectation management
      a. Provide guidance pertaining to diagnosis, prognosis, and related physical ability. Neuropsychological circuitry shows significant overlap between fear, pain perception, and disability. Multiple studies suggest that catastrophizing and fear-avoidant thoughts and behaviors may be larger predictions of disability level after an injury than the injury type or severity. Clinicians play an important role in the support, confrontation, and resolution of catastrophic thinking–related pain misperceptions (Silva et al., 2021).
      b. Encourage lifestyle integration of fundamental wellness practices to increase pain tolerance threshold and resilience, such as sleep hygiene, proper nutrition, comorbidity management, and so forth.
      c. Provide patient-applied active treatment instruction, such as the use of rest or activity, heat or ice, and compression and/or elevation.
   2. Pain psychology
      a. Cognitive–behavioral therapy
      b. Stress reduction
      c. Relaxation techniques and sleep optimization

d. Attention diversion
e. Goal setting
f. Pain and symptom diary
g. Catastrophizing management
h. Support groups
i. Guided imagery, biofeedback, focused virtual reality experiences
j. Physical therapy: guided, patient-specific stretching, strengthening, and proper body mechanics instruction for appropriate goal-oriented tasks
k. Manual therapies: osteopathic manipulation, acupuncture, massage, chiropractic
l. Durable medical equipment: Adaptive, ergonomic, and palliative devices or orthotics; transcutaneous electrical nerve stimulation unit
m. Gentle motion: tai chi, gentle stretching and strengthening, restorative or hatha yoga

B. *Non-opioid medication strategies* (Barclay & Nghiem, 2008; Caudill, 2009)

Special considerations: As is the case throughout CP treatment, a multipronged approach is preferred when considering the use of medications. Non-opioid medications should be optimized prior to initiating opioid medications for CP. This often requires the use of small doses of more than one type of medication class to maximize therapeutic effect while minimizing adverse effects. For all medications that follow, keep in mind the Beers Criteria List when prescribing to elderly patients (American Geriatrics Society, 2023).

1. Acetaminophen: for mild to moderate pain. Caution with liver disease, alcohol use, hepatitis, and use of other medications metabolized by the liver.
2. Nonsteroidal anti-inflammatory drugs (NSAIDs) and salicylates: For mild to moderate pain, may use in conjunction with acetaminophen. If one class fails, consider switching to another class of NSAIDs (e.g., switching from a nonselective cyclooxygenase inhibitor such as ibuprofen to a salicylic acid derivative or a selective cyclooxygenase inhibitor such as celecoxib). It is important to review the specific medication because dose and timing vary depending on the medication. Note the precautions associated with hypertension, coronary artery disease, congestive heart failure, diabetes, benign prostatic hypertrophy, and individuals older than 50 years of age. NSAIDs are contraindicated in patients who are pregnant or who have a history of gastrointestinal ulcer disease and chronic kidney disease or who are on a blood thinner.
3. Topical analgesic creams and patches: Appropriate for mild to moderate pain; may be used in conjunction with oral medications if not redundant in mechanism of action (i.e., don't use oral and topical NSAIDs concurrently). Dose varies and is dependent on analgesia desired and person's response. Examples include lidocaine 5% patches, up to three patches to the affected area at once for 12 hours within a 24-hour period, and lidocaine 4% cream or capsaicin cream, 0.025%–0.075%, applied to the affected area up to three to four times daily.
4. Antidepressants: The hormones implicated in depression are also part of the pain inhibition pathway in the CNS. Additionally, depression and CP are common synergistic comorbidities. As such, antidepressants may be a useful adjunctive therapy. Medications that increase serotonin and norepinephrine levels (serotonin–norepinephrine reuptake inhibitors [SNRIs] and tricyclic antidepressants [TCAs]) are especially indicated for CP treatment and neuropathic pain. Selective serotonin reuptake inhibitors (SSRIs) can be useful for mood symptoms comorbid with CP.

    TCAs are helpful for neuropathic pain disorders and associated sleep disturbances. A baseline electrocardiogram is indicated before initiating this classification of medication to assess for any conduction abnormalities because they can often prolong the QT interval. Start with a low dose (dosages for the indication of CP are typically lower than those used for depression) and titrate up over several weeks. Keep in mind the significant anticholinergic effects of these medications, which can limit use. The ones least likely to cause such effects are desipramine and nortriptyline.

    SNRIs may also be effective in the management of pain; duloxetine has a U.S. Food and Drug Administration (FDA) indication for musculoskeletal and neuropathic pain, and milnacipran has an FDA indication for fibromyalgia. Because SNRIs may cause an increase in blood pressure, the person's blood pressure should be well controlled before initiating an SNRI. Caution should be exercised with duloxetine in patients with alcohol use or risk of liver disease, given reports of hepatotoxicity. As with TCAs, SNRIs should be titrated. They should not be abruptly discontinued, given the risk for withdrawal signs and symptoms (may include but not limited to nausea, dizziness, irritability, and insomnia).
5. Anticonvulsants: These medications are commonly helpful for neuropathic pain, such as radiculopathy, diabetic neuropathy, and postherpetic neuralgia. Use with caution in renal insufficiency. Adjustments for renal impairment are indicated. Refer to reliable drug resources for dosing adjustment guidelines. Of note, gabapentin is gaining notoriety for abuse potential and misuse likelihood.
6. Other adjunctive medications: Muscle relaxants. Avoid carisoprodol (Soma®) because of abuse potential and the small margin of safety for overdose. In general, chronic use of muscle relaxants should be avoided for most types of CP; muscle relaxants are indicated primarily for spasticity rather than myofascial pain without spasticity. If they are prescribed for nonspastic CP, they should be prescribed for a limited time and with PRN administration instructions, not scheduled. For a time,

benzodiazepines were prescribed routinely as muscle relaxants. This practice has fallen out of favor because of the overdose potential, especially when combined with opioids for CP. It should be noted that benzodiazepines, baclofen, and carisoprodol can cause life-threatening abrupt discontinuation syndromes and therefore should be weaned. Also, cyclobenzaprine has a chemical structure similar to that of a TCA and has been implicated in contributing to serotonin syndrome.

C. *Opioid medication strategies*

Special considerations: Opioids pose a significant risk for adverse effects and have a relatively low margin of safety even when used as prescribed, and more so when used otherwise. More than 11.5 million Americans aged 12 or older reported misusing prescription opioids in 2016 (CDC, 2018). Opioid-related deaths in the Unites States have been at unprecedented high levels in recent years and have only increased since the COVID-19 pandemic, increasing 63% between 2019 and 2021 (Gomes et al., 2023). Demographic data shows that men aged 30-39 account for a large burden of these deaths and more recently is skewing younger (ages 15–19) (Gomes et al., 2023). Understanding this, it is important to appreciate the need to identify and support people at risk of substance related harms, especially younger men. It is also important to understand the overlap in evaluation and management of substance use disorders and CP because these conditions can coexist and may confound and exacerbate one another. Thus, the use of opioid risk evaluation and mitigation strategies (REMSs), initially and during treatment maintenance, is imperative. These strategies should routinely include—but are not limited to—the use of screening questionnaires, informed consent and treatment agreements (renewed at least annually), random testing for substances of abuse, participation in prescription drug monitoring programs (PDMPs), and provisions for overdose mitigation and rescue via naloxone.

1. Standards for prescribing controlled substances

    The clinician follows the accepted standards for prescribing controlled substances, which vary by state. Many facilities have policies and standard operating procedures around opioid prescribing, and these should be reviewed and followed as appropriate. Best-practice protocols will support clinic-wide consistency of REMS employment and opioid prescribing practices, precluding patients from "shopping" between multiple providers for increased access to opioids, and will encourage a single source for controlled substance prescriptions and dispensation to protect against dangerous redundant opioid exposure.

2. Initiating opioids

    The CDC published thorough guidelines for prescribing opioids in 2022. (Dowell, Ragan, Jones, et al., 2022). The full 2022 guidelines can be found at: https://www.cdc.gov/mmwr/volumes/71/rr/rr7103a1.htm?s_cid=rr7103a1.htm_w. A checklist for prescribers can be found at https://www.cdc.gov/drugoverdose/pdf/pdo_checklist-a.pdf.

    Along with the formal publication are numerous available educational materials, including information that is designed for patients and other non–health professionals. Key principles include the following:

    a. Opioids are not first-line or routine therapy for CP.
    b. Establish and measure goals for pain and functional improvement.
    c. Discuss benefits and risks and availability of non-opioid therapies with patient.
    d. Use immediate-release opioids when starting.
    e. Start low and go slow: Begin with the lowest appropriate dose and titrate gradually.
    f. When opioids are needed for acute pain, prescribe no more than needed (a 3- to 7-day supply is usually adequate unless severe trauma).
    g. Do not prescribe extended-release/long-acting opioids for acute pain.
    h. Follow up and reevaluate risk of harm; reduce dose or taper and discontinue if needed (**Figure 46-1**).
    i. Evaluate risk factors for opioid-related harms, which can be found at the National Institute on Drug Abuse (2021) website.
    j. Check state drug monitoring reports for high dosages and prescriptions from other providers.
    k. Use urine drug testing to identify prescribed substances and undisclosed use.
    l. Avoid concurrent benzodiazepine and opioid prescribing.
    m. Assess for and, if indicated, arrange treatment for OUD.

This chapter does not discuss specific opioids in depth, given that they are not first-line treatment for CP, and the complexity of their history, use, and risks warrant longer discussion. These authors do recommend that any professional involved in pain management be familiar with their use and history, as well as specific differences among opioids, such

---

FIGURE 46-1 Signs of Opioid Overdose

- Extreme sleepiness with an inability to awaken the person verbally or with vigorous movement (e.g., sternal rubbing)
- Slow respirations (<12 respirations/minute) and/or shallow breathing
- Vomiting
- Cyanosis of the digits and/or lips
- Constricted pupils
- Bradycardia and/or hypotension

Figure 46-1 Signs of opioid overdose

as mu agonism, synthetic properties, and mechanism of action (with the understanding that some have multiple mechanisms of action, such as tramadol). The advanced practice nurse should also be familiar with the screening, diagnosis, and treatment of OUD, including the use of medically assisted treatment with medications such as buprenorphine.

Detailed information about individual medications within the opioid family and related dosing and titration can be found at https://www.cdc.gov/drugoverdose/training/dosing/accessible/index.html and https://dailymed.nlm.nih.gov/dailymed/.

The use of a treatment agreement or opioid informed consent is strongly recommended (and may be required per facility policy). The use of the term *contract* should be avoided because it is misleading and may serve to deepen power dynamics that interfere with a collaborative patient–provider relationship. The goal of completing such an agreement should be education, expectation setting, and clarification of patient and provider roles and responsibilities (i.e., provider has a responsibility to ensure safe medication use, which may include tapering an opioid if risk or harm outweighs benefit, and the patient has the responsibility to participate in care and routine safety monitoring so that the provider may assess accurately).

3. Subsequent evaluations

Subsequent visits are determined by the clinician but initially may be monthly. More frequent visits may be required at the provider's discretion.

a. Consider safety screenings and complete as appropriate at each encounter. This may include urine toxicology (recommend at least annually once stable; more frequent at provider discretion), completion of state drug monitoring report in accordance with state and facility policy, screening for substance use, access to naloxone (It is recommended that all patients using opioids or with potential for exposure be provided with overdose education and naloxone prescription.), and ongoing monitoring of psychosocial well-being in general and/or in the context of opioid use via tools such as the Current Opioid Misuse Measure (COMM) (Butler et al., 2010).

   Special consideration for urine toxicology interpretation: Point-of-care screening in which substances of potential abuse are identified varies by facility. Clinicians should be familiar with facility testing limitations, confirmation protocols, and the metabolic pathway of the medications being evaluated in order to understand the significance of toxicology results.

b. Clinical encounters include an assessment of the following:
   i. Pain: PEG score and changes in pain since last encounter
   ii. Adverse events and side effects of therapy
   iii. Progress toward functional goals
   iv. Adherence to essential components of treatment agreement should be documented, with nonadherence to plan of care and documentation of minor or major agreement breaks noted on the problem list. Specific plans for addressing agreement breaks should be discussed and documented. For example, a setting may consider adopting the following approach: any patient with more than two major agreement breaks or three minor breaks will be referred for evaluation by a CP team to determine appropriate action to follow.

c. Refills of medications are documented in the electronic health record or paper chart, including date, name of opioid, dose, instructions for use, quantity prescribed, and number of refills. The patient brings all pain medication bottles to each and every visit at the request of the provider.

d. One primary provider writes prescriptions. In their absence, an alternate or covering provider is determined. This arrangement is reviewed with the patient.

e. Refills on controlled substances should be done during the visit, with only enough medication to last until the next visit.

f. Refills are not completed without an appointment or over the telephone.

g. Lost medications or stolen medications should not be replaced and should be recorded as a major agreement break. With rare exceptions, providers do not routinely refill lost or stolen medications. Exceptions by provider discretion require documentation of the rationale, and the incident must be recorded as a minor agreement break.

h. A treatment plan for addressing adverse effects should be discussed and documented.

4. Medication considerations
   a. Note contraindications to opioid therapy.
      i. Absolute contraindications
         a. Allergy to opioid agents
         b. Coadministration of drug capable of inducing life-threatening drug–drug interaction
         c. Active diversion of controlled substances
         d. Unwillingness or inability to comply with treatment plan
         e. Unwillingness to adjust at-risk activities that may result in serious injury/reinjury
      ii. Relative contraindications (prescribe with caution and more intensive monitoring)
         a. Meets criteria for current substance use disorder (e.g., as noted by the *Diagnostic and Statistical Manual of Mental Disorders*, 5th edition [American Psychiatric Association, 2013])

b. Acute psychiatric instability or high suicide risk
   c. History of intolerance, serious adverse effects, or lack of efficacy of opioid therapy
   d. Inability to manage opioid therapy responsibly (i.e., cognitive impairment, lack of stable and reliable caregiver or social support network)
   e. Severe social instability or inability to manage medications safely
   f. Sleep apnea and not on continuous positive airway pressure machine
   g. Advanced comorbidity or frail gestalt of overall health status that could further decrease the margin of safety of opioid use
 b. Coadministration of CNS depressants (alcohol, benzodiazepines, etc.), increasing the likelihood of respiratory depression and overdose
 c. Assess and address common adverse effects of opioid therapy: constipation, nausea and vomiting, itching, sweating, peripheral edema, urinary retention, myoclonus, hyperalgesia, dyspepsia, changes in cognition, perceptual or affective adverse effects, or sexual dysfunction.
 d. Indications to stop opioid therapy: Reduction or discontinuation of opioid should be considered if the risk of adverse effects outweighs the actual or potential benefit. Safety should be prioritized.
    i. Concerns around maintaining expectations outlined in opioid agreement/informed consent: These may include missed appointments/failure to engage in care, early refill requests, seeking medications from another provider or different pharmacy, and so forth.
    ii. Major agreement breaks include refusal of urine toxicology screen, lost or stolen medications, inappropriate drug screening results (with high-sensitivity confirmation, such as gas chromatography and a potential consultation with the lab toxicologist) indicating that the prescribed medication is absent despite patient statements of recent ingestion or that an illicit or inappropriate substance is present, patient is abusive to staff, pill count discrepancy, or request for pill count is refused.
    iii. Inappropriate use of alcohol or recreational drugs may be considered a major agreement break or cause for termination. If this is identified, consultation with addiction medicine/behavioral health and/or a specialty pain team should be offered and/or initiated.
    iv. Opioid therapy is discontinued if evaluation demonstrates a lack of efficacy, the patient desires to discontinue therapy, or the cause of pain has resolved.
    v. Opioid therapy is discontinued when there are serious safety issues as a result of treatment.
    vi. When opioid therapy is discontinued, the opioid is tapered and weaned off, unless there is dangerous or illegal behavior. Strategies for tapering and weaning have been suggested by the Medical Board of California (2023), the CDC (Dowell et al., 2022), and the VA/DoD (Opioid Therapy for Chronic Pain Work Group, 2017). Opioid therapy should be immediately discontinued for unsafe use of medications, diversion of prescription medication, or alteration or forgery of prescriptions. The provider should treat withdrawal symptoms with noncontrolled medications or refer for addiction counseling (Chou et al., 2009; Saxe et al., 2009).
    vii. If an opioid transition is warranted from one type of classic (full mu agonist) opioid to another, a dose reduction of 25%–75% should be applied to the morphine milliequivalents (MME) of the new opioid to account for a potential lack of cross-tolerance between the two opioids to protect against overdose. For more information on opioid MME and dosing, refer to the CDC website at https://www.cdc.gov/drugoverdose/training/dosing/accessible/index.html.
5. Referral to mental health and/or substance use services is recommended for the following indications:
   a. Patients with a past or current history of behaviors suggestive of substance use disorder. It is recommended to include this statement in the patient's treatment agreement.
   b. Patients with psychosocial comorbidities that hinder the treatment of pain
   c. Patients with a diagnosis of depression, anxiety, or other mental health disorders
   d. Provider's discretion: All patients may benefit from learning cognitive–behavioral techniques to improve self-care and function.
6. Consultation with pain specialist or addiction specialist is indicated in the following scenarios:
   a. Patients have significant chronic, substantiated pain with behaviors concerning for substance use.
   b. The patient's pain is not well controlled on current pain treatment plan and/or exceeds the established dose ceiling limits.
   c. The provider determines the need for consultation.
   d. The patient and/or treatment team feel the care planning is unsatisfactory to control pain and maintain functional goal.

All consultation is documented as part of the patient record. Not all patients have access to pain management specialists because of financial, insurance, location, availability, and transportation barriers. In these circumstances, review of the case with a CP team or review of the case with pain specialists by email or telephone consultation may be appropriate (Saxe et al., 2009).
   7. Buprenorphine
      a. Buprenorphine is a partial mu agonist medication within the opioid class. There are different formulations available for indications of OUD versus for pain. Buprenorphine is being used increasingly for CP as an alternative to full mu agonist opioids because of its reduced respiratory risks. The Consolidated Appropriations Act in 2023 eliminated the federal requirement for practitioners to have a waiver to prescribe medications like buprenorphine for OUD. All practitioners who have a current DEA registration that includes Schedule III authority may prescribe buprenorphine for OUD if permitted by state law (SAMHSA, 2023). It should be noted that only certain formulations of buprenorphine have a FDA indication for pain, but some other formulations are used off-label for the treatment of pain by some practitioners (Substance Abuse and Mental Health Services Administration [SAMHSA], 2022).
D. Medication cessations (transitions, withdrawal, and discontinuation syndromes)
   Abrupt medication discontinuation syndromes can range from uncomfortable to life threatening. Patients don't usually know the difference when in the midst of their subjective experience. It is the clinician's duty to properly educate and prepare patients for medication discontinuations and transitions. Particular attention and detailed care planning are indicated when transiting from one antidepressant to another to avoid serotonin syndrome and when switching from one opioid to another to avoid overdose due to a lack of cross-tolerance. Abrupt discontinuation of antidepressants, opioids, anticonvulsants, benzodiazepines, and muscle relaxants, such as carisoprodol and baclofen, can cause clinically severe symptoms. Withdrawal can be especially dangerous in the case of anticonvulsants, benzodiazepines, and muscle relaxants.

VI. Patient education and care plan implementation

A. Assist the patient and family in understanding and coping with CP and the steps of care in terms of the CP protocol.
   1. Provide verbal and written information regarding CP and nonpharmacologic and pharmacologic treatments.
   2. Assist the patient and family in obtaining all prior medical records and diagnostics, and facilitate the request for prior medical records.
B. Provide self-care strategies as mentioned in the section on nonpharmacologic management of CP.
C. Discuss management rationale for the following:
   1. Nonpharmacologic and non-opioid strategies as first-line treatment and progression to opioid as indicated
   2. Rationale for a dedicated CP team and protocol
D. Review the individual treatment agreement if the patient proceeds to the CP protocol.
   1. Discuss medication(s): dose; schedule of dosing; side effects of medications; and safety of activity on medication (e.g., driving or swimming), including risk of death if medications are used incorrectly or combined with substances or dangerous activity.
   2. Provide an explanation that one provider prescribes and one pharmacy dispenses, as well as an explanation of patient responsibility for managing medications safely, keeping appointments, and random urine screening.
   3. Provide education about and facilitation of the individual treatment plan or pain agreement (For a sample pain agreement go to https://store.samhsa.gov/sites/default/files/sma17-5053-6.pdf).
   4. Discuss overdose prevention, which includes ready access to drug and alcohol treatment services and management strategies that include access to emergency medical services and the administration of naloxone for patients and home co-habitants and caregivers. For additional information and educational resources, review the SAMHSA (2014) Opioid Overdose Toolkit at http://store.samhsa.gov/shin/content//SMA14-4742/Overdose_Toolkit.pdf.
   5. Discuss the need for documenting the consequences of nonadherence to the treatment plan, including discontinuation.
E. Encourage CP support groups.
F. Encourage mental health provider evaluation for ongoing support.

VII. CP support resources and tools

A. American Pain Society: http://www.ampainsoc.org
B. IASP: http://www.iasp.org
C. CDC Opioid Prescribing Guidelines: https://www.cdc.gov/opioids/healthcare-professionals/prescribing/guideline/index.html

References

American Geriatrics Society. (2023). Updated AGS Beers Criteria® for potentially inappropriate medication use in older adults. *Journal of the American Geriatrics Society, 71*(7), 2052–2081. https://doi.org/10.1111/jgs.18372

American Pain Foundation. (2008). Overview of American pain surveys: 2005–2006. *Journal of Pain & Palliative Care Pharmacotherapy, 22*(1), 33–38. doi:10.1080/15360280801989344

American Psychiatric Association. (2013). *Diagnostic and statistical manual of mental disorders* (5th ed.).

Barclay, L., & Nghiem, H. T. (2008). Primary care management of nonmalignant pain reviewed. *Medscape Multispecialty*. http://www.medscape.org/viewarticle/584508

Butler, S. F., Budman, S. H., Fanciullo, G. J., & Jamison, R. N. (2010). Cross validation of the current opioid misuse measure to monitor chronic pain patients on opioid therapy. *Clinical Journal of Pain, 26*(9), 770–776. doi:10.1097/AJP.0b013e3181f195ba

Caudill, M. A. (2009). *Managing pain before it manages you* (3rd ed.). Guilford Press.

Centers for Disease Control and Prevention. (2009). Prevalence and most common causes of disability among adults—United States, 2005. *Morbidity and Mortality Weekly Report, 58*(16), 421–426.

Centers for Disease Control and Prevention. (2018). *2018 Annual Surveillance Report of Drug-Related Risks and Outcomes—United States*. https://www.cdc.gov/drugoverdose/pdf/pubs/2018-cdc-drug-surveillance-report.pdf

Cheatle, M. D., Compton, P. A., Dhingra, L., Wasser, T. E., & O'Brien, C. P. (2019). Development of the revised Opioid Risk Tool to predict opioid use disorder in patients with chronic nonmalignant pain. *Journal of Pain, 20*(7), 842–851. doi:10.1016/j.jpain.2019.01.011

Chou, R., Fanciullo, G., Fine, P., Adler, J. A., Ballantyne, J. C., Davies, P., M. I. Donovan, Fishbain, D. A., Foley, K. M., Fudin, J., Gilson, A. M., Kelter, A., Mauskop, A., O'Connor, P. G., Passik, S. D., Pasternak, G. W., Portenoy, R. K., Rich, B. A., Roberts, R. G., ... American Pain Society–American Academy of Pain Medicine Opioids Guidelines Panel. (2009). Clinical guidelines for the use of chronic opioid therapy in chronic noncancer pain. *Journal of Pain, 10*(2), 113–130. doi:10.1016/j.jpain.2008.10.00

Daubresse, M., Chang, H., Yu, Y., Viswanathan, S., Shah, N. D., Stafford, R. S., Kruszewski, S. P., & Alexander, G. C. (2013). Ambulatory diagnosis and treatment of nonmalignant pain in the United States, 2000–2010. *Medical Care, 51*(10), 870–878. doi:10.1097/MLR.0b013e3182a95d86

Dowell, D., Ragan, K. R., Jones, C. M., Baldwin, G. T., Chou, R. (2022). CDC Clinical Practice Guideline for Prescribing Opioids for Pain—United States, 2022. MMWR Recomm Rep 2022;71(No. RR-3): 1–95. doi: http://dx.doi.org/10.15585/mmwr.rr7103a1

Federation of State Medical Boards of the United States, Inc (2005). Model policy for the use of controlled substances for the treatment of pain. *Journal of pain & palliative care pharmacotherapy, 19*(2), 73–78.

Fuchs-Lacelle, S., & Hadjistavropoulos, T. (2004). Development and preliminary validation of the Pain Assessment Checklist for Seniors With Limited Ability to Communicate (PACSLAC). *Pain Management in Nursing, 5*(2), 37–49. doi:10.1016/j.pmn.2003.10.001

Gomes, T., Ledlie, S., Tadrous, M., Mamdani, M., Paterson, J. M., & Juurlink, D. N. (2023). Trends in Opioid Toxicity-Related Deaths in the US Before and After the Start of the COVID-19 Pandemic, 2011-2021. JAMA network open, 6(7), e2322303. https://doi.org/10.1001/jamanetworkopen.2023.22303

Herr, K., Coyne, P. J., Key, T., Manworren, R., McCaffery, M., Merkel, S., Pelosi-Kelly, J., Wild, L., & American Society for Pain Management Nursing. (2006). Pain assessment in the nonverbal patient: Position statement with clinical practice recommendations. *Pain Management Nursing, 7*(2), 44–52. doi:10.1016/j.pmn.2006.02.003

Institute of Medicine. (2011). *Relieving pain in America: A blueprint for transforming prevention, care, education, and research*. http://www.iom.edu/~/media/Files/Report%20Files/2011/Relieving-Pain-in-America-A-Blueprint-for-Transforming-Prevention-Care-Education-Research/Pain%20Research%202011%20Report%20Brief.pdf

International Association for the Study of Pain. (2022). IASP revises its definition of pain for the first time since 1979. https://www.iasp-pain.org/wp-content/uploads/2022/04/revised-definition-flysheet_R2-1-1-1.pdf.

Krantz, M. J., Martin, J., Stimmel, B., Metha, D., & Haigney, M. C. P. (2009). QTc interval screening in methadone treatment. *Annals of Internal Medicine, 150*(6), 387–399. doi:10.7326/0003-4819-150-6-200903170-00103

Krebs, E. E., Lorenz, K. A., Bair, M. J., Damush, T. M., Wu, J., Sutherland, J. M., Asch, S. M., & Kroenke, K. (2009). Development and initial validation of the PEG, a three-item scale assessing pain intensity and interference. *Journal of General Internal Medicine, 24*(6), 733–738. doi:10.1007/s11606-009-0981-1

Kroenke, K., Spitzer R. L., & Williams J. B. (2001). The PHQ-9: validity of a brief depression severity measure. *Journal of General Internal Medicine, 16*(9), 606–613. doi:10.1046/j.1525-1497.2001.016009606.x

Medical Board of California (2023). *Guidelines for prescribing controlled substances for pain*. https://www.mbc.ca.gov/Download/Publications/pain-guidelines.pdf

Meghani, S. H., Polomano, R. C., Tait, R. C., Vallerand, A. H., Anderson, K. O., & Gallagher, R. M. (2012). Advancing a national agenda to eliminate disparities in pain care: directions for health policy, education, practice, and research. Pain medicine (Malden, Mass.), 13(1), 5–28. https://doi.org/10.1111/j.1526-4637.2011.01289.x

Morales, M. E., & Yong, R. J. (2021). Racial and Ethnic Disparities in the Treatment of Chronic Pain. Pain medicine (Malden, Mass.), 22(1), 75–90. https://doi.org/10.1093/pm/pnaa427

National Institute on Drug Abuse. (2017). *Overdose death rates, revised September 2017*. https://www.drugabuse.gov/related-topics/trends-statistics/overdose-death-rates

National Institute on Drug Abuse (2021). Opioid[SJ1] Risk Tool – OUD (ORT-OUD). https://nida.nih.gov/nidamed-medical-health-professionals/screening-tools-resources/opioid-risk-tool-oud-ort-oud

Nguyen, M., Ugarte, C., Fuller, I., Haas, G., & Portenoy, R. K. (2005). Access to care for chronic pain: racial and ethnic differences. *The Journal of Pain, 6*(5), 301–314. https://doi.org/10.1016/j.jpain.2004.12.008

Opioid Therapy for Chronic Pain Work Group. (2017). *VA/DoD clinical practice guideline for opioid therapy for chronic pain*. Version 3.0. Veterans Health Administration and Department of Defense.

Rikard, S. M., Strahan, A. E., Schmit, K. M., & Guy, G. P., Jr. (2023). Chronic Pain Among Adults—United States, 2019–2021. *MMWR. Morbidity and mortality weekly report, 72*(15), 379–385. https://doi.org/10.15585/mmwr.mm7215a1

Saxe, J. M., Smith, V., Ligon, E. D., McNerney, K., Hill, K., & Nierman, J. (2009). *Glide Health Services chronic nonmalignant pain management protocol* [Unpublished protocol]. San francisco: Glide Health Services.

Saxe, J. M., Smith, V., & McNerney, K. (2013). A blueprint to managing multiple chronic conditions and pain. *Journal of Family Practice, 62*(12), S1–S25.

Silva, M. J., Coffee, Z., Yu, C. H., & Martel, M. O. (2021). Anxiety and fear avoidance beliefs and behavior may be significant risk factors for chronic opioid analgesic therapy reliance for patients with chronic pain—results from a preliminary study. *Pain Medicine, 22*(9), 2106–2116. doi:10.1093/pm/pnab069

Spitzer, R. L., Kroenke, K., Williams, J. B., & Löwe, B. (2006). A brief measure for assessing generalized anxiety disorder: The GAD-7. *Archives of Internal Medicine, 166*(10), 1092–1097. doi:10.1001/archinte.166.10.1092

Substance Abuse and Mental Health Services Administration. (2014). *Opioid overdose toolkit.* http://store.samhsa.gov/shin/content//SMA14-4742/Overdose_Toolkit.pdf

Substance Abuse and Mental Health Services Administration. (2022). *Become a buprenorphine waivered practitioner.* https://www.samhsa.gov/medication-assisted-treatment/become-buprenorphine-waivered-practitioner

Substance Abuse and Mental Health Services Administration. (2023). *Waiver Elimination (MAT Act).* https://www.samhsa.gov/medications-substance-use-disorders/waiver-elimination-mat-act

Sullivan, M. J. L., Bishop, S. R., & Pivik, J. (1995). The pain catastrophizing scale: development and validation. *Psychological Assessment, 7*(4), 524–532.

Turk, D. (2006). Pain hurts—individuals, significant others and society! *American Pain Society Bulletin, 16*(1).

Yalcin, I., & Barrot, M. (2014). The anxiodepressive comorbidity in chronic pain. *Current Opinion in Anaesthesiology, 27*(5), 520–527. doi:10.1097/ACO.0000000000000116

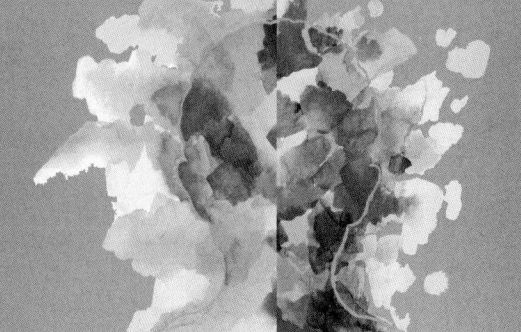

CHAPTER 47

Chronic Wound Care

Diana Roberts Mitchell and Eleanor Pascual

I. Introduction and general background

Chronic wound management by the advanced practice nurse (APN) is best achieved through a multidisciplinary team approach with an understanding of the impact on quality of life and overall health. Chronic wounds are present in approximately 2.5% of the U.S. population, with significant economic costs. Increasing rates of obesity, diabetes and an aging population will contribute to the growing challenge of managing this condition (Chandan, 2021). The classic definition of a chronic wound is a disruption in skin integrity and function that fails to progress through normal repair pathways (Lazarus et al., 1994). Underlying pathologies such as diabetes, venous and arterial insufficiency, lymphedema, vascular and autoimmune diseases, pressure injury, and inflammatory disorders are associated with chronic wounds. Chronic wounds are often referred to as *complex wounds* (Baranoski & Ayello, 2020).

Chronic wounds stall in the inflammatory stage of repair, whereas acute wounds proceed through the phases of healing (**Table 47-1**) in a timely, uncomplicated sequence, usually within a 3-month time frame (Bowers & Franco, 2020; Goldberg & Diegelmann, 2020). Surgical incisions, traumatic wounds, and burn injuries are examples of acute wounds that will heal by primary intention if free from complications of infection or dehiscence or adverse host conditions such as diabetes, vascular disorders, and compromised immune systems. In these settings, acute wounds often evolve into chronic wounds. Pressure injuries, dehisced surgical wounds, and venous and arterial ulcers typically heal by secondary intention (Bryant & Nix, 2016). A surgical intervention such as a myocutaneous flap procedure for a pressure injury may convert a previously chronic wound into an acute wound. Differentiating acute versus chronic and the phase of wound healing guides treatment approaches (Krasner, 2014).

Age, mobility, nutritional status, hydration, medications, tobacco, alcohol, and substance abuse are factors affecting the healing process. Comorbidities such as obesity, diabetes, cancer, vascular and respiratory diseases, chronic kidney disease, liver disease, and impaired immune responses will contribute to delayed wound healing. Psychosocial factors such as difficulties accessing care, housing, and nutritional support, as well as pain, stress, insomnia, dementia, depression, anxiety, and lack of social support, influence responses to treatment (Baranoski & Ayello, 2020; Krasner, 2014).

A. *Wound classifications: definitions and prevalence*
   1. Venous ulcers
      Venous disease due to reflux (valve incompetence) or obstruction (history of deep vein thrombosis) resulting in venous hypertension is the leading vascular disorder resulting in lower extremity ulceration. Venous leg ulcers comprise 60% to 80% of those affecting the lower extremity and affect an estimated 1% to 3% of the U.S. population (Bonkemeyer et al., 2019). Venous ulcers are often located in the gaiter area over the medial malleolus or mid-calf and typically have an irregular shape, shallow base, and large amount of exudate. Concurrent signs of venous disease include edema, varicose veins, atrophie blanche, lipodermatosclerosis, stasis dermatitis, and hemosiderin deposits (Wound, Ostomy, and Continence Nurse Society [WOCN], 2016). Patients may report limb discomfort and pain or a feeling of heaviness in their legs. Prolonged standing and sitting with legs dependent may increase pain and swelling. The most common risk factors for venous disease are age over 55 years, a family history of venous insufficiency, obesity, history of deep vein thrombosis (DVT), and pregnancy (Mathes, 2021). Chronic venous insufficiency may evolve into lymphedema, especially when untreated (Hamm, 2019).
   2. Arterial ulcers
      Arterial ulcers result from a reduced blood supply to the lower limb and account for 5% to 10% of lower extremity wounds. However, arterial insufficiency may complicate any ulcer etiology, such as

Table 47-1 Phases of Wound Healing Summary

Phases	Physiology
Hemostasis	Point of injury in which vasoconstriction occurs, followed by platelet activation and release of growth factors initiating the repair process
Inflammatory phase	Occurs within 24 hours to 4 days after injury and involves migration of neutrophils and macrophages supporting cell-mediated removal of bacteria and devitalized tissue
Proliferation	Occurs between post-injury day 4 and 21; fibroblasts migrate and proliferate, leading to collagen deposition and the formation of an extracellular matrix
Remodeling phase	Once the extracellular matrix is fully deposited, this phase may last years as the initial scar tissue is remodeled, type I collagen replaces type III collagen and is cross-linked, and scar tissue appears with approximately 80% of the original tensile strength

Data From Goldberg, S. R., & Diegelmann, R. F. (2020). What makes wounds chronic? *Surgical Clinics of North America, 100*(4), 681–693.

neuropathic diabetic foot ulcers, traumatic wounds, pressure injuries, or venous ulcers. Assessment of adequate vascular perfusion is critical in the care of lower extremity wounds to decrease the risk of limb loss and delayed healing. Arterial ischemia often causes severe pain, especially when the limb is elevated, and may disrupt sleep. Intermittent claudication, reproducible pain induced by exercise, may be present. The limb is frequently cool, with absent or diminished pulses. Dependent rubor and discoloration of the feet and toes may be present. Arterial ulcers present with a punched-out appearance; well-defined wound margins; and dry, necrotic tissue. The ulcer may extend to tendon, muscle, or bone. Edema is usually limited. Risk factors include smoking, diabetes, coronary artery disease, hypertension, and advanced age (Gupta et al., 2017).

3. Diabetic foot ulcers
Diabetes mellitus with poor glycemic control may lead to neuropathy and peripheral vascular disease, resulting in a diabetic foot ulcer. Improper foot care, callus formation, foot deformity, and poorly fitted footwear contribute to the risk of ulcer formation.

Approximately 54% of diabetic foot ulcers are attributed to neuropathy, 10% to ischemia, and 34% to a combination of these etiologies. Osteomyelitis is a frequent complication. An estimated 15% to 25% of individuals with diabetes will develop a foot ulcer during their lifetime, and 1% of these will end up with an amputation. Diabetic foot ulcers appear on the weight-bearing areas, the heel, the metatarsal heads, the lateral foot borders, the tips of the toes, and over the dorsum of clawed toes. Hypertrophic callus formation, fissures, Charcot foot deformity, hammer toes, necrosis, and dry gangrene are characteristics of diabetic foot ulcers.

Diabetic foot ulcers may occur at any age but are more prevalent in those 45 and older (Gupta et al., 2017; Oliver & Mutluoglu, 2021).

4. Pressure injuries
The terminology *pressure ulcer* was changed to *pressure injury* in 2016 by the National Pressure Injury Advisory Panel (NPIAP) to describe pressure damage to both intact and ulcerated skin. Pressure injuries are defined as localized skin or tissue injuries due to intense or prolonged pressure or in combination with friction and shearing forces on the skin (Gupta et al., 2017). These injuries commonly occur over bony prominences such as the sacrum, trochanters, and heels and are usually painful.

Appearance is based on depth of injury as classified by the European Pressure Ulcer Advisory Panel, NPIAP, and Pan Pacific Pressure Injury Alliance (2019):
- Stage I: nonblanchable erythema of intact skin
- Stage II: partial-thickness ulceration with exposed dermis
- Stage III: full-thickness skin loss
- Stage IV: full-thickness skin and tissue loss
- Unstageable pressure injury: obscured full-thickness skin and tissue loss
- Deep tissue injury: non-blanchable deep red, maroon, or purple discoloration

Risk factors for pressure injuries include impaired immobility, advanced age, impaired sensation, poor nutritional status, and body mass index (BMI) < 20, as well as chronic medical conditions such as diabetes, congestive heart failure, dementia, and stroke. In addition, prolonged surgery, pressure from a therapeutic or diagnostic device, and the use of vasopressors can increase the risk of developing a pressure injury.

An estimated 3 million adults annually are treated for pressure injuries in the United States (Mervis & Phillips, 2019). In 2019, hospital-acquired pressure injury (HAPI) costs were predicted to exceed $26.8 billion (Padula & Delarmente, 2019). The overall prevalence of pressure injuries in the United States from 2015 to 2019 ranged from 8.8% (in 2015) to 9.14% (in 2019) (VanGilder et al., 2021).

5. Atypical ulcers

Although the majority of wounds are of vascular etiology, approximately 20% to 23% of nonhealing wounds refractory to standard interventions are related to more complex causes, including inflammatory/autoimmune disorders, vasculopathies, malignancies, and metabolic and genetic disease (Baranoski & Ayello, 2020; Shanmugam et al., 2017). Some of the more common atypical chronic wounds are reviewed.

a. Vasculitic ulcers are due to inflammation and necrosis of the blood vessels caused by circulating antibody–antigen complexes depositing in the walls of blood vessels. The appearance varies based on the vessels involved and may range from small purpuric lesions to larger areas of necrosis. The skin lesions are often severely painful and associated with comorbidities of underlying infection, triggering medications, malignancies, rheumatoid arthritis, or connective tissue disease such as systemic lupus erythematosus and scleroderma. Cutaneous vasculitis usually presents on the lower extremities. Underlying systemic organ involvement may occur, affecting the kidneys, lungs, and gastrointestinal tract (Hamm, 2019; Shanmugan et al., 2017).

b. Pyoderma gangrenosum is not due to infection or gangrene but to an autoimmune disorder in which traumatic wounds, surgical sites, or small skin lesions evolve into inflamed, painful, necrosed ulcers, commonly with distinct violaceous borders. The ulcers exhibit pathergy— increasing in size with minimal trauma or debridement. This disorder is often associated with inflammatory bowel disease, arthritis, lymphomas, systemic lupus, and malignancies (Pompeo, 2016).

c. Malignant etiologies include basal and squamous skin cancer, melanoma, Marjolijn ulcers, cutaneous lymphomas, and fungating wounds in which metastatic spread from a tumor ulcerates the skin. Associated symptoms may include necrosis, malodor, bleeding, heavy microbial overgrowth, and pain (Vardhan et al., 2019). In addition, treatment of skin cancer may result in a chronic wound after radiation therapy. Radiation skin ulcers may manifest immediately following treatment or years later (Wei et al., 2018). Simple wounds in areas previously treated by radiation may evolve into chronic ulcers. These ulcers are frequently necrotic and lack healthy granulation (Seaman, 2017).

d. Calciphylaxis causes skin ulceration as a result of a metabolic disorder associated with secondary hyperparathyroidism. An estimated 1%–4% of patients on dialysis may develop this disorder. It is characterized by vascular and cutaneous calcification leading to necrotic ulcer formation. These wounds are severely painful and increase in size and ulceration without treatment. Calciphylaxis is associated with a high mortality rate, with less than 50% of patients surviving for over a year (Shanmugan et al., 2017).

II. Database

A. *Subjective*

1. Past medical history and risk factors: advanced age; *obesity*; malnutrition; immobility; diabetes; autoimmune disease; vascular disease; history of DVT; cancer; thyroid disease; respiratory disease; neurological disorders such as stroke or Parkinson disease; chronic kidney disease; history of trauma; past infections such as methicillin-resistant *Staphylococcus aureus* (MRSA), Lyme disease, or necrotizing fasciitis; dermatologic conditions such as psoriasis, bullous pemphigoid, stasis dermatitis, and fungal infections

2. Surgical history: surgical venous interventions, cardiovascular surgery, angioplasties, amputations, past surgical complications

3. Family history: diabetes, venous disease, arterial disease, lymphedema, sickle cell

4. Social history: social support network, caregiver support, access to transportation, nutrition, housing status, tobacco, alcohol, substance abuse, lifestyle activities (e.g., exercise, recreation)

5. Occupational history: prolonged standing, sitting, ability to work

6. Medications and allergies: past antibiotic therapy, medications influencing immune response and healing (anticoagulants; antibiotics, systemic and topical; anti-inflammatory drugs: ibuprofen, aspirin, dapsone; narcotics; anticonvulsants; corticosteroids; chemotherapeutic agents; hydroxyurea; angiotensin-converting enzyme I [ACE-I] antihypertensives; immunosuppressants; tumor necrosis factor alpha [TNF-α] inhibitors; T-cell inhibitors; disease-modifying antirheumatic drugs (DMARDs); hormones; diuretics; pentoxifylline; herbal supplements and vitamins (Beitz, 2017)

7. Review of systems:
   a. Constitutional: fever, chills, malaise, pain (location, severity, quality, timing, duration, interventions which offer relief), quality of sleep, appetite, weight loss, mental well-being, anxiety, depression, fatigue
   b. Cardiovascular: dependent or chronic edema, varicose veins, claudication, rest pain
   c. Respiratory: use of supplemental oxygen, shortness of breath
   d. Gastrointestinal: bowel habits (diarrhea, constipation, incontinence), liver disease, weight gain or loss, eating habits, nutritional supplements

e. Genitourinary: incontinence, dialysis
f. Musculoskeletal: activity levels, limitations to mobility, ability to ambulate, transition, reposition, assistive devices (e.g., cane, walker, wheelchair, Hoyer lift)
g. Neurologic: peripheral neuropathy, neuropathic pain, neurological deficits, paralysis, memory, mood
h. Skin: previous wounds or infectious disorders, rashes, dermatologic disorders, cysts, nodules, skin growths, pruritus, bleeding, bruising

B. Objective
1. Vital signs: Assess for changes from baseline. Monitor weight. Obtain pain assessment. Note that many elderly or immunocompromised patients do not exhibit fever with a cellulitic wound infection or sepsis. Pain may be absent or diminished in patients with neuropathy or deeply damaged necrotic wounds.
2. Respiratory assessment: Obtain pulse oximeter reading in patients with shortness of breath and/or labored respirations. Assess breath sounds in patients with new or increased congestion.
3. Cardiovascular: Assess arterial pulses with all extremity wounds and in patients with peripheral vascular disease or diabetes; assess for cyanosis, discoloration of extremities, pallor, mottling, temperature changes, edema, varicose veins; check for Stemmer's sign (**Box 47-1**) in patients with lower extremity edema.
4. Musculoskeletal: Assess range of motion; gait; and structural deformities such as contractures, amputations, and Charcot foot.
5. Neurologic: Assess mental status/orientation; assess for peripheral neuropathy with monofilament test.
6. Skin: Measure length, width, and depth of wound; note location and appearance—irregular shape is often characteristic of venous ulcers versus the punched-out annular shape of arterial ulceration. Note tissue damage—superficial, partial or full thickness. Assess tissue quality—tissue slough, eschar, blisters, bullae, hematomas, ecchymosis, granulation, epithelialization. Note exudate: amount, color, odor. Assess wound edges, periwound skin condition, spreading erythema, and any skin temperature changes (e.g., increased warmth or coolness). In full-thickness ulcers, note any underlying structures—tendon, bone. Gently probe if safe to do so; avoid if underlying arterial graft is present. Note any rashes, dry and scaly skin, dystrophic nails, nodules, and plaques.
7. Review of relevant laboratory findings:
a. Tissue swab culture report: Chronic wounds become colonized; culture reports may not reflect true infection and lead to misuse of systemic antibiotics. Use only in correlation with clinical signs of infection to target antibiotic therapy (**Box 47-2**).
b. Tissue biopsy: When warranted, a tissue biopsy culture with over 10^5 microorganisms is the gold standard for determining infection (Baranoski & Ayello, 2020) (**Box 47-3**). Review past biopsies that pertain to wound examination, such as those to rule out skin cancer and autoimmune skin disorders. Biopsies should be obtained only by providers with specialty training in obtaining the specimen correctly.

Box 47-2 Obtaining a Wound Culture

The quantitative swab culture identifies the bacterial species of the infection and is used to assist in selecting the appropriate antibiotic therapy.

The Levine Quantitative Swab Technique:

1. Use proper personal protective equipment (PPE), such as gloves, face shields, and nonporous gowns.
2. Gather all supplies needed:
   - Normal saline solution
   - 10-cc syringe
   - Sterile gauze (4 × 4)
   - Anaerobe and aerobic culture swab
   - Label with the correct patient information
   - Biohazard plastic bag for culture transport
3. Identify 1 cm of clean wound tissue to swab. Infection resides in viable tissue; do not swab eschar or periwound skin, which will lead to false results.
4. Cleanse the wound with preservative-free sterile saline or water.
5. Apply the swab and rotate with pressure over 1–2 cm of wound tissue for 5 seconds (trying to elicit fluid).
6. When tip is saturated, place in sterile container, avoiding contamination.
7. Transport within 2 hour to the laboratory to keep the specimen stable.
(Byrant & Nix, 2016)

Box 47-1 Assessing for Stemmer's Sign

The Stemmer's sign (or Kaposi–Stemmer sign) is a clinical indication of lymphedema. The clinician performs the test by pinching the skin at the base of the patient's second toe on the dorsal aspect of the foot or the middle finger of the hand. Skin that does not fold up into a tent is a positive Stemmer's sign and considered a sign of lymphedema (Hamm, 2019).

c. Imaging: Review or order as indicated: x-ray reports; arterial noninvasive studies, such as arterial ultrasound and ankle–brachial index (ABI) (**Table 47-2**); venous reflux studies; and magnetic resonance imaging (MRI) scans related to wound etiology, such as those to rule out osteomyelitis. Review any past wound photos to note wound evolution, and obtain current photos.

d. Lab findings: Complete blood count (CBC) with differential, platelet count, transferrin, erythrocyte sedimentation rate, creatinine and glomerular filtration rate, hemoglobin A1c, C-reactive protein (CRP), prealbumin, vitamin D level, zinc, coagulation labs, hepatitis panel. If suspected calciphylaxis, check calcium, phosphorus, and parathyroid hormone. If atypical ulcer, check immune panels: immunoglobulin (Ig)G, IgM, IgA, rheumatoid factor, hepatitis B, hepatitis C, HIV, cryoglobulins, antinuclear antibodies, antiphospholipid antibodies.

Box 47-3 Obtaining a Tissue Biopsy

Tissue biopsy is considered the gold standard for determining true wound infection and is indicated in wounds resistant to past antimicrobial therapies. Tissue biopsy for pathology is warranted in the diagnosis of atypical skin ulcers to rule out malignancies and autoimmune skin disorders such as vasculitis. However, tissue biopsy is an invasive procedure, and the risks versus benefits must be assessed. The procedure is performed by a trained provider (physician, advanced practice nurse, or physician assistant). A punch biopsy or scalpel may be used to obtain at least a 3-mm sample. Local injectable anesthesia may be provided with 1% preservative-free lidocaine. The open wound is cleansed with a preservative-free sterile solution, and a specimen is taken from viable granulation tissue. Bleeding should be controlled. The specimen is placed in a specimen container containing formalin and sent to the lab for processing (Bryant & Nix, 2016; WOCN, 2016).

III. Assessment

Based on findings of systems review, physical exam, imaging, and laboratory data, form diagnosis and differential diagnoses as indicated. Note any related diagnoses obtained from exams, such as malnutrition, edema, lymphedema, neuropathy, obesity, protein malnutrition, and failure to thrive (Seaman, 2010).

Table 47-2 Procedure for obtaining an ABI (Ankle-Brachial Index)

1. Place the patient in a supine position.
2. Using a doppler probe, search for the brachial pulse. Once audible, leave the doppler in place and inflate the cuff above the last brachial pulse sound. Slowly deflate the cuff until a brachial pulse sound is audible. Record the highest brachial pressure.
3. Place the blood pressure cuff above the malleoli. Place the Doppler probe at a 45-degree angle on the dorsalis pedis or posterior tibial artery.
4. Inflate the cuff until the pulse is no longer audible then slowly deflate the cuff while monitoring the return of the pulse signal. The first audible return of the dorsalis pedis is recorded as the ankle systolic pressure. The higher of the two systolic pressures in each leg is sued to calculate the ABI.
5. Calculate the ABI by dividing the higher of the two ankle pressures by the higher of the two brachial pressures.

ABI Value	Interpretation
> 1.3	Abnormally high range- results not reliable due to calcification of vessel wall TBI or TcPO2 indicated
0.90 to 1.3	Normal Range
0.75 - 0.90	Borderline perfusion disease
0.50 - 0.75	Severe disease
< 0.5	Severe ischemia, wound healing unlikely unless revascularization accomplished

Data from Baranoski, S. & Ayello, Elizabeth. (2020). Wound care essentials: Practice principles.

IV. Plan
A. *Multidisciplinary approach to care: Based on etiology and patient care needs, consult and work with team members in formulating the treatment plan. The patient, family members, and primary care providers are consulted foremost in developing treatment goals and plans (Couch, 2017). Additional team members/consultations may include the following:*
   1. Home Health: Patients who are homebound, require caregiver assistance, or have incapacitating disease states are eligible for home health nursing care. Consult with home health staff to formulate a plan to best meet patient needs in the home setting. Order pressure-relief mattresses, wheelchair and support devices as indicated.
   2. Dermatology: Consult on atypical wound management, patients requiring biopsy, malignant skin growth management, and autoimmune skin disorders. Consult on rashes and skin lesions not responding to standard therapy.
   3. Rheumatology: Obtain consultation on all autoimmune-related skin disorders
   4. Cardiovascular: Consult on ulcers with arterial or venous etiology, determine adequate flow for healing, and order appropriate compression garments or wraps in management of venous ulcers and lower extremity lymphedema.
   5. Podiatry: Obtain podiatry consult on all diabetic foot ulcers and wounds below the ankle.
   6. Infectious disease: Consult when wounds are growing resistant organisms, in patients with multiple antibiotic allergies, and in cases with infectious wound complications such as osteomyelitis.
   7. Nephrology: Consult on all patients with calciphylaxis. Consult nephrology when patients on dialysis or those with chronic kidney disease (CKD) require systemic antibiotic therapy.
   8. Orthopedics: Obtain consultation on ulcers complicated by osteomyelitis, complex hand ulcers, and joint complications.
   9. General surgery: Consult when a wound requires more debridement than can be safely performed in an outpatient clinic setting.
   10. Plastic surgery: Consult on wounds failing to close, potentially requiring graft or flap procedures; hypertrophic or keloid scar formation are additional consult indications.
   11. Physical therapy: Consult on strategies to increase patient mobility; ability to transfer; increase safety measures at home; improve gait; manage lymphedema; and obtain assistive mobility devices, custom-fit compression garments, and pneumatic pumps.
   12. Nutritionists: Consult for patients with signs of malnourishment, patients with special dietary needs, and patients with low or severely high body mass index.
   13. Social services: Obtain if patient lacks access to housing, transportation, or nutrition or if there are safety issues in the home. Report to social services and law authorities any patients with a positive screening or signs of domestic violence or abuse.
B. Diagnostic tests
   1. If suspected peripheral vascular disease in patients with diabetes or those with diminished pedal pulses and if therapeutic compression such as Unna boot application is planned, obtain an ABI. Noninvasive arterial doppler studies, including toe–brachial index (TBI), transcutaneous oxygen measurement (TCOM), and duplex ultrasounds provide information on perfusion in patients with arterial ulceration (Gupta et al., 2017). In patients with insufficient arterial flow to support wound healing, additional arterial testing such as arteriograms, CTA and MRA may be ordered in consult with vascular surgery prior to revascularization procedures. (Baranoski & Ayello, 2020).
   2. Tissue biopsy: If suspected atypical ulcer, obtain tissue biopsy for pathology. Biopsy wounds failing to progress or enlarging after 6–8 weeks of wound treatment. Obtain a biopsy for microbial studies in cases where antibiotic therapy based on swab culture and sensitivities fails to resolve infection (Baranoski & Ayello, 2020).
   3. Obtain additional lab work indicated in monitoring response to therapy: cultures, CBC, hemoglobin A1c, prealbumin, CRP, erythrocyte sedimentation rate.
   4. Obtain imaging as indicated: X-ray as an initial exam in assessing for osteomyelitis, MRI if indicated by x-ray or in patients with wounds probing to bone. Consult with orthopedics in obtaining a bone biopsy for directing treatment of osteomyelitis. Consult with vascular surgery regarding further vascular studies indicated, such as angiograms, venous reflux duplex imaging, or MRI scans. Obtain an immediate ultrasound of the lower extremity for any patient who exhibits symptoms of a DVT: acute swelling, pain, erythema of the calf, + Homan's sign (Thachil, 2014).
C. *Topical wound therapy*
   Choose dressings by the following criteria: promotion of moist healing, decrease of bioburden, decrease in pain, protection of wound bed, cost-effectiveness, ability of patient or caregiver to apply, and availability of materials needed. See **Table 47-3** for a list of topical care categories. Determine frequency of dressing changes based on wound condition, amount of exudate, and patient's access to assistance as needed. Plan reassessment of wound and topical treatment based on wound severity and risk of complications.
D. *Debridement*
   If the wound contains slough, eschar, or biofilm, debridement is indicated. **(Note that if the wound exhibits pathergy as characteristic of pyoderma gangrenosum, sharp and mechanical debridement is contraindicated until the autoimmune**

Table 47-3 Topical Wound Dressing Categories

Categories	Product Examples	Indications
Antimicrobials	Silver-based gels, alginates, hydrofibers and foams, silver sulfadiazine, Manuka honey–based gels, Manuka honey hydrocolloids and alginates, mupirocin, cadexomer iodine-based gels, sodium hypochlorite solutions and gels, hypochlorous acid, polyhexamethylene biguanide (PHMB), hypertonic saline gauze	Clinical signs of wound infection: odor, purulence, necrosis, increased size and exudate, swab cultures with heavy microbial growth correlated with wound assessment or tissue culture with greater than 10^6 colony growth
Bacteriostatic agents	Methylene blue, gentian violet foam composites, hydrophilic polyurethane foams combined with surfactants	Control of bioburden by inhibiting bacterial growth
Absorbent dressings	Hydrophilic polyurethane foams, polyvinyl foam, silicone foam, alginates, hydrofibers, polymer-based dressings	For heavily draining wounds, foams may be combined with antimicrobials or bacteriostatic agents.
Barrier dressings	Petrolatum-based ointments or impregnated gauze, hydrocolloids, zinc paste, transparent polyurethane films, foams	Decrease friction and pressure, provide protection, and promote moist healing.
Debriding agents	Manuka honey gel, granular zinc paste gel, enzymatic ointment, hydrocolloids	Enzymatic debriding ointments such as collagenase dissolve eschar. Applied daily over time, hydrocolloids may be used for autolytic debridement. Manuka honey and granular zinc provide mechanical debridement and assist in tissue slough removal.
Hydrogels	May be bacteriostatic, antimicrobial, or combined with collagen or other cell-growth–promoting factors	Provide moisture to dry wound beds and promote moist healing.
Matrix dressings	Include collagen powders; gels; and porcine, ovine, placental, extracellular matrix, and bioengineered skin substitutes	Used on granulation beds to promote a framework for re-epithelialization in stalled chronic wounds

reaction is under control. **Arterial ulcers should not be debrided unless revascularization has been performed and vascular testing indicates sufficient flow.**) Debridement methods include sharp surgical, enzymatic, mechanical, autolytic, ultrasound, pulsed lavage and biologic. Debridement should be performed only by clinicians with certified training in the procedure (Baranoski & Ayello, 2020).

E. *Medications*

Review medications for those that interfere with the healing process, and offer alternatives when possible. Consult with the primary care provider in reducing polypharmacy. Check wound cultures for sensitivities and review past antibiotic usage. Antibiotics are indicated if cellulitis is present. Topical steroids are beneficial in the short-term treatment of stasis dermatitis. Pentoxifylline may be used in patients with venous and arterial leg ulcers to improve flow by reducing viscosity (Beitz, 2017). Diuretics such as furosemide will not benefit patients with lower extremity ulcers due to lymphedema but may assist in managing patients with blistering leg ulcers related to edema caused by congestive heart failure (CHF).

F. *Nutritional support*

Encourage hydration with water (take into account patients with limited fluid restrictions, as in CHF and CKD). General recommendations are to increase intake of vegetables, protein, and whole fruit; avoid sugar and processed foods; and limit grains. Most patients will benefit from a quality multivitamin during the healing process; avoid iron supplementation unless iron-deficiency anemia is present. If malnourishment is present, consult with a nutritionist and consider high-caloric/high-protein liquid supplementation between meals, 1–2 times daily (Quain, 2015).

G. *Adjunctive therapies*

Consider specialized therapies when wound management does not achieve measurable results. These may include negative wound pressure therapy, hyperbaric oxygen therapy, platelet-rich plasma, growth factors, skin substitutes, ultraviolet light, and electrical stimulation. Review contraindications, weigh risks versus benefits, and employ under wound specialist supervision (Baranoski & Ayello, 2020).

H. Education

Discuss lifestyle factors affecting wound healing, such as underlying disease management, nutrition, and mobility. Provide written instructions on wound care, any additional diagnostic tests ordered, nutritional support, positioning, and physical therapy exercises as indicated. Demonstrate wound care procedures. Provide contact information for patient, family, and caregivers to provide support in the delivery of wound care. Develop a plan that includes ongoing reassessment of goals and interventions with patient, family, care providers, and multidisciplinary team members.

References

Baranoski, S., & Ayello, E. A. (2020). *Wound care essentials.* Wolters Kluwer.

Beitz, J. M. (2017). Pharmacologic impact (aka "Breaking Bad") of medications on wound healing and wound development: A literature-based overview. *Ostomy Wound Management, 63*(3), 18–28.

Bonkemeyer Millan, S., Gan, R. & Townsend, P. E. (2019). Venous ulcers: Diagnosis and treatment. *American Family Physician, 100*(5), 298–305.

Bowers, S., & Franco, E. (2020). Chronic wounds: Evaluation and management. *American Family Physician, 101*(3), 159–166.

Bryant, R. A., & Nix, D. P. (2016). *Acute & chronic wounds: Current management concepts* (5th ed.). Elsevier Mosby.

Chandan, K. (2021). Human wound and its bioburden: Updated 2020 compendium of estimates. *Advanced Wound Care, 10*(5), 281–292.

Couch, K. S. (2017). The expanding role of the nurse & NP in chronic wound care. *Today's Wound Clinic,* 10–11. Retrieved from http://www.todaysclinic.com

European Pressure Ulcer Advisory Panel, National Pressure Injury Advisory Panel, and Pan Pacific Pressure Injury Alliance. (2019). *Prevention and treatment of pressure ulcers/injuries: quick reference guide.* https://www.epuap.org/wp-content/uploads/2016/10/quick-reference-guide-digital-npuap-epuap-pppia-jan2016.pdf

Goldberg, S. R., & Diegelmann, R. F. (2020). What makes wounds chronic? *Surgical Clinics of North America, 100*(4), 681–693.

Gupta, S., Andersen, C., Black, J., de Leon, J., Fife, C., Lantis III, J. C., Niezgoda, J., Snyder, R., Sumpio, B., Tettlebacch, W., Treadwell, T., Weir, D., & Silverman, R. P. (2017). Management of chronic wounds: Diagnosis, preparation, treatment, and follow-up. *Wounds, 29*(Suppl. 9), S19–S36.

Hamm, R. L. (2019). *Wound diagnosis and treatment.* McGraw-Hill Education.

Krasner, D. L. (2014). *Chronic wound care: The essentials.* HMP Communications.

Lazarus, G. S., Cooper, D. M., Knighton, D. R., Margolis, D. J., Pecoraro, R. E., Rodeheaver, G., & Robeson, M. C. (1994). Definitions and guidelines for assessment of wounds and evaluation of healing. *Archives of Dermatology, 130*(4), 489–493.

Mathes, B.M. (2021). Clinical manifestations of lower extremity chronic venous disease. *UpToDate.* http://www.uptodate.com

Mervis, J. S., & Phillips, T. J. (2019). Pressure ulcers: Pathophysiology, epidemiology, risk factors, and presentation. *Journal of the American Academy of Dermatology, 81*(4), 881–890. https://doi.org/10.1016/j.jaad.2018.12.069

Oliver, T. I., & Mutluoglu, M. (2021). Diabetic foot ulcer. *StatPearls.* http://www.ncbi.gov/books/NBK537328/

Padula, W. V., & Delarmente, B. A. (2019). The national cost of hospital-acquired pressure injuries in the United States. *International Wound Journal, 16*(3), 634–640. https://doi.org/10.1111/iwj.13071

Pompeo, M. Q. (2016). Pyoderma gangrenosum: Recognition and management. *Wounds, 28*(1), 7–13.

Quain, A. M. (2015). Nutrition in wound management: A comprehensive overview. *Wounds, 27*(12), 327–335.

Seaman, S. (2010). *Comprehensive assessment of patients with chronic wounds.* SAWC Spring 2010 Pre-Conference Supplement. http://www.sawc.net

Seaman, S. (2017). Radiation-induced skin injury: A challenging issue in the outpatient wound clinic. *Today's Wound Clinic, 11*(11), 9–14.

Shanmugan, V. K., Angra, D., Rahimi, H., & McNish, S. (2017). Vasculitic and autoimmune wounds. *Journal of Vascular Surgery: Venous and Lymphedema Disorders, 5*(2), 280–292.

Thachil, J. (2014). Deep vein thrombosis. *Hematology, 19*(5), 309–310.

VanGilder, C. A., Cox, J., Edsberg, L. E., & Koloms, K. (2021, December). Pressure injury prevalence in acute care hospitals with unit-specific analysis: Results from the International Pressure Ulcer Prevalence (IPUP) survey database. *Journal of Wound, Ostomy, and Continence Nursing, 48*(6), 492–503.

Vardhan, M., Flaminio, Z., Sapru, S., Tilley, C. P., Fu, M. R., Comfort, C., Li, X., & Saxena, D. (2019). The microbiome, malignant fungating wounds, and palliative care. *Frontiers in Cellular and Infection Microbiology, 9,* 373. https://doi.org/10.3389/fcimb.2019.00373

Wei, J., Meng, L., Hou, X., Qu, C., Wang, B., Xin, Y., & Jiang, X. (2018). Radiation-induced skin reactions: Mechanism and treatment. *Cancer Management and Research, 11,* 167–177. https://doi.org/10.2147/CMAR.S188655

Wound, Ostomy, and Continence Nurse Society. (2016). *Core curriculum: Wound management.* Wolters Kluwer.

CHAPTER 48

Dementia

Nhat Bui and Jennifer Merrilees

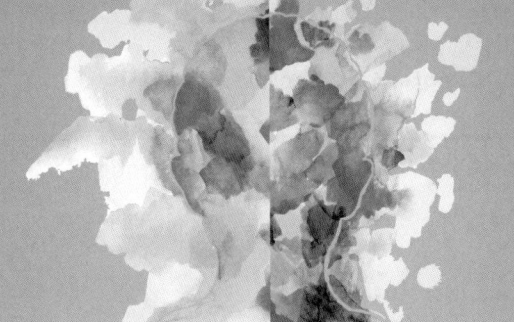

I. Introduction and general background

Dementia refers to diseases and conditions characterized by a decline in cognitive function such as difficulties with memory, language and problem solving and other thinking skills that negatively affects a person's ability to perform daily activities (Alzheimer's Association, 2023). Neurodegenerative diseases that cause dementia are typically due to a slowly progressive dysfunction and death of neurons in regions of the brain that support cognitive function. Cognitive impairment has been recategorized as a neurocognitive disorder that is either minor (cognitive impairment with no impact on daily function) or major (cognitive impairment that interferes with daily function). Presenting symptoms are varied and can include memory loss, executive dysfunction, speech and language changes, motor symptoms, and/or behavioral and emotional symptoms and other symptoms depending on where in the brain the process is occurring (Plassman et al., 2007).

Common causes of dementia include Alzheimer disease (AD), vascular dementia, frontotemporal dementia (FTD), and dementia with Lewy bodies (DLB). Other disorders that may be associated with dementia are Huntington disease, HIV/AIDS, Parkinson disease (PD), alcohol use, and head trauma. Rapidly progressive dementias are rare and include Creutzfeldt–Jakob disease. There are also nondegenerative causes of dementia, such as cerebrovascular disease, among others. For many individuals (especially those of older age), there are multiple types of pathology present. There is no cure for dementia, although current research aimed at the reversal or prevention of dementia is underway.

Although there is no single test for dementia, the evaluation is directed at clarifying the onset and progression of symptoms, ruling out reversible conditions, and specifying the likely underlying cause for the dementia (**Table 48-1**). Approximately 9% of patients have a potentially treatable cause of dementia (e.g., thyroid abnormality, vitamin deficiency, depression, delirium, medication side effects, and excessive use of alcohol and other substances). Thus, a comprehensive evaluation is critical to correctly identify and diagnose patients with dementia and initiate appropriate management (Clarfield, 2003).

There is significant variation in dementia incidence among ethnic and racial groups. The highest incidence of Alzheimer's or other dementias is in non-Hispanic Black and Hispanic older adults. It is lowest among Asian Americans and intermediate among Latinos, Pacific Islanders, and White Americans. It is projected that 38% of Black Americans, 35% of American Indians/Alaskan Natives, 32% of Latinos, 30% of White Americans, 28% of Asian Americans, and 25% of Pacific Islanders will develop dementia by 2040 (Mayeda et al., 2016). The difference in risk for dementia among racial and ethnic groups can be explained by socioeconomic disparities produced by the historic and continued marginalization of Hispanic and Black people. Structural racism influences access to quality health care, occupational safety, employment opportunities and environmental factors that increase risk for dementia as well as chronic conditions that are associated with developing dementia (Alzheimer's Association, 2023).

A. *Alzheimer disease (AD)*
  1. Definition and overview
     AD is the most common cause of dementia. Neuronal death is caused by the overaccumulation of amyloid plaques and neurofibrillary tangles. Although the sites of earliest damage in AD are the hippocampus and entorhinal cortex (areas important to memory function), the disease eventually affects multiple regions of the brain. The strongest risk factor for AD is advanced age, although prior head injury; family history of AD; and cardiovascular factors, such as hypertension, pose an increased risk for the development of AD. When AD occurs in a person younger than age 65, it is referred to as *early-age onset*, *younger onset*, or *early-onset AD*. Most cases of AD are not familial, although genetic risk increases in early-onset AD when a first-degree relative has AD and in the presence of certain genetic mutations.

Table 48-1 Possible Causes of Dementia (Partial List)

Neurodegenerative	Alzheimer disease, Down syndrome, Parkinson disease, dementia with Lewy bodies, frontotemporal dementia, multisystem atrophy, Huntington disease
Cerebrovascular	Vascular dementia, vasculitis
Prion associated	Creutzfeldt–Jakob disease, Gerstmann–Sträussler–Scheinker syndrome, fatal familial insomnia
Neurogenetic	Spinocerebellar ataxias, mitochondrial encephalopathies, Wilson disease
Infectious	Meningitis, encephalitis, leukoencephalopathy, neurosyphilis, Whipple disease, HIV
Toxic or metabolic	Systemic: thyroid, parathyroid, adrenal, liver, kidney, sarcoidosis, vitamin deficiencies, hypoxia/ischemia, drugs, alcohol, heavy metals
Other	Multiple sclerosis, neoplastic, hydrocephalus

2. Prevalence
More than one in nine people age 65 and older have AD, whereas one in three people age 85 and older have AD. People younger than 65 can also develop AD. While prevalence studies of early or younger onset AD are limited, researchers believe about 200,000 people have younger-onset dementia (Alzheimer's Association, 2023). More women than men have AD, largely because women typically live longer than men. It is estimated that a growing number of Americans will live into their 80s and 90s, resulting in even greater numbers of people with dementia. By 2050, the number of people age 65 and older with AD is projected to reach over 12 million people (Alzheimer's Association, 2023).

B. *Vascular dementia*
1. Definition and overview
Vascular dementia (also called *multi-infarct dementia*) is caused by cerebrovascular ischemia, cerebral small vessel disease, and lacunar infarcts in the brain (often referred to as *white-matter disease*). Cerebrovascular disease will be present in people with dementia but is rarely the only cause. The current model points toward a multifactorial cause of cognitive impairment as one ages, in which vascular factors such as atherosclerosis, infarcts, and amyloid angiopathy contribute alongside other neurodegenerative causes. Symptoms are similar to those of AD, although the onset may be more easily identified, and the progression of symptoms can be characterized by "stepwise" changes reflecting the occurrence of strokes. Risk factors include strokes, hypertension, hypercholesteremia, and diabetes. Vascular dementia may coexist with AD or DLB.

2. Prevalence
Vascular dementia is considered the second-most-common cause of dementia About 5-10% of people with dementia is caused by vascular dementia alone (Rizzi et al., 2014). It is more commonly a mixed pathology or co-occurring with a neurodegenerative disease such as Alzheimer's disease (Alzheimer's Association, 2023). It is due to vascular factors as people age, including presence of atherosclerosis, infarcts, and amyloid angiopathy that contribute to neurodegeneration (Wolters, 2019).

C. *Dementia with Lewy bodies (DLB)*
1. Definition and overview
The symptoms of DLB can be similar to those of AD, with several important distinctions. Core diagnostic criteria for DLB are as follows: recurrent visual hallucinations, parkinsonian signs (resting tremor, stiffness or rigidity, slowness of movement, shuffling gait), rapid eye movement (REM) sleep behavior disorder, and fluctuations in alertness and attention (McKeith, 2017). DLB is caused by the accumulation of Lewy bodies containing α-synuclein, which deposit within neurons and affect multiple brain regions, which is also seen in PD. DLB should be diagnosed when dementia occurs before or concurrently with parkinsonism. Although the term *Parkinson disease dementia* (PDD) can be used to describe dementia that occurs in the context of a well-established PD, generic terms such as *Lewy body disease* are often helpful and acceptable in clinical practice.

2. Prevalence
DLB is considered the third-most-common cause of dementia. It affects up to 5% of the general population and accounts for approximately 15-20% of all cases of dementia based on neuropathological studies (Kane, 2018)). Similar to other neurodegenerative diseases, the prevalence of DLB increases with age, with the average age of onset being 75 years (Hogan et al., 2016).

D. *Frontotemporal dementia (FTD)*
1. Definition and overview
FTD refers to a heterogeneous group of syndromes caused by focal damage to the frontal and anterior temporal lobes of the brain. The focal damage results in behavioral disorders, executive dysfunction, and language deficits. FTD is divided into two major subtypes: behavioral-variant frontotemporal dementia (bvFTD) and aphasia syndromes. The aphasia syndromes include a semantic variant and progressive nonfluent aphasia (PNFA). bvFTD is the

most common clinical subtype and is typically characterized by social disinhibition, impulsivity, apathy, loss of empathy, and executive dysfunction. The semantic variant is characterized by difficulty naming common objects, people, and words, with progressive trouble in identifying the meaning of those items they are trying to name. Complaints about fluency or speech rhythm and pronunciation occur with PNFA. Other FTD-related movement disorders include corticobasal degeneration, progressive supranuclear palsy, and motor neuron disease. Tau, TDP-43, and progranulin are proteins involved in cellular dysfunction and death that occur with FTD.

2. Prevalence
FTD typically presents in mid- to later life, with approximately 60% of people presenting between 45 and 64 years of age. The prevalence of FTD is 15 to 22 per 100,000 and 81 per 100,000 cases of dementia among people under the age of 65. FTD is more common than AD in patients under the age of 60 years and accounts for 20% of all patients with degenerative dementias. Population studies show nearly equal distribution by sex assigned at birth. FTD is frequently familial and hereditary, with up to 40% of affected individuals having a significant family history. Nongenetic risk factors are yet to be identified (Ratnavalli et al., 2002).

E. *Mixed dementia*
1. Definition and overview
Mixed dementia refers to the coexistence of one or more neurodegenerative and cerebrovascular disease pathologies. Older adults with AD pathology often have concurrent cerebrovascular disease pathologies, as well as other neurodegenerative diseases. Common combinations include AD and vascular dementia, AD with DLB, and AD with vascular dementia and DLB.

2. Prevalence
Advances in research have shown that the presence of mixed pathologies is relatively common. Evidence shows that mixed pathologies may account for a larger proportion of the variability of cognitive impairment in aging. About half of people with dementia have mixed pathology.

II. Database (may include but is not limited to)

A. *Subjective* (**Table 48-2**)
One of the most important steps in the evaluation of a person with suspected dementia is to obtain a description of the symptoms and associated features with the patient and an informant (someone who knows the patient well). It is critical to involve an informant to verify information: patients with dementia may have limited insight and may mask or downplay their deficits. The focus of the interview is aimed at onset, duration, and progression of symptoms and whether they represent a change from the patient's baseline abilities. Taking a careful history is critical to determine how the symptoms have progressed and the potential temporal relationships of related factors (e.g., medical conditions, medications, stroke events). It is important to understand the pattern and character of the deficits. Patients and families can be encouraged to maintain a log or journal to help in the evaluation of the person with suspected cognitive deficits. It can be helpful to start with general questions, such as "What are you concerned about?" The practitioner should then move to more specific questions, such as "What was the very first thing that was different or caused your concern?" and "How have the symptoms progressed—have they worsened, stayed the same, or improved?"

Most dementia conditions have a slow progression and an onset that can be hard to identify. In contrast, the rapidly progressive dementias (RPDs) can manifest in a much shorter time, sometimes over weeks to months. If RPD is suspected, the evaluation should be completed with referral to a specialist made promptly.

A careful review of medications (prescription and over the counter) should be conducted, paying attention to those with psychoactive properties or side effects. It is important that the patient bring all medications to the evaluation in order to clarify dosages and expiration dates and the patient's understanding of the purpose of, administration of, and adherence to the medications.

1. Alzheimer disease (AD)
    a. Patients with AD or their family members often report deficits in short-term memory, although memory loss is not always a primary cognitive deficit. Initial symptoms can also include non-amnestic symptoms, such as problems with word finding, visual–spatial deficits (getting lost), or executive dysfunction (organization and planning). Statements may include: "They seem more forgetful"; "They take longer to get things done"; "They are getting lost in familiar places"; "They repeat the same question multiple times"; "They cannot multitask as well as before"; "They cannot come up with the right word to use"; and "They may have trouble navigating the use of technology such as remembering how to access or the passwords to email, tablet, the computer, smart phone, or smart television control."
    b. Report of personality or behavioral changes: Apathy, anxiety, depression, anger/aggression, disinhibition, or irritability and mood swings. Common complaints may include "They are quieter"; "They don't engage in activities as in the past"; and "They anger easily now."
    c. Report of functional decline. See earlier discussion. Examples may include problems with completing tasks at work, paying bills late, forgetting appointments, misplacing personal items, diminished standards in personal hygiene and grooming (e.g., not showering as often, appearance that is unkempt, or wearing the same

Table 48-2 Features of Dementia

Syndrome	Symptoms	Onset	Areas of Brain Affected	Biochemical/ Protein	Possible Associated Symptoms	Progression
Alzheimer disease	Short-term memory loss, word-finding difficulty, visual–spatial difficulties (getting lost or disoriented)	Gradual; more common after age 65 but can occur earlier	Multiple areas; global atrophy on imaging	Deficits in acetylcholine/beta-amyloid and tau	Apathy, depression, diminished insight over time	Slowly progressive over 7–10 yr (or longer)
Dementia with Lewy bodies	Recurrent and well-formed visual hallucinations, fluctuating cognition, parkinsonian symptoms, visual–spatial deficits, short-term memory loss	Gradual	Multiple areas; global atrophy on imaging	Deficits in acetylcholine and dopamine/ alpha-synuclein	Rapid eye movement sleep behavior disorder, falls, anxiety	Slowly progressive
Vascular dementia	Dependent on the location of ischemia	May be sudden with identifiable onset and proceed in a stepwise manner	Cortical or subcortical changes on imaging		Irritability, apathy	Dependent on management of stroke risk factors
Frontotemporal dementia	Behavior and personality change: apathy, disinhibition, poor judgment, social misconduct, executive dysfunction	Gradual; before age 60	Frontal and anterior temporal lobes (anterior sections of the brain)	Deficits in serotonin/tau, Pick bodies, or TDP-43	Speech and language changes occur in the aphasic variant. Motor deficits occur in progressive supranuclear palsy, corticobasal degeneration, and amyotrophic lateral sclerosis (related disorders). Diminished insight early in disease (behavioral-variant frontotemporal dementia)	Progressive over 6–8 yr

clothes over again), and problems with driving (e.g., running through stop signs, driving too fast or slow, getting lost, new traffic violations or car accidents, and/or new dents and scrapes on the car).
   d. Report of risk factors for AD: Risk factors include advanced age, family history of AD, history of moderate and severe traumatic brain injury (with loss of consciousness or posttraumatic amnesia), cardiovascular disease risk factors, and previous diagnosis of mild cognitive impairment.
2. Vascular dementia
   a. Patient or family reports of deficits in short-term memory, finding the right word, difficulties with navigation, or problems with executive function (organization and planning)
   b. Report of personality or behavioral changes: apathy, depression, irritability, or anxiety
   c. Report of functional decline: See earlier examples in item 1 of this section.
   d. Report of a strokelike event that coincides with the previously mentioned cognitive, behavioral, and functional changes. It may be possible to identify a specific time point at which symptoms presented.
   e. A medical review may reveal the presence of vascular risk factors (hypertension, hypercholesteremia, or diabetes).
3. Dementia with Lewy bodies (DLB)
   a. Patient or family reports of fluctuating deficits in visual–spatial abilities, navigation, executive function (organization and planning), short-term memory, or finding the right word
   b. Report of personality or behavioral changes: Formed visual hallucinations are common (e.g., small people or animals, movement in one's peripheral vision), as well as the misperception of objects (e.g., mistaking a tree for the figure of a person). Other examples of behavioral changes may include delusions or paranoia (e.g., false beliefs about people stealing from them), daytime sleepiness, anxiety, apathy, and depression.
   c. Report of functional decline. See earlier examples in item 1 of this section.
   d. Report of motor symptoms suggestive of Parkinsonism (shuffling gait or dragging feet more while walking, bradykinesia, stiffness, and falls caused by tripping)
   e. Report of sleep changes suggestive of REM behavior disorder: Symptoms may include new onset of thrashing and moving while sleeping, arm and leg movements as if warding off an attack, dream enactment, hitting the bed partner during sleep, or falling out of bed during sleep.
4. Frontotemporal dementia (FTD)
   a. Report of executive dysfunction; poor judgment; and speech and language changes that may include loss of object and word meaning, or dysarthria. Common complaints may include "They have been making abnormal or risky decisions"; "They cannot seem to organize tasks"; "They don't know what certain words mean anymore"; and "Speech is halting, and it is hard to get words out."
   b. Report of personality and behavioral changes: apathy, disinhibition, impulsivity, social or personal misconduct, unusual eating behaviors, compulsions, and diminished empathy. Common complaints: "They have become a different person"; "They have been yelling at people"; "They don't care about things/don't care about me"; "They say they will do things but don't"; "They make suggestive comments to others"; "They talk to strangers more readily"; "They have become selfish or self-centered"; and "Eating behavior has changed [e.g., eats more, carbohydrate cravings, or engages in food fads]."
   c. Report of functional decline: Examples may include trouble with task completion, trouble maintaining a job, diminished abilities in managing financial and legal matters (showing poor judgment, making risky investments, unusual purchases, or giving away money), and diminished standards in hygiene and grooming.
   d. Report of motor symptoms suggestive of amyotrophic lateral sclerosis, corticobasal degeneration, or progressive supranuclear palsy (falls, weakness, or diminished ability to control limb movements)
   e. Report of a family history suggestive of FTD that may include dementia, behavioral disorders, or psychiatric disorders

B. Objective
 1. Mental status screening and evaluation
    a. Use a reliable and valid instrument. The Montreal Cognitive Assessment (MOCA) provides a brief screening of memory, language, executive function, and visual–spatial abilities. It is available in multiple languages and is free of charge.
    b. The MOCA, along with administration instructions, is available at http://www.mocatest.org.
    c. Comprehensive neuropsychological testing by a neuropsychologist may be necessary to accurately demonstrate the presence and character of deficits.
 2. Functional assessment
    a. A reliable and valid instrument that assists in comparing present with past performance in functional domains can be used in conjunction with the clinical interview.
    b. Functional abilities can be assessed in multiple domains, including occupational performance, finances, medication management, driving, use of computer, household tasks (e.g., housekeeping and cooking), and personal hygiene.

c. Examples of functional assessment instruments include the Functional Activities Questionnaire (Pfeffer et al., 1982) and the Instrumental Activities of Daily Living Scale (Lawton & Brody, 1969). Both tools are easy to administer and have good reliability and validity. A disadvantage of both tools is the reliance on self-report or informant report rather than direct observation of functional abilities.
d. An instrumental activities of daily living (ADLs) scale is available at http://consultgerirn.org or https://www.alz.org/careplanning/downloads/lawton-iadl.pdf.
e. Direct observation of a person's function can be accomplished with tools such as the Functional Activities Questionnaire in Older Adults With Dementia, the Texas Functional Living Scale, or the Executive Function Performance Test. Online assessments include the Barthel Index for ADLs, available at https://www.mdcalc.com/barthel-index-activities-daily-living-adl. In addition, occupational therapists can be helpful in the assessment of mobility, function, self-care, and swallowing.

3. Assessment of mood
   a. Evaluation should include an assessment for depression because mood disorders share similar features with neurodegenerative conditions. Depression can coexist with dementia, although its prevalence decreases with increased dementia severity.
   b. A commonly used screen is the Geriatric Depression Scale. Using a yes/no format, patients answer questions about their mood over the past week. A long version (30 items) and a short version (15 items) are available. Scoring guidelines are provided to rate the severity of depression.
   c. The Geriatric Depression Scale is available at http://consultgerirn.org.
   d. The Patient Health Questionnaires (PHQs) are mental health screening tools designed for use in the office practice setting. They are available at http://www.phqscreeners.com. For additional details about the PHQs, see Chapter 49, Depression in Adults.

4. Physical and neurologic examination
   a. The routine physical examination should be completed to identify the presence of any medical problems (e.g., hypertension or atrial fibrillation).
   b. The neurologic examination should include an assessment of mental status, cranial nerves, motor abilities, reflexes, coordination, and gait and balance and an assessment for focal neurologic signs.

5. Relevant diagnostic tests
   a. Laboratory screening routinely includes complete blood count (to rule out anemia and infection), serum chemistries, thyroid and liver function, and vitamin B_{12} (to rule out metabolic conditions). A rapid plasma reagin test (RPR) and/or folate level or homocysteine and methylmalonic acid may be warranted, depending on clinical findings and history. See **Table 48-3** for a summary of routine laboratory screening.
   b. Other tests may be indicated based on the history or physical examination (e.g., electrocardiography or electroencephalography).
   c. Biomarkers
      i. Brain imaging can help identify the degree and pattern of atrophy and may detect other causes for cognitive deficits (e.g., intracranial bleeding, space-occupying lesions, and hydrocephalus). The most common imaging techniques are magnetic resonance imaging (MRI) and computed tomography (CT). Functional brain imaging, such as positron emission tomography (PET), provides information on metabolic activity in the brain, although the data can be difficult to interpret. The U.S. Food and Drug Administration has approved newer techniques in PET imaging using special tracers that bind to amyloid and tau proteins. The amyloid PET imaging is now covered by most insurance plans, and current guidelines suggest that its use should always be in the context of an evaluation by a specialist because the results are difficult to interpret if not in conjunction with an appropriate workup.
      ii. Proteins in cerebrospinal fluid (CSF): Specialty laboratories can provide analysis of levels of β-amyloid and phosphorylated tau.

Table 48-3 Common Laboratory Screening in Assessment of Dementia

Laboratory Tests
Complete blood cell count
Serum electrolytes, including magnesium
Serum chemistry panel, including liver function
Thyroid function
Vitamin B_{12}
Folate acid level or homocysteine
Methylmalonic acid
Urinalysis
Serologic tests for syphilis*
Toxicology screening*
HIV*

* Based on clinical relevance.

d. Genetic testing: May be pursued if there is a family history, a known gene, and/or a desire for confirmation. The different types of dementia carry varying familial risk. Referral to a genetic counselor is typically indicated in order to clarify the presence of genetic risk and discuss the implications of genetic testing.

III. Assessment
A. *Determine the diagnosis.*
1. Major neurocognitive disorder or dementia is diagnosed when there are cognitive or behavioral (neuropsychiatric) symptoms that interfere with functional independence in complex instrumental activities of daily living (IADLs), represent a decline from previous levels of performance, and are not explained by delirium or major psychiatric disorder. The cognitive or behavioral impairment involves a minimum of two of the following domains: (a) impairment in the ability to remember new information; (b) impaired reasoning and ability to manage complex tasks; (c) impaired visuospatial abilities; (d) impaired language functions; or (e) changes in behavior, personality, or comportment (American Psychiatric Association, 2013).
2. Minor neurocognitive disorder or mild cognitive impairment is diagnosed when there is a subjective report and/or objective evidence of cognitive impairment and there is no decline in functional independence or ability to carry out IADLs. This may or may not precede the development of dementia. Schedule follow-up testing within 6 months to a year or as needed.

IV. Goals of clinical management
Desired outcomes for the patient with dementia are that (a) they remain as independent as possible in an environment that matches their functional abilities, (b) the dementia and comorbid conditions are well managed, and (c) their family members and caregivers are well supported. A balance between the patient's autonomy and the family's needs and their resources is a priority and often a constant challenge in navigating clinical management.

V. Plan
A. *Conduct further workup or provide referral to specialist as needed.*
Referrals are indicated when symptoms are atypical, occur in a younger patient, are suggestive of a rapidly progressive dementia, or are confounded by difficult psychiatric or behavioral disturbances. Referrals may be helpful when a second opinion is desired.
B. *Pharmacologic management*
1. There are several classes of medications used to treat disease symptoms or improve cognitive function and symptoms. They do not affect the underlying brain changes or alter the course of the disease.
2. There is an emerging class of disease modifying agents. As of 2023, the Food and Drug Administration (FDA) approved two infusion medications, that are monoclonal antibody therapy, called aducanumab and lecanemab. They remove beta amyloid protein from the brain, slowing cognitive and functional decline. They are approved for use in people with biomarker confirmed early-stage Alzheimer's disease. These are still not cures for Alzheimer's disease and not appropriate for all patients. Besides common potential side effects from infusions, the most concerning side effect is amyloid-related imaging abnormalities (ARIA) which is localized swelling or bleeding in or on the surface of the brain. Given that these agents are still new in clinical use, patients must consult a specialist and be monitored closely through the course of treatment (Alzheimer's Association, 2023).
3. Commonly used medications are outlined in **Table 48-4**. Discuss possible side effects of the acetylcholinesterase inhibitors, including gastrointestinal upset and vivid dreams. Slow titration of medication, use of the patch administration method, and administration of medication in the morning rather than at bedtime are common strategies to prevent these side effects. These medications are not indicated for patients with bradycardia; consider obtaining an electrocardiogram before initiation of therapy.
4. Review expected and realistic goals of treatment (e.g., treatment is for symptomatic improvement and not a cure or reversal of disease). Expected benefits may be a mild improvement in memory function, mood, and alertness. Higher doses are often indicated in DLB. It is recommended that 6–12 months of therapy are needed to adequately assess the benefit of therapy (California Workgroup on Guidelines for Alzheimer's Disease Management, 2008).
5. Dietary supplements and other medications: Ginkgo biloba, vitamin E, and estrogen have been considered as treatments for AD, although research has not provided compelling evidence in favor of these medications.
6. If the patient has vascular disease or mixed dementia, they should receive management and education regarding modification of cardiovascular risk factors.
C. *Nonpharmacologic management*
1. Conduct patient and family education.
   a. Discuss implications of diagnosis as it pertains to the patient's occupation and other responsibilities, especially driving.
   b. **DICE Model is helpful in identifying all the factors involved with a particular behavioral symptom (Kales)**
   c. Provide education, coaching and links to resources regarding dementia diagnosis, progression, and goals of care that aligns with the patient and family's values, culture, education, and abilities.

Table 48-4 Medications Used in the Treatment of Dementia

Drug	Indications	Possible Side Effects	Other Considerations
Cholinesterase inhibitors: donepezil (Aricept®), galantamine (Razadyne®, Reminyl®), rivastigmine (Exelon®)	Used primarily in Alzheimer's disease (AD) and dementia with Lewy bodies (DLB) to slow the breakdown of acetylcholine, a neurotransmitter important for memory. May be helpful in managing the hallucinations and fluctuating cognition of DLB.	Gastrointestinal (nausea, vomiting, diarrhea). Contraindicated in patients with bradycardia.	Obtain baseline electrocardiogram before initiation in patients with cardiovascular conditions. Rivastigmine available in patch form.
N-methyl-D-aspartate antagonist: memantine (Namenda®)	Used to reduce glutamate-mediated excitotoxicity that occurs with cell death. Approved for treatment of advanced AD (Mini-Mental Status Examination scores ≤ 15).	Constipation, dizziness, and headache	Not effective in frontotemporal dementia (FTD)
Selective serotonin reuptake inhibitors	Used to treat mood disorders in dementia as well as the behavioral symptoms in FTD	Gastrointestinal (nausea and diarrhea) and agitation	

  d. Support the value of maintaining physical activity and exercise. Physical exercise has been linked to improvement of mood, maintenance of mobility, decreased risk for falls, and possible improvement of cognition.
  e. Provide information regarding educational and supportive resources available in the community (see Resources and Tools at the end of the chapter for suggestions).
  f. Provide information about advance directives and durable power of attorney while the patient is in the early stages of disease and may have agency over their decisions. Make referrals for legal and financial advice, especially if there are concerns about the patient's judgment, decision making, or vulnerability. A formal evaluation for capacity may be warranted.
  g. Discuss participation in research. People with dementia and their caregivers find it very meaningful to participate in observational research as well as clinical trials of potentially beneficial new and emerging treatments. The National Institutes of Health maintains a listing of all clinical trials at http://www.clinicaltrials.gov. Refer to research programs based on patient and family's interest and eligibility.
2. Safety management
  a. Determine whether the patient is residing in a setting that best meets their functional and cognitive abilities. These decisions are specific and unique to each patient and family's situation, resources and abilities. Refer to social work, placement advisors or case managers to discuss options. Types of living situations range from living at home alone to living at home with supervision, board and care, assisted living, and memory care units.
  b. If wandering or getting lost is a concern, discuss strategies for maintaining safety and refer the patient and family to the MedicAlert + Alzheimer's Association Safe Return program (operated by the Alzheimer's Association). Discuss strategies for ensuring safety concerns (e.g., door alarms and supervision).
  c. Patients with dementia and their caregivers are vulnerable to abuse. Refer to adult protective services if there is concern for the well-being of the patient or the caregiver.
  d. Driving
    i. Depending on cognitive and motor findings, the patient can be requested to stop driving, complete a test of driving abilities through the department of motor vehicles, or be referred to a driver's safety course that will assess driving ability.
    ii. Reporting to the Department of Public Health and Department of Motor Vehicles of the diagnosis of dementia should be consistent with state laws; some states have mandatory reporting requirements.
3. Management of behavioral symptoms
Behavioral symptoms occur commonly in dementia and can contribute to caregiver distress. Behavioral symptoms are caused by structural changes in the brain, neurotransmitter depletion, changes in how the patient perceives and responds to

environmental stimuli, or a combination of all of these factors.
a. The first step in managing these symptoms is to discuss the character, frequency, and severity of the symptoms with the patient and caregiver. Describe the behavior specifically (e.g., not just "sundowning," but "behavior that changes in the evening and includes pacing, repetitive statements that this is not their house, pushing the caregiver away, and trying to open the front door to leave the house").
b. Identify whether the symptoms are hazardous, frustrating, or tolerable. Not all behaviors are problematic. For example, wandering is a beneficial form of exercise as long as the patient can engage in the activity safely. Other behaviors are hazardous, such as agitation and aggression that may be physically dangerous to the patient or the caregiver. Caregivers may need counseling and therapy to assist with coping with the stress involved in managing behavioral symptoms.
c. Develop an individualized plan of care for managing behavioral symptoms. Strategies for managing behavioral symptoms fall into five categories. In many cases, using a combination of interventions is necessary.
  i. *Environmental* refers to modifying the patient's environment. Examples include providing activities that are enjoyable for the patient and match their functional level without being overwhelming. For example, for patients vulnerable to sweepstakes offers in the mail, have mail diverted to a post office box where it can be screened before reaching the patient. If the patient is having disturbing visual illusions, remove the stimuli from the environment. Environmental strategies also include the use of communication techniques that match the patient's level of comprehension and that do not provoke an argument.
  ii. *Behavioral* refers to substituting a behavior that is more tolerable or safer than the current/prior behavior(s). Examples include substitution of sugar-free candy or nonalcoholic beverages for patients with food or drink cravings.
  iii. *Pharmacologic* refers to the use of a medication that specifically targets the behavior. Examples include a selective serotonin reuptake inhibitor to treat agitation. Antipsychotics can be used for delusions that are frightening and disabling for the patient. Their use is associated with an increased risk of death, and they should be used only in cases of severe agitation, aggression, or psychosis and in conjunction with an assessment for potential medical reasons for the behavior.
  iv. *Physical* refers to the use of a physical restraint or barriers to prevent patient movement. These strategies should only be considered as a last resort. It may be necessary to move the patient to a more protected and supportive environment, such as a memory care unit, in which the patient can move about in a secured setting.
  v. *Internal to the caregiver* refers to acknowledgment and acceptance by the caregiver of the behavior. Counseling and education regarding expected disease symptoms and progression, identification of strategies for effective behavior management, and obtaining respite and support from caregiving duties are examples of helpful interventions.
4. Follow-up care
  a. Follow-up assessment of the person with dementia is typically every 6 months to a year or sooner if needed and should include the following:
    i. An assessment of daily function to assess progression of disease and identify concerns of the patient or family
    ii. Cognitive status testing to assess progression of disease
    iii. Review for comorbid physical or neuropsychiatric conditions
    iv. Review of current medications to assess for therapeutic effectiveness and potential negative side effects
    v. Physical examination as appropriate
    vi. Continuation of patient and family education as needed and referrals for education and caregiver support as needed
5. Preparation for end-of-life care
  a. Explore the patient's and family's cultural values and preferences (per advance directives if available).
  b. Discuss goals for managing patient care regarding dementia and any comorbid conditions.
  c. Emphasize comfort measures (e.g., simplify medication regimen, maximize comfort for patient, and initiate referral for hospice care as indicated).

VI. Assessment and management of concomitant conditions

There are factors that may negatively affect the status of the patient with dementia and their caregiver. For example, depression has been shown to contribute to excess disability of the patient with dementia. Selective serotonin reuptake inhibitors are the ideal medication for treating depression (Swartz et al., 2000). Sudden changes in the patient's behavior may not be caused by advancing disease but may be delirium or a result of underlying acute medical change, such as pneumonia, urinary tract infection, constipation, or poorly controlled pain. Sudden changes warrant both a medical evaluation and a review of the patient's medications.

VII. Assessment of the status of the family caregiver

Family caregivers provide the bulk of care to people with dementia. The initial period of noticing changes in their loved ones, along with navigating the diagnostic evaluation and coping with the diagnosis. [ADD] The survival length of AD is typically 4 to 8 years following diagnosis, although some people live as long as 20 years with the disease. Over the disease trajectory, family caregivers provide an extensive range of assistance. Caregiving responsibilities may include a variety of tasks ranging from management of medications and appointments to decision making; money management; guarding the safety of the patient; locating and arranging for assistance via community resources and programs; hiring and supervising hired help; and assistance with walking, dressing, and other aspects of physical care. Dementia family caregiving is complex and individualized affected by various factors including social pressures, race, ethnicity, financial resources, supportive resources, and preparedness. The dementia caregiver is often associated with negative physical and emotional outcomes for the caregiver, although many express satisfaction and find meaning in their roles as caregivers (Yu, 2019). Children and teenagers often need the most support and education given the impact of being a caregiver at a young age as well as different life stages. Desired outcomes for family caregivers include the promotion of positive coping strategies and emotional and physical well-being.

A. *Assess the caregiver's physical and emotional health concerns.*
   1. Assess their level of strain. The Modified Caregiver Strain Index (CSI) is a 13-item survey designed to measure strain for certain aspects of caregiving, with higher scores indicative of greater strain. The CSI is available at http://consultgerirn.org.
   2. Assess for depression and anxiety. Consider tools such as the Geriatric Depression Scale or PHQ, as previously noted.
   3. Assess the caregiver's coping strategies for managing the strain of caregiving, and promote positive strategies (e.g., exercise, counseling).
   4. Validate and encourage the caregiver in identifying activities that are pleasurable for them and methods for incorporating these activities into their lifestyle.
   5. Refer to caregiver support groups, counseling, respite care, or other services.

B. *Provide assistance for children and teenagers dealing with a family member's dementia.*
   1. There are educational and supportive resources for children and teenagers coping with a family member's dementia:
      a. http://www.alz.org/living_with_alzheimers_just_for_kids_and_teens.asp
      b. https://dementiainmyfamily.org.au/
      c. https://www.caregivingyouthinstitute.org/
      d. http://www.alzheimers.org.uk/site/scripts/documents

VIII. Resources and tools

A. *Resources for all*
   1. The Alzheimer's Association is a national organization with local offices and can be a resource for all types of dementia (http://www.alz.org; 1-800-272-3900)
   2. https://www.communityresourcefinder.org
   3. Alzheimer's Disease Education and Referral Center, a service sponsored by the National Institute on Aging (http://www.alzheimers.org; 1-800-438-4380)
   4. Alzheimers.gov, sponsored by the U.S. Department of Health and Human Services
   5. Areas on Aging (https://eldercare.acl.gov/Public/About/Aging_Network/AAA.aspx)
   6. Family Caregiver Alliance (https://www.caregiver.org)
   7. Get Palliative Care: Palliative care directory (http://getpalliativecare.org)
   8. Disease specific associations (CurePSP, aFTD, lbda, naa.org)

B. *Resources for providers*
   1. Alzheimer's Association Facts and Figures 2023
   2. California Department of Public Health (CADPH)/California Alzheimer's Disease Center (CADC) Toolkit https://www.cdph.ca.gov/Programs/CCDPHP/DCDIC/CDCB/Pages/AlzheimersDiseaseProgram.aspx
   3. Center to Advance Palliative Care (CAPC) https://www.capc.org/training/best-practices-in-dementia-care-and-caregiver-support/
   4. Costa, P., Williams, T., & Somerfield, M. (1996). *Early identification of Alzheimer's disease and related dementias. Clinical practice guideline, Quick reference guide for clinicians* (AHCPR Publication No. 97-0703). Agency for Health Care Policy and Research.
   5. Guideline for Alzheimer's Disease Management: California Workgroup on Guidelines for Alzheimer's Disease Management http://www.alz.org/socal/images/professional_NATLguideline.pdf
   6. The Hartford Institute for Geriatric Nursing, College of Nursing, New York University. Contains best practice information on the care of older adults and multiple assessment tools with administration and scoring instructions. http://consultgerirn.org or www.hartfordign.org

References

Alzheimer's Association. (2023). 2023 Alzheimer's disease facts and figures. *Alzheimer's & Dementia*. https://www.alz.org/media/Documents/alzheimers-facts-and-figures.pdf

American Psychiatric Association. (2013). *Diagnostic and statistical manual of mental disorders* (5th ed.). https://doi.org/10.1176/appi.books.9780890425596

Clarfield A. M. (2003). The decreasing prevalence of reversible dementias: an updated meta-analysis. *Archives of internal medicine, 163*(18), 2219–2229. https://doi.org/10.1001/archinte.163.18.2219

Hogan, D. B., Fiest, K. M., Roberts, J. I., Maxwell, C. J., Dykeman, J, Pringsheim, T., Steeves, T., Smith, E. E., Pearson, D., & Jetté, N. (2016). The prevalence and incidence of dementia with Lewy bodies: A systematic review. *Canadian Journal of Neurological Science, 43*(2), S83–S95. https://doi.org/10.1017/cjn.2016.2

Kane, J. P. M., Surendranathan, A., Bentley, A., Barker, S. A. H., Taylor, J. P., Thomas, A. J., Allan, L. M., McNally, R. J., James, P. W., McKeith, I. G., Burn, D. J., & O'Brien, J. T. (2018). Clinical prevalence of Lewy body dementia. *Alzheimer's Research & Therapy, 10*(1), 19. https://doi.org/10.1186/s13195-018-0350-6

Lawton, M., & Brody, E. (1969). Assessment of older people: Self-maintaining and instrumental activities of daily living. *Gerontologist, 9*(3), 179–186.

Mayeda, E. R., Glymour, M. M., Quesenberry, C. P., & Whitmer, R. A. (2016). Inequalities in dementia incidence between six racial and ethnic groups over 14 years. *Alzheimer's & Dementia: The Journal of the Alzheimer's Association, 12*(3), 216–224. https://doi.org/10.1016/j.jalz.2015.12.007

McKeith, I. G., Boeve, B. F., Dickson, D. W., Halliday, G., Taylor, J. P., Weintraub, D., Aarsland, D., Galvin, J., Attems, J., Ballard, C. G., Bayston, A., Beach, T. G., Blanc, F., Bohnen, N., Bonanni, L., Bras, J., Brundin, P., Burn, D., Chen-Plotkin, A., Duda, J. E., ... Kosaka, K. (2017). Diagnosis and management of dementia with Lewy bodies: Fourth consensus report of the DLB Consortium. *Neurology, 89*(1), 88–100. https://doi.org/10.1212/WNL.0000000000004058

Pfeffer, R., Kurosaki, T., Harrah, C., Chance, J., & Filos, S. (1982). Measurement of functional activities in older adults in the community. *Journal of Gerontology, 37*(3), 323–329. https://doi.org/10.1093/geronj/37.3.32

Plassman, B. L., Langa, K. M., Fisher, G. G., Heeringa, S. G., Weir, D. R., Ofstedal, M. B., Burke, J. R., Hurd, M. D., Potter, G. G., Rodgers, W. L., Steffens, D. C., Willis, R. J., & Wallace, R. B. (2007). Prevalence of dementia in the United States: The aging, demographics, and memory study. *Neuroepidemiology, 29*(1–2), 125–132. https://doi.org/10.1159/000109998

Ratnavalli, E., Brayne, C., Dawson, K., & Hodges, J. R. (2002). The prevalence of frontotemporal dementia. *Neurology, 58*(11), 1615–1621. https://doi.org/10.1212/wnl.58.11.1615

Rizzi, L., Rosset, I., & Roriz-Cruz, M. (2014). Global epidemiology of dementia: Alzheimer's and vascular types. *BioMed Research International*, 2014, 908915. https://doi.org/10.1155/2014/908915

Segal-Gidan, F., Cherry, D., Jones, R., Williams, B., Hewett, L., Chodosh, J., & California Workgroup on Guidelines for Alzheimer's Disease Management (2011). Alzheimer's disease management guideline: update 2008. *Alzheimer's & Dementia: The Journal of the Alzheimer's Association, 7*(3), e51–e59. https://doi.org/10.1016/j.jalz.2010.07.005

Swartz, M., Barak, Y., Mirecki, I., Naor, S., & Weizman, A. (2000). Treating depression in Alzheimer's disease: Integration of differing guidelines. *International Psychogeriatrics, 12*(3), 353–358. https://doi.org/10.1017/s1041610200006451

Vann Jones, S., & O'Brien, J. (2014). The prevalence and incidence of dementia with Lewy bodies: A systematic review of population and clinical studies. *Psychological Medicine, 44*(4), 673–683. https://doi.org/10.1017/S0033291713000494

Wolters, F., & Ikram, A. (2019). Epidemiology of vascular dementia: Nosology in a time of epiomics. *Arteriosclerosis, Thrombosis, and Vascular Biology, 39*(8), 1542–1549. https://doi.org/10.1161/ATVBAHA.119.311908

Yu, D. S. F., Cheng, S. T., & Wang, J. (2018). Unravelling positive aspects of caregiving in dementia: An integrative review of research literature. *International journal of nursing studies, 79*, 1–26. https://doi.org/10.1016/j.ijnurstu.2017.10.008

CHAPTER 49

Depression

Beth Phoenix and Kathleen McDermott

I. Introduction and general background

A. Definition, overview, and epidemiology

The term *depression* may be used to describe a mood state, a clinical syndrome, or a distinct mental disorder. In a clinical context, *depression* refers to conditions characterized by persistent depressed mood accompanied by additional symptoms (see **Figure 49-1**). Depression can be expressed as discrete major depressive episodes or as persistent depressive disorder (also known as *dysthymia*), a condition characterized by depressive symptoms of varying severity that continue for at least 2 years. It can also occur as part of a bipolar mood disorder, in which depressive episodes alternate with manic or hypomanic episodes or where both manic–hypomanic and depressive symptoms are manifested during the same period of time (mixed episode).

Depression can appear similar to, or accompany, other psychiatric disorders, such as anxiety disorders, thought disorders, and substance abuse disorders. Thus, clinicians should be familiar with the current version of the *Diagnostic and Statistical Manual of Mental Disorders* (*DSM*) to distinguish depression from other psychiatric illnesses. As with all psychiatric illnesses, medical causes of depressive symptoms must be ruled out before determining a diagnosis of depression. Therefore, clinical evaluation should involve the assessment of biologic, psychological, and social factors.

The 12-month prevalence of major depressive disorder for U.S. adults has been estimated at 10.4%, with a lifetime prevalence of 20.6% (Hasin et al., 2018), so it is important for the primary care provider to screen for, assess, and treat depression. Although depression is comparable in prevalence to other disorders commonly seen in primary care, low rates of assessment and treatment persist (Siniscalchi et al., 2020). Initiatives to improve the quality of depression care in primary care settings have resulted in the development of depression care tool kits (e.g., MacArthur Initiative, 2009) and models to integrate behavioral healthcare services into primary care settings.

Depression is a significant public health problem—the World Health Organization (2017) ranks depression as the largest single contributor to global disability. Depression has a significant impact on public health for multiple reasons: it is widespread; it interferes with many aspects of functioning; the typical age of onset is in the teenage or young adult years; and the disorder can easily become chronic, particularly if treatment is not prompt and adequate. If depressive episodes are not adequately treated, the brain becomes sensitized to being in a depressed state, which is then more likely to recur in the future. This phenomenon, called *kindling*, may lead to depressive episodes that are more frequent, more severe, and of longer duration, with incomplete recovery between episodes. For this reason, it is important to prevent long-term morbidity through early diagnosis and aggressive treatment, with the goal of complete remission.

As well as causing suffering and impaired functioning, inadequately treated depression can exacerbate other health problems. Persons with depression are more likely to develop other chronic health conditions, experience premature mortality from health conditions such as cancer and diabetes, and use healthcare resources at a higher rate than others in the population (Sporinova et al., 2019). The relationship between medical morbidity and depression is likely bi-directional. The suffering and negative impacts on people's quality of life from chronic illness, such as pain and decreased activity, are associated with increased risk of depression. Persistent depression may negatively impact overall health by interfering with self-care behaviors and adherence to medical treatment. Depression and common medical conditions may share common causal mechanisms such as inflammatory mechanisms and dysregulation of physiologic stress responses (Herrera, et al., 2021).

In addition to the significant burden of depression-related disability, depression is also a significant cause

PHQ-9 Patient Depression Questionnaire

For initial diagnosis:

1. Patient completes PHQ-9 Quick Depression Assessment.
2. If there are at least 4 ✓s in the shaded section (including Questions #1 and #2), consider a depressive disorder. Add score to determine severity.

Consider Major Depressive Disorder
- if there are at least 5 ✓s in the shaded section (one of which corresponds to Question #1 or #2)

Consider Other Depressive Disorder
- if there are 2-4 ✓s in the shaded section (one of which corresponds to Question #1 or #2)

Note: Since the questionnaire relies on patient self-report, all responses should be verified by the clinician, and a definitive diagnosis is made on clinical grounds taking into account how well the patient understood the questionnaire, as well as other relevant information from the patient.
Diagnoses of Major Depressive Disorder or Other Depressive Disorder also require impairment of social, occupational, or other important areas of functioning (Question #10) and ruling out normal bereavement, a history of a Manic Episode (Bipolar Disorder), and a physical disorder, medication, or other drug as the biological cause of the depressive symptoms.

To monitor severity over time for newly diagnosed patients or patients in current treatment for depression:

1. Patients may complete questionnaires at baseline and at regular intervals (eg, every 2 weeks) at home and bring them in at their next appointment for scoring or they may complete the questionnaire during each scheduled appointment.
2. Add up ✓s by column. For every ✓: Several days = 1 More than half the days = 2 Nearly every day = 3
3. Add together column scores to get a TOTAL score.
4. Refer to the accompanying **PHQ-9 Scoring Box** to interpret the TOTAL score.
5. Results may be included in patient files to assist you in setting up a treatment goal, determining degree of response, as well as guiding treatment intervention.

Scoring: add up all checked boxes on PHQ-9

For every ✓ Not at all = 0; Several days = 1;
More than half the days = 2; Nearly every day = 3

Interpretation of Total Score

Total Score	Depression Severity
1-4	Minimal depression
5-9	Mild depression
10-14	Moderate depression
15-19	Moderately severe depression
20-27	Severe depression

PHQ9 Copyright © Pfizer Inc. All rights reserved. Reproduced with permission. PRIME-MD ® is a trademark of Pfizer Inc.

A2662B 10-04-2005

Figure 49-1 Patient Health Questionnaire-9 (PHQ-9)

Pfizer. (1999). *Patient Health Questionnaire-9 (PHQ-9)*. Retrieved from http://www.uspreventiveservicestaskforce.org/Home/GetFileByID/218

of premature mortality from suicide. Many adults who died by suicide visited their primary care provider within 1 month of their deaths, so familiarity with suicide risk factors is strongly recommended. The Suicide Assessment Five-Step Evaluation and Triage (SAFE-T) Pocket Card (U.S. Department of Health and Human Services, 2009) summarizes major risk factors for suicide (see **Table 49-1**) and provides guidance for assessing and managing suicide risk. The combination of severe depression and excessive alcohol consumption is implicated in a large proportion of deaths by suicide in the United States, making substance use assessment a critical part of depression evaluation.

Table 49-1 Suicide Risk Factors

Category of Risk	Examples
Suicidal behavior	<ul><li>History of prior suicide attempts</li><li>Self-injurious behavior</li></ul>
Current/past psychiatric disorders	<ul><li>Mood, psychotic, personality, and conduct disorders</li><li>Substance misuse</li><li>Comorbidities and recent onset increase risk</li></ul>
Key symptoms	<ul><li>Anhedonia</li><li>Impulsivity</li><li>Hopelessness</li><li>Anxiety/panic</li><li>Insomnia</li><li>Command hallucinations</li></ul>
Family history	<ul><li>Suicide attempts</li><li>Psychiatric disorders requiring hospitalization</li></ul>
Precipitants/ Stressors/ Interpersonal	<ul><li>Events leading to shame or despair (losses)</li><li>Persistent medical illness</li><li>Intoxication</li><li>Family turmoil</li><li>Abuse history</li><li>Social isolation</li></ul>
Change in treatment	<ul><li>Discharge from psychiatric hospitalization</li><li>Provider or treatment change</li></ul>
Access to firearms	

U.S. Department of Health and Human Services. (2009). *SAFE-T Pocket Card*. HHS Publication No. (SMA) 09-4432. Washington, D.C

Table 49-2 Depression Risk Factors

Other serious physical and mental health problems
Concurrent substance abuse or dependence
Family history of depression or suicide
Childhood depression or physical, emotional, or sexual abuse
Long-term use of certain medications
Personality traits, such as having low self-esteem and being overly dependent, self-critical, or pessimistic
Having recently given birth
Unemployment or low socioeconomic group
Female gender (increases risk of exposure to psychosocial stressors)
Poor social support
Negative life events, such as bereavement, new onset of illness, institutionalization, financial strain, work-related distress, or experience of discrimination
Physical inactivity
Unhealthy eating styles

The U.S. Preventive Services Task Force (USPSTF) recommends depression screening for adults with adequate systems in place to accurately diagnose depression and provide effective treatment (Siu, 2016). The USPSTF does not recommend specific screening tools but discusses instruments that have been studied for use with different populations, such as the Hospital Anxiety and Depression Scale (HADS), Geriatric Depression Scale (GDS), Edinburgh Postnatal Depression Scale (EPDS), and Patient Health Questionnaire for Adolescents (PHQ-A).

The following two questions, sometimes referred to as the Patient Health Questionnaire (PHQ)-2, are highly effective in identifying most cases of depression (Manea et al., 2016): "Over the past 2 weeks, have you felt down, depressed, or hopeless?" and "'Over the past 2 weeks, have you felt little interest or pleasure in doing things?" A positive response to either of these questions warrants a more thorough screening for depression. The Patient Health Questionnaire–9 (PHQ-9), a commonly used tool for depression screening and monitoring response to treatment, incorporates *DSM* diagnostic criteria for major depressive disorder (Figure 49-1).

II. Database

A. Subjective (**Table 49-2**)
   1. Past health history: depression; anxiety; other psychiatric illness; trauma history, including head trauma; chronic medical illnesses (e.g., HIV/AIDS, hepatitis C); physical disability; new serious health diagnosis; obstetric history; medication history, including current medications, medications or supplements taken in the past, and effect on depression
   2. Family history: depression, including death by suicide; other psychiatric illness; alcohol or other substance use disorder
   3. Occupational history: presence or absence of rewarding and meaningful work, work stress
   4. Personal and social history: support systems; substance use, including alcohol, nicotine, narcotics, and illicit drugs; relationship status; precipitating factors (stressors and losses)
   5. Review of systems: somatic complaints without focal findings, including headaches and other pain; anhedonia, depressed mood, hypersomnia or insomnia, psychomotor agitation or slowing; indecisiveness or decrease in concentration; fatigue or loss of energy; changes in appetite or weight; feeling guilty or poor self-esteem; suicidal thoughts or plans; irritability; pressured speech or thoughts; increase in goal-directed behaviors or risk-taking behaviors or in activities that have a high potential for negative consequences (e.g., buying sprees or

sexual indiscretions); expansive or euphoric mood; psychosis, including paranoia and auditory or visual hallucinations; and inability to engage in activities of daily living

B. *Objective*
 1. Physical examination findings
    a. Vital signs, including weight
    b. Thyroid examination
    c. Neurologic examination if indicated. Clinical assessment sometimes reveals that depressive symptoms are caused by an organic brain illness. Many discrete neurologic disorders (e.g., Parkinson disease, Alzheimer disease, cerebral vascular accidents, multiple sclerosis, traumatic brain and spinal cord injuries, dementias, and epilepsy) are associated with an increased risk of depression. Thus, a neurologic examination is often indicated in the physical assessment of depression.
    d. Mental status examination
       i. Appearance and behavior: Patient may demonstrate poor hygiene, poor eye contact, and inability to engage with interviewer.
       ii. Motor function: Patient may demonstrate motor slowing or agitation.
       iii. Affect: can vary from anxious or irritable to depressed with constricted affect
       iv. Mood: Use the patient's own description of mood.
       v. Language: Assess flow and volume. Speech may be quiet, with few words, and slow or may exhibit some nervous pressure.
       vi. Thought process: may be slow, evidenced by increased latency of response
       vii. Thought content: What are the patient's main concerns? The patient may have suicidal or homicidal thoughts with or without a plan to carry these out (these may indicate an emergency situation and must be carefully evaluated). Depressive symptoms may include obsessions, perseverations, paranoid ideas, feelings of depersonalization or unreality, and morbid thoughts. Psychotic depression may include auditory or visual hallucinations or delusions.
       viii. Cognition: Assess possible changes in all areas, including orientation, concentration, and memory; visuospatial skills; ability to abstract; and executive functioning.
       ix. Insight: Rated good, fair, or poor based on the patient's awareness of their depressive symptoms. Patients who are unsure or unaware that symptoms may be caused by depression are rated fair or poor.
       x. Judgment: Rated good, fair, or poor based on the patient's ability to gather and organize information to make plans and function well.
 2. Data from diagnostic tests: No single test is associated with a definitive diagnosis of depression; however, the following should be considered as part of a basic workup of depressive symptoms from other causes or of medical problems associated with depression:
    a. Complete blood count to rule out anemia
    b. Metabolic panel to rule out possible medical causes of depressive symptoms
    c. Thyroid-stimulating hormone and free T4 to rule out thyroid dysregulation
    d. Serum vitamin D, vitamin B_{12}, and folic acid levels to rule out vitamin deficiencies
    e. Drug of abuse screen to rule out co-occurring substance use disorders
    f. Hormone levels (gender specific) to rule out endocrine dysregulation

III. Assessment

A. *Determine the diagnosis (DSM-5; American Psychiatric Association, 2013)*
 1. Major depressive disorder: presence of five out of nine depressive symptoms, with one of the symptoms being depressed mood or anhedonia, occurring daily for at least 2 weeks
 2. Persistent depressive disorder (dysthymia): presence of three depressive symptoms (including depressed mood) for a duration of at least 2 years, with symptoms present more days than not
 3. Dysthymia with intermittent major depressive episodes ("double depression"): persistent depression with periods of more severe depressive symptoms
 4. Other psychiatric conditions that may explain the patient's presentation
    a. Bipolar disorder: if the patient currently meets the criteria for a depressive episode but also has a history of manic or hypomanic episodes characterized by sustained expansive, euphoric, or irritable mood with pressured speech or thoughts, with an increase in goal-directed behaviors or risk-taking activities (e.g., gambling with money that is meant to be used to pay rent) or with reduced need for sleep without feeling fatigue
    b. Thought disorder: presence of psychosis, disorganized thinking, or paranoia
    c. Anxiety disorder: when patient does not meet all criteria for a depressive disorder but may have some of the symptoms accompanied by disabling worry about things that are out of the patient's control
    d. Substance use disorder: if depressive symptoms are better accounted for by substance intoxication or withdrawal
    e. Other medical conditions that explain symptoms, including but not limited to thyroid or other endocrine disorders, dementia, anemia, and malnutrition
    f. Medication side effects. Various pharmacologic factors and physical disease states may be associated with the onset of depression. As such,

it is imperative to consider whether a person's depression is due to a general medical condition, or whether a medical condition may be an exacerbating factor. Since many neurologic and medical disorders can cause symptoms of depression, many patients first present to their primary care provider for care of these issues. Obtaining a thorough clinical and life history as well as consideration of the patient's current life situation are essential to ensure accurate diagnosis. A few notable medical conditions and pharmacologic factors that can cause depression include treatment with Interferon, adrenal and/or thyroid dysfunction, infectious mononucleosis, rheumatoid arthritis, Lupus, HIV, viral pneumonia, nutritional deficiencies, and sleep apnea. Habitual use of CNS depressant drugs like alcohol or withdrawal from stimulant drugs may also cause depressive symptoms.
   g. Bereavement: persistent feelings of grief associated with the loss of a loved one
5. Specifiers may be used if appropriate.
   a. Severity: mild, moderate, or severe, based on the impact depression has on the patient's functional ability, the intensity of distress caused by symptoms of depression, and the presence of suicidal thoughts
   b. Chronicity: single episode or recurrent
   c. With or without psychotic features, such as nihilistic delusions or ideas of reference
   d. With atypical features: Presence of weight gain and hypersomnia. Although "typical depression" is characterized by insomnia and weight loss, "atypical depression" is characterized by hypersomnia and weight gain. This specifier can be misleading because both types of depression are commonly seen in the primary care setting.
   e. In remission: partial (alleviation of some but not all symptoms) or full (complete alleviation of symptoms); early (< 6 months) or sustained (> 6 months)
   f. Other specifiers, including with anxious distress, with mixed features, with melancholic features, with catatonia, with peripartum onset, and with seasonal pattern
B. *Significance and motivation*
   Assess the significance of depression to the patient and significant others, including impact on work, relationships, and activities. Determine the patient's understanding of the diagnosis and willingness and ability to follow the treatment plan. Assess for the presence of social supports and other patient strengths that may influence the ability to recover from depression.

IV. **Goals of clinical management**
A. *Screening and diagnosing depression*
   Although the optimal timing and interval for screening for depression have not been established, the USPSTF suggests screening adults if they have not been screened or demonstrate known risk factors for depression (Siu, 2016).
B. *Treatment*
   1. Medication treatment
      Select a treatment plan that leads to sustained full remission of depressive symptoms. Complete remission should be determined by not only the relative absence of symptoms but also recovery of the patient's premorbid level of functioning and sense of well-being (Novick et al., 2017). Less than one-third of depressed patients achieve remission with their initial course of antidepressant treatment, and approximately another one-third will require several treatment regimens. Another one-third will fail to respond to two or more adequate trials of antidepressant monotherapy, which is considered treatment-resistant depression. Treatment resistance is associated with a range of comorbid physical and mental disorders, including substance abuse.

      Depression may remit without treatment in approximately one out of eight people (Mekonen et al., 2022). However, given the risks of untreated depression, such as an increased probability of future depressive episodes and persistent decrease in functioning, prompt individualized treatment is recommended (Oluboka et al., 2018). Because there is considerable variability across patients in response to antidepressant agents, patients should be monitored closely for therapeutic response and tolerability of the medication. All patients with depression need to be monitored for changes in condition, and treatment planning should involve not only a consideration of the severity and impact of depression but also the patient's health beliefs, as well as adherence to the treatment plan and ability to access components of the care plan.
   2. Treatment phases (see **Figure 49-2**)
      a. Acute phase: 0–16 weeks. Plan: Initiate treatment and monitor weekly for first month and at least once a month thereafter.
      b. Continuation phase: 16–20 weeks after symptom remission. Plan: Continue treatment, monitor every 2–3 months.
      c. Maintenance phase: 6 months symptom-free. Plan: Continue monitoring and treatment every 2–3 months.
      d. Discontinuation: Consider treatment discontinuation only after the patient has been symptom-free for 6–12 months. Because the risk of relapse is highest in the initial 2-month period following discontinuation of treatment, patients should continue to be monitored for several months. Patient education should include a review of early signs of depression, such as sleep disturbance and loss of interest in normal activities. Emphasize the importance of immediately resuming previously successful treatment in the event of a symptom relapse.

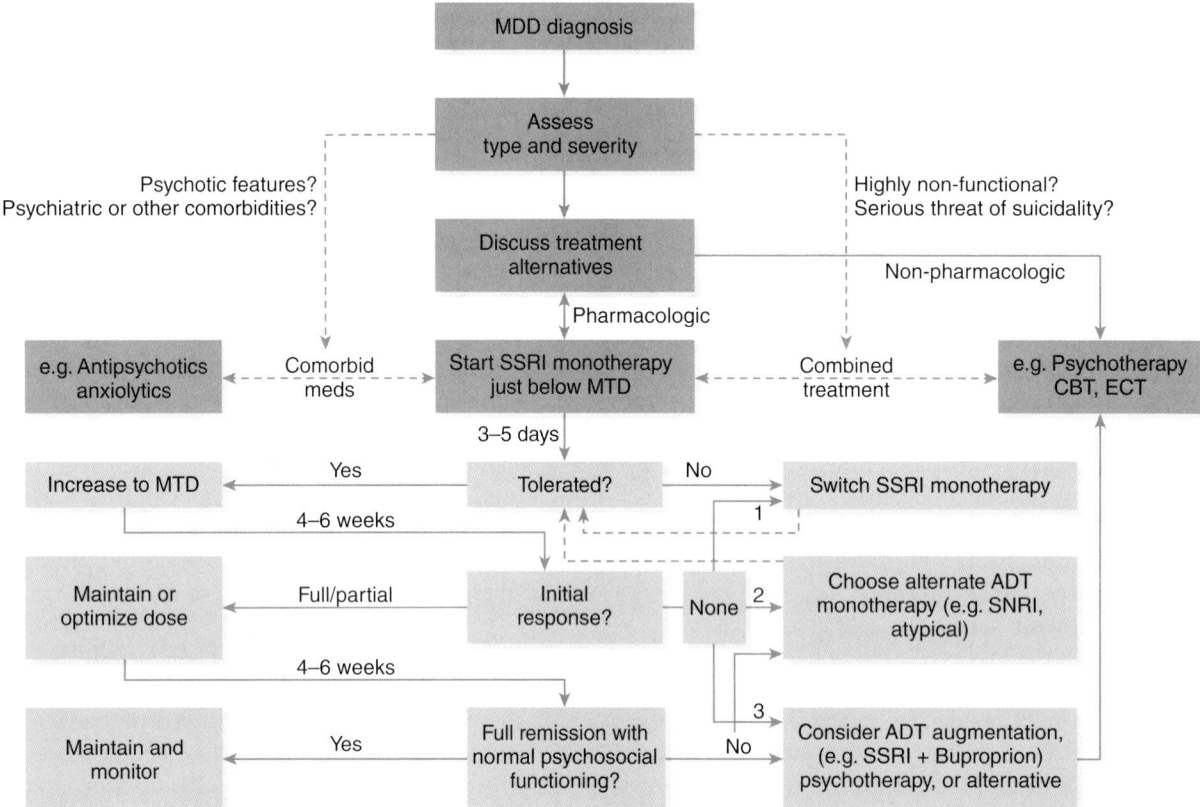

ADT, antidepressant treatment; CBT, cognitive behavioural therapy; ECT, electroconvulsive therapy; GI, gastrointestinal; MDD, major depressive disorder, MTD, minimum therapeutic dose, SNRI, serotonin norepinephrine reuptake inhibitor; SSRI, selective serotonin reuptake inhibitor.

Figure 49-2 Primary care treatment algorith for depression

Reproduced from Santarsieri D., Schwartz T.L. (2015). Antidepressant efficacy and side-effect burden: A quick guide for clinicians. *Drugs Context. 2015*; 4: 212290. doi: 10.7573/dic.212290

C. Patient adherence
Select an approach that maximizes patient adherence, including but not limited to cost, frequency of treatment, tolerability of treatment, and patient health beliefs.

V. Plan

A. *Diagnostic tests to rule out other causes of depressive symptoms*
Complete blood count with differential; complete metabolic panel, vitamin B_{12}, folate, thyroid-stimulating hormone, free T4; gamma-glutamyl transferase (GGT) or breathalyzer if alcohol use suspected; consider a drug of abuse screen and a more thorough toxicology screen (e.g., heavy metal screen) if indicated by history. HIV testing if indicated by history.

B. *Management (includes treatment, consultation, referral, and follow-up care)*
1. Medication management: Medication treatment should always include consideration of patient and family history of medication treatment for depression, cost and insurance coverage, past or anticipated side effects, and concurrent patient medications (**Figures 49-3, 49-4,** and **Table 49-3**)
2. Psychotherapy: For mild to moderate depression, psychotherapy has generally been found to be equal in efficacy to pharmacologic treatment, and the combination of medication and psychotherapy is more effective than either modality alone. Circumstances under which referral for psychotherapy should be considered as a first-line treatment option include patient preference and pregnancy and lactation. Even brief psychotherapy of six to eight sessions, such as cognitive–behavioral therapy and problem-solving therapy, can be effective in treating depression. Behavioral activation, in which patients are encouraged to increase their participation in interesting and enjoyable activities, is easy to administer in primary care settings and has shown efficacy in decreasing depressive symptoms (Cuijpers et al., 2019).
3. Combined treatment with antidepressants and psychological treatment is recommended for:
   a. Partial response to either treatment alone
   b. Patients with personality disorders or complex psychosocial problems
   c. Patients with a history of chronic or severe depression

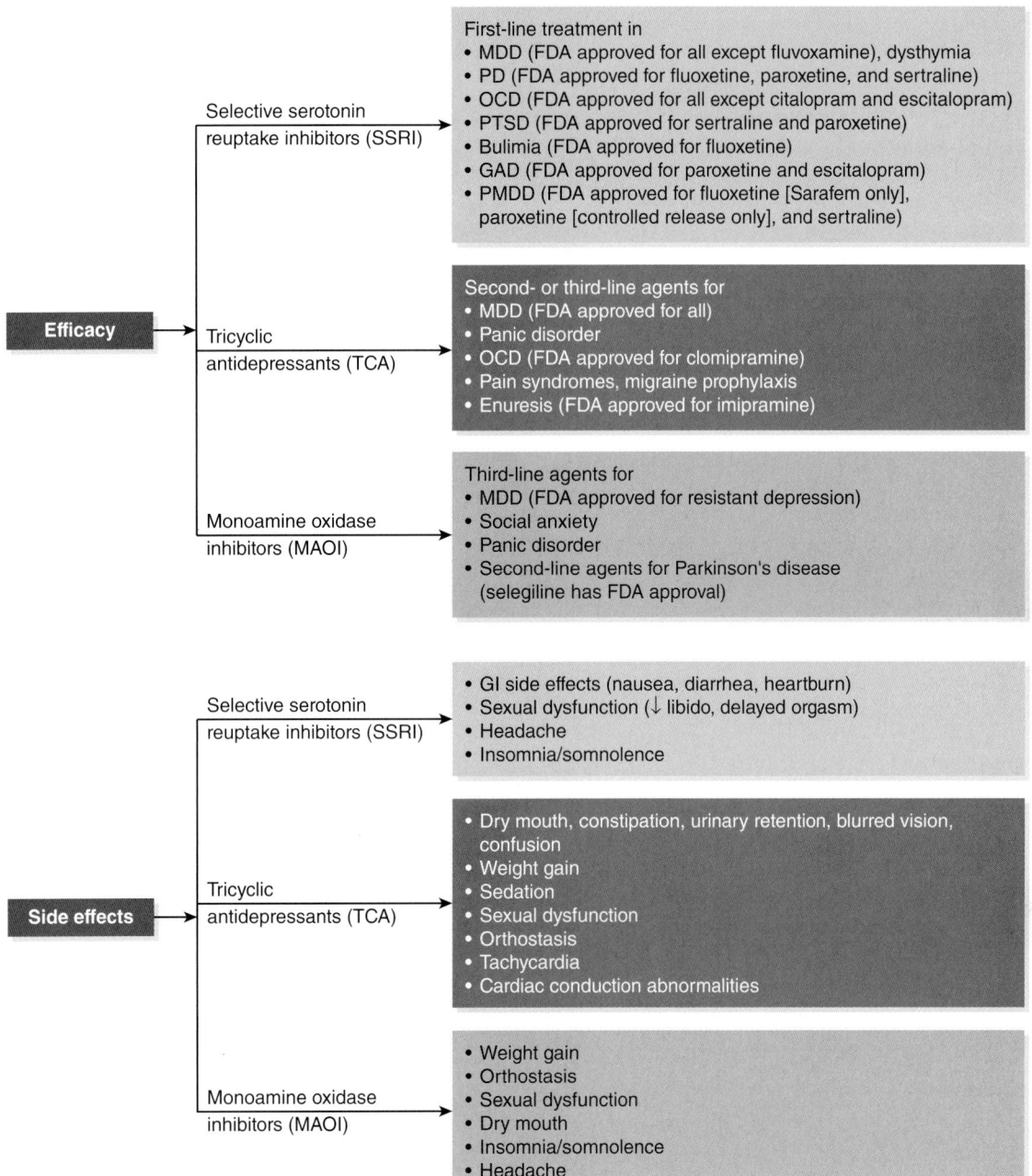

Figure 49-3 Overview of Antidepressant Classes

Data from Schatzberg, A. F., & DeBattista, C. (2019). *Manual of Clinical Psychopharmacology* (9th ed.). Washington, DC: American Psychiatric Association Publishing.

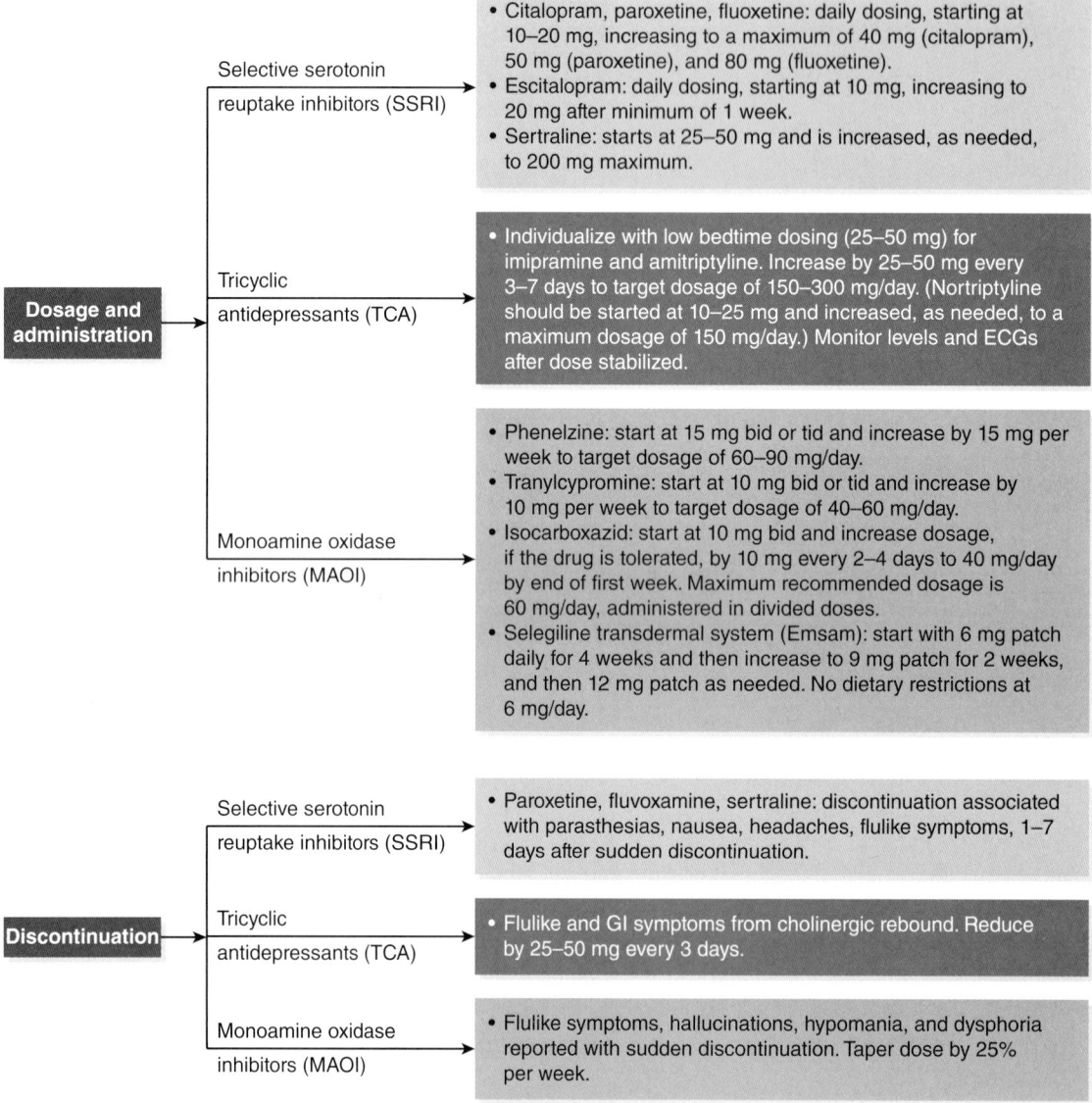

Figure 49-3 (Continued)

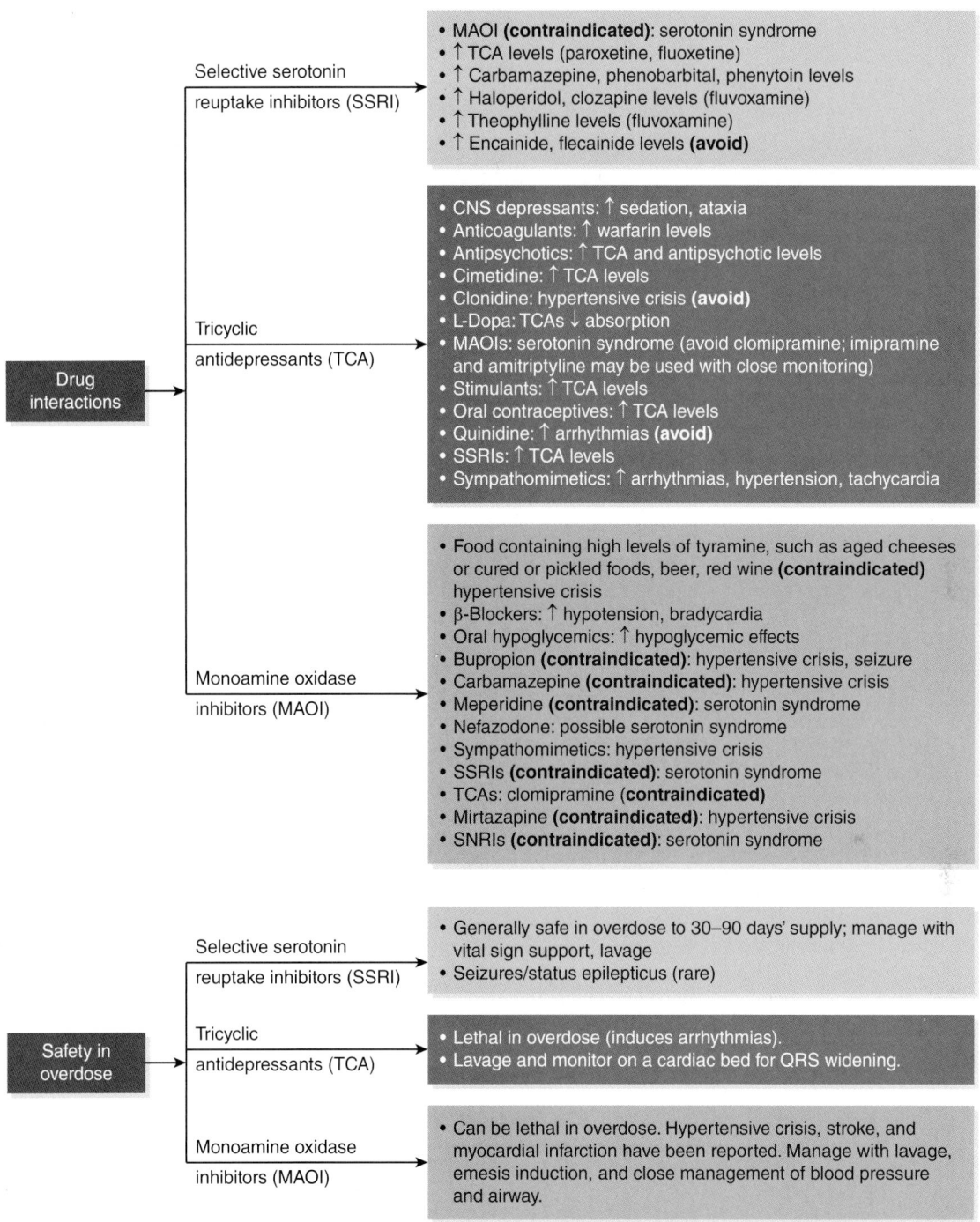

Figure 49-3 (Continued)

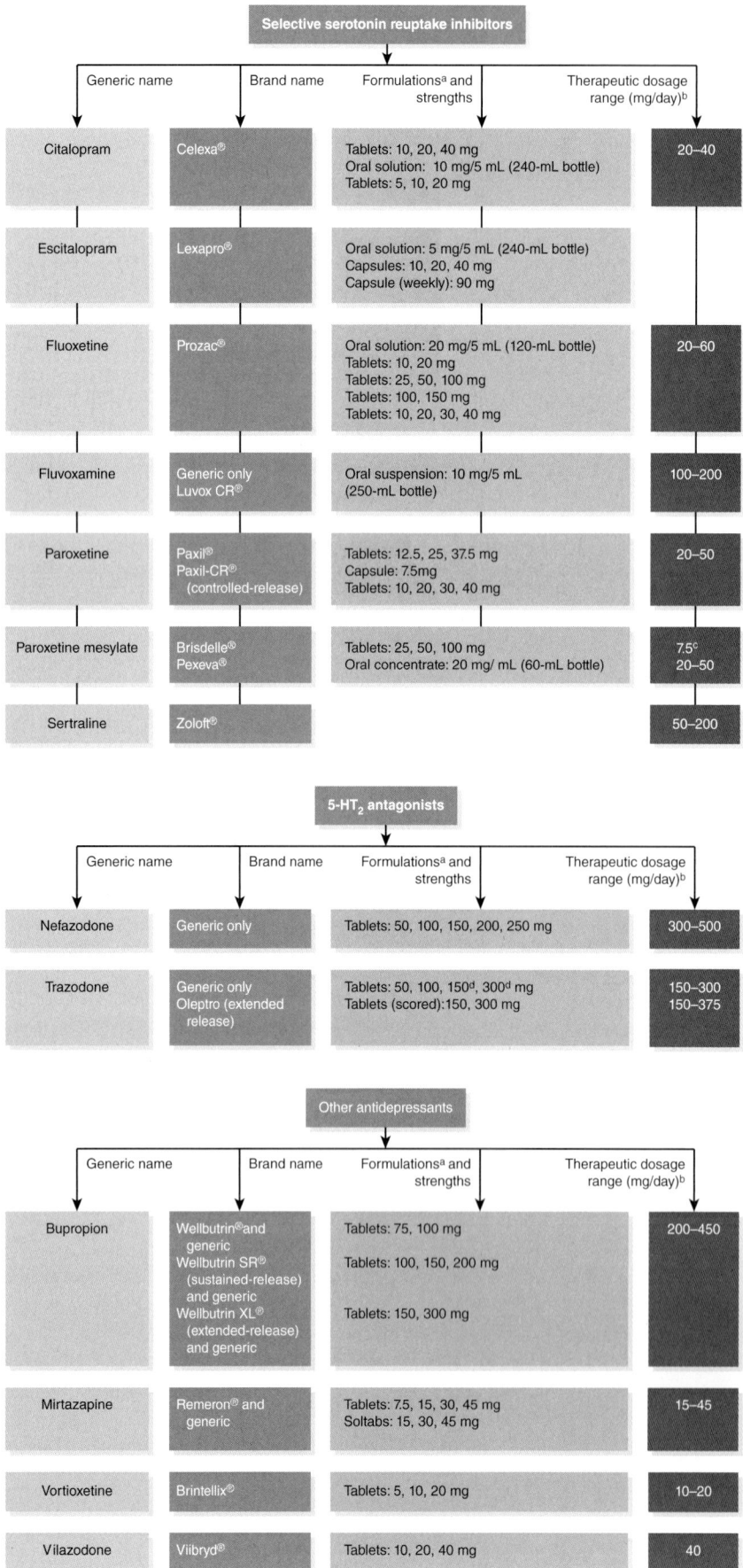

Figure 49-4 Antidepressant Names, Formulations and Strengths, and Dosages

Data from Schatzberg, A. F., & DeBattista, C. (2019). *Manual of Clinical Psychopharmacology* (9thed.). Washington, DC: American Psychiatric Association Publishing.

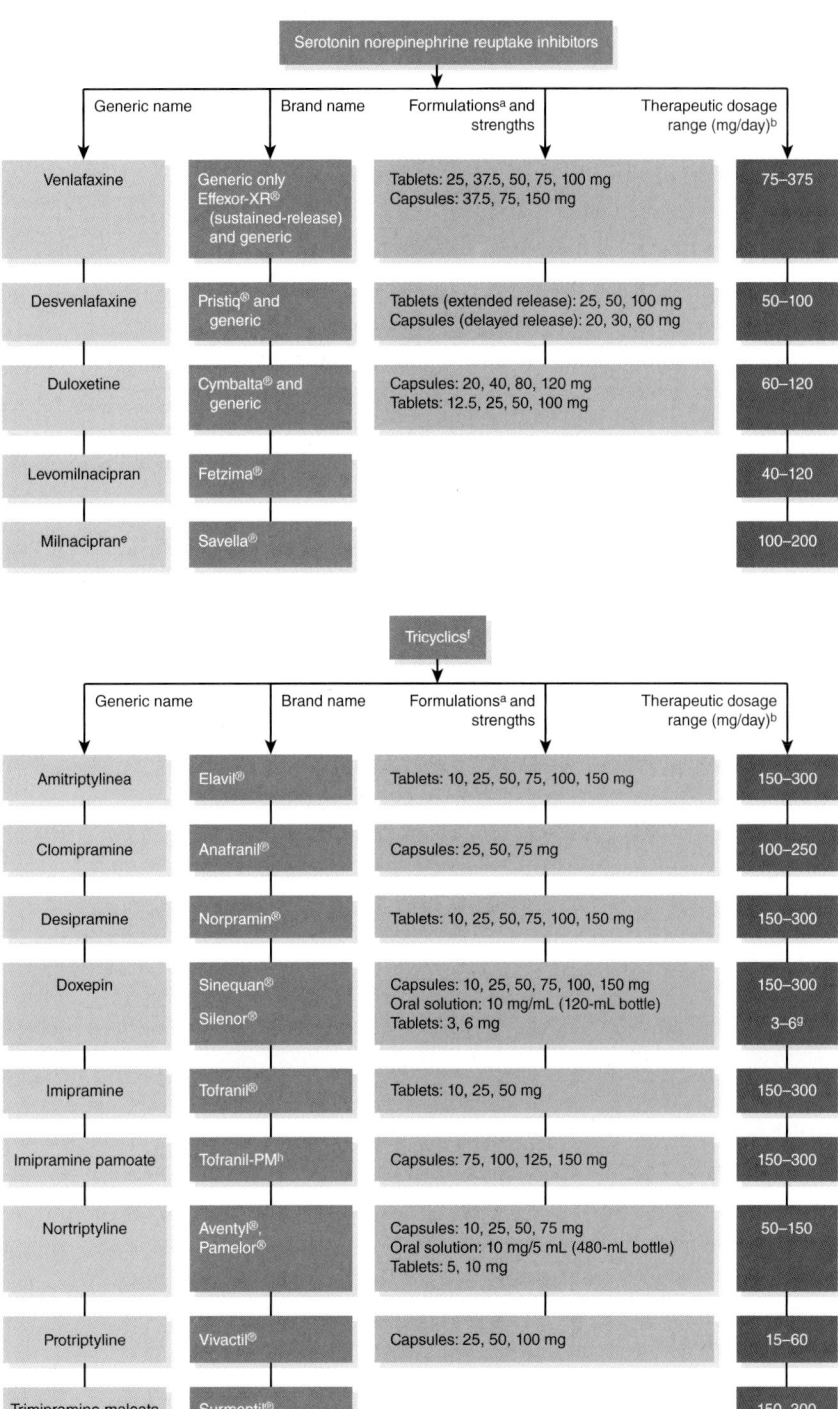

Figure 49-4 (Continued)

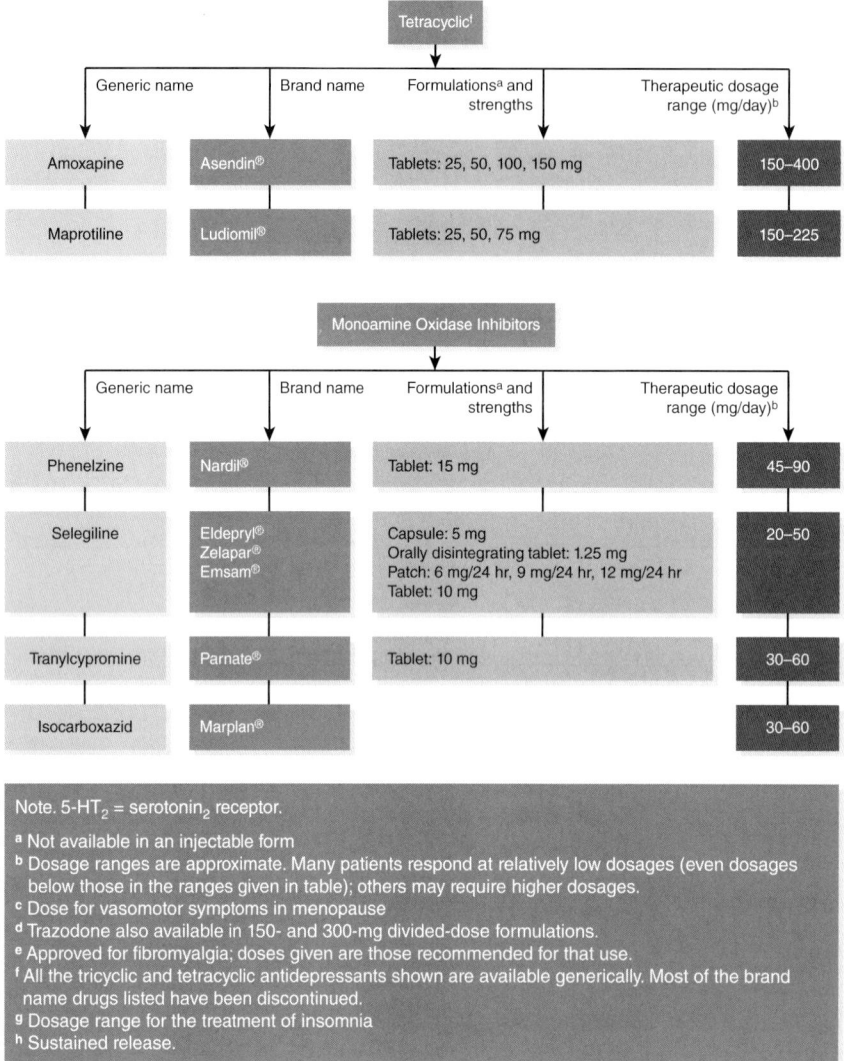

Figure 49-4 (Continued)

4. Referral to mental health or psychiatric specialty for evaluation or management: Refer patients with psychotic symptoms, suspicion of bipolar disorder or thought disorder, current or prior treatment-resistant depression, depressive symptoms that fail to improve despite several treatment trials, severe functional impairment, active suicidal ideation or plan, and concurrent psychiatric or neurologic disorder.

Patients may be referred to a psychiatric provider to determine the appropriateness of neuromodulation therapies. Commonly used neuromodulatory therapies that alter brain activity through electromagnetic stimulation include electroconvulsive therapy (ECT) and transcutaneous magnetic stimulation (TMS). ECT, which has been used for decades, is a rapid and effective treatment for unipolar depression but is not generally used as a first-line treatment because it requires general anesthesia and may result in side effects such as memory loss. TMS is an office-based procedure that uses electrical currents to stimulate target brain regions. Although not as effective as ECT, it compares favorably to antidepressant medications in effectiveness, is easier to administer, and is generally well tolerated.

C. *Patient education*
  1. Information: Provide verbal and written information regarding the following:
    a. The disease process, including but not limited to signs and symptoms and possible causes and risks, including self-harm
    b. The importance of treatment, including nonpharmacologic treatment, with the goal of complete and sustained remission of depression; expected treatment duration; and community resources to manage psychiatric crises
    c. Selection of written educational materials, including online resources, should consider the following:
      i. Patient educational and reading level
      ii. Availability of materials in patient's preferred language
      iii. Accuracy of information and freedom from commercial bias

Table 49-3 Antidepressant Side Effects (SEs): Classes, SEs, and Prescribing Considerations for Antidepression Treatment (ADT)

Class	Drugs	SE	Considerations
TCA	Imipramine, Amitriptyline, Doxepin, Desipramine, Nortriptyline	Weight gain, sedation, dry mouth, nausea, blurred vision, constipation, tachycardia	Generally, not first-line therapy because of increased anticholinergic and cardiotoxic SE
MAOI	Isocarboxazid, Phenelzine, Tranylcypromine, Selegiline	Weight gain, fatigue, sexual dysfunction, hypotension	Generally, not first-line therapy because of serotonin syndrome and hypertensive crises
SSRI	Fluoxetine, Paroxetine, Sertraline, Citalopram, Escitalopram	Headaches, GI distress, insomnia, fatigue, anxiety, sexual dysfunction, weight gain	Often first-line treatment because of safer SE profile. Subtle SE differences must be weighed by the prescriber.
SNRI	Venlafaxine, Desvenlafaxine, Duloxetine, Levomilnacipran	Nausea, insomnia, dry mouth, headache, increased blood pressure, sexual dysfunction, weight gain	SEs are similar to but may be slightly more frequent than with SSRI.
Atypical	Bupropion	Headache, agitation, insomnia, loss of appetite, weight loss, sweating	Increased seizure risk in patients with eating disorders or epilepsy. No sexual dysfunction or weight gain. May also help to quit smoking.
	Mirtazapine	Sedation, increased appetite, weight gain	Sedation may be less with higher dose. Much reduced nausea and sexual dysfunction compared with SSRI/SNRI. Some risk of reduced white blood cell count.
	Trazodone	Sedation, nausea, priapism (rare)	Lower risk of weight gain and sexual dysfunction but may cause priapism. Often used to induce sleep as a positive effect.
	Vilazodone	Nausea, diarrhea, insomnia	Better SE profile than most ADTs, with lower risk of sexual dysfunction or weight gain
	Vortioxetine	Nausea, diarrhea, dizziness	Similar SE profile to the SSRI. May have precognitive benefits in adults with MDD.

GI, gastrointestinal; *MAOI*, monoamine oxidase inhibitor; *MDD*, major depressive disorder; *SE*, side effect; *SNRI*, serotonin–norepinephrine reuptake inhibitor; *SSRI*, selective serotonin reuptake inhibitor; *TCA*, tricyclic antidepressant.

Reproduced from Santarsieri D., Schwartz T.L. (2015). Antidepressant efficacy and side-effect burden: A quick guide for clinicians. *Drugs Context*. 2015; 4: 212290. doi: 10.7573/dic.212290

2. Counseling
   a. Supportive counseling, focusing on problem solving and use of coping strategies
   b. Behavioral recommendations: regular exercise, especially aerobic exercise; balanced diet; presence of supportive relationships; increased engagement in pleasurable activities; avoidance of excessive use of alcohol or drugs; and sleep hygiene

VI. Self-management resources and tools

Brief educational or self-management interventions, such as manualized therapies and the use of interactive web-based or other computer programs based on cognitive–behavioral approaches, have been shown to improve depression outcomes for patients treated in primary care settings. Self-management, which is one of the core components of the collaborative care model for depression care, has demonstrated a variety of positive outcomes, including reduction in depressive symptoms and increased patient and provider satisfaction (Duggal, 2019).

A. Educational resources (books and websites)
   1. The National Institute of Mental Health (NIMH) Depression webpage (https://www.nimh.nih.gov/health/topics/depression) provides an overview of

depression-related conditions and includes links to multiple educational resources, such as brochures, shareable online resources, and multimedia information. NIMH publications on depression in Spanish can be found at https://www.nimh.nih.gov/health/publications/espanol/depression-listing.

2. There are many depression management self-help workbooks available, most of which are based on a cognitive–behavioral therapy approach. *Feeling Good: The New Mood Therapy* (Burns, 1980) is a classic in the field that uses a cognitive therapy approach to depression management. It is commonly used as self-guided treatment and in depression treatment programs. The Wellness Interventions for Life's Demands (WILD5) program uses a wellness-based approach to depression management that includes attention to sleep, exercise, nutrition, mindfulness, and social connectedness. More information about the program and its self-help workbooks is available at https://www.wild5wellness.com.

B. Community support groups

Multiple U.S.-based mental health support and advocacy organizations host educational resources and help users connect to services and peer support. These include the Depression and Bipolar Support Alliance (http://www.dbsalliance.org/), Mental Health America (https://mhanational.org/), the Anxiety and Depression Association of America (https://adaa.org/), and the National Alliance on Mental Illness (https://nami.org/Home).

C. Mobile apps

Digital technologies are increasingly being used to support depression self-management. Mobile apps allow users to monitor symptoms, access targeted education resources, set medication reminders, and in some cases, communicate with providers. Apps may be used as a delivery method for evidence-based treatment methods such as cognitive–behavioral or mindfulness-based therapies. Mobile apps are widely used by individuals to self-manage depressive symptoms, either alone or in combination with formal treatment, and the research base demonstrating that the use of well-designed mobile apps can decrease depressive symptoms is growing (Kerst et al., 2020).

However, the quality of the ever-increasing number mental health mobile apps on the market is quite variable. Many available apps are not designed or monitored by licensed mental health professionals and do not use evidence-based strategies for self-management. This has led to the development of multiple evaluation frameworks to assess the validity and potential usefulness of mental health apps, although most existing evaluation frameworks may not devote sufficient attention to issues related to diversity, equity, and inclusion (Ramos et al., 2021). The American Psychiatric Association has launched the App Advisor initiative (www.psychiatry.org/psychiatrists/practice/mental-health-apps) to help health professionals select the most useful and evidence-based mobile health resources for their patients.

References

American Psychiatric Association. (2013). *Diagnostic and statistical manual of mental disorders* (5th ed.).

Boland, R., & Verduin, M. (2022). *Kaplan & Saddock's synopsis of psychiatry* (12th ed.). Wolters Kluwer.

Burns, D. D. (1980). *Feeling good: The new mood therapy*. William Morrow.

Cuijpers, P., Quero, S., Dowrick, C., & Arroll, B. (2019). Psychological treatment of depression in primary care: recent developments. *Current Psychiatry Reports, 21*(12), 1–10. doi:10.1007/s11920-019-1117-x

Duggal, H. S. (2019). Self-management of depression: Beyond the medical model. *Permanente Journal, 23*(3), 18–295. doi:10.7812/TPP/18-295

Hasin, D. S., Sarvet, A. L., Meyers, J. L., Saha, T. D., Ruan, W. J., Stohl, M., & Grant, B. F. (2018). Epidemiology of adult DSM-5 major depressive disorder and its specifiers in the United States. *JAMA Psychiatry, 75*(4), 336–346. doi:10.1001/jamapsychiatry.2017.4602

Herrera, P. A., Campos-Romero, S., Szabo, W., Martínez, P., Guajardo, V., & Rojas, G. (2021). Understanding the relationship between depression and chronic diseases such as diabetes and hypertension: a grounded theory study. *International journal of environmental research and public health, 18*(22), 12130. https://doi.org/10.3390/ijerph182212130

Kerst, A., Zielasek, J., & Gaebel, W. (2020). Smartphone applications for depression: a systematic literature review and a survey of health care professionals' attitudes towards their use in clinical practice. *European Archives of Psychiatry and Clinical Neuroscience, 270*(2), 139–152. doi:10.1007/s00406-018-0974-3

MacArthur Initiative on Depression and Primary Care. (2009). *Depression management toolkit.* https://www.aetnabetterhealth.com/content/dam/aetna/medicaid/maryland/providers/pdfs/Macarthur%20Depression%20Toolkit.pdf.

Manea, L. Gilbody, S., Hewitt, C., North, A., Plummer, F., Richardson, R., Thombs, B. D., Williams, B., & McMillan, D. (2016). Identifying depression with the PHQ-2: A diagnostic meta-analysis. *Journal of Affective Disorders, 203*, 382–395. doi:10.1016/j.jad.2016.06.003

Mekonen, T., Ford, S., Chan, G. C. K., Hides, L., Connor, J. P., & Leung, J. (2022). What is the short-term remission rate for people with untreated depression? A systematic review and meta-analysis. *Journal of Affective Disorders, 296*, 17–25. doi:10.1016/j.jad.2021.09.046

Novick, D., Montgomery, W., Vorstenbosch, E., Moneta, M. V., Dueñas, H., & Haro, J. M. (2017). Recovery in patients with major depressive disorder (MDD): Results of a 6-month, multinational, observational study. *Patient Preference and Adherence, 11*, 1859–1868. doi:10.2147/PPA.S138750

Oluboka, Katzman, M. A., Habert, J., McIntosh, D., MacQueen, G. M., Milev, R. V., McIntyre, R. S., & Blier, P. (2018). Functional recovery in major depressive disorder: providing early optimal treatment for the individual patient. *International Journal of Neuropsychopharmacology*, 21(2), 128–144. doi:10.1093/ijnp/pyx081

Ramos, G., Ponting, C., Labao, J. P., & Sobowale, K. (2021). Considerations of diversity, equity, and inclusion in mental health apps: A scoping review of evaluation frameworks. *Behaviour Research and Therapy*, 147, 103990. doi:10.1016/j.brat.2021.103990

Santarsieri, D., & Schwartz, T. L. (2015). Antidepressant efficacy and side-effect burden: a quick guide for clinicians. *Drugs in Context*, 4, 212290. doi:10.7573/dic.212290

Schatzberg, A. F., & DeBattista, C. (2019). *Manual of Clinical Psychopharmacology* (9th ed.). American Psychiatric Association Publishing.

Siniscalchi, K. A., Broome, M. E., Fish, J., Ventimiglia, J., Thompson, J., Roy, P., Pipes, R., & Trivedi, M. (2020). Depression screening and measurement-based care in primary care. *Journal of Primary Care & Community Health*, 11, 2150132720931261. doi:10.1177/2150132720931261

Siu, A. L. (2016). Screening for depression in adults: U.S. Preventive Services Task Force recommendation statement. *JAMA*, 315(4), 380–387. doi:10.1001/jama.2015.18392

Sporinova, B., Manns, B., Tonelli, M., Hemmelgarn, B., MacMaster, F., Mitchell, N., Au, F., Ma, Z., Weaver, R., & Quinn, A. (2019). Association of mental health disorders with health care utilization and costs among adults with chronic disease. *JAMA Network Open*, 2(8), e199910. doi:10.1001/jamanetworkopen.2019.9910

U.S. Department of Health and Human Services. (2009). *SAFE-T Pocket Card* (HHS Publication No. [SMA] 09-4432). https://store.samhsa.gov/sites/default/files/d7/priv/sma09-4432.pdf.

World Health Organization. (2017). *Depression and other common mental disorders: Global health estimates.* https://apps.who.int/iris/handle/10665/254610

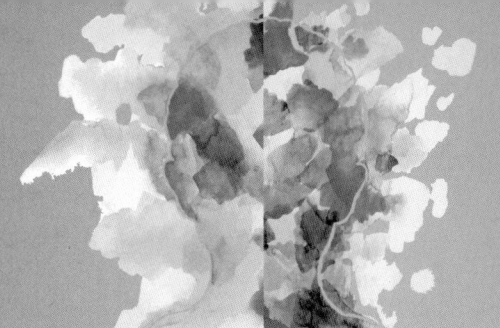

CHAPTER 50

Diabetes Mellitus

Anjali Asrani

I. Introduction and general background
Diabetes mellitus (DM) is a metabolic disorder characterized by hyperglycemia that results from decreased insulin secretion, insulin resistance, or both. There are several types of diabetes. The most common types are type 1, type 2, and gestational diabetes.
A. Prevalence and incidence
Approximately 537 million adults were living with diabetes worldwide in 2021. This figure represents 10.5% of the global population and is projected to increase to 783.2 million in 2045 (International Diabetes Federation, 2022). The United States is home to 37.3 million people living with diabetes. Of these, one-fifth are undiagnosed (Centers for Disease Control and Prevention [CDC], 2022). Type 1 diabetes (T1D) accounts for approximately 5%–10% of diagnosed diabetes cases, whereas type 2 diabetes (T2D) makes up the other 90%–95%. Of note, the incidence of both T1D and T2D is growing exponentially (American Diabetes Association [ADA], 2009).
B. Type 1 diabetes
1. Definition and overview
T1D is usually caused by an autoimmune process that destroys the β (beta) cells in the pancreas, thereby resulting in little or no insulin production. Individuals with T1D cannot live without administration of exogenous insulin. Although T1D is often associated with youth, it can develop at any age. T1D diagnosed in adulthood may also be called *latent autoimmune diabetes of the adult* (LADA). LADA can have a much slower progression from diagnosis to absolute insulin insufficiency and is frequently misdiagnosed as T2D. The presentation of T1D in children, on the other hand, is often acute, with 40%–60% of new-onset T1D presenting in diabetic ketoacidosis (DKA). There is also a subset of nonautoimmune diabetes caused by injury to the pancreas, resulting in insulin insufficiency (ADA, 2022).

C. Type 2 diabetes
1. Definition and overview
T2D is usually the result of insulin resistance, although it can eventually lead to decreased insulin production. T2D is thought to stem from a combination of complex environmental, socioeconomic, and genetic factors. Risk factors for T2D include age older than 35 years, higher body weight, sedentary lifestyle, family history of diabetes, history of gestational diabetes, delivery of a baby over 9 lb, lower socioeconomic status, and race or ethnicity (African Americans, Latinos, Native Americans, and Asian Americans/Pacific Islanders have a higher incidence). Although originally associated with adults, T2D is becoming more common in children and adolescents. According to the SEARCH for Diabetes in Youth Study (Dabelea et al., 2014), T2D in youth represents 50% of new-onset diabetes in youth. Moreover, ethnic minority youth in the United States are at higher risk for T2D when compared to their White peers.
D. Gestational diabetes
1. Definition and overview
Gestational diabetes occurs in 3%–12% of pregnancies. Pregnancy is an insulin-resistant state. Women with a history of gestational diabetes have a 40%–60% chance of developing T2D in the next 5–10 years after their pregnancy; therefore, they should have their blood sugar monitored periodically. For more in-depth information, see Chapter 33, Gestational Diabetes Mellitus: Early Detection and Management in Pregnancy.

II. Database
A. Subjective
1. History of presenting illness
a. Age of onset
b. Presenting signs and symptoms: Assess for classic signs or symptoms—weight gain or loss, polyuria, polydipsia, and/or polyphagia.

c. Growth and developmental history for children and youth
d. Routines: nutrition (food security, food diary, sugary beverages), exercise (type and duration), housing stability (access to refrigeration and cooking), and alcohol intake
e. Review of medication regimens, response to therapy, and adherence issues
f. Assessment of readiness for change, SMART (specific–measurable–attainable–realistic–timely) goal attainment, and barriers to self-care
g. Self-glucose monitoring: Assess trends of high and low values.
h. Hypoglycemia: Assess for awareness, frequency, and cause.
2. Past health history
   a. Medical illnesses: hypertension, metabolic syndrome, hyperlipidemia, thyroid disease, celiac, pancreatitis, pancreatic cancer, cystic fibrosis, hemochromatosis, Cushing syndrome, acromegaly, glucagonoma, higher body weight, and pheochromocytoma
   b. Diabetes-related complications: microvascular disease (retinopathy, nephropathy, neuropathy, including sensory and autonomic); macrovascular disease: cardiovascular disease (CVD), peripheral artery disease, and cerebrovascular disease
   c. Surgical history: pancreatic, liver, or gastric bypass surgery
   d. Trauma history: pancreatic trauma
   e. Obstetric and gynecological history: history of gestational diabetes or delivery of baby weighing more than 9 lb; contraception method
   f. Medication history: medications that increase blood glucose levels or interfere with the release of insulin (e.g., glucocorticoids, pentamidine, nicotinic acid, thyroid hormone, phenytoin, atypical antipsychotics, and thiazides); use of immune checkpoint inhibitors; any over-the-counter medications or herbs containing sugar (e.g., sweetened cough preparations)
3. Family history
   a. DM (type 1 or type 2)
   b. Metabolic syndrome
   c. Higher body weight
   d. Autoimmune disorders
   e. Other endocrine disorders
4. Occupational and educational history
   a. Education, preferred methods of learning, literacy level, and numeracy
   b. Occupation: type, ability to control environment as it relates to food intake and self-monitoring of blood glucose, work-related activity, work hours, and rest
   c. Days missed from school or work due to illness
5. Personal and social history
   a. Tobacco, alcohol, and drug use
   b. Diet history and 24-hour food and drink recall, food insecurity, household members who may influence cooking and food purchasing
   c. Exercise: type and duration
   d. Cultural history, living arrangements, housing, and psychosocial supports and problems
   e. Sexual history: partners and sexual activity; sexually transmitted infection prevention/condom use; contraception for individuals engaging in sexual practices that can lead to pregnancy
6. Review of symptoms
   a. Constitutional signs and symptoms: fatigue, weight loss, and polydipsia
   b. Skin, hair, and nails; slowed wound healing
   c. Eye, ear, nose, and throat; blurry vision; gum infections or dental disease
   d. Respiratory: shortness of breath
   e. Cardiac: chest pain
   f. Gastrointestinal: polyphagia and symptoms of gastroparesis
   g. Genitourinary: polyuria, recurrent genital yeast infections, sexual or erectile dysfunction
   h. Neurologic: decreased sensation or tingling and numbness in extremities
   i. Psychiatric: anxiety, depression, history of trauma, present or past use of antipsychotic medications

B. Objective
   1. Physical examination findings
      a. Height, weight, body mass index (BMI > 25 or > 23 in Asians)
      b. Vital signs, including orthostatic blood pressure if indicated
      c. Skin: acanthosis nigricans; fungal infections of feet or toenails; cracks in skin or wounds, especially hands and feet; lipohypertrophy at insulin injection sites
      d. Head, eyes, ears, nose, and throat: fundoscopic exam to assess for retinopathy, cataracts, vision test for blurry vision, teeth or gum inflammation, and poor dentition
      e. Thyroid: thyromegaly
      f. Lungs: crackles consistent with cardiovascular sequela
      g. Cardiac: blood pressure, irregular heartbeat, cardiomegaly, and murmurs
      h. Abdomen: hepatomegaly
      i. Vascular: peripheral pulses, bruits, and edema
      j. Neurologic: Sensory and motor strength; deep tendon reflexes (patellar and Achilles). Consider screening for functional performance.
      k. Foot examination: inspection (note calluses, lesions, edema, nail integrity, and any structural deformities); pulses in dorsalis pedis and posterior tibial; determination of proprioception, vibration, and 10-g monofilament sensation
   2. Supporting data from relevant diagnostic tests (**Table 50-1**)

Table 50-1 Diagnostic Criteria for Nongestational Diabetes

1. Hemoglobin A1C ≥ 6.5%
2. Fasting (minimum of 8 hours without food) plasma glucose ≥ 126 mg/dL
3. 2-hour plasma glucose ≥ 200 mg/dL following a 75-g oral glucose tolerance test
4. Random plasma glucose of 200 mg/dL in patients presenting with signs and symptoms of hyperglycemia

Diagnosis requires two abnormal tests in the absence of clear hyperglycemic symptoms and unequivocal testing. Two tests may be obtained from either the same sample or two separate test samples.

Data from American Diabetes Association. (2022). Standards of medical care in diabetes—2022. *Diabetes Care, 45* (Suppl. 1), S17.

Table 50-2 Clinical Interpretations of Plasma Glucose Concentrations

Glucose Concentration (mg/dL)	Clinical Interpretation
Fasting	
<100	Within the reference range
100–125	Impaired fasting glucose/prediabetes
≥126	Overt diabetes mellitus
2-hr post–challenge load (75-g oral glucose tolerance test)	
<140	Within the reference range
140–199	Impaired glucose tolerance/prediabetes
≥200	Overt diabetes mellitus

Data from American Diabetes Association. (2022). Standards of medical care in diabetes—2022. *Diabetes Care, 45* (Suppl. 1), S18–S19.

III. Assessment

A. *Type*
 1. Type 1 and type 2 diabetes: See Table 50-1 for the criteria of diagnosis and **Table 50-2** for the clinical interpretations of plasma glucose concentrations. Special tests may be obtained to assess for insulin production (e.g., C-peptide), as well as to confirm T1D immune-mediated beta cell destruction (e.g., islet cell autoantibodies and autoantibodies to insulin). Of note, some patients with T1D do not test positive for antibodies, and patients with injury to the insulin-producing cells caused by a secondary facture would test negative for autoantibodies. No matter the cause, pancreatic function, if in doubt, should be investigated because the treatment plan would then focus on insulin. If a primary care provider is in doubt about the type of diabetes, it is reasonable to consult with endocrine specialists (ADA, 2022; Patel & Marcerollo, 2010).
 2. Gestational diabetes
    a. There are two strategies but no clinical evidence to support one over the other. Testing should occur at 24–28 weeks of gestation.
       i. One-step strategy: 2-hour, 75-g oral glucose tolerance test, *or*
       ii. Two-step approach: 1-hour, 50-g (nonfasting) screen followed by a 3-hour, 100-g oral glucose tolerance test for those who screen positive
    b. Diagnosis of gestational diabetes mellitus (GDM) is made when values exceed the following:
       i. One step:
          - Fasting ≥ 92 mg/dL
          - 1 h: ≥180 mg/dL
          - 2 h: ≥153 mg/dL
       ii. Two step:
          - 1 h: ≥140 mg/dL, then proceed to step 2
          - 3 h: ≥140 mg/dL (ADA, 2022)

B. *Severity*
 Assess the severity of the disease via the presence or absence of end-organ complications, microvascular complications, and impact on basic and intermediate activities of daily living.

C. *Significance*
 Assess the significance of diabetes and any related complications to the patient and loved ones. This may include diabetes distress and patient concerns over the burden of living with diabetes. Diabetes Distress Assessment Scales can be used for evaluation (https://diabetesdistress.org/).

D. *Motivation and ability*
 Determine the patient's obstacles to and motivation for change via motivational interviewing techniques, and assess for support and barriers to achieving self-management goals. Motivational interviewing involves an approach that avoids instructing patients on what to do. Instead, the focus is on the practitioner trying to better understand a patient's values, concerns, and barriers and factors that drive their motivation for change. It's imperative that providers listen and communicate with empathy so they may better help patients find concrete ways to achieve their goals and move beyond obstacles for personal health management.

IV. Goals of clinical management

A. *Screening or diagnosing diabetes* (Tables 50-1, 50-2, and 50-3)

Choose a cost-effective approach for screening and diagnosing diabetes.
B. *Treatment*
Jointly develop a treatment plan with the patient that manages glucose and prevents complications in a safe and effective manner without causing hypoglycemia. Treatment goals should optimize quality of life and take the patient's preferences into account. Goals should always be adjusted and determined by multiple factors, including risk for hypoglycemia, disease duration, life expectancy, comorbidities, vascular complications, and resources and support systems available to the patient (ADA, 2022).

For all patients with diabetes, current guidelines should be used to address dyslipidemia and hypertension therapy goals. For patients meeting the criteria for antihypertensive therapy, consider angiotensin-converting enzyme inhibitors (ACEis) or angiotensin receptor blockers (ARBs), which convey renal protection and reduce the risk of progressive proteinuria. Once proteinuria has been detected, an ACEi, ARB, or a sodium/glucose cotransporter-2 inhibitor (SGLT2i; T2D only and with sufficient insulin production) should be started to slow the progression of nephropathy (ADA, 2022).

C. *Patient adherence*
Provide self-management education and support in order to maximize patient adherence. Providers should use motivational interviewing and problem-solving strategies to support patients and create a collaborative medication plan. National standards for diabetes self-management education (DSME) clearly state that goals should be patient centered, be personally relevant, and take into account the patient's lived experience (Haas et al., 2012). For example, patients should be educated about the action and side effects of each medication in a way that they can understand. Clinicians should choose medications in partnership with the patient, focusing on how these fit into each patient's work and home life and schedule in a safe and reasonable way. Patients must be given ample time to ask questions about medications outside of mere adherence. If patients do not meet A1c goals or do not pick up medications, clinicians must spend time conversing with the patient to identify obstacles and revise a joint plan.

D. *Prevention of complications*
For all types of diabetes, screening for kidney disease, retinopathy, and neuropathies is of great importance because glycemic management can reduce the risk of microvascular complications. Primary and secondary prevention of cardiovascular risk factors is also critical.

V. Plan

A. *Primary prevention: criteria screening of high-risk groups (Table 50-3)*
  1. Treatment guidelines for prediabetes: Individuals at high risk for developing T2D (prediabetes), defined as impaired fasting glucose (IFG) of 100–125 mg/dL, impaired glucose tolerance (IGT) of 140–199 mg/dL 2 hours post–glucose load, or an HbA1C of 5.7%–6.4%, should be referred to structured programs that emphasize lifestyle changes, including moderate weight loss (7% of body weight) and regular physical activity (150 min/wk, strength training 2×/wk) (ADA, 2022). In at-risk individuals younger than 60 years old, metformin therapy should be considered for the prevention of T2D. Ongoing monitoring for diabetes should be done at least annually. Modifiable cardiovascular disease (CVD) risk factors should be identified, and appropriate interventions are recommended (ADA, 2022). Refer to **Table 50-3** for criteria of high-risk groups.

B. *Diagnostics*
  1. Hemoglobin A1C every 3–6 months (depending on whether glycemia is at goal and use of continuous glucose monitoring [CGM])
  2. Annual urine albumin/creatinine ratio
  3. Creatinine, estimated glomerular filtration rate (eGFR), potassium

Table 50-3 Criteria for Testing for Diabetes or Prediabetes in Asymptomatic Adults

1. Testing should be considered in all adults who meet the following criteria and/or risk factors:
   - All adults ages 35+, regardless of other risk factors
   - Adults of any age with BMI of ≥ 25 kg.m^2 (or ≥ 3kg/m^2 in individuals with Asian ancestry)
   - Physical inactivity
   - First-degree relative with diabetes
   - High-risk race/ethnicity (e.g., African American, Latino, Native American, Asian American, Pacific Islander)
   - Women who delivered a baby weighing >9 lb or were diagnosed with gestational diabetes mellitus (GDM)
   - Hypertension (≥140/90 mmHg or on therapy for hypertension)
   - High-density lipoprotein (HDL) cholesterol level < 35 mg/dL (0.90 mmol/L) and/or a triglyceride level > 250 mg/dL (2.82 mmol/L)
   - Women with polycystic ovary syndrome
   - A1C ≥ 5.7%, impaired glucose tolerance (IGT), or impaired fasting glucose (IFG) on previous testing
   - Other clinical conditions associated with insulin resistance (e.g., higher body weight, acanthosis nigricans)
   - History of cardiovascular disease (CVD)

2. If results are normal, testing should be repeated at a minimum of 3-year intervals, with consideration of more frequent testing depending on initial results (e.g., those with prediabetes should be tested yearly) and risk status.

4. Annual lipid panel
5. Liver function tests if on thiazolidinedione medications and/or statins
6. B_{12} level if on metformin

C. Management *(includes treatment, consultation, referral, and follow-up care)*

Providers must first investigate the cause of the diabetes, especially if it is related to infection or medication use, and treat the patient accordingly. Patients initially presenting with T1D or ketosis-prone T2D may be hospitalized depending on their symptoms and degree of illness (e.g., diabetic ketoacidosis). The goal of treatment is to achieve near-normal blood glucose levels without significant hypoglycemia, attain and maintain reasonable body weight when relevant, and normalize lipids and blood pressure as indicated. All patients should be referred for diabetes education and dietary counseling that is tailored to their specific type of diabetes and individual concerns.

1. Medical nutrition therapy (MNT)
   a. Reduction in energy intake is a cornerstone of treatment in T2D and may be needed in T1D. MNT for both types of diabetes involves a distribution of carbohydrates that takes into consideration an individual's pharmacological treatment as well as the person's activity pattern. People with diabetes should consult with a dietician at diagnosis, with any significant changes in management, and on an annual basis.
   b. Of the macronutrients, carbohydrates (CHOs) have the most significant effect on blood glucose levels, so patients need to learn to identify a CHO and approximate appropriate portions of carbs for their treatment plan. Patients with no pancreatic function using multiple insulins may benefit from learning more exact estimations of CHOs or "carb counting" in order to safely dose their insulin. Recent evidence suggests that there are no ideal percentages for CHO, protein, and fat intake and that the individual MNT plan should be personalized and address current eating patterns as well as personal preferences, including cultural traditions. It is advisable that patients obtain most of their CHOs from whole foods, such as fruits, vegetables, whole grains, legumes, and other low-glycemic-index foods. Sucrose is allowable, but if used on a regular basis, it will replace more nutrient-dense food in the diet. Sugar-containing beverages should be avoided as much as possible because of their immediate effect on blood glucose levels and contribution to nonnutritive calories; they may also worsen CVD risk profiles. Consumption of lean proteins with carbohydrates can help to slow the digestion of carbohydrates and resultant rise in glucose (ADA, 2022).
   c. Sugar-sweetened beverages comprise a subset of carbohydrate intake, with regular consumption by half the U.S. population (Ogden et al., 2011). Added sugars are found in sodas, juices, lemonades, iced teas, sports and energy drinks, and blended coffees. The average can of soda has 7–10 teaspoons of sugar, which rapidly increases blood sugar and has far-reaching repercussions for the management of diabetes and weight. Patients should always be asked about sugar-sweetened beverage consumption and counseled on strategies for avoidance. Elimination of sugar-sweetened beverages can have a significant impact on lowering glucose.
   d. Fiber, saturated fat, and dietary cholesterol intake are as recommended for the general population. Newer studies show benefit from diets that are rich in unsaturated fatty acids (ADA, 2022).
2. Exercise
   a. Ideally, a minimum of 150 minutes/week of moderate-intensity aerobic physical activity (50%–70% of maximum heart rate) is advised. However, for patients who are sedentary, setting individualized activity goals can be more realistic and effective. For exercise rules and precautions, refer to **Table 50-4**.

Table 50-4 Exercise Rules and Precautions

Check glucose before and after exercise. Exercise increases the risk of hypoglycemia. If taking sulfonylureas, meglitinides, or insulin, carry fast-acting carbohydrates during exercise. Avoid vigorous exercise in the presence of ketosis.
Wear properly fitted footwear.
Before starting, screen for vascular or neurologic complications.
Caution in patients with retinopathy, neuropathy, and peripheral vascular disease.
High-risk patients should start slowly.
Carry identification that includes diagnosis and medication list.
Avoid exercise in extreme temperatures and humidity.
Use proper equipment.
Complete proper warm-up and stretching exercises.
Adequate hydration.
Stop for any pain, lightheadedness, or shortness of breath.

Data from American Diabetes Association. (2015). Standards of medical care in diabetes—2015. *Diabetes Care, 38*(Suppl. 1), S9.

b. Patients with T2D without contraindications should perform resistance training at least two to three times per week (ADA, 2022).
3. Setting SMART goals

Jointly setting goals for the plan of care is a cornerstone of diabetes management. Making plans for medication and/or lifestyle changes can be overwhelming and difficult to carry out for a variety of reasons. Working with patients to set tangible, self-identified goals can empower patients and be helpful in successfully enacting plans between appointments. Goals can focus on diet, exercise, medication, or some other area that addresses diabetes management. SMART goals should add beneficial behaviors and avoid a focus on restriction or deprivation. SMART goals are:

S—specific: tangible and focus on one specific action
M—measurable: include a metric that measures progress
A—achievable: attainable and realistic for the patient
R—relevant: directly addresses diabetes management
T—time bound: includes a time frame for starting the goal and measuring progress

Some examples of SMART goals using this framework above may be as follows: including vegetables in one meal per day for the next month; spending 1 hour every Saturday to organize medications into pill boxes for the next 6 weeks; cooking a family dinner once per week for the next 2 months; or start walking twice per week (every Wednesday and Saturday) for at least 10 minutes, for the next month. All goals should be individualized and identified jointly by the patient and provider.

4. Pharmacological therapy
   a. Prophylactic medications
      i. Aspirin (75–162 mg/day) is strongly recommended for patients with diabetes and prior history of stroke or myocardial infarction (MI) to reduce the risk of cardiovascular morbidity and mortality. The benefits of aspirin as a strategy for primary prevention in diabetes are less clear and can be outweighed by the risks of bleeding. An individualized approach is recommended when considering aspirin therapy as a primary prevention strategy in people with T1D and T2D who are 50–69 years old and have at least one additional major risk factor (i.e., family medical history of cardiovascular disease, hypertension, smoking, dyslipidemia, or albuminuria; ADA, 2022).
      ii. ACEis or ARBs for patients with hypertension or microalbuminuria; SGLT2is for proteinuria in patients with T2D who are not prone to ketosis (American Association of Clinical Endocrinology [AACE], 2020; ADA, 2022; Joslin Diabetes Center, 2020).
   b. Type 1 DM
      For T1D management, the mainstay of the treatment plan is insulin, preferably a basal/bolus regimen via injection or insulin pump. Dosing of total insulin for T1D is often 0.4–1.0 units/kg (ADA, 2022). According to the Diabetes Control and Complications Trial (DCCT) and the follow-up Epidemiology of Diabetes Interventions and Complications (EDIC) (National Diabetes Information Clearinghouse, 2009), it is well established that patients with T1D should check their blood glucose level and base insulin dosing on the amount of CHOs eaten and the corresponding blood glucose level. Current therapy for patients with T1D usually requires prandial injections of a rapid-acting insulin and a once- or twice-per-day long-acting basal insulin. This type of therapy is referred to as *basal/bolus therapy*, comprising multiple daily injections. Alternately, insulin pumps deliver continuous insulin via subcutaneous infusion. Patients with T1D should always be referred to endocrinology.
   c. Type 2 DM
      T2D management usually begins with lifestyle modification, exercise, and then oral agents. This treatment plan is, however, usually guided by the patient's hemoglobin A1C level, blood glucose levels, and comorbidities. If the patient is grossly hyperglycemic at presentation (e.g., A1c > 9%), then insulin is usually recommended. There are several algorithms for the treatment of T2D (AACE, 2020; ADA, 2022; Joslin Diabetes Center, 2020) (**Figure 50-1**).
   d. Oral agents (**Table 50-5**)
   e. Injectable (other than insulin) (**Table 50-6**)
   f. Insulins (**Tables 50-7**, **50-8**, and **50-9**)

All patients using insulin and at risk for hypoglycemia should have a prescription for glucagon. Both patients and those living in their households should be educated about treating severe hypoglycemia and how and when to use glucagon. Multiple preparations are available, including injectable and inhalable versions.

5. Self-monitoring of blood glucose (SMBG) and CGM
   According to the Joslin Diabetes Center (2020), "The frequency of SMBG should be individualized, based on factors such as glucose goals, medication changes, use of continuous glucose sensor, and patient motivation. Most patients with type 1 diabetes should monitor using SMBG or a Continuous Glucose Monitoring (CGM) device at least 4 to 6 times per day. . . . Most patients using intensive insulin therapy should ideally monitor before meals and bedtime, prior to exercise, when they suspect hypoglycemia, after treating hypoglycemia, and prior to driving. For patients with T2D, the frequency of monitoring is dependent upon such factors as mode of treatment, risk for hypoglycemia, and whether glycemia is at goal" (p. 8). All patients should be educated on their individualized glucose targets; actionable readings; and that the fact that any checks,

First-line therapy is metformin and comprehensive lifestyle modification. If A1c continues above goal, intensify therapy.				
If ASCVD Predominates	**If HF or CKD Predominates**	**Without Established ASCVD or CKD**		
		Compelling Need to Minimize Hypoglycemia	**Compelling Need to promote weight loss**	**If Cost is a Major Issue**
GLP-1 or SGLT2i (if eGFR adequate)	Preferable SGLT2i (if eGFR adequate). Otherwise, add GLP-1	Add GLP-1, SGLT2i, DPP-4, or TZD	Add GLP-1 or SGLT2i	Add sulfonylurea or TZD
If A1c above target ↓	*If A1c above target ↓*	*If A1c above target ↓*	*If A1c above target ↓*	*If A1c above target ↓*
Continue with addition of agent outlined above.	Avoid TZD in the setting of HF	Continue with addition of agents outlined above.	Continue with addition of agent outlined above.	Continue with addition of agent outlined above.
Add SGLT2i	Add DPP-4 (not saxagliptin) if not on GLP-1	*If A1c above target ↓*	*If A1c above target ↓*	*If A1c above target ↓*
Add sulfonylurea, DPP-4 if not on GLP-1, or TZD	Add sulfonylurea	Consider addition of basal insulin or sulfonylurea	Add DPP-4 (if not on GLP-1)	Consider lowest cost insulin, DPP-4 or SGLT2i
Add insulin	Add insulin			

Data from Melanie J. Davies, David A. D'Alessio, Judith Fradkin, Walter N. Kernan, Chantal Mathieu, Geltrude Mingrone, Peter Rossing, Apostolos Tsapas, Deborah J. Wexler, John B. Buse; Management of Hyperglycemia in Type 2 Diabetes, 2018. A Consensus Report by the American Diabetes Association (ADA) and the European Association for the Study of Diabetes (EASD). *Diabetes Care* 1 December 2018; 41 (12): 2669–2701. https://doi.org/10.2337/dci18-0033

Figure 50-1 Glucose-Lowering Medication in Type 2 Diabetes: Overall Approach

regardless of the reading, are positive steps in one's self-management plan. Guilt and shame should never be associated with glucose checks.

Fingerstick home glucose checks have been the primary means of self-monitoring of glucose for many patients. However, the role of technology in managing diabetes is expanding, and the advent of CGM provides an alternative avenue for SMBG. Continuous glucose monitors measure interstitial glucose levels and convert these readings to estimates of plasma levels. Numerous studies have found that consistent CGM use corresponds with a reduction in A1c and hypoglycemia in adults of all age groups. Continuous glucose monitors provide additional insights over fingerstick readings, including highlighting and analyzing glucose trends, sounding alarms at preset thresholds for hypo- and hyperglycemia, and monitoring glucose readings more frequently. Real-time glucose data can also serve as a teaching tool for patients to understand the connection between glucose levels, diet, and exercise. Continuous glucose monitors should be offered to all patients with T1D and any patient with T2D who is on hypoglycemic agents or who wishes to monitor their glucose more frequently (ADA, 2022; Joslin Diabetes Center, 2000). Insurance coverage of these devices is expanding.

There are several continuous glucose monitors with U.S. Food and Drug Administration (FDA) approval. At the time of publishing, the Dexcom and Freestyle Libre systems were the most widely used.

6. Prevention of hypoglycemia

Hypoglycemia is a side effect caused by treatment of diabetes with insulin or other hypoglycemic agents and needs to be minimized by the provider by optimizing treatment and empowering patients to understand their medications and take them safely. *Hypoglycemia* is defined as blood glucose levels below 70 mg/dL. Symptoms of hypoglycemia may include dizziness, sweating, hunger, confusion, imbalance, tachycardia, and irritability. Depending on the severity and degree of hypoglycemia, patients can be at risk for falls, motor vehicle accidents, seizures, coma, loss of consciousness, or death.

Table 50-5 Oral Agents*

Generic	Brand Name	Daily Dose (Min-Max)	Dosing (QD = daily; BID = twice a day; TID = three times a day)
Sulfonylureas (stimulate insulin production, may cause hypoglycemia)			
Glipizide	Glucotrol®	2.5–40 mg	QD-BID
Glipizide controlled release	Glucotrol XL®	2.5–20 mg	QD
Glimepiride	Amaryl®	1–8 mg	QD
Glyburide	Micronase®, DiaBeta®	1.25–20 mg	QD-BID
Micronized glyburide	Glynase®	0.75–12 mg	QD-BID
Meglitinide analogs (stimulate insulin production, may cause hypoglycemia)			
Repaglinide	Prandin®	0.5–16 mg	QID before meals
D-Phenylalanine derivative (stimulates insulin production, may cause hypoglycemia)			
Nateglinide	Starlix®	120–360 mg	TID before meals
Biguanides (increase insulin sensitivity and reduce glucose production by the liver)			
Metformin	Glucophage®	500–2,000 mg	QD-TID with meals
Metformin extended release	Glucophage XR® Glumetza®	500–2,000 mg	QD with a meal
Metformin	Riomet® (oral solution)	(5 cc = 500 mg) 500–550 mg	QD-TID with meals
Thiazolidinediones (increase insulin sensitivity, caution in patients with heart failure)			
Pioglitazone	Actos®	15–45 mg	QD
Alpha-glucosidase inhibitors (inhibit absorption of glucose, GI side effects common)			
Acarbose	Precose®	25–300 mg	TID with meals
Miglitol	Glyset®	25–300 mg	TID with meals
DPP-4 inhibitors (prevent the inactivation of incretins)			
Sitagliptin	Januvia®	100 mg	QD
Saxagliptin	Onglyza®	2.5–5 mg	QD
Linagliptin	Tradjenta®	5 mg	QD
Alogliptin	Nesina®	25 mg	QD
SGLT-2 inhibitors (reduce renal glucose reabsorption, increase glucose secretion in the urine)			
Canagliflozin	Invokana®	100–300 mg	Q a.m.
Dapagliflozin	Farxiga®	5–10 mg	Q a.m.
Empagliflozin	Jardiance®	10–25 mg	Q a.m.
Ertugliflozin	Steglatro®	5–15 mg	Q a.m.
GLP-1 receptor agonists (increase insulin release, reduce hepatic production of glucose, decrease appetite, and slow digestion)			
Semaglutide	Rybelsus®	3–14 mg	QD

Note: There are several combinations of various oral agents that are often available and may be appropriate to reduce cost and pill burden.

DPP-4, dipeptidyl peptidase 4; *GI*, gastrointestinal; *GLP-1*, glucagon-like peptide 1; *SLGT-2*, sodium-glucose transport protein 2.

Table 50-6 Injectable Agents (Non-Insulin)

GLP-1 receptor agonists

Semaglutide	Ozempic®*	0.25–2.0 mg	Weekly
Dulaglutide	Trulicity®	0.75–4.0 mg	Weekly
Liraglutide	Victoza®*	0.6–1.8 mg	QD
Tirzepitide	Mounjaro®*	2.5–15 mg	Weekly
Exenatide, immediate release	Byetta®	5–10 mcg	BID
Exenatide, extended release	Bydureon®	2 mg	Weekly
Lixisenatide	Adlyxin®	10–20 mcg	QD
Semaglutide	Wegovy®†	0.25–2.4 mg	Weekly
Liraglutide	Saxenda®†	0.6–3.0 mg	Daily

DPP-4, dipeptidyl peptidase 4; GLP-1, glucagon-like peptide 1.
* GLP-1 receptor agonists should not be combined with DPP-4s; people with diabetes should be offered to be titrated to the highest tolerable dose if weight loss is desired.
† Higher doses of semaglutide and liraglutide are approved for weight loss. May not be covered by insurance for a diagnosis of diabetes without higher body weight.

Table 50-7 Insulins*

Generic Name	Brand Name	Type	Onset	Peak	Duration
Lispro-aabc	Lyumjev®	Rapid	5–15 min	0.5–2 hr	2–5 hr
Aspart-niacinimide	Fiasp®	Rapid		0.5–2 hr	2–5 hr
Aspart	NovoLog®	Rapid	10–20 min	0.5–2.5 hr	2–5 hr
Lispro	Humalog®	Rapid	5–15 min	0.5–2.5 hr	2–5 hr
Glulisine	Apidra®	Rapid	5–15 min	0.5–2.5 hr	2–4 hr
Regular insulin	Novolin® R	Short acting	30–60 min	2–4 hr	5–8 hr
	Humulin® R	Same	Same	Same	Same
NPH	Novolin® N	Intermediate	1–3 hr	6–10 hr	16–24 hr
	Humulin® N	Same	Same	Same	Same
Glargine	Lantus®	Long acting	45 min–4 hr	None	Glargine
Detemir	Semglee®	Long acting	45 min–4 hr	None	24 hr
Glargine	Toujeo®	Long acting	6 hours	None	36 hr
Degludec	Tresiba®	Long acting	4 hours	None	42 hr

*Inhaled insulins (Afrezza) and concentrated injectable insulins (e.g., Toujeo u-300, Lyumjev U-200, Humalog U-200, and Humulin Regular u-500) are available yet less commonly used than the standard injectable insulins.

Medications should be selected that reduce the risk of hypoglycemia. For patients requiring insulin, providers should review the following:

a. Treatment of nonsevere hypoglycemia and the 15/15 rule: Glucose or another form of fast-acting CHO should be consumed to treat hypoglycemia. After 15 minutes, recheck glucose. If persistently hypoglycemic, repeat steps. Another snack with protein should be consumed to prevent recurrence.

b. All patients requiring insulin should have a prescription for glucagon. Family members and caregivers should be taught how to administer glucagon in the event of severe hypoglycemia.

Table 50-8 Combined Insulins

Premixed	Brand Name
Neutral protamine Hagedorn (NPH)/Regular	Novolin® 70/30
	Humulin® 70/30
	Humulin® 50/50
Lispro protamine/lispro	Humalog® Mix 75/25
Lispro protamine/lispro	Humalog® Mix 50/50
Aspart protamine/aspart	Novolog® Mix 70/30

Table 50-9 Combined Insulins and GLP-1 Receptor Agonists

Insulin	GLP-1RA	Brand Name	Dose
Degludec	Liraglutide	Xultophy 100/3.6®	10–50 units QD
Glargine	Lixisenatide	Soliqua 100/33®	15–60 units QD

GLP-1, glucagon-like peptide 1; *QD*, daily.

c. Assess the patient for hypoglycemia unawareness, which can indicate frequent hypoglycemia and a loss of associated symptoms.
d. Consider CGM therapy for all patients at risk for hypoglycemia, on insulin, and/or with hypoglycemia unawareness. CGM devices have the ability to alarm with impending and detected hypoglycemia.
e. Hypoglycemia treatment thresholds should be tailored to the individual. Some patients may require a higher threshold for treatment of hypoglycemia. For example, in certain geriatric patients, it may be appropriate to treat hypoglycemia of <100 mg/dL.
7. Self-management goals and clinical goals (**Table 50-10**)
8. Healthcare maintenance
    a. Immunizations
        i. Annual influenza vaccine
        ii. Pneumococcal 13-valent conjugate vaccine (PCV13): 1 dose for adults with diabetes ages 19–64
        iii. Pneumococcal 23-valent polysaccharide vaccine (PPCV23): 1 dose at least 8 weeks after PCV13, then another dose of PPSV23 at least 5 years later. One dose of PPSV23 after age 65.
        iv. Hepatitis B vaccine in adults 19–59 years old if unvaccinated, and consider if > 60 years old (Matthew & Jayne, 2015)

Table 50-10 Clinical Goals

	American Diabetes Association	American Association of Clinical Endocrinologists
Preprandial glucose	80–130	<110
2-hour postprandial glucose	<180	<140
Hemoglobin A1c	<7%, with a less stringent goal of 8% for selected populations	≤6.5% for most; less stringent for people with comorbidities and older adults
Blood pressure	<140/90; or <130/80 for patients with 10-year atherosclerotic cardiovascular disease (ASCVD) risk of ≥15% or existing ASCVD	<130/80; individualized based on age, comorbidities, and duration of disease
Lipids	Moderate-intensity statin should be used as primary prevention for patients 40–75 years of age with diabetes. High-intensity statin use should be considered for patients at higher risk or for secondary prevention. See Chapter 60, Lipid Disorders, for additional information.	Low-density lipoprotein (LDL) mg/dL: <100, moderate risk; <70, high risk
	Triglycerides: <150 mg/dL	Same
Urine albumin/creatinine ratio	<30 mg/g albumin/creatinine ratio	Same

Data from American Diabetes Association (2022); American Association of Clinical Endocrinologists and American College of Endocrinology—AACE Comprehensive Type 2 Diabetes Management Algorithm (2020).

v. Follow CDC guidelines for all other age-appropriate vaccine schedules.
vi. Smoking cessation counseling at every visit
9. Referrals and monitoring
Patients should be educated about potential complications from diabetes and how to prevent them. With this in mind, all people with diabetes should have the following referrals and monitoring:
   a. All patients with DM should be referred for DSME and support services.
   b. Patients with diabetes should be referred to an endocrinologist for the following reasons:
      i. Diagnosis of T1D
      ii. Starting an insulin pump
      iii. Recurrent diabetic ketoacidosis
      iv. Recurrent hypoglycemia
      v. Unable to adequately manage glucose or erratic blood glucose readings
   c. Women of childbearing age should receive preconception counseling and should be on reliable forms of contraception if pregnancy is not desired. Glucagon-like peptide-1 agonist (GLP1a) medications should only be used by women of childbearing age who are on reliable forms of contraception. Combined oral contraceptives should be avoided in patients with DM-related complications or who have had diabetes for 20 or more years (American College of Obstetricians and Gynecologists, 2019).
   d. Mental health referrals should be made as needed: Screen for depression, diabetes-related stress, anxiety, eating disorders, history of trauma and posttraumatic stress disorder (PTSD), and cognitive impairment when self-management is suboptimal.
   e. Dilated eye examination by an ophthalmologist annually. For people with T1D, first referral should occur 5 years after disease onset. For people with T2D, referral should occur at the initial visit. If exam is normal and glycemia is at goal, screening should be repeated every 1–2 years. Patients with GDM should be referred during the first trimester.
   f. Foot examination with 10-g monofilament at least annually. Patients with evidence of peripheral neuropathy or a history of ulcers or amputation should have a foot exam performed at each visit.
   g. Dental examination every 6 months with dentist
   h. Consider referral for sleep study and sleep apnea evaluation, especially in patients with T2D and higher body weight.
10. Patient education
   a. Sick-day guidelines
      i. Prevention of dehydration and ketosis
      ii. Adequate fluid and calorie intake
      iii. Alert patient to signs and symptoms of hypoglycemia and hyperglycemia.
      iv. Include patient's family and significant others in the plan.
   b. Concerns and feelings
   Assist the patient and significant others in expressing and coping with concerns and feelings related to the diagnosis of diabetes, its potential complications, and the management of this disease. Assist the patient in developing strategies to promote behavior change.
   c. Information: Provide verbal and/or written information regarding the following after you have assessed their preferred methods of learning:
      i. The diabetes disease process, including signs and symptoms of hyperglycemia and hypoglycemia, pathophysiology of T1D and T2D, and complications of diabetes
      ii. Diagnostic tests, including what they mean, frequency, and importance of testing
      iii. Medical management and side effects
      iv. Meal planning and exercise: how to incorporate these into the patient's lifestyle
      v. Rationale, action, use, side effects, and cost of therapeutic interventions, including medications
      vi. Self-glucose monitoring: what the parameters are and how to interpret the results for self-management decision making (ADA, 2022)
      vii. Adherence to long-term treatment plans
      viii. Prevention of complications, self-management strategies
      ix. Travel instructions, medical alert identification, and health maintenance

VI. Diabetes and Language

Language plays a powerful role in diabetes care, advocacy, and engagement. Words used by clinicians have the ability to facilitate engaged, respectful care, or alternately, their words may promote bias and shame and disengage patients. A task force composed of members from the American Association of Diabetes Educators (AADE) and the ADA published guidelines in 2017 that highlight the importance of language in diabetes care and call for language that is person first, free of bias or stigma, and strengths based; fosters collaboration; and is neutral and fact based (Dickensen et al., 2017

Language recommendations include using objective measures with a strengths-based framework. For example, instead of designating a patient or their diabetes as being "non-compliant" or "uncontrolled," an assessment should focus on whether a patient is at their glycemic goal, and elaborating on obstacles to meeting the individualized target. For example, "A1c is above goal of 7.0, with cost of medication and unreliable access to refrigeration contributing to intermittent insulin administration and hyperglycemia." Identifying obstacles helps to avoid focusing on personal failures, and helps to highlight areas where a patient may need additional, actionable support. Language should be person-first, and not reduce the person with their condition. In lieu of calling patients "diabetic," guidelines recommend referring to a "person with diabetes." Glucose "checks" help shift focus on gathering valuable data, and away from "testing" which implies a pass/fail mentality.

VII. Self-management resources and tools

There are numerous educational opportunities for individuals with diabetes, either online, by mail, or by telephone.
  A. *National Diabetes Education Program*
     The National Diabetes Education Program has publications available by mail or online that are geared toward different age groups (from teenagers to older adults) and ethnic backgrounds and are written in a variety of languages (http://ndep.nih.gov/).
  B. *American Diabetes Association*
     The ADA's website has extensive patient information online, brochures for purchase, and a hotline number for patients who want to speak with someone directly (http://www.diabetes.org).
  C. *Joslin Diabetes Center*
     The Joslin Diabetes Center has patient education online, brochures, and cookbooks for purchase, including some for children and teenagers, and has Spanish and Asian American websites (www.joslin.org).
  D. *Juvenile Diabetes Research Foundation International*
     The Juvenile Diabetes Research Foundation International provides online or printed information for adults, teenagers, and children and has links to Facebook, Twitter, and YouTube. In addition, it has links to community events, local chapters, and affiliates around the globe (http://www.jdrf.org).
  E. *Community support groups*
     There are numerous support groups for individuals with diabetes; in addition to those listed previously, others include the following:
     1. Defeat Diabetes Foundation, Inc.
        Find local support groups (http://www.defeatdiabetes.org/).
     2. American Diabetes Association
        Website has a link to community events and programs, including those geared toward specific ethnic groups (http://www.diabetes.org/).
     3. Diabetes Health
        Website links to multiple community events (www.diabeteshealth.com/)
  F. *Other resources*
     GLU (https://myglu.org/)
     TuDiabetes (www.tudiabetes.org/)
     DiabetesMine (www.healthline.com/diabetesmine)
     TCOYD—Taking Control of Your Diabetes (http://tcoyd.org/)
     Behavioral Diabetes Institute (www.behavioraldiabetesinstitute.org/)
     diaTribe (http://diatribe.org/)

References

American Association of Clinical Endocrinology. (2020). *AACE comprehensive type 2 diabetes management algorithm.* https://pro.aace.com/pdfs/diabetes/AACE_2019_Diabetes_Algorithm_03.2021.pdf

American College of Obstetricians and Gynecologists. (2019). *The use of hormonal contraception in women with coexisting medical conditions* (ACOG Practice Bulletin No. 206). https://oce-ovid-com.ucsf.idm.oclc.org/article/00006250-201902000-00041/HTML.

American Diabetes Association. (2009). *Diabetes statistics.* http://www.diabetes.org/diabetes-basics/diabetes-statistics/.

American Diabetes Association. (2022). Standards of medical care in diabetes—2022. *Diabetes Care, 45*(Suppl. 1), S17–S38. https://doi.org/10.2337/dc22-S002

Centers for Disease Control and Prevention. (2022). *Diabetes data and statistics.* https://www.cdc.gov/diabetes/data/index.html.

Dabelea, D., Rewers, A., Stafford, J. M., Standiford, D.A., Lawrence, J. M., Saydah, S., Imperatore, G., D'Agostino, R. B., Jr., Mayer-Davis, E. J., Pihoker, C., & SEARCH for Diabetes in Youth Study Group. (2014). Trends in the prevalence of ketoacidosis at diabetes diagnosis: The SEARCH for Diabetes in Youth Study. *Pediatrics, 133*(4), e938–e945. https://doi.org/10.1542/peds.2013-2795

Dickinson, J. K., Guzman, S. J., Maryniuk, M. D., O'Brian, C. A., Kadohiro, J. K., Jackson, R. A., D'Hondt, N., Montgomery, B., Close, K. L., & Funnell, M. M. (2017). The use of language in diabetes care and education. *Diabetes Care, 40*(12), 1790–1799. https://doi.org/10.2337/dci17-0041

Haas, L., Maryniuk, M., Beck, J., Cox, C. E., Duker, P., Edwards, L., et al. (2012). National standards for diabetes self-management education and support. *Diabetes Educator, 38*(5), 619–629. https://doi.org/10.1177/0145721712455997

International Diabetes Federation. (2022). *Facts and figures.* https://idf.org/aboutdiabetes/what-is-diabetes/facts-figures.html

Joslin Diabetes Center. (2020). *Clinical guidelines for adults with diabetes.* https://joslin-prod.s3.amazonaws.com/www.joslin.org/assets/2020-08/clinicalguidelinesformanagementofadultswithdiabetes.pdf

Matthew J. A., Jayne P. (2015) Adherence to guidelines for Hepatitis B, Pneumococcal, and Influenza Vaccination in patients with diabetes. *Clinical Diabetes, 33*(3), 116–122. https://doi.org/10.2337/diaclin.33.3.116

National Diabetes Information Clearinghouse. (2009). *DCCT and EDIC: The Diabetes Control and Complications Trial and follow-up study.* http://diabetes.niddk.nih.gov/dm/pubs/control/

Ogden, C. L., Kit, B. K., Carroll, M. D., & Park, S. (2011). *Consumption of sugar drinks in the United States, 2005–2008.* U.S. Department of Health and Human Services, Centers for Disease Control and Prevention, National Center for Health Statistics.

Patel, P., & Macerollo, A. (2010). Diabetes mellitus: Diagnosis and screening. *American Family Physician, 81*(7), 863–870.

CHAPTER 51

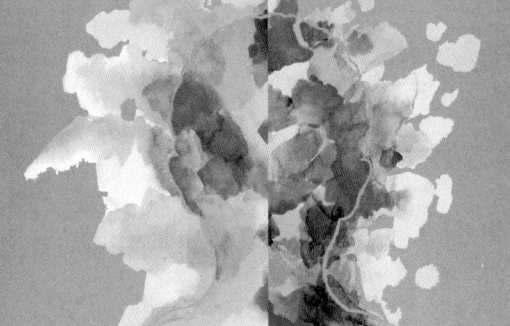

Epilepsy

Maritza López and Paul Garcia

I. Introduction and general background

This chapter provides information to help the primary care provider evaluate a patient with previously diagnosed epilepsy. *Epilepsy* refers to a group of conditions that are characterized by the recurrent risk of disturbances of cerebral function (seizures) because of excessive neuronal discharges in the brain occurring in a paroxysmal manner (Fisher et al., 2014). An epileptic seizure occurs when the cerebral cortex is rendered hyperexcitable (because of an increase in excitatory neurotransmission, a decrease in inhibitory neurotransmission, or a disturbance in brain circuitry) by any of a number of causes, including metabolic disturbances, injuries, strokes, tumors, and developmental abnormalities (Lowenstein, 2008). Depending on the site in the brain that is affected, the disturbance of function may result in a loss or impairment of consciousness, altered behavior, or an abnormality of motor or sensory function. When the cause of the disturbance is easily reversible (e.g., hyponatremia, hypoglycemia, alcohol withdrawal, medication toxicity, fever), the seizure is said to be "provoked," and the patient's condition is not considered epilepsy.

When the cause of the seizure is not readily reversible and seizures have occurred on more than one occasion, the chance for further seizures is high, and the patient is said to have epilepsy (Marks & Garcia, 1998). According to the International League Against Epilepsy (ILAE), epilepsy can be diagnosed when two or more unprovoked seizures recur after 24 hours, when a person has one unprovoked seizure but is at high risk of another, or if the person is diagnosed with an epilepsy syndrome (Fisher et al., 2014).

Epilepsy is a common condition in all medical practices, and all practitioners will be called on to care for patients with epilepsy. In the United States, an estimated 3 million people live with epilepsy, and 150,000 new cases are diagnosed each year (Centers for Disease Control and Prevention [CDC], 2023). About 1 in 26 people will develop epilepsy in their lifetime (England et al., 2012). People of all ages, genders, ethnicities, and socioeconomic backgrounds are affected by epilepsy. Although epilepsy can affect all populations, studies have shown that the prevalence of seizures is higher in patients with lower socioeconomic status in both developed and developing countries (de Boer et al., 2008). Furthermore, there appear to be disparities related to race/ethnicity and socioeconomic groups in both the United States (where universal insurance does not exist) and Canada (where health delivery is based on the premise of universality) (Burneo et al., 2009).

As a group, people with epilepsy face both medical and psychosocial challenges (including employment and educational barriers). This is exacerbated by stigma that is present to some extent in all cultures and populations (de Boer et al., 2008). It is important to consider the socioeconomic, psychological, and physical impact of epilepsy when caring for all patient groups to achieve optimal treatment outcomes. The lifetime risk of dying from a seizure-related cause is estimated to be as high as 20% (Hesdorffer & Tomson, 2013). Successful treatment of epilepsy both prolongs life and improves quality of life (Galanopoulou et al., 2012).

II. Database (may include but is not limited to)
A. Subjective
1. Seizure history
    a. Age of onset
    b. Description of seizures from patient and witnesses
    c. Most recent seizures: characteristics and frequency
    d. Any changes in seizure pattern (including characteristics and frequency)
    e. Triggering events (stress, fatigue, alcohol, sleep deprivation, and menstruation)
    f. Impairment of consciousness
    g. Any recent intervention, including paramedics, emergency department visits, or benzodiazepine use
    h. Any previous intervention, including surgery or medication changes

i. Previous diagnostic workup, including electroencephalogram (EEG) and magnetic resonance imaging (MRI); last visit with neurologist
2. Antiepileptic drugs (AEDs) and medications
   a. Name, formulation, strength, and dosing schedule. Note recent change from brand to generic or between different generics, as well as adherence to medication.
   b. Dose changes: drugs tried in the past, responses (therapeutic and toxic), and tolerability
   c. Signs and symptoms of AED toxicity, including blurred vision, diplopia, ataxia, somnolence or fatigue, confusion or mental slowing, and gastrointestinal upset
   d. Concomitant treatment for other conditions that may interact with AEDs (e.g., nonsteroidal anti-inflammatory drugs, antibiotics, oral contraceptives, anticoagulants, herbal supplements)
   e. Use of rescue medications, such as sublingual lorazepam, buccal midazolam, or rectal diazepam
3. Past medical history
   a. Head trauma, developmental and genetic disorders, and neurologic and psychiatric disorders
   b. Recent minor illnesses, especially gastrointestinal disorders with vomiting or fever
   c. Chronic illnesses (e.g., HIV/AIDS, cerebrovascular disease, cancer)
4. Family history (query both sides of the family) of seizures or epilepsy
5. Personal and social history
   a. Occupational history
   b. Habits: alcohol or substance use
   c. Sleep patterns (change in sleep patterns may provoke seizures)
   d. Stress and coping: recent stressors (can provoke seizures), coping strategies, and social support
   e. Recreational activities and safety: driving, swimming, climbing, other risky activities for patients with ongoing seizures, and use of helmets or other protective devices
6. Review of systems
   a. Skin: rash or jaundice
   b. Gastrointestinal: signs and symptoms of chemical hepatitis (e.g., nausea, vomiting, anorexia, abdominal pain, or malaise)
   c. Neurologic: full review of systems
   d. Psychiatric: Note affect and symptoms of active psychiatric disease.
   e. Weight gain or loss
B. Objective
1. Physical examination
   a. Temperature and blood pressure
   b. Cardiac (rule out cardiac origin)
   c. Neurologic examination
      i. Cranial nerves (special emphasis on nystagmus)
      ii. Cerebellar testing (special emphasis on gait disturbances and Romberg)
      iii. Focal motor signs and mental status
   d. Skin: rashes, signs of neurocutaneous syndrome (hypo-/hyperpigmented macules)
2. Diagnostic testing and workup
   a. Source (should be neurologist or epileptologist)
   b. Supporting documentation
      i. Abnormal EEG (not always present)
      ii. MRI: Although not always revealing, MRI remains the best modality to identify subtle but dangerous structural causes of seizures (e.g., small tumors or vascular malformations). A computed tomography (CT) scan can be obtained quickly at most institutions and thus is useful for visualizing acute structural causes such as hemorrhages or trauma; however, if CT is unrevealing, MRI is still necessary to exclude subtle structural causes (Ramli et al., 2015).

III. Assessment
A. *Determine the diagnosis. The following diagnoses should be considered for all patients presenting with seizures:*
   1. Epilepsy (**Table 51-1**)
   2. Cerebrovascular disease
   3. Cardiac arrhythmias with resulting cerebral hypoperfusion
   4. Syncope
   5. Nonepileptic (i.e., psychogenic) seizure
   6. Transient ischemic attack
   7. Migraine
   8. Alzheimer disease and other neurodegenerative disorders (can cause seizures in the geriatric population)
   9. Infection (may exacerbate seizures)
   10. Movement disorder
   11. Diabetes
B. *Severity*
   1. Determine if seizures are fully controlled.
   2. If seizures are not fully controlled, determine if the patient is at the maximum clinically tolerated dose of medication (regardless of serum levels).
   3. Assess for AED toxicity (**Table 51-2**).
C. *Significance*
   Assess the significance of the symptoms and chronic nature of this disorder to the patient and significant others (i.e., burden, quality of life, eagerness for surgical intervention).
D. *Patient adherence*
   Assess if the patient is able to adhere to the treatment plan (direct, open-ended inquiry; medication refill history).

IV. Goals of clinical management
A. *Achieve seizure-free status with lowest side-effect profile of AED therapy.*
B. *Attempt to arrive at AED monotherapy if possible.*

Table 51-1 Epilepsy Syndromes

	Generalized	Focal
	Seizures begin diffusely throughout the cerebral cortex.	Seizures arise from a discrete focus in cerebral cortex or limbic structures (hippocampus or amygdala).
Idiopathic (primary, without clear cause)	**Seizure types:** absence, myoclonic, tonic–clonic **Neurologic examination:** normal **Neuroimaging:** normal **EEG:** normal background with fast (3- to 6-Hz) generalized spike-and-wave discharges **Common examples:** childhood absence epilepsy, juvenile myoclonic epilepsy, epilepsy with generalized tonic–clonic seizures on awakening **Treatment:** valproate, ethosuximide (effective for absence seizures only), topiramate, lamotrigine, felbamate, levetiracetam, or zonisamide	**Seizure types:** simple partial (focal without impairment of consciousness), complex partial (focal with impairment of consciousness), or secondarily generalized tonic–clonic **Neurologic examination:** normal **Neuroimaging:** normal **EEG:** normal background with focal epileptiform discharges **Common examples:** benign childhood epilepsy with centrotemporal spikes (Rolandic epilepsy); benign epilepsy with occipital paroxysms **Treatment:** Often no medical treatment is necessary; all AEDs may be effective except ethosuximide.
Symptomatic (secondary; caused by an apparent or assumed brain lesion)	**Seizure types:** atypical absence, myoclonic, tonic, atonic, tonic–clonic **Neurologic examination:** diffuse or multifocal abnormalities **Neuroimaging:** diffuse or multifocal abnormalities common **EEG:** abnormal background with slow (<3-Hz) generalized or multifocal epileptiform discharges **Common examples:** Lennox–Gastaut syndrome, progressive myoclonus epilepsies **Treatment:** valproate, lamotrigine, levetiracetam, felbamate, rufinamide, topiramate, zonisamide, clobazam, ketogenic diet, corpus callosotomy, or vagus nerve stimulator	**Seizure types:** focal without impairment of consciousness, focal with impairment of consciousness, secondarily generalized tonic–clonic **Neurologic examination:** focal abnormalities or normal **Neuroimaging:** focal abnormalities common **EEG:** normal or abnormal background with focal or multifocal epileptiform discharges **Common examples:** temporal lobe epilepsy, frontal lobe epilepsy **Treatment:** carbamazepine, phenytoin, valproate, gabapentin, pregabalin, lacosamide, lamotrigine, levetiracetam, oxcarbazepine, topiramate, zonisamide (adjunct therapy—vigabatrin, pregabalin, perampanel, eslicarbazepine), or resective surgery

AED, antiepileptic drug; EEG, electroencephalogram.

Reproduced from "Management of seizures and epilepsy," 1998, *American Family Physician*. Copyright © 1998 American Academy of Family Physicians. All Rights Reserved; Modified from Marks, W. J., Jr., & Garcia, P. A. (1998). Seizures and epilepsy: Current management. *American Family Physician*, 57(7), 1589–1600.

C. Assist the patient in achieving optimal level of functioning with daily activities and quality of life while living with a chronic, often unpredictably relapsing disorder.

V. Plan
A. Screening: There are no screening tests or preventive strategies for epilepsy.
B. Diagnostic tests
1. Blood levels of AEDs: To assess for adherence or possible toxicity. Not all AEDs have defined "therapeutic ranges" (e.g., benzodiazepines and all AEDs released subsequent to valproic acid). Note that AED therapeutic ranges are only a rough guide; many patients require levels in the "toxic" range to achieve complete seizure control and tolerate these levels without significant clinical toxicity. Likewise, some patients may have their seizures controlled at blood levels below the usual therapeutic range. Routine blood level monitoring is not useful.
2. Complete blood count: Thrombocytopenia, anemia, and leukopenia secondary to AEDs. Obtain a baseline before initiating a new AED and in early phase of treatment or if patient is symptomatic.
3. Liver enzymes and liver function tests: Obtain a baseline before initiating a new AED and in early phase of treatment or if patient is symptomatic.

Table 51-2 Oral Antiepileptic Medications

Generic Name	Brand Name	Strengths Available* (mg)	Typical Adult Starting Dose†	Typical Increment and Rate of Ascension‡§	Most Common Dose-Related Adverse Effects	Non-Dose-Related and Idiosyncratic Reactions
Brivaracetam	Briviact®	10, 25, 50, 75, 100 mg; 10 mg/mL (oral solution); 50 mg/5 mL (IV solution)	50 mg BID	Increase to 100 mg BID, based on patient response and tolerability	Somnolence, dizziness, fatigue, nausea	Bronchospasm and angioedema, leukopenia, neutropenia, psychosis
Cannabidiol	Epidiolex®	100 mg/mL (oral solution)	2.5 mg/kg BID	Increase by 2.5 mg/kg BID weekly to a maximum of 12.5 mg/kg BID (may increase as often as QOD, if dictated by clinical circumstance)	Diarrhea, somnolence, anorexia, liver enzyme elevation	Rash, angioedema
Carbamazepine	Tegretol® Tegretol-XR® Carbatrol®	100, 200 100, 200, 400 100, 200, 300 mg	200 mg BID 200 mg BID 200 mg BID	200 mg/wk (dose TID-QID) 200 mg/wk 200 mg/wk	Dizziness, somnolence, ataxia, nausea, vomiting, diplopia, blurred vision	Hyponatremia, rash, Stevens–Johnson syndrome, leukopenia, aplastic anemia, agranulocytosis, transaminitis, hepatic failure
Cenobamate	Xcopri®	12.5, 25, 50, 100, 150, 200 mg	12.5 mg QD	Increase every other week to 25, 50, 100, 150, and then 200 mg QD. Max dose 400 mg/day.	Somnolence, dizziness, diplopia, confusion, hyperkalemia, ECG QT interval shortening > 20 ms	Severe rash, DRESS
Clobazam	Onfi®	2.5 mg/mL Tablet: 10 mg, 20 mg	10 mg BID	10 mg BID on week 1 then to 20 mg BID	Ataxia, dysarthria, constipation, drooling, lethargy, somnolence, urinary tract infection, cough, fever, aggressive behavior	Stevens–Johnson syndrome
Eslicarbazepine	Aptiom®	200, 400, 600, 800 mg	400 mg daily	Increments of 400 mg/wk to 800–1,200 mg/wk	Nausea, vomiting, ataxia, dizziness, headache, somnolence, fatigue, blurred vision, diplopia	Drug-induced eosinophilia, liver dysfunction, anaphylaxis, angioedema

Ethosuximide	Zarontin®	250 mg	250 mg QD to 250 mg BID	250 mg/wk	Anorexia, nausea, vomiting, drowsiness, headache, dizziness	Rash, Stevens–Johnson syndrome, hemopoietic complications, systemic lupus erythematosus (SLE)
Felbamate	Felbatol®	400, 600 mg	1,200 mg/day in 3 to 4 divided doses	600-mg increments every 2 weeks up to 2,400 mg/day	Photosensitivity, weight loss, abdominal pain, nausea/vomiting, dizziness, headache, insomnia	Stevens–Johnson syndrome, hematologic abnormalities (e.g., aplastic anemia, leukopenia), hepatic failure
Gabapentin	Neurontin®	100, 300, 400, 600, 800 mg	300 mg TID	300 mg/wk	Somnolence, dizziness, ataxia, fatigue	Rash, weight gain, behavioral changes, extremity edema
Lacosamide	Vimpat®	50, 100, 150, 200 mg	50 mg BID	100 mg/wk to max 400 mg/day	Dizziness, ataxia, vomiting, diplopia, nausea, vertigo	PR interval lengthening
Lamotrigine	Lamictal® Lamictal-XR®	25, 100, 150, 200 25, 50, 100, 200 mg	25 mg/day only for monotherapy (special considerations for polytherapy not addressed here)	25–50 mg/ 2 wk only for monotherapy (special considerations for polytherapy not addressed here)	Dizziness, ataxia, somnolence, headache, diplopia, blurred vision, nausea, vomiting, rash	Rash, Stevens–Johnson syndrome, transaminitis
Levetiracetam	Keppra® Keppra-XR®	250, 500, 750 500, 750 mg	500 mg BID	1,000-mg increments every 2 weeks up to 3,000 mg/day	Somnolence, asthenia, infection, dizziness	Depression, irritability
Oxcarbazepine	Trileptal® Oxtellar	150, 300, 600 mg	300 mg BID	600 mg every week up to 2,400 mg/day	Dizziness, somnolence, diplopia, fatigue, nausea, vomiting, ataxia, abnormal vision, abdominal pain, tremor, dyspepsia, abnormal gait	Stevens–Johnson syndrome, bone marrow suppression, hyponatremia
Perampanel	Fycompa®	2, 4, 6, 8, 10, 12 mg	2 mg orally	Increase by 2 mg daily per week. Max dose 12 mg QHS.	Backache, unsteady gait, ataxia, dizziness, headache, somnolence, psychiatric effects, fatigue	Psychiatric behavior, homicidal, suicidal thoughts

(*continues*)

Table 51-2 Oral Antiepileptic Medications *(continued)*

Generic Name	Brand Name	Strengths Available* (mg)	Typical Adult Starting Dose†	Typical Increment and Rate of Ascension‡§	Most Common Dose-Related Adverse Effects	Non–Dose-Related and Idiosyncratic Reactions
Phenobarbital		15, 30, 60, 100 mg	100 mg QD	15–30 mg/wk	Somnolence, cognitive and behavioral effects	Rash, Stevens–Johnson syndrome, hematopoietic complications, transaminitis, hepatic failure
Phenytoin	Dilantin®	30, 50, 100 mg	300 mg daily	25–30 mg/wk	Ataxia, diplopia, slurred speech, confusion	Rash, Stevens–Johnson syndrome, hematopoietic complications, gingival hyperplasia, coarsening of facial features, transaminitis, hepatic failure
Pregabalin	Lyrica®	25, 50, 75, 100, 150, 200, 225, 300 mg	75 mg BID or 50 mg TID	300 mg/wk to max 600 mg/day	Dizziness, somnolence, dry mouth, peripheral edema, ataxia, confusion, asthenia, abnormal thinking, blurred vision, incoordination, weight gain	Weight gain, skin rash
Rufinamide	Banzel®	200, 400 mg	400–800 mg/d in 2 divided doses	400–800 mg/day every 2 days to max 3,200 mg/day	Somnolence, dizziness, ataxia, headache, fatigue, nausea	Multiorgan hypersensitivity, QT interval shortening
Tiagabine	Gabitril®	4, 6, 8, 10, 12, 16 mg	4 mg daily	4 mg/wk (dose 2–4 times daily	Dizziness, nervousness, asthenia, confusion, tremor	

Topiramate	Topamax 1® Trokendi XR	25, 50, 100, 200 mg (25, 50, 100, 200 mg)	25 mg BID or 50 mg daily	Increase 50 mg/wk to 400 mg daily (same as above)	Somnolence, dizziness, ataxia, slurred speech, psychomotor slowing, cognitive problems, word-finding difficulty	Weight loss, transaminitis, nephrolithiasis
Valproate	Depakote® Depakote-ER®	125, 250, 500 mg 250, 500 mg	250 mg TID 500 mg daily	250 mg/wk Same as above	Nausea, vomiting, tremor, thrombocytopenia, weight gain	Transaminitis, hepatic failure, pancreatitis, rash, Stevens–Johnson syndrome, hair damage or loss
Vigabatrin	Sabril®	500	500 mg orally twice daily	500-mg increments at weekly intervals, depending on response, up to 1,500 mg twice daily	Weight increase, confusion, decreased coordination, blurred vision, diplopia, infection of ear, aggressive behavior, fatigue	Hepatic failure, visual field defect, psychiatric disorder, suicidal thoughts.
Zonisamide	Zonegran®	25, 50, 100 mg	100 mg/day	200 mg/day every 2 wk to max 400 mg/day	Somnolence, anorexia, dizziness, headache, nausea, agitation/irritability	Stevens–Johnson syndrome, oligohydrosis, hyperthermia, nephrolithiasis

BID, twice a day; *DRESS*, drug rash with eosinophilia and systemic symptoms; *ECG*, electrocardiogram; *IV*, intravenous; *QD*, every day; *QHS*, every night at bedtime; *QID*, four times a day; *QOD*, every other day; *TID*, three times a day.

*Strengths listed are for tablet or capsule formulations of the brand-name agents.

[†]Initiation doses for some agents vary, depending on concomitant medications, body weight, age of patient, and other factors; consult prescribing information for each drug. Doses are for nonurgent initiation of medication; clinical circumstances may necessitate higher initial doses and accelerated titration. See prescribing information for pediatric doses, which are based on body weight and often must be administered more frequently than in adults.

[‡]Rate of ascension may need modification, depending on seizure frequency and occurrence of adverse effects. Note that phenytoin may be increased in 25-mg increments by using a halved 50-mg Dilantin® Infatab® tablet or by 30 mg using a 30-mg Dilantin Kapseal® capsule.

[§]For children and adults with swallowing impairments, check with your pharmacy to see whether tablets can be crushed or if oral solutions/suspensions are available.

Data from "Management of seizures and epilepsy." 1998, American Family Physician. Copyright © 1998 American Academy of Family Physicians. All Rights Reserved; Marks, W. J., Jr., & Garcia, P. A. (1998). Seizures and epilepsy: Current management. *American Family Physician*, *57*(7), 1589–1600. Additional medication information was obtained from: http://www.micromedexsolutions.com/micromedex2/librarian/ © 2015 Truven Health Analytics Inc. Reviewed by Brian Aldredge, PharmD UCSF Epilepsy Center. Acknowledgment: Robin Taylor, NP, authored prior edition. Schachter, S. C. (2021, November 9). Antiseizure medications: Mechanism of action, pharmacology, and adverse effects. *UpToDate*. Retrieved December 31, 2021, from https://www.uptodate.com/contents/antiseizure-medications-mechanism-of-action-pharmacology-and-adverse-effects

Table 51-3 Medication Treatment Strategies for Patients With Epilepsy

Establish an epilepsy syndrome diagnosis for each patient (Table 51-1).

Select medications appropriate for that epilepsy syndrome (Table 51-1).

Among the syndrome-appropriate medications, choose the agent best suited for the particular patient, based on patient and medication characteristics (Table 51-2).

Initiate and titrate the medication at doses, increments, and rates appropriate for that medication to enhance tolerability (Table 51-2).

Ascend the medication, regardless of serum levels, until complete seizure control is achieved or until persistent, unacceptable side effects occur.

If satisfactory seizure control is not achieved, transition the patient to another agent appropriate for the epilepsy syndrome being treated. Attempt to arrive at antiepileptic drug monotherapy for each patient.

If trials with one or two agents fail to achieve acceptable results, refer the patient to an epilepsy specialist for consultation.

Reproduced from "Management of seizures and epilepsy," 1998, *American Family Physician*. Copyright © 1998 American Academy of Family Physicians. All Rights Reserved; Modified from Marks, W. J., Jr., & Garcia, P. A. (1998). Seizures and epilepsy: Current management. *American Family Physician, 57*(7), 1589–1600.

Some AEDs can cause elevated liver enzymes, but this is not common or clinically significant and usually does not require discontinuation of the AED.
4. Consider other tests if diagnosis is in question (electrolytes, glucose, creatinine, rapid plasma reagin [RPR], electrocardiogram, tilt-table [to rule out syncope], video-EEG telemetry).

C. *Medication management (Tables 51-2 and 51-3)*
In order to prescribe the best individualized medication or combination of medications, one must consider several factors, including seizure classification, adverse drug reactions, comorbid conditions, interaction with other medications, gender (childbearing status), and cost (Kanth et al., 2021).

D. *Surgical management*
Patients who continue to have seizures in spite of adequate trials of medications may be considered for surgery. According to Rugg-Gunn et al. (2020), 30%–40% of patients with focal epilepsy may become seizure-free with surgical intervention. In addition to curative resective brain surgery, several other types of surgeries may be considered. Palliative surgery, such as neuromodulation devices or corpus callosotomy, may also be offered. To be considered for surgery, patients should be referred to an epilepsy specialist at a comprehensive epilepsy center offering a full complement of treatment options.

E. *Referral guidelines*
Refer to neurologist or epileptologist in the following scenarios:
1. Diagnosis of epilepsy is in question.
2. Seizures are uncontrolled on one AED at maximum tolerated dose.
3. Complete seizure control, but with bothersome or intolerable AED side effects
4. AED withdrawal: Consider after 2–3 years of seizure control.
5. Pregnant woman with a seizure disorder

F. *Patient education*
1. Provide verbal and written information about the etiology and treatment of epilepsy.
2. Discuss the importance of adherence to medication regimes, emphasizing that the maximum tolerated dose is one increment below the dose at which the patient experiences side effects (Alldredge, 2013).
3. Review the importance of lifestyle issues for seizure control: regular sleep–wake schedule, minimal or modest alcohol intake, and maintenance of hydration.

VI. **Self-management resources**

A. *Epilepsy Foundation*
An excellent resource for patient and families can be found at http://www.epilepsy.com. This site is sponsored by the Epilepsy Therapy Project and the Epilepsy Foundation. The individuals involved with this site are among the top epilepsy experts in the country. A wide variety of resources are available on diagnosis, treatment, clinical trials, and support for family and caregivers.

The website is also a good resource for patients and families to identify local Epilepsy Foundation affiliates throughout the country. These local affiliates can help direct patients and families to additional local resources (e.g., advocacy, job training, support groups).

The website also has a function called Nile—The New Seizure Diary App, which allows patients and families to enter seizures, medications, and side effects. It can be used to set alerts so that patients remember to take their medications at the proper times.

The website also has a section for healthcare professionals, with more sophisticated information that is highly accurate and carefully reviewed: http://professionals.epilepsy.com/homepage/index.html.

B. *Seizure tracker*

Seizure Tracker is a website that allows patients to enter data on medication dosages, seizure frequencies, use of rescue medications, and so forth, then share this information with healthcare providers of their choosing. https://seizuretracker.com.

C. *Citizens United for Research in Epilepsy (CURE)*

CURE is an organization that promotes awareness and education of epilepsy and raises funds for research on epilepsy. http://www.cureepilepsy.org/.

References

Alldredge, B. K. (2013). Seizure disorders. In M. Kimble, B. K. Alldredge, R. L. Corelli, M. E. Ernst, B. J. Guglielmo, P. A. Jacobson, W. A. Kradjan, & B. R. Williams (Eds.), *Koda-Kimble & Young's applied therapeutics: The clinical use of drugs* (10th ed., 1387–1418). Baltimore: Wolters Kluwer Health/Lippincott Williams & Wilkins.

Burneo, J. G., Jette, N., Theodore, W., Begley, C., Parko, K., Thurman, D. .J, Wiebe, S, Task Force on Disparities in Epilepsy Care, & North American Commission of the International League Against Epilepsy. (2009). Disparities in epilepsy: Report of a systematic review by the North American Commission of the International League Against Epilepsy. *Epilepsia*, 50(10), 2285–2295. https://doi.org/10.1111/j.1528-1167.2009.02282.x

Centers for Disease Control and Prevention. (2023, October 6). *Epilepsy*. https://www.cdc.gov/epilepsy/data/index.html

de Boer, H. M., Mula, M., & Sander, J. W. (2008). The global burden and stigma of epilepsy. Epilepsy and Behavior, 12(4), 540–546. https://doi.org/10.1016/j.yebeh.2007.12.019

England, M. J., Liverman, C. T., Schultz, A. M., & Strawbridge, L. M. (2012). Epilepsy across the spectrum: Promoting health and understanding. A summary of the Institute of Medicine report. *Epilepsy & Behavior*, 25(2), 266–276. https://doi.org/10.1016/j.yebeh.2012.06.016

Fisher, R., Acevedo, C., Arzimanoglou, A., Bogacz, J., Cross, H., Elger, C. E., Engel, J., Forsgren, L., French, J. A., Glynn, M., Hesdorffer, D. C., Lee, B. I., Mathern, G. W., Moshé, S. L., Perucca, E., Scheffer, I. E., Tomson, T., Watanabe, M., & Wiebe, S. (2014). A practical clinical definition of epilepsy. *Epilepsia*, 55(4), 415–482. https://doi.org/10.1111/epi.12550

Galanopoulou, A., Buckmaster, P. S., Staley, K., Moshé, S. L., Perucca, E., Engel J., Jr., Löscher, W., Noebels, J. L., Pitkänen, A., Stables, J., White, H. S., O'Brien, T. J., Simonato, M., American Epilepsy Society Basic Science Committee, & International League Against Epilepsy Working Group on Recommendations for Preclinical Epilepsy Drug Discovery. (2012). Identification of new epilepsy treatments: Issues in preclinical methodology. *Epilepsia*, 53(3), 571–582. https://doi.org/10.1111/j.1528-1167.2011.03391.x

Hesdorffer, D., & Tomson, T. (2013). Sudden unexpected death in epilepsy. Potential role of antiepileptic drugs. *CNS Drugs*, 27(2), 113–119. https://doi.org/10.1007/s40263-012-0006-1

Kanth, K. M., Clark, S., & Britton, J. W. (2021). Antiseizure medication therapy. In G. D. Cascino, J. I. Sirven, & W. O Tatum (Eds.), *Epilepsy* (pp. 179–216). Wiley Blackwell. doi.org:10.1002/9781119431893.ch11

Lowenstein, D. H. (2008). Seizures and epilepsy. In A. S. Fauci, E. Braunwald, D. L. Kasper, S. L. Hauser, D. L. Longo, J. L. Jameson, & J. Loscalzo (Eds.), *Harrison's principles of internal medicine online* (17th ed., 988–994). McGraw-Hill.

Marks, W. J., Jr., & Garcia, P. A. (1998). Management of seizures and epilepsy. *American Family Physician*, 57(7), 1589–1600.

Ramli, N., Rahmat, K., Lim, K. S., & Tan, C. T. (2015). Neuroimaging in refractory epilepsy. Current practice and evolving trends. *European Journal of Radiology*, 84(9), 1791–1800. https://doi.org/10.1016/j.ejrad.2015.03.024

Rugg-Gunn, F., Miserocchi, A., & McEvoy, A. (2020). Epilepsy surgery. *Practical Neurology*, 20(1), 4–14. https://doi.org/10.1136/practneurol-2019-002192

Schachter, S. C. (2021, November 9). Antiseizure medications: Mechanism of action, pharmacology, and adverse effects. *UpToDate*. https://www.uptodate.com/contents/antiseizure-medications-mechanism-of-action-pharmacology-and-adverse-effects

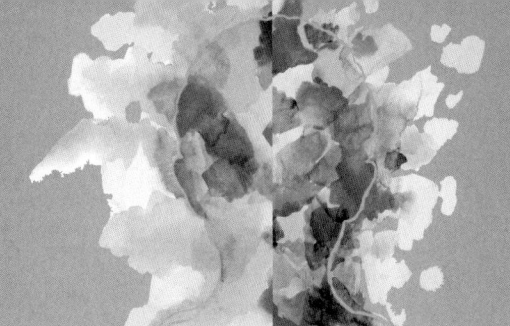

CHAPTER 52

Gastroesophageal Reflux Disease

Elizabeth Gatewood

I. Definition and overview

Gastroesophageal reflux disease (GERD) is defined as a condition that develops when the reflux of the stomach contents into the esophagus causes troublesome symptoms and/or complications (Vakil et al., 2006). It is the most common gastrointestinal (GI) diagnosis recorded during outpatient clinic visits in the United States (Katz et al., 2022; Peery et al., 2012). GERD affects 19 million adults, accounting for 5,235,107 outpatient visits and 325,666 emergency department visits annually (Peery et al., 2019; Practice Parameters Committee of the American College of Gastroenterology, 2008; Wang & Sampliner, 2008). Prevalence is estimated at 18.1%–27.8% in North America, 8.8%–25.9% in Europe, and 2.5%–7.8% in East Asia, with increasing prevalence in North America and East Asia (El-Serag et al., 2014). Over 50% of the general population in the United States reports regular heartburn, with about one-third reporting regurgitation symptoms in the last week (Cohen et al., 2014). GERD has a significant impact on mental and physical quality of life (Badillo & Fancis, 2014). Globally, GERD is associated with a number of factors, including age > 50, higher body weight, tobacco smoking, NSAID or aspirin use, lower income, and lower educational level (Eusebi et al., 2018).

A. Significance and complications

Recognizing and treating GERD are important, not only for symptomatic management but also to avoid the complications of esophagitis, Barrett's esophagus, and esophageal carcinoma (Clarrett & Hachem, 2018). Approximately 5.6% of the population in the United States has Barrett's esophagus (Spechler & Souza, 2014). Barrett's esophagus occurs when the normal squamous epithelium in the tubular esophagus is replaced by columnar epithelium. This can occur when normal esophageal mucosa is exposed repeatedly to stomach acid. Barrett's esophagus is an identifiable precursor for esophageal dysplasia and esophageal adenocarcinoma, which is one of the fastest-rising cancers in the Western population (Qumseya et al., 2019). The worldwide incidence of esophageal cancer is 65.8 cases per 1,000 patient-years in those with high-grade dysplasia. The risk with low-grade dysplasia is 16.98 cases per 1,000 patient-years compared to 5.98 cases without dysplasia (Hauser et al., 2014). The mortality rate from esophageal adenocarcinoma is high and has increased in frequency by a factor of 7 in the United States in the past four decades (Spechler & Souza, 2014). Additional complications associated with GERD include esophagitis, esophageal ulceration, and esophageal strictures. Extra-esophageal symptoms of GERD are common, with chest pain being the most common symptom, followed by pulmonary and head and neck complaints (Durazzo et al., 2020). Respiratory manifestations, such as chronic cough, shortness of breath, and exacerbation of asthma, are commonly seen in GERD (Gaude, 2009). Laryngitis, tonsillitis, and dental erosion are common head and neck complaints (Durazzo et al., 2020). These symptoms may be present in the absence of classic GERD symptoms, making the diagnosis difficult.

B. Pathophysiology and etiology of GERD

In normal individuals (i.e., those who do not have GERD), four mechanisms protect the esophageal epithelium from being damaged by reflux of gastric contents (Hauser et al., 2014):

1. A competent lower esophageal sphincter (LES), which acts as a barrier to reflux
2. Effective movement of contents through the esophagus
3. Secondary peristalsis, which sweeps refluxed material back into the stomach and closes the LES

4. The acid-neutralizing effect of swallowed saliva and mucous present in the upper GI (UGI) tract

There are multiple mechanisms that lead to GERD, including (1) motor abnormalities, resulting in decreased esophageal motility, and (2) anatomical factors, such as a hiatal hernia and higher body weight (Argyrou et al., 2018). Esophageal dysmotility is associated with a great many illnesses, including rheumatologic and endocrine disorders. Altered gastric motility may be associated with a weak LES or transient LES relaxation, weak or disordered esophageal peristalsis, or delayed gastric emptying. GERD is sometimes the first symptom in young women with scleroderma, CREST (calcinosis, Raynaud phenomenon, esophageal dysmotility, sclerodactyly, and telangiectasia) syndrome, or mixed connective tissue disorders. Motility is further affected by structural factors that increase abdominal pressure (hiatal hernia, pregnancy, weight gain, higher body weight, and tight clothing) and by hormonal influences (progesterone, cholecystokinin, secretin, and low gastrin). These cause the LES to be unable to prevent stomach acid from coming in contact with the esophageal mucosa, and prolonged contact with the acid leads to erosion. Local esophageal damage can also be caused by increased gastric acid secretion or the retrograde passage of bile and pancreatic juice. Mucosal injury further decreases the rate of passage of the bolus of food through the UGI tract. Additional factors that decrease the flow of acid and food through the UGI tract include reduced saliva, increased hydrochloric acid, and decreased mucosal blood flow. Hormonal influences can cause transient LES relaxation, excess acid production, and decreased UGI tract motility (**Table 52-1**). There is also a genetic component to GERD, though research does not yet indicate the significance for treatment (Argyrou et al., 2018).

II. Database (may include but is not limited to)
A. *Subjective*
1. Past medical history
   a. Peptic ulcer disease (associated with a hypersecretory state)
   b. Obesity (body mass index [BMI] > 29) causes increased pressure on the stomach and lower esophagus, causing more acid to reflux. It also causes delayed gastric emptying. Incidence of symptoms rises progressively with total body weight (El-Serag & Thrift, 2021)
   c. Gallbladder disease may cause symptoms similar to GERD.
   d. Pregnancy can exacerbate reflux because of hormonal influences and increased pressure on the upper digestive tract.
   e. Neurologic disease, such as a stroke or brain tumor, or any condition that affects neural pathways
   f. Diabetes can cause gastroparesis, which in turn causes increased reflux.
   g. Collagen-vascular disease (scleroderma, mixed connective tissue disease, and systemic lupus erythematosus) can cause collagen to replace muscle in the GI tract resulting in loss of motility and dysfunction
   h. Noncardiac chest pain
   i. Chronic cough, recurrent infections, or asthma
   j. Laryngitis or hoarseness

Table 52-1 Gastroesophageal Reflux Disease (GERD) Common Etiologies

Causative Factor	Clinical Examples
Motility disorders	Esophageal dysmotility caused by diminished peristalsis: rheumatologic and endocrine disorders, such as Sjögren syndrome, scleroderma, CREST (calcinosis, Raynaud phenomenon, esophageal dysmotility, sclerodactyly, and telangiectasia) syndrome, or mixed connective tissue disorders Altered gastric motility, including a weak lower esophageal sphincter or transient lower esophageal sphincter relaxation, weak or disordered esophageal peristalsis, and delayed gastric emptying seen with gastroparesis or gastric outlet obstruction
Local damage	Increased gastric acid secretion or the retrograde passage of bile and pancreatic juices that cause damage to the esophageal mucosa
Change in resistance to gastric acid	Factors that decrease the flow of acid and food through the upper gastrointestinal tract, such as reduced saliva (Sjögren syndrome, anticholinergic medications, age), increased hydrochloric acid (stress response or gastrinoma), or decreased mucosal blood flow (radiation therapy or ischemia).
Structural and physiologic changes	Associated with the following conditions: hiatal hernia, obstructive sleep apnea, weight gain, higher body weight, pregnancy, or wearing tight clothing
Hormonal influences	Progesterone, cholecystokinin, secretin, and low gastrin

k. Dental erosions
l. Cerebral palsy and other neurodevelopmental disabilities
m. Medications: aspirin, nonsteroidal anti-inflammatory drugs, hormones, vitamins (vitamin C, iron, potassium), adrenergics, anticholinergics, antibiotics (tetracyclines and clindamycin), statins, nitrates, benzodiazepines, angiotensin-converting enzyme (ACE) inhibitors, bisphosphonates, calcium channel blockers, warfarin, corticosteroids (MacFarlane, 2018)
2. Family history
   a. Peptic ulcer disease, GI cancer, gallbladder disease
   b. Diabetes, rheumatologic, and other endocrine disorders
3. Personal and social
   a. Current life stressors: Stress can reduce the esophageal perception thresholds for pain (Mizyad et al., 2009).
   b. Diet
      i. Certain foods and drinks may trigger GERD, with patients often self-adjusting their diets based on symptoms. Currently, it is thought that spicy foods may have a slower digestion rate and require longer to clear. Ingestion of alcohol exacerbates symptoms by decreasing LES pressure. Studies of other foods, such as chocolate, carbonated beverages, and mint, have not demonstrated improved symptoms with avoidance. Therefore, current guidelines call for individual patients with GERD to avoid those foods and habits that worsen their symptoms (Katz et al., 2022; Sethi & Richter, 2017).
      ii. Large meals and late-night eating are known provoking factors for GERD.
4. Review of systems
   a. Gastrointestinal
      i. Pain: The typical symptom is *heartburn*, a retrosternal burning sensation originating in the subxiphoid region and spreading upward into the chest occurring 30–60 minutes after meals. In severe episodes, there are esophageal spasms or noncardiac chest pain. The pain can radiate into the neck, shoulders, and back.
      ii. Dysphagia, episodes of choking (can present as coughing with eating)
      iii. Regurgitation of gastric contents into the mouth
      iv. Nausea and vomiting (vomiting can be seen with GERD, although not a common associated symptom)
      v. Aggravating factors for these symptoms
         a. Position (lying down, especially postprandial reclining; bending over and lifting heavy objects)
         b. Wearing tight clothing or belts
         c. Individual provoking factors (as noted previously, this may include tobacco, alcohol, caffeine, and certain foods)
      b. Ear, nose, and throat: chronic sore throat, early morning hoarseness
      c. Mouth: complaint of bad breath (halitosis)
      d. Cardiac: Chest pain—full cardiac review of systems is indicated, and cardiac etiology must be ruled out. The symptoms of GERD may mimic cardiac disease, and the reverse is also true.
      e. Pulmonary: cough (especially nocturnal cough), wheezing (shortness of breath is not typically seen with GERD)
B. *Objective*
   1. Physical examination
      a. General: appearance, mood, development, nourishment; note tight clothing if present
      b. Weight, BMI
      c. Ear, nose, and throat: dentition changes, tooth decay, and pharyngeal erythema
      d. Cardiac examination: should be normal in a patient with GERD
      e. Chest examination: wheezing, adventitious sounds
      f. Abdominal examination: higher body weight, epigastric tenderness, distention, and tympanic bowel sounds
      g. Rectal examination: stool hemoccult

III. Assessment

A. *Determine the diagnosis*
   GERD is most commonly diagnosed by history and presenting symptoms. The following diagnoses should be considered for all patients presenting with symptoms of GERD:
   1. Cardiac disease or angina (should be excluded before beginning GI evaluation) (Katz et al., 2022)
   2. Esophageal stricture or mass
   3. Esophageal motility disorder
   4. Esophageal spasm
   5. *Helicobacter pylori* infection
   6. Gastroparesis
   7. Peptic ulcer disease
   8. Zollinger–Ellison syndrome
B. *Severity*
   Assess the severity of the disease, including duration of symptoms and risk for complications of untreated or undertreated GERD. The diagnosis of GERD is currently subdivided into:
   1. Erosive disease (ERD)
   2. Nonerosive disease (NERD)
C. *Significance and motivation*
   Assess the significance of the symptoms to the patient and explain the often chronic nature of this disorder. Determine the motivation and ability of the patient to follow through with the treatment plan, which can involve significant modification of weight, habits, food choices, and timing of meals.

IV. Goals of clinical management
A. *Screening for complications*
Patients with alarm symptoms or signs such as dysphagia, GI bleed (hematemesis, hematochezia, melena), iron-deficiency anemia, persistent vomiting, weight loss, new onset at age >65, or GI cancer in a first-degree relative require diagnostic studies, including endoscopy.

B. *Treatment*
Initial treatment of patients with GERD focuses on lifestyle modification. Pharmacological treatment of GERD focuses on decreasing the symptoms through decreased acidity. The two mainstays of medication treatment are proton pump inhibitors (PPIs) and H2-receptor antagonists (H2RAs; H2 blockers).
  1. Medical management is designed to promote gastric emptying, augment the resting tone of the LES, and favorably alter the nature of refluxed material through nonpharmacologic and pharmacologic means.
  2. Treatment aims to assist the patient in the management of GERD symptoms and enhance lifestyle modification.

The goal is to prevent recurrence of symptoms and disease and prevent complications.

C. *Prevention of complications*
These include the following: Barrett's esophagus, adenocarcinoma, esophagitis, dysphagia caused by esophageal strictures, narrowing or spasm, ulcers, persistent pain, and bleeding.

V. Plan
A. *Screening*
There are no screening tests available for the early detection or prevention of GERD. However, there are preventive measures that can be taken. These include maintaining normal body weight, reducing stress, tobacco cessation, and avoiding eating large fatty meals before bedtime.

B. *Diagnostic tests*
  1. Laboratory tests: complete blood count, stool for occult blood
  2. Electrocardiogram if chest pain is present. Perform or refer for additional cardiology diagnostic studies if angina is suspected or cannot be ruled out.
  3. UGI series: If dysphagia is present, consider UGI series to rule out a stricture or mass.
  4. According to the 2022 Practice Guideline for the Diagnosis and Management of GERD (Katz et al., 2022), endoscopy is indicated in the following circumstances:
     a. Alarm signs or symptoms, such as persistent vomiting; hematemesis; evidence of GI blood loss; involuntary weight loss; progressive dysphagia; anemia; evidence of GI bleeding; chest pain proven to be of noncardiac etiology; or a mass, stricture, or ulcer found on imaging studies
     b. Patients with chest pain without heartburn who have had adequate evaluation to exclude heart disease
     c. Unrelenting symptoms despite 8 weeks of therapy or return of symptoms when PPIs are discontinued
     d. Chronic GERD with three or more risk factors for Barrett's esophagitis (male sex, age > 50 years, white race, tobacco smoking, higher body weight, and family history of Barrett's esophagitis or esophageal adenocarcinoma in a first-degree relative)
     e. Recurrent symptoms after antireflux surgery
     f. Endoscopy is ideally performed 2–4 weeks after stopping PPI.
  5. Special studies
     Additional evaluation includes tests to measure reflux and more precisely evaluate the motility of the esophagus and stomach (gastric emptying study, manometry with a 24-hour pH study, and endoscopy with biopsy). A gastric emptying study may reveal decreased gastric emptying, which can cause functional dyspepsia. A manometry with pH study can quantify the amount of reflux that a patient has in 24 hours and also measures the pressure in the upper and lower esophageal sphincters. These tests characterize GERD more precisely and also provide evidence for determining if the patient is an appropriate surgical candidate.

C. *Management*
A stepwise approach to the management of GERD is appropriate. Lifestyle modification followed by medications is often enough to relieve symptoms. For those with persistent symptoms, a referral to a specialist is appropriate. Next steps may include promotility therapy, followed by antireflux surgery.
  1. Lifestyle modifications (Badillo & Francis, 2014)
     a. Mechanical measures: Raise the head of the bed 8–10 inches. Maintain an upright posture for a minimum of 30–60 minutes after eating.
     b. Dietary measures
        i. Do not eat within 3 hours of bedtime.
        ii. Avoid those foods/beverages that seem to aggravate symptoms (alcohol, spicy foods).
     c. Smoking cessation
     d. Weight loss when BMI is >29 or when there has been a recent weight gain
     e. Stress management
  2. Pharmacologic measures
     Initial pharmacologic treatment of GERD is influenced by the frequency and severity of symptoms and whether the patient is thought to have ERD (erosive reflux disease) or NERD (nonerosive reflux disease). Excellent documentation exists showing that PPIs are more effective and relieve symptoms more rapidly than H2RAs (Maret-Ouda, Markar, & Lagergen, 2020).
     a. *For mild symptoms*: Patients with infrequent symptoms often respond well to antacids. Liquid or chewable preparations: take 1 and 3 hours after meals and at bedtime until symptoms resolve.

b. *For mild to moderate symptoms*: H2RAs can be effective and are less expensive than PPIs. They work by blocking histamine-induced stimulation of gastric parietal cells. H2RAs are most effective when given as a divided dose twice daily.

Clinicians who use a "step-down approach" to the treatment of GERD often begin treatment with PPIs rather than with H2RAs. Clinicians who prefer a "step-up" approach begin with H2RAs.

c. For moderate to severe symptoms or for the suspicion or diagnosis of erosive reflux, the treatment of choice is a PPI. PPIs are potent inhibitors of gastric acid secretion, working by turning off the pumps in parietal cells. All PPIs seem to be equally effective, although side-effect profiles may differ for the individual patient. The initial selection of a particular PPI is often determined by insurance company formularies. There are many preparations on the market, and the reader is encouraged to consult information for each agent. Most PPIs are given once daily, 30–60 minutes before the first meal of the day. Dosage can be increased to twice daily if needed or given at bedtime if nighttime symptoms are an issue. PPI treatment should achieve resolution of symptoms and complete healing of the esophagus in 8 weeks. If symptoms recur within 6 months, chronic therapy may be needed with either daily or twice-daily dosing of a PPI. Patients who do have resolution of symptoms can continue taking PPIs or H2RAs on an as-needed basis. H2RAs can be added to PPIs to control nighttime symptoms, but it should be noted that H2RAs can exhibit waning effectiveness over time (tachyphylaxis) within a relatively short time. Concerns regarding the side effects of long-term use of PPIs have resulted in some patients being discontinued abruptly (Vaezi et al., 2017). These risks should be discussed with the patient, along with the benefits of PPI therapy, in order to make an appropriate treatment decision. Some studies have demonstrated an association between long-term use of PPIs and adverse conditions, including infections, osteoporosis, malabsorption of vitamins and minerals, heart attacks, and strokes. These studies are not considered definitive by the American Association of Gastroenterology because of their flaws and lack of proof of cause and effect (Katz et al., 2022). Other studies, including a recent randomized controlled trial (RCT), have demonstrated safety with PPI use over a 3-year period of time (Moayyedi et al., 2019). The American Association of Gastroenterology supports the use of PPIs for GERD based on their risk–benefit profile (Katz et al., 2022). It is important, however, to discuss this with your patient prior to prescribing.

See **Table 52-2** for a list of side effects associated with GERD medications. Serious side effects can be associated with H2RAs, but these are rare. Long-term PPI use has been associated with multiple safety concerns, although research has not consistently demonstrated a causal relationship. PPIs are also associated with an increased risk of *Clostridium difficile* and other enteric infections and may be contraindicated in patients at high risk for these infections. PPIs have also been associated with malabsorption of minerals and vitamins, including magnesium, calcium, and vitamin B_{12}.

3. Promotility therapy
   a. For patients with slow gastric emptying, consider using prokinetics/antiemetics:
      i. Metoclopramide (Reglan®), 10 mg three to four times daily: This agent increases the rate of gastric and esophageal emptying by stimulating the smooth muscle of the intestine. The potential side effects of metoclopramide should be reviewed with the patient before initiating treatment. The most serious, although infrequent, side effects include tardive dyskinesia, agranulocytosis, supraventricular tachycardia, hyperaldosteronism, and neuroleptic malignant syndrome.
      ii. Cisapride (Propulsid®), 10 mg four times daily before meals and at bedtime: Given its risk for potentially life-threatening arrhythmias, this agent is now only available for limited-access protocol use by gastroenterologists. It is very effective in enhancing gastric emptying and generally has fewer side effects than metoclopramide.
      iii. For nausea, one can use ondansetron (Zofran®) or promethazine (although the latter often produces drowsiness).
      iv. Domperidone has been found to be effective but is not approved for GERD by the U.S. Food and Drug Administration.
   b. For patients with gastroparesis who do not respond to medications, consider a referral to a tertiary medical center for a gastric stimulator.
4. Surgical options

The most common surgical procedure performed for GERD is the Nissen fundoplication. This surgery may be indicated in a small number of patients with severe reflux who do not respond to PPIs or who may have reasons, such as drug side effects, for preferring surgical management. An alternate surgical intervention is a partial fundoplication (anterior and posterior). For all procedures, the patient must undergo a detailed evaluation by a gastroenterologist before surgery can be considered. Presurgical evaluation includes endoscopy, UGI series, and esophageal manometry with a 24-hour pH study. Outcomes comparing the surgical

Table 52-2 Commonly Used Gastroesophageal Reflux Disease (GERD) Medications*

Medication Category With Examples	Initial Dose	Maintenance Dose	Precautions
Antacids			Use with caution in renal impairment. Many drug interactions, especially with higher doses (e.g., antipsychotics, anticonvulsants, and calcium channel blockers).
Aluminum hydroxide and magnesium hydroxide (Alamag OTC, Maalox®)	5–10 mL or 2–4 tablets 1–3 hours after meals and at bedtime	PRN according to symptoms	
Calcium carbonate and magnesium hydroxide (Mylanta® Gelcaps, Mylanta® Supreme, or Rolaids® Extra Strength)	Same as above	Same as above	Constipation is a frequent side effect.
H2-receptor antagonists			Many adverse reactions, including cardiac arrhythmias, reversible confused state, and increased prolactin levels. Use with caution in renal impairment (creatinine clearance < 50). Monitor for vitamin B_{12} deficiency with long-term use.
Famotidine (Pepcid®)	20 mg twice daily; take second dose in the evening or at bedtime	20 mg at bedtime	
Nizatidine (Axid®)	150 mg twice daily or 300 mg daily (taken in the evening or at bedtime if single dose)	150 mg daily	
Proton pump inhibitors (PPIs)	Usually prescribed for 8 weeks for initial treatment		Check for drug interactions; caution if hepatic impairment. Consider Mg at baseline and ongoing if long-term use. Take before breakfast. If twice-daily dosing, take second dose before evening meal. No dose adjustment required for renal impairment.
Omeprazole (Prilosec®)	20–40 mg daily	20–40 mg daily	Take 30 minutes before a meal.
Lansoprazole (Prevacid®)	15–30 mg daily	15–30 mg daily	Take 30 minutes before a meal.
Pantoprazole (Protonix®)	20–40 mg daily	20–40 mg daily	Take at least 1 hour before a meal.
Rabeprazole (AcipHex®)	20 mg daily	20 mg daily	
Esomeprazole (Nexium®)	40 mg daily	40 mg daily	
Dexlansoprazole (Dexilant®)	30 mg daily	30 mg daily	

OTC, over the counter; *PRN*, as needed.

* Reflects suggested dosages for GERD. Dosages for erosive esophagitis and other esophageal disorders may vary.

interventions demonstrate comparable decreases in reflux scores, with significant improvement compared to PPIs (Amer et al., 2018). The most common side effect is dysphagia, which can persist years after surgery. Partial fundoscopy has less risk of dysphagia (a common side effect) than full fundoplication (Amer et al., 2018).

The surgical treatment of choice for the patient with higher body weight is bariatric surgery.

D. Follow-up
1. Follow-up should take place approximately 4–6 weeks after initiating treatment or sooner if symptoms increase in severity. Assess adherence to treatment plan.
2. Gastroenterology consult is indicated if symptoms worsen, complications occur, or symptoms are refractory to treatment. If no response to treatment, consider esophagogastroduodenoscopy (EGD) and/or UGI series.
3. Assess for side effects of medications.

E. Patient education
1. Assist the patient and family to voice their concerns and develop coping strategies with respect to the disease process and its management.
2. Provide verbal and written information about the pathophysiology of GERD and its treatment. The National Institutes of Health has a very good handout that is available for distribution. See the website in the following section.
3. Discuss what the patient can expect with diagnostic testing, including preparation and aftercare.
4. Explain the therapeutic benefits and side effects of any prescribed treatment. Discuss the duration of treatment.
5. Stress that follow-up is recommended in person or by telephone/video visit to monitor treatment response and make appropriate treatment regimen changes.

VI. Self-management resources
A. The National Institutes of Health
   The National Institutes of Health has multiple brochures for patients. Refer to the website http://digestive.niddk.nih.gov/ddiseases/pubs/gerd/.
B. The Mayo Clinic
   The Mayo Clinic also has excellent resources: http://www.mayoclinic.com/health/gerd/DS00967.

References

Amer, M. A., Smith, M. D., Khoo, C. H., Herbison, G. P., & McCall, J. L. (2018). Network meta-analysis of surgical management of gastro-oesophageal reflux disease in adults, *British Journal of Surgery*, 105(11), 1398–1407. https://doi.org/10.1002/bjs.10924

Argyrou, A., Legaki, E., Koutserimpas, C., Gazouli, M., Papaconstantinou, I., Gkiokas, G., & Karamanolis, G. (2018). Risk factors for gastroesophageal reflux disease and analysis of genetic contributors. *World Journal of Clinical Cases*, 6(8), 176–182. https://doi.org/10.12998/wjcc.v6.i8.176

Badillo, R., & Francis, D. (2014). Diagnosis and treatment of gastroesophageal reflux disease. *World Journal of Gastrointestinal Pharmacology and Therapeutics*, 5(3), 105–112. https://doi.org/10.4292/wjgpt.v5.i3.105

Clarrett, D. M., & Hachem, C. (2018). Gastroesophageal reflux disease (GERD). *Missouri Medicine*, 115(3), 214–218.

Cohen, E., Bolus, R., Khanna, D., Hays, R. D., Chang, L., Melmed, G. Y., Khanna, P., & Spiegel, B. (2014). GERD symptoms in the general population: Prevalence and severity versus care-seeking patients. *Digestive Diseases and Sciences*, 59(10), 2488–2496. https://doi.org/10.1007/s10620-014-3181-8

Durazzo, M., Lupi, G., Cicerchia, F., Ferro, A., Barutta, F., Beccuti, G., Gruden, G., & Pellicano, R. (2020). Extra-esophageal presentation of gastroesophageal reflux disease: 2020 update. *Journal of Clinical Medicine*, 9(8), 2559. https://doi.org/10.3390/jcm9082559

El-Serag, H. B., Sweet, S., Winchester, C. C., & Dent, J. (2014). Update on the epidemiology of gastro-oesophageal reflux disease: A systematic review. *Gut*, 63(6), 871–880. https://doi.org/10.1136/gutjnl-2012-304269

El-Serag, H. B., & Thrift, A. P. (2021). Obesity and gastroesophageal reflux disease. In J. E. Richter, D. O. Castell, D. A. Katzka, P. O. Katz, A. Smout, S. Spechler, & M. F. Vaezi (Eds.), *The Esophagus* (pp. 624–632). John Wiley & Sons. https://doi.org/10.1002/9781119599692.ch36

Eusebi, L. H., Ratnakumaran, R., Yuan, Y., Solaymani-Dodaran, M., Bazzoli, F., & Ford, A. C. (2018). Global prevalence of, and risk factors for, gastro-oesophageal reflux symptoms: A meta-analysis. *Gut*, 67(3), 430–440. https://doi.org/10.1136/gutjnl-2016-313589

Gaude, G. S. (2009). Pulmonary manifestations of gastroesophageal reflux disease. *Annals of Thoracic Medicine*, 4(3), 115–123. https://doi.org/10.4103/1817-1737.53347

Hauser, S. C., Oxentanko, A. S., & Sanchez, W. (2014). *Mayo Clinic gastroenterology and hepatology board review*. Mayo Clinic Scientific Press.

Katz, P. O., Gerson, L. B., & Vela, M. F. (2022). ACG clinical guideline for the diagnosis and management of gastroesophageal reflux disease. *American Journal of Gastroenterology*, 117, 27–56. https://doi.org/10.14309/ajg.0000000000001538

MacFarlane, B. (2018). Management of gastroesophageal reflux disease in adults: A pharmacist's perspective. *Integrated Pharmacy Research & Practice*, 7, 41–52. https://doi.org/10.2147/IPRP.S142932

Maret-Ouda, J., Markar, S. R., & Lagergren, J. (2020). Gastroesophageal reflux disease: A review. *JAMA*, 324(24), 2536–2547. https://doi.org/10.1001/jama.2020.21360

Mizyed, I., Fass, S. S., & Fass, R. (2009). gastro-oesophageal reflux disease and psychological comorbidity. *Alimentary pharmacology & therapeutics*, 29(4), 351–358.

Moayyedi, P., Eikelboom, J. W., Bosch, J., Connolly, S. J., Dyal, L., Shestakovska, O., Leong, D., Anand, S. S., Störk, S., Branch, K. R. H., Bhatt, D. L., Verhamme, P. B., O'Donnell, M., Maggioni, A. P.,

Lonn, E. M., Piegas, L. S., Ertl, G., Keltai, M., Bruns, N. C., ... COMPASS Investigators. (2019). Safety of proton pump inhibitors based on a large, multi-year, randomized trial of patients receiving rivaroxaban or aspirin. *Gastroenterology, 157*(3), 682–691.e2. https://doi.org/10.1053/j.gastro.2019.05.056

Peery, A. F., Crockett, S. D., Murphy, C. C., Lund, J. L., Dellon, E. S., Williams, J. L., Jensen, E. T., Shaheen, N. J., Barritt, A. S., Lieber, S. R., Kochar, B., Barnes, E. L., Fan, Y. C., Pate, V., Galanko, J., Baron, T. H., & Sandler, R. S. (2019). Burden and cost of gastrointestinal, liver, and pancreatic diseases in the United States: Update 2018. *Gastroenterology, 156*(1), 254–272.e11. https://doi.org/10.1053/j.gastro.2018.08.063

Peery, A. F., Dellon, E. S., Lund, J., Crockett, S. D., McGowan, C. E., Bulsiewicz, W. J., Gangarosa, L. M., Thiny, M. T., Stizenberg, K., Morgan, D. R., Ringel, Y., Kim, H. P., DiBonaventura, M. D., Carroll, C. F., Allen, J. K., Cook, S. F., Sandler, R. S., Kappelman, M. D., & Shaheen, N. J. (2012). Burden of gastrointestinal disease in the United States: 2012 update. *Gastroenterology, 143*(5), 1179–1187.e3. https://doi.org/10.1053/j.gastro.2012.08.002

Qumseya, B. J., Bukannan, A., Gendy, S., Ahemd, Y., Sultan, S., Bain, P., Gross, S. A., Iyer, P., & Wani, S. (2019). Systematic review and meta-analysis of prevalence and risk factors for Barrett's esophagus. *Gastrointestinal Endoscopy, 90*(5), 707–717.e1. https://doi.org/10.1016/j.gie.2019.05.030

Sethi, S., & Richter, J. E. (2017). Diet and gastroesophageal reflux disease: Role in pathogenesis and management. *Current Opinion in Gastroenterology, 33*(2), 107–111. https://doi.org/10.1097/MOG.0000000000000337

Spechler, S. J., & Souza, R. F. (2014). Barrett's esophagus. *New England Journal of Medicine, 371*, 836–845. https://doi.org/10.1056/NEJMra1314704

Vaezi, M. F., Yang, Y.-X., & Howden, C. W. (2017). Complications of proton pump inhibitor therapy. *Gastroenterology, 153*(1), 35–48. https://doi.org/10.1053/j.gastro.2017.04.047

Vakil, N., van Zanten, S. V., Kahrilas, P., Dent, J., Jones, R., & Group, G. C. (2006). The Montreal definition and classification of gastroesophageal reflux disease: A global evidence-based consensus. *Official Journal of the American College of Gastroenterology, 101*(8), 1900–1920. https://doi.org/10.1111/j.1572-0241.2006.00630.x

Wang, K. K., & Sampliner, R. (2008). Practice Parameters Committee of the American College of Gastroenterology, Updated guidelines 2008 for the diagnosis, surveillance and therapy of Barrett's esophagus. *American Journal of Gastroenterology, 103*(3), 788–797. https://doi.org/10.1111/j.1572-0241.2008.01835.x

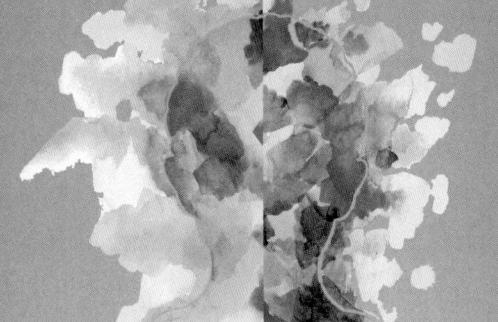

CHAPTER 53

Geriatric Syndromes

Courtney Gordon

I. Introduction and general background

Geriatric syndromes are defined as common conditions frequently seen in older adults that cannot be classified into a single disease but have a significant impact on well-being and overall quality of life. They are complex conditions more frequently seen among older adults that are multifactorial in etiology and require a multidisciplinary approach to effectively manage and treat. Despite popular belief, these syndromes are not part of the normal aging process and are only associated with aging. The geriatric syndromes discussed in this chapter include many of the conditions commonly seen in primary care practice settings caring for older adults. Those syndromes are frailty, sensory impairment, falls, urinary incontinence, and delirium.

A. Frailty
  1. Definition and overview
     Frailty is an increasingly recognized geriatric syndrome that has a tremendous impact on the older individual, their family, and society as a whole (Theou et al., 2011). Frailty is a condition made up of many different components. Presenting complaints commonly include decreased energy, poor appetite and inability to consume adequate nutrition, weight loss, weakness, and decreased physical activity. It is a chronic syndrome that is progressive in nature, developing along a continuum of severity. Frailty is associated with a high risk for poor clinical outcomes because of the inability to recover from stressors. These adverse clinical outcomes often include falls, functional impairment, loss of independence, and mortality. The main goal is prevention of frailty by maintaining muscle mass and activity level in older adults, as well as adequate nutritional intake.
  2. Prevalence
     Frailty tends to be more prevalent in the presence of any stressors to the body. Stressors in older adults can include many factors. Common factors seen in the primary care setting of older adults include infections, dehydration, new medications or medication changes, mental health disorders, any change in living arrangements (e.g., experiencing homelessness or moving), food insecurity, change of caregivers or lack of caregiving support, or recent serious illness requiring hospitalization.

B. Sensory impairment
  1. Definition and overview
     Both visual and hearing impairments greatly affect the quality of life of older adults. Other sensory impairments that are commonly seen in advanced age include changes in taste and smell. Along with sensory impairments comes social isolation, depression, anxiety, loss of independence, greater risk of falls, and functional decline.

     Visual impairment is defined as visual acuity of less than 20/40. Blindness is defined as visual acuity of less than 20/200 (Durso & Sullivan, 2013). There are many common eye conditions older adults are likely to develop as they age that result in worsening visual acuity. Those include but are not limited to cataracts, age-related macular degeneration, glaucoma, and diabetic retinopathy.

     Hearing impairment has a substantial negative impact on the way people are able to communicate. It has also been linked to an increased incidence of cognitive deterioration, increased falls, and gait disorders, particularly in older adults. Presbycusis is defined as age-related hearing loss. There are many reasons why older adults suffer from hearing loss, and it is important to recognize the different types of hearing loss and the typical clinical presentation to help guide diagnosis. The most common type in older adults is sensorineural hearing loss. Sensorineural hearing loss is caused by damage to the inner ear and is permanent. Other types of hearing loss are classified as conductive or mixed. A common cause of hearing loss that is fixable is cerumen impaction. By removing the cerumen, hearing should improve.

Various infections can also cause hearing loss in older adults, and some individuals may have an autoimmune inner ear disease that can contribute to hearing loss, such as systemic lupus erythematous, Crohn disease, and ulcerative colitis, to name a few. Diabetes mellitus can affect the vasculature of the cochlea, leading to hearing loss. Ototoxic medications like aminoglycoside antibiotics, antimalarial medications, platinum-based chemotherapy agents, loop diuretics, and nonsteroidal anti-inflammatory drugs can all worsen hearing loss as well. Acoustic neuroma, Meniere disease, trauma (Injury from puncturing the ear canal with an external device), and radiation can all also contribute to hearing loss in the older adult.

2. Prevalence

Both visual and hearing impairments increase in incidence as people age. These impairments have a substantial impact on the quality of life of the older adult, as well as the medical system. Chronic eye conditions are one of the most common reasons for office visits among those 65 years and older (Durso & Sullivan, 2013).

Hearing loss is one of the most common chronic conditions affecting people over the age of 65. The prevalence of hearing loss is 20%–40% in adults aged 50 years or older and more than 80% for those aged 80 years or older (Chou et al., 2011).

C. *Falls*

1. Definition and overview

Significant morbidity and mortality are associated with falls in older adults. The prognosis worsens in people with repetitive and frequent falls. Falls and gait disorders, like all geriatric syndromes, play an important role in the quality of life of older adults. Depression and confusion are often seen in older adults who suffer from falls. People often are forced to move out of their homes into residential facilities as a result of frequent falls, gait disorders, and the resultant risk of injury to themselves in the home. The fear of falling can also create stress for individuals and their families. The fear of falling has been shown to increase overall fall risk. One of the major consequences of fear of falling is the restriction and avoidance of activities (Delbaere et al., 2004).

2. Prevalence

Falls are the most common event that, in turn, causes loss of independence in older adults. More than one-third of community-living adults older than 65 years fall each year. The incidence increases for those individuals over the age of 80 and those who reside in residential facilities.

Approximately 10% of falls result in a major injury, such as a fracture, soft tissue injury, or traumatic brain injury (Tinetti & Kumar, 2010).

D. *Urinary incontinence*

1. Definition and overview

Urinary incontinence is defined as any involuntary leakage or loss of urine. Urinary incontinence is a syndrome that can result from different medical conditions and the usage of certain medications. Leading risk factors for urinary incontinence include being female, cognitive impairment, abdominal surgery, higher body weight, impaired mobility, and increasing age. Incontinence has a substantial impact on an individual's quality of life as well as financially on the healthcare system. An estimated $12 billion is spent annually on incontinence supplies, medications, and caregiver time (Williams et al., 2014). The different types of urinary incontinence include functional incontinence, stress incontinence, urge incontinence, overflow incontinence, and mixed incontinence. Please refer to Chapter 25, Urinary Incontinence in Persons Assigned Female at Birth, for more detailed information.

2. Prevalence

Urinary incontinence increases in incidence with age and is more common in women than men. Approximately 15%–30% of healthy older adults experience some urinary leakage. The prevalence is nearly 50% among frail community dwellers and between 50% and 75% among institutionalized older adults (Williams et al., 2014). Incontinence often goes unreported or underreported by older adults, likely in some part because of feelings of embarrassment and social stigma. Urinary incontinence, like falls, is thought to be one of the main reasons persons are moved out of their homes and into residential nursing facilities. It can be a great burden on caregivers and negatively affects quality of life for the older adult experiencing urinary incontinence. Urinary incontinence is associated with a 30% increase in functional decline and a twofold increased risk of falls, depressive symptoms, and nursing home placement (Goode et al., 2010).

E. *Delirium*

1. Definition and overview

Like the previous syndromes, delirium is multifactorial and important to recognize in the older adult population because individuals experiencing delirium are at an increased risk for poor clinical outcomes, and it is considered a medical emergency. Key features include an acute onset, a fluctuating course, and waxing and waning of symptoms. Although it is typically described as a transient syndrome, some cases of delirium have been reported to last as long as a few weeks to months. Delirium is often misdiagnosed as dementia, especially in the acute care setting. It is important to remember that most dementias typically present gradually and progressively over many months to years, unlike delirium, which occurs suddenly and changes often over the course of 24 hours. However, a major predisposing factor for the development of delirium is underlying cognitive impairment, so older adults often can have both delirium and dementia. Other predisposing factors for delirium include depression or anxiety, coexisting medical conditions, drugs/medications, environmental changes, electrolyte disturbances, infection, injury and change in functional status, poor appetite, and sensory impairment. Three different forms of delirium exist—hyperactive, hypoactive, and mixed. In hyperactive delirium, the individual is very anxious and agitated, has difficulty sleeping, and can be aggressive with staff and caregivers. Hypoactive delirium is often missed in the acute setting because the main symptoms are that the patient is more lethargic and sleepy than their baseline. Mixed delirium is common and is a combination of the two (Wong et al., 2010).

2. Prevalence

Delirium is a common occurrence in older adults and is associated with high morbidity and mortality. It is important for clinicians to recognize symptoms of delirium and make a diagnosis quickly. Delirium is associated with functional decline and immobility, which result in further complications of care. Delirium is the most common complication among hospitalized older adults (Witlox et al., 2010). On admission to the hospital, the prevalence of delirium can range from 10% to 40% of older adults. Patients admitted to the intensive care unit (ICU) have an even higher incidence of 70%–87% (Williams et al., 2014). The prevalence of delirium at the end of life is also reported to be quite high as well, upward of 80%–85% (Durso & Sullivan, 2013). Delirium complicates hospital stays for at least 20% of the 12.5 million patients 65 years of age or older who are hospitalized each year and increases hospital costs by $2,500 per patient; about $6.9 billion of Medicare hospital expenditures are attributable to delirium (Inouye, 2006).

II. Database

A. *Subjective*

1. Frailty

Subjective data are obtained from a detailed history from the older adult if they are able to provide information, as well as from any family members or caregivers who are present. Family members or caregivers typically complain that the person is overall slowing down. The individual seems weaker or more tired than usual. Persons often complain of having no energy and feeling as if everything is a burden.

2. Sensory impairment

Older adults with visual impairments often will have various complaints. It is important to do a thorough, detailed history to decipher what requires attention from an ophthalmologist or specialist versus what can be handled safely in the outpatient setting. Some questions to consider include the following: Does the person now require reading glasses? Do they have associated pain? Is their vision blurred? What is the time frame for loss of vision?

Hearing-loss data are often reported from family members and caregivers who find the person is not hearing as well or has a noticeable change. Hearing loss that is associated with age is gradual and can span many years. Common complaints from persons are not being able to hear well in large crowds; for example, when dining in a restaurant, they might have difficulty engaging in conversations because of an inability to hear well and to distinguish sounds. Hearing loss is often considered by older adults and family members as a normal part of aging and not something that can be fixed. Often, this is not the case. As a clinician, it is important to ask about the nature of the hearing loss; the timing (days, months, years); and any associated symptoms, such as ear pain, ringing, drainage, or dizziness. If they have already been examined and have hearing aids, are they wearing them appropriately? Do they know how to care for the hearing aids?

3. Falls

During the detailed history, it is important to ask if the older adult has had any previous falls, balance issues, or recent changes in vision. What medications is the person taking? Are they feeling more depressed or anxious, suffering from dizziness, and/or do they have any associated pain? These factors all contribute to an increased risk for falls. By targeting risk factors, interventions can be made, with the goal of decreasing the incidence of falls.

4. Urinary incontinence

A thorough history of urinary incontinence must include gaining information from the older adult and caregivers about the frequency, duration, and severity of symptoms. Older adults are often reluctant to discuss urinary incontinence because of feelings of embarrassment, so sensitivity regarding questioning is important. Questions should include the following: Do you ever leak urine when you cough or sneeze? Do you have problems making it to the bathroom in time? If yes, why do you have difficulty? Do you find yourself getting up frequently during the night to urinate?

5. Delirium

A clinical diagnosis of delirium is made after a detailed history, a cognitive assessment, and a physical and neurological exam. Knowing a person's cognitive status at baseline is important to determine any fluctuations or subtle changes. Obtaining a detailed history from family members and caregivers is vital to ascertain any recent changes in mental status. It is important for clinicians to note the timing of the change in mental status and the course thus far. Additionally, identify any preceding factors such as new medications, change in physical environment, or injury. It is important to diagnose delirium because it can be a medical emergency and may improve quickly with treatment.

B. *Objective: physical examination*

1. Frailty

a. Pertinent physical exam findings may include:
   i. Head, eyes, ears, nose, and throat (HEENT)—temporal wasting, dry mucous membranes
   ii. Cardiovascular—tachycardia or other arrhythmias

iii. Weight loss and poorly fitting clothes
2. Sensory impairment
   a. Measure visual acuity using the Snellen chart.
   b. Examine whether the older adult's pupils respond to light.
   c. Assess visual fields via confrontation and extraocular motility.
   d. Examine the outer parts of the eye (lids, lashes, and brows)
   e. With an ophthalmoscope, assess the lens for opacities; the optic disc for increased cupping or pallor, arteriovenous narrowing, nicking, and/or copper and silver wiring; and the maculae for hemorrhages, exudates, and drusen.
   f. When assessing hearing, it is imperative to examine with an otoscope and observe the ear canal as well as the tympanic membrane. Cerumen can occlude the ear canal, resulting in significant hearing loss and discomfort, and can be easily removed, providing relief. When inspecting the ear canal, look for any tumors, cysts, polyps, or foreign bodies that might impair hearing. It is important to look for any perforation of the tympanic membrane or significant thickening of the membrane, which can worsen hearing. Examinations with otoscopes and ophthalmoscopes can be particularly challenging in patients with dementia, so extra time and careful explanation of the exam process are recommended.
   g. When assessing hearing, clinicians can perform tuning fork tests, such as the Weber and Rinne tests, to differentiate the type of hearing loss in the older adult.
3. Falls
   a. Examine footwear and clothing, which can impede safety.
   b. Obtain orthostatic vital signs.
   c. Assess cognitive status with a validated tool such as the MOCA included in this chapter (**Figures 53-1**).
   d. Check visual acuity (see previous section on sensory impairment).
   e. Pertinent physical exam findings can include:
      i. HEENT—Nystagmus and other ocular deficiencies contributing to the risk for falls. Ears impacted with cerumen, contributing to dizziness and falls. Examine mouth to look for moist mucous membranes. Dry membranes are an indicator of dehydration, which can contribute to falls.
      ii. Cardiovascular—Assess for arrhythmias and other cardiac abnormalities that can cause syncope and falls. Assess both carotid arteries for bruits.
      iii. Musculoskeletal—Examine for strength and any movement disorders that can contribute to falls.
   f. There are several validated tests that measure balance and mobility in the older adult, but these are often not practical to perform in a busy clinic setting. The Timed Up-and-Go test and the functional reach test, however, are fairly easy to use and take relatively little time (**Table 53-1**).
4. Urinary incontinence
   a. Older adults or their caregivers can complete a voiding or bladder diary, which the clinician can use to review episodes of incontinence regarding timing and frequency. Patients or their caregivers write down the time of urination; the amount; and any additional comments, such as what they were doing, for example, coughing, sneezing, or sleeping.
   b. Physical exam is less useful for initial assessment of urinary incontinence than the detailed history (Goode et al., 2010). However, a thorough physical exam should include:
      i. Cardiovascular—A thorough cardiovascular assessment looking for signs of fluid overload associated with congestive heart failure, which can contribute to incontinence. Assess for elevated jugular venous pressure, arrhythmias, increased edema to extremities, and shortness of breath.
      ii. Abdominal—Palpate the bladder for fullness and if there is any associated pain or tenderness. Examine the abdomen for any constipation, which can contribute to incontinence.
      iii. A rectal exam should be done, particularly for men, to assess for enlarged prostate, masses, or fecal impaction.
      iv. For women, assess for prolapse or atrophy, as well as a cystocele or rectocele, which can contribute to incontinence, as well as any masses.
5. Delirium
   a. Clinicians should use the Confusion Assessment Method (CAM; Inouye et al., 1990), Mini-cog, Montreal Cognitive Assessment (MOCA) (Figure 53-1), or another validated tool to help determine cognitive status (Durso & Sullivan, 2013). These tests assess for cognitive changes, attention span, organization, and level of consciousness.
   b. The CAM is simple to use and also comes in an ICU format for patients admitted to ICUs. It is easily administered at the bedside.
   c. It is important to perform MOCA at routine follow-up visits in the outpatient setting to assess baseline cognitive functioning and therefore be able to identify any changes.
   d. Pertinent physical exam findings may include:
      i. Cardiovascular—Assess for cardiac arrhythmias, such as atrial fibrillation, bradycardia, tachycardia, or congestive heart failure (CHF) exacerbation, that could be the source of the delirium.
      ii. Abdominal—Assess for distention, pain, and bowel sounds. Acute abdominal pain

Figure 53-1 Montreal Cognitive Assessment (MOCA).

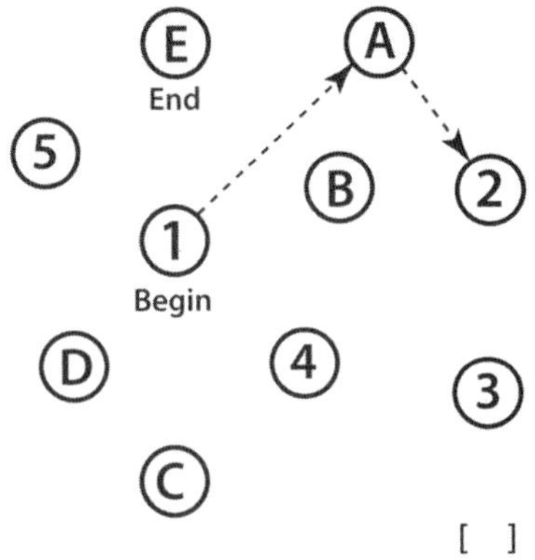

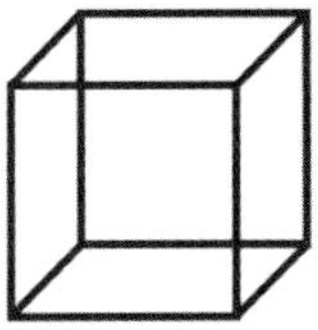

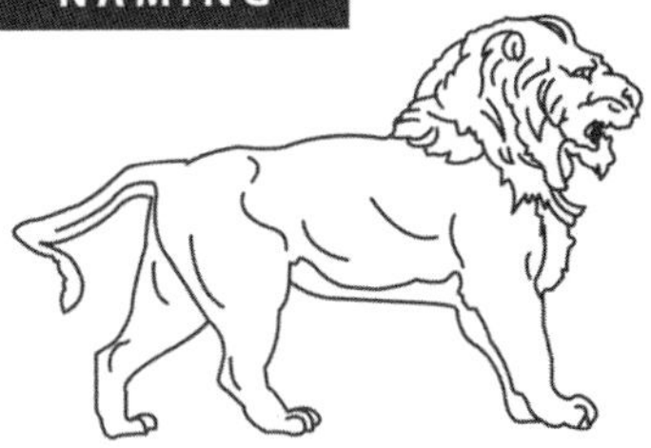

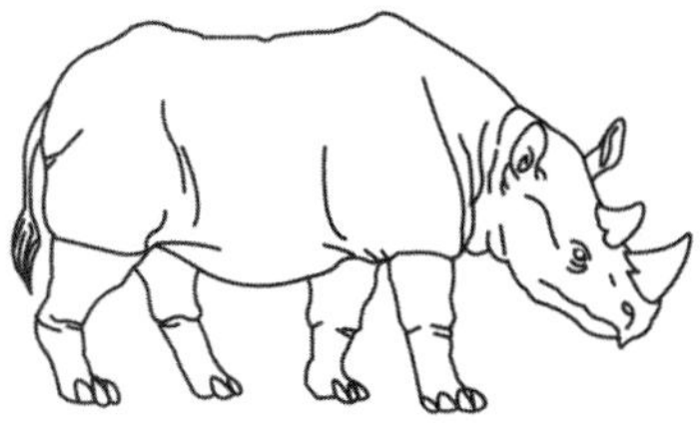

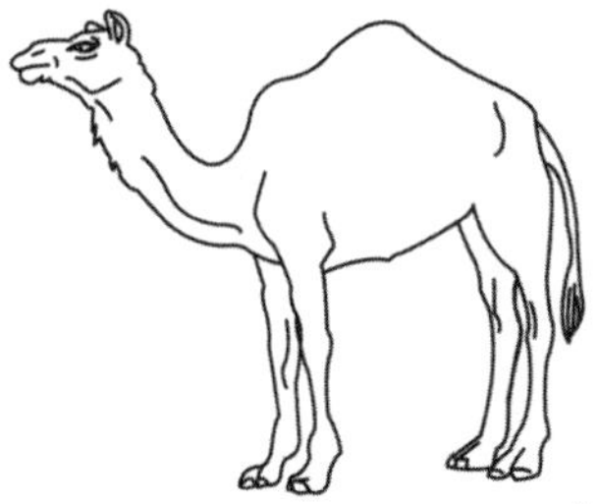

Copyright Z. Nasreddine, MD. Reproduced with permission. Copies are available at www.mocatest.org

Table 53-1 Special Maneuvers

Timed Up-and-Go Test The most frequently recommended screening test for mobility, takes less than 1 minute to administer	This test measures an older adult's strength and balance. Patient should stand from a chair without using arms to push up. Patient walks across the exam room and turns around. Patient walks back to chair and sits down again without using arms. Inability to do this test within 15 seconds indicates an increased fall risk. Patient is also graded on a scale of 1 to 5 regarding muscle strength, balance, and gait abnormalities while performing test.
Functional Reach Test	This test is performed with a leveled yardstick secured to the wall just above the patient's waist. Patient being tested stands with shoulders perpendicular to the wall, makes a fist, and extends the arm as far forward as possible along the wall without losing balance or taking a step. Test should be done without shoes or socks. The distance reached is measured using the yardstick. Patient should accomplish 6 inches or greater. Inability to do so is an indicator to pursue further testing and assessment for functional decline.

Data from Tinetti, M. E., & Kumar, C. (2010). The patient who falls. "It's always a trade-off." *JAMA, 303*(3), 258–266.

and constipation can cause delirium in the older adult.

iii. Neurological—Focus attention on mental status, which might show hyperalertness or lethargy. Assess mood, which can be agitated, anxious, or more confused. Assess grip strength and motor skills to rule out stroke.

III. Assessment
A. Frailty

The use of a comprehensive geriatric assessment allows clinicians to care for frail older adults. This allows clinicians to address the different components of frailty. A team-based approach including physicians, advanced practice providers, nurses, pharmacists, therapists, and dietitians has been shown to have positive effects when treating older adults. The focus of assessment in frailty is to eliminate or treat any underlying stressors that are contributing to frailty.

According to the American Geriatric Society, a person must have three or more characteristics in order to be classified as having frailty (Durso & Sullivan, 2013):
1. Weight loss—more than 10 lb unintentionally in the past year
2. Exhaustion—sensation that everything takes an enormous effort to complete
3. Slowness—time to walk 15 feet
4. Low activity level—uses less than 270 kcal/week
5. Weakness—can calculate with grip-strength measurement

A clinician should be able to recognize any precipitating causes of frailty and address these to promote functional improvement and decrease decline in status. It is important to assess nutritional status and note any impairments in older adults' instrumental activities of daily living (IADLs) and activities of daily living (ADLs). ADLs are basic activities of daily living that persons do to function during the day: eating, bathing, toileting, transferring (walking), and continence. IADLs are things that are not considered to be necessary for fundamental functioning but do allow an individual to live independently in the community, and are important to overall quality of life and also impact someone's sense of self and identity. IADLs include preparing meals, housework, managing medications, and taking medications.

B. Sensory impairment

It is important to recognize normal changes in the aging eye versus an acute or progressive visual problem. In all adults, presbyopia develops as a result of the lens becoming less flexible and losing the ability to accommodate. Older adults have an inability to focus their eyes on objects that are near. Most older adults will require reading glasses in their lifetime in order to clearly see objects that are near. Common ocular disorders to identify and/or to be suspicious of and refer to an ophthalmologist are dry eyes (keratoconjunctivitis sicca), cataracts, glaucoma, retinopathy, and macular degeneration.

Some predisposing factors of hearing impairment cannot be changed, such as genetic predisposition, sex, and aging of the cochlea. Other factors can be modified, such as removal of cerumen impaction, reduction of exposure to noise, and cessation of ototoxic medications. Clinicians must be able to differentiate the different types of hearing loss in older adults.

C. Falls

Often, falls are not a result of one single action but rather a culmination of events leading up to the fall. There are many risk factors for falling in the older adult population that clinicians should be aware of. These include balance impairment, previous falls, decreased muscle strength, visual impairment, more than four medications or the use of a psychoactive medication, gait impairment, depression, anxiety, dizziness, functional limitations, age greater than 80 years, female sex, low body weight, urinary incontinence, cognitive impairment, arthritis, diabetes, and pain (Tinetti & Kumar, 2010).

D. *Urinary incontinence*

Once the cause and type of urinary incontinence the older adult is experiencing are identified, steps can be made to treat and correct contributing factors. Management of urinary incontinence should focus on the individual's goals and issues that are most problematic to the older adult in order to improve quality of life.

E. *Delirium*

The diagnosis of delirium is primarily clinical and based on careful observation of key features. Key clinical features include acute onset and fluctuating course, inattention, disorganized thinking, altered level of consciousness, disorientation, memory impairment, perceptual disturbances, increased or decreased psychomotor activity, and disturbance of the sleep–wake cycle (Wong et al., 2010).

A useful mnemonic to help identify reversible causes of delirium is listed in **Table 53-2**.

IV. Goals of clinical management

A. *Screening*
1. Thorough screening to determine geriatric syndrome
2. It is important to choose screening and diagnostic tools that are cost-effective and patient appropriate.

B. *Treatment*
1. Select a safe and effective treatment plan based on diagnosis of geriatric syndrome as well as patient's goals of care.

C. *Patient adherence*
1. Select an approach that maximizes patient adherence, and continue to monitor patient adherence throughout treatment.

V. Plan

A. *Frailty*
1. Diagnostic studies (**Table 53-3**)
2. Treatment/patient and caregiver education
   a. Prevention is key.
   b. Causes of frailty should be treated in order to prevent the human and economic burden associated with this syndrome (Theou et al., 2011).
   c. Immobility is often a precursor to worsening frailty, so making sure the older adult remains physically active is important. Maintaining muscle mass and strength through routine exercises, including stretching and weight resistance, has been shown to be beneficial (Theou et al., 2011).
   d. Counseling patients and caregivers on adequate nutrition and caloric intake is important. Depending on the case, supplemental protein might be used.
   e. Counsel patients, family members, and caregivers on the availability of community support systems (e.g., Meals on Wheels or other home delivery food options).

B. *Sensory impairment*
1. Diagnostic studies are sometimes needed in the assessment and treatment of sensory impairments. When pursuing diagnostic studies, it is important to review the goals of care and what will be done with the results of the studies obtained. Occasionally, a computed tomography (CT) scan/magnetic resonance imaging (MRI) of the brain might be used if there is concern for a stroke or head injury contributing to impairment.

Table 53-2 Delirium Mnemonic

D	Drugs	Any changes to prescription regimen. Any new medications, adjustments in dosage, and interactions with other medications and foods.
E	Electrolyte disturbances	Dehydration, thyroid abnormalities, sodium and potassium deficiencies
L	Lack of drugs	Withdrawal from medications, poor pain control resulting from inefficient prescribing and treatment, withdrawal from alcohol or other drugs
I	Infection	Urinary tract and respiratory infections are the most commonly seen infections in older adults.
R	Reduced sensory input	Poor vision and inability to hear, as well as changes in smell, taste, and touch
I	Intracranial	Stroke, hemorrhage, brain injury, infectious process of the brain
U	Urinary	Urinary retention, incontinence, and infection. Also includes fecal incontinence and impaction.
M	Myocardial	Myocardial infarction, congestive heart failure, arrhythmias

Data from Durso, S., & Sullivan, G. (Eds.). (2013). *Geriatrics review syllabus: A core curriculum in geriatric medicine* (8th ed.). New York: American Geriatrics Society.

Table 53-3 Geriatric Syndromes and Labs/Imaging

Labs/Imaging to Obtain	Geriatric Syndrome	Rationale
Complete blood count	Frailty Falls Urinary incontinence Delirium	Assess for anemia and/or elevated white count, which could indicate an infectious process contributing to these particular geriatric syndromes.
Serum electrolyte	Frailty Falls Urinary incontinence Delirium	Assess for hypo-/hyperkalemia, hypo-/hypernatremia, and dehydration, which can contribute to these particular geriatric syndromes.
Renal panel	Frailty Falls Urinary incontinence Delirium	Assess kidney functioning to determine if kidney injury, failure, or disease is contributing to these particular geriatric syndromes.
Thyroid panel	Frailty Delirium	Assess for hyper-/hypothyroidism. Hyperthyroidism can contribute to weight loss and frailty. Uncontrolled hyper-/hypothyroidism can lead to delirium.
Urinalysis, urine culture	Frailty Falls Urinary incontinence Delirium	If concern for infectious process that is treatable and often contributes to frailty, falls, increased urinary incontinence, and delirium. Especially helpful in patients with dementia who cannot express symptoms of infection.
Albumin, prealbumin	Frailty	Indicator of protein intake and overall nutritional state
Serum glucose	Falls Delirium	Assess for hypoglycemia, which can lead to falls and delirium in the older adult.
Vitamin B_{12}	Falls Delirium	Low levels are associated with proprioceptive problems, contributing to falls and increased confusion resulting in delirium.
Vitamin D	Falls	High risk for fractures from fall if level is low
Electrocardiogram	Falls Delirium	Evaluate for abnormal rhythm or cardiac pathology contributing to syncope, resulting in a fall or delirium.
Computed tomography (CT) scan/magnetic resonance imaging (MRI) brain	Sensory impairment Falls Delirium	If concern for stroke, bleed, or injury to the head, which can contribute to sensory impairment, falls, and/or delirium
Ultrasound of bladder	Urinary incontinence	To assess volume of urine inside the bladder. A postvoid residual is often done in the hospital setting to examine for urinary retention. This test is rarely needed in the ambulatory setting.
Renal ultrasound	Urinary incontinence	Evaluate for kidney disease and problems with the urinary tract
CT abdomen/pelvis	Urinary incontinence	Evaluate for obstructions, tumors, cysts
Arterial blood gas	Delirium	If concern for hypoxia, poor perfusion contributing to delirium
Toxicology	Falls Delirium	Assess for presence of illegal substances contributing to falls and delirium
Electroencephalogram	Sensory impairment Falls Delirium	If concern for seizure activity contributing to sensory impairment, falls, and/or delirium

2. Treatment/patient and caregiver education
   a. By identifying the visual condition affecting the older adult, steps can be taken to fix the problem or allow the patient to accommodate to new visual changes. For example, dry eyes tend to be a common complaint in older adults. The use of nonprescription artificial tears can help alleviate dry eyes. The use of warm compresses can be helpful as well.
   b. Encourage patients to have an annual eye exam.
   c. Provide education regarding a safe visual environment in the home, particularly focusing on adequate lighting. Older adults lose the ability to see well in dim light.
   d. Treatments for common conditions like cataracts, age-related macular degeneration, glaucoma, and diabetic neuropathy vary with the diagnosis, so recognizing the condition can then allow you to guide treatment.
   e. Depending on the cause of the hearing loss, some conditions can be helped with medical and or surgical intervention.
   f. To better assess hearing, refer to an audiologist for formal audiometric testing and assistance with obtaining hearing aids and other devices that can amplify hearing, such as a pocket talkers, if appropriate. There are many devices, such as amplified telephones, visual alarm systems, and vibrating alarm clocks, available to help older adults navigate hearing loss and adjust to their living environment.
   g. Adaptive techniques, such as teaching family members or caregivers to speak directly in front of the person and using low tones, have been shown to be beneficial. Older adults lose the ability to hear high-pitched tones.

C. *Falls*
   1. Diagnostic studies (Table 53-3)
   2. Treatment/patient and caregiver education
      a. Fall prevention strategies are important. Collaborate with families and institutions if the person is residing in a facility to promote an environment that is safe and reduces the risk of falls.
      b. Need to individualize treatment plans for patients based on cause of falls.
      c. Treat any modifiable risk factors that can contribute to falls, for example, correcting visual impairment and ensuring the older adult has appropriate footwear.
      d. Medication reduction and physical therapy have been shown to be helpful in reducing further falls (Cameron et al., 2010).
      e. Clinicians should work along with physical therapist colleagues to establish an exercise program for older adults.
      f. Manage postural hypotension by titrating medications, optimizing fluid intake, and teaching behavioral strategies to reduce incidents.
      g. Provide vitamin D supplement when appropriate to reduce the risk of fractures from falls.

D. *Urinary incontinence*
   1. Diagnostic studies (Table 53-3)
   2. Treatment/patient and caregiver education
      a. Initiate behavioral targeted therapies as well as medications or, at times, surgical intervention when appropriate based on type of urinary incontinence. Make referral to urology and/or urogynecology if needed.
      b. It is also important to recognize medications that contribute to worsening of urinary incontinence and remove those if this can be done safely. Common medications include alpha-blockers, antipsychotics, loop diuretics, narcotics, and tricyclic antidepressants.
      c. Treat comorbid conditions contributing to urinary incontinence, such as diabetes mellitus and dementia.
      d. Behavioral modifications include timed voiding, for example, having the patient empty the bladder every 2 hours, and pelvic muscle training, which involves the use of Kegel exercises to strengthen the pelvic floor and surrounding muscles.
      e. Medications can be used to treat some types of urinary incontinence. Anticholinergic drugs are the most commonly prescribed medications for incontinence, and it is important to recognize the side effects of these medications in older adults, which can be quite problematic. Some of these side effects include confusion, constipation, dry eyes and mouth, and falls. Other agents often prescribed are antimuscarinics, such as oxybutynin, tolterodine, trospium, and fesoterodine. Alpha-blockers and tricyclic antidepressants have also been used.
      f. Devices such as pessaries can be trialed in women who suffer from organ prolapse resulting in overflow incontinence. It is important to recognize that pessaries do require some care from the individual, so they are often not appropriate for older adults with cognitive impairment.
      g. Several different surgical interventions can also be used if the patient is deemed a surgical candidate. Appropriate referrals are needed to specialists. Please refer to Chapter 25, Urinary Incontinence in Persons Assigned Female at Birth, for more detailed treatment regimens.

E. *Delirium*
   1. Diagnostic studies (Table 53-3)
   2. Treatment/patient and caregiver education
      a. After accurate diagnosis of delirium, steps can be taken to reduce complications and provide treatment.
      b. It is important to identify and treat any reversible conditions contributing to delirium.
      c. Attempt to prevent further complications and decline by reducing medications where appropriate.

d. Nonpharmacologic strategies include correcting any sensory impairment (see the section on sensory impairment for details); avoiding physical restraints, including foley catheters, that keep patients from being mobile; sleep hygiene; reorientation; and environment optimization.
e. Pharmacologic strategies are useful for severe cases of delirium where the person's safety and well-being or the safety and well-being of caregivers or staff are at risk. Pharmacologic treatment strategies include the use of an antipsychotic such as Haldol; atypical antipsychotics such as risperidone, olanzapine, or quetiapine; a benzodiazepine such as lorazepam; and/or an antidepressant such as trazodone (Inouye, 2006). The same geriatric principles apply when prescribing these medications: starting low and going slow, meaning start with a low dose and titrate up slowly if needed to achieve the desired response.
f. It is important to always weigh the goals of care for the individual being treated with the invasiveness of procedures and tests, and also the patient's own care goals and preferences.

VI. Online resources for clinicians, patients, and caregivers
A. AARP (http://www.aarp.org)
B. Alzheimer's Association (http://www.alz.org)
C. American Geriatrics Society (http://www.americangeriatrics.org)
D. American Geriatrics Society Beers Criteria (http://geriatricscareonline.org/ProductAbstract/american-geriatrics-society-updated-beers-criteria-for-potentially-inappropriate-medication-use-in-older-adults/CL001)
E. Family Caregiver Alliance (http://www.caregiver.org)
F. Gerontological Advanced Practice Nurses Association (https://www.gapna.org)
G. John A. Hartford Foundation (http://www.jhartfound.org)
H. The Hartford Institute for Geriatric Nursing, College of Nursing, New York University (http://consultgerirn.or/ or www.hartfordign.org)
   1. The Hartford Institute Assessment Tools Try This (http://www.hartfordign.org/practice/try_this)
I. The Hospital Elder Life Program (http://www.hospitalelderlifeprogram.org/about)
J. Medicare (http://www.medicare.gov)
K. National Institute on Aging (http://nia.nih.gov)
L. U.S. Preventive Services Task Force: Falls Prevention in Older Adults: Counseling and Preventive Medication (http://www.uspreventiveservicestaskforce.org/Page/Topic/recommendation-summary/falls-prevention-in-older-adults-counseling-and-preventive-medication)
M. Centers for Disease Control and Prevention: Older Adult Fall Prevention (http://cdc.gov/falls)

References

Cameron, I. D., Murray, G. R., Gillespie, L. D., Robertson, M. C., Hill, K. D., Cumming, R. G., & Kerse, N. (2010). Interventions for preventing falls in older people in nursing care facilities and hospitals. *Cochrane Database of Systematic Reviews, 2010*(1), CD005465. doi:10.1002/14651858.CD005465.pub2

Chou, R., Dana, T., Bougatsos, C., Fleming, C., & Beil, T. (2011). Screening adults aged 50 years or older for hearing loss: A review of the evidence for the U.S. Preventive Services Task Force. *Annals of Internal Medicine, 154*(5), 347–355.

Delbaere, K., Crombez, G., Vanderstraeten, G., Willems, T., & Cambier, D. (2004). Fear-related avoidance of activities, falls, and physical frailty. A prospective community-based cohort study. *Age and Ageing, 33*(4), 368–373.

Durso, S., & Sullivan, G. (Eds.). (2013). *Geriatrics review syllabus: A core curriculum in geriatric medicine* (8th ed.). American Geriatrics Society.

Goode, P. S., Burgio, K. L., Richter, H. E., & Markland, A. D. (2010). Incontinence in older women. *JAMA, 303*(21), 2172–2181.

Inouye, S. K. (2006). Delirium in older persons. *New England Journal of Medicine, 354*(11), 1157–1165.

Inouye, S., van Dyck, C., Alessi, C., Balkin, S., Siegal, A., & Horwitz, R. (1990). Clarifying confusion: The Confusion Assessment Method. *Annals of Internal Medicine, 113*(12), 941–948.

Theou, O., Stathokostas, L., Roland, K. P., Jakobi, J. M., Patterson, C., Vandervoort, A. A., & Jones, G. R. (2011, April 4). The effectiveness of exercise interventions for the management of frailty: A systematic review. *Journal of Aging Research*, 1–19.

Tinetti, M. E., & Kumar, C. (2010). The patient who falls. "It's always a trade-off." *JAMA, 303*(3), 258–266.

Williams, B., Chang, A., Ahalt, C., Chen, H., Conant, R., Landefeld, S., Ritchie, C., & Yukawa, M. (Eds.). (2014). *Current diagnosis & treatment: Geriatrics* (2nd ed.). McGraw-Hill Education.

Witlox, J., Eurelings, L. S., de Jonghe, J. F. M., Kalisvaart, K. J., Eikelenboom, P., & van Gool, W. A. (2010). Delirium in elderly patients and the risk of postdischarge mortality, institutionalization, and dementia: A meta-analysis. *JAMA, 304*(4), 443–451.

Wong, C. L., Holroyd-Leduc, J., Simel, D. L., & Straus, S. E. (2010). Does this patient have delirium? Value of bedside instruments. *JAMA, 304*(7), 779–786.

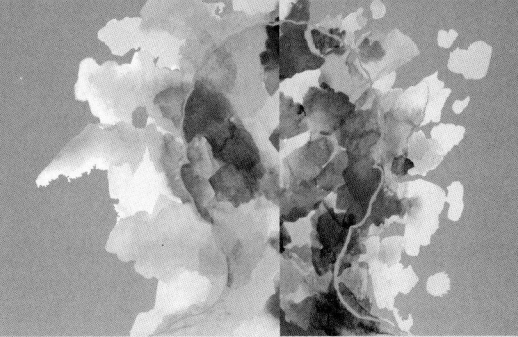

CHAPTER 54

Heart Failure

Lisa Guertin

I. Introduction and general background

Heart failure is a common condition seen in the primary care setting. It is a clinical syndrome that can occur suddenly or over time and arises from cardiac derangements within the pericardium, myocardium, or endocardium and/or structural abnormalities of the vessels or valves.

A. Definition and overview

Heart failure, as defined by the American College of Cardiology (ACC) and American Heart Association (AHA), is a complex clinical syndrome that results from any structural or functional impairment of ventricular filling or ejection of the blood (Heidenreich et al., 2022). Heart failure is a clinical diagnosis based on the presentation of symptoms, which typically include dyspnea, fatigue, fluid retention, and exercise intolerance.

Heart failure can involve the left ventricle, right ventricle, or both ventricles. Left ventricular heart failure occurs when the left ventricle is unable to pump sufficiently to meet the body's demands. The myocardial muscle may be too weak and thin to eject the blood from the ventricle, or the myocardial muscle may be too thick and stiff, causing inadequate ventricular filling. Both forms of heart failure cause elevated left ventricular filling pressures.

The symptoms of left ventricular failure predominantly include dyspnea and fatigue. Dyspnea arises from pulmonary edema. Pulmonary edema occurs from the ineffective ejection of blood from the left ventricle, causing elevated left atrial pressures, resulting in fluid backup in the pulmonary vasculature and, ultimately, the lungs. Subsequently, the persistent increased pulmonary volume and pressure can begin to affect the right ventricle. Fatigue arises from the inability of the ventricles to eject enough blood to meet the needs of the body, causing decreased forward flow and, ultimately, decreased cardiac output. However, the symptom of fatigue occurs in both left and right ventricular failure. Signs of right ventricular failure include peripheral edema, ascites, and hepatic and splenic congestion, predominantly arising from systemic venous fluid congestion. Three major clinical subsets of heart failure are systolic, diastolic, and mildly reduced. Systolic heart failure, called heart failure with reduced ejection fraction (HFrEF), occurs when the heart loses its ability to contract normally and the ejection fraction (EF) falls to ≤40%. As systolic heart failure progresses, the ventricle may become dilated. Reduced contractile function causes increased end-systolic and end-diastolic volumes, dilating the ventricle. This condition is called dilated cardiomyopathy (DCM). DCM is largely categorized into two etiologies: ischemic or nonischemic. Ischemic disease is the predominant cause of left ventricular systolic failure in the United States. There are multiple causes of nonischemic cardiomyopathy, including but not limited to familial, alcohol induced, cardiotoxicity as a result of medications, infectious diseases, inflammatory diseases, rheumatologic disorders, thyroid disease, some muscular dystrophies, long-standing poorly controlled hypertension, and valvular heart disease.

Diastolic heart failure is abnormal filling of the left or right ventricle caused by impaired myocardial relaxation or stiffness of the heart muscle. Common causes of diastolic heart failure are chronic hypertension with left ventricular hypertrophy and restrictive, infiltrative, and hypertrophic cardiomyopathies. Fifty percent of patients with heart failure have a preserved EF (Heidenreich et al., 2022). Heart failure with preserved EF (HFpEF) includes those patients with an EF of ≥50%.

Heart failure with mildly reduced EF (HFmrEF) is defined as an EF between 41% and 49%. These patients have been identified in retrospective analysis of randomized controlled trials because they have generally been excluded. Data suggests these patients may follow the trajectory of HFrEF and benefit from treatment (Heidenreich et al., 2022).

The New York Heart Association (NYHA) and American College of Cardiology Foundation/American Heart Association (ACCF/AHA) have complementary classifications and staging for defining the functional status and severity of heart failure. NYHA classifications are as follows (Criteria Committee of the American Heart Association, 1994):
1. Class I: No symptoms, with or limitations in ordinary activities.
2. Class II: Slight, mild limitation of activity; the patient is comfortable at rest or with mild exertion.
3. Class III: Marked limitation of any activity; the patient is comfortable only at rest.
4. Class IV: Severe limitations; any physical activity causes discomfort, and symptoms occur at rest.

The ACCF/AHA staging of heart failure are as follows (Heidenreich et al., 2022):
1. Stage A: Patients at high risk for developing heart failure but without structural heart disease or symptoms of heart failure.
2. Stage B: Structural heart disease but without signs or symptoms of heart failure.
3. Stage C: Structural heart disease with prior or current symptoms of heart failure.
4. Stage D: Refractory heart failure requiring specialized interventions.

B. *Prevalence and incidence*

The AHA estimates ~6 million Americans over the age of 20 have heart failure, occurring more frequently in men and in those over the age of 60 (Virani et al., 2021). The prevalence is expected to increase 46% by the year 2030 (Virani et al., 2021).

Multiple risk factors contribute to heart failure, including but not limited to coronary disease, hypertension, diabetes, obesity, and smoking (Virani et al., 2021). It is important to note that 33.3% of adults in the United States have at least one risk factor (Virani et al., 2021). Racial disparities exist; Black and Hispanic individuals have more heart failure risks than Whites (Virani et al., 2021). Although survival after a heart failure diagnosis has improved, mortality is 42.3% at 5 years and greater in Black individuals (Virani et al., 2021). According to the AHA, the estimated annual cost of heart failure to the nation is expected to increase to $69.8 billion by 2030 (Virani et al., 2021).

II. **Database (may include but is not limited to)**
A. *Subjective*
 1. Past health history
    a. Medical history: hypertension; coronary artery disease (myocardial infarction [MI]); arrhythmia; valvular heart disease including aortic or pulmonic stenosis, mitral or tricuspid stenosis, or mitral or aortic regurgitation; congenital heart disease; unhealthy amount of body fat; peripheral vascular disease; diabetes; obstructive sleep apnea; hyperlipidemia; anemia; thyroid disease; peripartum myopathy; other hormonal disorders; systemic lupus erythematosus; scleroderma; sarcoidosis; amyloidosis; infectious diseases, including HIV; Chagas disease; viral endocarditis and myocarditis; and malignancies requiring medications such as anthracycline, trastuzumab (Herceptin), high-dose cyclophosphamide, toxoids, mitomycin-C, 5-fluorouracil, and the interferons or other nonchemotherapy cardiotoxic medications (Yancy et al., 2013).
    b. Surgical history: Cardiac surgeries, including valve replacements, myectomy, and coronary artery bypass. Endovascular procedures such as stent placement, ethanol, or radiofrequency ablation.
    c. Medication history: Some categories of medications used in heart failure may have an adverse effect. For example, calcium channel blockers (harmful) and beta-blockers are negative inotropes. However, beta-blockers should not be excluded from the treatment regimen because they remain part of guideline directed medical therapy for the treatment of systolic heart failure. Antiarrhythmic medications and inotropes may be proarrhythmic. Thiazolidinediones and nonsteroidal anti-inflammatories can cause fluid retention. Other cardiotoxic medications.
 2. Family history: Atherosclerosis, MI, cerebrovascular accident (CVA), peripheral arterial disease, sudden cardiac death, arrhythmias, conduction disease (often requiring pacemakers or internal cardioverter defibrillators [ICDs]), heart failure, or cardiomyopathy
 3. Occupational and educational history
    a. Exposures to chemicals or toxins
    b. Level of education
    c. Ability to work; days missed from work or school
 4. Personal and social history
    a. Alcohol, cocaine, methamphetamine, and intravenous drug use
    b. Diet: Adherence to a heart-healthy and low-sodium diet
    c. Exercise: Assess the distance able to ambulate without stopping because of fatigue or shortness of breath, the ability to climb stairs, and participation in routine exercise or sedentary lifestyle.
    d. Activities of daily living: Ability to perform routine tasks without fatigue or shortness of breath.
    e. Culture and cultural practices
    f. Living situation
 5. Review of symptoms
    a. Constitutional signs and symptoms: Recent hospitalizations, fever, chills, rigors, fatigue, weight gain or loss. Weight loss is concerning because it is a poor prognostic indicator of heart failure.
    b. Respiratory: dyspnea with or without exertion, orthopnea, paroxysmal nocturnal dyspnea, and productive or nonproductive cough

c. Cardiac: chest pain, palpitations, edema, syncope, and presyncope
d. Gastrointestinal: anorexia, nausea, early satiety, increasing abdominal girth, and abdominal discomfort
e. Genitourinary: sexual dysfunction, sexually transmitted disease exposure, and urination patterns
f. Endocrine: heat or cold intolerance
g. Neurologic: lightheadedness, dizziness, frequent naps or inability to stay awake, decreased concentration, memory loss, and signs of transient ischemic attack (TIA) or CVA
h. Psychiatric: anxiety and/or depression

B. Objective
1. Physical examination findings
   a. Height, weight, body habitus, and general appearance
   b. Vital signs:
      i. Blood pressure: Assess for blood pressure abnormalities, including hyper- or hypotension and orthostatic blood pressures.
      ii. Pulse: Assess the rate, evaluating for tachycardiac and bradycardia, and the strength and regularity throughout. Assess the character of the carotid upstroke.
   c. Skin: pallor, cyanosis, cool temperature
   d. Thyroid/neck: goiter and/or bruits
   e. Lungs: tachypnea, rales, wheezing, ability to speak full sentences
   f. Cardiac: arrhythmia; elevated jugular venous pressure; additional heart sounds, such as S3 gallop, S4, or murmur; laterally displaced point of maximum impulse (PMI); heaves, lifts, and thrills; and edema (abdominal, peripheral, or sacral)
   g. Abdomen: increased abdominal girth indicating ascites (fluid wave, shifting dullness), abdominal tenderness, hepatomegaly, and hepatojugular reflux lasting longer than 10 seconds with sustained abdominal pressure

III. Assessment

A. *Determine the diagnosis.*
   Heart failure is a clinical diagnosis that is largely based on findings from the history and physical examination. Diagnostic testing is important and useful in confirming the diagnosis, the underlying etiology, and the severity of the disease.
   1. Differential diagnosis
      a. Chronic obstructive pulmonary disease
      b. Asthma
      c. Pulmonary embolism
      d. Interstitial lung disease
      e. Pneumonia
      f. Sleep apnea
      g. Pulmonary artery hypertension
      h. Myocardial ischemia
      i. Valvular heart disease
      j. Atrial fibrillation or other arrhythmia
      k. Anemia or other blood dyscrasias
      l. Venous insufficiency or thrombosis
      m. Cirrhosis
      n. Gastrointestinal disorders
      o. Renal disease or failure
      p. Endocrine disorders such as thyroid disease
      q. Deconditioning
      r. Depression
      s. Unhealthy amount of body fat
      t. Adverse effects from medications

B. *Severity*
   1. Assess the severity of the disease based on the NYHA classifications and/or ACCF/AHA heart failure staging.

C. *Motivation and ability*
   1. Determine the patient's willingness and ability to adhere to a treatment plan.
   2. Evaluate the patient's social supports and resources for success in the outpatient setting.

IV. Goals of clinical management

A. *Select and implement a treatment plan that appropriately manages heart failure in a beneficial and cost-effective manner.*
B. *Implement an evidence based treatment plan that enables patients' adherence.*
C. *Relieve symptoms.*
D. *Prevent/decrease admissions to an acute care facility.*
E. *Improve survival.*

V. Plan

A. *Diagnostic tests*
   1. Noninvasive testing
      a. General laboratory studies: complete blood count (CBC) with differential, basic metabolic panel, calcium, magnesium, liver tests, fasting glucose, urinalysis, lipid panel, iron studies, and thyroid-stimulating hormone (Heidenreich et al., 2022)
      b. Additional testing: hemochromatosis genetic test, HIV, rheumatologic diseases, amyloidosis, and pheochromocytoma (Yancy et al., 2013)
      c. Cardiac-specific laboratory studies: Natriuretic peptide—B-type natriuretic peptide (BNP) and N-terminal pro-B-type natriuretic peptide (NT pro-BNP)—can be useful in patients with dyspnea and to assess the severity of the disease (Yancy et al., 2013). It is important to consult the laboratory performing the test to obtain the normal range of laboratory values. Additionally, there are multiple factors that may cause an elevated BNP and NT pro-BNP; these include conditions that cause myocardial strain, acute renal failure, age, female sex, and liver cirrhosis. Having an elevated amount of body fat can lower the BNP or NT pro-BNP value.

d. Electrocardiogram: left ventricular hypertrophy, evidence of prior MI, arrhythmia, conduction problems, and axis deviation
e. Chest radiograph: cardiomegaly, pulmonary congestion
f. Echocardiogram: ventricular size, function, wall motion, atrial size, valvular function, and hemodynamic values
g. Cardiovascular magnetic resonance may be appropriate for the initial evaluation of heart failure and may be helpful in assessing myocardial perfusion, viability, and fibrosis imaging (Patel et al., 2013).
h. For evaluation of ischemic disease, consider noninvasive stress echocardiography, single-photon emission computed tomography (CT) (Heidenreich et al., 2022), or CT coronary angiography to evaluate for coronary artery disease in patients with low to intermediate pretest probability (McDonagh et al., 2021).
i. Additional testing may be required based on the findings from initial tests.
2. Invasive testing
a. Right-heart catheterization may be useful in determining volume status, hemodynamic values, and intracardiac filling pressures to assess specific therapeutic questions (Yancy et al., 2013).
b. Continuous hemodynamic monitoring with pulmonary artery catheter to guide treatment in patients who have persistent symptoms, hypotension, worsening renal function, and vasoactive medications can be useful (Heidenreich et al., 2022).
c. Coronary angiogram is recommended if the etiology of heart failure is concerning for ischemic heart disease and the patient is a candidate for revascularization (Patel et al., 2013).
d. Endomyocardial biopsy (EMB) may be useful in the diagnosis and management of acute-onset, unexplained cardiomyopathy that does not respond to the usual standard of practice. Furthermore, EMB plays a role in suspected infiltrative disease that presents either as unexplained hypertrophic cardiomyopathy or as restrictive disease (Bennett et al., 2013).

B. Management (includes treatment, consultation, referral, and follow-up care)
1. Acute heart failure: Immediate intervention of oxygen and arrange hospital admission. Depending on the severity, emergency response may be required and the patient may therefore be admitted via the emergency department. The patient may require ventilator support, intravenous diuretics, ultrafiltration, intravenous inotropes, vasopressors, vasodilators, or mechanical support (National Institute for Health and Care Excellence [NICE], 2014).
2. Chronic heart failure
a. Treatment is often performed in a progressive, stepwise approach. A referral to cardiology should be initiated on diagnosis (**Figure 54-1**).
b. The focus of stage A heart failure management is on risk modification, including hypertension control, diabetes control, and lipid management to control atherosclerosis and unhealthy amount of body fat.
c. Stage B heart failure management includes stage A management plus intervention for structural heart disease. Special considerations should be given to patients with stage B heart failure, a history of MI and/or revascularization, and structural heart disease.
d. The development of symptoms classifies patients as stage C. Stage C heart failure management is multifaceted and aims at reducing morbidity and mortality through self-care and pharmacologic strategies. ICD implantation may be appropriate for this group of patients for either primary or secondary prevention. Additionally, cardiac resynchronization therapy (CRT) may be indicated for a subset of patients.
e. Stage D heart failure patients are considered refractory, and the disease progresses despite implementation of guideline directed therapy (strategies in stages A, B, and C). These patients may require intravenous inotropic support or other advanced therapies, such as mechanical circulatory support or heart transplantation.
f. Lifestyle modification
   i. Smoking cessation
   ii. Alcohol cessation or restriction
   iii. Illicit drug use cessation
   iv. Exercise: At least 150 min to 300 min of moderate-intensity aerobic physical activity or 75 min to 150 min of vigorous-intensity aerobic physical activity a week (Piercy & Troiano, 2018). Referral to cardiac rehabilitation. Lack of improvement after a training program portends a poor prognosis (Tang & Francis, 2010).
   v. Diet: Sodium restriction in patients who are symptomatic. Less than 3 g/daily sodium restriction improved NYHA class and lower extremity edema; 1.5 g/daily is difficult to achieve and can improve quality of life, but it remains unclear whether clinical outcomes are improved (Heidenreich et al., 2022).
   vi. Free water: Restrict daily intake to 1.5–2 L to treat hyponatremia secondary to vasopressin secretion (McDonagh et al., 2021).
g. Weight and blood pressure monitoring: Document weight and blood pressure daily, at the same time every day; monitor trends. Provide parameters that indicate when the patient should contact the provider regarding weight gain, evidence of volume overload, and blood pressure.
h. Healthcare maintenance
   i. Annual and age-appropriate vaccinations
   ii. Age-appropriate cancer screening

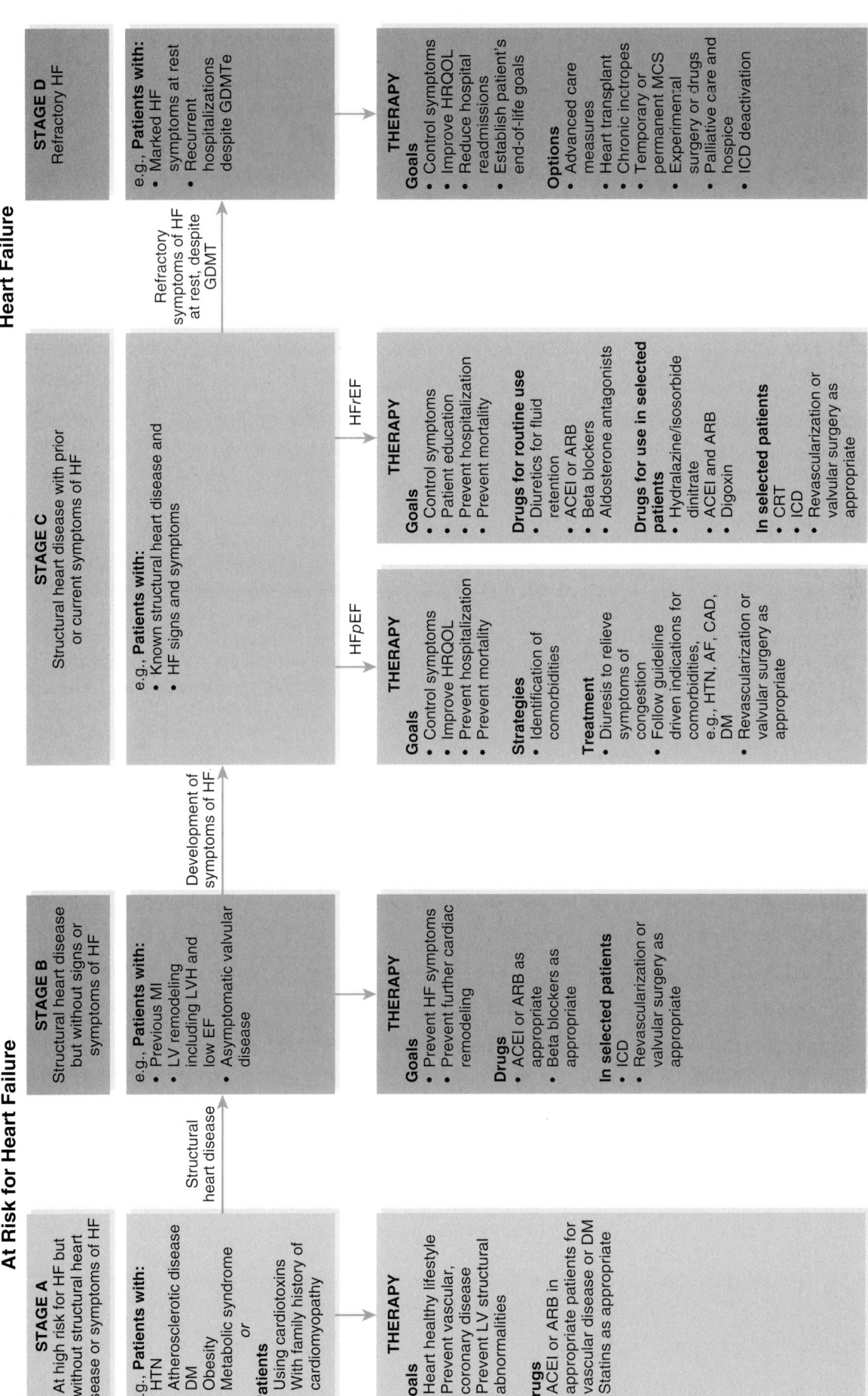

Figure 54-1 Heart failure risk

ACE-I, angiotensin-converting enzyme inhibitor; DMT, guideline-determined medical therapy.

Reproduced from Yancy, C. W., Jessup, M., Bozkurt, B., Butler, J., Casey, D. E., Jr., Drazner, M. H., et al. (2013). 2013 ACCF/AHA guideline for the management of heart failure: A report of the American College of Cardiology Foundation/American Heart Association task force on practice guidelines. *Journal of the American College of Cardiology, 62*(16), e147–e239.

iii. Dental care
iv. Medic alert information
i. Treatment of other illnesses/conditions that may be causative or contributory to heart failure
   i. Other cardiac diseases (coronary artery disease, valvular disease, tachyarrhythmias)
   ii. Diabetes (see Chapter 50, Diabetes Mellitus)
   iii. Hypertension (see Chapter 57, Hypertension)
   iv. Dyslipidemia (see Chapter 60, Lipid Disorders)
   v. Unhealthy amount of body fat (see Chapter 63, Obesity)
   vi. Sleep apnea
   vii. Thyroid disorders (see Chapter 65, Thyroid Disorders)
   viii. Infection
   ix. Anemia: Absorption of oral iron supplements is decreased; intravenous iron infusion may be necessary.
   x. Inflammation or inflammatory processes
j. Pharmacologic therapy
   i. Guideline directed medical therapy (GDMT) for HFrEF includes angiotensin-converting enzyme inhibitor (ACE-I) or angiotensin receptor blocker (ARB) or angiotensin receptor–neprilysin inhibitor (ARNI), beta-blocker, aldosterone antagonist, and sodium-glucose cotransporter 2 (SGLT2) inhibitor. When a patient is unable to tolerate ACE-Is, ARBs, and ARNIs or needs additional afterload reduction, hydralazine and nitrates are used.
   ii. HFpEF management predominantly consists of controlling comorbidities, which include hypertension (see Chapter 57, Hypertension, for the related guidelines) and myocardial ischemia. Symptom management with the judicious use of diuretics (Table 54-2). Aldosterone antagonists are indicated as a class IIb recommendation in patients with HFpEF with an EF of ≥45% and elevated BNP or with hospitalization within the past year. Must have an estimated glomerular filtration rate of >30, serum creatinine of <2.5 mg/dL, and potassium of <5.0 mEq/L (Yancy et al., 2017). There is emerging evidence supporting the use of ARB or ARNI and SGLT2i in the treatment of HFpEF. ARB and ARNI are a class IIb recommendation and SGLT2i is a class IIa recommendation.
   iii. Volume retention
   iv. Heart rhythm and rate control
   v. Hypertension (see Chapter 57, Hypertension, for the related guidelines)
   vi. Start at a low dose and titrate up as patient tolerates until the maximum safe dosage allowable. See **Box 54-1** for medication approaches for HFrEF.

Box 54-1 Medication Management for Systolic Heart Failure With Low Ejection Fraction (EF)

1. Angiotensin-converting enzyme inhibitor (ACE-I) (**Table 54-1**)
   a. Provides left ventricular reverse remodeling and survival benefit
   b. ACE-I intolerance includes dry, irritating cough that is often dose related. May also cause angioedema.
   c. Monitor electrolytes and renal function closely after initiation of treatment and dosage adjustments.
2. Angiotensin receptor blockers (ARBs) (Table 54-1)
   a. Provides survival benefit and reduces the incidence of heart failure. It can be an alternative to ACE-I or initiated with the goal of transitioning to an ARNI.
   b. Monitor electrolytes and renal function closely after initiation of treatment and dosage adjustments. May cause angioedema.
3. Angiotensin receptor–neprilysin inhibitor (ARNI) (Table 54-1)
   a. Enhances natriuresis, myocardial relaxation, and anti-remodeling; decreases hospitalization and mortality in NYHA class II–III heart failure.
   b. Must wash out ACE-I for 36 hours prior to initiation.
   c. Use caution in patients because it may lead to hypotension, renal insufficiency, and angioedema.
   d. Monitor fluid status after initiation. With increased natriuresis, may require diuretic adjustments.
4. Hydralazine in conjunction with a nitrate (Table 54-1)
   a. Can be used if the patient is unable to tolerate ACEs, ARBs, and ARNIs; it can also be used as adjunctive therapy in NYHA class III–IV heart failure in patients requiring additional afterload reduction.
5. Aldosterone antagonists (Tables 54-1 and 54-2)
   a. Recommended for patients with persistent symptoms with NYHA class II–IV heart failure and EF of ≤35%.
   b. Monitor electrolytes and renal function closely after initiation of treatment and dosage adjustments.
6. Beta-blockers (Table 54-1)
   a. Can provide improvement in EF as well as anti-ischemic properties and reduces mortality.
   b. Should not be initiated in low-output heart failure and volume overload.
7. Sodium-glucose cotransporter 2 (SGLT2) inhibitor (Table 54-1)
   a. Recommended for patients, without or without diabetes, with NYHA class II–IV heart failure and EF of ≤40%.

b. Reduces heart failure hospitalizations, decreases cardiovascular death, and slows the decline of estimated glomerular filtration rate.
c. Enhances natriuresis/diuresis.
d. May cause fungal urinary tract infection and euglycemic ketoacidosis, especially with poor oral intake.
8. Diuretic therapy (**Table 54-2**)
    a. Indicated for patients to control volume retention.
    b. Monitor electrolytes and renal function closely after initiation of treatment and dosage adjustments.
9. Ivabradine
    a. Class IIa recommendation for NYHA class II–III patients to reduce heart failure hospitalizations. Indicated when heart rate is >70 bpm at rest.
    b. Provides heart rate reduction by inhibition in the sinoatrial node.
    c. Can be given with beta-blockers, but the patient must be on maximal beta-blocker dose before the heart rate assessment.
10. Digoxin
    a. Remains controversial in the patient population with systolic heart failure.
    b. Digoxin can be used in patients as adjunctive therapy if they remain symptomatic despite guideline-directed management.
    c. Digoxin should be avoided in patients with sinus node or atrioventricular node conduction disease (Yancy et al., 2013).
    d. Monitor digoxin levels to ensure they remain in a low therapeutic range and do not become toxic. Higher serum concentrations have been associated with increased mortality (Heidenreich et al., 2022).
11. Amiodarone and dofetilide
    a. The only recommended antiarrhythmic medications to have neutral effects on mortality in patients with heart failure (Heidenreich et al., 2022).
    b. Prior to starting and after initiation of amiodarone, monitor thyroid-stimulating hormone and baseline pulmonary function test.
    c. Monitor for signs of amiodarone-induced pulmonary fibrosis, liver dysfunction, and thyroid toxicity.
12. Antithrombotics
    a. Use is based on the CHA2DS2-VACs score for arrhythmia and dilated cardiomyopathy because of an increased risk of left ventricular thrombus (Yancy et al., 2013).
    b. Choose an appropriate, approved, and individualized antithrombotic agent for the patient.
13. Harmful in NYHA class II–IV heart failure
    a. Thiazolidinediones.
    b. Calcium channel blockers (CCBs): The nondihydropyridine CCBs have negative inotropic properties and are considered harmful in patients with a low EF and therefore are not recommended. Amlodipine is the only CCB that may be considered in the management of hypertension or ischemic heart disease in patients with heart failure because it has neutral effects on morbidity and mortality (Yancy et al., 2013).
    c. Nonsteroidal anti-inflammatory drugs (NSAIDs) and cyclooxygenase 2 (COX-2) inhibitors.

k. ICD device therapy is recommended as primary prevention for patients with DCM or ischemic heart disease; patients with an EF of <35% and NYHA class II or higher heart failure or with an EF of <30% and NYHA class I heart failure; or those who are on guideline directed therapy and are at risk of sudden cardiac death (McMurray et al., 2012). CRT is recommended for patients with an EF of <35%, those in sinus rhythm with a QRS duration of 150 ms or greater, and those with left bundle branch (LBBB) morphology (Heidenreich et al., 2022).

For patients with NYHA classification II and III heart failure, a CardioMEMS device may be implanted to monitor changes in pulmonary artery pressures and heart rate. This information can inform decision making earlier in heart failure hemodynamic changes and reduce heart failure hospitalizations. However, the cost-effectiveness of the device needs to be considered.

l. Palliative and end-of-life care
    i. Palliative care can facilitate discussions regarding advanced care planning and is indicated in patients with NYHA Class III–IV heart failure (Teuteberg & Teuteberg, 2016).
    ii. Consider for patients who have advanced persistent symptoms at rest despite pharmacologic therapy
    iii. Recurrent heart failure hospitalizations
    iv. Recurrent ICD shocks
    v. Poor quality of life, including little or no ability to conduct activities of daily living
    vi. Need for continuous intravenous inotropic support
    vii. Further advanced heart failure therapy is not clinically indicated or is unwanted
    viii. Consider hospice referral.

Table 54-1 Guideline-Determined Medical Therapy (GDMT)

Drug	Initial Dose
Angiotensin-Converting Enzyme (ACE) Inhibitors	
Captopril	6.25 mg three times daily
Enalapril	2.5 mg twice daily
Fosinopril	5–10 mg daily
Lisinopril	2.5–5 mg daily
Perindopril	2 mg daily
Quinapril	5 mg twice daily
Ramipril	1.25–2.5 mg daily
Trandolapril	1 mg daily
Angiotensin Receptor Blockers (ARBs)	
Candesartan	4–8 mg daily
Losartan	25–50 mg daily
Valsartan	20–40 mg twice daily
Angiotensin Receptor–Neprilysin Inhibitor (ARNIs)	
Sacubitril/valsartan	24 mg/26 mg or 49 mg/51 mg twice daily (dose determined by maximal tolerated dose of ACE or ARB)
Hydralazine and Isosorbide Dinitrate	
Fixed-dose combination	37.5 mg hydralazine/20 mg isosorbide dinitrate three times daily
Hydralazine and isosorbide dinitrate	Hydralazine 25–50 mg, three or four times daily, and isosorbide dinitrate 20–30 mg, three or four times daily
Aldosterone Antagonists	
Spironolactone	12.5–25 mg daily
Eplerenone	25 mg daily
Beta-Blockers	
Bisoprolol	1.25 mg daily
Carvedilol	3.125 mg twice daily
Carvedilol CR	10 mg daily
Metoprolol succinate extended release	12.5–25 mg daily
Sodium-Glucose Cotransporter 2 (SGLT2) Inhibitor	
Dapagliflozin	10 mg daily
Empagliflozin	10 mg daily

Data from Maddox T. M., Januzzi J. L., Allen L. A., Breathett K., Butler J., Davis L. L., Fonarow G. C., Ibrahim N. E., Lindenfeld J., Masoudi F. A., Motiwala S. R., Oliveros E., Patterson, H. J., Walsh M. N., Wasserman A., Yancy C. W., & Youmans Q. R. (2021). 2021 Update to the 2017 ACC Expert Consensus Decision Pathway for Optimization of Heart Failure Treatment: Answers to 10 Pivotal Issues About Heart Failure With Reduced Ejection Fraction. *Journal of the American College of Cardiology, 77*(6), 772–810. https://doi.org/10.1016/j.jacc.2020.11.022; McDonagh, T. A., Metra, M., Adamo, M., Gardner, R. S., Baumbach, A., Böhm, M., Burri, H., Butler, J., Čelutkienė, J., Chioncel, O., Cleland, J. G. F., Coats, A. J. S., Crespo-Leiro, M. G., Farmakis, D., Gilard, M., Heymans, S., Hoes, A. W., Jaarsma, T., Jankowska, E. A., ... ESC Scientific Document Group. (2021). 2021 ESC Guidelines for the diagnosis and treatment of acute and chronic heart failure. *European Heart Journal, 42*(36), 3599–3726. https://doi.org/10.1093/eurheartj/ehab368; Heidenreich, P. A., Bozkurt, B., Aguilar, D., Allen, L. A., Byun, J. J., Colvin, M. M., Deswal, A., Drazner, M. H., Dunlay, S. M., Evers, L. R., Fang, J. C., Fedson, S. E., Fonarow, G. C., Hayek, S. S., Hernandez, A. F., Khazanie, P., Kittleson, M. M., Lee, C. S., Link, M. S., ... Yancy, C. W. (2022). 2022 AHA/ACC/HFSA Guideline for the Management of Heart Failure: A Report of the American College of Cardiology/American Heart Association Joint Committee on Clinical Practice Guidelines. *Circulation, 145*(18), e895–e1032. https://doi.org/10.1161/CIR.0000000000001063; Yancy C. W., Jessup M., Bozkurt B., Butler J., Casey D. E., Colvin M. M., Drazner M. H., Filippatos G. S., Fonarow G. C., Givertz M. M., Hollenberg Steven M., Lindenfeld JoAnn, Masoudi Frederick A., McBride Patrick E., Peterson Pamela N., Stevenson Lynne Warner, & Westlake Cheryl. (2017). 2017 ACC/AHA/HFSA Focused Update of the 2013 ACCF/AHA Guideline for the Management of Heart Failure. *Journal of the American College of Cardiology, 70*(6), 776–803. https://doi.org/10.1016/j.jacc.2017.04.025

Table 54-2 Loop Diuretics

Drug	Initial Dose
Loop Diuretics	
Bumetanide	0.5–1 mg once or twice daily
Furosemide	20–40 mg once or twice daily
Torsemide	10–20 mg daily
Thiazide Diuretics	
Chlorothiazide	250–500 mg once or twice daily
Chlorthalidone	12.5–25 mg daily
Hydrochlorothiazide	25 mg once or twice daily
Indapamide	2.5 mg daily
Metolazone	2.5 mg daily
Aldosterone Antagonists (Potassium-Sparing Diuretics)	
Amiloride	5 mg daily
Spironolactone	12.5–25 mg daily
Triamterene	50–75 mg twice daily
Sequential Nephron Blockade (Administration of Thiazide Diuretic 30–60 Minutes Prior to Loop Diuretic)	
Metolazone	2.5–10 mg daily + loop diuretic
Hydrochlorothiazide	25–100 mg once or twice daily + loop diuretic
Chlorothiazide	500–1,000 mg daily + loop diuretic

Data from Heidenreich, P. A., Bozkurt, B., Aguilar, D., Allen, L. A., Byun, J. J., Colvin, M. M., Deswal, A., Drazner, M. H., Dunlay, S. M., Evers, L. R., Fang, J. C., Fedson, S. E., Fonarow, G. C., Hayek, S. S., Hernandez, A. F., Khazanie, P., Kittleson, M. M., Lee, C. S., Link, M. S., ... Yancy, C. W. (2022). 2022 AHA/ACC/HFSA Guideline for the Management of Heart Failure: A Report of the American College of Cardiology/American Heart Association Joint Committee on Clinical Practice Guidelines. *Circulation, 145*(18), e895–e1032. https://doi.org/10.1161/CIR.0000000000001063 and Yancy C. W., Jessup M., Bozkurt B., Butler J., Casey D. E., Colvin M. M., Drazner M. H., Filippatos G. S., Fonarow G. C., Givertz M. M., Hollenberg Steven M., Lindenfeld JoAnn, Masoudi Frederick A., McBride Patrick E., Peterson Pamela N., Stevenson Lynne Warner, & Westlake Cheryl. (2017). 2017 ACC/AHA/HFSA Focused Update of the 2013 ACCF/AHA Guideline for the Management of Heart Failure. *Journal of the American College of Cardiology, 70*(6), 776–803. https://doi.org/10.1016/j.jacc.2017.04.025

---

ix. Advanced directives and durable power of attorney should be in place.

m. Appropriate follow-up for interventions implemented or anticipated implementation.

n. Collaborate with prescribing providers regarding the ongoing treatment plan as well as elimination of the medications or treatments that cause or exacerbate heart failure.

C. *Patient education and support*
1. The patient must be able to adhere to the treatment plan and have adequate resources to comply effectively with the regimen. Instituting the plan may take time. The patient and patient's support system must have an understanding of the treatment regimen, disease progression, and potential complications, which will require ongoing education. Anticipate barriers to the treatment plan because this may prevent future complications.
2. It is also important to provide both verbal and written information to the patient and the patient's support system. This information should include but is not limited to heart failure education, symptoms, prognosis, complications, and disease management. The patient should be referred to social services in order to ensure that a full spectrum of resources is available. Social services are useful in providing emotional support for both the patient and the patient support system to improve coping skills and provide any additional financial resources.

VI. **Self-management resources and tools**

A. *Patient education*
1. AHA (https://www.heart.org/en/health-topics/heart-failure). The AHA has print and online education materials and online videos. Websites are available in Spanish, Chinese, Vietnamese, and English.
2. Centers for Disease Control and Prevention (https://www.cdc.gov/heartdisease/materials_for_patients.htm)
3. Medline Plus from the National Library of Medicine and National Institutes of Health (https://medlineplus.gov/heartfailure.html). Provides an interactive tutorial in English and Spanish and extensive resources for aspects of the disease.
4. Heart Failure Matters (https://www.heartfailurematters.org). This is an interactive, multilingual educational website containing animations, videos, and tools for patients with heart failure. It is available in English, French, German, and Spanish. It has a family and caregiver section and links to a variety of other related websites.
5. HeartFailure.org (https://www.heartfailure.org). Provides online education as well as additional links to other resources.
6. Million Hearts (https://millionhearts.hhs.gov/learn-prevent/recipes.html). This is a website from the U.S. Department of Health and Human Services that provides heart-healthy recipes.
7. Heart Failure Society of America (https://hfsa.org/patient). Provides information about heart failure risk factors, symptoms, and stages, as well as tools and additional resources for patients and caregivers.

B. *Community support groups*
1. Local healthcare institutions may be a resource for support groups in the area.

2. The AHA (https://www.heart.org/) offers a variety of community events and support groups for individuals with heart disease.
3. Mended Hearts (https://mendedhearts.org) is an organization for individuals with heart disease. Patients must pay to join. Mended Hearts offers group meetings, hospital visiting programs, an annual convention, educational resources, and various events. Patients can join a local chapter.

References

Bennett, M. K., Gilotra, N. A., Harrington, C., Rao, S., Dunn, J. M., Freitag, T. B., Halushka, M. K., & Russell, S. D. (2013). Evaluation of the role of endomyocardial biopsy in 851 patients with unexplained heart failure from 2000–2009. *Circulation. Heart Failure*, 6(4), 676–684.

Criteria Committee of the American Heart Association. (1994). *Nomenclature and criteria for diagnosis of diseases of the heart and great vessels* (9th ed.). Little Brown.

Heidenreich, P. A., Bozkurt, B., Aguilar, D., Allen, L. A., Byun, J. J., Colvin, M. M., Deswal, A., Drazner, M. H., Dunlay, S. M., Evers, L. R., Fang, J. C., Fedson, S. E., Fonarow, G. C., Hayek, S. S., Hernandez, A. F., Khazanie, P., Kittleson, M. M., Lee, C. S., Link, M. S., ... Yancy, C. W. (2022). 2022 AHA/ACC/HFSA guideline for the management of heart failure: a report of the American College of Cardiology/American Heart Association Joint Committee on Clinical Practice Guidelines. *Circulation*, 145(18), e895–e1032. doi:10.1161/CIR.0000000000001063

Maddox, T. M., Januzzi, J. L., Allen, L. A., Breathett, K., Butler, J., Davis, L. L., Fonarow, G. C., Ibrahim, N. E., Lindenfeld, J., Masoudi, F. A., Motiwala, S. R., Oliveros, E., Patterson, H. J., Walsh, M. N., Wasserman, A., Yancy, C. W., & Youmans, Q. R. (2021). 2021 update to the 2017 ACC Expert Consensus Decision Pathway for Optimization of Heart Failure Treatment: Answers to 10 pivotal issues about heart failure with reduced ejection fraction. *Journal of the American College of Cardiology*, 77(6), 772–810. doi:10.1016/j.jacc.2020.11.022

McDonagh, T. A., Metra, M., Adamo, M., Gardner, R. S., Baumbach, A., Böhm, M., Burri, H., Butler, J., Čelutkienė, J., Chioncel, O., Cleland, J. G. F., Coats, A. J. S., Crespo-Leiro, M. G., Farmakis, D., Gilard, M., Heymans, S., Hoes, A. W., Jaarsma, T., Jankowska, E. A., ... ESC Scientific Document Group. (2021). 2021 ESC guidelines for the diagnosis and treatment of acute and chronic heart failure. *European Heart Journal*, 42(36), 3599–3726. doi:10.1093/eurheartj/ehab368

McMurray, J. J., Adamopoulos, S., Anker, S. D., Auricchio, A., Bohm, M., Dickstein, K., Falk, V., Filippatos, G., Fonseca, C., Gomez-Sanchez, M. A., Jaarsma, T., Køber, L., Lip, G. Y. H., Maggioni, A. P., Parkhomenko, A., Pieske, B. M., Popescu, B. A., Rønnevik, P. K., Rutten, F. H. ... ESC Committee for Practice Guidelines. (2012). ESC guidelines for the diagnosis and treatment of acute and chronic heart failure 2012: The task force for the diagnosis and treatment of acute and chronic heart failure 2012 of the European Society of Cardiology. Developed in collaboration with the Heart Failure Association (HFA) of the ESC. *European Heart Journal*, 33(14), 1787–1847.

National Institute for Health and Care Excellence. (2014). *Acute heart failure: diagnosis and management*. http://www.nice.org.uk/guidance/cg187

Patel, M. R., White, R. D., Abbara, S., Bluemke, D. A., Herfkens, R. J., Picard, M., Shaw, L. J., Silver, M., Stillman, A. E., Udelson, J., American College of Radiology Appropriateness Criteria Committee, & American College of Cardiology Foundation Appropriate Use Criteria Task Force. (2013). 2013 ACCF/ACR/ASE/ASNC/SCCT/SCMR appropriate utilization of cardiovascular imaging in heart failure: A joint report of the American College of Radiology Appropriateness Criteria Committee and the American College of Cardiology Foundation Appropriate Use Criteria Task Force. *Journal of the American College of Cardiology*, 61(21), 2207–2231.

Piercy, K. L., & Troiano, R. P. (2018). Physical activity guidelines for Americans from the US Department of Health and Human Services. *Circulation: Cardiovascular Quality and Outcomes*, 11(11), e005263. doi:10.1161/CIRCOUTCOMES.118.005263

Tang, W. H. W., & Francis, G. S. (2010). The year in heart failure. *Journal of the American College of Cardiology*, 55(7), 688.

Teuteberg, J., J., & Teuteberg, W., G. (2016). *Palliative care for patients with heart failure*. American College of Cardiology. https://www.acc.org/Latest-in-Cardiology/Articles/2016/02/11/08/02/Palliative-Care-for-Patients-With-Heart-Failure

Virani, S. S., Alonso, A., Aparicio, H. J., Benjamin, E. J., Bittencourt, M. S., Callaway, C. W., Carson, A. P., Chamberlain, A. M., Cheng, S., Delling, F. N., Elkind, M. S. V., Evenson, K. R., Ferguson, J. F., Gupta, D. K., Khan, S. S., Kissela, B. M., Knutson, K. L., Lee, C. D., Lewis, T. T., ... Tsao, C. W. (2021). Heart disease and stroke statistics—2021 update. *Circulation*, 143(8), e254–e743. doi:10.1161/CIR.0000000000000950

Yancy, C. W., Jessup, M., Bozkurt, B., Butler, J., Casey, D. E., Colvin, M. M., Drazner, M. H., Filippatos, G. S., Fonarow, G. C., Givertz, M. M., Hollenberg, S. M., Lindenfeld, J., Masoudi, F. A., McBride, P. E., Peterson, P. N., Stevenson, L. W., & Westlake, C. (2017). 2017 ACC/AHA/HFSA focused update of the 2013 ACCF/AHA guideline for the management of heart failure. *Journal of the American College of Cardiology*, 70(6), 776–803. doi:10.1016/j.jacc.2017.04.025

Yancy, C. W., Jessup, M., Bozkurt, B., Butler, J., Casey, D. E., Jr., Drazner, M. H., Fonarow, G. C., Geraci, S. A., Horwich, T., Januzzi, J. L., Johnson, M. R., Kasper, E. K., Levy, W. C., Masoudi, F. A., McBride, P. E., McMurray, J. J., Mitchell, J. E., Peterson, P. N., Riegel, B., ... American Heart Association Task Force on Practice Guidelines. (2013). 2013 ACCF/AHA guideline for the management of heart failure: A report of the American College of Cardiology Foundation/American Heart Association task force on practice guidelines. *Journal of the American College of Cardiology*, 62(16), e147–e239. doi:10.1016/j.jacc.2013.05.019

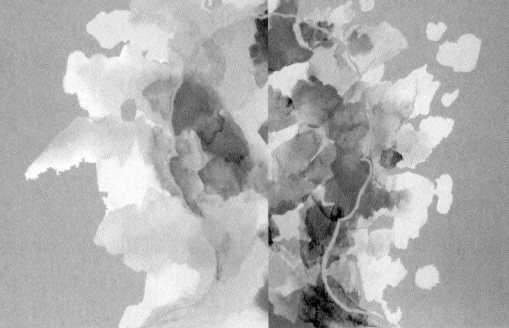

CHAPTER 55

Herpes Simplex Virus

Natalie L. Wilson and Geraldine Collins-Bride

I. Introduction and general background

Herpes simplex viruses (HSVs) cause the sexually transmitted infections (STIs) more commonly referred to as *herpes*. The infections from HSV are categorized into two serotypes: herpes simplex virus 1 (HSV-1) and herpes simplex virus 2 (HSV-2). HSV-1 primarily affects oral and ocular cells and is associated with mild to severe symptoms and illnesses. HSV-2 primarily causes genital lesions. Although they both can occur in both mucosal areas, HSV-1 predominantly prefers the trigeminal ganglion, and HSV-2 prefers the sacral ganglion. However, because of the transmission route of oral-to-genital contact, HSV-1 and HSV-2 can be found interchangeably on the mucosa of the oral and genital sites. HSV-1 anogenital herpetic infections have become more prominent in younger women and men who have sex with men (MSM). Genital herpes infections are often asymptomatic, and transmission occurs as a result of persons being unaware of their infection or being unaware of viral shedding while asymptomatic. Millions of people have been exposed to HSV globally. Genital herpes is a chronic viral infection transmitted from human to human (direct skin-to-skin contact causing lesions).

HSVs belong to the *Herpesviridae* family of viruses, which have central double-stranded DNA enclosed in an icosapentahedral capsid, surrounded by a group of tegument proteins encapsulated in a bilayer envelope of membrane proteins and glycoproteins. HSV-1 and HSV-2 are a part of the alpha-herpes virus subfamily; these viruses are known to establish latency in neurons. During infection, the virus binds to the host cell membrane, forming a fusion pore through which the viral nucleocapsid and tegument proteins are delivered into the host cell (Connolly et al., 2021).

The virus causes a recurring vesicular eruption of the skin or mucous membrane surfaces that have had prior contact exposure. HSV nucleocapsid contains viral DNA and proteins, which help the viral DNA and the proteins into the human cell and then use the proteins to incorporate into the human DNA. The viral DNA then attaches to the human DNA and uses the normal transcription process to replicate many herpes virions until the cells rupture and release the virions. The other pathway for active infection is that the HSV is dormant while incorporated with human DNA, and the human cell reproduces with the virus, without replication and cellular lysis.

Similar to other herpes viruses, after initial infection, a latent state is established that can be followed by reactivation of the virus and recurrent local disease. After the replication period in the epithelium, the virus will infect the epithelium interface with neurons termini of the peripheral nervous system. The viral nucleocapsids are transported to the neuronal cell bodies. The viral genome and HSV-1 chromosome enter the neuronal nuclei and establish a latent reservoir for the lifetime of the host (Singh & Tscharke, 2020). The course of disease, however, varies among individuals from asymptomatic to recurrent clinical presentations. Most people are asymptomatic, which contributes to silent transmission even when there are no signs of infection. Genital herpes increases the risk of HIV transmission and acquisition. Management of genital HSV should address the chronic nature of the disease rather than focusing solely on the treatment of acute episodes of genital lesions (Centers for Disease Control and Prevention [CDC], 2021). There are no current vaccines for HSV-1 and HSV-2 approved by the U.S. Food and Drug Administration (FDA; Rice, 2021). Therefore, HSV-1 and HSV-2 have infected a large fraction of the human population, with transgenerational persistence of the virus. Each year in the United States, there are approximately 776,000 HSV primary infections (Cole, 2020).

A. *Types of HSV*
  1. HSV-1
     HSV-1 is responsible for most of the infections in the face and upper body. Oral and perioral lesions, often referred to by the public as "cold sores" or "fever blisters," are common presentations. HSV-1 prefers

the trigeminal ganglion. HSV-1 can also infect mucous membranes or abraded skin at any site, including the ocular, genital, and labial areas. Serious manifestations of HSV disease, such as encephalitis and meningitis, are rare in the immunocompetent patient. Primary HSV-1 infection is widespread and commonly transmitted in childhood, with 60% of individuals infected prior to the age of 50. Globally, up to 212 million people are living with genital HSV-1 infection (Looker et al., 2015).

2. HSV-2

HSV-2 is responsible for most genital skin infections. HSV-2 prefers the sacral ganglion. Most cases of recurrent genital herpes are caused by HSV-2, although seroprevalence trends show that the percentage of genital herpes caused by HSV-1 is increasing (Tuddenham et al., 2022; Workowski et al., 2021). A total of 20%–25% of the adult population has serologic evidence of HSV-2 infection (Fleming et al., 1997). An estimated 492 million people aged 15–49 years worldwide (95% uncertainty interval [UI], 430.4–610.6 million) are living with HSV-2 infection, with the highest infection rates being among women (James et al., 2020). Subclinical viral shedding is common in the first few years after the primary HSV infection and then becomes less frequent—from 25% of days in the first year after infection to 4% of days in later years. The majority of genital infections are acquired during contact with persons unaware that they have the infection and who are asymptomatic when transmission occurs. In addition, individuals may not attribute symptoms such as vulvar rashes, irritation, or fissures to genital herpes ulcers. Thus, subclinical viral shedding and unrecognized mild symptoms are key factors in both horizontal (partner-to-partner) and vertical (parent-to-newborn) transmission (Samies et al., 2021; Stephenson-Famy & Gardella, 2014).

HSV-2 infection is an important risk factor for HIV (Malekinejad et al., 2021) acquisition and transmission. Persons with dual HIV and HSV infections are more likely to shed both viruses from open herpes ulcers caused by HSV-2, explaining the increased risk of HIV transmission from individuals with HSV-2 infections (Mujugira et al., 2011). Conversely, the likelihood of horizontal acquisition of HIV infection significantly increases from twofold to three- or fourfold in persons with HSV infection as a result of open herpes lesions coming into contact with the bodily fluids of an HIV-infected partner (Freeman et al., 2006).

3. Neonatal HSV

In the United States, there is an incidence rate of 5–33 per 100,000 live births (i.e., 1,500 cases) annually (Pinninti & Kimberlin, 2018). Although HSV-2 had previously caused the majority of neonatal herpes cases in the United States, the shift in sexual preferences to oral sex has increased the genital transmission of HSV-1 to the neonate, making it the predominate strain in this group (Looker et al., 2015; Pinninti & Kimberlin, 2018). Neonatal infection with HSV is associated with high neonatal morbidity, with poor neurologic outcomes for disseminated disease, and mortality. The risk for transmission to the neonate exposed to HSV (HSV-1 or HSV-2) in the birth canal is 85%, the risk for postnatal infection from direct cutaneous contact is 10%, and the risk via utero exposure is 5%. Transmission of HSV is associated with the type of HSV (HSV-1 or HSV-2), type of infection (primary, nonprimary, recurrent), the serologic status of the mother, the delivery route, fetal membranes, and the use of scalp electrodes during delivery. The highest risk of transmission is when there are inadequate protective immunoglobulins (e.g., immunoglobulin G [IgG]) to HSV to protect the infant from HSV crossing the placenta. A previous infection of either HSV-1 or HSV-2 (i.e., nonprimary) will pose a lesser risk to an infant due to cross-protection of IgG. Reactivation of HSV-2 or HSV-1 during pregnancy is the most common form of HSV infection in pregnancy. This is difficult to detect because of asymptomatic shedding of the virus. However, the presence of a lesion with recurrent HSV is associated with a 10- to 30-fold increase in the risk of transmission to a neonate (Stephenson-Famy & Gardella, 2014).

According to the 2021 CDC treatment guidelines for STIs (Workowski et al., 2021), pregnant people without known genital herpes should be counseled to abstain from vaginal intercourse during the third trimester with partners known or suspected of having genital herpes. In addition, pregnant people without known orolabial herpes should be advised to abstain from receptive oral sex during the third trimester with partners known or suspected to have orolabial herpes. In pregnant people with active genital lesions at the time of delivery, a cesarean delivery is recommended. Suppressive acyclovir treatment for recurrent genital herpes is recommended starting at 36 weeks' gestation. Most genital herpes infections during pregnancy are recurrent and therefore present a lower risk of transmission to the neonate, 50%–60% with primary infections versus <3% for recurrent infections (Pinninti & Kimberlin, 2018). Antiviral prophylaxis is effective in reducing the frequency of cesarean delivery among women who have recurrent genital herpes, lowering the risk of a recurrence at delivery (Stephenson-Famy & Gardella, 2014; Workowski et al., 2021). Routine HSV-2 screening is not recommended in pregnant people. Treatment may not protect against transmission to neonates in all cases. There is no mandatory reporting of neonatal HSV.

Management of genital herpes should focus on the chronic infection versus treatment of acute episodic outbreaks of genital lesions. Counsel patients who use light-based treatment with selective photothermolysis for keloids or hair removal that, although rare, outbreaks of HSV can be stimulated in the treatment area. Have antivirals available for self-treatment (Zaouak et al., 2019).

B. *Clinical presentations: primary, nonprimary first-episode, and recurrent HSV*
   1. Primary infection
      This is the first clinical episode of genital herpes in an individual *without antibodies* to HSV-1 or HSV-2. Primary infection can be severe, with painful genital ulcers and systemic symptoms such as fever, myalgias, malaise, and tender inguinal lymphadenopathy. Lesions classically appear as vesicles or pustules that open in 12–24 hours to form shallow ulcers. Symptoms usually occur within a few weeks after infection and resolve within 2 weeks (**Figure 55-1**). Complications of HSV infection are more likely in primary infection and can include aseptic meningitis, sacral autonomic nervous system dysfunction, and disseminated lesions.
   2. Nonprimary first-episode infection
      This is the first clinical episode of herpes in an individual *with serologic evidence of prior infection* with either HSV-1 or HSV-2. The clinical presentation is usually less severe compared to primary infection, with fewer local lesions, mild to no systemic symptoms, and a shorter duration of symptoms (Corey et al., 1983; Kimberlin & Rouse, 2004).
   3. Recurrent infection
      After the primary episode, the median numbers of symptomatic recurrences are 1.3 for HSV-1 and 4.0 for HSV-2. Recurrent clinical episodes of herpes are typically less severe than primary and nonprimary first episodes and resolve within 5–10 days. Systemic symptoms are uncommon (Tuddenham et al., 2022). Triggers that may cause recurrent disease include acute illness, stress, sunlight, fatigue, menstrual periods, and unknown factors. Fifty percent of patients with recurrent episodes experience prodromal symptoms, such as sensitivity to touch (hyperesthesia), local tingling or itching, and peripheral nerve pain (Kimberlin & Rouse, 2004). A smaller number of patients develop frequent recurrences of HSV outbreaks that can cause both physical and emotional distress. For individuals who experience six or more outbreaks yearly, suppressive antiviral therapy should be offered (Workowski et al., 2021). Although the medical complications from recurrent infection are uncommon, the psychosocial and psychosexual impacts can cause significant distress for patients.
   4. Asymptomatic infection
      In asymptomatic infections, an individual has serum antibodies, yet there is no history of clinical outbreaks. Unrecognized mild symptoms of HSV-2 are common, however, and may account for nearly two-thirds of individuals with what appears to be asymptomatic infection (Workowski et al., 2021).

II. Database
A. *Subjective*
   1. Past medical history and situational factors (may include but are not limited to)
      a. History of similar ulcer eruption (i.e., location of lesion and duration of the outbreaks). Note results of culture if done previously.
      b. History of contact exposure to individual with known HSV infection

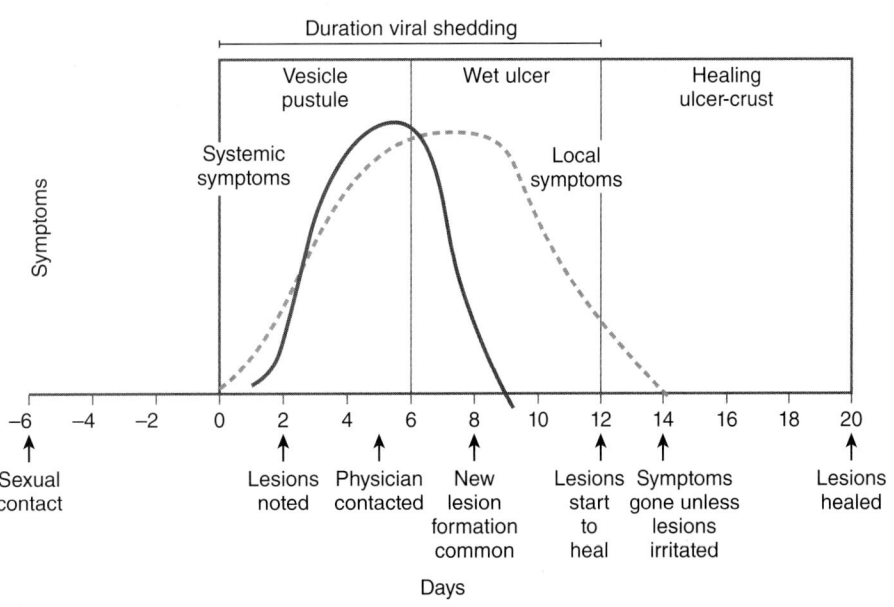

Figure 55-1 Genital HSV Counseling Topics.

Centers for Disease Control and Prevention. (2021). 2021 Sexually Transmitted Diseases: Treatment guidelines. Retrieved from https://www.cdc.gov/std/treatment-guidelines/herpes.htm

c. History of stimulus known to trigger eruption: sunlight, menses, fever, other illnesses, stress, and increased sexual activity
d. History of rash, eczema, and erythema multiforme
e. History of immunocompromise: HIV/AIDS, leukemia, lymphoma, other malignancies, autoimmune diseases, and posttransplant patients
f. History of sexual practices, including oral–genital contact: Ask, "Which body parts do you use for sex (penis/vagina, anus, mouth)?"
g. History of STIs
h. Current pregnancy
2. Occupational history
a. Exposure history
b. Type of profession (e.g., healthcare worker and dentist [herpetic whitlow])
c. Contacts and personal protection
3. Symptomatology
a. Fever, headache, malaise, myalgias, and tender lymph nodes
b. Burning pain, tingling, hyperesthesia, or itching of involved skin and mucous membranes define the prodromal symptoms of recurrent infection, which precede the outbreak of lesions by a few hours to up to 2 days.
c. Depending on the site of infection
i. Genital lesions: dysuria, urinary retention, sacral or genital paresthesias, rectal tenesmus, and constipation
ii. Oral lesions: facial paresthesias, mouth pain (gingivostomatitis), difficulty eating, and visual disturbances or pain
d. No symptoms
B. Objective
1. Vital signs: fever infrequent, most common in primary infection or with secondary complications, such as aseptic meningitis
2. Skin: tender, single, or clustered vesicles, pustules, or ulcers on a clean erythematous base. Ulcers may appear crusted over in the period before resolution. Lesions most frequently occur in or around the mouth, on the vulva, on the penile glans or shaft, or in the perianal area. Ulcers may occur on distal fingers (herpetic whitlow), especially in healthcare workers.
3. Eye: unilateral conjunctivitis, blepharitis with vesicles on the lid margin, keratitis with dendritic lesions or with punctuate opacities on ophthalmic examination
4. Mouth: small ulcers located on the soft palate, buccal mucosa, tongue, or floor of the mouth
5. Lymph: may have tender, nonfluctuant regional lymphadenopathy, especially in primary outbreaks
6. Genitourinary: May see urethral, vaginal, or rectal discharge, depending on severity of involvement. Internal lesions may be challenging to observe, and HSV DNA may be negative. If rectal involvement, on anoscopy, may see either ulcerations (not distinct lesions) and/or swollen, inflamed mucosa. HSV lesions may be found inside the foreskin, labia, vagina, or rectum.

III. Assessment
A. *Determine the diagnosis*
1. Primary
2. Nonprimary first episode
3. Recurrent
4. Asymptomatic
5. Other conditions that may explain the patient's presentation:
a. Infectious genital ulcer diseases: syphilis, chancroid, lymphogranuloma venereum, granuloma inguinale, or monkeypox
b. Noninfectious genital ulcers: Behçet syndrome, Crohn's disease, or fixed drug eruption
c. Mucopurulent cervical discharge: chlamydia, gonorrhea, or mycoplasmas
d. Vulvar rashes: allergic contact dermatitis (especially poison oak or poison ivy vulvitis), impetigo, psoriasis
e. Orolabial ulcers: aphthous stomatitis
f. Herpes zoster
g. Other etiologies of proctitis
B. *Severity*
Assess the severity of the infection, including diagnosis of complications:
1. Urine retention resulting from bladder neck spasm
2. Proctitis, particularly in MSM
3. Constipation
4. Difficulty eating solid foods
5. Secondary bacterial infections caused by *Streptococci* or *Staphylococci*
6. Erythema multiforme
7. Herpes keratitis
8. Disseminated herpes
9. Aseptic meningitis
10. Neonatal herpes
11. Emotional stress and psychological morbidity, especially seen with recurrent genital HSV

IV. Goals of clinical management
A. *Choose a cost-effective approach for diagnosing HSV infection.*
B. *Select a treatment plan that addresses the patient's symptom severity, frequency of recurrence, transmission risk to uninfected partner, and cost.*
C. *Select an approach that maximizes patient adherence, with consideration to frequency of dosing and pill burden.*
D. *Provide an education plan that empowers patients to cope with a chronic, recurrent STI through self-management resources.*

V. Plan
A. *Screening*
1. The American Academy of Family Physicians (AAFP, 2017) and the U.S. Preventive Services Task

Force (USPSTF) (Bibbins-Domingo et al., 2016) recommend against routine serologic screening for the general population and for pregnant people. Counseling about the risks and benefits of serologic screening should be discussed and offered to select groups of patients, including patients who may have HSV-infected sex partners and HIV-positive patients (AAFP, 2017; Bibbins-Domingo et al., 2016). HSV serologic testing should be considered for persons presenting for evaluation of STIs, especially for those persons with multiple sex partners, persons with HIV infection, and MSM at increased risk for HIV acquisition (AAFP, 2017; Feltner et al., 2016).

B. Diagnostic tests
1. HSV viral culture by nucleic acid amplification testing (NAAT) or culture if active lesions are present
   The gold standard for diagnosis of HSV if an active lesion is present is a NAAT or culture. Viral culture is highly specific (>99%), but sensitivity depends on the stage of the lesion. Sensitivity is highest (90%) when lesion vesicles are scraped and the base of an ulcer can be sampled. As lesions start to heal, the culture sensitivity decreases rapidly (sensitivity at ulcer stage = 70% and at crust stage = 30%) (Corey et al., 1983). Determination of the type of HSV infection predicts recurrence risk (50% with HSV-2, 10% with HSV-1) but otherwise is not necessary or helpful. This mostly gives assurance and confirmation to the patient.
2. HSV polymerase chain reaction (PCR)
   PCR is highly sensitive but has a significantly increased cost. PCR is now approved by the FDA for testing of anogenital specimens, but cost prohibits this method of testing in the majority of clinical settings. Use ulcer scrapings or aspiration of vesicle fluid. PCR should be used to detect HSV in spinal fluid in cases where central nervous system infection is suspected. PCR amplicons can be typed to determine the cause of the infection—HSV-1, HSV-2, or both. Viral shedding is intermittent; therefore, culturing older lesions may fail to detect HSV by NAAT, or culture may not indicate the absence of HSV.
3. Cytology (Pap or Tzanck)
   Cytology is no longer recommended because of its low sensitivity and specificity.
4. Type-specific herpes virus serology
   Antibodies to HSV-1 and HSV-2 can be detected anywhere from 3 weeks to 3 months after infection and remain indefinitely. HSV immunoglobulin M (IgM) testing for HSV-1 or HSV-2 is not useful because of positivity during recurrent genital or oral herpes episodes. Testing may be clinically useful in the following cases:
   a. To rule out an HSV diagnosis if the serology result is negative at least 6 weeks after the primary HSV episode
   b. To determine primary herpes infection if the patient is seronegative during the primary initial symptoms with conversion to seropositive after 6 weeks from the onset of the outbreak
   c. In asymptomatic patients who have a sex partner with genital herpes
   d. For patients at increased risk for STIs (i.e., multiple sex partners, HIV infection, transgender women, and MSM at increased risk for HIV acquisition) who request comprehensive STI screening (Workowski et al., 2021)
5. Diagnostic tests as necessary to rule out etiologies other than HSV infection, including syphilis serology to rule out primary or secondary syphilis and monkeypox culture to rule out monkeypox disease.
6. All persons with genital herpes should be screened for HIV.

C. Management
1. Preventive
   a. Use barrier protection during mucosal contact with persons with a known or suspected active herpes lesion, such as condoms and dental dams.
   b. Avoid or decrease exposure to known recurrence triggers (i.e., illness, stress, sunlight/light therapy, multiple sex partners, and fatigue).
   c. Friction from sexual intercourse can also trigger a recurrence. Use water-based lubricants and moisturizers that can help prevent irritation and micro-tearing of the skin.
   d. Antiviral medications used to treat or suppress recurrent outbreaks or prophylactic therapy of an infected person to prevent horizontal transmission to an uninfected partner
2. Symptomatic
   a. Initial genital herpes
      Newly acquired genital herpes can be distressing for the patient. It is important to assure the patient that there are treatment options and to counsel the patient to avoid transmission to partners. The presentation can be prolonged, with severe, painful, and pruritic shallow ulcerations with an erythematous discrete border, possibly with neurologic involvement. It is also common for persons who had a mild initial episode to have severe recurrent infections. Therefore, it is critical that the person receives antiviral medications during the first episode of genital herpes.
   b. Recurrent HSV-2
      Patients with symptomatic recurrence of genital lesions should receive therapy to reduce the frequency of recurrences or episodically to shorten the duration of genital lesions. Some persons with infrequent recurrent outbreaks may benefit from antiviral therapy, and options for treatment should be discussed, weighing the risks and benefits of suppressive versus episodic treatment, using person-centered care. Treatment does decrease the risk of transmitting HSV-2 to susceptible partners.
      Recurrent genital herpes can be reduced by 70%–80% with suppressive therapy and reduce

subclinical viral shedding, improving quality of life (Fife et al., 2006; Tyring et al., 2002). In discordant couples in which a partner has a history of genital HSV-2 infection, treatment decreases the rate of HSV-2 transmission. Encourage sexual partners to consider suppressive antiviral therapy as part of a comprehensive strategy for preventing transmission, along with barrier protection and avoidance of sex during a recurrence of genital herpes. Providers should have a discussion with patients annually to assess whether they want to continue suppressive therapy.
    c. HIV infection
    People living with HIV infection (PLWH) may have severe episodes of genital, perianal, or oral herpes. HSV shedding is increased among PLWH, and lesions can be extensive, painful, and atypical. The recommended therapy for the first-episode genital HSV is the same as that for persons without HIV infections. Treatment courses may need extension based on immunological and viral status. Therapy decreases the clinical manifestation of HSV for suppression or recurrent episodes. For those in advanced stages of HIV (i.e., AIDS), there is a high risk for genital ulcer disease for the first 6 months of treatment with antiretroviral therapy (ART). This can be mitigated using suppressive antiviral therapy for 6 months and can be continued, but it does not reduce the risk for HIV or HSV-2 transmission. Discordant HIV partners at risk for HSV or HIV should receive counseling for HIV prevention with preexposure prophylaxis (PrEP). For severe HSV, initiating therapy with intravenous acyclovir might be necessary.
    d. Treatment options
        i. Sitz bath or cool compresses
        ii. Topical anesthetic or viscous lidocaine as needed
        iii. Fiber diet or stool softeners to prevent constipation as needed
        iv. Nonsteroidal anti-inflammatory medications to reduce pain
        v. Antiviral medications for primary or recurrent outbreaks (**Table 55-1**)
        vi. Essential oils for antiherpetic activity (Schnitzler, 2019)
  3. Criteria for consultation or specialty referral
    a. Generalized involvement
    b. Any complications present
    c. Pregnancy
  4. Follow-up
    a. As medically indicated for patients with primary herpes, depending on the severity of the infection
    b. Follow-up is not medically necessary with infrequent recurrent outbreaks, although some patients may require follow-up visits to focus on counseling and education.
    c. Patients on suppressive therapy should be re-evaluated every 12 months.
D. *Patient education*
  1. Goal: Educate on the clinical course of the disease, emphasizing risk factors for HSV transmission. Address concerns and feelings to help patients cope with herpes as a chronic disease.
    Counseling plays a significant role in patients diagnosed with genital HSV. The following topics should be discussed when counseling persons with genital HSV infection:
    - The natural history of the disease, with emphasis on the potential for recurrent episodes, asymptomatic viral shedding, and the attendant risks of sexual transmission
    - The effectiveness of suppressive therapy for persons experiencing a first episode of genital herpes in preventing symptomatic recurrent episodes
    - Use of episodic therapy to shorten the duration of recurrent episodes
    - Importance of informing current sex partners about genital herpes and informing future partners before initiating a sexual relationship
    - Potential for sexual transmission of HSV to occur during asymptomatic periods (asymptomatic viral shedding is more frequent in genital HSV-2 infection than genital HSV-1 infection and is most frequent during the first 12 months after acquiring HSV-2)
    - Importance of abstaining from sexual activity with uninfected partners when lesions or prodromal symptoms are present
    - Effectiveness of daily use of valacyclovir in reducing risk for transmission of HSV-2 and the lack of effectiveness of episodic or suppressive therapy in persons with HIV and HSV infection in reducing risk for transmission to partners who might be at risk for HSV-2 acquisition
    - Effectiveness of male latex condoms, which, when used consistently and correctly, can reduce (but not eliminate) the risk of genital herpes transmission (Martin et al., 2009)
    - HSV infection in the absence of symptoms (type-specific serologic testing of the asymptomatic partners of persons with genital herpes is recommended to determine whether such partners are already HSV seropositive or whether risk for acquiring HSV exists)
    - Risk for neonatal HSV infection
    - Increased risk for HIV acquisition among HSV-2–seropositive persons who are exposed to HIV (suppressive antiviral therapy does not reduce the increased risk for HIV acquisition associated with HSV-2 infection) (Mujugira et al., 2011)
    Asymptomatic persons who receive a diagnosis of HSV-2 infection by type-specific serologic testing

Table 55-1 Drug Treatment of Herpes Simplex Infections

First Clinical Episode		
	Acyclovir 400 mg orally 3×/day for 7–10 days OR	Treatment can be extended if healing is incomplete after 10 days of therapy.
	Famciclovir 250 mg orally 3×/day for 7–10 days OR	
	Valacyclovir 1 gm orally 2×/day for 7–10 days OR	

Suppressive Therapy Recurrent HSV-2		
	Acyclovir 400 mg orally 2×/day OR	Acyclovir 200 mg orally 5×/day is effective but is not recommended because of the frequency of dosing.
	Valacyclovir 500 mg orally 1×/day; OR	Valacyclovir 500 mg once a day might be less effective than other valacyclovir or acyclovir dosing regimens for persons who have frequent recurrences (i.e., ≥10 episodes/year).
	Famciclovir 250 mg orally 2×/day	

Episodic Therapy for Recurrent Genital		
	Acyclovir 800 mg orally 2×/day for 5 days; or Acyclovir 800 mg orally 3×/day for 2 days	
	Famciclovir 1 gm orally 2×/day for 1 day Famciclovir 500 mg orally once, followed by 250 mg 2×/day for 2 days Famciclovir 125 mg orally 2×/day for 5 days	
	Valacyclovir 500 mg orally 2×/day for 3 days; or Valacyclovir 1 gm orally 1×/day × 5 days	

Treatment of HSV-2 in Persons Living With HIV Infection		
Daily Suppressive Therapy	Acyclovir 400–800 mg orally 2–3×/day Famciclovir 500 mg orally 2×/day Valacyclovir 500 mg orally 2×/day	
Episodic Therapy	Acyclovir 400 mg orally 3×/day Famciclovir 500 mg orally 2×/day for 5–10 days Valacyclovir 500 mg orally 2×/day for 5–10 days	

Daily Suppression for Genital Herpes in Pregnant People		
	Acyclovir 400 mg orally 3×/day	
	Valacyclovir 500 mg orally 2×/day	

Note: Intravenous acyclovir therapy should be provided for patients with severe primary HSV disease or complications that necessitate hospitalization (e.g., disseminated infection, pneumonitis, or hepatitis) or central nervous system complications (e.g., meningitis or encephalitis). The recommended regimen is acyclovir, 5–10 mg/kg body weight intravenously every 8 hours for 2–7 days or until clinical improvement is observed, followed by oral antiviral therapy to complete at least 10 days of total therapy.

Workowski, K. A., Bachmann, L. H., Chan, P. A., Johnston, C. M., Muzny, C. A., Park, I., . . . Bolan, G. A. (2021). Sexually Transmitted Infections Treatment Guidelines, 2021. MMWR Recomm Rep, 70(4), 1-187

*Intravenous acyclovir therapy should be provided for patients with severe primary HSV disease or complications that necessitate hospi-talization (e.g., disseminated infection, pneumonitis, or hepatitis) or central nervous system complications (e.g., meningitis or encephalitis). The recommended regimen is acyclovir, 5–10 mg/kg body weight intravenously every 8 hours for 2–7 days or until clinical improvement is observed, followed by oral antiviral therapy to complete at least 10 days of total therapy.

should receive the same counseling messages as persons with symptomatic infection. In addition, such persons should be educated about the clinical manifestations of genital herpes.

Pregnant people and women of childbearing age who have genital herpes should inform the providers who care for them during pregnancy and those who will care for their newborn infant about their infection. Persons with HSV-1 genital herpes infection should be educated that the risk for recurrent genital herpes and genital shedding is lower with HSV-1 compared to HSV-2. HSV-1 suppression with therapy should be used only with frequent recurrences, especially if it causes substantial psychosocial distress. Counsel people who become pregnant to inform their obstetrician about their HSV diagnosis.

Reproduced from Centers for Disease Control and Prevention. (2021). *2021 sexually transmitted diseases: Treatment guidelines.* https://www.cdc.gov/std/treatment-guidelines/herpes.htm

VI. Self-management resources and tools
  A. Patient education
      1. Basic fact sheet that address frequently asked questions by patients about HSV infection can be printed from the CDC website: http://www.cdc.gov/std/herpes/stdfact-herpes.htm.
      2. Herpes Resource Center (http://herpes-foundation.org/herpes-resource-center/)
      3. American Sexual Health Association (http://ashastd.org; https://www.youtube.com/ashastd)
      4. National Institute of Allergy and Infectious Disease (http://niaid.nih.gov)
  B. Community support groups
      1. The Herpes Resource Center has an affiliated network of local support (HELP) group for people concerned about HSVs (http://herpesresourcecenter.com).

References

American Academy of Family Physicians. (2017). Serologic screening for genital herpes infection: recommendation statement. *American Family Physician, 95*(12).

Bibbins-Domingo, K., Grossman, D. C., Curry, S. J., Davidson, K. W., Epling, J. W., Jr., García, F. A., Kemper, A. R., Krist, A. H., Kurth, A. E., Landefeld, C. S., Mangione, C. M., Phillips, W. R., Phipps, M. G., Pignone, M. P., Silverstein, M., & Tseng, C. W. (2016). Serologic screening for genital herpes infection: US Preventive Services Task Force recommendation statement. *JAMA, 316*(23), 2525-2530. doi:10.1001/jama.2016.16776

Centers for Disease Control and Prevention. (2021). 2021 Sexually Transmitted Diseases: Treatment Guidelines. Retrieved from https://www.cdc.gov/std/treatment-guidelines/STI-Guidelines-2021.pdf

Cole, S. (2020). Herpes simplex virus: Epidemiology, diagnosis, and treatment. *Nursing Clinics of North America, 55*(3), 337–345. doi:10.1016/j.cnur.2020.05.004

Connolly, S. A., Jardetzky, T. S., & Longnecker, R. (2021). The structural basis of herpesvirus entry. *Nature Reviews Microbiology, 19*(2), 110–121. doi:10.1038/s41579-020-00448-w

Corey, L., Adams, H. G., Brown, Z. A., & Holmes, K. K. (1983). Genital herpes simplex virus infections: Clinical manifestations, course and complications. *Annuals of Internal Medicine, 98*(6), 958–972.

Feltner, C., Grodensky, C., Ebel, C., Middleton, J. C., Harris, R. P., Ashok, M., & Jonas, D. E. (2016). Serologic screening for genital herpes: An updated evidence report and systematic review for the US Preventive Services Task Force. *JAMA, 316*(23), 2531–2543. doi:10.1001/jama.2016.17138

Fife, K. H., Warren, T. J., Ferrera, R. D., Young, D. G., Justus, S. E., Heitman, C. K., & Burroughs, S. M. (2006). Effect of valacyclovir on viral shedding in immunocompetent patients with recurrent herpes simplex virus 2 genital herpes: A US-based randomized, double-blind, placebo-controlled clinical trial. *Mayo Clin Proceedings, 81*(10), 1321–1327. doi:10.4065/81.10.1321

Fleming, D. T., McQuillan, G. M., Johnson, R. E., Nahmias, A. J., Aral, S. O., Lee, F. K., & St Louis, M. E. (1997). Herpes simplex virus type 2 in the United States, 1976 to 1994. *New England Journal of Medicine, 337*(16), 1105–1111. doi:10.1056/NEJM199710163371601

Freeman, E. E., Weiss, H. A., Glynn, J. R., Cross, P. L., Whitworth, J. A., & Hayes, R. J. (2006). Herpes simplex virus 2 increases HIV acquisition in men and women: A systematic review and meta-analysis of longitudinal studies. *AIDS, 20*, 73–83.

James, C., Harfouche, M., Welton, N. J., Turner, K. M., Abu-Raddad, L. J., Gottlieb, S. L., & Looker, K. J. (2020). Herpes simplex virus: Global infection prevalence and incidence estimates, 2016. *Bulletin of the World Health Organization, 98*(5), 315–329. doi:10.2471/blt.19.237149

Kimberlin, D. W., & Rouse, D. J. (2004). Clinical practice. Genital herpes. *New England Journal of Medicine, 350*(19), 1970–1977. doi:10.1056/NEJMcp023065

Looker, K. J., Magaret, A. S., May, M. T., Turner, K. M., Vickerman, P., Gottlieb, S. L., & Newman, L. M. (2015). Global and regional estimates of prevalent and incident herpes simplex virus type 1 infections in 2012. *PLoS One, 10*(10), e0140765. doi:10.1371/journal.pone.0140765

Malekinejad, M., Barker, E. K., Merai, R., Lyles, C. M., Bernstein, K. T., Sipe, T. A., DeLuca, J. B., Ridpath, A. D., Gift, T. L., Tailor, A., & Kahn, J. G. (2021). Risk of HIV acquisition among men who have sex with men infected with bacterial sexually transmitted infections: A systematic review and meta-analysis. *Sexually Transmitted Diseases, 48*(10), e138–e148. doi:10.1097/OLQ.0000000000001403

Mujugira, A., Magaret, A. S., Baeten, J. M., Celum, C., & Lingappa, J. (2011). Risk factors for HSV-2 infection among sexual partners of HSV-2/HIV-1 co-infected persons. *BMC Research Notes, 4*, 64. doi:10.1186/1756-0500-4-64

Pinninti, S. G., & Kimberlin, D. W. (2018). Neonatal herpes simplex virus infections. *Seminars in Perinatology, 42*(3), 168–175. doi:10.1053/j.semperi.2018.02.004

Rice, S. A. (2021). Release of HSV-1 cell-free virions: Mechanisms, regulation, and likely role in human-human transmission. *Viruses*, *13*(12), 2395. https://www.mdpi.com/1999-4915/13/12/2395

Samies, N. L., James, S. H., & Kimberlin, D. W. (2021). Neonatal herpes simplex virus disease: Updates and continued challenges. *Clinics in Perinatology*, *48*(2), 263–274. doi:10.1016/j.clp.2021.03.003

Schnitzler, P. (2019). Essential oils for the treatment of herpes simplex virus infections. *Chemotherapy*, *64*(1), 1–7. doi:10.1159/000501062

Singh, N., & Tscharke, D. C. (2020). Herpes simplex virus latency is noisier the closer we look. *Journal of Virology*, *94*(4). doi:10.1128/JVI.01701-19

Stephenson-Famy, A., & Gardella, C. (2014). Herpes simplex virus infection during pregnancy. *Obstetrics and Gynecology Clinics of North America*, *41*(4), 601–614. doi:10.1016/j.ogc.2014.08.006

Tuddenham, S., Hamill, M. M., & Ghanem, K. G. (2022). Diagnosis and treatment of sexually transmitted infections: A review. *JAMA*, *327*(2), 161–172. doi:10.1001/jama.2021.23487

Tyring, S. K., Baker, D., & Snowden, W. (2002). Valacyclovir for herpes simplex virus infection: long-term safety and sustained efficacy after 20 years' experience with acyclovir. *Journal of Infectious Diseases*, *186*(Suppl 1), S40–46. doi:10.1086/342966

Workowski, K. A., Bachmann, L. H., Chan, P. A., Johnston, C. M., Muzny, C. A., Park, I., Reno, H., Zenilman, J. M., & Bolan, G. A. (2021). Sexually transmitted infections treatment guidelines, 2021. *MMWR Recommendations and Reports*, *70*(4), 1–187. doi:10.15585/mmwr.rr7004a1

Zaouak, A., Benmously, R., Hammami, H., & Fenniche, S. (2019). A case of herpes simplex virus reactivation after fractional ablative carbon dioxide laser to treat a burn scar. *Journal of Cosmetic and Laser Therapy*, *21*(3), 145–146. doi:10.1080/14764172.2018.1481513

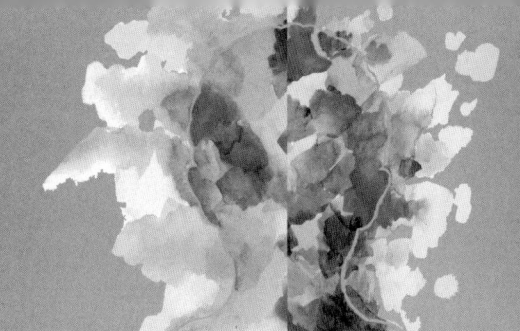

CHAPTER 56

HIV Infection in Adolescents and Adults

Christopher Berryhill Fox

I. Introduction and general background

Since the first cases of acquired immunodeficiency syndrome (AIDS) were diagnosed in 1981, there have been significant scientific advances in the understanding of the biology, natural history, and clinical management of human immunodeficiency virus (HIV) infection. Far from the bleak years of the early epidemic, when HIV was poorly understood and responsible for significant morbidity and premature mortality, HIV infection is now a manageable chronic condition in primary care.

Both the U.S. Department of Health and Human Services (DHHS) and the HIV Medical Association of the Infectious Diseases Society of America (IDSA) publish evidence-based guidelines identifying best practices in the clinical management of HIV (Panel on Antiretroviral Guidelines for Adults and Adolescents [PAGAA], 2021; Thompson et al., 2020). This chapter reviews and summarizes current DHHS and IDSA guidelines for generalist advanced practice nurses who provide primary care to people living with HIV (PLWH). Generalist primary care providers can screen for and diagnose new HIV infections, order initial laboratory assessments, start and follow antiretroviral therapy (ART) in consultation with HIV experts, diagnose and manage HIV-associated comorbidities, and provide HIV-specific healthcare maintenance and disease prevention.

Antiretroviral pharmacology is the cornerstone of HIV clinical management but can be intimidating to generalist primary care providers because of the sheer number of agents and combination regimens available. This chapter does not include an extensive discussion of antiretroviral drug classes, specific agents, or regimens. However, generalists do play an important role in antiretroviral stewardship, particularly in the management of drug–drug interactions. Given the high prevalence of polypharmacy in HIV primary care, drug–drug interactions frequently encountered in primary care are highlighted throughout the chapter.

Similarly, the chapter includes only basic content on ART initiation and management. The recommended initial regimens in the DHHS antiretroviral management guidelines change frequently and are easily accessible online (http://clinicalinfo.hiv.gov). Complex ART management is best done in consultation with an HIV specialist. The National HIV Curriculum, a free website from the University of Washington, provides an overview of ART for advanced practice nurses who are interested in enriching their HIV knowledge (https://www.hiv.uw.edu). In addition, the National Clinician Consultation Center is an excellent resource for ART management consultation (https://nccc.ucsf.edu).

A. *HIV stigma*

Since the beginning of the epidemic, PLWH and their caregivers, families, and friends have experienced stigma and discrimination. Following the American Nurses Association (2015) *Code of Ethics*, advanced practice nurses have an obligation to respect human dignity by addressing and combating HIV stigma at all levels, from individual attitudes to structural systems. Person-first language should be used when referring to PLWH rather than stigmatizing terms like *positives*. Advanced practice nurses should also resist attitudes that judge PLWH as somehow deserving of HIV infection because of their individual risk factors, race, ethnicity, or sexual orientation. Similarly, PLWH should be affirmed for their desires to have a full life, including having children and being sexually active.

B. *Epidemiology*

HIV is the virus that causes AIDS. There are two types of HIV: HIV-1 and HIV-2. HIV-1 is the most prevalent globally and, without treatment, typically progresses to death within 8–10 years. HIV-2 occurs mostly in West Africa and has a slower clinical progression (Hønge et al., 2019). This chapter focuses exclusively on HIV-1, and use of the term *HIV* should be understood as referring to HIV-1.

HIV is transmitted through certain bodily fluids: semen, preseminal fluid (or preejaculate), rectal secretions, vaginal secretions, blood, and breast milk. Transmission occurs when an infected fluid enters the body of an HIV-uninfected person via a mucous membrane (particularly the rectal or vaginal mucosa) or the bloodstream. Vertical transmission, now rare in the United States, can occur during pregnancy, labor, delivery, or breastfeeding. Nonvertical HIV exposures that carry the highest risk for transmission are parenteral (blood transfusion; sharing injection drug use [IDU] equipment, e.g., needles and syringes; and percutaneous, e.g., as a needle stick during a medical procedure) and sexual (specifically anal and penile-vaginal sex) (Patel et al., 2014). Oral sex carries a low risk of HIV transmission, and exposures through biting, spitting, throwing bodily fluids, and sharing sex toys have negligible risk (Centers for Disease Control and Prevention [CDC], 2020b; Patel et al., 2014; Pretty et al., 1999).

AIDS represents the advanced stages of HIV infection and is characterized by the progressive depletion of CD4 T lymphocytes (often called *T cells* or *CD4 cells*), resulting in life-threatening opportunistic infections (OIs) and certain malignancies. For the purpose of disease surveillance, the Centers for Disease Control and Prevention (CDC, 2014) developed a case definition for AIDS that has been revised several times to reflect advances in testing, diagnosis, and treatment of HIV. The current case definition of AIDS includes all HIV-infected people with CD4 counts of ≤200 cells/mm^3 or a diagnosis of certain AIDS-defining illnesses (**Table 56-1**).

The CDC has been tracking cases of AIDS since 1981 when the first cases of *Pneumocystis carinii* (later renamed *Pneumocystis jiroveci*) pneumonia began appearing in young, otherwise healthy gay men (CDC, 1981). In addition to surveillance of AIDS cases, the CDC has fully established an HIV incidence surveillance system to effectively track trends in new infections. Confidential name-based reporting systems have been implemented in all 50 states, the District of Columbia, and six U.S. dependent areas (American Samoa, Guam, the Northern Mariana Islands, Puerto Rico, the Republic of Palau, and the U.S. Virgin Islands) (CDC, 2021a). There is typically a 1–2 year lag in the reporting of CDC surveillance data.

1. HIV prevalence and incidence in the United States
   The CDC (2021a) estimates that as of 2019 (the last year for which data are available), there were 1.2 million PLWH aged 13 years or older in the United States and dependent areas. Approximately 12% of PLWH had not been diagnosed and were unaware of their infections. There was an estimated incidence of 36,740 new HIV infections, with an incidence rate of 13.2 per 100,000, a decreasing trend overall, although some groups have increasing HIV incidence rates.

2. HIV and men who have sex with men (MSM)
   The term *MSM* is used clinically and in public health to describe a diverse group of people whose sexual behavior is independent of sexual orientation. The term may encompass cisgender men, transgender men (if defined based on gender identity), or transgender women (if defined based on sex assigned at birth) (Worksowski et al., 2022). HIV has disproportionately affected gay, bisexual, and other MSM since the early epidemic, and the trend has continued. Although less than 4% of the cisgender male population is MSM, this group accounted for 69% of all diagnosed HIV cases in 2019 (CDC, 2021a).

Table 56-1 AIDS-Defining Illnesses in Adolescents and Adults

Candidiasis of bronchi, trachea, or lungs
Candidiasis of esophagus
Cervical cancer, invasive
Coccidioidomycosis, disseminated or extrapulmonary
Cryptococcosis, extrapulmonary
Cryptosporidiosis, chronic intestinal (>1 month duration)
Cytomegalovirus disease (other than liver, spleen, or nodes), onset at age > 1 month
Cytomegalovirus retinitis (with loss of vision)
Encephalopathy attributed to HIV
Herpes simplex: chronic ulcers (>1 month duration) or bronchitis, pneumonitis, or esophagitis
Histoplasmosis, disseminated or extrapulmonary
Isosporiasis, chronic intestinal (>1 month duration)
Kaposi sarcoma
Lymphoma, Burkitt (or equivalent term)
Lymphoma, immunoblastic (or equivalent term)
Lymphoma, primary, of brain
Mycobacterium avium complex or *Mycobacterium kansasii*, disseminated or extrapulmonary
Mycobacterium tuberculosis of any site, pulmonary, disseminated, or extrapulmonary
Mycobacterium, other species or unidentified species, disseminated or extrapulmonary
Pneumocystis jirovecii (previously known as *Pneumocystis carinii*) pneumonia
Pneumonia, recurrent
Progressive multifocal leukoencephalopathy
Salmonella septicemia, recurrent
Toxoplasmosis of brain
Wasting syndrome attributed to HIV

Centers for Disease Control and Prevention. (2014). Revised surveillance case definition for HIV infection—United States, 2014. *Morbidity and Mortality Weekly Report, 63*(3), 1–10. http://www.cdc.gov/mmwr/pdf/rr/rr6303.pdf

With the exception of MSM age 55 and older, HIV incidence rates in MSM decreased during 2015–2019, perhaps due to increased access to preexposure prophylaxis (PrEP) and antiretroviral treatment for HIV (CDC, 2021a).

3. HIV and Black Americans

There are significant racial and ethnic disparities in HIV incidence, prevalence, and survival in the United States, particularly among Black Americans, the race most effected by HIV. Although Black Americans comprised 13% of the U.S. population in 2019, the group accounted for 40% of confirmed HIV cases (CDC, 2021a). Black Americans also had the highest HIV death rate in 2019, at 16.1 per 100,000—a dramatic contrast from the death rates of white Americans (2.5 per 100,000) and Latinx Americans (4.5 per 100,000) (CDC, 2021a).

Young Black American MSM are the subgroup most affected by HIV. Black MSM have a one-in-two lifetime risk of HIV infection and comprised 51% of new infections among all MSM ages 13–24 in 2019 (CDC, 2021a; Hess et al., 2017). Black cisgender women had the highest incidence of non-MSM new HIV infections in the United States in 2019, with an incidence rate more than 12 times that of white cisgender women and 4 times that of Latinas (CDC, 2021a).

The particular impact of HIV on Black communities and individuals arises from complex factors, including structural racism, poverty and lower wages, and decreased access to health care (Adimora et al., 2014). The mass incarceration of Black American men has also played a role. Prison environments have a high risk for HIV transmission because of the high HIV prevalence, sexual activity and IDU while in prison, and lack of access to harm-reduction supplies like clean needles and condoms (Valera et al., 2017). Geography is another important factor because many Black Americans live in the U.S. South, the epicenter of the current U.S. HIV epidemic, although HIV racial disparities are widespread across the county.

4. HIV and U.S. geography

Historically, most PLWH have been clustered in major metropolitan areas in three states: California, New York, and Florida. Currently, the South, a region comprising 16 states and the District of Columbia, has emerged as the geographical area most impacted by HIV in the United States, with 53% of new HIV infections and 48% of deaths of PLWH in 2019 (CDC, 2021a).

The South's HIV epidemic is partly a matter of challenged resources. The region has high poverty rates, HIV provider shortages, a largely suburban and rural population with difficulty accessing healthcare services over long distances, and a less developed healthcare infrastructure (Adimora et al., 2014). The South also has a concentration of states with restrictive Medicaid programs that did not expand after the passage of the Affordable Care Act of 2010 (Kaiser Family Foundation, 2021).

In addition to resource problems, the South's political culture has contributed to the regional HIV epidemic. Although the region is politically heterogeneous, widespread homophobia and HIV stigma exist in the South's public institutions. Many governmental jurisdictions have enacted laws and policies that obstruct HIV prevention services, such as fact-based sex education in public schools and needle-exchange programs, or have restricted access to general sexual health services, leading to increased rates of sexually transmitted infections, which, in turn, have increased HIV incidence (Adimora et al., 2014).

5. HIV and people who inject drugs

The U.S. opioid epidemic has fueled new HIV diagnoses among people who inject drugs in recent years, starting with a notable cluster of 181 cases identified in rural Scott County, Indiana, during 2014–2015 (Peters et al., 2016). Since then, many clusters related to IDU have emerged in various locations, both urban and rural.

Although IDU with opioids is prominent, injection of methamphetamine and other substances also accounts for new cases. In 2019, IDU was a risk factor for 3,976, or about 11% of, new HIV cases in the United States and dependent areas (CDC, 2021a).

6. HIV and cisgender women

Although incidence rates have decreased in recent years, cisgender women continue to be affected by HIV in the United States and dependent areas, particularly Black cisgender women as mentioned previously. In 2019, cisgender women comprised 23% of PLWH and represented 19% of new cases. Heterosexual contact accounted for the majority of new cases among cisgender women overall. However, IDU accounted for 40% of new cases among American Indian/Alaska Native cisgender women and 36% of white cisgender women (CDC, 2021a).

7. HIV and older adults

As the population ages, older adults now comprise the largest age group of PLWH in the United States. As of 2019, PLWH age 50 or older accounted for 52% of all diagnosed HIV infections, with about 1 in 10 individuals with diagnosed HIV infection age 65 or older (CDC, 2021a).

The graying of the HIV epidemic in the United States reflects increased survival from ART, as well as infection with HIV later in life. Older adults may be unaware of their HIV risk or may have never been offered testing by a healthcare provider due to a perception of low risk. Compared to their younger counterparts, older adults are more likely to be diagnosed late in disease progression (CDC, 2020a).

8. HIV and transgender people

The CDC (2021a) tracks HIV in transgender populations, although the quantity and quality of the data are limited by gaps in recordkeeping and reporting in the U.S. healthcare system. The transgender subgroup most affected by HIV is male-to-female transgender women, with 11,032 diagnosed cases in 2019, followed by 462 cases among female-to-male transgender men and 201 cases among people with other gender identities (such as genderqueer, nonbinary, or Two-Spirit).

Although the number of transgender PLWH is small compared to the overall epidemic, transgender groups experienced sharply increased rates of new HIV cases over 2015–2019, with a 23% increase among ages 25–34 and a 22% increase among ages 35–44. As a group, transgender women, in particular, face multiple challenges that increase HIV risk, including transphobia and gender-based violence, mistrust of the healthcare system or poor access to gender-affirming care, and employment and housing discrimination leading to survival sex work (Sevelius et al., 2011).

9. HIV and the global epidemic

Globally, there have been 78 million people infected with HIV since the start of the epidemic, resulting in 35 million deaths (United Nations Joint Programme on HIV/AIDS [UNAIDS], 2021). UNAIDS estimates that there was a total of 38 million PLWH globally in 2020, with the majority of cases (55%) in eastern and southern Africa. Heterosexual sex is the main mode of transmission in this region, with cisgender women experiencing roughly 60% of new infections in 2019. Among countries globally, South Africa has the highest burden of HIV, with approximately 5.3 million PLWH.

Deaths from AIDS-related causes peaked globally in 2004 and have now fallen 61% with advances in prevention and treatment, as well as increased access to ART. In 2020, 87% of PLWH globally were accessing ART (UNAIDS, 2021).

New HIV infections around the globe decreased 30% from 2010 to 2019. In 2020, there were 1.5 million new HIV infections, compared to 2.1 million in 2010 (UNAIDS, 2021). Despite this downward trend, certain groups remain highly vulnerable to new HIV infections, including adolescent and young women, MSM, transgender people, sex workers, persons who inject drugs (PWIDs), and individuals who are incarcerated.

At the time of publication, the full impacts of the COVID-19 pandemic and global climate crisis on the HIV pandemic were unknown. However, the emergence of these crises has strained political and healthcare delivery systems and may have widespread, lasting consequences on HIV incidence, prevalence, morbidity, and mortality. In the coming years, epidemiologists will better illuminate the intersection of HIV with these global crises.

C. *Pathogenesis and natural history of HIV infection*

1. Acute HIV infection

Acute HIV infection is characterized by an initial burst of viremia from rapidly replicating virus, along with a marked depletion of CD4 T-helper lymphocytes (or CD4 cells), the primary host cell of the virus (**Figure 56-1**). After infection, HIV disseminates throughout the body. Within days to weeks, approximately 40%–90% of newly infected people will experience a nonspecific, self-limiting viral syndrome or seroconversion illness characterized by fever, generalized maculopapular rash, lymphadenopathy, and pharyngitis (PAGAA, 2021). Due to the high levels of replicating virus, transmission of HIV to uninfected partners via sex or needle-sharing is more likely during this phase of infection. Vertical transmission is more likely as well.

HIV enters a host CD4 cell by attaching and binding to chemokine coreceptors CCR5 or CXCR4 on the cell surface. Once in the cell cytoplasm, HIV enzymes reverse-transcribe viral RNA into viral DNA. Viral DNA enters the host cell nucleus and integrates into the cell's genome. This process allows HIV to use the machinery of the host cell as a factory for replicating virus while simultaneously destroying the host cell.

In addition to CD4 cells, HIV can enter and integrate into the genomes of other cells with CD4 or chemokine coreceptors. including dendritic cells, monocytes, macrophages, astrocytes, and the epithelial cells of nephrons. Once integrated, HIV persists as a latent viral reservoir in the host genome indefinitely. This reservoir maintains the presence of HIV in the body even if an individual is taking effective ART (Sung & Margolis, 2018).

2. Clinical latency

After acute HIV infection, a period of clinical latency follows as the virus becomes somewhat controlled by the body's innate and acquired immune systems, including the development of neutralizing antibodies, which occur within about 3 months after primary infection (PAGAA, 2021). The period of latency is characterized by a moderate recovery of CD4 cells and a marked reduction in viremia that maintains some constancy, also known as a *viral set point* (Figure 56-1). Although PLWH experience few symptoms during this phase of infection, the virus continues to actively replicate, and there is persistent immune activation and inflammation in the body.

The gut plays a large role in HIV immunopathogenesis. The lamina propria of the gut wall is rich in lymphoid tissue and contains large numbers of CCR5-expressing CD4 cells. During acute HIV infection, gut-associated lymphoid tissues are a primary site of viral replication, leading to rapid CD4 cell destruction in this region, as well as apoptosis of enterocytes in the lamina propria. The physical and immunologic barrier in the gut wall weakens, allowing for microbial translocation, or the movement of bacterial products from the lower digestive tract lumen to the body's systemic blood circulation,

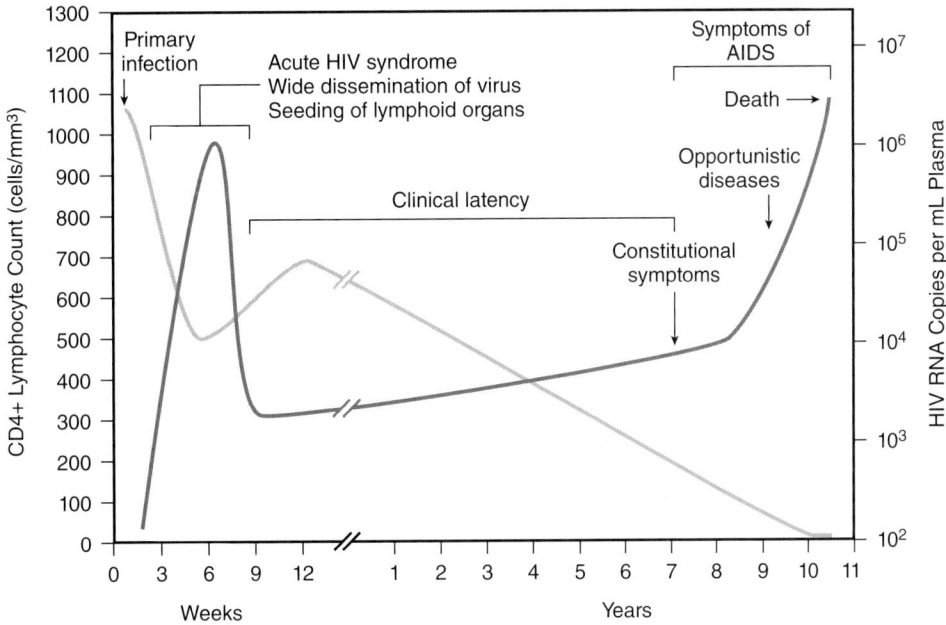

Figure 56-1 Typical course of HIV infection.

During the period after primary infection, HIV disseminates widely in the body, and an abrupt decrease in CD4 T-helper lymphocytes in the peripheral circulation occurs. An immune response to HIV ensues, with a decrease in detectable viremia. A period of clinical latency follows, during which CD4 T-helper lymphocyte counts continue to decrease, until they fall to a critical level, below which there is a substantial risk of opportunistic infections.

Sigve. June 3, 2011. https://commons.wikimedia.org/w/index.php?curid=15383502

although without causing bacteremia. Sometimes referred to as "leaky gut," the permeability of the gut wall and the translocation of microbes is responsible for much of the chronic immune activation and inflammation associated with HIV that persists during clinical latency. The gut also becomes a site of low-level viral replication. Both chronic inflammation and low-level viral replication persist, even in the setting of ART (Pérez et al., 2019).

If HIV infection goes unrecognized, CD4 cells will progressively deplete over a period of months to years (on average, 8–10 years) as cells are destroyed and production decreases. High levels of viremia are associated with more rapid depletion of CD4 cells and more rapid clinical progression. The loss of CD4 cells eventually leads to immune system failure and death from HIV, usually as a result of an AIDS-related illness (Figure 56-1).

D. Antiretroviral therapy

Currently recommended ART regimens are potent and effective in suppressing HIV replication but cannot eradicate HIV in host cells. Successful HIV treatment requires lifelong therapy and adherence to ART. Incomplete or intermittent adherence to ART can result in the failure to fully suppress HIV replication and lead to the development of HIV–drug-resistant virus (PAGAA, 2021).

Since the first combined ART regimens were introduced in the mid-1990s, there have been significant improvements in ART potency, tolerability, and frequency of dosing. Current regimens recommended for initial treatment consist of a combination of two or three agents. Many regimens are now available as once-daily, single-tablet regimens, which simplify therapy and support adherence by reducing pill burden. In 2021, the U.S. Food and Drug Administration (FDA) approved the first long-acting injectable ART regimen of intramuscular cabotegravir and rilpivirine, which may further improve adherence.

PLWH who are highly experienced with ART may have complicated salvage regimens composed of three or more agents, selected based on known viral resistance, tolerability, potential for toxicity, and clinical judgment. There are now three agents — the postattachment inhibitor ibalizumab, the gp120-attachment inhibitor fostemsavir, and the capsid inhibitor lenacapavir — that are reserved for PLWH who have high treatment experience, including virologic failure with agents from more commonly used classes (PAGAA, 2021).

Historically, the initiation of ART has been guided by CD4 T-lymphocyte counts. Current evidence-based guidelines recommend ART for all, regardless of the pretreatment CD4 T-lymphocyte count (**Table 56-2**). This recommendation is based on evidence from randomized controlled trials and observational studies that show a reduction in mortality for both AIDS-defining illnesses and non–AIDS-defining illnesses (e.g., cardiovascular, liver, or kidney disease) in individuals who are started on ART at higher pretreatment CD4 cell counts (PAGAA, 2021; Strategies for Management of Antiretroviral Therapy [SMART] Study Group et al., 2006).

E. The HIV care continuum

The HIV care continuum, also called the *treatment cascade*, is a useful model for evaluating HIV care at both the population and individual levels. The continuum describes a series of steps to identify, engage, and retain PLWH in medical care—starting with diagnosis, then moving in order to receipt of care, retention in care, and achievement of viral suppression (CDC, 2019). The most recent prevalence-based care continuum for the United States and dependent areas indicates that only 57% of individuals with HIV infections were virally suppressed in 2019 (**Figure 56-2**) (CDC, 2021a). Advanced practice nurses play an essential role in improving health outcomes of PLWH along all steps of the HIV care continuum by diagnosing new infections and immediately linking patients to medical care. Once patients are engaged in care, rapid initiation of ART and viral load (VL) suppression improves individual health outcomes and prevents further transmission of HIV.

F. HIV and common comorbidities

The success of ART has significantly reduced deaths from AIDS-defining illnesses, leading to a near-normal life expectancy for many PLWH (Marcus et al., 2020). As a result, HIV primary care increasingly involves the management of comorbidities. Chronic conditions such as cardiovascular disease (CVD), non–AIDS-defining malignancies, type 2 diabetes mellitus (T2DM), chronic obstructive pulmonary disease, osteoporosis, thromboembolic disease, liver disease, renal disease, and neurocognitive dysfunction are now the most common causes of morbidity and mortality in PLWH (Antiretroviral Therapy Cohort Collaborative, 2017). Improved survival for PLWH has increased the prevalence of older adults (age $\geq$ 50 years) living with HIV who have multiple chronic conditions complicated by HIV infection and treatment. Improvements in life expectancy of PLWH beyond those that can be achieved with the use of ART depend on optimal management of multiple comorbidities.

Many evidence-based guidelines for managing chronic diseases do not address the nuances of HIV infection in the management of comorbidities. To address this gap in the recommendations, the IDSA has developed guidelines for managing comorbid conditions commonly

Table 56-2 Initiating Antiretroviral Therapy in Treatment-Naive Adults and Adolescents

Antiretroviral therapy (ART) is recommended for all people living with HIV (PLWH) to reduce morbidity and mortality **(AI)** and to prevent the transmission of HIV to others **(AI)**.

- ART should be initiated immediately (or as soon as possible) after diagnosis in order to increase the uptake of ART and linkage to care, decrease the time to viral suppression for individual patients, and improve the rate of virologic suppression among PLWH **(AII)**.
- When initiating ART, it is important to educate patients regarding the benefits of ART and deploy strategies to optimize care engagement and treatment adherence **(AIII)**.

Rating of Recommendations: A = Strong; B = Moderate; C = Optional.
Rating of Evidence: I = Data from randomized controlled trials; II = Data from well-designed nonrandomized trials or observational cohort studies with long-term clinical outcomes; III = Expert opinion.

Panel on Antiretroviral Guidelines for Adults and Adolescents. (2021). *Guidelines for the use of antiretroviral agents in HIV-1-infected adults and adolescents.* U.S. Department of Health and Human Services. https://clinicalinfo.hiv.gov/sites/default/files/guidelines/documents/AdultandAdolescentGL.pdf

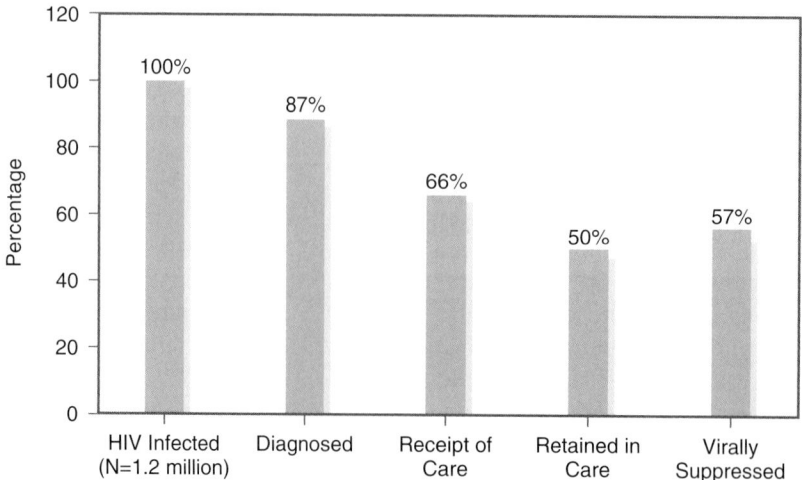

Figure 56-2 HIV/AIDS Care Continuum in the United States, 2011

Centers for Disease Control and Prevention. (2014). Vital Signs: HIV diagnosis, care, and treatment among persons living with HIV—United States, 2011. *Morbidity and Mortality Weekly Report, 63*(47), 1113–1117. Accessed at http://www.cdc.gov/mmwr/pdf/wk/mm6347.pdf

seen in PLWH (Thompson et al., 2020). The following sections highlight recommendations that are most relevant to advanced practice nurses in primary care.

1. HIV and cardiovascular disease

   Despite effective ART, PLWH have an increased risk of CVD compared to the general population, including a higher risk of atherosclerotic cardiovascular disease (ASCVD) events such as myocardial infarction. In a retrospective study of an urban population, sudden cardiac death occurred at a rate four times higher in PLWH compared to individuals without HIV infection (Narla, 2021). The higher cardiovascular risk in HIV infection is complex and multifactorial, with contributions from chronic HIV-related inflammation and immune activation, adverse effects of ART, and the prevalence of traditional cardiovascular risk factors: hypertension, dyslipidemia, metabolic syndrome, diabetes, chronic kidney disease (CKD), and cigarette smoking (Hsue, 2019). A metanalysis of smoking prevalence in Western high-income countries found that smoking rates in PLWH were 2.5 times higher than those in the general population (Park et al., 2016). Smoking cessation should be encouraged in all PLWH who smoke.

   Addressing ASCVD risk in HIV requires attention to the characteristics of specific agents when managing ART. Some antiretroviral (ARV) agents, particularly the protease inhibitor (PI) class, are more associated with dyslipidemia and increased ASCVD risk than others. If possible, PIs should be avoided in PLWH who have high ASCVD risk (PAGAA, 2021). In addition, the nucleoside reverse transcriptase inhibitor (NRTI) abacavir has been associated with an increased risk of myocardial infarction, although studies have presented conflicting data. Despite this uncertainty, experts recommend caution when including abacavir in an ART regimen for an individual with high ASCVD risk or complete avoidance of abacavir if possible. Current DHHS guidelines describe the characteristics of other specific agents in regard to ASCVD risk (PAGAA, 2021).

   Mitigating ASCVD risk in HIV also requires attention to traditional cardiovascular risk factors. The American College of Cardiology's widely used ASCVD Risk Estimator (https://tools.acc.org/ASCVD-Risk-Estimator-Plus), which provides a 10-year ASCVD risk estimate, underestimates ASCVD risk in chronic inflammatory conditions like HIV infection. Thus, the most recent guidelines for primary prevention of ASCVD from the American College of Cardiology and American Heart Association identify HIV as a risk-enhancing clinical factor that may warrant an upward revision of the patient's 10-year ASCVD risk when determining the need for statin therapy or other aggressive ASCVD risk-reduction measures. Unfortunately, there is not a simple formula for accurately adjusting the estimated 10-year ASCVD risk in PLWH. Adults living with HIV who have low, borderline, or intermediate ASCVD risk may benefit from coronary artery calcium assessment via computed tomography (CT) scan before deciding to initiate or intensify statin therapy (Arnett et al., 2019).

   Special attention should be paid to drug–drug interactions when initiating and titrating antihypertensives, anticoagulants, and antiplatelet medications for PLWH. For example, lovastatin and simvastatin are contraindicated in patients on ART regimens that contain PIs or the pharmacokinetic enhancer cobicistat, which is a component of some ARV combination tablets (PAGAA, 2021).

2. HIV and T2DM

   The prevalence of T2DM in PLWH is 3%–15% in the United States, which is comparable to the prevalence of T2DM in the general population (CDC, 2020c; Hsu et al., 2021). Some studies report a higher incidence of T2DM in PLWH compared to people without HIV, but others do not (Hsu et al., 2021). ART, particularly exposure to some older PI and NRTI agents that are no longer used, has been implicated in the development of T2DM. More recently, investigators have reported evidence of weight gain and the development of obesity after exposure to the integrase strand transfer inhibitor (INSTI) class, particularly in cisgender women (Bourgi et al., 2020). The impact of INSTIs on weight gain may occur more frequently in certain agents (e.g., dolutegravir) or when an INSTI is included in a regimen containing the NRTI drug tenofovir alafenamide. Research regarding weight gain due to ART and the development of T2DM is ongoing.

   Hemoglobin A1c (Hgb A1c) is not recommended as a screening test for T2DM by IDSA because of the poor reliability of Hgb A1c in the setting of ART, either over- or under-estimating plasma glucose levels (Thompson et al., 2020). Instead, fasting plasma glucose is the preferred screening test for T2DM in PLWH. Hgb A1c is still a useful tool for monitoring treatment of T2DM in PLWH, but it should be interpreted cautiously. Some experts suggest that a lower Hgb A1c target may be needed (Monroe et al., 2015).

   At this time, treatment goals, lifestyle modification, and clinical management of T2DM are the same as for the general population. When managing T2DM in PLWH, attention should be paid to drug–drug interactions. In particular, the INSTI agents dolutegravir and bictegravir, both included in recommended initial regimens by DHHS, increase metformin blood levels and may increase adverse effects, requiring careful monitoring or dose adjustments (PAGAA, 2021).

3. HIV and malignancies

   There are three AIDS-defining cancers: Kaposi sarcoma, non-Hodgkin lymphoma, and cervical cancer (Table 56-1). Rates of Kaposi sarcoma and non-Hodgkin lymphoma have decreased with the wide use of ART, whereas rates of cervical cancer have not (Panel on Opportunistic Infections in Adults and Adolescents with HIV [POIAAH], 2021). PLWH also have an increased risk of non–AIDS-defining cancers that are virally mediated or related to specific health behaviors: lung cancer (tobacco), hepatocellular carcinoma (hepatitis B and C, heavy alcohol use, and fatty liver), and anal cancer (human papilloma virus).

Recommendations for cancer screening for PLWH, compared to the general population, vary depending on the type of cancer. Cervical cancer screening in PLWH with a uterus differs from the current U.S. Preventive Services Task Force (USPSTF) recommendations for initiation of screening, frequency of screening, and management of abnormal cytology (**Table 56-3**). Screening recommendations for breast, colorectal, lung, and prostate cancer in PLWH are the same as recommendations for the general population. There are currently no evidence-based guidelines for anal cancer screening in PLWH, although some experts recommend annual cytology for all adults via an anal Pap smear if referral to high-resolution anoscopy is available for evaluation and treatment of abnormal findings (POIAAH, 2021).

4. HIV and renal disease

The spectrum of renal disease in HIV includes acute kidney injury and glomerular diseases (HIV-associated nephropathy), as well as CKD. HIV is a well-known risk factor for CKD. Other risk factors for CKD in PLWH include older age, female sex, comorbid diabetes or hypertension, IDU, lower CD4 cell count, history of acute kidney injury, and higher HIV RNA levels (Wyatt, 2017).

Exposure to specific antiretroviral agents is also a risk factor for CKD. Tenofovir, a backbone component of most DHHS-recommended initial regimens, has been implicated in HIV medication–associated kidney injury (PAGAA, 2021). The formulation of most concern is tenofovir disoproxil fumarate (TDF). Kidney injury with TDF can be acute, presenting as proximal tubular dysfunction, or chronic, with declines in glomerular filtration rate related to cumulative exposure to the drug. Tenofovir alafenamide (TAF), an oral prodrug of tenofovir, has less kidney toxicity compared to TDF and is now a component of several once-daily, single-tablet regimens. Recommendations for renal dose adjustments for specific antiretroviral agents are found in the DHHS treatment guidelines (PAGAA, 2021). Comprehensive clinical practice guidelines for the management of CKD in PLWH have been published (Lucas et al., 2014).

5. HIV and bone disease

Low bone mineral density (BMD) is highly prevalent in PLWH, and bone fractures in PLWH age 50 and older occur more frequently compared to age-matched peers without HIV (Gonciulea et al., 2017; Thomsen et al., 2020). The etiologies of low BMD are multifactorial and include traditional risks as well as HIV-specific risk factors such as chronic inflammation and osteoclast activation, ART-associated bone loss, and HIV/hepatitis C virus (HCV) coinfection. Following the initiation of ART, a 2%–6% decrease in BMD occurs over the first 2 years of therapy (Carr et al., 2020).

All ART regimens have been implicated in bone loss, with tenofovir having the strongest association (Carr et al., 2020). As in renal disease, the TAF formulation of tenofovir is associated with less bone toxicity compared to TDF. The IDSA recommends that all postmenopausal cisgender women and cisgender men age ≥50 receive baseline bone densitometry by DXA, noting that there is currently poor evidence to guide bone densitometry for transgender or other gender-diverse individuals regardless of gonadal or hormone status (Thompson et al., 2020) (Table 56-3).

6. HIV and viral hepatitis

Chronic viral hepatitis is more prevalent in PLWH because of the similar routes of transmission (sexual transmission and IDU) of hepatitis and HIV. Coinfection with chronic hepatitis B virus (HBV) or HCV results in a more rapid progression to fibrosis and cirrhosis and an increased risk of hepatocellular carcinoma (HCC). Both HBV and HCV may complicate the treatment of HIV because of the hepatotoxicity associated with ART.

HIV/HBV coinfected patients have higher levels of HBV viremia and a lower likelihood of clearing infection after acute HBV infection. All HIV-infected patients without evidence of immunity to HBV should be vaccinated (**Table 56-4**).

There are three antiretroviral drugs from the NRTI class with activity against HBV: lamivudine, emtricitabine, and tenofovir. Some are available alone or in a fixed-dose combination. HBV and HIV must be treated concurrently with ART that is active against both infections.

Special precaution should be taken when initiating ART for an individual with HIV/HBV coinfection. The return to immune competence as CD4 cell counts increase can lead to reactivation of HBV-related liver disease. Liver transaminases must be followed more closely when initiating ART in HIV/HBV coinfected patients (POIAAH, 2021).

The treatment of HCV has evolved significantly over the last decade, leading to astounding treatment efficacy, improved tolerability, and decreased adverse events. Studies of HCV direct-acting antiviral agents (DAAs) have shown that these drugs are safe in HIV/HCV coinfection and have similar efficacy compared to the HCV-monoinfected population. There are multiple drug–drug interactions between DAAs and antiretroviral agents.

I. Introduction and general background

Table 56-3 Healthcare Maintenance and Disease Screening for People Living With HIV

Test	Frequency	Comments
Anal cancer screening	Consider for all adults at entry to care and annually based on risk	■ There are no national guidelines for anal cancer screening, but some experts recommend screening with anal cytology or high-resolution anoscopy (HRA) **(CIII)**. ■ Annual digital anorectal exam may also be considered **(BIII)**. ■ Anal Pap smears should not be performed if there is no access to HRA for evaluation of abnormal results.
Bone densitometry (DXA)	Baseline at age ≥ 50 years for postmenopausal cisgender women and cisgender men	■ People living with HIV (PLWH) have an increased prevalence of osteopenia and osteoporosis and an increased risk of fragility fractures compared to the general population. ■ There is insufficient evidence for bone density screening for transgender or nonbinary PLWH. Consider screening according to national guidelines based on sex at birth or based on individual risk factors, including hormone therapy.
Breast cancer screening	According to national guidelines	■ Cancer screening guidelines for the general population apply to PLWH.
Cervical cancer screening	<30 years old: Screen at time of initial diagnosis. If normal, repeat in 12 months **(BII)**. If 3 consecutive normal Pap smears, repeat every 3 years. ≥30 years old: Pap testing only: At baseline and every 12 months **(BII)**. If results of the 3 consecutive Pap tests are normal, recommend follow-up Pap tests every 3 years **(BII)**. Co-testing with human papillomavirus (HPV): At baseline. If Pap normal and HPV negative, follow-up co-testing every 3 years **(BII)**. If Pap normal and HPV positive, repeat in 12 months. If either positive, refer for colposcopy.	■ PLWH who have a cervix have a higher prevalence of HPV infection and an increased incidence of cervical cancer compared to the general population. ■ Begin screening at sexual debut regardless of the mode of HIV transmission (e.g., sexual, perinatal exposure) but no later than 21 years old. ■ Co-testing with HPV test is not recommended for persons with HIV ≥30 years old. ■ PLWH ≥65 years should continue screening indefinitely, unless they have low life expectancy.
Chest radiograph	Baseline	■ For PLWH who have a history of latent *Mycobacterium tuberculosis* infection or a history and exam suggestive of preexisting lung disease.
Colorectal cancer screening	According to national guidelines	■ Cancer screening guidelines for the general population apply to PLWH.
Cytomegalovirus immunoglobulin G (IgG)	Consider at entry to care for certain individuals	■ There is discordance in the guidelines. The U.S. Department of Health and Human Services (DHHS) suggests clinicians may screen in PLWH who have a low likelihood of cytomegalovirus seropositivity, which includes people who have not had men who have sex with men (MSM) sex, injected drugs, or had exposure to child daycare settings **(AIII)**. The Infectious Diseases Society of America (IDSA) does not recommend screening any asymptomatic PLWH.

(continues)

Table 56-3 Healthcare Maintenance and Disease Screening for People Living With HIV *(continued)*

Test	Frequency	Comments
Dilated retinal examination	Annually when CD4 < 100 cells/mm^3	■ Screen for HIV-related retinopathy and asymptomatic cytomegalovirus (CMV).
Fasting plasma glucose	At entry to care and annually	■ Fasting plasma glucose should also be checked after initiating or modifying antiretroviral therapy. ■ Hemoglobin A1c is not recommended as a screening test for type 2 diabetes mellitus because of poor reliability, but it may be used to monitor treatment in PLWH who already have diabetes.
Gonorrhea and chlamydia	At entry to care; more frequently based on exposure risk	■ Nucleic acid amplification tests (NAATs) are sensitive and preferred for both genital and extragenital specimens, provided that they are processed in a laboratory that has been Clinical Laboratory Improvement Amendments certified for the assay. ■ Screen all anatomical sites based on exposure history: oropharyngeal, vaginal, urine, and rectal. Swabs are preferred for vaginal specimens. Urine is preferred for persons with a penis. ■ Triple-site screening is preferred for all MSM. ■ Consider screening PLWH with multiple sex partners every 3–6 months.
Hepatitis A IgG	At entry to care	■ Vaccination is recommended for MSM, PWIDs, and individuals with chronic liver disease **(AIII)**. ■ Reassess IgG 1 month after completing vaccination. ■ If antibody negative and CD4 count ≤ 200 cells/mm^3, wait until CD4 recovery before vaccinating **(BIII)**.
Hepatitis B serologies (hepatitis B surface antibody [anti-HBs], core antibody [anti-HBc], and surface antigen [HBsAg])	At entry to care	■ Screening includes anti-HBs, core anti-HBc, and HBsAg. ■ Presence of anti-HBs > 10 mIU/mL indicates immunity. ■ Isolated positive anti-HBc (no detected anti-HBs or HBsAg) likely indicates distant hepatitis B infection. Most individuals with isolated anti-HBc have negative hepatitis B virus (HBV) DNA, so routine DNA testing is not recommended. ■ All PLWH should be vaccinated against hepatitis B. See Table 56-4.
Hepatitis C antibody	At entry to care regardless of exposure risk; annually or more frequently for individuals at increased risk	■ Individuals at increased risk for hepatitis C infection include sexually active MSM and PWIDs.
Immunizations		■ See Table 56-4.
Liver ultrasonography	Every 6 months for PLWH with cirrhosis or chronic hepatitis B infection	■ PLWH who have chronic hepatitis B infection are at increased risk of hepatocellular carcinoma regardless of cirrhosis status. ■ Perform screening with liver ultrasonography, with or without alpha-fetoprotein.
Lung cancer screening	According to national guidelines	■ Cancer screening guidelines for the general population apply to PLWH.
Measles titer	At entry to care	■ For individuals who have unknown immunity. ■ Immunity can be generally assumed for PLWH born before 1957, documented vaccination status, or prior evidence of serologic immunity. ■ PLWH born before 1960 may have been received an inadequate vaccine. May consider a booster measles, mumps, rubella (MMR) dose in lieu of serology.

Test	Frequency	Comments
Mycobacterium tuberculosis infection screening, tuberculin skin test (TST) or interferon-gamma release assay (IGRA)	At entry to care regardless of CD4 count or risk exposure **(AII)**; annual screening for individuals who continue to have risk of exposure **(AIII)**	<ul><li>PLWH who have latent *M. tuberculosis* infection (LTBI) have a 3%–16% annual risk of active disease.</li><li>Routine use of both TST and IGRA is not recommended.</li><li>TST: Criteria for a positive skin test include ≥5-mm induration at 48–72 hours.</li><li>IGRA: Has advantages over TST for LTBI screening in adults with HIV, including single patient visit to conduct test; results available in 24 hours; does not cross-react in patients who have been previously immunized with the bacillus Calmette-Guerin (BCG) vaccine; and has higher specificity (92%–97%) compared to TST. Disadvantages include cost and limited data on PLWH.</li><li>Rescreen after stating ART when CD4 ≥ 200 cells/mm^3 and previous LTBI screening was negative.</li></ul>
Prostate cancer	According to national guidelines	<ul><li>Cancer screening guidelines for the general population apply to PLWH.</li></ul>
Serum lipids	At entry to care and annually	<ul><li>May be fasting or random</li><li>Lipid evaluation is also recommended after initiating or modifying antiretroviral therapy (ART).</li></ul>
Serum testosterone level	Only in specific clinical scenarios	<ul><li>For cisgender men who have fatigue, weight loss, decreased libido, erectile dysfunction, depression, or evidence of low bone mineral density</li><li>Fasting morning specimen is preferred.</li><li>Calculate free and total serum testosterone levels.</li></ul>
Syphilis, using local testing protocol	At entry to care and annually; more frequent screening (every 3–6 months) for those with multiple sex partners	<ul><li>Nontreponemal tests (Venereal Disease Research Laboratory [VDRL] and rapid plasma regain [RPR]) are sensitive and specific in PLWH. They should be confirmed with a treponemal test such as fluorescent treponemal antibody absorbed (FTA-ABS) or *Treponema pallidum* particle agglutination (TP-PA).</li><li>Some labs may use enzyme immunoassays (EIAs) or chemiluminescence immunoassays (CIAs) in syphilis testing algorithms, followed by a reflexed quantitative, nontreponemal test if the EIA or CIA is positive.</li></ul>
Trichomonas vaginalis	At entry to care	<ul><li>All PLWH having vaginal sex</li><li>There is increased risk of HIV transmission and pelvic inflammatory disease in untreated trichomoniasis.</li><li>NAAT swab testing is the preferred method.</li></ul>
Varicella IgG	At entry into care	<ul><li>Screen if no known history of chicken pox or shingles.</li></ul>

Rating of Recommendations: A = Strong; B = Moderate; C = Optional.
Rating of Evidence: I = Data from randomized controlled trials; II = Data from well-designed nonrandomized trials or observational cohort studies with long-term clinical outcomes; III = Expert opinion.

Data from Thompson, M. A., Horberg, M. A., Agwu, A. L., Colasanti, J. A., Jain, M. K., Short, W. R., Singh, T., & Aberg, J. A. (2020). Primary care guidance for persons with human immunodeficiency virus: 2020 update by the HIV Medicine Association of the Infectious Diseases Society of America. *Clinical Infectious Diseases*. https://doi.org/10.1093/cid/ciaa1391; Panel on Antiretroviral Guidelines for Adults and Adolescents. (2021). *Guidelines for the use of antiretroviral agents in HIV-1-infected adults and adolescents*. U.S. Department of Health and Human Services. https://clinicalinfo.hiv.gov/sites/default/files/guidelines/documents/AdultandAdolescentGL.pdf; Panel on Opportunistic Infections in Adults and Adolescents with HIV. (2021). *Guidelines for the prevention and treatment of opportunistic infections in adults and adolescents with HIV: Recommendations from the Centers for Disease Control and Prevention, the National Institutes of Health, and the HIV Medicine Association of the Infectious Diseases Society of America*. U.S. Department of Health and Human Services. http://aidsinfo.nih.gov/contentfiles/lvguidelines/adult_oi.pdf

Table 56-4 Immunizations for People Living With HIV

All people living with HIV (PLWH) should be immunized according to the Centers for Disease Control and Prevention (CDC) Advisory Committee on Immunization Practices (ACIP) immunization schedule. In general, the immune response to vaccines in PLWH is not as robust compared to HIV-noninfected populations. Some clinicians may defer vaccines if CD4 count is expected to increase to ≥200 cells/mm^3 after initiating antiretroviral therapy (ART). Some vaccines should not be deferred regardless of CD4 count. Close contacts of persons with HIV should receive all age-appropriate vaccines, with the exception of live oral polio virus and smallpox vaccines.

Vaccines that are contraindicated in PLWH

- Bacillus Calmette-Guerin (BCG)
- Live attenuated intranasal influenza (LAIV4)
- Oral polio virus (OPV)
- Smallpox (ACAM2000® version only)
- Typhoid oral vaccine (Ty21a)

Live vaccines that can be administered when CD4 counts are >200 cells/mm^3

Vaccine	Comments
Measles, mumps, and rubella (MMR)	■ PLWH are at increased risk for severe complications if infected with measles. ■ Newly diagnosed adults without acceptable evidence of measles immunity should receive the MMR vaccine unless they have evidence of severe immunosuppression (CD4 counts ≤ 200 cells/mm^3). If necessary, separate components of the vaccine can be given.
Varicella (VAR)	■ People born in the United States before 1980 do not need to receive VAR. ■ No studies have evaluated the vaccine in PLWH. ■ VAR may be considered in varicella seronegative PLWH aged ≥8 years with CD4 counts ≥ 200 cells/mm^3. ■ Do not administer during pregnancy. ■ Dosing schedule is 2 doses 3 months apart.
Yellow fever (YF)	■ YF vaccination is safe in PLWH without severe immunosuppression (CD4 counts ≥ 200 cells/mm^3). ■ Less immunogenic in PLWH
Zoster vaccine, live (ZVL)	■ No longer recommended by ACIP because of the superior efficacy of the recombinant zoster vaccine (RZV; Shingrix®) ■ If RZV is not available, ZVL should not be used in PLWH with CD4 counts ≤ 200 cells/mm^3.

Vaccines that can be administered at any CD4 cell count

Inactivated, recombinant, subunit, polysaccharide, and conjugate vaccines and toxoids are safe and can be administered to all PLWH.

Vaccine	Comments
Hepatitis A (HAV)	■ ACIP recommends for all PLWH ■ May use 2-dose HAV series (Havrix®, Vaqta®) or 3-dose HAV-HBV series (Twinrix®) ■ Schedules are the same as those for the general population.
Hepatitis B (HBV)	■ Vaccinate all PLWH without evidence of immunity. ■ Screen for HBV status prior to vaccination. Screening includes surface antibody (anti-HBs), core antibody (anti-HBc), and surface antigen (HBsAg). See Table 56-3. ■ Immunity is indicated by anti-HBs ≥ 10 mIU/mL. ■ An individual with anti-HBs <10 mIU/mL at 1–2 months is considered a nonresponder **(BIII)**. ■ PLWH have a lower magnitude and duration of immunity following vaccination compared to HIV-uninfected people.

I. Introduction and general background

Vaccine	Comments
	▪ Early vaccination (while CD4 > 350 cells/mm^3) is recommended, but vaccination should not be deferred based on CD4 count **(AIII)**. ▪ Recombinant 3-dose vaccines (Energix-B®, Recombivax-HB®), the 3-dose HAV-HBV (Twinrix®) series, or the 2-dose Heplisav-B® can be used. ▪ Anti-HBs should be obtained 1–2 months after completion of a vaccine series. ▪ PLWH without an adequate vaccine response can receive a repeat vaccination series, either single-dosed **(BIII)** or double-dosed **(BI)**. ▪ Isolated positive anti-HBc (with negative anti-HBs and negative HBsAg) likely represents past infection with loss of anti-HBs. These individuals should be revaccinated with a single standard dose of HBV vaccine, followed by an anti-HBs titer check in 1–2 months. Immunity is indicated by anti-HBs ≥ 10 mIU/mL. If anti-HBs is < 10 mIU/mL, repeat a full series, followed by another titer check **(AII)**.
Hemophilus influenzae type B (Hib)	Only indicated for PLWH who have other indications, such as asplenia or hematopoietic stem cell transplant.
Human papillomavirus (HPV)	▪ PLWH ages 9–26 years should receive a 3-dose series of the HPV 9-valent recombinant vaccine (Gardasil 9®) regardless of the age when they received their initial dose. ▪ Do not administer during pregnancy ▪ Vaccination of PLWH ages 26–45 years can be considered based on shared decision making.
Influenza inactivated (IIV) or influenza recombinant (RIV4)	▪ Indicated annually for all adolescent and adult PLWH regardless of age or comorbid conditions.
Meningococcal serogroups A, C, W, Y (MenACWY)	▪ Recommended by ACIP because of growing evidence that PLWH are at greater risk for infection with these serogroups. ▪ ACIP recommends a 2-dose series MenACWY (Menactra®, Menveo®, or MenQuadfi®) at least 8 weeks apart, followed by a booster every 5 years.
Meningococcal serogroup B (MenB)	▪ Not routinely recommended for PLWH. Only recommended in outbreak situations or in individuals with asplenia or other specific conditions.
Mpox	▪ ACIP recommends a 2-dose Mpox series (JYNNEOS®) at least 1 month apart for all people age 18 years at risk for Mpox during an outbreak.
Pneumococcal vaccines (PCV13, PCV15, PCV20, and PPSV23)	▪ Administration recommendations are based on previous receipt of pneumococcal vaccines. ▪ No history of pneumococcal vaccination or history unknown: 1 dose of PCV15 (Vaxneuvance®) or PCV20 (Prevnar 20®). If PCV15 is used, administer 1 dose of PPSV23 (Pneumovax®) at least 1 year later. An interval of at least 8 weeks can be considered for severely immunocompromised individuals. ▪ History of a single dose of PCV13 (Prevnar®): Administer 1 dose of PPSV23 at least 8 weeks after PCV13, then a second dose of PPSV23 at least 5 years after first PPSV23. At age ≥ 65 years, administer 1 dose of PPSV23 at least 5 years after most recent dose of PPSV23. There should be only one PPSV23 dose after age 65. ▪ History of PPSV23 alone: Administer 1 dose of PCV15 or PCV20 at least 1 year after PPSV23 dose. ▪ There is currently no evidence to guide the administration of PCV15 or PCV20 subsequent to a completed PCV13/PPSV23 series.
Respiratory syncytial virus (RSV)	All individuals age ≥ 60 years.
SARS-CoV-2 (COVID-19)	▪ At the time of publication, COVID-19 vaccination with any of the available vaccines that have received emergency U.S. Food and Drug Administration (FDA) approval or approval is recommended for all adult PLWH. ▪ Refer to up-to-date guidance from Centers for Disease Control and Prevention (CDC) regarding future immunization recommendations.

(continues)

Table 56-4 Immunizations for People Living With HIV (continued)

Vaccine	Comments
Tetanus and diphtheria toxoids and acellular pertussis (Tdap) or Tetanus and diphtheria toxoids (Td)	Boost every 10 years.
Zoster recombinant (RZV)	■ Two doses of RZV (Shingrix®), given 2–6 months apart, should be administered to all PLWH age ≥ 19 years old. ■ A shorter vaccine schedule of 2 doses, given 1–2 months apart, can be considered for PLWH with significant immunosuppression. ■ Administration timing should take into account an individual's level of immunosuppression and the likelihood of having an adequate vaccine response. Delaying administration in PLWH with severe immunocompromise or unstable disease may be warranted.

Rating of Recommendations: A = Strong; B = Moderate; C = Optional.
Rating of Evidence: I = Data from randomized controlled trials; II = Data from well-designed nonrandomized trials or observational cohort studies with long-term clinical outcomes; III = Expert opinion.

Data from Anderson, T. C., Masters, N. B., Guo, A., Shepersky, L., Leidner, A. J., Lee, G. M., Kotton, C. N., & Dooling, K. L. (2022). Use of recombinant zoster vaccine in immunocompromised adults aged ≥19 years: Recommendations of the Advisory Committee on Immunization Practices - United States, 2022. *Morbidity and Mortality Weekly Report*, 71(3), 80–84. https://doi.org/10.15585/mmwr.mm7103a2; Centers for Disease Control and Prevention. (2022). Recommended adult immunization schedule for ages 19 years or older, United States, 2022. https://www.cdc.gov/vaccines/schedules/downloads/adult/adult-combined-schedule.pdf; Kobayashi, M., Farrar, J. L., Gierke, R., Britton, A., Childs, L., Leidner, A. J., Campos-Outcalt, D., Morgan, R. L., Long, S. S., Talbot, H. K., Poehling, K. A., & Pilishvili, T. (2022). Use of 15-Valent Pneumococcal Conjugate Vaccine and 20-Valent Pneumococcal Conjugate Vaccine Among U.S. Adults: Updated Recommendations of the Advisory Committee on Immunization Practices - United States, 2022. *Morbidity and Mortality Weekly Report*, 71(4), 109–117. https://doi.org/10.15585/mmwr.mm7104a1; MacNeil, J. R., Rubin, L. G., Patton, M., Ortega-Sanchez, I. R., & Martin, S. W. (2016). Recommendations for use of meningococcal conjugate vaccines in HIV-infected persons—Advisory Committee on Immunization Practices, 2016. *Morbidity and Mortality Weekly Report*, 65(43), 1189–1194. https://doi.org/10.15585/mmwr.mm6543a3; Panel on Opportunistic Infections in Adults and Adolescents with HIV. (2021). *Guidelines for the prevention and treatment of opportunistic infections in adults and adolescents with HIV: Recommendations from the Centers for Disease Control and Prevention, the National Institutes of Health, and the HIV Medicine Association of the Infectious Diseases Society of America.* U.S. Department of Health and Human Services. http://aidsinfo.nih.gov/contentfiles/lvguidelines/adult_oi.pdf

Recommendations for concomitant use of DAAs and antiretrovirals are available in the DHHS guidelines (PAGAA, 2021) and through the American Association for the Study of Liver Diseases and IDSA (2021).

II. HIV testing

A. Rationale

Twelve percent of Americans with HIV do not know that they are infected (CDC, 2021a), which has led the DHHS to identify increasing awareness of HIV serostatus as a Leading Health Indicator in *Healthy People 2030* (Office of Disease Prevention and Health Promotion, n.d.). In addition, diagnosing HIV infections as quickly as possible is a strategy of the U.S. federal government's multiagency plan to end the HIV epidemic by 2030 (Office of Infectious Disease and HIV/AIDS Policy, 2021).

Early detection of HIV infection benefits patients by creating an opportunity to initiate ART, thereby preventing further immune destruction, with its resulting morbidity and mortality. Knowledge of HIV serostatus also has major public health implications: individuals with HIV who do not know their serostatus are the source of approximately 38% of new HIV transmissions in the United States (Li et al., 2019). A person with unsuppressed virus is significantly more likely to transmit virus to a sexual or needle-sharing partner. Individuals with acute HIV infection may have very high levels of HIV. Individuals may also unknowingly facilitate viral transmission by participating in high-risk behaviors that they would otherwise avoid if they were aware of their HIV serostatus.

In a nationwide survey of Americans, the top reasons that individuals gave for never receiving an HIV test were lack of perceived risk (#1) and lack of a recommendation for testing by a doctor (#2) (Kaiser Family Foundation, 2009). Therefore, it is incumbent on clinicians to discuss HIV risk with patients and offer routine testing.

B. National screening recommendations

As of 2006, the CDC recommends screening all patients ages 13–64 years, except in settings of low undiagnosed HIV prevalence (defined as <0.1%, or less than 1 in every 1,000 HIV tests is positive). The USPSTF et al. (2019) recommend screening all patients ages 15–65 years (Grade A recommendation), with screening of younger adolescents or older adults based on HIV risk.

1. Consent process for HIV screening: Historically, HIV testing involved separate written informed consent and extensive counseling. This process was found to be a barrier to testing and is no longer recommended. Both the CDC (2006) and the

USPSTF et al. (2019) recommend opt-out consent: a patient must specifically decline testing. Opt-out testing has been codified in the laws of many states; however, clinicians should refer to specific laws regarding consent requirements in their state of practice. A summary of these laws is available at the Center for HIV Law & Policy. See the Resources section.
   2. Repeat screening: The CDC recommends repeat screening at least yearly for patients at high risk for HIV infection (Branson et al., 2006). The USPSTF et al. (2019) state that there is insufficient evidence to make a recommendation, but it is reasonable to screen high-risk patients more frequently. Patients at high risk include:
      a. People who inject drugs and their sex partners
      b. People who exchange money or drugs for sex
      c. Anyone with an HIV-infected partner
      d. People with more than one sex partner
      e. People who have a sex partner who has multiple partners
   3. Specific recommendations for MSM: The CDC recommends that sexually active MSM be screened for HIV at least annually. Clinicians may consider screening MSM at high risk every 3–6 months, depending on individual risk factors like multiple sex partners or substance use, local HIV prevalence, and availability of testing (DiNenno et al., 2017).
   4. HIV screening in pregnancy: The CDC (2006) and the USPSTF et al. (2019) have published specific recommendations for HIV screening in pregnancy, which are available online. See the Resources section.
C. *Screening tests*
   1. HIV screening tests: HIV testing technology is divided into "generations," with fourth-generation assays preferred for screening today. Fourth-generation assays (referred to as *combination*, *combo*, or *HIV Ab/Ag*) differentiate between HIV-1 and HIV-2, as well as detect both HIV immunoglobulin M (IgM) antibodies and the HIV p24 antigen, which appears about 14–20 days after infection (Branson et al., 2014). These newer generations of assays are now widely available; however, clinicians may need to verify the generation of assay used at their specific clinical sites.
   2. Rapid testing: Rapid testing offers the advantage of a result within 20 minutes or less. A rapid fourth-generation test (HIV Ab/Ag combination test) is preferred because rapid HIV antibody-only tests rely on second-generation assays that may not detect HIV for weeks to months after infection (Branson et al., 2014).
   3. HIV VL testing: HIV RNA is detectable by current assays approximately 10 days after infection (Branson et al., 2014). Because of the variability of HIV viremia, RNA VL testing is not approved by the FDA for the diagnosis of HIV. However, VL testing is appropriate to identify HIV in any patient with recent HIV risk and presentation of signs and symptoms consistent with acute retroviral syndrome (ARS). During this phase of infection, when plasma HIV RNA VLs are reliably high, VL testing may detect evidence of HIV before antibody or antigen tests become reactive. For this reason, HIV RNA testing is also used in scenarios when an HIV Ab/Ag test is indeterminant.
   4. HIV screening during PrEP: The CDC (2021b) now recommends HIV screening with both an HIV Ab/Ag *and* an HIV RNA PCR (either quantitative or qualitative assay) for individuals who are currently or recently using antiretroviral agents for PrEP. The recommendation is based on data from the HPTN 083 Study, which identified a diagnosis delay of up to 1–4 months on average for individuals on PrEP (Marzinke et al., 2021).
D. *Linkage to care and partner services*
   Once diagnosed with HIV, immediate linkage of the patient to medical care is essential. Clinicians should also initiate conversations about partner disclosure as soon as possible. Partners of individuals with new HIV diagnoses are at particular risk for infection, and if not already infected, they are prime candidates for HIV prevention services such as PrEP and postexposure prophylaxis (PEP).

   Patients may opt for self-disclosure to partners; dual disclosure (patient discloses to partners with a clinician or counselor available in the room to provide support and information); or third-party anonymous notification, in which a trained public health worker notifies partners of exposure and offers testing services without identifying the original patient. Clinicians should contact local public health authorities to check for availability of this service.

III. **Database**
A. *Subjective*
   1. Medical history
      a. Obtain documentation of positive HIV antibody test. If HIV infection cannot be confirmed, repeat the HIV antibody test.
      b. ARS: review for past symptoms consistent with ARS, which may help to identify the approximate date of HIV infection.
      c. Obtain past CD4 counts (absolute and percentage), CD4 nadir, and HIV VLs.
      d. AIDS-defining illnesses and HIV-related conditions: OIs, malignancies, thrush, hairy leukoplakia, herpes simplex virus, herpes zoster outbreaks, anemia, thrombocytopenia, recurrent bacterial skin infections, and cervical or anal cancer
      e. Antiretroviral history:
         i. Prescribed regimens: List all past regimens and antiretroviral components of regimens, side effects, and adverse events.

ii. Document start and stop dates for each regimen or component and changes in HIV VL.
iii. Document results of HIV resistance assays: genotype, phenotype, resistance archive, and tropism assays. Obtain past medical records to confirm information.
iv. Review past adherence issues with ART, such as medication intolerance, depression or other mental illness, low health literacy, inadequate social support, active substance use, homelessness, or nondisclosure of HIV status.
f. Other medications and allergies: Complete a medication reconciliation of all prescribed and over-the-counter medications, supplements, and herbal therapies
g. History of transfusion of blood, platelets, or serum products between 1975 and 1985; history of artificial insemination from an anonymous donor
h. Comorbid conditions: risk factors or history of CVD, diabetes, lung disease, kidney disease, liver disease, malignancies, and osteoporosis
i. Psychiatric/behavioral: mood disorders, anxiety and panic disorders, posttraumatic stress disorder, other severe mental illness, suicidal ideation or past suicide attempts, and history of psychiatric hospitalizations
j. Sexually transmitted diseases: history of past infections and treatment: gonorrhea, chlamydia, chancroid, syphilis, trichomoniasis, herpes simplex virus (HSV), HBV, HCV, and human papilloma virus (HPV)
k. Active or latent tuberculosis infection (LTBI): results of tuberculin skin tests (TSTs) or interferon-gamma release assay (IGRA). If patient has a history of LTBI, record date, treatment, and chest X-ray (CXR) results
l. Immunization status (Table 56-4)
m. Individuals assigned female sex at birth: last menstrual period, previous abnormal Pap smears, genital condyloma, recurrent vaginal yeast infections, pelvic inflammatory disease, gravid and para status, mammograms, and BMD screening
n. Individuals assigned male sex at birth: genital or anal condyloma, abnormal anal Pap smear results and treatment, and BMD screening
o. Foreign travel or residence in areas endemic for specific organisms (e.g., southwestern United States: coccidioidomycosis; Ohio and Indiana: histoplasmosis)
p. Other risk factors for opportunistic infections: cat ownership and consumption of uncooked beef are risks for toxoplasmosis.
2. Personal and social
a. Age, sex assigned at birth, gender identity, race, and ethnicity
b. Sexual history:
i. Number and gender(s) of partners
ii. Sexual practices: anal, penile-vaginal, oral, or other practices
iii. Use of condoms or other barrier methods, and other strategies for decreasing risk of HIV transmission
c. History of tobacco use:
i. If cigarettes, age at onset, number of cigarettes per day, and pack-year history
ii. If currently smoking, review past attempts to quit smoking and interest in smoking cessation.
d. Substance use, including alcohol, cocaine, methamphetamine, heroin, marijuana, poppers (amyl nitrate), and other substance use:
i. Type and mode of ingestion
ii. If IDU, injection practices and use or access to clean injection equipment
iii. Relationship between substance use and sexual activity
e. Social support, relationships, and housing:
i. Patient's emotional response to diagnosis
ii. Disclosure of HIV status to sex partners, family, and friends and level of support
iii. History of homelessness or unstable housing
iv. Any past or current relationships with HIV service organizations or other support services
f. History of intimate partner violence (IPV) or sexual assault
g. History of incarceration
3. Family history
a. Malignancies, neurologic diseases, osteoporosis, atherosclerotic disease, and history of early coronary heart disease (i.e., myocardial infarction in first-degree relative before age 55 in males and before age 65 in females)
4. Review of systems
a. General: usual body weight, fever or drenching sweats, unintentional weight loss of more than 10%, and persistent fatigue or anorexia
b. Dermatologic: persistent skin rashes, recurrent outbreaks of HSV, easy bruising or bleeding, red- to violet-colored papular or macular lesions, pruritic papules
c. Lymph nodes: rapid or asymmetrical lymph node swelling or a change in the size of a node or tender lymph nodes
d. Ear, nose, and throat: oral lesions or sores, periodontal disease, caries; painful or sensitive teeth
e. Eyes: decreased visual acuity or vision loss
f. Pulmonary: cough, dyspnea, and hemoptysis
g. Cardiac: chest pain, murmurs, palpitations
h. Gastrointestinal: diarrhea, nausea, emesis, bloating, rectal pain, rectal lesions or discharge, bright red blood per rectum.

i. Genitourinary and gynecologic: genital lesions or sores, dysuria, vaginal discharge, pelvic pain, penile discharge, testicular pain or masses, contraception, use of barrier methods during sexual activity
j. Anorectal: rectal pain or discharge
k. Musculoskeletal: weakness, arthralgia, myalgia, and risks for osteoporosis.
l. Neurologic: persistent or severe headaches, changes in cognition, memory loss, confusion or forgetfulness, seizures, weakness, pain or numbness in hands or feet
m. Psychiatric: depression, anxiety, and insomnia
5. Family history: CVD, diabetes, renal disease, alcohol and substance use disorders, malignancies, HIV, depression, and emotional or physical abuse

B. *Objective*
1. General appearance and body habitus: wasting or unintentional weight loss, obesity, fat redistribution syndromes (dorsocervical fat pad, gynecomastia, or visceral fat accumulation), lipoatrophy (loss of subcutaneous fat in face and extremities), frailty
2. Height, weight, blood pressure, waist circumference, and baseline SpO$_2$ resting and with exercise
3. Skin: tinea, onychomycosis, folliculitis, seborrheic dermatitis, bruising or petechiae, herpes, molluscum contagiosum, condyloma, Kaposi sarcoma lesions (purplish macular, papular, or nodular lesions; discrete and well circumscribed; do not blanch with compression)
4. Lymph nodes: completed examination for presence of lymphadenopathy, defined as >1 cm in two or more noncontiguous extrainguinal sites, one of which may be cervical. Assess for asymmetry and consistency of node.
5. Eyes: visual acuity and visual field testing. Examine for lesions on lids or sclera, funduscopic exam for hemorrhage, exudate, or cotton wool spots.
6. Oropharynx: ulcerations on tongue or mucous membranes. White coating on tongue or oropharynx (oral candidiasis), fringed lesions on lateral border or dorsum of tongue (hairy leukoplakia), inflammation or receding of gingiva (periodontal disease).
7. Cardiovascular: heart exam, pulses, and presence of lower extremity edema
8. Chest: lung exam
9. Breast: nodules or nipple discharge
10. Abdomen: enlargement of spleen or liver, masses, or tenderness
11. Genitourinary: discharge, lesions, masses, condyloma, HSV, Pap smear of cervix if present
12. Anorectal: ulcers, fissures, digital rectal exam, anoscopy, and anal Pap smear
13. Neurologic: screening exam, including mental status examination. Standard Mini Mental State Examination is not sensitive for detecting HIV-associated neurocognitive disorders. Montreal Cognitive Assessment is preferred (Fazeli et al., 2017).

IV. Assessment
A. *Determine the diagnosis*
1. HIV antibody testing
2. Plasma HIV RNA (VL)
B. *Staging of disease and HIV–drug-resistance testing*
1. CD4 lymphocyte count
2. Clinical assessment for OIs
3. Genotypic resistance assays on all ARV-naive patients at entry into care, regardless of whether ART will be initiated immediately
C. *Motivation and ability*
HIV is associated with significant stigma and disparities in healthcare outcomes. Common barriers to engaging and retaining patients in care include untreated mental illness, active substance use, nondisclosure of HIV status, transportation, childcare issues, houselessness or unstable housing, joblessness, health insurance, food insecurity, and lack of social support. During initial visits, allow time to establish a therapeutic relationship, identify the patient's priorities and preferences for care, and address actual and potential barriers to care.

V. Goals of clinical management
A. *Treatment goals (PAGAA, 2021)*
1. Reduce HIV-associated morbidity and prolong the duration and quality of survival.
2. Restore and preserve immunologic function.
3. Durably and maximally suppress plasma HIV VL.
4. Prevent transmission of HIV.
B. *Healthcare maintenance*
C. *Support adherence to ART and retention in care*
D. *Prevention of new infections*

VI. Plan
A. *Initial laboratory and diagnostic tests*
1. Order initial laboratory and diagnostic studies (**Table 56-5**).
B. *Management*
1. Initiate HIV-specific and routine healthcare maintenance for age and gender (Tables 56-3 and 56-4).
2. Initiate ART: Initial recommended regimens for HIV change frequently based on data from clinical trials, cohort studies, and the experience of clinicians and community members actively engaged in HIV patient care. Clinicians should review the most current treatment recommendations (https://aidsinfo.nih.gov/guidelines) and/or consult with an HIV expert prior to initiating an ART regimen.
   The DHHS (PAGAA, 2021) antiretroviral guidelines provide recommended initial regimens for most people. These are regimens studied in randomized controlled trials that have shown to be optimally effective, tolerable, and easy to use. The guidelines also identify other initial regimens that may be used in certain clinical situations. These alternatives have disadvantages, such as reduced potency, tolerability, or toxicity profiles. However, an alternative regimen may be the best regimen for a specific patient.

Table 56-5 Laboratory Studies to Perform at Antiretroviral Therapy Initiation and During Monitoring of Therapy

Laboratory Test	Frequency and Comments
HIV-1 antibody test	■ HIV infection should be confirmed in all patients entering care, either through documentation or laboratory testing. Repeat an HIV antibody test if HIV diagnosis has not been confirmed.
CD4 T-cell count, absolute and percentage	■ At entry into care and every 3–6 months prior to initiation of antiretroviral therapy (ART). ■ Every 3–6 months after initiation of ART or if CD4 cell count < 300 cells/mm^3 ■ Every 6–12 months after 2 years on ART with consistently suppressed viral load (VL). Some experts recommend annual CD4 cell count if VL is durably suppressed for >2 years. ■ Routine monitoring of lymphocyte subsets (e.g., CD8) other than CD4 absolute and percentage is not recommended.
HIV RNA viral load (VL)	■ Most important indicator of initial and sustained response to ART ■ VL suppression is defined as a VL persistently below the lower limits of detection for the assay used (HIV RNA < 20 to 75 copies/mL). ■ Measured at entry into care, at initiation of therapy, and on a regular basis thereafter ■ Repeating VL while not on therapy is optional. **(CIII)**
HIV resistance testing	■ At entry into care and regardless of decision to initiate ART ■ HIV-drug resistance has been demonstrated in 6%–16% of transmitted HIV-1 infections, commonly to nonnucleoside reverse transcriptase inhibitors (NNRTIs) and nucleoside reverse transcriptase inhibitors (NRTIs). ■ Genotypic testing is the preferred initial resistance assay to guide therapy in antiretroviral-naive patients.
HLA-B*5701	■ At entry into care or prior to starting an ART regimen containing abacavir to reduce the risk of hypersensitivity reaction ■ An abacavir hypersensitivity reaction is a multiorgan clinical syndrome occurring in the first few weeks of abacavir initiation in 5%–8% of patients positive for haplotype HLA-B*5701. ■ Re-challenge with abacavir after this clinical syndrome can cause a life-threatening hypersensitivity reaction. ■ Patients who test HLA-B*5701 positive *should not* be prescribed abacavir, and their positive HLA-B*5701 results should be recorded as an abacavir allergy in the medical record.
Coreceptor tropism assays	■ Perform if a C-C chemokine receptor type 5 (CCR5) antagonist is being considered as part of an ART regimen. **(AI)** ■ Tropism assay screens for HIV resistance to either CCR5 and/or CXCR4 virus. ■ Requires HIV-1 plasma RNA of >1,000 copies/mL ■ Consult with HIV specialist prior to ordering to determine need for assay and interpretation of results.
Hepatitis B virus (HBV) serology	■ At entry into care and as clinically indicated (Table 56-3)
Hepatitis C virus (HCV) serology	■ At entry into care and as clinically indicated (Table 56-3)
Complete blood count with white blood count differential	■ At entry into care and every 3–6 months once ART initiated and when clinically indicated ■ Anemia of chronic disease, leukopenia, and thrombocytopenia are manifestations of untreated advanced HIV. ■ Zidovudine causes anemia. Review complete blood cell count every 2–8 weeks after initiation of zidovudine.

Laboratory Test	Frequency and Comments
Basic chemistry panel	- At entry into care, every 3–6 months prior to initiation of ART, and every 3–6 months or as clinically indicated after initiation of ART. - Some experts suggest monitoring the phosphorus levels of patients on tenofovir.
Aspartate transaminase (AST), alanine transaminase (ALT), total bilirubin	- At entry into care, every 6–12 months prior to initiation of ART, and with any ART modification - Once on ART, every 3–6 months and as clinically indicated
Fasting plasma glucose	- At entry into care and annually if normal - At time of initiation of ART or modification of ART
Fasting lipid profile	- At entry into care, prior to initiation of ART, and as clinically indicated - Consider every 4–5 weeks after starting new ART regimen that affects lipids
Glucose-6-phosphate dehydrogenase (G6PD)	- Screen once at entry to care or before starting oxidant drugs. - G6PD is a genetic variation that predisposes to hemolytic anemia if oxidative drugs are prescribed. - Patients should be tested for G6PD deficiency before administration of dapsone or primaquine. An alternative agent should be used in patients found to have G6PD deficiency.
Toxoplasma gondii, Toxo immunoglobulin G (IgG)	- At entry into care for exposure to *T. gondii* - If seronegative, counsel on prevention of new *Toxoplasma* infections. Avoid eating raw or undercooked meat. If the patient owns a cat that goes outdoors, recommend frequent litter changes and thorough handwashing after changing litter box. - Retest for Toxo IgG if CD4 falls to <100/mm^3 to determine need for primary prophylaxis for toxoplasmosis.
Urinalysis	- At entry to care, prior to initiating or modifying ART, and annually - At least every 6 months for individuals on tenofovir disoproxil fumarate (TDF)
Pregnancy test	- Prior to initiation of ART, when starting or modifying ART, and as clinically indicated

Rating of Recommendations: A = Strong; B = Moderate; C = Optional.
Rating of Evidence: I = Data from randomized controlled trials; II = Data from well-designed nonrandomized trials or observational cohort studies with long-term clinical outcomes; III = Expert opinion.

Data from Panel on Antiretroviral Guidelines for Adults and Adolescents. (2021). *Guidelines for the use of antiretroviral agents in HIV-1-infected adults and adolescents*. U.S. Department of Health and Human Services. https://clinicalinfo.hiv.gov/sites/default/files/guidelines/documents/AdultandAdolescentGL.pdf; Thompson, M. A., Horberg, M. A., Agwu, A. L., Colasanti, J. A., Jain, M. K., Short, W. R., Singh, T., & Aberg, J. A. (2020). Primary care guidance for persons with human immunodeficiency virus: 2020 Update by the HIV Medicine Association of the Infectious Diseases Society of America. *Clinical Infectious Diseases*. https://doi.org/10.1093/cid/ciaa1391

3. Initiate antimicrobial prophylaxis to prevent first episode of HIV-related OIs as indicated (**Table 56-6**).
4. Provide screening and counseling for prevention of HIV transmission.
5. Identify and manage chronic comorbid conditions.
6. Refer patients with illnesses of unclear etiology or evidence of HIV-drug resistance to HIV specialist.
7. Refer to social worker or local AIDS service organization for case management services: housing, mental health and substance abuse treatment, health insurance, eligibility for federally funded AIDS programs, transportation to clinic appointments, childcare, and parenting needs.

C. *Management considerations specific to cisgender women living with HIV*
   1. Reproductive counseling and contraception: Desire for pregnancy should be discussed with all people with childbearing potential. When constructing an ART regimen for a cisgender woman desiring pregnancy, clinicians should avoid agents with teratogenic potential and be mindful of the pharmacokinetic characteristics of pregnancy on individual antiretroviral components. If a cisgender woman does not desire pregnancy, provide preconception counseling and initiate discussions regarding contraception. Cisgender women with HIV can use all forms of contraceptive options, although hormonal options should be checked for drug–drug interactions with antiretroviral agents. The DHHS guidelines provide more details (PAGAA, 2021).
   2. Pregnancy: The landmark AIDS Clinical Trials Group 076 study demonstrated the safety and efficacy of ART in pregnant cisgender women for the prevention of perinatal transmission of HIV (Connor et al., 1994). The use of ART and avoidance of breastfeeding by PLWH have virtually eliminated perinatal

Table 56-6 Prophylaxis to Prevent First Episode of Opportunistic Infections in Adults and Adolescents

Pathogen	Indication	Preferred Therapies	Alternative Therapies
Coccidioidomycosis	■ New positive immunoglobulin (Ig)M or IgG serology in a disease-endemic area and CD4 count < 250 cells/mm^3 **(BIII)**	■ Fluconazole 400 mg PO daily **(BIII)**	
Histoplasmosis	■ Individuals with CD4 count ≤ 150 cells/mm^3 and high risk because of occupation or living in a hyperendemic community (prevalence >10 cases/100 patient years) **(BI)**	■ Itraconazole 200 mg PO daily **(BI)**	
Latent *Mycobacterium avium* infection (LTBI)	■ Positive screening test without evidence of active infection **(AI)** ■ Positive screening without treatment for prior active or latent infection **(AI)** ■ Close contact with a person with infectious tuberculosis, regardless of screening test result **(AI)**	■ Isoniazid (INH) 300 mg plus pyridoxine 25–50 mg PO daily for 9 months **(BII)**	■ Rifapentine (dose-adjusted based on weight) PO plus INH 900 mg PO plus pyridoxine 50 mg PO once weekly for 12 weeks **(AIII)**; only recommended for persons on raltegravir- or elvitegravir-based ART regimens; or ■ Rifampin 600 mg PO daily for 4 months **(BI)**; or ■ Consult with experts or public health authorities if the person was exposed to drug-resistant tuberculosis. **(AIII)**
Malaria	■ Persons traveling to disease-endemic regions	■ Recommendations for people with HIV are the same as those for uninfected individuals.	
Mycobacterium avium complex (MAC) disease	■ CD4 count < 50 cells/mm^3, as follows: ■ Not recommended if starting ART **(AII)** ■ Recommended if on ART but not fully suppressed **(AI)** ■ Rule out active disease before starting prophylaxis	■ Azithromycin 1,200 mg PO once weekly **(AI)** or ■ Clarithromycin 500 mg PO BID **(AI)** or ■ Azithromycin 600 mg twice weekly **(BIII)**	■ Rifabutin, dosing based on current ART regimen **(BI)** ■ Rule out active tuberculosis before starting rifabutin.
Pneumocystis pneumonia (PJP)	■ CD4 count < 200 cells/mm^3 **(AI)** or ■ CD4 < 14% **(BIII)** or ■ CD4 count ≥ 200 cells/mm^3 but < 250 cells/mm^3 if unable to initiate ART and monitor CD4 count every 3 months **(BIII)**	■ Trimethoprim/sulfamethoxazole (TMP-SMX) double-strength (DS) 1 tablet PO daily **(AI)**, or ■ TMP-SMX single-strength (SS) 1 tablet PO daily **(AI)**	■ TMP-SMX DS 1 tablet 3 times weekly **(BI)** or ■ Dapsone 100 mg PO daily or ■ Dapsone 50 mg PO BID or ■ Atovaquone 1,500 mg PO daily See the DHHS OI guidelines for additional alternatives (POIAAH, 2021).

Pathogen	Indication	Preferred Therapies	Alternative Therapies
Toxoplasma gondii encephalitis	■ *Toxoplasma* IgG positive with CD4 count < 100/mm^3 **(AII)** ■ Regimens effective against toxoplasmosis are also effective for *Pneumocystis jirovecii* pneumonia (PJP) prophylaxis.	■ TMP-SMX DS 1 tablet PO daily **(AII)**	■ TMP-SMX DS 1 tablet 3 times weekly **(BIII)** or ■ TMP-SMX 1 SS daily **(BIII)** or ■ Dapsone 50 mg PO daily plus pyrimethamine 50 mg and leucovorin 25 mg once weekly **(BI)** See the U.S. Department of Health and Human Services opportunistic infection guidelines (cited as table source) for additional alternatives.

- TMP-SMX DS once daily also confers protection against toxoplasmosis and many respiratory bacterial infections; lower dose also likely confers protection.
- Patients should be tested for glucose-6-phosphate dehydrogenase (G6PD) before administration of dapsone or primaquine. Alternative agents should be used in patients found to have G6PD deficiency.

Rating of Recommendations: A = Strong; B = Moderate; C = Optional.
Rating of Evidence: I = Data from randomized controlled trials; II = Data from well-designed nonrandomized trials or observational cohort studies with long-term clinical outcomes; III = Expert opinion.

Data from Panel on Opportunistic Infections in Adults and Adolescents with HIV. (2021). *Guidelines for the prevention and treatment of opportunistic infections in adults and adolescents with HIV: Recommendations from the Centers for Disease Control and Prevention, the National Institutes of Health, and the HIV Medicine Association of the Infectious Diseases Society of America.* U.S. Department of Health and Human Services. http://aidsinfo.nih.gov/contentfiles/lvguidelines/adult_oi.pdf

transmission of HIV in countries where access to HIV care and access to clean water for infant formula are available. All pregnant PLWH should be referred to a specialist in HIV perinatology for management. Early and consistent adherence to ART and maintenance of virologic suppression are crucial during pregnancy in order to prevent transmission to the fetus. DHHS has published specific guidelines on antiretroviral management during pregnancy, which include recommended ART regimens (Panel on Treatment of Pregnant Women with HIV Infection and Prevention of Perinatal Transmission, 2021). Many new parents struggle with ART adherence postpartum. Providers should assess adherence and offer support frequently.

3. ART regimen considerations in cisgender women: The goals of treatment for cisgender women are the same as for other adults and adolescents, and cisgender women generally respond well to ART. In recent years, concerns have emerged about cisgender women and significant weight gain associated with integrase inhibitors, particularly dolutegravir and bictegravir, which are components of the DHHS-recommended initial ART regimens (PAGAA, 2021). A pooled analysis of eight studies by Sax et al. (2020) found that although weight gain is common for all people after initiating antiretrovirals because of the return-to-health phenomenon, weight gain following initiation of integrase inhibitors appears heightened in cisgender women, particularly Black cisgender women. The mechanism is unknown. The analysis did not reveal significant elevations of hyperglycemia, blood pressure, or low-density lipoprotein (LDL) cholesterol among individuals with ≥10% weight gain compared to individuals gaining less weight at 96 weeks after ART initiation. At this time, the data are not clear enough to make specific recommendations about avoiding integrase inhibitors in cisgender women.

4. Postmenopausal cisgender women with HIV: Cisgender women with HIV have an increased incidence of osteopenia and osteoporosis at an earlier age and an increased risk of fragility fractures. Clinicians may want to consider avoiding ART regimens that are associated with a greater decrease in BMD when selecting a regimen for postmenopausal women (PAGAA, 2021). Attention should also be paid to antiretroviral drug–drug interactions when starting hormone replacement therapy to manage menopausal symptoms.

D. *Management considerations specific to transgender PLWH*
1. Terminology: *Transgender* refers to a "person whose gender identity or gender expression differs from the sex they were assigned at birth" (Office of AIDS Research, 2021). Some individuals may identify as gender-fluid or nonbinary, and terminology is evolving. Transgender people may participate in a variety of social, legal, psychological, and medical processes to affirm their gender identities. Some transgender individuals may pursue surgery or use hormones to enhance feminine or masculine physical characteristics—although some may not.

2. Addressing barriers to care: Transgender PLWH may experience difficulty engaging in HIV care and adhering to ART as a result of past negative experiences with healthcare providers; prioritization of gender-affirming health care over HIV management; concerns about drug–drug interactions with antiretrovirals; or the impacts of stigma and discrimination, such as unstable housing or poor access to monetary resources (PAGAA, 2021). To combat stigma, healthcare settings should affirm transgender patients through appropriate staff training, gender-inclusive registration materials and restroom facilities, and use of the patient's correct gender when addressing or referring to the patient. Gender-affirming hormone therapy and ART management should be integrated, and adherence to ART should never be presented as a prerequisite for obtaining hormone therapy (Poteat, 2016). Clinicians without experience in providing hormone therapy to transgender individuals should consult with providers who have clinical expertise in this area. Clinicians caring for transgender PLWH should make use of community agencies providing support services for transgender individuals and refer patients to those agencies.
   a. Drug–drug interactions and gender-affirming hormones: In general, there are no significant drug–drug interactions between sex hormones and antiretroviral agents. Interactions that do exist, such as with certain nonnucleoside reverse transcriptase inhibitors, protease inhibitors, and pharmacokinetic enhancers, can usually be managed by adjusting the hormone dose. Transgender people on hormone therapy should be reassured that ART will not affect their development of desired sex characteristics.
3. Healthcare maintenance: Preventive healthcare for transgender PLWH is based on health risks and sex assigned at birth. In transgender women, digital rectal examinations and prostate cancer screening may be indicated based on age, other risk factors, and shared decision making by the provider and patient. In transgender men, pelvic examination, cervical Pap smear, and mammography based on recommended guidelines should be provided.

E. *Prevention of new infections*
1. Treatment as prevention: PLWH have a central role in the prevention of HIV transmission at the individual and population levels. All PLWH should be counseled that there is *zero risk* of sexual HIV transmission if they achieve and maintain viral suppression (defined as a VL < 200 copies/mL), which is also known as *treatment as prevention*. Four key prevention studies—HTPN 052, Opposites Attract, PARTNER 1, and PARTNER 2—have provided solid scientific support for treatment as prevention for both heterosexual and homosexual sex (Bavinton et al., 2018; Cohen et al., 2016; Rodger et al., 2019). There were no linked transmissions of HIV among the 146,535 total sex acts between serodifferent individuals (one partner with HIV and the other without) in these four studies.
2. Undetectable = Untransmittable: The Prevention Access Campaign has created the public health initiative "Undetectable = Untransmittable" or "U=U" to promote the understanding of treatment as prevention and thereby reduce HIV stigma and empower PLWH. The campaign is now endorsed by the CDC, the National Institutes of Health, and over 1,025 other HIV organizations from 102 countries (Eisinger et al., 2019; McCray, 2019; Prevention Access Campaign, 2021; World Health Organization, 2018). U=U applies to sexual HIV transmission risk only.
3. Role of the provider in supporting HIV prevention: A consortium of U.S. governmental and nonprofit HIV service organizations has produced recommendations for HIV prevention in clinical care settings with PLWH (CDC et al., 2014). These recommendations encourage providers to consider contextual issues—individual, structural, social, ethical, and legal—when working with PLWH. In conversations with patients about HIV prevention, providers should be sensitive, respectful, and culturally appropriate and empower patients to engage in HIV prevention without blaming or shaming. Providers must acknowledge that patients have the right and responsibility to make HIV prevention decisions for themselves.

   Above all, providers must support patients in treatment adherence and engagement in care in order to achieve viral suppression. Support includes linking patients to care; providing referrals for services such as food assistance, housing, transportation to medical visits, and medication adherence counseling; and development of healthcare systems, such as the medical home model, that provide patients with wraparound care.

   Providers should discuss HIV risk behaviors with patients at every visit. Through education, counseling, and shared decision making, providers can support PLWH in setting realistic goals for HIV prevention using evidence-based risk-reduction strategies. Providers should offer specific healthcare services that reduce the risk of HIV transmission, such as condom distribution, referrals to syringe exchanges, screening for sexually transmitted infections, family planning care, and referral to treatment for substance use or psychiatric illness.
4. Legal concerns: PLWH often have questions and fears regarding the legal ramifications of their HIV serostatus. Laws regarding HIV serostatus disclosure vary by state. Clinicians can become familiar with these laws at the website of the Center for HIV Law and Policy (https://www.hivlawandpolicy.org).

F. *Patient education*

HIV education should be conducted over several visits to provide basic information on HIV treatment, prevention of secondary transmission, and indications for ART. It is important to emphasize that HIV is a chronic, manageable disease and that improved quality of life can be expected if individuals are engaged in care and motivated to take ART. There are several excellent websites that can provide resources and guidance in HIV/AIDS patient and provider education. See the Resources section.

VII. Resources

A. *General information*
1. AIDS.gov: Gateway for HIV/AIDS information and resources from the U.S. federal government, aimed at both clinicians and patients. https//aids.gov
2. Centers for Disease Control and Prevention's HIV/AIDS Website: Fact-based information, statistical data, education, prevention tools, and clinician resources. https://www.cdc.gov/hiv/default.html
3. Henry J. Kaiser Family Foundation's HIV/AIDS website: Policy analysis, global and national HIV/AIDS data, and links to patient resources, including Spanish-language patient information. https://www.kff.org/hivaids

B. *Clinical management*
1. AIDS*info*: Portal for HIV/AIDS clinical guidelines, education materials, and research information from the DHHS. https://hivinfo.nih.gov
2. AIDS Education and Training Center (AETC): National network of HIV experts who provide guidelines, training materials, webinars, clinical consultation, and technical assistance for healthcare providers caring for PLWH. Administered by the Ryan White HIV/AIDS Program of the Human Resources and Services Administration. https://aidsetc.org
3. Human Resources and Services Administration HIV/AIDS Bureau: The government agency, part of the DHHS, that is responsible for administering the Ryan White Care Program, the source of federal funding for HIV medical care, treatment, and support services. https://hab.hrsa.gov
4. National Clinician Consultation Center: Rapid phone and online consultation on HIV/AIDS management, PEP, PrEP, perinatal HIV/AIDS, and HIV testing from HIV-expert clinicians at the University of California, San Francisco. Consultation services available nationwide. https://nccc.ucsf.edu
5. National HIV Curriculum: Educational site with HIV prevention and management learning modules from the University of Washington and the AETC. Free continuing education available. https://www.hiv.uw.edu
6. Center of Excellence for Transgender Health: Resources and guidelines for transgender patient care from the University of California, San Francisco. https://prevention.ucsf.edu/transhealth
7. HIVE: Preconception and perinatal HIV/AIDS resources for patients, their partners, and healthcare providers. https://hiveonline.org

C. *HIV medications*
1. University of Liverpool HIV Drug Interactions Portal: Simple, searchable database of HIV-drug interactions. https://hiv-druginteractions.org
2. Stanford University HIV Drug Resistance Database: Resource for analyzing HIV-drug resistance. https://hivdb.stanford.edu

D. *Patient education and advocacy*
1. AVERT.org: Large online compendium of HIV/AIDS education materials, produced by AVERT, an international HIV/AIDS charity based in the United Kingdom. https://www.avert.org
2. Prevention Access Campaign: Health equity initiative with news, information, and resources for the Undetectable=Untransmittable (U=U) campaign. https://preventionaccess.org
3. HIV Nightline: Free, confidential emotional support and information on HIV/AIDS. Open nightly from 5 p.m. to 5 a.m. Pacific Standard Time. Nationwide toll-free: 1-800-628-9240. https://www.sfsuicide.org/hotlines
4. Center for HIV Law and Policy: Comprehensive resource for legal and policy issues related to HIV, including individual state criminalization laws. https://www.hivlawandpolicy.org

E. *Consumer media*
1. *The Body*: Online HIV resource featuring information, news, advocacy, and personal perspectives. Features a Spanish-language version. https://www.thebody.com
2. *Positively Aware*: Glossy print and online magazine covering HIV news and advocacy. Includes patient-friendly annual HIV and HCV drug guides. https://www.positivelyaware.com
3. *POZ*: Glossy print and online magazine covering the lives people living with HIV. Includes news, personal profiles, investigative features, and online communities. https://www.poz.com

F. *Professional organizations*
1. Association of Nurses in AIDS Care (ANAC): National organization of nurses dedicated to HIV/AIDS advocacy and patient care. Offers HIV specialty credentialing, professional development, networking, and an annual national conference. Publishes the *Journal of the Association of Nurses in AIDS Care*. https://www.nursesinaidscare.org
2. American Academy of HIV Medicine (AAHIVM): National organization for HIV care providers, offering membership and HIV specialty credentialing to advanced practice nurses. Publishes *HIV Specialist* magazine. https://aahivm.org

References

Adimora, A. A., Ramirez, C., Schoenbach, V. J., & Cohen, M. S. (2014). Policies and politics that promote HIV infection in the Southern United States. *AIDS, 28*(10), 1393–1397. doi:10.1097/qad.0000000000000225

American Association for the Study of Liver Diseases & Infectious Diseases Society of America. (2021). *HCV guidance: Recommendations for testing, managing, and treating hepatitis C.* https://www.hcvguidelines.org/

American Nurses Association. (2015). *Code of ethics for nurses with interpretive statements.* https://www.nursingworld.org/coe-view-only

Antiretroviral Therapy Cohort Collaboration (2017). Survival of HIV-positive patients starting antiretroviral therapy between 1996 and 2013: A collaborative analysis of cohort studies. *The Lancet HIV, 4*(8), e349–e356. doi:10.1016/S2352-3018(17)30066-8

Arnett, D. K., Blumenthal, R. S., Albert, M. A., Buroker, A. B., Goldberger, Z. D., Hahn, E. J., Himmelfarb, C. D., Khera, A., Lloyd-Jones, D., McEvoy, J. W., Michos, E. D., Miedema, M. D., Muñoz, D., Smith, S. C., Jr. Virani, S. S., Williams, K. A., Sr, Yeboah, J., & Ziaeian, B. (2019). 2019 ACC/AHA guideline on the primary prevention of cardiovascular disease: A report of the American College of Cardiology/American Heart Association Task Force on Clinical Practice Guidelines. *Circulation, 140*(11), e596–e646. doi:10.1161/CIR.0000000000000678

Bavinton, B. R., Pinto, A. N., Phanuphak, N., Grinsztejn, B., Prestage, G. P., Zablotska-Manos, I. B., Jin, F., Fairley, C. K., Moore, R., Roth, N., Bloch, M., Pell, C., McNulty, A. M., Baker, D., Hoy, J., Tee, B. K., Templeton, D. J., Cooper, D. A., Emery, S., ... Opposites Attract Study Group. (2018). Viral suppression and HIV transmission in serodiscordant male couples: An international, prospective, observational, cohort study. *The Lancet HIV, 5*(8), e438–e447. doi:10.1016/S2352-3018(18)30132-2

Bourgi, K., Jenkins, C. A., Rebeiro, P. F., Palella, F., Moore, R. D., Altoff, K. N., Gill, J., Rabkin, C. S., Gange, S. J., Horberg, M. A., Margolick, J., Li, J., Wong, C., Willig, A., Lima, V. D., Crane, H., Thorne, J., Silverberg, M., Kirk, G., ... North American AIDS Cohort Collaboration on Research and Design (NA-ACCORD). (2020). Weight gain among treatment-naïve persons with HIV starting integrase inhibitors compared to non-nucleoside reverse transcriptase inhibitors or protease inhibitors in a large observational cohort in the United States and Canada. *Journal of the International AIDS Society, 23*(4), e25484. doi:10.1002/jia2.25484

Branson, B. M., Handsfield, H. H., Lampe, M. A., Janssen, R. S., Taylor, A. W., Lyss, S. B., Clark, J. E., & Centers for Disease Control and Prevention (CDC) (2006). Revised recommendations for HIV testing of adults, adolescents, and pregnant women in health-care settings. *MMWR. Recommendations and reports: Morbidity and mortality weekly report. Recommendations and reports, 55*(RR-14), 1–CE4.

Branson, B. M., Owen, S. M., Wesolowski, L. G., Bennett, B., Werner, B. G., Wroblewski, K. E., & Pentella, M. A. (2014, June 27). *Laboratory testing for the diagnosis of HIV infection: Updated recommendations.* Centers for Disease Control and Prevention and Association of Public Health Laboratories. https://stacks.cdc.gov/view/cdc/23447

Carr, A., Grund, B., Schwartz, A. V., Avihingsanon, A., Badal-Faesen, S., Bernadino, J. I., Estrada, V., La Rosa, A., Mallon, P., Pujari, S., White, D., Wyman Engen, N., Ensrud, K., Hoy, J. F., & International Network for Strategic Initiatives in Global HIV Trials START Bone Mineral Density Substudy Group. (2020). The rate of bone loss slows after 1-2 years of initial antiretroviral therapy: Final results of the Strategic Timing of Antiretroviral Therapy (START) bone mineral density substudy. *HIV Medicine, 21*(1), 64–70. doi:10.1111/hiv.12796

Centers for Disease Control and Prevention. (1981). Pneumocystis pneumonia—Los Angeles. *Morbidity and Mortality Weekly Report, 30*(21), 250–251.

Centers for Disease Control and Prevention. (2014). Revised surveillance case definition for HIV infection—United States, 2014. *Morbidity and Mortality Weekly Report, 63*(3), 1–10. http://www.cdc.gov/mmwr/pdf/rr/rr6303.pdf

Centers for Disease Control and Prevention. (2019). *Understanding the HIV care continuum* [Fact sheet]. https://www.cdc.gov/hiv/pdf/library/factsheets/cdc-hiv-care-continuum.pdf

Centers for Disease Control and Prevention. (2020a). *HIV and older adults* [Fact sheet]. https://www.cdc.gov/hiv/pdf/group/age/olderamericans/cdc-hiv-older-americans.pdf

Centers for Disease Control and Prevention. (2020b). *HIV transmission.* https://www.cdc.gov/hiv/basics/transmission.html

Centers for Disease Control and Prevention. (2020c). *National diabetes statistics report, 2020.* https://www.cdc.gov/diabetes/pdfs/data/statistics/national-diabetes-statistics-report.pdf

Centers for Disease Control and Prevention. (2021a). *HIV surveillance report, 2019.* https://www.cdc.gov/hiv/pdf/library/reports/surveillance/cdc-hiv-surveillance-report-2018-updated-vol-32.pdf

Centers for Disease Control and Prevention. (2021b). *Preexposure prophylaxis for the prevention of HIV infection in the United States—2021 update: A clinical practice guideline.* https://www.cdc.gov/hiv/pdf/risk/prep/cdc-hiv-prep-guidelines-2021.pdf

Centers for Disease Control and Prevention, Health Resources and Services Administration, National Institutes of Health, American Academy of HIV Medicine, Association of Nurses in AIDS Care, International Association of Providers of AIDS Care, the National Minority AIDS Council, & Urban Coalition for HIV/AIDS Prevention Services. (2014). *Recommendations for HIV prevention with adults and adolescents with HIV in the United States, 2014.* http://stacks.cdc.gov/view/cdc/26062

Cohen, M. S., Chen, Y. Q., McCauley, M., Gamble, T., Hosseinipour, M. C., Kumarasamy, N., Hakim, J. G., Kumwenda, J., Grinsztejn, B., Pilotto, J. H., Godbole, S. V., Chariyalertsak, S., Santos, B. R., Mayer, K. H., Hoffman, I. F., Eshleman, S. H., Piwowar-Manning, E., Cottle, L., Zhang, X. C., ... HPTN 052 Study Team. (2016). Antiretroviral therapy for the prevention of HIV-1 transmission. *New England Journal of Medicine, 375*(9), 830–839. doi:10.1056/NEJMoa1600693

Connor, E. M., Sperling, R. S., Gelber, R., Kiselev, P., Scott, G., O'Sullivan, M. J., VanDyke, R., Bey, M., Shearer, W., & Jacobson, R. L. (1994). Reduction of maternal-infant transmission of human immunodeficiency virus type 1 with zidovudine treatment. Pediatric AIDS Clinical Trials Group Protocol 076 Study Group. *The New England Journal of Medicine, 331*(18), 1173–1180. doi:10.1056/NEJM199411033311801

DiNenno, E. A., Prejean, J., Irwin, K., Delaney, K. P., Bowles, K., Martin, T., Tailor, A., Dumitru, G., Mullins, M. M., Hutchinson, A. B., & Lansky, A. (2017). Recommendations for HIV screening of gay, bisexual, and other men who have sex with men—United States, 2017. *Morbidity and Mortality Weekly Report, 66*(31), 830–832. doi:10.15585/mmwr.mm6631a3

Eisinger, R. W., Dieffenbach, C. W., & Fauci, A. S. (2019). HIV viral load and transmissibility of HIV infection: Undetectable equals untransmittable. *JAMA, 321*(5), 451–452. doi:10.1001/jama.2018.21167

Fazeli, P. L., Casaletto, K. B., Paolillo, E., Moore, R. C., Moore, D. J., & The HNRP Group. (2017). Screening for neurocognitive impairment in HIV-positive adults aged 50 years and older: Montreal Cognitive Assessment relates to self-reported and clinician-rated everyday functioning. *Journal of Clinical and Experimental Neuropsychology*, 39(9), 842–853. doi:10.1080/13803395.2016.1273319

Gonciulea, A., Wang, R., Althoff, K. N., Palella, F. J., Lake, J., Kingsley, L. A., & Brown, T. T. (2017). An increased rate of fracture occurs a decade earlier in HIV+ compared with HIV– men. *AIDS*, 31(10), 1435–1443. doi:10.1097/QAD.0000000000001493

Hess, K. L., Hu, X., Lansky, A., Mermin, J., & Hall, H. I. (2017). Lifetime risk of a diagnosis of HIV infection in the United States. *Annals of Epidemiology*, 27(4), 238–243. doi:10.1016/j.annepidem.2017.02.003

Hønge, B. L., Petersen, M. S., Jespersen, S., Medina, C., Té, D., Kjerulff, B., Engell-Sørensen, T., Madsen, T., Laursen, A. L., Wejse, C., Krarup, H., Møller, B. K., Erikstrup, C., & Bissau HIV Cohort Study Group. (2019). T-cell and B-cell perturbations identify distinct differences in HIV-2 compared with HIV-1-induced immunodeficiency. *AIDS (London, England)*, 33(7), 1131–1141. doi:10.1097/QAD.0000000000002184

Hsu, R., Brunet, L., Fusco, J. S., Mounzer, K., Vannappagari, V., Henegar, C. E., Van Wyk, J., Curtis, L., Lo, J., & Fusco, G. P. (2021). Incident type 2 diabetes mellitus after initiation of common HIV antiretroviral drugs. *AIDS*, 35(1), 81–90. doi:10.1097/QAD.0000000000002718

Hsue, P. Y. (2019). Mechanisms of cardiovascular disease in the setting of HIV infection. *Canadian Journal of Cardiology*, 35(3), 238–248. doi:10.1016/j.cjca.2018.12.024

Kaiser Family Foundation. (2009). *Survey brief: Views and experiences with HIV testing in the U.S.* https://www.kff.org/wp-content/uploads/2013/01/7926.pdf

Kaiser Family Foundation. (2021). *Status of state Medicaid expansion decisions* [Interactive online map]. https://www.kff.org/medicaid/issue-brief/status-of-state-medicaid-expansion-decisions-interactive-map/

Li, Z., Purcell, D. W., Sansom, S. L., Hayes, D., & Hall, H. I. (2019). Vital signs: HIV transmission along the continuum of care—United States, 2016. *Morbidity and Mortal Weekly Report*, 68(11), 267–272. doi:10.15585/mmwr.mm6811e1

Lucas, G. M., Ross, M. J., Stock, P. G., Shlipak, M. G., Wyatt, C. M., Gupta, S. K., Atta, M. G., Wools-Kaloustian, K. K., Pham, P. A., Bruggeman, L. A., Lennox, J. L., Ray, P. E., Kalayjian, R. C., & HIV Medicine Association of the Infectious Diseases Society of America. (2014). Clinical practice guideline for the management of chronic kidney disease in patients infected with HIV: 2014 update by the HIV Medicine Association of the Infectious Diseases Society of America. *Clinical Infectious Diseases*, 59(9), e96–e138. doi:10.1093/cid/ciu617

Marcus, J. L., Leyden, W., Anderson, A. N., Hechter, R., Horberg, M. A., Haihong, H., Lam, J. O., Towner, W. J., Yuan, Q., & Silverberg, M. J. (2020, March 8–11). *Increased overall life expectancy but not comorbidity-free years for people with HIV* [Abstract]. Conference on Retroviruses and Opportunistic Infections, Boston, Massachusetts, United States. https://www.croiconference.org/abstract/increased-overall-life-expectancy-but-not-comorbidity-free-years-for-people-with-hiv

Marzinke, M. A., Grinsztejn, B., Fogel, J. M., Piwowar-Manning, E., Li, M., Weng, L., McCauley, M., Cummings, V., Ahmed, S., Haines, C. D., Bushman, L. R., Petropoulos, C., Persaud, D., Adeyeye, A., Kofron, R., Rinehart, A., St Clair, M., Rooney, J. F., Pryluka, D., Coelho, L., ... Eshleman, S. H. (2021). Characterization of human immunodeficiency virus (HIV) infection in cisgender men and transgender women who have sex with men receiving injectable cabotegravir for HIV prevention: HPTN 083. *Journal of Infectious Diseases*, 224(9), 1581–1592. doi:10.1093/infdis/jiab152

McCray, E. (2019, August 30). *Dear health department and CBO grantees* [Open letter]. https://58b1608b-fe15-46bb-818a-cd15168c0910.filesusr.com/ugd/de0404_966c29f826d4481abf8bba0690bdd439.pdf

Monroe, A. K., Glesby, M. J., & Brown, T. (2015). Diagnosing and managing diabetes in HIV-infected patients: Current concepts. *Clinical Infectious Diseases*, 60(3), 453–462. doi:10.1093/cid/ciu779

Narla, V. A. (2021). Sudden cardiac death in HIV-infected patients: A contemporary review. *Clinical Cardiology*, 44(3), 316–321. doi:10.1002/clc.23568

Office of AIDS Research. (2021). *Glossary of HIV/AIDS-related terms 2021* (9th ed.). U.S. Department of Health and Human Services. https://clinicalinfo.hiv.gov/sites/default/files/glossary/Glossary-English_HIVinfo.pdf

Office of Disease Prevention and Health Promotion. (n.d.). Increase knowledge of HIV status— HIV02. *Healthy People 2030*. U.S. Department of Health and Human Services. https://health.gov/healthypeople/objectives-and-data/browse-objectives/sexually-transmitted-infections/increase-knowledge-hiv-status-hiv-02

Office of Infectious Disease and HIV/AIDS Policy. (2021, June 2). *Ending the HIV epidemic: About ending the HIV epidemic in the U.S.: Overview*. U.S. Department of Health and Human Services. https://www.hiv.gov/federal-response/ending-the-hiv-epidemic/overview

Panel on Antiretroviral Guidelines for Adults and Adolescents. (2021). *Guidelines for the use of antiretroviral agents in HIV-1-infected adults and adolescents*. U.S. Department of Health and Human Services. https://clinicalinfo.hiv.gov/sites/default/files/guidelines/documents/AdultandAdolescentGL.pdf

Panel on Opportunistic Infections in Adults and Adolescents With HIV. (2021). *Guidelines for the prevention and treatment of opportunistic infections in adults and adolescents with HIV: Recommendations from the Centers for Disease Control and Prevention, the National Institutes of Health, and the HIV Medicine Association of the Infectious Diseases Society of America*. U.S. Department of Health and Human Services. http://aidsinfo.nih.gov/contentfiles/lvguidelines/adult_oi.pdf

Panel on Treatment of Pregnant Women with HIV Infection and Prevention of Perinatal Transmission. (2021). *Recommendations for the use of antiretroviral drugs in pregnant women with HIV infection and interventions to reduce perinatal HIV transmission in the United States*. U.S. Department of Health and Human Services. https://clinicalinfo.hiv.gov/en/guidelines/perinatal

Park, L. S., Hernández-Ramírez, R. U., Silverberg, M. J., Crothers, K., & Dubrow, R. (2016). Prevalence of non-HIV cancer risk factors in persons living with HIV/AIDS: A meta-analysis. *AIDS*, 30(2), 273–291. doi:10.1097/QAD.0000000000000922

Patel, P., Borkowf, C. B., Brooks, J. T., Lasry, A., Lansky, A., & Mermin, J. (2014). Estimating per-act HIV transmission risk: A systematic review. *AIDS*, 28(10), 1509–1519. doi:10.1097/QAD.0000000000000298

Pérez, P. S., Romaniuk, M. A., Duette, G. A., Zhao, Z., Huang, Y., Martin-Jaular, L., Witwer, K. W., Théry, C., & Ostrowski, M. (2019). Extracellular vesicles and chronic inflammation during HIV infection. *Journal of Extracellular Vesicles*, 8(1), 1687275. doi:10.1080/20013078.2019.1687275

Peters, P. J., Pontones, P., Hoover, K. W., Patel, M. R., Galang, R. R., Shields, J., Blosser, S. J., Spiller, M. W., Combs, B., Switzer, W. M.,

Conrad, C., Gentry, J., Khudyakov, Y., Waterhouse, D., Owen, S. M., Chapman, E., Roseberry, J. C., McCants, V., Weidle, P. J., ... Indiana HIV Outbreak Investigation Team. (2016). HIV infection linked to injection use of oxymorphone in Indiana, 2014–2015. *New England Journal of Medicine, 375*(3), 229–239. doi:10.1056/NEJMoa1515195

Poteat, T. (2016, June 17). *Transgender health and HIV.* UCSF Transgender Care and Treatment Guidelines. https://transcare.ucsf.edu/guidelines/hiv

Pretty, I. A., Anderson, G. S., & Sweet, D. J. (1999). Human bites and the risk of human immunodeficiency virus transmission. *American Journal of Forensic Medical Pathology, 20*(3), 232–239. doi:10.1097/00000433-199909000-00003

Prevention Access Campaign. (2021). *Risk of sexual transmission of HIV from a person living with HIV who has an undetectable viral load: Messaging primer & consensus statement.* https://www.preventionaccess.org/consensus

Rodger, A. J., Cambiano, V., Bruun, T., Vernazza, P., Collins, S., Degen, O., Corbelli, G. M., Estrada, V., Geretti, A. M., Beloukas, A., Raben, D., Coll, P., Antinori, A., Nwokolo, N., Rieger, A., Prins, J. M., Blaxhult, A., Weber, R., Van Eeden, A., ... PARTNER Study Group. (2019). Risk of HIV transmission through condomless sex in serodifferent gay couples with the HIV-positive partner taking suppressive antiretroviral therapy (PARTNER): Final results of a.m.lticentre, prospective, observational study. *Lancet, 393*(10189), 2428–2438. doi:10.1016/S0140-6736(19)30418-0

Sax, P. E., Erlandson, K. M., Lake, J. E., Mccomsey, G. A., Orkin, C., Esser, S., Brown, T. T., Rockstroh, J. K., Wei, X., Carter, C. C., Zhong, L., Brainard, D. M., Melbourne, K., Das, M., Stellbrink, H. J., Post, F. A., Waters, L., & Koethe, J. R. (2020). Weight gain following initiation of antiretroviral therapy: Risk factors in randomized comparative clinical trials. *Clinical Infectious Diseases, 71*(6), 1379–1389. doi:10.1093/cid/ciz999

Sevelius, J. M., Keatley, J., & Gutierrez-Mock, L. (2011). HIV/AIDS programming in the United States: Considerations affecting transgender women and girls. *Women's Health Issues, 21*(Suppl. 6), S278–S282. doi:10.1016/j.whi.2011.08.001

Strategies for Management of Antiretroviral Therapy (SMART) Study Group, El-Sadr, W. M., Lundgren, J., Neaton, J. D., Gordin, F., Abrams, D., Arduino, R. C., Babiker, A., Burman, W., Clumeck, N., Cohen, C. J., Cohn, D., Cooper, D., Darbyshire, J., Emery, S., Fätkenheuer, G., Gazzard, B., Grund, B., Hoy, J., ... Rappoport, C. (2006). CD4+ count-guided interruption of antiretroviral treatment. *New England Journal of Medicine, 355*(22), 2283–2296. doi:10.1056/NEJMoa062360

Sung, J. M., & Margolis, D. M. (2018). HIV persistence on antiretroviral therapy and barriers to a cure. *Advances in Experimental Medicine and Biology, 1075,* 165–185. doi:10.1007/978-981-13-0484-2_7

Thompson, M. A., Horberg, M. A., Agwu, A. L., Colasanti, J. A., Jain, M. K., Short, W. R., Singh, T., & Aberg, J. A. (2020). Primary care guidance for persons with human immunodeficiency virus: 2020 update by the HIV Medicine Association of the Infectious Diseases Society of America. *Clinical Infectious Diseases, 73*(11), e3572–e3605. doi:10.1093/cid/ciaa1391

Thomsen, M. T., Wiegandt, Y. L., Gelpi, M., Knudsen, A. D., Fuchs, A., Sigvardsen, P. E., Kühl, J. T., Nordestgaard, B., Køber, L., Lundgren, J., Hansen, A. E., Kofoed, K. F., Jensen, J. B., & Nielsen, S. D. (2020). Prevalence of and risk factors for low bone mineral density assessed by quantitative computed tomography in people living with HIV and uninfected controls. *Journal of Acquired Immune Deficiency Syndromes, 83*(2), 165–172. doi:10.1097/QAI.0000000000002245

United Nations Joint Programme on HIV/AIDS. (2021). *Fact sheet 2021: Preliminary UNAIDS 2021 epidemiological estimates.* https://www.unaids.org/sites/default/files/media_asset/UNAIDS_FactSheet_en.pdf

U.S. Preventive Services Task Force, Owens, D. K., Davidson, K. W., Krist, A. H., Barry, M. J., Cabana, M., Caughey, A. B., Curry, S. J., Doubeni, C. A., Epling, J. W., Jr. Kubik, M., Landefeld, C. S., Mangione, C. M., Pbert, L., Silverstein, M., Simon, M. A., Tseng, C. W., & Wong, J. B. (2019). Screening for HIV infection: US Preventive Services Task Force recommendation statement. *JAMA, 321*(23), 2326–2336. doi:10.1001/jama.2019.6587

Valera, P., Chang, Y., & Lian, Z. (2017). HIV risk inside U.S. prisons: A systematic review of risk reduction interventions conducted in U.S. prisons. *AIDS Care, 29*(8), 943–952. doi:10.1080/09540121.2016.1271102

Workowski, K. A., Bachmann, L. H., Chan, P. A., Johnston, C. M., Muzny, C. A., Park, I., Reno, H., Zenilman, J. M., & Bolan, G. A. (2021). Sexually Transmitted Infections Treatment Guidelines, 2021. *MMWR. Recommendations and reports : Morbidity and mortality weekly report. Recommendations and reports, 70*(4), 1–187. doi:10.15585/mmwr.rr7004a1

World Health Organization. (2018, 20 July). *Viral suppression for HIV treatment success and prevention of sexual transmission of HIV* [Departmental news]. https://www.who.int/news/item/20-07-2018-viral-suppression-for-hiv-treatment-success-and-prevention-of-sexual-transmission-of-hiv

Wyatt, C. M. (2017). Kidney disease and HIV infection. *Topics in Antiviral Medicine, 25*(1), 13–16.

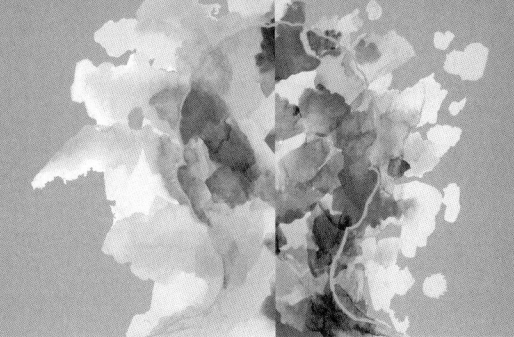

CHAPTER 57

Hypertension

Sarah Goodman

I. Introduction and definition

Hypertension (HTN) is one of the most common conditions seen in primary care and is also considered one of the most significant preventable causes of disease and death, primarily because of its association with heart disease, stroke, and renal failure (James et al., 2014). Most patients with HTN have additional risk factors, including dyslipidemias, glucose intolerance or diabetes, a family history of early cardiovascular events, higher body weight, and/or cigarette smoking (Weber et al., 2014). In some communities, fewer than 50% of all patients with HTN have adequately controlled blood pressure (BP) (Weber et al., 2014).

A. Prevalence

The Centers for Disease Control and Prevention (CDC) reported that the prevalence of HTN in 2017–2018 among U.S. adults aged 18 and over was approximately 45.4%, with higher rates among men (51.0%) compared with women (39.7%) (CDC, 2020). The prevalence does increase with age and is highest among older adults and among non-Hispanic Black adults at 57.1% (CDC, 2020).

The World Health Organization (WHO, 2021) considers HTN to be the main attributable risk factor for death due to cardiovascular disease (CVD) worldwide. According to a 2021 WHO report, 32% of all global deaths were due to CVD. The prevalence of HTN is greatest in middle- and low-income countries with larger populations and poorer access to health care (WHO, 2013).

B. Definition

HTN is a continuous and independent risk factor for CVD, and the presence of additional risk factors (elevated total cholesterol, high-density lipoprotein cholesterol < 35, smoking, diabetes, and left ventricular hypertrophy are the most significant) compounds the risk from HTN. Elevated systolic BP (SBP) and diastolic BP (DBP) are each considered important risk factors.

According to the 2017 definitions published by the American College of Cardiology/American Health Association (ACC/AHA), the definition of HTN is a BP of ≥130 mm Hg systolic or ≥80 mm Hg diastolic. The diagnosis must be made using an average of ≥2 BP readings on ≥2 occasions (ACC, 2018). Diastolic HTN is a stronger cardiovascular risk factor and more common before the age of 50 than systolic HTN. However, systolic HTN is more common after the age of 50 than diastolic HTN. DBP may actually decrease with aging, whereas SBP increases with aging. This is most likely a result of the progressive stiffening of the arterial circulation that occurs with aging (Weber et al., 2014).

C. Classification and treatment goal recommendations

Over time, the recommendations for both diagnosing and treating HTN have varied. In 2004, the seventh report of the Joint National Committee (JNC) on Prevention, Detection, Evaluation, and Treatment of High Blood Pressure (JNC 7) categorized BP as follows: (1) normal (<120 systolic and <80 diastolic), (2) pre-HTN (120–139 systolic or 80–89 diastolic), (3) HTN stage 1 (140–159 systolic or 90–99 diastolic, and (4) HTN stage 2 (≥160 systolic or ≥100 diastolic). The eighth JNC report in 2014 specifically focused on evidence to support the need to initiate antihypertensive pharmacologic therapy at specific BP thresholds and whether there is evidence to support adjusting pharmacologic treatment to specified BP goals (James et al., 2014).

In 2017, the ACC/AHA published guidelines lowered the definition of HTN to ≥130/≥80 mm Hg because of growing evidence of the direct relationship between BP and cardiovascular risk (ACC, 2021). The 2017 ACC/AHA categorized BP as follows: (1) normal BP, (2) elevated BP, (3) HTN stage 1, and (4) HTN stage 2 (ACC, 2021) (**Table 57-1**). The designation of "elevated BP" is meant to identify those individuals at high risk of developing frank HTN who may benefit from adapting lifestyle modifications that either lower

Table 57-1 2017 American College of Cardiology/American Health Association (ACC/AHA) Guidelines for High Blood Pressure in Adults

BP Category	Pressure Ranges	Recommendations
Normal BP	<120/<80 mm Hg	Promote healthy lifestyle; reassess BP annually.
Elevated BP	120–129/<80 mm Hg	Start with nonpharmacologic therapy; reassess BP in 3–6 months.
Stage 1 hypertension	130–139/80–89 mm Hg	**ASCVD or 10-year CVD risk ≥ 10%:** Start with both nonpharmacologic and pharmacologic therapy. Reassess BP in 1 month. If at goal, reassess every 3–6 months. If not at goal, assess for adherence and consider intensification of therapy. **No ASCVD and 10-year CVD risk < 10%:** Start with nonpharmacologic therapy; reassess BP in 3–6 months. If not at goal, consider initiation of pharmacologic therapy.
Stage 2 hypertension	≥140/≥90 mm Hg	Start with both nonpharmacologic and pharmacologic therapy. Reassess BP in 1 month. If at goal, reassess every 3–6 months. If not at goal, assess for adherence and consider intensification of therapy.

ASCVD, atherosclerotic cardiovascular disease; *BP*, blood pressure; *CVD*, cardiovascular disease.

© 2021 American College of Cardiology Foundation; *New guidance on blood pressure management in low-risk adults with stage 1 hypertension*. Retrieved from https://www.acc.org/latest-in-cardiology/articles/2021/06/21/13/05/new-guidance-on-bp-manage-ment-in-low-risk-adults-with-stage-1-htn#:~:text=The%202017%20AHA%2FACC%20guidelines,%2F%3C80%20mm%20Hg).

BP or slow the rate of progression (ACC, 2018). This stage should be viewed as a warning and an incentive for care providers to strongly counsel these individuals regarding lifestyle modifications.

In 2021, the AHA released new guidance regarding the management of stage 1 HTN with a low 10-year risk for atherosclerotic cardiovascular disease (ASCVD) compared to those with ASCVD or a high 10-year CVD risk. The ASCVD Risk Calculator is published by the ACC/AHA and determines the 10-year risk of heart disease or stroke for adult patients (Goff et al., 2014). Even for someone with a low ASCVD risk score, the ACC/AHA guidelines recognize the potential long-term effects of HTN, hence the additions to the BP guidelines in 2021 (ACC, 2021).

Of note, "white coat" HTN (elevated BP in a clinical setting but normal BP at home) and masked HTN (elevated BP at home, but normal in a clinical setting) are also associated with increased risk of ASCVD, although not as high as the risk with sustained HTN (Tientcheu et al., 2015).

II. Database (may include but is not limited to)
A. *Subjective*
  1. Most patients are asymptomatic.
     a. Although most patients are asymptomatic, some may experience headaches, dizziness, blurred vision, tinnitus, chest pain, shortness of breath, nausea, vomiting, extremity swelling, or anxiety, which may be unrelated to actual elevated BP or be caused by end-organ damage.
  2. The following symptoms suggest secondary causes for HTN.
     a. Muscle cramps, polyuria, weakness, and excessive thirst: primary aldosteronism (rare)
     b. Headache, pallor, palpitations, sweating, and flushing: pheochromocytoma (very rare)
     c. Hirsutism, easy bruising, swollen face, and symptoms of diabetes mellitus: Cushing syndrome (rare)
     d. Severe chest pain radiating to back: aortic dissection or aneurysm (common)
     e. Claudication: coarctation of aorta (rare to be found late in life)
     f. Snoring and daytime fatigue: sleep apnea (common)
     g. Palpitations, insomnia, anxiety, and weight loss: hyperthyroidism (common) (See Chapter 65, Thyroid Disorders, for details.)
  3. Symptoms suggestive of target-organ damage
     a. Exertional chest pain, shortness of breath, orthopnea, peripheral edema, and paroxysmal nocturnal dyspnea: coronary artery disease or heart failure
     b. Fatigue, pruritus, or peripheral edema: renal failure
     c. Syncopal episodes or dizziness, memory loss, motor weakness, speech difficulties, or other focal neurologic findings: cerebrovascular disease
     d. Claudication and sudden loss of vision: peripheral arterial disease
  4. Past health history
     a. History and workup of HTN (When was patient first told they had high BP?); course of treatment and complications, including medications tried and failed or with adverse effects
     b. Diabetes, lipid abnormalities, gout, cardiovascular and cerebrovascular disease, and renal disease
     c. Use of prescribed or over-the-counter drugs and illicit drugs that may influence BP or interfere with the effectiveness of an antihypertensive drug

(e.g., hormonal contraceptives, steroids, nonsteroidal anti-inflammatory drugs, alcohol, cocaine, amphetamines, appetite suppressants or other "diet" supplements, tricyclic antidepressants, monoamine oxidase inhibitors, or decongestants [pseudoephedrine and phenylpropanolamines or analogues]) (**Table 57-2**)
       d. Dietary supplement use, including products containing "herbal ecstasy," ma huang/ephedra, ergot-containing products, and St. John's wort
       e. If higher weight, note history of weight gain.
    5. Family history: history of HTN, stroke, sudden cardiac death, diabetes, heart failure, renal disease, or other CVD
    6. Personal and social history: habits
       a. Alcohol use: Chronic use and withdrawal elevate BP.
       b. Recreational drug use, especially cocaine and amphetamines; anabolic steroids; recent withdrawal from narcotics
       c. Diet: includes sodium intake or "hidden sodium" in canned or prepared foods, vegetable and fruit intake, fat and cholesterol intake
       d. Exercise: type, frequency, and level of exercise
       e. Tobacco use: not a cause of HTN but is an additional risk factor for CVD, and withdrawal may be associated with elevated BP
       f. May affect responsiveness to certain medications (see pharmacologic treatment section)
       g. Emotional stress, including impact of racism or white supremacy, poverty, social support system, family and living situation, employment and work-related stress, ability to obtain and pay for healthcare services, access to resources to maintain the patient's desired level of health, and educational level/ literacy (which may affect understanding of treatment recommendations, and/or ability to read patient handouts)
B. Objective
    1. Physical examination
       a. Vital signs, including BP, should be taken after the patient has been sitting quietly for at least 5 minutes with arm resting on a flat surface and feet on the floor. The patient should have emptied their bladder prior to measuring BP. Additionally, the patient should not have used caffeine, tobacco, or alcohol or exercised for at least 30 minutes before the BP measurement. The initial evaluation should include a BP measurement in both arms. At least two measurements should be obtained, with the average of the two recorded. Periodic standing BP measurements are recommended for those at risk for postural BP changes or with such symptoms and when adding or changing medications. A proper-size cuff is essential; the cuff bladder should encircle at least 80% of the arm to ensure an accurate BP reading (U.S. Department of Health and Human Services [USDHHS], 2004).
       b. Complete a fundoscopic evaluation for arteriovenous nicking, arteriolar narrowing, papilledema, hemorrhages, or exudates.
       c. Assess neck for carotid bruits, distended veins, and enlarged thyroid.
       d. Evaluate the heart for precordial heave, thrills, rate, murmurs, or other extra sounds, such as S3 and S4.
       e. Auscultate the lungs for adventitious sounds (e.g., crackles and wheezing).
       f. Evaluate the abdomen for bruits, enlarged kidneys, or striae.
       g. Assess the extremities for diminished or absent peripheral arterial pulses, edema, or femoral artery bruits.
       h. Neurologic assessment as baseline and for evaluation of abnormal sensory, motor, and cognitive findings suggestive of target-organ damage.
    2. Diagnostic tests
       a. Laboratory: urinalysis (for proteinuria or hematuria suggesting end-organ damage or secondary HTN), fasting blood glucose or hemoglobin A1C (for hyperglycemia suggesting diabetes), hematocrit (for anemia suggesting other disease or polycythemia), serum potassium (may affect medication choice and/or suggest etiology of end-organ damage), creatinine and estimated glomerular filtration rate (may affect medication choice or suggest end-organ damage or secondary HTN), calcium (may be associated with renal disease and thyroid disease), thyroid-stimulating hormone (TSH) and free L-thyroxine (FT4) (for hyperthyroidism), and fasting lipid profile (associated risk factor)
       b. Twelve-lead electrocardiogram (as baseline and/or for evidence of arrhythmias, conduction defects, ischemia and/or infarct, and/or left ventricular hypertrophy)
       c. If secondary HTN is suspected based on the patient's presentation, other tests should be included (**Table 57-3**).

III. Assessment

A. *Determine the diagnosis* (Table 57-1) (AHA, 2021).
B. *Severity*
    1. Assess severity based on level of BP and presence or absence of other risk factors or other compelling diseases.
       a. Hypertensive emergencies are characterized by severe elevations in BP (>180/120 mm Hg) and complicated by evidence of impending or progressive target-organ dysfunction. They require immediate BP reduction (not necessarily to normal) to prevent or limit target-organ damage (e.g., intracerebral hemorrhage or acute myocardial infarction).
       b. Hypertensive urgencies are those situations associated with severe elevations in BP without progressive target-organ dysfunction (USDHHS, 2004).

Table 57-2 Common Substances Associated With Hypertension in Humans

Prescription Drugs	Illicit Drugs and Other "Natural Products"	Food Substances	Chemical Elements and Other Industrial Chemicals
Cortisone and other steroids: (both corticosteroids and mineralocorticoids), adrenocorticotropic hormone (ACTH)	Cocaine and cocaine withdrawal	Sodium chloride	Lead
Estrogens (usually just oral contraceptive agents with high estrogenic activity)	Ma huang, "herbal ecstasy," and other phenyl propanolamine analogues	Ethanol	Mercury
Nonsteroidal anti-inflammatory drugs	Nicotine and withdrawal	Licorice	Thallium and other heavy metals
Phenylpropanolamines and analogues	Anabolic steroids	Tyramine-containing foods (with monoamine oxidase inhibitors)	Lithium salts, especially the chloride
Cyclosporine and tacrolimus	Narcotic withdrawal	Caffeine	
Erythropoietin	Methylphenidate		
Sibutramine	Phencyclidine		
Ketamine	Ketamine		
Desflurane	Ergotamine and other ergot-containing herbal preparations		
Carbamazepine	St. John's wort		
Bromocriptine			
Metoclopramide			
Antidepressants (especially venlafaxine)			
Buspirone			
Clonidine (abrupt withdrawal) with or without the simultaneous initiation of beta-adrenergic blocking agents			
Pheochromocytoma: beta-adrenergic blocking agent without alpha-blocker first; glucagon			
Clozapine			
Weight-loss drugs			

U.S. Department of Health and Human Services. (2004). *Seventh report of the Joint National Committee on Prevention, Detection, Evaluation, and Treatment of High Blood Pressure (JNC 7)* (NIH Publication no. 0405230) (p. 59). Washington, DC: National Institutes of Health, National Heart, Lung, and Blood Institute, National High Blood Pressure Education Program, U.S. Department of Health and Human Services. Retrieved from http://www.nhlbi.nih.gov/guidelines/hypertension/jnc7full.htm

Table 57-3 Screening Tests for Identifiable Causes of Hypertension

Diagnosis	Diagnostic Test
Chronic kidney disease	Estimated glomerular filtration rate
Coarctation of the aorta	Computerized tomography angiography
Cushing syndrome and other glucocorticoid excess states, including chronic steroid therapy	History; dexamethasone suppression test
Drug induced or related	History and drug screening
Pheochromocytoma	24-hour metanephrine and normetanephrine
Primary aldosteronism and other mineralocorticoid excess states	24-hour urinary aldosterone level or specific measurements of other mineralocorticoids
Renovascular hypertension	Doppler flow study; magnetic resonance angiography
Sleep apnea	Sleep study with O_2 saturation
Thyroid or parathyroid disease	Thyroid-stimulating hormone, serum parathyroid hormone

U.S. Department of Health and Human Services. (2004). *Seventh report of the Joint National Committee on Prevention, Detection, Evaluation, and Treatment of High Blood Pressure (JNC 7)* (NIH Publication no. 0405230). Washington, DC: National Institutes of Health, National Heart, Lung, and Blood Institute, National High Blood Pressure Education Program, U.S. Department of Health and Human Services. Retrieved from http://www.nhlbi.nih.gov/guidelines/hypertension/jnc7full.htm

C. *Significance and patient's motivation and ability*
Assess the significance of this diagnosis to the patient and to significant others. Additionally, assess patient's understanding of HTN and willingness and ability to follow a treatment plan, including lifestyle modifications. This assessment should be made on an ongoing basis throughout follow-up visits.

IV. Goals of clinical management
A. *Public health goal*
Reduce cardiovascular and renal morbidity and mortality.
B. *Individual's goal related to self-management and patient adherence*
Choose a plan, including medications, lifestyle modifications, and follow-up, that is tailored to the patient.
C. *BP goal (see Section I.C for BP goals for different groups of affected individuals)*

V. Plan and management
A. *Lifestyle modification*
This is the first step in counseling and treating patients with elevated BP and stage 1 HTN and is an essential component of treatment for stage 2 HTN. In patients with elevated BP or stage 1 HTN, lifestyle modifications may be definitive therapy. For other stages of HTN, lifestyle modification may reduce the number and doses of antihypertensives required to reach goal BP, as well as decrease the risk of or delay progression to end-organ damage.
1. Weight
   a. Weight loss of as little as 10 lb (4.5 kg) reduces BP or prevents HTN in many overweight individuals (USDHHS, 2004).
2. Diet
   a. There is strong evidence that consuming a diet that emphasizes vegetables, fruits, whole grains, low-fat dairy, poultry, fish, legumes, nontropical vegetable oils, and nuts and limits intake of sweets, sugar-sweetened beverages, and red meats can benefit BP lowering (Eckel et al., 2013). The Dietary Approaches to Stop Hypertension (DASH) diet and the American Heart Association (AHA) diet are consistent with these recommendations and generally recommended (AHA, 2021; Heller, 2015).
   b. Strong evidence also exists for consuming no more than 2,400 mg of sodium daily, and reducing further to 1,500 mg/day is associated with greater BP reduction. Even reducing sodium intake by at least 100 mg a day, although not ideal, can lower BP (Eckel et al., 2013).
3. Alcohol
   Alcohol intake should be limited to 1 oz or less daily of ethanol (two drinks) in men) and no more than 0.5 oz (one drink) in women (AHA, 2021).
4. Exercise
   Regular aerobic activity often lowers BP in adults. Three to four sessions a week of approximately 40 minutes each involving moderate to vigorous intensity exercise are recommended (Eckel et al., 2013).
5. Tobacco abstinence
   For overall cardiovascular risk reduction, smoking cessation is essential and should be a major focus of counseling for providers.
6. Other lifestyle modifications or alternative treatments
B. *Pharmacologic treatment* (**Table 57-4**)
Reducing elevated BP with medications has been shown in numerous studies to decrease the incidence of cardiovascular mortality and morbidity.
1. Factors to be considered in the selection of therapy
   a. Cost of medication
   b. Metabolic and subjective side effects
   c. Potential drug–drug interactions
   d. Concomitant diseases that may be beneficially or adversely affected by the antihypertensive agent chosen

Table 57-4 Commonly Used Antihypertensive Medications*

Class of Drug	Drug Name	Usual Dose Range (mg/day)	Usual Daily Frequency	Mechanism	Comments
Thiazide diuretics	Chlorthalidone	12.5–25	1	Decreased plasma volume and extracellular fluid volume; decreased cardiac output initially, followed by decreased total peripheral resistance with normalization of cardiac output. Long-term effects include slight decreases in extracellular fluid volume.	For thiazide and loop diuretics, lower doses and dietary counseling should be used to avoid metabolic changes (e.g., potassium, sodium losses). Check electrolytes 1–2 weeks after initiating these medications.
	Chlorothiazide	125–500	1–2		
	Hydrochlorothiazide	12.5–50	1		
	Indapamide	1.25–2.5	1		
	Polythiazide	2–4	1		
	Metolazone (Zaroxolyn)	2.5–5.0	1		
Loop diuretics	Bumetanide	0.5–2	2	See thiazides.	Higher doses may be needed for patients with renal impairment or congestive heart failure. Ethacrynic acid is the only alternative for patients with allergy to thiazide and sulfur-containing diuretics.
	Ethacrynic acid	50–100	1–2		
	Furosemide	10–80	2		
	Torsemide	2.5–10	1		
β-Blockers	Atenolol	25–100	1	Decreased cardiac output and increased total peripheral resistance; decreased plasma renin activity; atenolol, betaxolol, bisoprolol, and metoprolol are cardioselective.	Selective agents also inhibit in higher doses (e.g., all may aggravate asthma).
	Betaxolol	5–20	1		
	Bisoprolol	2.5–10	1		
	Metoprolol	50–200	1–2		
	Metoprolol extended release	25–100	1		
	Nadolol	40–120	1		
		40–160	2		
	Propranolol	60–180	1		
	Propranolol long acting	10–40	2		
β-Blockers with intrinsic sympathomimetic activity	Acebutolol	200–800	2	See β-blockers. Acebutolol is cardioselective.	Use intrinsic sympathomimetic activity agents for those with bradycardia who must receive β-blockers.
	Penbutolol	10–40	1		
	Pindolol	10–40	2		

Angiotensin-converting enzyme inhibitors (ACEIs)	Benazepril	10–40	1	Block formation of angiotensin II by cleaving angiotensin I, thereby promoting vasodilation and reducing the circulation of aldosterone, which results in decreased sodium and water retention. They also increase bradykinin and vasodilatory prostaglandins.	Diuretic doses should be reduced or discontinued before starting ACEIs whenever possible to prevent excessive hypotension. May cause hyperkalemia in patients with renal impairment or in those receiving potassium-sparing agents. Can cause acute renal failure in patients with severe bilateral renal artery stenosis or severe stenosis in artery in a solitary kidney.
	Captopril	25–100	2		
	Enalapril	5–20	1–2		
	Fosinopril	10–40	1		
	Lisinopril	10–40	1		
	Moexipril	7.5–30	1		
	Perindopril	4–8	1		
	Quinapril	10–80	1		
	Ramipril	2.5–2.0	1		
	Trandolapril	1–4	1		
Angiotensin II receptor blockers	Candesartan	8–32	1	Blocks the angiotensin II receptor, thus inhibiting the action of angiotensin II, as noted previously. Bradykinin levels are not altered, so there is a lower incidence of an associated dry cough than with ACEIs.	See ACEIs.
	Eprosartan	400–800	1–2		
	Irbesartan	150–300	1		
	Losartan	25–100	1–2		
	Olmesartan	20–40	1		
	Telmisartan	20–80	1		
	Valsartan	80–320	1–2		
Calcium channel blockers	Amlodipine	2.5–10	1	Block inward movement of calcium ion across cell membranes and cause smooth muscle relaxation.	Dihydropyridines—more potent peripheral vasodilators than other calcium channel blockers and, as such, may cause more dizziness, headache, flushing, peripheral edema, and tachycardia. All can reduce sinus rate and produce heart block, especially in combination with other antihypertensives.
	Diltiazem (Sutters, 2015)	180–360	1		
	Cardizem SR®*	180–360	1		
	Cardizem CD®*	180–480	1		
	Dilacor XR®*	180–540	1		
	Tiazac SA®*	2.5–2.0	1		
	Felodipine	2.5–5	2		
	Isradipine	20–40	2		
	Nicardipine	30–60	2		
	Nicardipine SR	30–120	2		
	Nifedipine XL	17–34	1		
	Nisoldipine	180–480	1–2		
	Verapamil (long acting and sustained release) (Sutters, 2015)				

*"In some patients treated once daily, the antihypertensive effect may diminish toward the end of the dosing interval (trough effect). Blood pressure (BP) should be measured just prior to dosing to determine if satisfactory BP control is obtained" (USDHHS, 2004, p. 11).

Data from James, P. A., Oparil, S., Carter, B. L., Cushman, W. C., Dennison-Himmelfarb, C., Handler, J., et al. (2014). 2014 evidence-based guidelines for the management of high blood pressure in adults: Report from the panel members appointed to the Eighth Joint National Committee (JNC 8). *JAMA, 311*(5), 507–520. doi: 10.1001/jama.2013.284427. Sutters, M. (2015). Chapter 11: Systemic hypertension. In M. A. Papadakis, S. McPhee, & M. W. Rabow (Eds.), *Current medical diagnosis and treatment* (54th ed.). New York: McGraw-Hill Education.

2. General treatment guidelines
   a. In the general population, initial pharmacologic treatment should include a thiazide-type diuretic, calcium channel blocker (CCB), angiotensin-converting enzyme inhibitor (ACEI), or angiotensin receptor blocker (ARB) (James et al., 2014).
   b. If goal BP is not reached within a month of treatment, add another agent from those listed previously (CCB, ACEI, ARB, or thiazide diuretic). Note: Do not use an ACEI and ARB in the same patient. Continue to assess BP regularly and adjust treatment regimen to desired BP goal.
   c. If goal BP is not reached with two drugs, add a third from the list (CCB, ACEI, ARB, or thiazide diuretic). Note: Do not use an ACEI and ARB in the same patient.
   d. If goal BP is not reached with titration of drugs from this list because of a contraindication or the need to use more than three drugs, other antihypertensive medications (from other classes) may be used.
   e. Consider referral to a hypertensive specialist if goal BP is not reached using four medications and after a careful review of patient's compliance with medication and lifestyle modifications (James et al., 2014).
   f. Simplify the regimen to once-daily dosing if possible for greater adherence.
   g. In some patients on once-daily dosing, there may be a trough effect: waning of effectiveness of medications at the end of the dosing interval. Therefore, it is best to measure the BP just before the next dose to determine the need for dosage adjustment (USDHHS, 2004).
   h. In stage 2 HTN, consider starting therapy with two drugs, either as separate prescriptions or in fixed-dose combinations, because this increases the likelihood of reaching the BP goal more promptly than with one agent (USDHHS, 2004).
   i. "Start low and go slow" when initiating medication in an elderly patient to reduce the risk of orthostatic hypotension, which is a risk for falls. Counsel patients to change positions slowly, such as from seated to standing, in order to avoid orthostatic hypotension.

C. Patient education
   It is essential that this be done in the language in which the patient is fluent (oral and written) and at a reading level appropriate to the patient's education. When in doubt, aim at a sixth-grade or lower level of reading.
   1. Provide oral and written information on cardiovascular risk factors associated with HTN and the long-term prognosis of HTN if untreated.
   2. Elicit the patient's concerns regarding the diagnosis, including their acceptance of the diagnosis.
   3. Provide the patient with a written copy of their BP reading at each visit. If possible, provide a wallet card that contains multiple readings.
   4. Come to a mutual agreement with the patient on the BP goal.
   5. Provide specific, preferably written, information on lifestyle modifications that you are recommending for this patient.
   6. Be sure to underscore the importance of the need to continue treatment to maintain a normal BP.
   7. Explain that most individuals with HTN are usually asymptomatic, so the patient will not usually be able to tell if the BP is elevated or not based on symptoms.
   8. Have the patient repeat their understanding of the treatment regimen before the end of the visit.
   9. Include in the patient education cautions regarding the use of cold preparations and over-the-counter analgesics (e.g., pseudoephedrine, nonsteroidal anti-inflammatory drugs, respectively).
   10. Encourage the use of validated home BP-monitoring devices for interested and able patients, especially those with refractory HTN. Offer a prescription for a BP cuff to any patient whose health plan covers a monitor.

D. Follow-up and monitoring
   1. Laboratory follow-up
      a. Check serum electrolytes 1–2 weeks after starting a diuretic.
      b. Check serum potassium and creatinine 2–4 weeks after starting an ACEI.
      c. Check serum electrolytes and creatinine at least annually for all patients on antihypertensive medications.
   2. Have the patient bring in all medications to each follow-up visit.
   3. Challenges reaching target BP goal
      a. Consider nonadherence to medication or lifestyle recommendations, including excessive sodium intake or increased alcohol intake.
      b. Consider use of over-the-counter medications or illicit drugs.
      c. Evaluate for high levels of stress or psychiatric conditions that can affect BP, such as anxiety or panic disorders.
      d. Screen for secondary causes for HTN.
      e. Always maintain an attitude of empathetic concern and genuine interest in developing the best possible, workable plan for the patient as a partner in treatment.

References

American College of Cardiology. (2018). *2017 guideline for high blood pressure in adults.* https://www.acc.org/Latest-in-Cardiology/ten-points-to-remember/2017/11/09/11/41/2017-Guideline-for-High-Blood-Pressure-in-Adults

American College of Cardiology. (2021). *New guidance on blood pressure management in low-risk adults with stage 1 hypertension.* https://www.acc.org/Latest-in-Cardiology/Articles/2021/06/21/13/05/New-Guidance-on-BP-Management-in-Low-Risk-Adults-with-Stage-1-HTN

American Heart Association. (2021). *The American Heart Association diet and lifestyle recommendations.* https://www.heart.org/en/healthy-living/healthy-eating/eat-smart/nutrition-basics/aha-diet-and-lifestyle-recommendations

Centers for Disease Control and Prevention. (2020). *Hypertension prevalence among adults aged 18 and over: United States, 2017–2018.* https://www.cdc.gov/nchs/products/databriefs/db364.htm#:~:text=The%20prevalence%20of%20hypertension%20increased,hypertension%20by%20age%20was%20observed.

Eckel, R. H., Jakicic, J. M., Ard, J. D., de Jesus, J. M., Houston Miller, N., Hubbard, V. S., Lee, I. M., Lichtenstein, A. H., Loria, C. M., Millen, B. E., Nonas, C. A., Sacks, F. M., Smith, S. C., Jr., Svetkey, L. P., Wadden, T. A., Yanovski, S. Z., Kendall, K. A., Morgan, L. C., Trisolini, M. G., ... American College of Cardiology/American Heart Association Task Force on Practice Guidelines (2013). 2013 AHA/ACC guideline on lifestyle management to reduce cardiovascular risk: A report of the American College of Cardiology/American Heart Association Task Force on Practice Guidelines. *Circulation, 129*(25, Suppl. 2), S76–S99. doi:10.1161/01.cir.0000437740.48606.d1.

Goff, D. C., Lloyd-Jones, D. M., Bennett, G., Coady, S., D'Agostino, R. B., Gibbons, R., et al. (2014) 2013 ACC/AHA guideline on the assessment of cardiovascular risk: a report of the American College of Cardiology/American Heart Association Task Force on Practice Guidelines. Journal of the American College of Cardiology, 63(25, Part B):2935–2959. doi: 10.1016/j.jacc.2013.11.005

Heller, M. (2015). *The DASH diet eating plan.* http://dashdiet.org/default.asp.

James, P. A., Oparil, S., Carter, B. L., Cushman, W. C., Dennison-Himmelfarb, C., Handler, J., Lackland, D. T., LeFevre, M. L., MacKenzie, T. D., Ogedegbe, O., Smith Jr., S. C., Svetkey, L. P., Taler, S. J., Townsend, R. R., Wright Jr., J. T., Narva, A. S., & Ortiz, E. (2014). 2014 evidence-based guidelines for the management of high blood pressure in adults: Report from the panel members appointed to the Eighth Joint National Committee (JNC 8). *JAMA, 311*(5), 507–520. doi:10.1001/jama.2013.284427

Sutters, M. (2015). Systemic hypertension. In M. A., Papadakis, S., McPhee, & M. W., Rabow (Eds.), *Current medical diagnosis and treatment* (54th ed., pp. 435–467). McGraw-Hill Education.

Tientcheu, D., Ayers, C., Das, S. R., McGuire, D. K., de Lemos, J. A., Khera, A., Kaplan, N., Victor, R., & Vongpatanasin, W. (2015, November 17). Target organ complications and cardiovascular events associated with masked hypertension and white-coat hypertension: Analysis from the Dallas Heart Study. *Journal of the American College of Cardiology, 66*(20), 2159–2169. doi:10.1016/j.jacc.2015.09.007

U.S. Department of Health and Human Services. (2004). *Seventh report of the Joint National Committee on Prevention, Detection, Evaluation, and Treatment of High Blood Pressure (JNC 7)* (NIH Publication No. 0405230). National Institutes of Health, National Heart, Lung, and Blood Institute, National High Blood Pressure Education Program, U.S. Department of Health and Human Services. http://www.nhlbi.nih.gov/guidelines/hypertension/jnc7full.htm

Weber, M. A., Schriffin, E. L., White, W. B., Mann, S., Lindholm, L. H., Kenerson, J. G., Flack, J. M., Carter, B. L., Materson, B. J., Ram, C. V., Cohen, D. L., Cadet, J. C., Jean-Charles, R. R., Taler, S., Kountz, D., Townsend, R. R., Chalmers, J., Ramirez, A. J., Bakris, G. L., ... Harrap, S. B. (2014). Clinical practice guidelines for the management of hypertension in the community: A statement by the American Society of Hypertension and the International Society of Hypertension. *Journal of Clinical Hypertension, 16*(1), 14–26. doi:10.1111/jch.12237

World Health Organization. (2013). *A global brief on hypertension: Silent killer, global public health crisis* (Document No. WHO/DCO/WHD/2013.2). http://www.who.int/cardiovascular_diseases/publications/global_brief_hypertension/en/

World Health Organization. (2021). *Cardiovascular diseases (CVDs).* https://www.who.int/news-room/fact-sheets/detail/cardiovascular-diseases-(cvds)

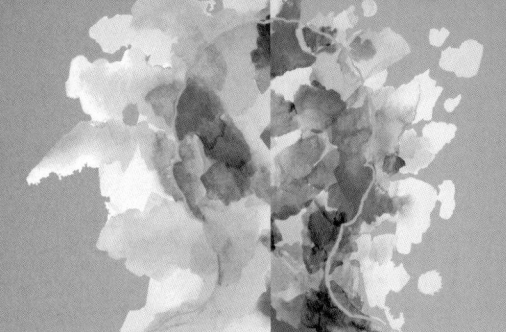

CHAPTER 58

Intimate Partner Violence (Domestic Violence)

Jessica Draughon Moret and JoAnne Saxe

I. Introduction and general background

Intimate partner violence (IPV) is a serious, preventable public health problem affecting more than 40 million Americans during their lifetime (Smith et al., 2018). The term *IPV* encompasses multiple types of relationships and multiple types of violence. IPV is defined as "physical or sexual violence (use of physical force) or threat of such violence; or psychological/emotional abuse and/or coercive tactics when there has been prior physical and/or sexual violence" (Saltzman et al., 2002, p. 11). An intimate partner can be a current or former spouse or other romantic or sexual partner (Breiding et al., 2014). Therefore, in addition to physical violence, the term *IPV* includes teen dating violence, stalking, intimate partner sexual assault, and reproductive coercion.

IPV is associated with many acute and chronic negative health outcomes, including intimate partner homicide (Matias et al., 2020; Spencer & Stith, 2020). Sharps and colleagues' landmark study shows that over 40% of female-identified intimate partner homicide victims in 11 cities accessed health care in the 12 months prior to their murder (Sharps et al., 2001). Clinicians should be aware of the scope of IPV, both its impact on individual patients' health and society.

A. *Types of IPV*

The National Intimate Partner and Sexual Violence Survey (NISVS) collects population-based data in the United States, generating the most accurate and reliable incidence and prevalence estimates for IPV in the following categories (Smith et al., 2018):

1. *Physical violence* includes but is not limited to acts of hitting, slapping, shoving, grabbing, and biting and also includes denying a partner medical care or forcing them to ingest alcohol or drugs.
2. *Sexual violence* includes forcible penetration (insertive or receptive) and any nonconsensual sexual act proscribed by federal, tribal, or state law, including when a person lacks capacity to consent (Department of Justice, Office of Violence Against Women [DOJ], 2021). Sexual violence may also include reproductive coercion: behaviors attempting to control a person's reproductive decision making, for example, birth control sabotage or pregnancy coercion (Moore et al., 2010).
3. *Stalking* is a pattern of interaction that is unwanted by the target and includes harassment or threats resulting in fear or safety concerns. It may include digital harassment or cyber-harassment.
4. *Psychological aggression* includes expressive aggression and coercive control:
   a. *Expressive aggression* may also be termed *emotional abuse* and involves name-calling, insulting, or diminishing one's abilities,
   b. *Coercive control* includes behaviors intended to control or threaten. This may include tracking the person's whereabouts, social isolation from family or friends or other sources of emotional support, or economic abuse—controlling access to finances and/or financial resources (e.g., employment).

IPV categories are not mutually exclusive; they often present together as a complex, ongoing pattern of abuse. Although all states have legislation defining IPV, those definitions vary across states. In most state laws addressing IPV, the relationship necessary for a charge of domestic assault or abuse generally includes a spouse, former spouse, persons currently residing together or those who have within the previous year, or persons who share a common child (DOJ, n.d.).

In the United States, IPV is also commonly referred to as *domestic violence*. This is a more imprecise term because "domestic" could be misconstrued as violence against any member of a household (e.g., elder abuse, child abuse). The DOJ defines domestic violence to include children or other family members (DOJ, n.d.), whereas IPV is more specific to the dynamics of power and control inherent in current or former romantic or sexual relationships.

B. IPV prevalence and incidence

The NISVS data from the 2015 data year related to intimate partner–perpetrated violence, including reports of lifetime and past-year incidence (based on when the data were collected; indicates between 2014 and 2015), are summarized next. The NISVS does not specify whether respondents are cis- or trans-, only whether they identify as female or male. Of all people reporting a lifetime experience of IPV, 71.1% of women and 55.8% of men experienced the first episode before the age of 25 (Smith et al., 2018).

1. Sexual violence

   One in 5 women, or 18.3% of all women, and 1 in 10 men, or 10.9% of all men, report having experienced unwanted sexual acts perpetrated by an intimate partner during their lifetime. This includes full and attempted forced penetration, sexual coercion, and drug- or alcohol-facilitated violations. The past-year incidence of intimate partner sexual violence includes 2.4% of women and 1.6% of men.

2. Stalking

   One in 10 women (10.4%) and 2.2% of men report stalking victimization. The past-year incidence of intimate partner stalking includes 2.2% of women and 0.8% of men.

3. Physical violence

   Almost 1 in 3 women (30.6%) and 1 in 3 men (31.5%) in the United States have experienced physical violence by their intimate partner during their lifetime. Of these people, 1 in 5 women (21.4%) and 1 in 7 men (14.9%) have experienced severe violence, characterized by being hit by a fist or other object, beaten, or slammed against something hard. A past-year incidence of physical violence was reported by 2.9% of women and 3.8% of men.

4. Psychological aggression

   The survey also reports that 1 in 3 of all men and women have experienced psychological aggression by an intimate partner in their lifetime.

C. IPV consequences

The most severe outcome of IPV is death. In 2017, 42% of female-identified and 7% of male-identified homicide victims were killed by intimate partners (Petrosky et al., 2020). There are far-reaching psychological, physical, sexual and reproductive, and societal sequelae.

1. Mental health sequelae

   IPV significantly co-occurs with depression (Bacchus et al., 2018; World Health Organization [WHO], 2013), acute and posttraumatic stress disorders (WHO, 2013), substance use (Bacchus et al., 2018; WHO, 2013), and suicidal ideation (Ellsberg et al., 2008).

2. Physical health sequelae

   According to the NISVS data, 24.3% of women and 13.8% of men have been a victim of *severe* physical violence, and 15% of women and 4% of men have sustained injuries (Breiding et al., 2014). Aside from acute physical injury, IPV is associated with chronic pain (WHO, 2013), chronic stress, chronic immune system activation and inflammation (Goldberg et al., 2021), accelerated cellular aging (Humphreys et al., 2012), and cardiovascular disease risk (Chandan et al., 2020).

3. Reproductive health sequelae

   Reproductive health is affected through diminished control over sexual and reproductive health decisions (Moore et al., 2010), unplanned pregnancies (Moore et al., 2010; Taillieu & Brownridge, 2010; WHO, 2013), preterm labor (Silverman et al., 2006; WHO, 2013), low-birth-weight neonates (Silverman et al., 2006; WHO, 2013), and maternal morbidity and mortality (Silverman et al., 2006).

4. Costs to society

   Lifetime costs of IPV in the United States are over $100K for women and $23K for men (Centers for Disease Control and Prevention [CDC], 2021). The total cost to society of lost wages, productivity, medical services for injuries, and the legal system was estimated at $3.6 trillion (CDC, 2021). Costs are generally higher when IPV is ongoing or occurred within the past 12 months (Bonomi et al., 2009; Fishman et al., 2010; Jones et al., 2006). Variation exists as to whether these costs return to baseline over time (Fishman et al., 2010) or remain elevated even when abuse ceased more than 5 years in the past (Bonomi et al., 2009).

D. Risk factors

Although there are some specific populations that may experience heightened risk for IPV, the annual incidence and lifetime prevalence of IPV is such that a broad commitment to universal education of all patients regarding healthy relationships and IPV is key. Research shows that women who speak to a healthcare provider about abuse are 4 times more likely to access additional IPV interventions (McCloskey et al., 2006).

Any of the following findings—solely or in combination—may indicate that a patient is experiencing IPV and warrant additional investigation.

- Medical records indicating repeated visits or previous injuries
- Injuries in various stages of healing
- Clothing that does not match the season—for example, long sleeves in summer, which may be worn to hide bruising
- Documented history of IPV
- A history with inconsistent descriptions of injuries
- If accompanied by a partner, the partner answers for the patient or declines to leave the room.

- Vague and nonspecific responses to questions
- A history of anxiety, depression, sleeplessness, fatigue, or chronic somatic complaints

E. *Population considerations*

IPV often falls under the umbrella term *gender-based violence*. The U.S. Agency for International Development (USAID) defines gender-based violence as follows:

> Violence that is directed at an individual based on his or her biological sex, gender identity, or perceived adherence to socially defined norms of masculinity and femininity. It includes physical, sexual and psychological abuse; threats; coercion; arbitrary deprivation of liberty; and economic deprivation, whether occurring in public or private life. (USAID, 2012, p. 6)

Therefore, anyone who identifies as a historically marginalized gender- or sexual- identity is at increased risk for experiencing all forms of gender-based violence. This includes (but is not limited to) cis-women, lesbian, gay, bisexual, trans-women, trans-men, queer, intersex (gay, lesbian, bisexual, transgender, queer, intersex, and asexual [LGBTQI+]) people, or anyone socialized as a woman.

Any additional historically marginalized identity (i.e., intersectionality) may heighten an individual person's risk of experiencing IPV—the interaction of two or more "identities" is greater than the risk associated with the sum of the components (Crenshaw, 1989). These historically marginalized and socially constructed identities (e.g., race, class, and gender) combine synergistically. Anyone who is at risk for gender-based violence is at higher risk for IPV if they also hold an additional historically marginalized identity, for example, Black, Indigenous, and people of color (BIPOC); the poor; the disabled; or the otherwise disenfranchised. Any discrimination or lack of access to resources may place a person at higher risk (Burton et al., 2021). For example, a person who has immigrated to the United States may experience language barriers or, depending on documentation status, fear of police involvement and may therefore choose not to disclose IPV to their healthcare provider (regardless of whether the provider practices in a state with mandated reporting for IPV). Without additional history and physical data, it is impossible to identify a patient experiencing IPV just by looking at them. Providers must be aware that IPV can affect anyone from any race, class, and gender and commit to performing routine IPV assessment for all patients. Specific information about the risks of IPV for the three following "invisible" identities is provided to illustrate this point. Providing additional information about these three identities does not mean that other historically marginalized identities are free from increased risk.

1. LGBTQI+

    People from the LGBTQI+ community experience IPV at higher rates. Half of all people who identify as transgender experience IPV during their lifetime (James et al., 2016). Moreover, 61% of bisexual women, 44% of lesbian women, 37% of bisexual men, and 26% of homosexual men report IPV in their lifetime (Walters et al., 2013).

2. Women with disabilities

    People with disabilities are more likely to experience IPV (Basile et al., 2016; Breiding & Armour, 2015; Scherer et al., 2016; Smith, 2008). The increased risk of IPV among women with disabilities may be due to physical dependence on an intimate partner combined with structural risk factors, such as poverty, and isolation (Breiding & Armour, 2015; Hassouneh-Phillips & Curry, 2002).

3. Women living with HIV

    Women living with HIV experience IPV at rates slightly higher than the national average (55%; Machtinger et al., 2012). IPV also affects the health of women living with HIV; they are more likely to be lost to follow-up (Siemieniuk et al., 2013), are less likely to be prescribed antiretroviral therapy, are less likely to adhere to antiretroviral therapy (Hatcher et al., 2015), and have faster disease progression to AIDS (Anderson et al., 2018).

F. *Screening*

The goal of screening or secondary prevention typically is to identify disease processes early before signs or symptoms are present. In the context of IPV, the "symptoms" are what is assessed with screening. The goal of screening or universal assessment for IPV is for patients to understand that healthcare providers care what happens to them, that IPV is a sign of an unhealthy relationship, that the patient is not alone in their experience of IPV, and that there is help and to provide a safe environment to discuss the signs of an unhealthy relationship. The goal is *not* disclosure or for the patient to leave the violent relationship.

The U.S. Preventive Services Task Force (USPSTF) recommends screening all women of reproductive age for IPV and referral of women who screen positive for additional support (Curry et al., 2018). The USPSTF states there is limited evidence to support a recommendation for routine screening of men and the elderly for IPV. Best practice includes universal assessment for IPV in a private place, communicating the limits of confidentiality—whether the clinician is a mandated reporter of IPV—and the use of a valid and reliable screening tool (Paterno & Draughon, 2016). There are multiple well-researched screening tools with acceptable sensitivity and specificity for identifying recent (past 12 months) and ongoing IPV (Feltner et al., 2018; Rabin et al., 2009). For example:

- Abuse Assessment Screen (AAS; Laughon et al., 2008)
- Humiliation, Afraid, Rape, Kick (HARK; Sohal et al., 2007)
- Hurt, Insulted, Threaten, Scream (HITS; Sherin et al., 1998)

Table 58-1 Sample Script for Routine Intimate Partner Violence Screening With Use of the Abuse Assessment Screen

Part of Script	Example Language
Normalizing statement	Next I am going to ask you questions about intimate partner violence. These are questions we ask all of our patients.
Mandatory reporting (if applicable)	Before I ask you these questions, I do need to tell you that I am a mandated reporter of intimate partner violence. What that means is that if you answer yes to any of the following questions, I will have to file a report with the police on your behalf.
Normalizing statement	We know that all couples argue. When you and your partner argue…
Abuse Assessment Screen (AAS)	1. Within the last year, have you been pushed, shoved, slapped, hit, kicked, choked, or otherwise physically hurt by your partner or ex-partner? 2. Since you've been pregnant, have you been hit, slapped, kicked, or otherwise physically hurt by someone? 3. Within the last year, has anyone forced you to have sexual activities that you did not want? 4. Are you afraid of anyone?
Negative Screen	Thank you for answering. We like to make sure women know this is a safe place to discuss intimate relationships.
Positive Screen	Thank you for sharing with me; I know it can be difficult to talk about these topics.
Additional empowering statements	I believe you. This was not your fault. No one deserves to be treated this way. There is help.

Reproduced from Paterno, Mary T, and Jessica E Draughon. "Screening for Intimate Partner Violence." *Journal of midwifery & women's health* vol. 61,3 (2016): 370-5. doi:10.1111/jmwh.12443. Copyright 2016 by the American College of Nurse Midwives. Reprinted with permission

- Slapped, Threatened, and Throw (things) (STaT; Paranjape & Liebschutz, 2003)

See **Table 58-1** for a sample screening script using the AAS. A "yes" to any item on a screening tool is considered a positive screen for IPV.

Screening fits nicely within the Confidentiality, Universal Education and Empowerment, and Support (CUES) intervention developed over the past decade in collaboration with Futures Without Violence (2018). CUES is an effective and structured intervention (Futures Without Violence, 2021) to assist healthcare providers in talking with their patients about IPV. CUES has been shown to increase disclosures of IPV and decrease negative health sequelae in multiple settings (Decker et al., 2012; Ghandour et al., 2015; Miller et al., 2011, 2015, 2016, 2017).

1. Confidentiality: Communicate *first* any limits to confidentiality. As of this writing, California, Nebraska, and North Dakota all require healthcare providers to report incidences of IPV to law enforcement. Patients deserve to know whether they may safely disclose IPV to their healthcare provider, and the consequences of said disclosure, at the opening of any conversation about IPV. As with screening, ensure that all conversations about IPV are held in private without anyone else present—this includes small children who may repeat what they hear at inopportune times.
2. Universal education and empowerment: Provide education to all patients about healthy relationships and healthy conflict within relationships. Futures Without Violence has developed safety cards (which fold up to the size of a business card) to be used as a prompt for key topics to guide the conversation. This information is freely available on the organization's website.
3. Support: In the event that a patient chooses to disclose IPV, first, validate the patient's experience and courage in disclosing IPV to you. Then provide a warm referral to your local IPV advocate resources. A warm referral may entail making the call to the IPV advocate center and potentially remaining with the patient while they speak with the advocate (Chamberlain & Levenson, 2013). Warm referrals increase the likelihood of follow-up.

The published recommendations state screening (and/or CUES) should be performed on an annual basis for all women of reproductive age (Curry et al., 2018), upon entry to prenatal care, at least once per trimester, and at the postpartum visit (American College of

Box 58-1 Considerations Specific to Pregnant People

- Estimates of IPV during pregnancy vary widely from 1.5% to 67% (Mojahed et al., 2021).
- Unplanned pregnancy is associated with increased risk of IPV (Yakubovich et al., 2018).
- The severity of violence may increase during pregnancy (American College of Obstetricians and Gynecologists, 2012).
- Pregnancy-associated homicide is a major contributor to maternal mortality (Cliffe et al., 2019).

Obstetricians and Gynecologists, 2012). Pregnancy presents a time of increased demands on any relationship; risks to note in pregnant people are highlighted in (**Box 58-1**). If a patient seeks care specifically for injuries related to IPV, the visit will have a different goal than if IPV is disclosed as part of universal screening and/or CUEs.

II. The focused IPV assessment and database (may include but is not limited to)

A. *Subjective*

It is important to document what the patient reports as close to verbatim as possible. Use direct quotes, and do not sanitize their language. Information in the patient's narrative may include the identity of the person the patient reports inflicting their injuries, the circumstances surrounding the event, any past history of violence, the nature of the injuries, and use of any threats or weapons.

B. *Objective*

Perform a complete head-to-toe examination or focused evaluation as indicated by history or report of injuries. Document the character and extent of all physical injuries, including areas of pain and tenderness, even if there is no obvious bruising or injury. Use a body map to note where injuries are located. If photography is available, it is appropriate to photograph injuries. If using a ruler or other scale in photographs, be sure to take a photograph both with and without the ruler.

Additional components of the physical examination are listed in **Table 58-2**.

III. Treatment

Evaluate the extent of injuries and the need for immediate medical intervention. See **Table 58-3** for potential diagnoses. Also assess for immediate safety concerns—for example, if the abuser is the person who drove the patient to the appointment or if the patient reports feeling unsafe to leave the office and/or return home. A trained IPV advocate or licensed clinical social worker is an appropriate member of the interprofessional care team to call upon for assistance in managing immediate safety concerns.

Table 58-2 Physical Examination

Components of the Physical Examination
Assess general appearance: Level of distress
Vital signs
Other physical examination data: 1. Look carefully for multiple abrasions and contusions to different anatomic sites and multiple injuries in various stages of healing. 2. Most accidents involve the extremities, whereas intimate partner violence injuries often involve protected areas: the face, neck, chest, breasts, abdomen, genitalia, or anus.
Mental status examination: Evaluate mood, orientation, and thought processes.

Table 58-3 Assessment

Diagnoses
Determine the diagnosis (not mutually exclusive). 1. History of prior intimate partner violence (IPV) 2. Recent IPV without observable injury 3. Current history of IPV with observable injury   a. Report as required by state regulations

Determine the *International Classification of Diseases* (ICD) codes for IPV, which are divided into four categories (Rudman, 2000):
1. Adult maltreatment and abuse (995–981)
2. The primary diagnosis (underlying reason for admittance)
3. Modifier codes that provide details (E-codes)
4. History codes that provide information on previous incidents (V-codes)
 	
With ICD-10 implementation, code 995 will be replaced with T74 (confirmed) and T76 (suspected), and the coding will include the following (Women's Preventive Services Initiative, 2021):
   a. Suspected or confirmed
   b. Type of abuse, for example:
      i. Physical abuse
      ii. Sexual abuse (rape, sexual assault)
      iii. Psychological abuse (bullying and intimidation, intimidation through social media)
   c. Encounter type (initial encounter, subsequent encounter, sequela encounter)

IV. Goals of clinical management

The goals in managing patients reporting IPV depend on the nature of the disclosure and whether injuries are present.

V. Plan
A. When IPV is disclosed as part of universal screening and/or the CUES intervention, provide support as noted under Section F, Screening.
B. When IPV is the chief complaint:
   1. Assess, document, and treat injuries as indicated by health history and your focused physical assessment.
   2. Diagnostic testing: Obtain radiographs, computed tomography, or magnetic resonance imaging based on the extent of injury. Treat as indicated.
   3. Address immediate safety concerns in collaboration with the interprofessional team.
   4. Refer the patient to a clinician and/or forensic nursing program with specific training in IPV assessment. Forensic examiners have additional training in documenting injuries and obtaining in-depth IPV histories. Just as with other complicated disease processes, specialty consultation is appropriate and encouraged when available.
C. When sexual assault co-occurs with the reported incident of IPV:
   1. Ensure the patient is medically stable.
   2. Provide postexposure prophylaxis for pregnancy (Haeger et al., 2018) and sexually transmitted infections (STIs) (Workowski et al., 2021), including chlamydia, gonorrhea, trichomonas, hepatitis, human papillomavirus (HPV), and HIV (Dominguez et al., 2016), as appropriate.
   3. Depending on local jurisdiction time limits, it may be appropriate to refer the patient to a forensic nursing program for additional treatment and intervention. Time limits generally range from 72–120 hours after the assault. Forensic nursing care typically includes written and photographic documentation and physical trace evidence collection with or without coordination with law enforcement, according to patient preference.

VI. Self-management resources and tools
A. *Educational resources and support*
   Provide patient education brochures or frequently-asked-question documents as part of the universal empowerment and education portion of the CUES intervention. Provide warm referrals to appropriate community agencies and support groups for people experiencing IPV (e.g., local shelters), statewide coalitions and helplines (e.g., Jane Doe in Massachusetts, APIADV in San Francisco, CA), and national resources such as the following:
   1. National Domestic Violence Hotline (1-800-799-SAFE, 1-800-799-7233, or http://www.thehotline.org)
   2. National Dating Abuse Helpline and Love Is Respect (1-866-331-9474, text 77054, or http://www.loveisrespect.org)
   3. National Sexual Assault Hotline (1-800-656-HOPE or 1-800-656-4673)
B. *Safety planning resources*
   1. The evidence-based (Decker et al., 2020; Glass et al., 2021; Koziol-McLain et al., 2018) mobile phone application "MyPlan" may help patients to prioritize safety decisions within their relationships. It is available from the major app stores and at https://www.myplanapp.org/.
   2. A customizable safety plan for patients can be found at http://www.domesticviolence.org/personalized-safety-plan/.
C. *Resources for reducing stigma and increasing awareness of intimate partner violence*
   Resources for reducing stigma and increasing awareness of domestic violence can be found at http://www.nomore.org. Social media and campaign efforts may be appropriate for use within the clinic setting and to promote open disclosure with anticipatory guidance.
D. *Other services and resources*
   1. National Sexual Violence Resource Center (http://www.nsvrc.org)
   2. National Center for Victims of Crime's Stalking Resource Center (http://www.victimsofcrime.org/our-programs/stalking-resource-center)
   3. National Coalition of Anti-Violence Programs (http://www.avp.org/about-avp/coalitions-a-collaborations/82-national-coalition-of-anti-violence-programs)
   4. National Online Resource Center on Violence Against Women (http://www.vawnet.org/)
   5. Rape, Abuse, and Incest National Network (http://www.rainn.org), hotline at 1-800-656-HOPE

References

American College of Obstetricians and Gynecologists. (2012). Committee Opinion No. 518: Intimate partner violence. *Obstetrics and Gynecology, 119*(2 Pt. 1), 412–417. doi:10.1097/AOG.0b013e318249ff74

Anderson, J. C., Campbell, J. C., Glass, N. E., Decker, M. R., Perrin, N., & Farley, J. (2018). Impact of intimate partner violence on clinic attendance, viral suppression and CD4 cell count of women living with HIV in an urban clinic setting. *AIDS Care, 30*(4), 399–408. doi:10.1080/09540121.2018.1428725

Bacchus, L. J., Ranganathan, M., Watts, C., & Devries, K. (2018). Recent intimate partner violence against women and health: A systematic review and meta-analysis of cohort studies. *BMJ Open, 8*(7), e019995. doi:10.1136/bmjopen-2017-019995

Basile, K. C., Breiding, M. J., & Smith, S. G. (2016). Disability and risk of recent sexual violence in the United States. *American Journal of Public Health, 106*(5), 928–933. doi:10.2105/AJPH.2015.303004

Bonomi, A. E., Anderson, M. L., Rivara, F. P., & Thompson, R. S. (2009). Health care utilization and costs associated with physical and nonphysical-only intimate partner violence. *Health Services Research*, 44(3), 1052–1067. doi:10.1111/j.1475-6773.2009.00955.x

Breiding, M. J., & Armour, B. S. (2015). The association between disability and intimate partner violence in the United States. *Annals of Epidemiology*, 25(6), 455–457. doi:10.1016/j.annepidem.2015.03.017

Breiding, M. J., Smith, S. G., Basile, K. C., Walters, M. L., Chen, J., & Merrick, M. T. (2014). Prevalence and characteristics of sexual violence, stalking, and intimate partner violence victimization—National Intimate Partner and Sexual Violence Survey, United States, 2011. *Surveillance Summaries: Morbidity and Mortality Weekly Report*, 63(8), 1–18.

Burton, C. W., Gilpin, C. E., & Draughon Moret, J. (2021). Structural violence: A concept analysis to inform nursing science and practice. *Nursing Forum*, 56(2), 382–388. doi:10.1111/nuf.12535

Centers for Disease Control and Prevention. (2021, November 2). *Preventing intimate partner violence*. https://www.cdc.gov/violenceprevention/intimatepartnerviolence/fastfact.html

Chamberlain, L., & Levenson, R. (2013). *Addressing intimate partner violence, reproductive and sexual coercion: a guide for obstetric, gynecologic, reproductive health care settings* (3rd ed.). Futures Without Violence.

Chandan, J. S., Thomas, T., Bradbury-Jones, C., Taylor, J., Bandyopadhyay, S., & Nirantharakumar, K. (2020). Risk of cardiometabolic disease and all-cause mortality in female survivors of domestic abuse. *Journal of the American Heart Association*, 9(4), e014580. doi:10.1161/JAHA.119.014580

Cliffe, C., Miele, M., & Reid, S. (2019). Homicide in pregnant and postpartum women worldwide: A review of the literature. *Journal of Public Health Policy*, 40(2), 180–216. doi:10.1057/s41271-018-0150-z

Crenshaw, K. (1989). Demarginalizing the intersection of race and sex: A black feminist critique of antidiscrimination doctrine, feminist theory and antiracist politics. *University of Chicago Legal Forum*, 140, 139–167.

Curry, S. J., Krist, A. H., Owens, D. K., Barry, M. J., Caughey, A. B., Davidson, K. W., Doubeni, C. A., Epling, J. W., Grossman, D. C., Kemper, A. R., Kubik, M., Kurth, A., Landefeld, C. S., Mangione, C. M., Silverstein, M., Simon, M. A., Tseng, C. W., & Wong, J. B. (2018). Screening for intimate partner violence, elder abuse, and abuse of vulnerable adults: US Preventive Services Task Force final recommendation statement. *Journal of the American Medical Association*, 320(16), 1678–1687. doi:10.1001/jama.2018.14741

Decker, M. R., Frattaroli, S., McCaw, B., Coker, A. L., Miller, E., Sharps, P., Lane, W. G., Mandal, M., Hirsch, K., Strobino, D. M., Bennett, W. L., Campbell, J., & Gielen, A. (2012). Transforming the healthcare response to intimate partner violence and taking best practices to scale. *Journal of Women's Health*, 21(12), 1222–1229. doi:10.1089/jwh.2012.4058

Decker, M. R., Wood, S. N., Kennedy, S. R., Hameeduddin, Z., Tallam, C., Akumu, I., Wanjiru, I., Asira, B., Omondi, B., Case, J., Clough, A., Otieno, R., Mwiti, M., Perrin, N., & Glass, N. (2020). Adapting the myPlan safety app to respond to intimate partner violence for women in low and middle income country settings: App tailoring and randomized controlled trial protocol. *BMC Public Health*, 20(1), 808. doi:10.1186/s12889-020-08901-4

Department of Justice, Office of Violence Against Women. (n.d.). *Domestic violence*. https://www.justice.gov/ovw/domestic-violence#dv

Department of Justice, Office of Violence Against Women. (2021). *Sexual assault*. https://www.justice.gov/ovw/sexual-assault#sa

Dominguez, K. L., Smith, D., Vasavi, T., Crepaz, N., Lang, K., Heneine, W., McNicholl, J. M., Reid, L., Freelon, B., Nesheim, S. R., Huang, Y., & Weidle, P. L. (2016). *Updated guidelines for antiretroviral postexposure prophylaxis after sexual, injection drug use, or other nonoccupational exposure to HIV—United States, 2016*. Centers for Disease Control and Prevention. https://www.cdc.gov/hiv/pdf/programresources/cdc-hiv-npep-guidelines.pdf

Ellsberg, M., Jansen, H. A. F. M., Heise, L., Watts, C. H., Garcia-Moreno, C., & WHO Multi-country Study on Women's Health and Domestic Violence against Women Study Team. (2008). Intimate partner violence and women's physical and mental health in the WHO multi-country study on women's health and domestic violence: An observational study. *The Lancet*, 371(9619), 1165–1172. doi:10.1016/S0140-6736(08)60522-X

Feltner, C., Wallace, I., Berkman, N., Kistler, C. E., Middleton, J. C., Barclay, C., Higginbotham, L., Green, J. T., & Jonas, D. E. (2018). Screening for intimate partner violence, elder abuse, and abuse of vulnerable adults: evidence report and systematic review for the US Preventive Services Task Force. *Journal of the American Medical Association*, 320(16), 1688–1701. doi:10.1001/jama.2018.13212

Fishman, P. A., Bonomi, A. E., Anderson, M. L., Reid, R. J., & Rivara, F. P. (2010). Changes in health care costs over time following the cessation of intimate partner violence. *Journal of General Internal Medicine*, 25(9), 920–925. doi:10.1007/s11606-010-1359-0

Futures Without Violence. (2018). *CUES: An evidence-based intervention*. https://ipvhealth.org/health-professionals/educate-providers/

Futures Without Violence. (2021, January 21). *The evidence behind CUES: An intervention to address intimate partner violence in health settings*. https://ipvhealth.org/wp-content/uploads/2021/08/Evidence-for-CUES_1.28.21.pdf

Ghandour, R. M., Campbell, J. C., & Lloyd, J. (2015). Screening and counseling for intimate partner violence: A vision for the future. *Journal of Women's Health*, 24(1), 57–61. doi:10.1089/jwh.2014.4885

Glass, N. E., Clough, A., Messing, J. T., Bloom, T., Brown, M. L., Eden, K. B., Campbell, J. C., Gielen, A., Laughon, K., Grace, K. T., Turner, R. M., Alvarez, C., Case, J., Barnes-Hoyt, J., Alhusen, J., Hanson, G. C., & Perrin, N. A. (2021). Longitudinal impact of the myPlan app on health and safety among college women experiencing partner violence. *Journal of Interpersonal Violence*, 37(13–14), NP11436–NP11459. doi:10.1177/0886260521991880

Goldberg, X., Espelt, C., Porta-Casteràs, D., Palao, D., Nadal, R., & Armario, A. (2021). Non-communicable diseases among women survivors of intimate partner violence: Critical review from a chronic stress framework. *Neuroscience and Biobehavioral Reviews*, 128, 720–734. doi:10.1016/j.neubiorev.2021.06.045

Haeger, K. O., Lamme, J., & Cleland, K. (2018). State of emergency contraception in the U.S., 2018. *Contraception and Reproductive Medicine*, 3, 20. doi:10.1186/s40834-018-0067-8

Hassouneh-Phillips, D., & Curry, M. A. (2002). Abuse of women with disabilities. *Rehabilitation Counseling Bulletin*, 45(2), 96–104. doi:10.1177/003435520204500204

Hatcher, A. M., Smout, E. M., Turan, J. M., Christofides, N., & Stöckl, H. (2015). Intimate partner violence and engagement in HIV care and treatment among women: A systematic review and meta-analysis. *AIDS*, 29(16), 2183–2194. doi:10.1097/QAD.0000000000000842

Humphreys, J., Epel, E. S., Cooper, B. A., Lin, J., Blackburn, E. H., & Lee, K. A. (2012). Telomere shortening in formerly abused and never abused women. *Biological Research for Nursing*, 14(2), 115–123. doi:10.1177/1099800411398479

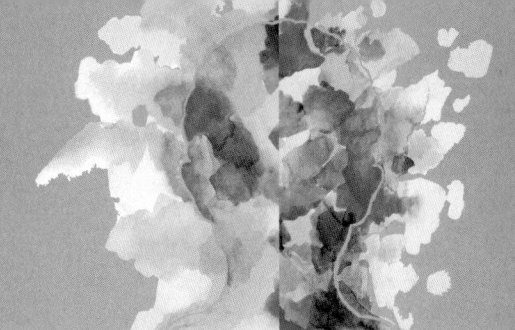

CHAPTER 59

Irritable Bowel Syndrome

Elizabeth Gatewood

I. Introduction and general background

Irritable bowel syndrome (IBS) is a "functional gastrointestinal disorder," a disorder of intestinal motility and visceral sensory perception. It is a syndrome related to clinically recognized signs and symptoms that cluster together (Drossman, 2016). There are no structural or biochemical causes associated with IBS. Although often associated primarily with the lower intestinal tract, the signs and symptoms of IBS can be found along the entire gastrointestinal (GI) tract. The biopsychosocial model recognizes the impact and intersection of psychosocial factors on physiology, which result in the clinical presentation of functional GI disorders (Engel, 1981). This model supports the multimodal treatments currently recommended (Hadjivasilis et al., 2019).

IBS is defined as a functional bowel disorder in which recurrent abdominal pain is associated with a change in bowel habits (constipation, diarrhea, or a mix), as well as symptoms of abdominal bloating/distention (Lacy & Patel, 2017). This constellation of symptoms led to the development of the Rome Criteria, which was done in conjunction with the World College of Gastroenterology in Rome, Italy, in 1998 (Rome I), 1999 (Rome II), 2006 (Rome III), and most recently in 2016 (Rome IV) (Rome Foundation, n.d.). The Rome criteria are used to aid in the diagnosis of IBS and create standardization, allowing for research. Recently the Rome Foundation Board of Directors proposed a modification to differentiate clinical criteria (Drossman & Tack, 2022). The aim of these clinical criteria is to reduce unnecessary studies and improve the patient–provider relationship by allowing for earlier diagnosis.

The following is a list of the Rome IV criteria for IBS diagnosis: recurrent abdominal pain or discomfort on average at least 1 day per month in the last 6 months, associated with two of the following features:
- Related to defecation
- Associated with change in frequency of stool
- Associated with a change in the form of stool (Lacy & Patel, 2017)

Other common characteristics include abdominal bloating and distention. These are not, however, required to make a diagnosis of IBS (Moayyedi et al., 2019).

Within IBS, there are four subtypes:
- IBS with predominant constipation (IBS-C)
- IBS with predominant diarrhea (IBS-D)
- IBS with mixed bowel habits (IBS-M)
- IBS unclassified (IBS-U)

The IBS-U category is for patients who meet the criteria but do not fall into one of the previous groups. Part of the diagnosis is appropriately identifying the subtype. Diagnosis of IBS can be made if all other diagnoses, structural or metabolic, have been eliminated. One must keep in mind that symptom expression differs among patients and may be any combination of these factors.

The revised clinical criteria proposed include four components:
- Qualitative: The qualitative features of the Rome IV criteria must be met.
- "Bothersomeness": The symptoms are severe enough to interfere with the patient's quality of life.
- Frequency: The revised clinical criteria do not include frequency as a requirement.
- Duration: Symptoms have been present for 8 weeks (instead of 6 months).

Although these new clinical criteria have been proposed and voted on by the Board, it is important to note that the newly proposed clinical criteria have not yet been validated and are still undergoing research. They are important to note, however, so that clinicians feel empowered to diagnose and treat patients earlier.

A. *Epidemiology*
1. Prevalence
   The prevalence of IBS varies but globally is around 11% (Black & Ford, 2020). When looked at more regionally, prevalence rates are around 7% in Asian and Middle Eastern areas; 11.8%–14.0% in North American, northern European, and Australian studies; and 15%–21% in southern European, African,

and South American regions (Black & Ford, 2020). There are multiple potential reasons for these variations, including differences in methodology between studies, lack of data or information (little is known about IBS in many African countries), and potential cultural differences. There is large variation in where and how many patients seek advice and treatment for symptoms of IBS, with studies ranging from 10%–80% of patients seeking care (Black & Ford, 2020; Corsetti & Whorwell, 2017; Shin et al., 2020). Patients often seek information from friends, family, and the internet prior to seeking advice from healthcare providers.

2. Impact

The burden of IBS is significant to the individual and society. It is associated with a lower quality of life, loss of income, and burden on family. Additionally, direct and indirect costs are substantial, including costs of healthcare use and absenteeism from work (Black & Ford, 2020). It is estimated that approximately $8 billion is spent per year in the United States on the care of patients with IBS (Hauser et al., 2008). Annually, IBS accounts for 3.5 million physician visits, 2.2 million prescriptions, and 35,000 hospitalizations annually (Hauser et al., 2014).

3. Risk factors

Globally, female sex confers greater risk, with a ratio of 1.67:1 (Lovell & Ford, 2012), with many studies citing a 2:1 ratio. These numbers may be somewhat inflated because females seek medical care more frequently than males; thus, the number of males with IBS may not be accurately reported. There is no significant difference based on age or socioeconomic status (Lovell & Ford, 2012). It tends to present in early adulthood (Mayer, 2008). Although IBS seems to have a familial component, a confirmed genetic risk has not been clearly established because of conflicting research (Black & Ford, 2020).

IBS has been associated with psychiatric comorbidities and can be exacerbated by stress, anxiety, and depression. In some cases, the onset of symptoms can occur after acute inflammatory conditions of the GI tract, such as postinfection IBS. Food sensitivities and allergies may also have a role, although formal food allergy testing is generally not recommended. There are many proposed theories related to the pathophysiology of these connections.

B. Pathophysiology

The pathophysiology of IBS is multifactorial and not fully understood. There are many possible mechanisms and causative factors. It is likely that a genetic predisposition triggered by an event result in a patient's development of IBS (Black & Ford, 2020). The most common explanations include postinfection, food intolerance, inflammation, serotonin (5-hydroxytryptamine [5-HT]) alterations, and lower pain thresholds (Black & Ford, 2020; Hadjivasilis et al., 2019). The brain–gut axis helps to explain the interactions between these various mechanisms.

Postinfection IBS is well established, with an incidence of approximately 10% 1 year after infection. Being female and having concurrent anxiety or depression increase the risk of ongoing IBS. Potentially abnormal 5-HT metabolism, increased permeability, and chronic immune activation may be underlying mechanisms contributing to IBS (Card et al., 2018).

Patients with IBS often note specific foods that trigger their symptoms. Over the years, research has helped identify specific foods that lead to inflammation and symptoms. Short-chain carbohydrates that are characterized by limited absorption, high osmotic activity, and intense bacterial fermentation—fermentable oligosaccharides, disaccharides and monosaccharides, and polyols (FODMAPS)—have been identified as irritants, leading to diets that restrict these components (Gibson, 2017; Murray et al., 2014). Avoidance of these has shown alleviation of symptoms in up to 75% of patients (Werlang et al., 2019).

In some patients, IBS seems to be associated with activation of the immune system, inflammation, intestinal permeability, and visceral hypersensitivity (Hadjivasilis et al., 2019; Matricon et al., 2012; Ohman & Simrén, 2010; Yuan et al., 2003). Although the mechanisms are not exactly clear, this reaction has been confirmed in multiple studies. Patients with IBS can have hypersensitivity throughout the entire digestive tract.

The enteric nervous system (ENS) is located in the digestive tract. More than 90% of the body's 5-HT and 50% of the dopamine are produced in the GI tract by the ENS (Raskov et al., 2016). Patients with IBS have shown significantly higher levels of 5-HT, which has also been correlated with the severity of abdominal pain (Cremon et al., 2011). Alterations in 5-HT release seem to affect the subtype of IBS, with patients with IBS-C having a decrease of 5-HT release and postinfection patients with IBS-D having an increased release. This 5-HT metabolism may be influenced by genetic factors. Medications that affect 5-HT receptors can have positive effects on IBS symptoms, further supporting the influence of 5-HT (Black & Ford, 2020).

The possible role of altered microbes is thought to be a potential contributor to the common symptom of abdominal distension. Observational studies have shown that patients with IBS have different intestinal microbes (Tap et al., 2017). Further, there has been some evidence of relief with fecal transplants and probiotics, which alter the intestinal microbes (Asha & Khalil, 2020; Ianiro et al., 2019).

The complex pathophysiology contributes to the varying patient presentations and broad treatments for patients with IBS. Developing good patient rapport is key to supporting the management of IBS.

II. Database (may include but is not limited to)
A. *Subjective findings*
 1. Past medical history
    a. Abdominal surgeries
    b. Substance abuse
    c. Thyroid disease
    d. Food sensitivities, especially lactose intolerance
    e. Carcinoid syndrome: causes profound diarrhea
    f. Gastroesophageal reflux disease frequently seen in patients with slow overall motility
    g. Medications prone to altering GI motility, such as opiates, stimulants, or laxatives
 2. Family history: IBS, inflammatory bowel disease, colon cancer, diabetes, and thyroid disease
 3. Psychosocial history
    a. Habits: alcohol, tobacco, or illicit drug use
    b. Situational stressors, coping mechanisms, and social support systems
    c. Exercise and physical activity: Sedentary lifestyle is commonly seen in patients with constipation and other bowel motility disorders.
    d. Diet history: Note typical diet, foods that trigger symptoms, amount of water and caffeine intake, use of artificial sweeteners (sorbitol, saccharin, or NutraSweet), use of chewing gum, and fiber intake.
 4. Review of systems
    a. Fever, chills, weight gain or loss, and fatigue
    b. Changes in skin, hair, nails, and other symptoms suggestive of thyroid disease
    c. Lower abdominal pain relieved with defecation, particularly in the left lower quadrant
    d. Constipation, diarrhea, or alternating diarrhea and constipation
    e. Bloating (upper and lower intestinal tract) and gas
    f. Frequency of stools and presence of mucus or blood in the stool (*patients with IBS typically do not have blood in the stool*)
    g. Anxiety, depression, and other psychiatric symptoms
    h. Nausea, vomiting, dyspepsia, and other upper GI symptoms
B. *Objective findings*
 1. Physical examination: A full physical examination is recommended, with particular attention to:
    a. Vital signs (note any orthostatic changes), and weight
    b. Thyroid examination
    c. Abdominal examination, noting bowel sounds, any masses, and tenderness (especially in the left lower quadrant)
    d. Pelvic examination noting any uterine or adnexal enlargement
    e. Mental status examination, noting appearance, behavior, mood, affect, and thought content

III. Assessment
A. *Determine the diagnosis*

Historically, IBS is a diagnosis of exclusion. There is some current debate that IBS should not only be a diagnosis of exclusion. It is important to rule out other causes of abdominal symptoms and complaints. The diagnostic and management approaches to patients with IBS focus on careful history and physical examination skills, in addition to building a strong therapeutic alliance with the patient to help understand the underlying disorder and symptom-based treatment. Diagnostic evaluations should be individualized to the patient's presenting symptoms to avoid unnecessary and expensive procedures.

The following diagnoses should be considered for all patients presenting with suspected IBS:
 1. Bacterial infections
 2. Colon cancer
 3. Diverticulosis and diverticulitis
 4. Eating disorders
 5. Adhesions
 6. Fecal incontinence
 7. Ovarian tumors, endometriosis, and adnexal cysts (based on organs present)
 8. Inflammatory bowel disease
 9. Atypical colitis, microscopic colitis, lymphocytic colitis, or eosinophilic gastroenteritis
 10. Thyroid disease, diabetes, and other endocrine disorders
 11. Celiac disease
 12. Depression, anxiety, and other mental health disorders
 13. Pelvic floor dysfunction caused by pelvic floor damage
 14. Carcinoid syndrome

B. *Severity*

Assess the severity of the disease.

C. *Significance*

Assess the significance of the symptoms and chronic nature of the disorder to the patient and significant others.

IV. Goals of clinical management
A. *Assist the patient to achieve optimal level of functioning with daily activities and quality of life.*
B. *Assist the patient with management strategies, including medications, stress relief, dietary recommendations, and psychosocial support.*
C. *Prevent pain by performing adequate pain assessments and referring to pain management for assistance if needed.*

V. Plan
A. *Screening*

There are no screening tests available for early detection or prevention of IBS.

Chapter 59 Irritable Bowel Syndrome

B. Diagnostic studies
   Based on symptoms and history
   1. Diet diary: The diet diary is an essential initial diagnostic tool for IBS management. The diary helps both the patient and the clinician to make associations between symptoms and foods. It also engages the patient in a meaningful way as a partner in both the diagnostic and treatment processes. The diary should note the time of meals and snacks; the type and quantity of foods eaten; and associated GI symptoms before or after food consumption, noting the time frame of symptom development.
   2. For recommended first- and second-line symptom-based diagnostic testing, see **Tables 59-1** and **59-2**.

Table 59-1 Initial Symptom-Based Diagnostic Workup for Irritable Bowel Syndrome*

Diarrhea-Predominant Symptoms	Constipation-Predominant Symptoms	Upper Gastrointestinal-Predominant Symptoms
Stool sample: culture and sensitivity, ova and parasites, and *Clostridium difficile* ■ To rule out bacterial and parasitic infections	Complete blood count with differential ■ To look for evidence of anemia seen with malignancies, inflammatory bowel disease (IBD), and other systemic disease ■ To look for leukocytosis seen with IBD and infections	Upper gastrointestinal series with a small bowel follow-through ■ To rule out structural abnormality or adhesions; also, to evaluate transit time with constipation and diarrhea
Stool sample for *Giardia* ■ To rule out *Giardia lamblia* infection. Increased risk in individuals with immunocompromise and those with a recent travel history.	Thyroid-stimulating hormone ■ To rule out hypothyroid disorders	Abdominal sonogram ■ To rule out gallstones
Stool sample for fecal occult blood ■ To rule out malignancy, IBD, and other systemic causes of intestinal bleeding	Plain abdominal film (also called a *flat plate of the abdomen*) ■ To look for a bowel obstruction or ileus, adhesions, and pseudo-obstruction	Serum liver function tests ■ To evaluate liver health and rule out hepatitis, cirrhosis, and other liver diseases
Stool sample for fecal fat/pancreatic elastase ■ Seen with malabsorption and pancreatic insufficiency	Stool sample for fecal occult blood ■ To rule out malignancy, IBD, and other systemic causes of intestinal bleeding	Serum lipase and amylase ■ To rule out pancreatitis
Complete blood count with differential ■ To look for evidence of anemia seen with malignancies, IBD, and other systemic disease ■ To look for leukocytosis seen with IBD and infections	Serum potassium and calcium ■ To rule out hypokalemia and hypercalcemia, both associated with constipation	
Erythrocyte sedimentation rate ■ Nonspecific marker of IBD and malignancy		
Fasting blood sugar ■ To rule out diabetes mellitus, which can present with diarrhea because of diabetic gastroenteropathy		
Thyroid-stimulating hormone ■ To rule out hyperthyroid disorders		
Electrolytes (depending on severity of symptoms) ■ To look for electrolyte disturbances seen with severe diarrhea and malabsorption		

*This is an exhaustive workup. Diagnostics should be ordered based on the individual patient's presentation and in collaboration with the patient.

Data from American College of Gastroenterology Task Force on Irritable Bowel Syndrome. (2009); World Gastroenterology Organization Global Guideline. (2009). Irritable bowel syndrome: A global perspective, 1–20.

Table 59-2 Second-Line Symptom-Based Diagnostic Workup for Irritable Bowel Syndrome

Diarrhea-Predominant Symptoms	Constipation-Predominant Symptoms	Upper Gastrointestinal–Predominant Symptoms
Celiac serologies (tissue transglutaminase immunoglobulin A [IgA] most sensitive) ■ To rule out celiac sprue disease	Colonoscopy or flexible sigmoidoscopy with a barium enema ■ To rule out mucosal (atypical colitis) or structural abnormalities	Endoscopy ■ To rule out celiac disease, gastric or duodenal ulcer, and gastroesophageal reflux disease with esophageal spasm
Repeat stool sample for ova and parasites and *Clostridium difficile* ■ To rule out a recurrent bacterial infection or *C. difficile*, commonly seen with recent history of antibiotic use	Abdominal and pelvic computerized tomography scan ■ To rule out cancer and other pathologic conditions	
Allergy testing (controversial) ■ To look for food allergies		
Endoscopy ■ To rule out celiac disease by taking small bowel biopsies looking for villous blunting with diarrhea, bloating, and pain		

Data from American College of Gastroenterology Task Force on Irritable Bowel Syndrome. (2009); World Gastroenterology Organization Global Guideline. (2009). Irritable bowel syndrome: A global perspective, 1–20.

---

3. Alarm symptoms warranting a gastroenterology referral include:
   a. Short history of symptoms
   b. Unintended weight loss
   c. Family history of colon cancer, celiac disease, or inflammatory bowel disease
   d. Rectal bleeding or abnormal stool studies
   e. Unexplained anemia
   f. Anorexia
   g. Blood in the stool
   h. Severe unrelenting diarrhea or constipation
   i. Nocturnal symptoms
   j. Onset in patients older than 50 years
   k. Palpable abdominal or rectal mass

C. Management

The mainstay of any treatment regimen for patients with suspected or confirmed IBS is, first and foremost, to build a therapeutic alliance with the patient. The underpinnings of this alliance include careful listening, validation of symptoms, and compassion for the distress that symptoms may cause for the patient. Such an alliance provides a platform for working with the patient through the symptom-based diagnostic and treatment process.

There are few studies that offer convincing evidence of effectiveness in curing the IBS symptom complex (Akehurst & Kaltenthaler, 2001). Current treatment guidelines focus on symptom-based treatment management (Hadjivasilis et al., 2019; Moayyedi et al., 2017).

1. For patients with diarrhea-prominent symptoms:
   a. Antidiarrheal agents
      i. Loperamide: 4 mg orally for the initial dose and then 2 mg up to 16 mg/day, as needed, to reduce stool frequency
      ii. Eluxadoline: 75–100 mg twice a day depending on tolerability. Check baseline creatinine and estimated glomerular filtration rate [eGFR].
   b. Bile acid sequestrants
      i. Cholestyramine: 4 g PO daily, twice a day; maximum dose 24 g/day; produced as powder
   c. 5-hydroxytryptamine (serotonin) 3 receptor antagonists
      i. Alosetron: 0.5–1 mg by mouth twice a day. Start 0.5 mg twice a day × 4 weeks and then can increase to a maximum of 2 mg/day. Note: Limited access in the United States.
2. For constipation-prominent symptoms:
   a. High-fiber diet with the addition of dietary fiber, psyllium, or Benefiber® (i.e., 1 heaping tablespoon in 8 oz of fluids taken by mouth one to two times per day with plenty of water). Also, add insoluble fiber (see list mentioned previously). Insoluble fiber helps the stool absorb water to facilitate passage of stool and prevent constipation.

b. Laxatives
  i. Polyethylene glycol (Miralax®), 18 g mixed in 8 oz of liquid one to two times per day, is very effective for constipation, but patients may continue to experience bloating and abdominal pain.
  ii. Bisacodyl (Dulcolax®): 5- to 15-mg tablets as a single dose; may take up to 30 mg if complete bowel evacuation is needed; 10-mg suppository as a single daily dose prn.
  iii. Senna or cascara tablets: 8.6 mg, 1–2 tablets by mouth prior to bedtime. Long-term use of senna may cause melanosis coli (MC) (dark pigment deposits in the lining of the large intestine). If this occurs, senna should be discontinued. MC will resolve around 1 year after discontinuation (Yang et al., 2020).
c. Chloride channel activator that increases intestinal fluid secretion and intestinal motility:
  i. Lubiprostone (Amitiza®): 8 mcg orally twice daily, for women aged 18 and older
  ii. Linaclotide (Linzess®): 290 mcg by mouth daily. Long-term safety profile is unknown. *Consultation with GI specialist is recommended.*
d. Increase oral fluids: Water is best, followed by low-sugar-content fluids.
e. Physical activity: Assist the patient in developing a regular daily exercise and activity plan. Physical activity has been shown to promote healthier bowel motility and overall better mental and physical health.

3. For abdominal pain:
  a. Antispasmodic agents
    i. Dicyclomine (Bentyl®): 20 mg orally four times per day prn. Can titrate up to a maximum of 160 mg per day.
    ii. Hyoscyamine: 0.125–0.25 mg orally, three to four times daily, prn pain. Take before food. Maximum dosage is 1.5 mg in 24 hours. Because of anticholinergic properties, use these medications with caution in the geriatric population.
  b. Low-dose tricyclic antidepressants (help to reduce visceral sensation): particularly beneficial for patients with IBS-D; amitriptyline 25 mg orally at bedtime, may titrate up to 100 mg at bedtime
  c. Serotonin reuptake inhibitor: Particularly beneficial for patients with IBS-C or concurrent anxiety of depression
  d. Pain management: Suggest nonpharmacologic measures first, such as relaxation, acupuncture, and meditation. Avoid the use of narcotic analgesics because of their addiction potential and GI side effects.

4. For abdominal bloating:
  a. Diet: All patients should try a *low-FODMAP diet* (Halmos, 2014). FODMAPs are short-chain sugars that are poorly absorbed by the small intestine (**Table 59-3**). Other dietary restrictions include limiting dairy products; carbonated beverages; caffeine; alcohol; red meats; artificial fats; and sugars, such as honey, high-fructose corn syrup, and artificial sweeteners (sorbitol-containing products).
    It can be overwhelming to restrict all these foods and substances at once. Often, selecting one or two food groups to eliminate and monitoring the effect is a reasonable approach to begin the dietary modification process. Referral to a nutritionist may also be helpful.
  b. Probiotics: Probiotics have been found to alleviate IBS symptoms with limited side effects. Products containing *Lactobacillus* reduced abdominal pain and flatulence and improved quality of life. General symptoms were improved with *Bifidobacterium*. Preparations with multiple strains may be beneficial (Asha & Khalil, 2020).

5. Other
  a. Fecal microbe transplantation: This is a new, recent treatment option that is being used in IBS with success (El-Salhy & Mazzawi, 2018). Patients receive either fresh or frozen stool from a donor, who can be identified by the family or obtained from a donor stool bank. It is usually completed via colonoscopy.

D. Follow-up
Reevaluate the patient in 4–6 weeks after initial treatment program and evaluation are done. If symptoms persist, consider changing treatment regimen or obtaining further diagnostic testing as indicated based on predominant symptoms. The following are recommendations for further testing after the initial evaluation, which are often done by a gastroenterologist.

1. Refractory constipation: Evaluate colonic transit time, pelvic floor function, and adhesions by considering the following additional tests:
  a. Colonic transit test
  b. Anorectal manometry
  c. Rectal sensation testing and emptying study
2. Refractory diarrhea: Evaluate for bacterial overgrowth, laxative abuse, atypical colitis, carcinoid syndrome, and increased colonic transit.
  a. Stool chemistry for surreptitious laxative abuse
  b. Duodenal aspirate for bacterial overgrowth
  c. Colonic biopsies for microscopic or collagenous colitis
  d. Urinary 5-hydroxy indoleacetic acid for carcinoid syndrome
  e. Small bowel transit study for increased transit
3. Pain: Evaluate small or large intestine for obstruction, intermediate obstruction, cancer, or adhesions.
  a. Plain abdominal radiograph for obstruction and intermediate obstruction
  b. Computed tomography (CT) scan of the abdomen for cancer and obstruction
  c. CT enterography for cancer, obstruction, and colitis
  d. Upper GI series with a small bowel follow-through for adhesions; can also evaluate transit time

Table 59-3 FODMAP Diet

	High FODMAP foods	Low FODMAP alternatives
Vegetables	Artichoke, asparagus, cauliflower, garlic, green peas, mushrooms, onion, sugar snap peas	Aubergine/eggplant, beans (green), bok choy, green capsicum (bell pepper), carrot, cucumber, lettuce, potato
Fruits	Apples, apple juice, cherries, dried fruit, mango, nectarines, peaches, pears, plums, watermelon	Cantaloupe, kiwifruit, mandarin, orange, pineapple, blueberry
Dairy & alternatives	Cow's milk, custard, evaporated milk, ice cream, soy milk (made from whole soybeans), sweetened condensed milk, yoghurt	Almond milk, brie/camembert cheese, feta cheese, hard cheeses, lactose-free milk, soy milk (made from soy protein)
Protein sources	Most legumes/pulses, some marinated meats/poultry/seafood, some processed meats	Eggs, firm tofu, plain cooked meats/poultry/seafood, tempeh
Breads & cereals	Wheat/rye/barley based breads, breakfast cereals, biscuits and snack products	Oats, quinoa flakes, quinoa/rice/corn pasta, rice cakes (plain), sourdough spelt bread, wheat/rye/barley free breads
Sugars, sweeteners & confectionery	High fructose corn syrup, honey, sugar free confectionery	Dark chocolate, maple syrup, rice malt syrup, table sugar
Nuts & seeds	Cashews, pistachios	Macadamias, peanuts, pumpkin seeds/pepitas, walnuts

Department of Gastroenterology, Monash University. Table reproduced with permission from Monash University (monashfodmap.com). Download the Monash University FODMAP Diet App for a comprehensive food guide containing the FODMAP ratings and serving sizes for hundreds of different foods and beverages. Available on iOS and Android.

E. Patient education
1. Assist the patient and family in verbalizing their concerns and coping strategies with respect to the disease process and management.
2. Provide verbal and written information about the pathophysiology of IBS and treatment.
3. Discuss what the patient can expect with diagnostic testing, preparation, and after-care.
4. Explain the therapeutic benefits and side effects of any prescribed treatment.
5. Reassure the patient that assistance is available when needed.
6. Emphasize the importance of stress management and good mental health in coping with this disorder.

VI. Self-management e-resources
A. *The National Institutes of Health has multiple brochures for patients with IBS.*
   (http://digestive.niddk.nih.gov/ddiseases/pubs/ibs/)
B. *Irritable Bowel Syndrome Association*
   (http://www.ibsgroup.org/ibsassociation)
C. *IBS FODMAP Dieting Guide*
   (http://www.ibsdiets.org/fodmap-diet/fodmap-food-list/)

References

Akehurst, R., & Kaltenthaler, E. (2001). Treatment of irritable bowel syndrome: A review of randomized controlled trials. *Gut, 48*(2), 272–282. doi:10.1136/gut.48.2.272

Asha, M. Z., & Khalil, S. F. H. (2020). Efficacy and safety of probiotics, prebiotics and symbiotic in the treatment of irritable bowel syndrome. *Sultan Qaboos University Medical Journal, 20*(1), e13–e24. doi:10.18295/squmj.2020.20.01.003

Black, C. J., & Ford, A. C. (2020). Global burden of irritable bowel syndrome: Trends, predictions and risk factors. *Nature Reviews Gastroenterology & Hepatology, 17*(8), 473–486. doi:10.1038/s41575-020-0286-8

Card, T., Enck, P., Barbara, G., Boeckxstaens, G. E., Santos, J., Azpiroz, F., Mearin, F., Aziz, Q., Marshall, J., & Spiller, R. (2018). Post-infectious IBS: Defining its clinical features and prognosis using an internet-based survey. *United European Gastroenterology Journal, 6*(8), 1245–1253. doi:10.1177/2050640618779923

Corsetti, M., & Whorwell, P. (2017). The global impact of IBS: Time to think about IBS-specific models of care? *Therapeutic Advances in Gastroenterology, 10*(9), 727–736. doi:10.1177/1756283X17718677

Cremon, C., Carini, G., Wang, B., Vasina, V., Cogliandro, R. F., De Giorgio, R., Stanghellini, V., Grundy, D., Tonini, M., De Ponti, F., Corinaldesi, R., & Barbara, G. (2011). Intestinal serotonin release, sensory neuron activation, and abdominal pain in irritable bowel syndrome. *The American Journal of Gastroenterology, 106*(7), 1290–1298. doi:10.1038/ajg.2011.86

Drossman, D. A. (2016). Functional gastrointestinal disorders: History, pathophysiology, clinical features, and Rome IV. *Gastroenterology, 150*(6), 1262-1279.e2. doi:10.1053/j.gastro.2016.02.032

Drossman, D. A., & Tack, J. (2022). Rome Foundation clinical diagnostic criteria for disorders of gut-brain interaction. *Gastroenterology, 162*(3), 675–679. doi:10.1053/j.gastro.2021.11.019

El-Salhy, M., & Mazzawi, T. (2018). Fecal microbiota transplantation for managing irritable bowel syndrome. *Expert Review of Gastroenterology & Hepatology, 12*(5), 439–445. doi:10.1080/17474124.2018.1447380

Engel, G. L. (1981). The clinical application of the biopsychosocial model. *Journal of Medicine and Philosophy, 6*(2), 101–124. doi:10.1093/jmp/6.2.101

Gibson, P. R. (2017). History of the low FODMAP diet. *Journal of Gastroenterology and Hepatology, 32*(Suppl. 1), 5–7. doi:10.1111/jgh.13685

Hadjivasilis, A., Tsioutis, C., Michalinos, A., Ntourakis, D., Christodoulou, D. K., & Agouridis, A. P. (2019). New insights into irritable bowel syndrome: From pathophysiology to treatment. *Annals of Gastroenterology, 32*(6), 554–564. doi:10.20524/aog.2019.0428

Halmos, E., Power, V., Shepherd, S., Gibson, P. R., & Muir, J. G. (2014). A diet low in FODMAPs reduces symptoms of irritable bowel syndrome. *Gastroenterology, 146*(1), 67–75. doi:10.1053/j.gastro.2013.09.046

Hauser, S. C., Oxentenko, A. S., & Sanchez, W. (2014). *Mayo Clinic gastroenterology and hepatology board review* (4th ed.). Mayo Clinic Scientific Press.

Hauser, S. C., Pardi, D. S., & Poterucha, J. J. (2008). *Mayo Clinic gastroenterology and hepatology board review* (3rd ed.). Mayo Clinic Scientific Press.

Ianiro, G., Eusebi, L. H., Black, C. J., Gasbarrini, A., Cammarota, G., & Ford, A. C. (2019). Systematic review with meta-analysis: Efficacy of faecal microbiota transplantation for the treatment of irritable bowel syndrome. *Alimentary Pharmacology & Therapeutics, 50*(3), 240–248. doi:10.1111/apt.15330

Lacy, B. E., & Patel, N. K. (2017). Rome Criteria and a diagnostic approach to irritable bowel syndrome. *Journal of Clinical Medicine, 6*(11), 99. doi:10.3390/jcm6110099

Lovell, R. M., & Ford, A. C. (2012). Global prevalence of and risk factors for irritable bowel syndrome: A meta-analysis. *Clinical Gastroenterology and Hepatology, 10*(7), 712-721.e4. doi:10.1016/j.cgh.2012.02.029

Matricon, J., Meleine, M., Gelot, A., Piche, T., Dapoigny, M., Muller, E., & Ardid, D. (2012). Review article: Associations between immune activation, intestinal permeability and the irritable bowel syndrome. *Alimentary Pharmacology & Therapeutics, 36*(11–12), 1009–1031. doi:10.1111/apt.12080

Mayer, E. A. (2008). Clinical practice. Irritable bowel syndrome. *New England Journal of Medicine, 358*(16), 1692–1699. doi:10.1056/NEJMcp0801447

Moayyedi, P., Eikelboom, J. W., Bosch, J., Connolly, S. J., Dyal, L., Shestakovska, O., Leong, D., Anand, S. S., Störk, S., Branch, K. R. H., Bhatt, D. L., Verhamme, P. B., O'Donnell, M., Maggioni, A. P., Lonn, E. M., Piegas, L. S., Ertl, G., Keltai, M., Bruns, N. C., … COMPASS Investigators. (2019). Safety of proton pump inhibitors based on a large, multi-year, randomized trial of patients receiving rivaroxaban or aspirin. *Gastroenterology, 157*(3), 682–691.e2. doi:10.1053/j.gastro.2019.05.056

Moayyedi, P., Mearin, F., Azpiroz, F., Andresen, V., Barbara, G., Corsetti, M., Emmanuel, A., Hungin, A. P. S., Layer, P., Stanghellini, V., Whorwell, P., Zerbib, F., & Tack, J. (2017). Irritable bowel syndrome diagnosis and management: A simplified algorithm for clinical practice. *United European Gastroenterology Journal, 5*(6), 773–788. doi:10.1177/2050640617731968

Murray, K., Wilkinson-Smith, V., Hoad, C., Costigan, C., Cox, E., Lam, C., Marciani, L., Gowland, P., & Spiller, R. C. (2014). Differential effects of FODMAPs (fermentable oligo-, di-, mono-saccharides and polyols) on small and large intestinal contents in healthy subjects shown by MRI. *American Journal of Gastroenterology, 109*(1), 110–119. doi:10.1038/ajg.2013.386

Ohman, L., & Simrén, M. (2010). Pathogenesis of IBS: Role of inflammation, immunity and neuroimmune interactions. *Nature Reviews Gastroenterology & Hepatology, 7*(3), 163–173. doi:10.1038/nrgastro.2010.4

Raskov, H., Burcharth, J., Pommergaard, H.-C., & Rosenberg, J. (2016). Irritable bowel syndrome, the microbiota and the gut-brain axis. *Gut Microbes, 7*(5), 365–383. doi:10.1080/19490976.2016.1218585

Rome Foundation. (n.d.). *Rome IV criteria*. https://theromefoundation.org/rome-iv/rome-iv-criteria/

Shin, A., Ballou, S., Camilleri, M., Xu, H., & Lembo, A. (2020). Information- and healthcare seeking behaviors in patients with irritable bowel syndrome. *Clinical Gastroenterology and Hepatology, 18*(12), 2840–2842. doi:10.1016/j.cgh.2019.09.020

Tap, J., Derrien, M., Törnblom, H., Brazeilles, R., Cools-Portier, S., Doré, J., Störsrud, S., Le Nevé, B., Öhman, L., & Simrén, M. (2017). Identification of an intestinal microbiota signature associated with severity of irritable bowel syndrome. *Gastroenterology, 152*(1), 111–123.e8. doi:10.1053/j.gastro.2016.09.049

Werlang, M. E., Palmer, W. C., & Lacy, B. E. (2019). Irritable bowel syndrome and dietary interventions. *Gastroenterology & Hepatology, 15*(1), 16–26.

Yang, N., Ruan, M., & Jin, S. (2020). Melanosis coli: A comprehensive review. *Gastroenterología y Hepatología, 43*(5), 266–272.

Yuan, Y. Z., Tao, R. J., Xu, B., Sun, J., Chen, K. M., Miao, F., Zhang, Z.-W., & Xu, J.-Y. (2003). Functional brain imaging in irritable bowel syndrome with rectal balloon-distention by using fMRI. *World Journal of Gastroenterology, 9*(6), 1356–1360. doi:10.3748/wjg.v9.i6.135

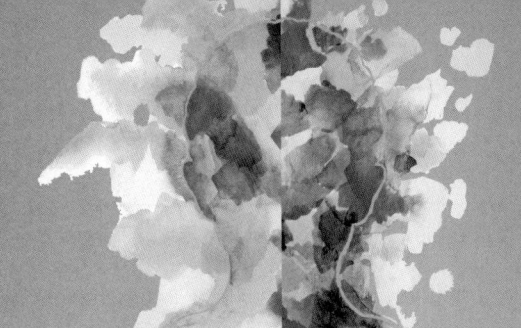

CHAPTER 60

Lipid Disorders

Lewis Fannon and J.V. Gatewood

I. Introduction and general background

Cardiovascular disease (CVD) is the leading cause of death worldwide (Heron, 2021; Sandesara et al., 2019). Numerous studies have demonstrated the positive correlation between higher cholesterol levels, particularly low-density lipoprotein cholesterol (LDL-C) levels, and higher atherosclerotic cardiovascular disease (ASCVD) risk (Ference et al., 2017). For this reason, the identification and management of lipid disorders are critical to mitigating cardiovascular risk, especially among patients already diagnosed with other risk factors, such as hypertension, diabetes mellitus, cigarette smoking, higher body weight, sedentary lifestyle, and family history of early coronary heart disease (Sandesara et al., 2019).

Lipid metabolism involves several types of lipoproteins and lipid–protein complexes, including LDL-C and high-density lipoprotein cholesterol (HDL-C), which are responsible for transporting cholesterol and triglycerides (TGs) within endogenous and exogenous pathways. They are responsible for lipid synthesis and delivery, as well as reverse cholesterol transport. This physiology is not discussed in detail here; however, it is important to underscore that different lipoproteins fulfill different roles (Đukanović et al., 2021).

The primary role of LDL-C is to carry cholesterol to extrahepatic cells. Any excess can result in atherogenesis, the formation of fatty plaques in the arteries. In contrast, HDL-C transports cholesterol from extrahepatic cells to the liver, where it has antiatherogenic, anti-inflammatory, and antioxidant properties. Higher levels of HDL-C are associated with lower cardiovascular risk, although it is important to note that this is true only up to around 120–130 mg/dL in women and 80–90 mg/dL in men, at which point risk can increase (Liu et al., 2022; Yang et al., 202). It is also important to remember that these pathways rely on normal hepatic and intestinal function for normal dietary cholesterol and TG absorption (Đukanović et al., 2021).

A. Definition and overview

Lipid disorders are defined by elevations in serum lipids (cholesterol, phospholipids, or TGs). The phospholipids include LDL-C, HDL-C, very-low-density lipoprotein (VLDL-C), intermediate-density lipoprotein (IDL-C), and chylomicrons.

Lipid disorders fall into two main categories: (1) primary (genetic or inherited) disorders of lipid metabolism and (2) secondary lipid disorders that are the result of other diseases (Yanai, 2021). For many patients, the causes of lipid disorders may be multifactorial, with both primary and secondary etiologies involved (**Box 60-1**).

B. Prevalence

Approximately 94 million Americans, or 38.1% of the U.S. adult population, had TC levels ≥ 200 mg/dL between 2015 and 2018 (Centers for Disease Control and Prevention [CDC], 2021; Virani et al., 2021). Asian Americans and Hispanic/Latinx Americans had the highest TCs levels among U.S. adults ≥20 years of age between 2015 and 2018, whereas non-Hispanic Black males had the lowest TC levels among U.S. adults (Virani et al., 2021). Interestingly, adult females had a higher TC prevalence than their male counterparts (Virani et al., 2021). Hyperlipidemia accounts for an estimated $26.4 billion annually in healthcare expenditures, with prescription medications and outpatient primary care visits accounting for two-thirds of total expenses (Virani et al., 2021). Low-income adults, African Americans, and Mexican Americans are disproportionately affected by dyslipidemia as age increases (Yandrapalli et al., 2019). This is especially important to note, given that the U.S. demographic is shifting toward an older population.

C. Diagnostic classifications

1. Inherited disorders of LDL-C metabolism
   Definition and overview: Primary or genetic disorders of lipid metabolism are less common than other types of dyslipidemia, but they are often responsible for the most severe forms of dyslipidemia. These disorders may be monogenic or polygenic. The most common form of monogenic hyperlipidemia is familial hypercholesterolemia, which affects approximately 1 in 200 Americans

Box 60-1 Definitions

1. Hyperlipidemia: A medical term for abnormally high levels of lipids in the blood, which include cholesterol and TGs. Can refer to multiple disorders that involve higher-than-normal lipid levels in the blood.
2. Dyslipidemia: Commonly used to describe any imbalance of lipids, such as cholesterol, LDL-C, TGs, and HDL-C. Refers to lipid levels that are either higher or lower than the normal range for those blood fats.
3. Hypercholesterolemia: An elevation of total cholesterol (TC) and/or LDL-C or non–HDL-C (defined as the subtraction of HDL-C from TC) in the blood. A type of hyperlipidemia (Verbeek et al., 2018).
4. Hypertriglyceridemia: An elevation of TGs in the blood.

Box 60-2 Hyperlipidemia

Hyperlipidemia is most commonly caused by a polygenic inheritance pattern. The manifestations of the disorder are influenced in large part by secondary factors such as higher (central) body weight and composition of the daily diet.

(Virani et al., 2021). Heritable forms of hyperlipidemia may result in elevated LDL-C with normal TG levels or elevated TGs in isolation (see Section C.2. Hypertriglyceridemia) (**Box 60-2**). Most are rare outside of certain specific demographic groups.

Primary disorders resulting in elevated LDL-C and normal TGs:
a. Familial hypercholesterolemia
b. Familial defective *ApoB-100*
c. Autosomal-dominant hypercholesterolemia resulting from mutations in *PCSK9*
d. Autosomal-recessive hypercholesterolemia
e. Sitosterolemia
f. Polygenic hypercholesterolemia
g. Elevated plasma levels of lipoprotein(a)

2. Hypertriglyceridemia
   a. Hypertriglyceridemia is generally believed to be an independent risk factor for CVD, but the amount of excess risk is small. Elevated levels of TGs are also associated with lower levels of HDL-C because of related metabolic pathways (Koo et al., 2021).
   b. May be primary, secondary, or multifactorial in origin. In general, possible genetic involvement should be considered when TGs start to exceed 500 mg/dL (Grundy et al., 2019).
   c. Primary lipid disorders causing elevated TGs and normal LDL-C:)
      i. Familial chylomicronemia
      ii. Apolipoprotein A-V (apoA-V) deficiency
      iii. Glycosylphosphatidylinositol anchored high-density lipoprotein binding protein 1 (GPIHBP1) deficiency
      iv. Hepatic lipase deficiency
      v. Familial dysbetalipoproteinemia
      vi. Familial hypertriglyceridemia: autosomal-dominant disorder that causes moderately elevated TG levels
      vii. Familial combined hyperlipidemia
   d. Secondary causes of hypertriglyceridemia include higher body weight, type 2 diabetes with poor glycemic control, nephrotic syndrome, hypothyroidism, pregnancy, and medications. Associated medications, some of them quite common, include tamoxifen, beta-blockers, immunosuppressives, HIV antiretrovirals, and retinoids.
   e. Very high levels of TGs are associated with pancreatitis. In patients with hypertriglyceridemia, additional factors associated with pancreatitis include poorly controlled diabetes, heredity, excessive alcohol use, and drug- or diet-induced hypertriglyceridemia.

3. Secondary disorders of lipoprotein metabolism
   a. Type 2 diabetes is one of the most important secondary causes of hyperlipidemia in primary care (Nuovo, 1999).
   b. Other secondary causes include:
      i. Excessive alcohol use
      ii. Hypothyroidism
      iii. Higher body weight
      iv. Pregnancy
      v. Cholestatic liver disease
      vi. Nephrotic syndrome
      vii. Immunoglobulin excess
      viii. Tobacco use (smoking)
      ix. Age
      x. Sedentary lifestyle
      xi. Medications: beta-blockers, thiazide diuretics, oral estrogens, steroid hormones, antiretrovirals, retinoids, and some atypical antipsychotics

D. *Treatment of hypercholesterolemia for secondary prevention*
   1. This includes treatment for patients with known Atherosclerotic Cardiovascular Disease (ASCVD). ASCVD includes the following: acute coronary syndrome (ACS)—within last 12 months, history of myocardial infarction (MI)—other than recent ACS mentioned above, history of ischemic stroke, (cerebrovascular disease), or symptomatic peripheral artery disease (PAD).

E. *Treatment of hypercholesterolemia for primary prevention*
   1. This includes providing treatment (usually statins) with the aim of avoiding the development of ASCVD (Grundy, 2019).

II. Database
A. Subjective
1. Past health history
   a. ASCVD: including cerebrovascular disease (CVD): acute coronary syndrome, history of myocardial infarction (MI), angina, peripheral vascular disease, abdominal aortic aneurysm.
       i. Premature CAD should raise suspicion for primary lipid disorders.
   b. Hypertension
   c. Excessive alcohol use
   d. Hypothyroidism
   e. Higher body weight
   f. Pregnancy
   g. Cholestatic liver disease
   h. Nephrotic syndrome
   i. Immunoglobulin excess
   j. Pancreatitis
   k. Diabetes mellitus
   l. Injuries: Patellar tendon—in the presence of hyperlipidemia, the tendon becomes mechanically less effective and more prone to injury.
   m. Other risk factors/diseases: Especially consider those with an inflammatory component that can cause dyslipidemia and atherosclerotic problems, which include (Hill & Bordoni, 2022):
       - Psoriasis
       - Crohn's disease
       - Inflammatory bowel disease
       - Chronic obstructive pulmonary disease
       - Depression
       - Chronic pain
       - Pediatric alopecia areata
       - Chronic kidney disease
2. Medications
   a. Medications that can promote hyperlipidemia: oral estrogens, steroid hormones, protease inhibitors, and some atypical antipsychotics.
   b. Common medications that can promote hypertriglyceridemia include beta-blockers, tamoxifen, immunosuppressives, HIV antiretrovirals, and retinoids.
3. Family history
   a. First-degree relative(s) with dyslipidemia.
   b. First-degree relative(s) with premature CAD (e.g., before age 55 in men and 65 in women).
   c. Family history of hyperlipidemia, familial hypercholesterolemia (or other known genetic issues in the family), special diets/ethnic ways of eating that were part of the patient's history and may be relevant to the discussion around lipids
4. Personal/social history and health-related behaviors
   a. High dietary saturated fat and cholesterol intake
   b. Excess total calorie intake
   c. Sedentary lifestyle
   d. Tobacco use (current and former)
   e. Excess alcohol use
   f. Exercise habits
   g. Social supports: May include families, spouses, parents, other relatives, and friends). This is important information to consider if an illness requires a lot of support. Where that support comes from is always an important consideration.
B. Objective
1. Physical exam
   a. Most cases of hypercholesterolemia will lack specific *symptoms* unless the hypercholesterolemia has been quite long-standing. However, there can be some specific physical exam *findings*, which may include the following (Gibson, 2013):
       i. Vital signs: high blood pressure
       ii. Skin: xanthelasma, or xanthelasma palpebrarum (yellow papular lesion on or by the corners of the eyelids next to the nose), peripheral skin breakdown (weeping, unhealing wounds)
       iii. Head, ears, eyes, nose, and throat (HEENT): Eyes—arcus senilis (white discoloration of the peripheral cornea), lipemia retinalis (the presence of "cream-colored" blood vessels, which can be seen with fundoscopic exam in patients with TG levels in excess of 2,000 mg/dL)
       iv. Heart and lungs: S4 heart sounds, rales (due to congestive heart failure caused by ischemia or MI)
           Extremities: xanthoma (thickening of tendons due to accumulation of cholesterol); reduced femoral, posterior tibial, and dorsalis pedis pulses; femoral bruit (due to PAD)
   b. Diagnostic tests
       i. Lipid panel reference ranges (adu): The CDC has used the American College of Cardiology/American Heart Association (ACC/AHA) 2018 Guidelines (Grundy, 2019) to

> **Special note: Talking about diet!**
>
> Any more people are frequently on a diet of some sort that may not even be for weight loss. There's keto, Atkins, vegan, mediteranean, vegetarian, DASH, etc. These can look VERY different from one another. Try not to be judgmental about people's dietary choices until you (the clinician) have seen lab results, etc. Different things work for different people, so at least try to be encouraging and praise the patient for being more mindful about what they're putting in their mouths! Also, keep in mind that weight can be a very loaded topic for some people and can be often linked to early life trauma. In summary: BE A GOOD LISTENER.

recommend "optimal cholesterol levels." Per the guidelines, these "goals" may be different for specific populations such as those with diabetes, certain age categories, or other risk factors In general, reference ranges for adults are as follows (refer to Grundy et al., 2019; CDC, 2023 for the information on specific populations):
- a. TC: About 150 mg/dL
- b. LDL ("bad") cholesterol: About 100 mg/dL.
- c. HDL ("good") cholesterol: At least 40 mg/dL in men and 50 mg/dL in women
- d. TGs: Less than 150 mg/dL
- e. Very high TGs: ≥ 500 mg/dL

ii. Risk calculators: The ACC ASCVD Risk Estimator Plus is the most commonly used risk calculator. These Pooled Cohort Equations have been validated in large community-based U.S. populations. The ACC ASCVD Risk Estimator Plus can be found at: https://tools.acc.org/ascvd-risk-estimator-plus/#!/calculate/estimate

III. Assessment
A. Determining diagnosis
1. Hyperlipidemia (pure, mixed, or unspecified)
2. Hypertriglyceridemia
3. Secondary causes of lipid disorders (e.g., type 2 diabetes with diabetic hyperlipidemia or hyperlipidemia due to steroid use).

B. Severity
1. Assess the severity of the disease and the need to treat based on history, physical, diagnostics, and calculated risk estimates using the ACC ASCVD Risk Estimator Plus (ACC, n.d.).

C. Significance
1. Assess significance to patient. This takes into account that the patient never exists in a vacuum but always as part of a "system." Unless the entire "system" is addressed, good outcomes cannot be expected.
2. Consider significance to caregivers and family, which in some cases will be huge (e.g., if the patient still lives with family, their needs must be taken into account for good outcomes to occur).

D. Motivation
1. Assess patient's preferences and willingness to adhere to recommended treatment plan. If the patient is unwilling or unable to follow recommendations, then alternate plans must be created. If possible, including the patient in all planning discussions is essential.

IV. Goals of clinical management
A. Screening
1. Use cost-effective and evidence-based tools to identify patients at elevated risk for CVD events (see above).

B. Treatment
1. Reduce risk of CVD events in those most susceptible.

C. Patient adherence
1. Develop a plan that fits patient preferences and ability to adhere to treatment. A good way to ensure adherence is to include the patient and caregiver(s) in the decision-making process. Always seek this input before developing any plan!

V. Plan
A. Screening
1. There is no clear consensus among experts as to when clinicians should start screening their patients for hyperlipidemia.
2. The 2018 AHA/ACC (Grundy et al., 2019) guidelines recommend that clinicians screen all adults over the age of 20 years old for baseline LDL-C levels in an effort to determine ASCVD risk (Grundy et al., 2019).
   a. The ACC/AHA Guidelines 2018 represents the class of recommendation (COR) as well as the level of evidence (LOE) on their tables as well as their algorithms. The COR represents the strength and estimated magnitude of benefit relative to risk. The LOE is a rating of the quality of the scientific evidence that supports the recommendation (Grundy et al., 2019) (**Table 60-1** and **Table 60-2**).
3. The U.S. Preventive Services Task Force (USPSTF) recently updated its recommendations in August of 2022 (USPSTF, 2022). The new recommendations are generally consistent with the 2016 recommendations that they replaced and that shifted the question of "who should be screened and how often" to "who should be prescribed statin therapies."
4. The USPSTF recommends screening all adults aged 40 years or older who meet the following criteria: (1) no known history of CVD; (2) no known symptoms of CVD; and (3) one or more risk factors for CVD, including diabetes, hypertension, noncoronary atherosclerosis, family history of CVD before the age of 55 in first-degree male relatives or age 65 in first-degree female relatives, tobacco use history, high body weight, sedentary lifestyle, or dyslipidemia (USPSTF, 2016). These recommendations do not include those with familial hypercholesterolemia or LDL-C levels greater than 190 mg/dL.

B. Diagnostics
1. Evaluate for primary causes.
   a. Severe Hypertriglyceridemia: Suspect primary cause if fasting plasma triglycerides ≥500 mg/dL.
   b. Elevated LDL-C: If levels greater than 95th percentile, suspect primary hyperlipidemia.
   c. Molecular studies: rarely indicated, given diagnosis is usually clinical and differentiation between specific types of primary hyperlipidemias rarely informs management.
2. Evaluate for secondary causes
   a. Diabetes: fasting glucose and/or hemoglobin A1c

Table 60-1 Recommendations for Measurement of Low-Density Lipoprotein Cholesterol (LDL-C) and Non–High-Density Lipoprotein Cholesterol (HDL-C)

COR	LOE	Recommendations
I	B-NR	1. In adults who are 20 years of age or older and not on lipid-lowering therapy, measurement of either a fasting or a nonfasting plasma lipid profile is effective in estimating ASCVD risk and documenting baseline LDL-C.
I	B-NR	2. In adults who are 20 years of age or older and in whom an initial nonfasting lipid profile reveals a triglycerides level of 400 mg/dL or higher (≥4.5 mmol/L), a repeat lipid profile in the fasting state should be performed for assessment of fasting triglyceride levels and baseline LDL-C.
IIa	C-LD	3. For adults with an LDL-C level less than 70 mg/dL (<1.8 mmol/L), measurement of direct LDL-C or modified LDL-C estimate is reasonable to improve accuracy over the Friedewald formula.
IIa	C-LD	4. In adults who are 20 years of age or older and without a personal history of ASCVD, but with a family history of premature ASCVD or genetic hyperlipidemia, measurement of a fasting plasma lipid profile is reasonable as part of an initial evaluation to aid in the understanding and identification of familial lipid disorders.

Reproduced from Grundy S, Stone N, Bailey A, et al. 2018 AHA/ACC/AACVPR/AAPA/ABC/ACPM/ADA/AGS/APhA/ASPC/NLA/PCNA Guideline on the Management of Blood Cholesterol. J Am Coll Cardiol. 2019 Jun, 73 (24) e285–e350. https://doi.org/10.1016/j.jacc.2018.11.003

Table 60-2 Applying Class of Recommendation and Level of Evidence to Clinical Strategies, Interventions, Treatments, or Diagnostic Testing in Patient Care* (Updated August 2015)

CLASS (STRENGTH) OF RECOMMENDATION

CLASS I (STRONG) — Benefit >>> Risk

Suggested phrases for writing recommendations:
- Is recommended
- Is indicated/useful/effective/beneficial
- Should be performed/administered/other
  - Comparative-Effectiveness Phrases[†]: Treatment/strategy A is recommended/indicated in preference to treatment B
  - Treatment A should be chosen over treatment B

CLASS IIa (MODERATE) — Benefit >> Risk

Suggested phrases for writing recommendations:
- Is reasonable
- Can be useful/effective/beneficial
- Comparative Effectiveness Phrases[†]:
  - Treatment/strategy A is probably recommended/indicated in preference to treatment B
  - It is reasonable to choose treatment A over treatment B

CLASS IIb (WEAK) — Benefit ≥ Risk

Suggested phrases for writing recommendations:
- May/might be reasonable
- May/might be considered
- Usefulness/effectiveness is unknown/unclear/uncertain or not well established

CLASS III: No Benefit (MODERATE) — Benefit = Risk
(Generally, LOE A or B use only)

Suggested phrases for writing recommendations:
- Is not recommended
- Is not indicated/useful/effective/beneficial
- Should not be performed/administered/other

(continues)

Table 60-2 Applying Class of Recommendation and Level of Evidence to Clinical Strategies, Interventions, Treatments, or Diagnostic Testing in Patient Care* (Updated August 2015) *(continued)*

CLASS (STRENGTH) OF RECOMMENDATION

CLASS III: Harm (STRONG) — Risk > Benefit

Suggested phrases for writing recommendations:
- Potentially harmful
- Causes harm
- Associated with excess morbidity/mortality
- Should not be performed/administrated/other

LEVEL (QUALITY) OF EVIDENCE[‡]

LEVEL A
- High-quality evidence[‡] from more than 1 RCT
- Meta-analyses of high-quality RCTs
- One or more RCTs corroborated by high-quality registry studies

LEVEL B-R (Randomized)
- Moderate-quality evidence[‡] from 1 or more RCTs
- Meta-analyses of moderate-quality RCTs

LEVEL B-NR (Nonrandomized)
- Moderate-quality evidence[‡] from 1 or more well-designed, well-executed nonrandomized studies, observational studies, or registry studies
- Meta-analyses of such studies

LEVEL C-LD (Limited Data)
- Randomized or nonrandomized observational or registry studies with limitations of design or execution
- Meta-analyses of such studies
- Physiological or mechanistic studies in human subjects

LEVEL C-EO (Expert Opinion)
Consensus of expert opinion based on clinical experience

COR and LOE are determined independently (any COR may be paired with any LOE).

A recommendation with LOE C does not imply that the recommendation is weak. Many important clinical questions addressed in guidelines do not lend themselves to clinical trials. Although RCTs are unavailable, there may be a very clear clinical consensus that a particular test or therapy is useful or effective.

* The outcome or result of the intervention should be specified (an improved clinical outcome or increased diagnostic accuracy or incremental prognostic information).

[†] For comparative-effectiveness recommendations (COR I and IIa; LOE A and B only), studies that support the use of comparator verbs should involve direct comparisons of the treatments or strategies being evaluated.

[‡] The method of assessing quality is evolving, including the application of standardized, widely used, and preferably validated evidence grading tools: and for systematic reviews, the incorporation of an Evidence Review Committee.

COR indicates Class of Recommendation; EO. expert opinion; LD. limited data; LOE. Level of Evidence; NR, nonrandomized; R. randomized; and RCT, randomized controlled trial.

Reproduced from Grundy S, Stone N, Bailey A, et al. 2018 AHA/ACC/AACVPR/AAPA/ABC/ACPM/ADA/AGS/APhA/ASPC/NLA/PCNA Guideline on the Management of Blood Cholesterol. *J Am Coll Cardiol. 2019 Jun, 73* (24) e285–e350. https://doi.org/10.1016/j.jacc.2018.11.003

---

  b. Excessive alcohol use: Alcohol Use Disorders Identification Test (AUDIT-c) (Bush et al., 1998)
  c. Hypothyroidism: thyroid panel
  d. Nephrotic syndrome and chronic renal insufficiency: urine protein and serum creatinin
  e. Hepatitis and cholestasis: liver function test
  f. Drugs: careful medication reconciliation
 3. Patient monitoring
  a. Office visit check-in and lipid panels every 6–12 months to ensure adherence and efficacy of therapy. It is necessary to not eat or drink anything besides water for 9–12 hours so as not to skew the results of the lipid panel (mainly the TG levels) (Hill & Bordoni, 2022; Grundy et al., 2019).
C. Management
 1. Lifestyle modification should be the initial component of any management plan and should include low refined carbohydrates; healthy proteins; moderate amounts of fruit; and moderate- to high-intensity

physical activity encompassing approximately 30 minutes per day, most days of the week, always taking into account any physical or medical limitations that require accommodation.
2. Before initiating therapy for any type of lipid disorder, evaluate and treat for hypothyroidism and nephrotic syndrome, perform liver function tests to check for any prior liver dysfunction because statins may exacerbate this issue (Hill & Bordoni, 2022), and perform urinalysis for albuminuria.
3. Even for patients with suspected or known primary hyperlipidemias, management should always involve continued evaluation and treatment of secondary causes.
4. Inherited disorders of LDL-C metabolism
   a. Statins and a second therapy (usually absorption inhibitor and/or bile acid sequestrant, niacin, omega-3s) are generally required at a minimum. In some cases, particularly for patients with homozygous familial hypercholesterolemia, additional agents are required.
   b. Apheresis, a method for removing LDL-C from the blood, can also be used when pharmacologic therapy is not enough.
5. Hypertriglyceridemia
   a. The two categories of hypertriglyceridemia consist of moderate hypertriglyceridemia (fasting or nonfasting TGs 175–499 mg/dL [2.0–5.6 mmol/L]) and severe hypertriglyceridemia (fasting TGs ~500 mg/dL [~5.6 mmol/L]).
   b. In moderate hypertriglyceridemia, the additional TGs are carried by VLDL-C, which, like LDL-C, is atherogenic and is often accompanied by other atherogenic factors. It is important to include nonpharmacologic steps in the initial assessment, using tools such as lifestyle modification and the identification of secondary factors that can increase the possibility of hypertriglyceridemia (diabetes, liver or kidney disease, and hypothyroidism). Many medications can cause an increase in TGs, so a medication review is always appropriate (**Table 60-3**). These medications can include the following: oral estrogens, Tamoxifen, raloxifene, retinoids, immunosuppressive drugs (cyclosporine, sirolimus, tacrolimus), beta blockers, interferon, atypical antipsychotic drugs, protease inhibitors, thiazide diuretics, glucocorticoids, rosiglitazone, bile acid sequestrants, l-asparaginase, and cyclophosphamide (Grundy et al., 2019). Moderate hypertriglyceridemia is often responsive to these non-pharmacologic actions.
   c. Those with severe hypertriglyceridemia are also at risk of developing acute pancreatitis caused by the increase in chylomicrons associated with

Table 60-3 Recommendations for Hypertriglyceridemia

COR	LOE	Recommendations
I	B-NR	1. In adults 20 years of age or older with moderate hypertriglyceridemia (fasting or nonfasting triglycerides 175 to 499 mg/dL [2.0 to 5.6 mmol/L]), clinicians should address and treat lifestyle factors (obesity and metabolic syndrome), secondary factors (diabetes mellitus, chronic liver or kidney disease and/or nephrotic syndrome, hypothyroidism), and medications that increase triglycerides.
IIa	B-R	2. In adults 40 to 75 years of age with moderate or severe hypertriglyceridemia and ASCVD risk of 7.5% or higher, it is reasonable to reevaluate ASCVD risk after lifestyle and secondary factors are addressed and to consider a persistently elevated triglyceride level as a factor favoring initiation or intensification of statin therapy.
IIa	B-R	3. In adults 40 to 75 years of age with severe hypertriglyceridemia (fasting triglycerides ≥ 500 mg/dL [≥ 5.6 mmol/L]) and ASCVD risk of 7.5% or higher, it is reasonable to address reversible causes of high triglyceride and to initiate statin therapy.
IIa	B-NR	4. In adults with severe hypertriglyceridemia (fasting triglycerides ≥ 500 mg/dL [‡5.7 mmol/L]), and especially fasting triglycerides ≥ 1,000 mg/dL (11.3 mmol/L]), it is reasonable to identify and address other causes of hypertriglyceridemia), and if triglycerides are persistently elevated or increasing, to further reduce triglycerides by implementation of a very low-fat diet, avoidance of refined carbohydrates and alcohol, consumption of omega-3 fatty acids, and, if necessary to prevent acute pancreatitis, fibrate therapy.

Reproduced from Grundy S, Stone N, Bailey A, et al. 2018 AHA/ACC/AACVPR/AAPA/ABC/ACPM/ADA/AGS/APhA/ASPC/NLA/PCNA Guideline on the Management of Blood Cholesterol. *J Am Coll Cardiol. 2019 Jun, 73* (24) e285–e350. https://doi.org/10.1016/j.jacc.2018.11.003

the increased VLDL-C. Severe hypertriglyceridemia most often has a genetic component but can also be associated with the lifestyle, diet, medication, and secondary factors mentioned earlier. Depending on the ASCVD risk assessment, statins may be an appropriate option (Table 60-3).

    d. Many patients with severe hypertriglyceridemia may best be served by regular follow-up with a cardiologist or lipid specialist.

6. Primary Prevention Strategies
   a. Both the U.S. Preventive Services Task Force and the AAC/AHA Task Force on Clinical Practice Guidelines have published similar recommendations for using statins for the primary prevention of cardiovascular disease. Both groups also offer recommendations for additional specific populations that, for the sake of brevity, will not be discussed here.
   b. Diet and lifestyle modifications are always the first line of prevention.
   c. Statin Use for the Primary Prevention of Cardiovascular Disease in Adults: U.S. Preventive Services Task Force Recommendation Statement (USPSTF, 2022)
      i. Generally consistent with the 2016 recommendation
      ii. Developed using the pooled cohort equations (PCEs), along with additional risk factors
      iii. The USPSTF "recommends that clinicians prescribe a statin for the primary prevention of CVD for adults aged 40 to 75 years who have 1 or more CVD risk factors (i.e. dyslipidemia, diabetes, hypertension, or smoking) and an estimated 10-year risk of a cardiovascular event of 10% or greater" (USPSTF, 2022, p. 747). For those in this population who have an estimated 10-year risk of 7.5%–10%, statins should be offered in conjunction with shared decision making (USPSTF, 2022) (**Table 60-4**).
      iv. Statin use was associated with a decrease in all-cause mortality and CVD events. The benefits appear to be present across diverse demographic and clinical populations.
      v. There was no clear dose response with regard to lipid-lowering effect. Most of the studies used to develop the recommendations used a moderate intensity of statin dose.
      vi. These recommendations apply to adults 40 years or older who do not already have CVD or signs or symptoms of CVD.
      vii. Recommendations do not apply to adults with an LDL-C level of >190 mg/dL (4.92 mmol/L) or known familial hypercholesterolemia.
      viii. Review of available data showed convincing evidence that the harms of statin use in adults aged 40–75 years are small.
   d. 2018 Guideline on the Management of Blood Cholesterol: A Report of the American College of Cardiology/American Heart Association Task Force on Clinical Practice Guidelines (Grundy et al., 2019)
      i. This guideline is a full revision of the 2013 ACC/AHA Guideline on the Treatment of Blood Cholesterol to Reduce Atherosclerotic Cardiovascular Risk in Adults (Stone et al., 2013).
      ii. As with the 2013 guidelines, specific attention is placed on shared decision making between the patient and provider.
      iii. In addition to the risk factors used in the PCEs, other "risk-enhancing factors" are taken into consideration.

Table 60-4 Very High Risk for Future ASCVD Events*

Major ASCVD Events
Recent acute coronary syndrome (within the past 12 months)
History of myocardial infarction (other than recent acute coronary syndrome event listed above)
History of ischemic stroke
Symptomatic peripheral arterial disease (history of claudication with ankle brachial index <0.89, or previous revascularization or amputation)

High-Risk Conditions
Age ≥65 years
Heterozygous familial hypercholesterolemia
History of prior coronary artery bypass surgery or PCI outside of the major ASCVD event(s)
Diabetes mellitus
Hypertension
Chronic kidney disease (eGFR 15-59 mL/min/1.73 m^2)
Current smoking
Persistently elevated LDL-C (LDL-C ≥100 mg/dL (≥2.6 mmol/L)) despite maximally tolerated statin therapy and ezetimibe
History of congestive heart failure

*Very High Risk includes a history of multiple ASCVD events or one major ASCVD event and multiple high-risk conditions.

Reproduced from Grundy S, Stone N, Bailey A, et al. 2018 AHA/ACC/AACVPR/AAPA/ABC/ACPM/ADA/AGS/APhA/ASPC/NLA/PCNA Guideline on the Management of Blood Cholesterol. *J Am Coll Cardiol.* 2019 Jun, 73 (24) e285–e350. https://doi.org/10.1016/j.jacc.2018.11.003

iv. Statins are recommended for primary prevention in patients with severe hypercholesterolemia and in adults 40–75 years of age with either diabetes mellitus or at very high risk for future ASCVD events (**Figure 60-1**).
v. The intensity of statin therapy is divided into three categories: high-intensity, moderate-intensity, and low-intensity with corresponding decreases in LDL-C levels
vi. Characteristics that create very high risk for future ASCVD events can be used as shared decision-making tools for those unsure about therapy or that may be at low to intermediate risk stratifications.
vii. In specific circumstances, non-statin medications such as ezetimibe, bile acid sequestrants, or PCSK9 inhibitors may be useful when combined with statin therapy (Grundy et al., 2019).

7. Treatment of hypercholesterolemia for secondary prevention.
    a. Diet and lifestyle modifications are always the first line of prevention.
    b. The AHA has a web-based campaign called "Healthy for Good" that focuses on an easy-to-understand approach that emphasizes three components: Eat smart. Move more. Be well.
        i. Eat smart: a wide variety of fruits and vegetables, along with whole grains, healthy sources of protein (mostly plants such as legumes and nuts, fish and seafood, low-fat or nonfat dairy, and if you eat meat and poultry, ensuring it is lean and unprocessed), liquid nontropical vegetable oils, minimally processed foods, minimized intake of added sugars, foods prepared with little or no salt, limited or preferably no alcohol intake, and low saturated fat (**Figure 60-2**.)

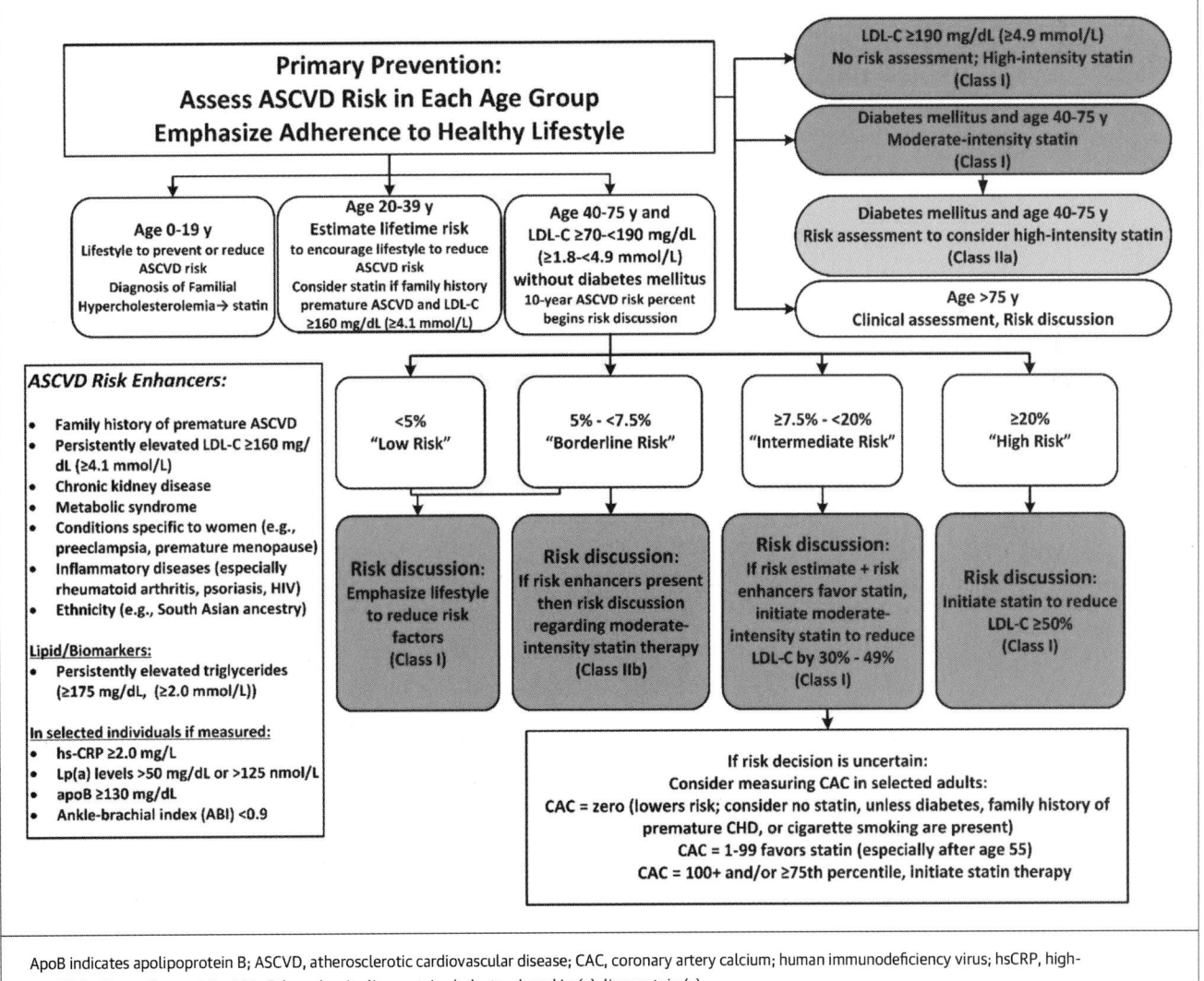

Figure 60-1 Primary prevention.

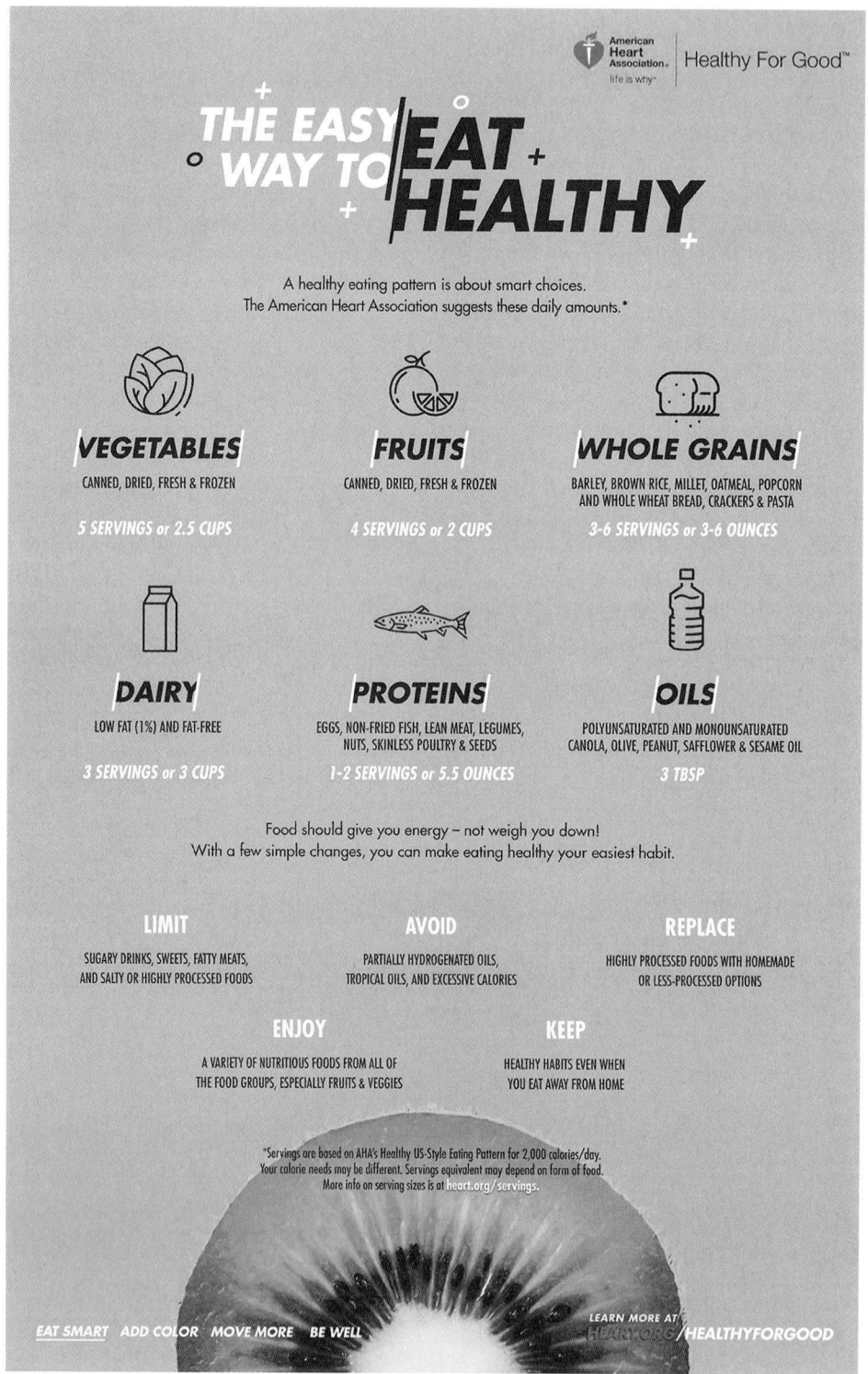

Figure 60-2 The Easy Way to Eat Healthy.

Reprinted with permission https://www.heart.org/en/healthy-living/healthy-eating/eat-smart/nutrition-basics/what-is-a-healthy-diet-recommended-serving-infographic ©American Heart Association, Inc.

ii. Move more: Work toward a goal of at least 150 minutes of moderate physical activity or 75 minutes of vigorous physical activity (or an equal combination of both) each week.

iii. Be well: Make sure to practice good self-care. This includes getting good sleep, practicing mindfulness, managing stress, keeping mind and body fit, and connecting socially.

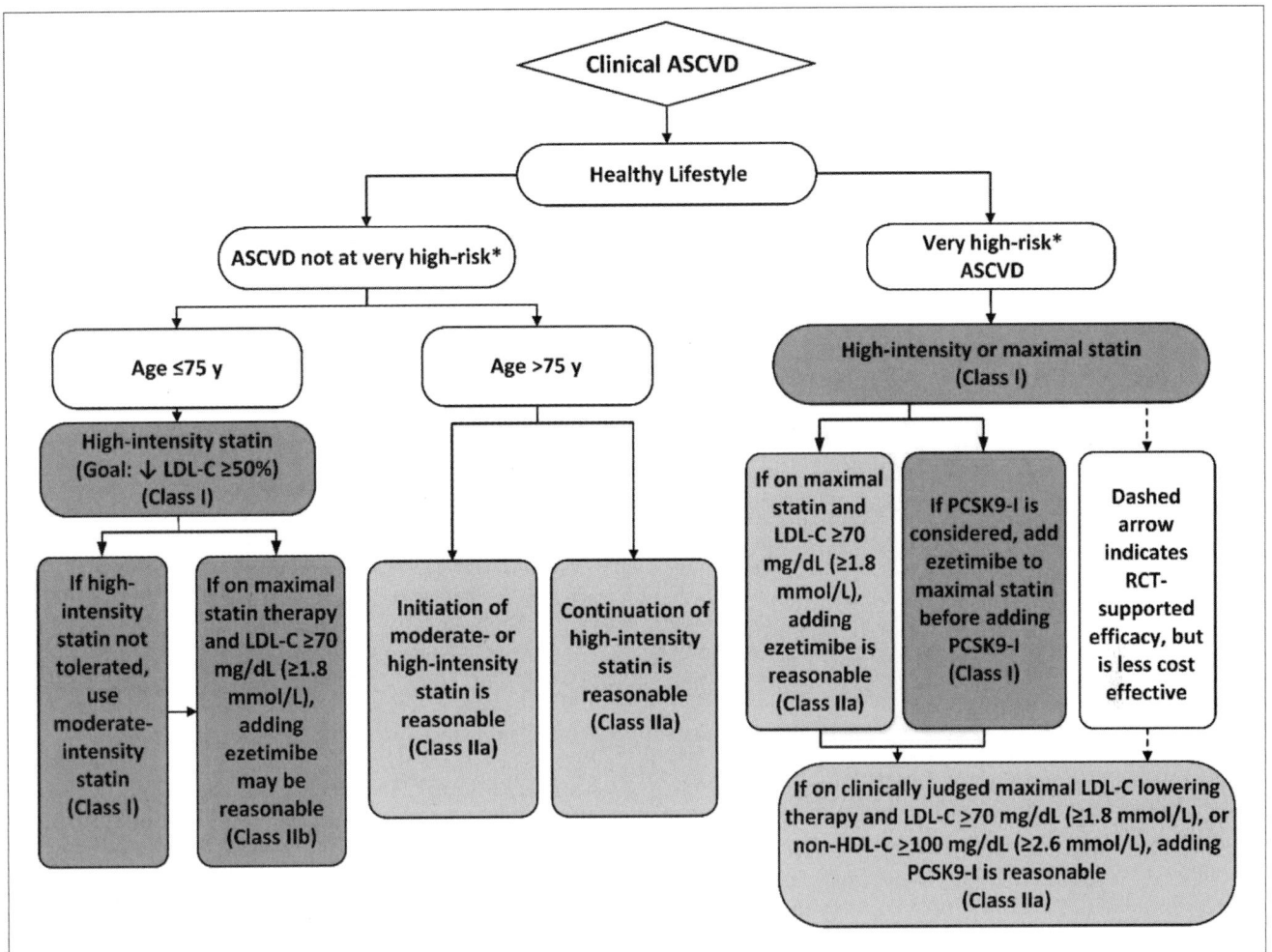

Figure 60-3 Secondary prevention in patients with clinical ASCVD.

Reproduced from Grundy S, Stone N, Bailey A, et al. 2018 AHA/ACC/AACVPR/AAPA/ABC/ACPM/ADA/AGS/APhA/ASPC/NLA/PCNA Guideline on the Management of Blood Cholesterol. *J Am Coll Cardiol. 2019 Jun, 73 (24) e285–e350.* https://doi.org/10.1016/j.jacc.2018.11.003

    c. The ACC/AHA 2018 Guidelines also present information on secondary prevention of ASCVD using pharmacologic strategies (Grundy et al., 2019). (**Figure 60-3**).
        i. Check baseline liver enzymes and TSH prior to initiating statin therapy.
        ii. Most patients with existing ASCVD are treated with statins (secondary prevention) (Grundy et al., 2019).
        iii. In some circumstances, non-statin medications such ezetimibe, bile acid sequestrants, or PCSK9 inhibitors, may prove useful in combination with statin therapy (Grundy et al., 2019).
    d. Continued Monitoring: ACC/AHA 2018 Guidelines Recommendation on Continued Monitoring.

8. Interprofessional team use and referral
    a. Endocrine: Consider for refractory hyperlipidemia or difficult-to-treat hyperlipidemias related to diabetes, higher body weight, or thyroid disease.
    b. Cardiology: Especially when there are hereditary disorders or when cholesterol levels remain uncontrolled despite frontline management.
    c. Registered Dietician/Nutritionist: For overweight patients, weight loss through diet and physical activity
    d. Tobacco cessation: The importance of tobacco cessation in reducing cardiovascular risk cannot be understated. For patients who use tobacco, motivational interviewing, nicotine replacement, pharmacologic therapy, and group support should be considered and offered as appropriate at each encounter.

VI. Resources and self-management tools
A. Patient education and online resources
1. Centers for Disease Control and Prevention: Resources for the public on the risks of high cholesterol and strategies for lifestyle modification and treatment. https://www.cdc.gov/cholesterol/about.htm
2. American Heart Association. *Prevention and Treatment of High Cholesterol (Hyperlipidemia) (AHA, 2023b).* Information on diet, exercise and other lifestyle changes to benefit cardiovascular health. https://www.heart.org/en/health-topics/cholesterol
3. American College of Cardiology ASCVD Risk Estimator Plus. https://tools.acc.org/ascvd-risk-estimator-plus/#!/calculate/estimate/
4. U.S. Preventive Services Task Force full report on Statin Use for the Primary Prevention of Cardiovascular Disease in Adults. https://www.uspreventiveservicestaskforce.org/uspstf/recommendation/statin-use-in-adults-preventive-medication#fullrecommendationstart
5. Characteristics of Common Lipid Lowering Medications and Common Side Effects Associated with Statin Use.

References

American College of Cardiology. (n.d.): *ASCVD Risk Estimator Plus.* https://tools.acc.org/ascvd-risk-estimator-plus/#!/calculate/estimate/

American Heart Association. (2014a). *The American Heart Association's diet and lifestyle recommendations.* https://www.heart.org/en/healthy-living/healthy-eating/eat-smart/nutrition-basics/aha-diet-and-lifestyle-recommendations

American Heart Association. (2014b). *Heart360.* https://www.heart360.org/Default.aspx?cid=9ea5cba5ffa4c87aab69dcac799a03de

Bush, K., Kivlahan, D. R., McDonell, M. B., Fihn, S. D., & Bradley, K. A. (1998). The AUDIT alcohol consumption questions (AUDIT-C): An effective brief screening test for problem drinking. Ambulatory care quality improvement project (ACQUIP). *Archives of Internal Medicine, 158*(16), 1789–1795. doi:10.1001/archinte.158.16.1789

Centers for Disease Control and Prevention. (2011). *High cholesterol facts.* https://www.cdc.gov/cholesterol/facts.htm

D'Agostino, R. B., Sr., Vasan, R. S., Pencina, M. J., Wolf, P. A., Cobain, M., Massaro, J. M., & Kannel, W. B. (2008). General cardiovascular risk profile for use in primary care: The Framingham Heart Study. *Circulation, 117*(6), 743–753. doi:10.1161/CIRCULATIONAHA.107.699579

Đukanović, N., Obradović, S., Zdravković, M., Đurašević, S., Stojković, M., Tosti, T., Jasnić, N., Đorđević, J., & Todorović, Z. (2021). Lipids and antiplatelet therapy: Important considerations and future perspectives. *International Journal of Molecular Sciences, 22*(6), 3180. doi:10.3390/ijms22063180

Durrington, P. (2003). Dyslipidaemia. *Lancet, 362*(9385), 717–731. doi:10.1016/S0140-6736(03)14234-1

Ference, B. A., Ginsberg, H. N., Graham, I., Ray, K. K., Packard, C. J., Bruckert, E., Hegele, R. A., Krauss, R. M., Raal, F. J., Schunkert, H., Watts, G. F., Borén, J., Fazio, S., Horton, J. D., Masana, L., Nicholls, S. J., Nordestgaard, B. G., van de Sluis, B., Taskinen, M. R., Tokgözoglu, L., ... Catapano, A. L. (2017). Low-density lipoproteins cause atherosclerotic cardiovascular disease. 1. Evidence from genetic, epidemiologic, and clinical studies. A consensus statement from the European Atherosclerosis Society Consensus Panel. *European Heart Journal, 38*(32), 2459–2472. doi:10.1093/eurheartj/ehx144

Gibson, C.M., (2013): *High Cholesterol Physical Exam.* https://www.wikidoc.org/index.php/High_cholesterol_physical_examination

Grundy, S. M., Stone, N. J., Bailey, A. L., Beam, C., Birtcher, K. K., Blumenthal, R. S., Braun, L. T., de Ferranti, S., Faiella-Tommasino, J., Forman, D. E., Goldberg, R., Heidenreich, P. A., Hlatky, M. A., Jones, D. W., Lloyd-Jones, D., Lopez-Pajares, N., Ndumele, C. E., Orringer, C. E., Peralta, C. A., ... Yeboah, J. (2019). 2018 AHA/ACC/AACVPR/AAPA/ABC/ACPM/ADA/AGS/APhA/ASPC/NLA/PCNA Guideline on the Management of Blood Cholesterol: A Report of the American College of Cardiology/American Heart Association Task Force on Clinical Practice Guidelines. *Circulation 139*(25), e1082–e1143. doi:10.1161/CIR.0000000000000625

Hill, M. F., & Bordoni, B. (2023). Hyperlipidemia. *In StatPearls.* StatPearls Publishing. https://www.ncbi.nlm.nih.gov/books/NBK559182/

Kochanek, K. D., Xu, J. Q., Murphy, S. L., Miniño, A. M., & Kung, H. C. (2011). Deaths: Final data for 2009. *National Vital Statistics Reports, 60*(3), 1–116.

Koo, B. K., Park, S., Han, K. D., & Moon, M. K. (2021). Hypertriglyceridemia Is an independent risk factor for cardiovascular diseases in Korean adults aged 30-49 years: A Nationwide Population-Based Study. *Journal of Lipid and Atherosclerosis, 10*(1), 88–98. https://doi.org/10.12997/jla.2021.10.1.88

Liu, C., Dhindsa, D., Almuwaqqat, Z., Ko, Y. A., Mehta, A., Alkhoder, A. A., Alras, Z., Desai, S. R., Patel, K. J., Hooda, A., Wehbe, M., Sperling, L. S., Sun, Y. V., & Quyyumi, A. A. (2022). Association Between High-Density Lipoprotein Cholesterol Levels and Adverse Cardiovascular Outcomes in High-risk Populations. *JAMA cardiology, 7*(7), 672–680. https://doi.org/10.1001/jamacardio.2022.0912

Natesan, V., & Kim, S. J. (2021). Lipid metabolism, disorders and therapeutic drugs—review. *Biomolecules & Therapeutics, 29*(6), 596–604. doi:10.4062/biomolther.2021.122

National Heart, Lung, and Blood Institute. (2014). *Heart & vascular diseases.* http://www.nhlbi.nih.gov/health/resources/heart

Nuovo, J. (1999). Hyperlipidemia in patients with type-2 diabetes. *American Family Physician, 59*(6), 1666–1671. https://www.aafp.org/pubs/afp/issues/1999/0315/p1666.html

Sandesara, P. B., Virani, S. S., Fazio, S., & Shapiro, M. D. (2019). The forgotten lipids: Triglycerides, remnant cholesterol, and atherosclerotic cardiovascular disease risk. *Endocrine Reviews, 40*(2), 537–557. doi:10.1210/er.2018-00184

Stone, N. J., Robinson, J. G., Lichtenstein, A. H., Merz, C. N. B., Blum, C. B., Eckel, R. H., Goldberg, A. C., Gordon, D., Levy, D., Lloyd-Jones, S. M., McBride, P., Sanford Schwartz, J., Shero, S. T., Smith Jr., S. C., Watson, K., Wilson, P. W. F., & American College of Cardiology/American Heart Association Task Force on Practice Guidelines (2014). 2013 ACC/AHA guideline on the treatment of blood cholesterol to reduce atherosclerotic cardiovascular risk in adults: A report of the American College of Cardiology/American Heart Association Task Force on Practice Guidelines.

Circulation, 129(25, Suppl. 2), S1–S45. doi:10.1016/j.jacc.2013.11.002

U.S. Preventive Services Task Force. (2008). *Lipid disorders in adults (cholesterol, dyslipidemia): Screening.* http://www.uspreventiveservicestaskforce.org/Page/Topic/recommendation-summary/lipid-disorders-in-adults-cholesterol-dyslipidemia-screening

US Preventive Services Task Force. (2016). Final Recommendation Statement. *Statin Use for the Primary Prevention of Cardiovascular Disease in Adults: Preventive Medication.* JAMA. 316(19): 1997–2007. https://jamanetwork.com/journals/jama/fullarticle/2584058

U.S. Preventive Services Task Force. (2022). Final Recommendation Statement. *Statin Use for the Primary Prevention of Cardiovascular Disease in Adults: Preventive Medication.* JAMA. 328(8): 746–753. https://www.uspreventiveservicestaskforce.org/uspstf/recommendation/statin-use-in-adults-preventive-medication

Verbeek, R., Hoogeveen, R. M., Langsted, A., Stiekema, L. C. A., Verweij, S. L., Hovingh, G. K., Wareham, N. J., Khaw, K. T., Boekholdt, S. M., Nordestgaard, B. G., & Stroes, E. S. G. (2018). Cardiovascular disease risk associated with elevated lipoprotein(a) attenuates at low low-density lipoprotein cholesterol levels in a primary prevention setting. *European heart journal, 39*(27), 2589–2596. https://doi.org/10.1093/eurheartj/ehy334

Virani, S. S., Alonso, A., Aparicio, H. J., Benjamin, E. J., Bittencourt, M. S., Callaway, C. W., Carson, A. P., Chamberlain, A. M., Cheng, S., Delling, F. N., Elkind, M. S. V., Evenson, K. R., Ferguson, J. F., Gupta, D. K., Khan, S. S., Kissela, B. M., Knutson, K. L., Lee, C. D., Lewis, T. T., ... American Heart Association Council on Epidemiology and Prevention Statistics Committee and Stroke Statistics Subcommittee. (2021). Heart disease and stroke statistics—2021 update: A report from the American Heart Association. *Circulation,* 143, e254–e743. doi:10.1161/CIR.0000000000000950

Vodnala, D., Rubenfire, M., & Brook, R., (2012). Secondary causes of dyslipidemia. *American Journal of Cardiology, 110*(6), 823–825. doi:10.1016/j.amjcard.2012.04.062.

Yanai, H., & Yoshida, H (2021). Secondary dyslipidemia: Its treatments and association with atherosclerosis. *Global Health & Medicine,* 3(1), 15–23. https://doi.org/10.35772/ghm.2020.01078

Yandrapalli, S., Nabors, C., Goyal, A., Aronow, W. S., & Frishman, W. H. (2019). Modifiable risk factors in young adults with first myocardial infarction. *Journal of the American College of Cardiology,* 73(5), 573–584. doi:10.1016/j.jacc.2018.10.084

Yang, H. S., Jeong, H. J., Kim, H., Hwang, H. K., Hur, M., & Lee, S. (2022). Sex-specific unshaped relationships between high-density lipoprotein cholesterol levels and 10-year major adverse cardiovascular events: A nationwide cohort study of 5.7 million South Koreans. *Annals of Laboratory Medicine,* 42(4), 415–427.

CHAPTER 61

Low Back Pain

H. Kate Lawlor and Brandon Sessler

I. Introduction and general background

The lumbosacral spine is the fulcrum of the body. Its skeletal structure, muscles, and ligaments bear the stressors of bending over, straightening up, lifting, carrying, and supporting the body's weight. So, it is not surprising that up to 60% of the U.S. population will experience low back pain (LBP) at some time during their adult lives (van Tulder et al., 2002). After upper respiratory infections, back pain is the next most common reason to seek nonemergency care (Atlas & Deyo, 2001). The differential diagnosis for LBP is lengthy, and a precise diagnosis cannot be made in more than 80% of cases (Chou et al., 2007), yet 80% of episodes of LBP in a primary care setting will spontaneously improve in 1–2 weeks, and 90% resolve within 6 weeks. The diagnostic challenge is to identify those patients who require a more extensive or urgent evaluation, those who present with "red flags" at their initial evaluation.

The differential diagnosis for LBP includes both muscular and focal spine disorders (e.g., disc herniation, spinal fracture, and spinal stenosis), regional nonspinal disorders (e.g., pelvic inflammatory disease, aortic aneurysm, and kidney stones), and systemic diseases (e.g., ankylosing spondylitis and metastatic cancer). Even if anatomic defects like narrowed disk space or the vertebral osteophytes of degenerative arthritis are found on x-rays, causality cannot be absolutely assumed because these defects are also common in asymptomatic patients and increase in frequency with age (Ehrlich, 2003). In fact, more than one-third of asymptomatic individuals older than age 60 will have evidence of disc herniation or spinal stenosis on specialized imaging (Ehrlich, 2003).

Table 61-1 lists the potential causes of LBP grouped by category. The most common causes are pain due to mechanical or degenerative processes. The most frequent sources of pain in these categories are lumbar-sacral strain and symptomatic herniated disc (Chou et al., 2007). The obligation for the clinician is to promptly identify those other patients whose pain may be due to urgent causes ("red flags"); that is, patients who warrant imaging or other evaluative procedures on their presenting visit (**Table 61-2**). These "red flags" may include ankylosing spondylitis, cord compression, a compression fracture, cancer, or cauda equina syndrome (see description in the following section) (Chou et al., 2007).

Back pain may also be the presenting symptom in other serious medical problems, including abdominal aortic aneurysm, peptic ulcer disease, kidney stones, and pancreatitis.

The following guidelines review the history, physical exam, and diagnostic tests necessary to differentiate more urgent causes of back pain (the "red flags") from mechanical and degenerative causes. For most patients, the history and physical exam are sufficient to identify the "red flags" that suggest more serious disorders (Chou et al., 2007).

II. Database (may include but is not limited to)
A. *Subjective*
  1. History of present illness
     a. Onset and duration (intermittent vs. constant)
     b. Circumstances when first occurred (trauma? work related?)
     c. Location and radiation of pain: Atypical location, such as mid-back, is more common in cancer. Pain that is localized to the mid-buttock may or may not be due to a spinal problem. Occasionally, this buttock pain is due to piriformis syndrome (PS), which is inflammation or spasm of the piriformis muscle that follows overuse or athletic injury. Because the muscle overlies the sciatic nerve, irritation of the piriformis muscle can cause the same sciatic nerve entrapment symptoms (see Section II.B.1.g.iii) as lumbosacral disorders. Thus, it is often difficult to differentiate.

Table 61-1 Most Common Causes of Low Back Pain

I. Mechanical (74%)
   A. Poor back or core abdominal muscle tone (may be secondary to higher body weight, pregnancy, or deconditioning)
   B. Chronic postural or lumbar-sacral strain

II. Structural/Degenerative (17%)
   A. Degenerative joint disease (osteoarthritis, degenerative disc disease, facet process) (10%)
   B. Sacroiliitis
   C. Scoliosis, kyphosis
   D. Disc protrusion or herniation (4%)
   E. Spinal stenosis (narrowing of spinal canal) (3%)
   F. Osteoporosis
   G. Piriformis syndrome
   H. Cauda equina syndrome (characterized by lower extremity weakness and sensory loss, saddle anesthesia of the perineum, urinary retention, or urinary or fecal incontinence—a surgical emergency)

III. Trauma (6%)
   A. Fall
   B. Work-related injury
   C. Compression fracture due to fall, osteoporosis, or chronic steroid use (4%)
   D. Subluxation of facet joint (2%)

IV. Inflammatory Diseases (0.93%)
   A. Ankylosing spondylitis (or other spondyloarthropathies)
   B. Rheumatoid arthritis

V. Infection (0.07%)
   A. Osteomyelitis
   B. Urinary tract infection (from indwelling catheter)
   C. Tuberculosis
   D. Intravenous drug abuse

VI. Cancer (1%)
   A. Multiple myeloma
   B. Metastatic cancer of prostate, breast, and lung
   C. Spinal cord tumors

VII. Visceral Disease (1%)
   A. Dissecting abdominal aneurysm (usually history of hypertension)
   B. Renal disease
   C. Pelvic disease

VIII. Psychogenic
   A. Tension/stress related
   B. Malingering (more often in setting of worker's compensation claim)

Data from Atlas, S., & Deyo, R. (2001). Evaluating and managing acute low back pain in the primary care setting. *Journal of General Internal Medicine*, 16, 120–131.

---

d. Quality and severity of pain: use specific descriptors and pain severity scale.
e. Progression of symptoms over time: Symptoms lasting >3 months represent "chronic" LBP.
f. Aggravating and alleviating factors
g. Worse with bending, lifting, prolonged standing, or sitting (most common with mechanical back pain)
h. Worse in morning: if pain less than 30 minutes after waking or shifting positions, suggests degenerative changes of vertebrae.
i. Relief with activity; worse with rest (typical of facet arthrosis or ankylosing spondylitis)
j. Relief with sitting or bending forward (suggestive of spinal stenosis)
k. Worse with cough, bowel movement, or sneezing (suggests disc pathology)
l. Complaints of urinary retention or incontinence from loss of sphincter function, bilateral motor weakness of lower extremities, and decrease in sensation over buttocks or perineum ("saddle anesthesia") suggest cauda equina syndrome,

Table 61-2 History and Physical Examination Findings Associated With Increased Likelihood of Serious Spine Condition ("Red Flags")

Disorder	History	Physical Exam/Studies for Diagnosis
All	- Failure to improve > 6 weeks - No relief with bed rest	
Cancer	- Age > 50 yr - Previous history of cancer (esp. multiple myeloma) - Unexplained weight loss of >10 lb in 6 months - Failure to improve after 1 month; worse at night - No relief with bed rest	- Lymphadenopathy - Plain lumbar-sacral (LS) spine films - Magnetic resonance imagining (MRI) - Elevated erythrocyte sedimentation rate (ESR)
Fracture	- Age > 50 yr; especially >70 yr - Weight < 125 lb - History of cancer (causes lytic metastases) - History of smoking (increased risk of osteoporosis) - History of significant trauma (fall from height, motor vehicle accident, or direct blow) - History of osteoporosis - Long-term steroid use (causes decreased bone density) - Substance abuse (increased risk of falls; alcohol use)	- Vertebral point tenderness - Visible on plain LS spine film
Vertebral Infection	- Fever, chills - Pain increased at rest - Recent skin or genital-urinary infection (history of indwelling catheter) - Intravenous drug use - Immunosuppression	- Fever > 100°F - Tenderness over a spinous process - MRI - Elevated ESR, positive C-reactive protein, elevated white blood count
Ankylosing Spondylitis	- Male > female; <45 years old - Positive family history of irritable bowel disease (IBD), ankylosing spondylitis - Pain > 3 mo; especially buttock pain - Pain in latter part of night; morning stiffness - Pain improved with exercise - May be associated with IBD, psoriasis, uveitis, plantar fasciitis, or Achilles tendinitis	- May be decreased chest expansion - Decreased spinal flexibility in sideways, frontal, and backward motions - May be sacroiliac (SI) joint tenderness - May be radiologic evidence of sacroiliitis on anteroposterior pelvic plain films - Elevated ESR, positive C-reactive protein - 90% + histocompatibility complex HLA-B27
Cauda Equina Syndrome	- Urinary retention or incontinence - Bowel incontinence - Progressive leg/foot weakness - Sensory loss in lower extremity(ies)	- Saddle anesthesia of perineum - Diminished anal sphincter tone - Severe unilateral or bilateral leg/foot weakness - Bladder distension - MRI - **Is surgical emergency**
Herniated Disc	- Back pain with leg pain in an L4, L5, or S1 nerve root distribution	- Positive straight leg raise test - MRI if symptoms > 1 month - Consider electromyelogram (EMG), nerve conduction studies (NCS)
Spinal Stenosis	- Radiating leg pain - Older age	- Consider MRI if symptoms > 1 month - Consider electromyogram (EMG)/nerve conduction studies (NCS)

Data from Atlas, S., & Deyo, R. (2001). Evaluating and managing acute low back pain in the primary care setting. Journal of General Internal Medicine, 16, 120–131. and Chou, R., Quaseem, A., Snow, V., et al. (2007). Diagnosis and treatment of low back pain: A joint clinical practice guideline from the American College of Physicians and the American Pain Society. Annals of Internal Medicine, 147(7), 478–491.

a surgical emergency—usually due to a massive, centrally herniated disc causing compression of nerve roots of lower cord segments.
- m. Associated signs and symptoms
  - i. Constitutional symptoms: fever, malaise, weight loss (each suggests a more serious concern)
  - ii. Ocular: painful, inflamed, or gritty eye (uveitis is associated with ankylosing spondylitis)
  - iii. Neurologic
    - a. Sciatica: A burning pain that radiates down the posterior or lateral aspect of one or both legs past the knee is 85% sensitive for S1–S2 nerve root irritation (Atlas & Deyo, 2007)
    - b. Sharp back pain when coughs or sneezes (indicative of disc compression)
    - c. Leg pain with standing or walking (neurogenic claudication); relief with sitting (suggests spinal stenosis)
    - d. Leg or foot weakness; gait disturbance; urinary retention or urinary incontinence; bowel incontinence (these symptoms in the aggregate suggest cauda equina syndrome resulting from cord compression, a surgical emergency)
  - iv. Abdominal: pain or diarrhea (inflammatory bowel disease can be associated with ankylosing spondylitis)
  - v. Genitourinary: dysuria, urinary frequency or urgency, recent indwelling catheter use (suggests urinary tract infection), pyelonephritis may present with flank pain and fever. Vaginal discharge and pelvic pain suggests pelvic infection.
  - vi. Vascular: chest pain or throbbing abdominal pain (LBP with these symptoms may signal an abdominal aortic aneurysm)
  - vii. Skin: history of psoriasis (associated with ankylosing spondylitis) or recent skin infection (may cause spinal infection)
  - viii. Psychologic: recent sleep disturbances, depressed or anxious mood, diminished participation in social activities (may signal depression)
- n. Patient's concern/theory about of source of symptoms
2. Past health history
   - a. Prior spinal diagnoses, fractures or surgery, history of current or previous cancers
   - b. Previous radiologic or imaging studies of spine; prior bone density testing
   - c. Medications
     - i. Used for back pain (especially opiates: dosage and frequency)
     - ii. Prescription (steroid use can be risk factor for osteoporosis and compression fractures)
     - iii. Over the counter
     - iv. Herbal/alternative
3. Family history
   - a. Disc disease
   - b. Osteoporosis
   - c. Rheumatoid arthritis, ankylosing spondylitis
   - d. Vascular disease
   - e. Scoliosis
   - f. Osteoarthritis
4. Occupational
   - a. Physical requirements of job
   - b. How many hours worked per week
   - c. Number of hours spent in prolonged sitting (risk factor for PS and deconditioning)
   - d. Recent job injury
   - e. Prior ergonomic assessments performed and results
   - f. Current worker's compensation claim or permanent disability
   - g. Job satisfaction
5. Personal/social (factors that may predict poorer or delayed resolution)
   - a. Other pending litigation: occupational or trauma
   - b. Impact of pain on activities of daily living (ADLs) or current relationships
   - c. History of depression
   - d. Outstanding disability claims
   - e. Previous worker's compensation claim(s)
   - f. Habits
     - i. Smoking (risk factor for osteoporosis)
     - ii. Injectable drug use (risk factor for spinal infection)
     - iii. Alcohol use (be alert to increased use for self-medicating pain)
     - iv. Recreational drug use
   - g. Interventions attempted to relieve pain, and results
     - i. Medications: (aspirin [acetylsalicylic acid, or ASA]; nonsteroidal anti-inflammatory drugs [NSAIDs], either oral or topical; acetaminophen [Tylenol]; and opioids)
     - ii. Herbal products
     - iii. Chiropractic care
     - iv. Physical therapy
     - v. Application of heat or cold
     - vi. Massage
     - vii. Acupuncture

B. *Objective*
   1. Physical exam: Patient should be undressed. Exam should include but is not limited to:
      - a. Height (loss of height suggests disc degeneration, kyphosis, or compression fracture)
      - b. Weight (unexplained weight loss may suggest cancer; low body weight is a risk factor for osteoporosis; high body weight is a risk factor for osteoarthritis)
      - c. Age (>50 yr at greater risk for cancer; >75 yr at greater risk for osteoporosis)

d. Gender (males at greater risk for ankylosing spondylitis; females >30 yr are largest population for PS)
e. Vital signs, including temperature (fever > 100°F suggests infection)
f. Spine (performed with patient unclothed, in gown and underwear)
   In the absence of a history suggestive of a serious condition, systemic disease, and/or illness not localized to the back region (Table 61-1), a focused spine and neurologic exam as described next should be an adequate screening exam to rule out serious or urgent causes of LBP, unless any "red flags" (Table 61-2) are identified (Ehrlich, 2003).
   i. Inspection: look for changes in normal spine curvature that may occur with muscle spasm, scoliosis, hyperkyphosis, or ankylosing spondylitis.
   ii. Standing: assess symmetry and posture
   iii. Palpation: assess for bone tenderness versus muscle spasm. With patient forward flexed, assess for lateral curvature and rotation of the spine, which suggests scoliosis. Frontal curve could signal hyperkyphosis. Palpate the area over the piriformis muscle at the sciatic notch if the patient complains of buttock pain. Eliciting tenderness with deep palpation suggests that the source of the patient's pain may be PS, not lumbar-sacral disorders.
   iv. Range of motion: assess flexibility and complaints of pain. Ask which movement causes the most pain. (Flexion causes increased pressure on the disc; extension loads the facet joints [facet arthrosis] and narrows the diameter of the spinal canal [spinal stenosis]; lateral bending causes increased pain if disc is herniated.)
   v. Gait: check heel and toe walking separately (heel walk involves the anterior tibialis and L4 and L5 innervation; toe walk uses the gastrocnemius and S1 innervation).
   vi. Measure leg length (difference of >2 cm causes significant postural alteration that can result in LBP).
g. Focused neurological exam
   i. Comparative strength testing of lower extremities
   ii. Reflex testing of lower extremities
   iii. Straight leg raises (SLR): screen for nerve root irritation, most commonly due to a herniated disc in the L5 or S1 nerve roots. While patient is supine, the affected leg should be elevated by the clinician with the ankle dorsiflexed and the knee fully extended. A (+) response ("sciatica") reproduces sharp or burning pain when the limb is raised to 30–70 degrees. This occurs in the setting of disc herniation or degenerative conditions causing neural foraminal stenosis and, less often, PS. The earlier the onset of pain during the test and the greater the severity, the more specific is the result. The SLR test is 64%–98% sensitive but is less specific (11%–61%) for lumbosacral disc herniation (McGee, 2007). Additionally, sciatic symptoms that occur down the opposite leg during testing usually indicate a large disc herniation. Sciatica resulting from spinal stenosis is more common in older patients, and pain is often bilateral (see **Table 61-3** for exam findings associated with impingement of specific nerve roots). Pain that is limited to the back or the hip during the SLR is considered a negative test. A negative test argues against disc herniation of the L4–S1 area. If positive SLR or "red flag" findings are present, the clinician needs to proceed with a more detailed neurologic exam of the lower extremities, as described in Section h.
      Much less L4 and minimal L2 or L3 disc movement occurs during the SLR test, so it is less useful in detecting disc herniation above L4. Flexing the knee with the patient in a prone position may reproduce the back and anterior thigh pain of upper lumbar disc herniation (Goroll & Mulley, 2014).
h. Expanded neurologic exam (to be done if symptoms or neurologic findings suggest a "red flag")
   i. Comparative muscle strength testing of upper and lower extremities: knee, great toe, and ankle dorsiflexion
   ii. Dermatomal sensation testing of lower extremities and feet
   iii. Measure circumference of thighs and calves: difference of >2 cm may indicate neurologic involvement of limb with smaller muscle mass.
   iv. If complaints and exam findings are consistent with cauda equine syndrome (severe unilateral or bilateral leg weakness, urinary retention/distended bladder, or fecal incontinence), check for perineal saddle anesthesia and diminished anal sphincter tone.
i. Systemic exam
   a. Eye exam: if complaints of eye pain or irritation. Anterior uveitis can be associated with ankylosing spondylitis.
   b. Pulmonary exam (chest expansion decreased in ankylosing spondylitis)
   c. Cardiac exam: Note evidence of aortic valve incompetence (can occur in ankylosing

Table 61-3 Neurologic Testing of Lumbosacral Nerve Impairment

Nerve Root	Motor Strength	Reflex	Sensory Area
L1	Hip flexion	None	Groin
L2	Hip flexion	None	Anterior thigh
L3	Knee extension	Patellar	Knee
L4	Ankle dorsiflexion	Patellar	Medial calf
L5	First toe dorsiflexion	Babinski	Web space between first and second toe
S1	Plantar flexion of foot, knee flexors or hamstrings	Achilles	Lateral foot
S2	Knee flexors, hamstrings	Knee flexor	Posterior thigh
S3–S4	External anal sphincter	Anal reflex, rectal tone	Perianal area

Reproduced from Papadakis, M., & McPhee, S. (Eds.). (2019). Low back pain. In Current Medical Diagnosis and Treatment (58th ed.). New York: McGraw-Hill Education.

spondylitis); include testing for aortic bruits to assess if aortic aneurysm is suspected as the source of LBP.
  d. Urinary exam: Assess for distended bladder (saddle anesthesia and/or diminished anal sphincter tone with fecal incontinence and urinary retention suggests cauda equina syndrome, a surgical emergency).
  e. Genitourinary exam: Note any pelvic tenderness or masses or cervical motion tenderness or discharge (suggests pelvic inflammatory disease in females); urethral discharge or dysuria (can be associated with ankylosing spondylitis); and prostate enlargement, tenderness, or masses (can signal infection or prostate cancer).
  f. Abdominal exam: Pulsatile mass near umbilicus suggests an aortic aneurysm.
  g. Rectal exam: Check for saddle anesthesia of the perineum or diminished anal sphincter tone if suspicion of cauda equina syndrome.
C. Diagnostic tests (may include, but not limited to)
  1. Radiographs: Basic x-ray findings are poorly correlated with specific symptoms and are not sensitive for important abnormalities (Chou et al., 2007). In addition, in several studies of asymptomatic individuals, disc degeneration was a common finding that increased with age (Atlas & Deyo, 2001). Therefore, plain x-rays of the spine have a very low sensitivity and specificity in the majority of cases and should not be obtained for patients with nonspecific LBP unless a "red flag" is present or pain has persisted for greater than 6 weeks.
    It is often difficult to convince a patient that an x-ray of their spine will not yield meaningful information unless their symptoms or findings include "red flags." Lumbar films not only frequently cause overdiagnosis of vertebral pathology, leading to unnecessary invasive interventions, but also excessive radiation. The average radiation exposure from lumbar radiography is 75 times higher than that from one chest x-ray (Chou et al., 2011).
    a. Only consider plain radiograph of the lumbosacral spine when:
      i. There are "red flags" in the patient's history or physical exam (Table 61-2).
      ii. Back pain is primarily in the high lumbar or thoracic regions (pain here is suggestive of a compression fracture or metastatic tumor).
      iii. The patient has not improved after a 6-week course of conservative therapy.
    b. Consider pelvic radiograph to look for sacroiliitis if suspicion of ankylosing spondylitis based on patient's history or exam (Chou et al., 2007).
    c. Consider chest x-ray if findings suggestive of abdominal aortic aneurysm.
    d. Referral to an orthopedic surgeon who specializes in the spine or a neurosurgeon is warranted for advanced radiographic studies—computerized tomography (CT) and/or magnetic resonance imaging (MRI)—in the following situations:
      i. If severe or progressive neurologic deficits
      ii. If suspicion of infection, tumor, or cauda equina syndrome, urgent study is warranted.
      iii. If sciatic symptoms suggest disc herniation or spinal stenosis
        a. Treat with a course of conservative care first (see Section IV.A), which may be sufficient (Atlas & Deyo, 2001).
        b. If surgery is likely to be needed for unimproved symptoms of disc herniation or spinal stenosis, consider referral to orthopedic surgeon specializing in the spine or a neurosurgical specialist *before*

advanced studies are ordered because the specialist may have a particular preferred test.

e. Despite frequent patient requests for imaging, its utility is largely limited to situations in which an interventional procedure is likely. Again, to emphasize this important point: in 22%–26% of *asymptomatic* adults, disc herniations are seen on MRI. Asymptomatic patients over age 60 have an incidence of spinal stenosis of up to 21% (Jarvik & Deyo, 2002). Patient education is important to explain the risk of unnecessary radiation and to underscore the frequency of false-positive results.

2. Routine blood and urine testing is unnecessary. Select tests may be helpful if a particular pathology is suspected:
   a. Erythrocyte sedimentation rate (ESR): if question of malignancy, ankylosing spondylitis, or suspicion of infection
   b. Complete blood count (CBC): may be used as screening test for neoplasms, infections, or inflammatory processes
   c. Prostate-specific antigen (PSA): if suspicion of metastatic prostate cancer
   d. Urinalysis: if question of urinary tract disease
   e. C-reactive protein: as screen for vertebral infection or ankylosing spondylitis
   f. HLA-B27: This may be used as a screen for ankylosing spondylitis (rate of reliability as a screen differs markedly among ethnic populations; strongest association with ankylosing spondylitis is in Caucasians) (Khan, 2002).
   g. Serum calcium and vitamin D level if concern of osteoporosis
   h. Alkaline phosphatase

3. Electromyography and nerve conduction studies should be reserved for use by specialists in recalcitrant or complex cases.

4. Prognosis is improved by surgery when there is an anatomic lesion that can be corrected and symptoms are neurologic. Refer for surgical evaluation under the following circumstances:
   a. Suspicion of cauda equina syndrome
   b. Deformity
   c. Fracture
   d. Cancer
   e. Suspicion of infection
   f. No improvement in neurologic symptoms after 3 months of conservative therapy

III. Assessment

More than 85% of cases of acute LBP presenting to a primary provider *cannot* reliably be attributed to a specific disease or spinal abnormality (Chou et al., 2007) but will recover within 6 weeks of conservative therapy as described in the plan, Section IV (Papadakis & McPhee, 2019).

A. Determine if evidence of nerve impingement is a result of disc herniation or spinal stenosis (Table 61-4).

B. Determine if presence of "red flags" suggests more serious pathology (cancer, infection, inflammatory condition, fracture; Table 61-2).

C. If no "red flags" are present, even if there is evidence of simple nerve impingement (i.e., sciatica but no evidence of cauda equina), treat as mechanical musculoskeletal back pain or PS, if presentation suggests it, and follow plan outlined in Section IV.

D. Determine if medical-legal issues concerning possible worker's compensation or disability claim are present. If there are medical-legal issues, refer to an occupational or spine specialist.

IV. Plan

A. *Acute LBP (acute: <1–6 weeks; may include sciatica but no "red flags")*

1. Physical measures: In a synthesis of 17 randomized controlled trials of nonpharmacologic therapies for LBP (Chou & Huffman, 2007b) and reviews of databases and randomized controlled trials from 2008 to 2016 (Qaseem et al., 2017), only the following interventions showed evidence of efficacy:

   a. Bed rest only if sciatic or muscle symptoms make walking/sitting difficult. Limit use of bed rest for only debilitating pain; bed rest for >48 hours is not only of no value, but it contributes to counterproductive deconditioning (Ehrlich, 2003).

   b. Patient contact should be made at 1 week, 2–4 weeks, and 6 weeks to assess expected improvement in pain. Any worsening of pain or new/worsening of neurologic losses should be evaluated promptly.

   c. Avoid prolonged sitting or standing; get up at regular intervals (every 30 minutes) to walk and stretch the paraspinal muscles.

   d. Activity modification as warranted by pain level/location. Avoid heavy lifting and extreme spinal flexion.

   e. Local application of moist heat may offer relief.

   f. If suspicion of PS, provide referral to physical therapist for training in stretching and strengthening of hip abductors, external rotators, and extensors.

   g. Spinal manipulation by an osteopathic doctor (DO) and gentle massage may be helpful in producing short-term improvements in pain. Patients should not undergo spinal manipulation if they have radicular symptoms or do back exercises not specifically designed for them because symptoms may be aggravated.

   h. Other nonpharmacologic therapies, such as acupuncture, back schools, low-level laser, lumbar supports, traction, transcutaneous electrical nerve stimulation (TENS) units, and ultrasonography, lack reliable evidence of

effectiveness in managing acute LBP. There have been no peer-reviewed studies that evaluate the effect of different mattresses or pillows on pain intensity.
2. Medications: In a review of 51 randomized controlled trials for the treatment of LBP from the Cochrane Central Registry of Controlled Trials (Chou & Huffman, 2007a):
   a. Non-Steroidal Anti-inflammatory Drugs (NSAIDs), such as Motrin, Naprosyn, Indocin, and Celebrex, were superior to placebo for global improvement of back pain with or without sciatica. No one agent was found to be superior to any other drug in the same class. Topical NSAIDs like diclofenac (brand name: Voltaren Arthritis Pain Gel) are available over the counter (OTC). Diclofenac has been approved by the U.S. Food and Drug Administration (FDA) to treat osteoarthritis of the knee, wrist, and hand. It has *not* been evaluated for use in the treatment of LBP, hip pain, or shoulder pain. Back pain due to arthritis may respond to topical NSAIDs. The treatment is a dime-sized dose of gel, which may be rubbed into the affected area up to 4 times/day. Topical NSAIDs only deliver a fraction of the systemic concentration of active medication found in oral OTC and prescription NSAIDs, so they are safer as a first pharmacologic agent to try for relief and are appropriate for use in patients with heart, kidney, or peptic ulcer disease.
   b. There was no evidence that acetaminophen (Tylenol) was any more effective than placebo (Qaseem et al., 2017), but clinicians may suggest it at dosages up to 4 g/day for patients who cannot tolerate NSAIDs.
   c. There was insufficient evidence to judge the independent benefit of ASA.
   d. Muscle relaxants (e.g., diazepam, tizanidine, cyclobenzaprine, baclofen): Use for <2 weeks; reserved for patients whose pain cannot be controlled alone by NSAIDs or acetaminophen because of *true* muscle spasm. Most effective when combined with NSAID or acetaminophen.
   e. Cannabidiol (CBD) is becoming popular as a source of pain relief and relaxation. As long as it is not sold in combination with THC (the source of the "high" in marijuana), CBD should not have any cognitive side effects. It has not been evaluated in peer-reviewed studies for its comparative effects on pain relief.
   f. The decision to prescribe antidepressants, anti-epileptic drugs, or epidural steroid injections for patients with sciatica should be left to a specialist. However, they were not shown to offer any independent, sustained pain relief.
   g. Opioid analgesics offered moderate benefits in relieving pain not controlled by NSAIDs or acetaminophen. Their use should be limited to <1 week and reserved for patients whose pain cannot be controlled by oral NSAIDs with nonpharmacologic agents or skeletal muscle relaxants or those who should not take these medications for other medical reasons. In a recent set of guidelines on the appropriate use of opioids, the Centers for Disease Control and Prevention (CDC) recommended that they only be used when other agents had failed and that they should be used at the lowest possible dose for the shortest period of time (Dowell et al., 2022).
3. For guidelines on returning to work, see Becker and Childress (2019).
4. File a "Physician's First Report of Injury" if symptoms are due to a work-related injury.

B. *Subacute LBP (6 weeks–3 months)*
  1. Physical measures (Chou & Huffman, 2007a)
     a. Intermittent bed rest (of no more than 48 hours at a time) only if radicular symptoms persist
     b. Modify activity as needed to control symptoms.
     c. Low-stress aerobic exercise (walking, swimming) as tolerated; avoid heavy lifting, prolonged sitting, and standing
     d. Refer workers with LBP beyond 6 weeks to a comprehensive rehabilitation program. Effective programs are multidisciplinary and involve case management, education about keeping active, behavioral treatment, and participation in an exercise program. Exercise training by physical therapist or DO for improvements in posture, core stability training, physical conditioning, and activity modification to decrease physical strain are keys for ongoing management (Papadakis & McPhee, 2019). Current guidelines contraindicate spinal manipulation in people with severe or progressive neurologic deficits. There is insufficient evidence to recommend for or against any *specific* type of exercise program or its frequency.
     e. Mindfulness-based stress reduction and acupuncture both have moderate-quality evidence to support their use (Qaseem et al., 2017).
     f. Local heat or cold if either provides relief
     g. There is insufficient evidence to recommend for or against herbal medicine, yoga, laser therapy, and diathermy.
     h. Lumbar corsets ("back belts"), traction, TENS unit use, traction, taping, and ultrasonography have failed to demonstrate benefit in numerous controlled trials.
  2. Medications (Chou & Huffman, 2007b; Qaseem et al., 2017)
     a. Topical NSAIDs like diclofenac (Voltaren Gel) have not been studied as a pain control agent for LBP but may offer relief.
     b. Nonnarcotic analgesics only (e.g., NSAIDs) unless contraindicated. Again, no single NSAID is superior to any other in controlling pain and symptoms.

c. Short-term use of skeletal muscle relaxants may offer some benefit if skeletal muscle spasm persists.
d. Opioids should be avoided because of risk of dependency or abuse, unless a brief course (1–2 weeks) is needed for severe pain.
e. Evidence is insufficient to consider tricyclic antidepressants, antiseizure agents, CBD, or systemic corticosteroids.
3. Conditioning (after initial pain has subsided)
   a. Biofeedback
   b. Conditioning training by physical therapist, DO, or other health professional to improve core muscle strength. More rigorous conditioning regimens are associated with the best outcomes (Chou et al., 2007).
   c. Ergonomic evaluation of the workplace if symptoms suggest aggravation by work activities
   d. Continue to check in by phone or visit to evaluate recovery and reinforce the need for conditioning. Remind patients that most symptoms of back pain resolve on their own.
4. Referral for specialty evaluation (Atlas & Deyo, 2001)
   a. Refer to a specialist for consideration of epidural steroid injections if sciatic pain (suggesting disc herniation) remains incapacitating during the latter period of conservative therapy. Pain relief will be short term (averaging 3–6 weeks) but may help patients to manage the pain during the period between the "end" of conservative therapy and the point of surgical decision making.
   b. Refer for surgical evaluation if a patient with sciatica has not improved after 4–12 weeks of conservative therapy and/or imaging with MRI or CT shows pathology in an area that corresponds to symptoms.
   c. Refer for diagnostic/specialty evaluation if new "red flag" symptoms appear while the patient is being treated with conservative therapy.
   d. Refer for evaluation by specialist if symptoms are caused by a workplace injury or the patient plans to file a disability claim.
5. For guidelines on returning to work, see Becker and Childress (2019).
6. Patient education (see web-based sample patient education in **Figure 61-1**).
7. Career counseling: Consider referral for vocational evaluation if patient's work repeatedly produces back pain despite conditioning and the patient is not amenable to surgical correction.

C. *Recurrent or chronic LBP (>3 months)*
1. Appropriate to do radiologic and/or imaging studies and/or blood tests if not resolved yet, especially if pain arose from work setting
2. Refer to appropriate specialist for consideration of intra-articular joint injection of glucocorticoids.

Cochrane research comparing 24 studies of patient education found that for patients with acute and subacute low back pain, there **is strong evidence that patients who received a 2.5-hour oral education session in addition to their usual care had better outcomes than people who only received their usual care**. Further, shorter educational sessions or providing only written information by itself without an in-person educational reinforcement did not seem to be effective (Cochrane Collaboration, 2023).
The contents of Figure 61-1, patient educational pieces are current as of February 2022.
1. patient.info/bones-joints-muscles/back-and-spine-pain/lower-back-pain
2. update.com/contents/low-back-pain-in-adults-beyond-the-basics
3. From the American Academy of Family Physicians: https://familydoctor.org/condition/low-back-pain/
4. From the National Institute of Arthritis and Musculoskeletal and Skin Diseases: niams.nih.gov/health-topics/back-pain/diagnosis-treatment-and-steps-to-take

Figure 61-1 Web-based samples of patient education materials for low back pain.
Data from Cochrane Central Registry of Controlled Trials .Individual patient education for low-back pain, https://www.cochrane.org/CD004057/BACK_individual-patient-education-for-low-back-pain

3. Refer to specialist for further evaluation/management if neurologic losses remain present despite compliance with conservative therapy.
4. Physical measures (Chou et al., 2007)
   a. Modify activity to control symptoms; avoid heavy lifting and prolonged sitting/standing.
   b. Low-stress aerobic exercise
   c. Massage
   d. Yoga as long as no radicular (sciatic) symptoms
   e. Manipulation by DO may be helpful as long as no sciatic symptoms are present.
   f. Acupuncture may offer additive short-term pain relief.
   g. Patient-specific exercises and activities per physical therapist or DO to improve core muscle strength and posture may reduce the likelihood of recurrence.
   h. Exercising in warm water can be effective analgesic. Do not do any exercises that increase the pain.
   i. Encourage return to work and activities of daily living (ADLs) as tolerated.
   j. A regular program of daily walking and low-stress aerobic activities once pain has resolved helps develop core muscle support.
5. Medications (Chou & Huffman, 2007b; Qaseem et al., 2017)
   a. Nonnarcotic analgesics only (NSAIDs)
   b. Consider tramadol or duloxetine as second-line medication therapy if inadequate relief with NSAIDs.

c. Opioids as last-choice treatment option only after other medications have failed or if they are contraindicated. Avoid extended-release and long-acting formulations. Recent evidence suggests that longer-term use of opioids (3–6 months) produces a lower level of pain relief (.5 at 3–6 months vs. 1 at 1–3 months) as well as a higher incidence of side effects. Risks and a planned exit strategy should be discussed with the patient (Dowell et al., 2022).
6. Referrals:
   a. Refer to a pain management specialist or physiatrist who specializes in the spine if insufficient relief with previously described measures and no evidence of structural disorder or discogenic cause of pain on imaging.
   b. Refer to an orthopedic surgeon who specializes in the spine or a neurosurgeon if no relief in symptoms by 12 weeks or if radicular symptoms persist.
7. Career counseling: Consider referral for vocational evaluation if the patient's work repeatedly produces back pain despite conditioning and the patient is not amenable to surgical correction.
8. Mental health support: There is strong evidence that several psychosocial factors correlate with the development of chronic back pain. Because strategies aimed at addressing these risk factors have not been individually evaluated, it is reasonable to refer the patient to a mental health professional trained in cognitive–behavioral therapy.
9. Conditioning
   a. Biofeedback, massage, yoga, Pilates, acupuncture, spinal manipulation, TENS, ultrasound, superficial heat, lumbar support, or taping did *not* prove efficacious after 12 weeks.
   b. Interdisciplinary rehabilitation is most effective when presented at the patient's worksite if the LBP involves a work-related injury (Chou & Huffman, 2007a).
   c. Conditioning training by physical therapist or DO
   d. Ergonomic evaluation of workplace if symptoms suggest aggravation by work activities and evaluation not already conducted
10. Patient education (Figure 61-1) and see section IV.B.d-h, and Section IV.C.4.
11. Summary treatment recommendations for patients with acute (<6 weeks), subacute (6–12 weeks), or chronic LBP (>12 weeks) who do not have any "red flags" in their presentation are summarized in **Figure 61-2**. Because it is difficult to predict the course and duration of an episode of LBP, it is important for the clinician to check in regularly with the patient who is still symptomatic and make treatment decisions jointly, reinforcing that 80% of cases of LBP will resolve spontaneously within 6 weeks of onset (Chou et al., 2007).

This research reviewed a collection of controlled trials, databases, and systematic reviews published from January 2008 through November 2016 involving adult patient populations (>18 years) diagnosed with acute, subacute, or chronic lower back pain (LBP) who both had or did not have radicular symptoms or symptomatic spinal stenosis. The quality of the evidence and the strength of the recommendation are noted for each intervention considered.

Recommendation #1: Given that most patients with acute or subacute LBP improve over time regardless of treatment, clinicians and patients should select nonpharmacologic treatment with superficial heat (moderate-quality evidence), massage, acupuncture, or spinal manipulation (low-quality evidence). If pharmacologic treatment is desired, clinicians and patients should select nonsteroidal anti-inflammatory drugs (NSAIDs) or skeletal muscle relaxants (moderate-quality evidence; grade: strong recommendation). There was no evidence that acetaminophen was any better than a placebo in pain relief or function through week 4. (Moderate-quality evidence showed that skeletal muscle relaxants provided short-term pain relief up to day 7.)

Recommendation #2: For patients with chronic LBP, clinicians and patients should initially select nonpharmacologic treatment with exercise, multidisciplinary rehabilitation, acupuncture, mindfulness-based stress reduction (moderate-quality evidence), tai chi, yoga, motor control exercise, progressive relaxation, electromyography biofeedback, low-level laser therapy, operant therapy, cognitive–behavioral therapy, or spinal manipulation (low-quality evidence). If pharmacological therapy is needed, NSAIDs had a moderate effect in improving pain and function, tramadol had a moderate effect in improving pain and a small effect in improving function, and duloxetine and buprenorphine both had small effects on pain and function. Opioids should be the last resort if needed for pain (grade: strong recommendation).

Recommendation #3: In patients with chronic LBP who have had an inadequate response to nonpharmacologic therapy, clinicians and patients should consider pharmacologic therapy with NSAIDs as first-line therapy and tramadol or duloxetine as second-line therapy. Clinicians should only consider opioids as an option in patients who have failed the aforementioned treatments and only if the potential benefits outweigh the risks for individual patients and after a discussion of known risks and realistic benefits is held with one's patient (grade: weak recommendation; moderate-quality evidence). In the presence of radicular LBP, exercise has been shown to improve pain and function (small effect).

High-Value Care: Clinicians should reassure patients that acute or subacute LBP usually improves over time regardless of treatment and should avoid prescribing costly and potentially harmful drugs. Systemic steroids were *not* shown to provide benefit and should not be prescribed for patients with acute or subacute LBP, even with radicular symptoms. For treatment of chronic LBP, clinicians should

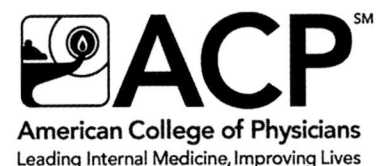

Summary of the American College of Physicians Guideline on Noninvasive Treatments for Acute, Subacute, or Chronic Low Back Pain

Disease/Condition	Low back pain
Target Audience	All clinicians
Target Patient Population	Adults with acute, subacute, or chronic low back pain
Interventions Evaluated	Pharmacologic interventions: NSAIDs, nonopioid analgesics, opioid analgesics, tramadol and tapentadol, antidepressants, SMRs, benzodiazepines, corticosteroids, antiepileptic drugs Nonpharmacologic interventions: interdisciplinary or multicomponent rehabilitation; psychological therapies; exercise and related interventions, such as yoga or tai chi; complementary and alternative medicine therapies, including spinal manipulation, acupuncture, and massage; passive physical modalities, such as heat, cold, ultrasound, transcutaneous electrical nerve stimulation, electrical muscle stimulation, interferential therapy, short-wave diathermy, traction, LLLT, lumbar supports/braces
Outcomes Evaluated	Pain, function, health-related quality of life, work disability/return to work, global improvement, number of back pain episodes or time between episodes, patient satisfaction, adverse effects

Benefits	Acute low back pain
	  Pharmacologic
	    NSAIDs: improved pain and function (small effect)
	    SMRs: improved pain (small effect)
	  Nonpharmacologic
	    Heat wrap: improved pain and function (moderate effect)
	    Massage: improved pain and function (at 1 but not 5 wk) (small to moderate effect)
	    Acupuncture: improved pain (small effect)
	    Spinal manipulation: improved function (small effect)
	
	Chronic low back pain
	  Pharmacologic
	    NSAIDs: improved pain (small to moderate effect) and function (no to small effect)
	    Opioids: improved pain and function (small effect)
	      Tramadol: improved pain (moderate effect) and function (small effect)
	      Buprenorphine (patch or sublingual): improved pain (small effect)
	    Duloxetine: improved pain and function (small effect)
	  Nonpharmacologic
	    Exercise: improved pain and function (small effect)
	    Motor control exercise: improved pain (moderate effect) and function (small effect)
	    Tai chi: improved pain (moderate effect) and function (small effect)
	    Mindfulness-based stress reduction: improved pain and function (small effect)
	    Yoga: improved pain and function (small to moderate effect, depending on comparator)
	    Progressive relaxation: improved pain and function (moderate effect)
	    Multidisciplinary rehabilitation: improved pain (moderate effect) and function (no to small effect)
	    Acupuncture: improved pain (moderate effect) and function (no to moderate effect, depending on comparator)
	    LLLT: improved pain and function (small effect)
	    Electromyography biofeedback: improved pain (moderate effect)
	    Operant therapy: improved pain (small effect)
	    Cognitive behavioral therapy: improved pain (moderate effect)
	    Spinal manipulation: improved pain (small effect)
	
	Radicular low back pain
	  Exercise: improved pain or function (small effect)

Harms	Generally poorly reported
	
	Pharmacologic
	  NSAIDs: increased adverse effects compared with placebo and acetaminophen (COX-2–selective NSAIDs decreased risk for adverse effects compared with traditional NSAIDs)
	  Opioids: nausea, dizziness, constipation, vomiting, somnolence, and dry mouth
	  SMRs: increased risk for any adverse event and central nervous system adverse events (mostly sedation)
	  Benzodiazepines: somnolence, fatigue, lightheadedness
	  Antidepressants: increased risk for any adverse event
	
	Nonpharmacologic
	  Poorly reported, but no increase in serious adverse effects

Figure 61-2 Summary of American College of Physicians' guidelines on noninvasive treatment for acute, subacute, or chronic pain. From Qaseem et al. (2017).

Reproduced from Qaseem, A. Wilt, T. et. al. (2017) Noninvasive treatments for acute, subacute and chronic low back pain; a clinical practice guideline from the American College of Physicians. Annals of Internal Medicine 166 (7) 513-530.

select therapies that have the fewest harms and lowest costs. Clinicians should avoid prescribing costly therapies and those with substantial potential harms, such as long-term opioids, and pharmacologic therapies that were not shown to be effective, such as tricyclic antidepressants and selective serotonin reuptake inhibitors.

Because the vast majority of cases of uncomplicated LBP resolve within 12 weeks, even if there is evidence of nerve root irritation, a major question still exists: When is the risk of spinal surgery clinically warranted in patients with LBP?

Historically, randomized trials comparing surgical to nonsurgical treatment of herniated discs have demonstrated small short-term differences in favor of surgery, but long-term outcomes comparing the two interventions remain controversial. In a widely referenced study (Lurie et al., 2014) that followed 1,244 patients for 8 years (2000–2008), the effectiveness of surgery versus nonoperative care (usual care included use of NSAIDs, active physical therapy, and education/counseling with home exercise instruction) was evaluated for the diagnosis of disc herniation as confirmed by a positive SLR test, complaints of radicular symptoms for at least 6 weeks, and visible disc herniation at a corresponding level on imaging. There were 501 participants in the randomized cohort and 743 participants in the observational group. Patients were evaluated at 6 weeks, 3 and 6 months, and annually thereafter. Primary outcome measures were changes from baseline on entrance to the study, bodily pain, physical function, and disability indices. Secondary outcomes were patient-reported self-improvement, work status, satisfaction with current symptoms, and sciatic severity.

Significantly, there was much "crossover" by patients in the nonoperative groups, who ended up choosing surgery. In both cohorts combined, 820 (66%) of patients initially randomized to or selecting nonoperative treatment received surgery at some point during the 8-year study period.

In patients with a herniated disc confirmed by imaging and leg symptoms persisting for at least 6 weeks, surgery was slightly superior to nonoperative treatment in relieving symptoms and improving function. In the longitudinal analysis, patients who had surgery outperformed the nonoperative group in all outcome measurements at 6 weeks. The nonoperative group showed substantial improvement over time. At year 8, 54% of the nonoperative group reported being satisfied with their symptoms, and 73% were satisfied with their care. This improvement was equivalent to the surgical group and was sustained with no degradation between years 4 and 8.

The risks of surgery included the following:
1. Number of deaths: Four deaths occurred, evenly distributed between the two groups. No perioperative deaths occurred; one death occurring 90 days after surgery was judged by the hospital's institutional review board to be the consequence of a comorbidity.
2. Surgical complications: Of all surgical patients, 3.2% experienced a dural tear requiring reoperation. Only six patients required a transfusion intraoperatively or postoperatively.
3. Repeat surgeries: Of the patients who had surgery, 15% required repeat surgery by year 8 for recurrent herniation at the same level. The rate of reoperation was not significantly different between the randomized and observational cohorts. However, differences in their characteristics were not described, and how much time passed between the two surgeries is not noted, so the significance and cost of these complications are unknown.

D. *Follow-up care to prevent recurrence after initial symptoms have resolved*

Because relapses in back pain are common—approaching 75% (Goroll & Mulley, 2014)—and the societal burden of chronic pain is large, strategies to prevent acute back pain from becoming chronic have been investigated. Agency for Healthcare Research and Quality (AHRQ, 2016) have synthesized the evidence on prevention:
1. Both reports emphasized the importance of clinician education and support in explaining the usually benign course of LBP, even though symptoms may persist for more than 1 month. Written materials reinforcing the clinician's message are useful to provide as a supplement.
2. Although both analyses determined that it is important to resume physical activity quickly after the acute pain has resolved, both concluded that there is insufficient evidence to recommend for or against the routine use of *specific* exercise interventions to prevent back pain.
3. Consider encouraging the patient to attend a community-based exercise program or gym program to support the performance of exercises and obtain the benefits of peer support in strengthening core musculature, reducing the likelihood of recurrence.
4. Other nonpharmacologic interventions listed in Section IV.A.1.h were not found to offer additional benefit or relief.
5. It has not been verified that a reduction in risk factors (i.e., higher body weight and smoking) will prevent the recurrence of back pain, although it intuitively seems a reasonable expectation.
6. The physical measures listed earlier in Section IV.C.4 for chronic LBP have not been validated as either preventing or not preventing recurring episodes of LBP.
7. The earlier recommendations for agents to avoid in treating LBP also apply in preventing recurrences of LBP.

8. Consult or refer for evaluation by an orthopedic spine surgeon or neurosurgeon if:
    a. Symptoms consistent with cauda equina syndrome
    b. Lower limb weakness or sensory losses
    c. Progressive neurologic deficit
    d. Presence of "red flags" (symptoms suggestive of cancer, bone infection, or ankylosing spondylitis require referral to other appropriate specialists)
    e. Severe spinal deformity
    f. Abnormal findings on MRI or CT
    g. Failure to secure relief of symptoms or worsening of symptoms *after 12 weeks* of conservative measures described previously

References

Agency for Healthcare Research and Quality. (2016) *Non-invasive treatments for low back pain: Current state of the evidence.* http://effectivehealthcare.ahrq.gov/products/back-pain-treatment/clinician

Atlas, S., & Deyo, R. (2001). Evaluating and managing acute low back pain in the primary care setting. *Journal of General Internal Medicine, 16*(2), 120–131. doi:10.1111/j.1525-1497.2001.91141.x

Becker, B., & Childress, M. (2019). Nonspecific low back pain and return to work. *American Family Physician, 100*(11), 697–708.

Chou, R., & Huffman, L. (2007a). Medications for acute and chronic low back pain: A review of the evidence for an American Pain Society/American College of Physicians Clinical Practice Guideline. *Annals of Internal Medicine, 147*(7), 505–514. doi:10.7326/0003-4819-147-7-200710020-00008

Chou, R., & Huffman, L. (2007b). Nonpharmacologic therapies for acute and chronic low back pain: A review of the evidence for an American Pain Society/American College of Physicians Clinical Practice Guideline. *Annals of Internal Medicine, 147*(7), 492–504. doi:10.7326/0003-4819-147-7-200710020-00007

Chou, R., Quaseem, A., Owens, D., Shekelle, S., & Clinical Guidelines Committee of the American College of Physicians. (2011). Diagnostic imaging for low back pain: advice for high-value health care from the American College of Physicians. *Annals of Internal Medicine, 154*(3), 181–189. doi:10.7326/0003-4819-154-3-201102010-00008

Chou, R., Quaseem, A., Snow, V., Casey, D., Cross, J. T., Jr., Shekelle, P., Owens, D. K., Clinical Efficacy Assessment Subcommittee of the American College of Physicians, American College of Physicians, & American Pain Society Low Back Pain Guidelines Panel. (2007). Diagnosis and treatment of low back pain: A joint clinical practice guideline from the American College of Physicians and the American Pain Society. *Annals of Internal Medicine, 147*(7), 478–491. doi:10.7326/0003-4819-147-7-200710020-00006

Cochrane Collaboration. (2023). *Individual patient education for low-back pain.* https://www.cochrane.org/CD004057/BACK_individual-patient-education-for-low-back-pain

Dowell, D., Ragann, K. R., Jones, C. M., Baldwin, G. T., & Chou, R. (2022). CDC clinical practice guideline for prescribing opioids for pain-United States, 2022. *MMWR Recommendations and Reports, 71*(3), 1–95. doi:10.15585/mmwr.rr7103a1

Ehrlich, G. (2003). Back pain. *Journal of Rheumatology, 30*(67), 26–31.

Goroll, A. H., & Mulley, A. (2014). *Primary care medicine* (7th ed.). Wolters Kluwer Health.

Jarvik, J. G., & Deyo, R. (2002). Diagnostic evaluation of low back pain with emphasis on imaging. *Annals of Internal Medicine, 137*(7), 586–597. doi:10.7326/0003-4819-137-7-200210010-00010

Khan, M. A. (2002). Update on spondyloarthropathies. *Annals of Internal Medicine, 136*(12), 896–907. doi:10.7326/0003-4819-136-12-200206180-00011

Luke, A., & Ma, B. (2019) Low back pain. In M. Papadakis, S. McPhee & M. Rabow (Eds.), *Current medical diagnosis and treatment* (58th ed., pp 1698, Table 41-2). McGraw-Hill Education.

Lurie, J., Tosteson, T., Tosteson, A., Zhao, W., Morgan, T. S., Abdu, W. A., Herkowitz, H., & Weinstein, J. N. (2014). Surgical versus non-operative treatment for lumbar disc herniation: Eight-year results for the Spine Patients Outcomes Research Trial (SPORT). *Spine, 39*(1), 3–16. doi:10.1097/BRS.0000000000000088

McGee, S. (2007). The leg. In S. McGee (Ed.), *Evidence-based physical diagnosis* (2nd ed., pp.786, Box 60-4). Saunders Elsevier.

Qaseem, A., Wilt, T., McLean, R. M., Forciea, M. A., Clinical Guidelines Committee of the American College of Physicians, Denberg, T. D., Barry, M. J., Boyd, C., Dobbin Chow, R., Fitterman, N., Harris, R. P., Humphrey, L. L., & Vijan, S. (2017). Noninvasive treatments for acute, subacute and chronic low back pain: A clinical practice guideline from the American College of Physicians. *Annals of Internal Medicine, 166*(7), 513–530. doi:10.7326/M16-2367

van Tulder, M., Koes, B., & Bombardier, C. (2002). Low back pain. *Best Practice and Research. Clinical Rheumatology, 16*(5), 761–765. doi:10.1053/berh.2002.0267

CHAPTER 62

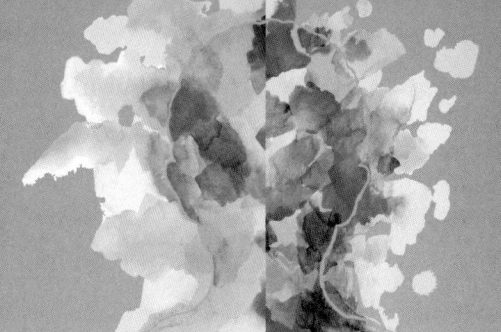

Nonalcoholic Fatty Liver Disease (NAFLD)

Miranda Surjadi

I. Introduction and general background

The liver is the largest solid organ in the body, weighing approximately 1–1.5 kg. The majority of cells in the liver consist of hepatocytes. Hepatocytes are responsible for the synthesis of serum proteins (albumin, coagulation factors, and many hormonal and growth factors), the production of bile, the regulation of nutrients, and metabolism and conjugation of lipophilic compounds for excretion in the bile or urine. Although there are many causes of liver diseases, one of the most common is nonalcoholic fatty liver disease (NAFLD). NAFLD is the most common chronic liver disease, affecting approximately one-quarter of the U.S. population (American Liver Foundation, 2023). Of those adults diagnosed with NAFLD, there is a smaller proportion who have nonalcoholic steatohepatitis (NASH), which is a more progressive form of fatty liver disease, typically diagnosed by liver biopsy. There are certain comorbidities associated with NAFLD and NASH, which include higher body weight, diabetes, hyperlipidemia, and metabolic syndrome (Chalasani et al., 2018). Potential long-term complications of NAFLD and NASH include compensated and decompensated cirrhosis (Chalasani et al., 2018).

A. NAFLD, NAFL, and NASH

1. Definitions

   NAFLD encompasses the entire spectrum of fatty liver disease, ranging from nonalcoholic fatty liver (NAFL) to NASH, and is a common cause of elevated liver enzymes (Chalasani et al., 2018). To define NAFLD, there needs to be evidence, by liver biopsy or imaging, of hepatic steatosis or fat in the liver that is greater than or equal to 5% of the total liver. In addition, all other causes of fatty liver disease must be excluded, such as alcoholic liver disease (Chalasani et al., 2018). NAFL is the presence of hepatic steatosis without liver cell injury. In contrast, NASH is the presence of hepatic steatosis with hepatocyte injury (ballooning hepatocytes on liver biopsy). NASH is more likely to progress to cirrhosis and liver failure (Chalasani et al., 2018).

2. NAFLD/NASH prevalence and high-risk groups

   NAFLD and NASH are very common liver diseases worldwide, and the rate of NAFLD continues to increase. In a meta-analysis investigating the global prevalence of NAFLD, Younossi and colleagues (2016) used imaging to estimate that approximately 25% of the world population has NAFLD. In the United States, the prevalence is also approximately 25% of the population (American Liver Foundation, 2023). Of those who have NAFLD, the prevalence of NASH is approximately 20% (American Liver Foundation, 2023).

   There are comorbidities associated with NAFLD and NASH where the prevalence is greatest, and most are metabolic in nature. The most common conditions associated with NAFLD are higher body weight, type 2 diabetes mellitus (T2DM), dyslipidemia, metabolic syndrome, and polycystic ovary syndrome (PCOS) (Chalasani et al., 2018). Higher body weight is the most common risk factor for NAFLD. With the growing epidemic of higher body weight, there is a similar growth of NAFLD. Sasaki and colleagues (2014) found that greater than 95% of people with severely high body weight who undergo bariatric surgery have NAFLD. Globally, in people with T2DM, over 50% also have NAFLD, a rate that is two times higher than that of the general population (Younossi et al., 2019). In people with dyslipidemia (high triglycerides, low high-density lipoprotein [HDL]), Assy and colleagues (2000) found the prevalence of NAFLD to be 50% in those who attended specialty lipid clinics. Finally, in people with PCOS, the prevalence of NAFLD was found to be about 24% (Romanowski et al., 2015).

3. Natural history
People with NAFLD who have evidence of advanced fibrosis, either by imaging or biopsy, have a higher incidence of progression to cirrhosis (Chalasani et al., 2018). The most common cause of death in people with NAFLD is cardiovascular disease (Chalasani et al., 2018). NASH is a more progressive form of NAFLD and is more likely to result in cirrhosis and decompensated liver disease. NASH is now the second-most-common reason for liver transplantation, according to Pais and colleagues (2016), behind chronic hepatitis C. Additionally, NAFLD and NASH are now the third-most-common cause of hepatocellular carcinoma (HCC) or liver cancer (Mohamad et al., 2015). To differentiate between NAFL and NASH, a liver biopsy is still considered the gold standard (Younossi et al., 2018).
4. Screening
According to the American Association for the Study of Liver Diseases (AASLD), routine screening for NAFLD is not currently recommended (Chalasani et al., 2018). Similarly, no screening guidelines are put forth by the U.S. Preventive Services Task Force (USPSTF). In contrast, the European Association for the Study of the Liver (EASL), European Association for the Study of Diabetes (EASD), and European Association for the Study of Obesity (EASO) (EASL et al., 2016) have put forth recommendations for screening for NAFLD in those with persistently elevated liver enzymes. Additionally, those with higher body weight and metabolic syndrome should be screened for NAFLD with serological liver enzymes and/or ultrasound (EASL et al., 2016). In high-risk individuals (age >50 years, T2DM, and metabolic syndrome), case finding for NASH is recommended (EASL et al., 2016) because of its progressive nature.

Despite the fact that the AASLD does not recommend routine screening for NAFLD in the general population, there should be a high index of suspicion for NAFLD in someone with T2DM and other metabolic conditions. Initial evaluation of NAFLD includes the exclusion of alcoholic fatty liver disease and other common liver diseases.

II. Database (may include but is not limited to)
A. *Subjective*
  1. NAFLD/NASH
     a. Past health history
        i. Comorbidities—established associations: type 2 diabetes mellitus, hyperlipidemia, higher body weight, metabolic syndrome, PCOS
        ii. Comorbidities—other conditions: hypothyroid, obstructive sleep apnea, hypopituitarism, hypogonadism, pancreatoduodenal resection, psoriasis
        iii. Exclude other causes of fatty liver: excessive alcohol intake, chronic hepatitis C, medication side effects, Wilson disease, lipodystrophy, Reye syndrome, starvation, acute fatty liver of pregnancy, and parenteral nutrition.
        iv. Medication history: hepatotoxic medications, such as tuberculosis (TB) medications, methotrexate, statins, and so forth
     b. Family history
        i. T2DM, hyperlipidemia, higher weight, metabolic syndrome, PCOS
        ii. Hepatocellular carcinoma
     c. Personal/social history
        i. Diet history
        ii. Exercise history
        iii. Alcohol use, drug use
     d. Immunizations
        i. Hepatitis A vaccine
        ii. Hepatitis B vaccine
     e. Review of systems
        i. Constitutional signs and symptoms: fatigue
        ii. Skin, hair, and nails: itching, bruising
        iii. Ear, nose, and throat: jaundice
        iv. Chest: gynecomastia
        v. Cardiac: shortness of breath, chest pain, palpitations
        vi. Abdomen: abdominal pain, abdominal distention, nausea, vomiting, clay-colored stools
        vii. Genitourinary: dark urine
        viii. Musculoskeletal: joint pain
        ix. Extremities: pedal edema
        x. Neurological: confusion, tremors, sleep–wake cycle disturbances
B. *Objective*
  1. Physical exam findings: Patients with NAFLD are generally clinically stable and asymptomatic. If they have cirrhosis, they may have physical exam findings (**Table 62-1**).
  2. Supporting data from relevant laboratory/diagnostic tests: to evaluate liver disease and exclude other types of common liver diseases (**Tables 62-2** and **62-3**)
     a. Liver function tests (LFTs): Aspartate aminotransferase (AST) and alanine aminotransferase (ALT) are generally elevated in people with NAFLD and NASH. However, some people with NAFLD present with normal AST and ALT. AST and ALT elevation are generally markers of liver inflammation and not specific for NAFLD or NASH.
     b. Markers of liver function: Platelets, albumin, prothrombin time (PT)/international normalized ratio (INR), total bilirubin. These tests are usually normal in people with NAFLD and NASH unless they have cirrhosis.
     c. Comorbidities: Hemoglobin A1c and lipid panel.

Table 62-1 Physical Examination Findings

Associated Findings (may or may not include):

Vital signs: Total body weight, blood pressure

General appearance: lethargy (hepatic encephalopathy)

Skin/hair: jaundiced, pruritus, bruising (cirrhosis)

Eyes: icteric sclerae (cirrhosis)

Chest/Lungs: spider nevi, gynecomastia, crackles (cirrhosis due to portal hypertension)

Cardiovascular: increased jugular venous pressure (cirrhosis due to portal hypertension)

Abdomen: ascites, fluid wave, caput medusae, hepatomegaly, splenomegaly (cirrhosis)

Extremities: palmar erythema, pedal edema (cirrhosis)

Neurological: asterixis, tremors, behavioral changes (hepatic encephalopathy)

III. Assessment

A. Determine the diagnosis

When NAFLD is suspected in a patient, it is important to exclude other etiologies of hepatic steatosis and rule out common causes of chronic liver disease. There also needs to be evidence of hepatic steatosis, either by imaging or through a liver biopsy. Elevated liver enzymes (AST, ALT) are commonly seen in someone with NAFLD but are not universally present.

1. Other conditions that may explain the patient's elevated LFTs
   a. Autoimmune hepatitis: antinuclear antibody (ANA)/anti–smooth muscle antibody positive; chronic necroinflammatory liver disease of unknown etiology
   b. Viral hepatitis: chronic hepatitis B virus (HBV) and chronic hepatitis C virus (HCV) (**Table 62-3**)
   c. Primary biliary cirrhosis: antimitochondrial antibody positive in 95%; chronic cholestatic liver

Table 62-2 Common Liver Tests

Function	Test	Definition	Clinical Implications	Comments
Marker of hepatocellular injury	Aspartate aminotransferase (AST)	Found mainly in hepatocytes. Released into bloodstream when there is liver injury	■ Increased in viral hepatitis ■ AST:ALT ratio of 2:1 in alcoholic hepatitis	Found in liver, heart, skeletal muscle, brain
Marker of hepatocellular injury	Alanine aminotransferase (ALT)	Found mainly in hepatocytes. Released into bloodstream when there is liver injury	■ Increased in viral hepatitis ■ ALT > AST in chronic viral hepatitis.	Found in liver
Marker of cholestatic injury	Alkaline phosphatase	Canicular enzyme that plays a role in bile production	■ Increased in hepatobiliary disease, bone disease, pregnancy, hyperparathyroidism	Found in liver, bone, intestine, and placenta
Marker of cholestatic injury	Bilirubin	Breakdown product of hemolysis. Taken up by liver cells and conjugated to water-soluble product. Excreted in bile	■ Elevations may indicate hepatic or extrahepatic disorder.	Hepatitis and cirrhosis cause conjugated hyperbilirubinemia
Marker of liver function	Albumin	Major component of plasma proteins. Liver synthesizes albumin.	■ Decreased in cirrhosis from chronic liver disease ■ Also decreased in nephrotic syndrome, malabsorption, protein-losing enteropathy	Indication of severity of liver disease
Marker of liver function	Platelets		■ Decreased in patients with cirrhosis	
Marker of liver function	Prothrombin time	Liver produces clotting factors I, II, V, VII, and X. Prothrombin time depends on the activity of these clotting factors.	■ Increased in cirrhosis from chronic liver disease	

Table 62-3 Common Liver Diseases Serologic Tests, Viral Hepatitides

Test	Clinical Implications	Comments
Hepatitis B surface antigen (HBsAg)	■ If positive for 6 months or more, denotes chronic infection.	
Hepatitis B core antibody immunoglobulin G (IgG anti-HBc)	■ Past exposure to hepatitis B virus (HBV)	
Hepatitis B core antibody immunoglobulin M (IgM anti-HBc)	■ Acute exposure to HBV ■ Reactivation of chronic infection	
Hepatitis B surface antibody (HBsAb)	■ Immunity to HBV	Vaccine-induced immunity will not have positive anti-HBc.
Hepatitis B DNA (HBV DNA)	■ Active viral replication	May be present in inactive disease state, but usually <2,000 IU/mL
Hepatitis B E antigen (HBeAg)	■ Active viral replication	May be negative in those with a pre–core mutant HBV
Hepatitis C Antibody (HCV Ab)	■ Detects antibodies to hepatitis C virus (HCV)	Positive in patients who have been exposed to hepatitis C
HCV RNA	■ Determines HCV viral load and determines if HCV RNA is undetectable	Positive in patients with chronic hepatitis C Useful in monitoring response to HCV therapy

disease more common in women age 50 and older
  d. Hemochromatosis: Elevated iron and ferritin; most common genetic disorder in the Caucasian population. The extent of liver injury is associated with the accumulation of hepatic iron.
  e. Wilson disease: autosomal-recessive defect of cellular copper export; decreased ceruloplasmin
  f. Alpha-1 antitrypsin deficiency: genetic disorder that affects lungs and liver
  g. Primary sclerosing cholangitis: chronic biliary duct inflammation; associated with inflammatory bowel disease
B. Severity
  1. Assessment of hepatic steatosis in people with NAFLD
    a. Liver biopsy: Most reliable for identifying the presence of hepatic steatosis (NAFLD) and/or steatohepatitis (NASH). A biopsy will also show the degree of fibrosis or scarring of the liver. To evaluate someone with suspected NAFLD and another type of liver disease, a liver biopsy is often preferred because it can determine the diagnosis. Liver biopsy is also the most invasive assessment, and its use is limited by cost and procedure-related side effects (Chalasani et al., 2018).
    b. Imaging modalities
      i. Magnetic resonance (MR) imaging: able to quantify hepatic steatosis either by spectroscopy or proton density fat fraction (Dulai et al., 2016; Idilman et al., 2020).
      ii. Ultrasonography (US) and computed tomography (CT) do not reliably predict liver histology in someone with NAFLD (Musso et al., 2011).
  2. Assessment of hepatic fibrosis in people with NAFLD
    a. Liver biopsy: Most reliable in determining degree of fibrosis in someone with suspected NAFLD. It should be considered in those with NAFLD who are at risk of having steatohepatitis (NASH) or advanced liver disease.
    b. Noninvasive tools
      i. Imaging: FibroScan and MR elastography (MRE) are both able to measure liver stiffness in people with suspected NAFLD (Imajo et al., 2016).
      ii. Clinical decision tools: NAFLD fibrosis score (NFS), FIB-4 index, aspartate aminotransferase to platelet ratio index (APRI), and FibroMeter and FibroSure
        • The NFS calculator: https://www.mdcalc.com/nafld-non-alcoholic-fatty-liver-disease-fibrosis-score

- NFS is based on variables: body mass index (BMI), presence of diabetes, age, platelet count, albumin, AST, ALT
- FIB-4 calculator: https://www.mdcalc.com/fibrosis-4-fib-4-index-liver-fibrosis
- FIB-4 is based on variables: AST, ALT, platelet counts, and age.
- APRI calculator: https://www.hepatitisc.uw.edu/page/clinical-calculators/apri
- FibroMeter and FibroSure are both blood tests used to evaluate liver fibrosis using blood biomarkers. FibroMeter is used more commonly in Europe, whereas FibroSure is used in the United States. Imajo and colleagues (2016) reported that the NFS and FIB-4 are better than the APRI and as good as MRE for predicting hepatic fibrosis in patients with NAFLD with more advanced liver disease (stage 3 or 4 fibrosis on Metavir score).

3. Assessment of cirrhosis

   At stage 4 fibrosis, it is assumed the person has cirrhosis of the liver or advanced scarring of the liver. If a patient has stage 4 fibrosis or cirrhosis, then the next step is to assess the severity of cirrhosis and determine if the patient has compensated or decompensated cirrhosis. Compensated cirrhosis refers to intact liver function (normal platelets, albumin, total bilirubin, PT/INR). Decompensated liver disease is manifested by a history of ascites, pedal edema, encephalopathy, and/or variceal bleeding. These patients should be referred to a liver transplant center for evaluation and treatment.

   a. Calculate the Model for End-Stage Liver Disease (MELD) score (Organ Procurement and Transplantation Network, n.d.). Allocation calculators: https://www.unos.org/transplantation/allocation-calculators/
   b. If the MELD score is 10 or greater, refer to liver transplant center.

C. *Significance*

   Assess the significance of the problem to the patient and significant others. Discuss treatment of NAFLD or NASH in addition to comorbidities as appropriate.

D. *Motivation and ability*

   Determine the patient's willingness and ability to follow the treatment plan.
   1. Consider food insecurity and housing insecurity when making recommendations about diet and exercise.
   2. Discuss factors that may hinder the patient from adhering to a low-fat diet or increased exercise. Problem-solve with your patients if they have difficulty accessing fresh produce or fruits.
   3. Educate patients on how to read food labels.

IV. Goals of clinical management

A. *NAFLD*
   1. Lifestyle interventions: diet, exercise, and weight loss
   Losing at least 5% of body weight has shown improvement in hepatic steatosis.
   Losing more than 7% of body weight was associated with improvement in liver histology and fibrosis (Musso et al., 2012).
   In the meta-analysis by Musso and colleagues (2012) of randomized, controlled trials (RCTs), weight reduction was done by caloric restriction in the diet or in addition to increased exercise. Both dietary changes and exercise are recommended for patients with NAFLD to achieve weight-loss goals.

   a. Diet: Decreasing calories by at least 30% is recommended to improve hepatic steatosis.
   b. Exercise: RCTs that assess the efficacy of exercise alone (without diet) in achieving improved liver histology and fibrosis are lacking in evidence. (Chalasani et al., 2018). The optimal duration of exercise and intensity of exercise have not been determined. St George and colleagues (2009) determined that those who exercised more than 150 minutes/week had a more pronounced reduction of serum aminotransferases, which was independent of weight loss.

   2. Pharmacologic interventions: Medications for fatty liver disease that are aimed at improving liver disease are reserved for those with liver biopsy–proven NASH with the presence of fibrosis (Chalasani et al., 2018).

B. *NASH*
   1. Lifestyle interventions: See NAFLD section.
   2. Pharmacologic interventions:

   a. Metformin: Provides some improvement in serum aminotransferases and insulin resistance but does not improve liver histology. Metformin is not recommended for the treatment of NASH in adult patients (Chalasani et al., 2018; Musso et al., 2010).
   b. Thiazolidinediones: Pioglitazone (45 mg/day) in patients with NASH with T2DM improves insulin sensitivity, serum aminotransferases, hepatic steatosis, and ballooning on liver histology (Belfort et al., 2006).

   Aithal and colleagues (2008) showed that pioglitazone (30 mg/day) is beneficial in patients with NASH without diabetes. Because of a lack of evidence, the use of pioglitazone should be reserved for those with liver biopsy–proven NASH only.

   c. Vitamin E: Vitamin E at a dose of 800 IU/day decreases serum aminotransferases and improves steatosis and ballooning on liver histology in patients with liver biopsy–proven NASH without diabetes (Sanyal et al., 2010). Treatment duration of vitamin E is not to exceed 2 years because the long-term safety of vitamin E is currently unknown. Additionally, vitamin E is not recommended in patients with NAFLD without a liver biopsy or those with NASH and T2DM.
   d. Obeticholic acid (OCA) and elafibranor: Both are currently in phase 3 registration trials for

patients with NASH. OCA at 25 mg/day was shown to improve steatohepatitis and fibrosis in phase 2 trials (Neuschwander-Tetri, 2020). Both medications are currently still in phase 3 trials and have not been approved by the U.S. Food and Drug Administration to treat NASH.

C. Management of comorbidities
  1. Cardiovascular disease and dyslipidemia: People with NAFLD are at high risk for cardiovascular morbidity and mortality. People with NAFLD may often present with high triglycerides, in addition to high low-density lipoprotein (LDL) and low HDL (Pais et al., 2016).

     Treatment of dyslipidemia with statins in patients with elevated aminotransferases (presumed to have NAFLD) results in improvement in cardiovascular outcomes (Athyros et al., 2010). Patients with NASH or NAFLD are not at higher risk for serious liver injury from statins. Statins are safe for use in patients with NAFLD and NASH cirrhosis but should be avoided in patients with decompensated cirrhosis (Chalasani et al., 2018).
  2. Diabetes: People with T2DM and concurrent NAFLD should be encouraged to maintain hemoglobin A1c at levels recommended by the American Diabetes Association (ADA, 2022).

V. Plan
A. HCC screening/surveillance
  The AASLD guidelines recommend starting HCC screening in patients with NAFLD and NASH with cirrhosis (Chalasani et al., 2018). HCC screening should be done with abdominal ultrasound every 6 months. Measurement of alpha-fetoprotein (AFP) is optional but not necessary for screening, and AFP alone is not recommended as a screening tool, unless in rare cases where imaging is not available. Imaging is the necessary technique for HCC screening.
B. Diagnostic tests
  1. NAFLD is often found incidentally on routine blood tests showing elevated serum aminotransferases and/or fatty liver on imaging. The gold standard for diagnosing NAFLD or NASH is by liver biopsy, which reveals cells that show hepatic steatosis or steatohepatitis. Patients with NAFLD or NASH are typically asymptomatic but often have comorbidities such as high body weight, T2DM, hyperlipidemia, and metabolic syndrome.
     a. LFTs: Complete blood count (CBC), complete metabolic panel, coagulation tests (PT/INR)
     b. Tests to rule out other causes of liver disease that could be causing elevated serum aminotransferases: hepatitis B serologies (hepatitis B surface antigen [HbsAg], hepatitis B core antibody [HBcAb], hepatitis B surface antibody [HBsAb]), HACV antibody (HCV Ab), ANA, iron studies, antimitochondrial antibody (AMA), anti–smooth muscle antibody, ceruloplasmin, alpha-1 antitrypsin (A1AT)
     c. Comorbidities of diabetes and hyperlipidemia: hemoglobin A1c, lipid panel
     d. Ruling out alcohol use
     e. Imaging—MRE, FibroScan to look for hepatic steatosis
     f. Fibrosis testing: Newer and noninvasive tests for fibrosis testing are preferable to liver biopsy if available. Some blood test markers (e.g., FibroSure) are becoming more widely available.
     g. Liver biopsy is still considered the gold standard but is limited in use because of cost, invasiveness, and potential for complications. It is recommended to pursue a liver biopsy for diagnosis if there are two or more possible liver etiologies. Liver biopsy is also recommended if there is a high suspicion for NASH (Chalasani et al., 2018).
C. Monitoring of NAFLD
  1. NAFLD/NASH
     a. Laboratory monitoring: in 3–6 months with labs; should include liver panel, A1c, and lipid panel after initial visit and every 6 months afterward
     b. Imaging: Ultrasound every 6 months if there is presence of cirrhosis; routine imaging is not recommended in patients with NAFLD/NASH without cirrhosis.
  2. Who and when to refer to specialist:
     a. A patient with NASH and cirrhosis who is a potential candidate for liver transplantation
     b. Patients with NAFLD or NASH with advanced fibrosis or cirrhosis
     c. Children or adolescents with NASH
     d. Management of NASH with pharmacological therapy
     e. Assessing the need for liver biopsy in someone with suspected NASH
     f. Patients with NAFLD or NASH and a possible second etiology of liver disease
  3. Patients with NAFLD/NASH cirrhosis:
     a. HCC surveillance with AFP and ultrasound every 6 months
     b. Variceal screening with endoscopy every 1–3 years
     c. Monitor MELD score every 3–6 months: INR, total bilirubin, albumin, creatinine, AST, ALT, platelets (see https://optn.transplant.hrsa.gov/data/allocation-calculators/meld-calculator/). Refer to liver transplant/liver specialist when appropriate for evaluation and treatment (if MELD > 10).
     d. Vaccinate for hepatitis A and B.
     e. Patient education: Avoid alcohol, adhere to low-salt diet, avoid raw fish/shellfish, avoid nonsteroidal anti-inflammatories, and limit acetaminophen (maximum of 2,000 mg daily).

VI. Self-management resources and tools
A. Patient education
  1. AASLD, http://www.aasld.org
  2. American Liver Foundation, http://www.liverfoundation.org/

References

Aithal, G. P., Thomas, J. A., Kaye, P. V., Lawson, A., Ryder, S. D., Spendlove, I., Austin, A. S., Freeman, J. G., Morgan, L., & Webber, J. (2008). Randomized, placebo-controlled trial of pioglitazone in nondiabetic subjects with nonalcoholic steatohepatitis. *Gastroenterology*, 135(4), 1176–1184.

American Diabetes Association, Professional Practice Committee. (2022). 6. Glycemic targets: *Standards of medical care in diabetes—2022*. *Diabetes Care*, 45 (Suppl. 1), S83–S96. doi:10.2337/dc22-S006

American Liver Foundation. (2023). *Nonalcoholic fatty liver disease (NAFLD)*. https://liverfoundation.org/liver-diseases/fatty-liver-disease/nonalcoholic-fatty-liver-disease-nafld/

Assy, N., Kaita, K., Mymin, D., Levy, C., Rosser, B., & Minuk, G. (2000). Fatty infiltration of liver in hyperlipidemic patients. *Digestive Diseases and Sciences*, 45(10), 1929–1934.

Athyros, V. G., Tziomalos, K., Gossios, T. D., Griva, T., Anagnostis, P., Kargiotis, K., Pagourelias, E. D., Theocharidou, E., Karagiannis, A., Mikhailidis, D. P., & GREACE Study Collaborative Group. (2010). Safety and efficacy of long-term statin treatment for cardiovascular events in patients with coronary heart disease and abnormal liver tests in the Greek Atorvastatin and Coronary Heart Disease Evaluation (GREACE) Study: A post-hoc analysis. *The Lancet*, 376(9756), 1916–1922. doi:10.1016/S0140-6736(10)61272-X

Belfort, R., Harrison, S. A., Brown, K., Darland, C., Finch, J., Hardies, J., Balas, B., Gastaldelli, A., Tio, F., Pulcini, J., Berria, R., Ma, J. Z., Dwivedi, S., Havranek, R., Fincke, C., DeFronzo, R., Bannayan, G. A., Schenker, S., & Cusi, K. (2006). A placebo-controlled trial of pioglitazone in subjects with nonalcoholic steatohepatitis. *New England Journal of Medicine*, 355(22), 2297–2307.

Chalasani, N., Younossi, Z., Lavine, J. E., Charlton, M., Cusi, K., Rinella, M., Harrison, S. A., Brunt, E. M., & Sanyal, A. J. (2018). The diagnosis and management of nonalcoholic fatty liver disease: Practice guidance from the American Association for the Study of Liver Diseases. *Hepatology*, 67(1), 328–357. doi:10.1002/hep.29367

Dulai, P. S., Sirlin, C. B., & Loomba, R. (2016). MRI and MRE for non-invasive quantitative assessment of hepatic steatosis and fibrosis in NAFLD and NASH: Clinical trials to clinical practice. *Journal of Hepatology*, 65(5), 1006–1016.

European Association for the Study of the Liver (EASL), European Association for the Study of Diabetes (EASD), & European Association for the Study of Obesity (EASO). (2016). EASL–EASD–EASO clinical practice guidelines for the management of non-alcoholic fatty liver disease. *Diabetologia*, 59(6), 1121–1140. doi:10.1007/s00125-016-3902-y

Idilman, I. S., Li, J., Yin, M., & Venkatesh, S. K. (2020). MR elastography of liver: Current status and future perspectives. *Abdominal Radiology*, 45(11), 3444–3462.

Imajo, K., Kessoku, T., Honda, Y., Tomeno, W., Ogawa, Y., Mawatari, H., Fujita, K., Yoneda, M., Taguri, M., Hyogo, H., Sumida, Y., Ono, M., Eguchi, Y., Inoue, T., Yamanaka, T., Wada, K., Saito, S., & Nakajima, A. (2016). Magnetic resonance imaging more accurately classifies steatosis and fibrosis in patients with nonalcoholic fatty liver disease than transient elastography. *Gastroenterology*, 150(3), 626–637.e7.

Mohamad, B., Shah, V., Onyshchenko, M., Elshamy, M., Aucejo, F., Lopez, R., Hanouneh, I. A., Alhaddad, R., & Alkhouri, N. (2015). Characterization of hepatocellular carcinoma (HCC) in non-alcoholic fatty liver disease (NAFLD) patients without cirrhosis. *Hepatology International*, 10(4), 632–639.

Musso, G., Cassader, M., Rosina, F., & Gambino, R. (2012). Impact of current treatments on liver disease, glucose metabolism and cardiovascular risk in non-alcoholic fatty liver disease (NAFLD): A systematic review and meta-analysis of randomised trials. *Diabetologia*, 55(4), 885–904. doi:10.1007/s00125-011-2446-4

Musso, G., Gambino, R., Cassader, M., & Pagano, G. (2010). A meta-analysis of randomized trials for the treatment of nonalcoholic fatty liver disease. *Hepatology*, 52(1), 79–104.

Musso, G., Gambino, R., Cassader, M., & Pagano, G. (2011). Meta-analysis: Natural history of non-alcoholic fatty liver disease (NAFLD) and diagnostic accuracy of non-invasive tests for liver disease severity. *Annals of Medicine*, 43(8), 617–649.

Neuschwander-Tetri, B. A. (2020). Therapeutic landscape for NAFLD in 2020. *Gastroenterology*, 158(7), 1984–1998.e3.

Organ Procurement and Transplantation Network. Policies Available from https://optn.transplant.hrsa.gov/. Accessed November 1, 2022.

Pais, R., Sidney Barritt, A., Calmus, Y., Scatton, O., Runge, T., Lebray, P., Poynard, T., Ratziu, V., & Conti, F. (2016). NAFLD and liver transplantation: Current burden and expected challenges. *Journal of Hepatology*, 65(6), 1245–1257.

Romanowski, M. D., Parolin, M. B., Freitas, A. C. T., Piazza, M. J., Basso, J., & Urbanetz, A. A. (2015). Prevalence of non-alcoholic fatty liver disease in women with polycystic ovary syndrome and its correlation with metabolic syndrome. *Arquivos de Gastroenterologia*, 52(2), 117–123.

Sanyal, A. J., Chalasani, N., Kowdley, K. V., McCullough, A., Diehl, A. M., Bass, N. M., Neuschwander-Tetri, B. A., Lavine, J. E., Tonascia, J., Unalp, A., Van Natta, M., Clark, J., Brunt, E. M., Kleiner, D. E., Hoofnagle, J. H., & Robuck, P. R. (2010). Pioglitazone, Vitamin E, or Placebo for Nonalcoholic Steatohepatitis. *New England Journal of Medicine*, 362(18), 1675–1685.

Sasaki, A., Nitta, H., Otsuka, K., Umemura, A., Baba, S., Obuchi, T., & Wakabayashi, G. (2014). Bariatric surgery and non-alcoholic fatty liver disease: Current and potential future treatments. *Frontiers in Endocrinology*, 5, 164–164.

St George, A., Bauman, A., Johnston, A., Farrell, G., Chey, T., & George, J. (2009). Effect of a lifestyle intervention in patients with abnormal liver enzymes and metabolic risk factors. *Journal of Gastroenterology and Hepatology*, 24(3), 399–407. doi:10.1111/j.1440-1746.2008.05694.x

Younossi, Z. M., Golabi, P., de Avila, L., Paik, J. M., Srishord, M., Fukui, N., Qiu, Y., Burns, L., Afendy, A., & Nader, F. (2019). The global epidemiology of NAFLD and NASH in patients with type 2 diabetes: A systematic review and meta-analysis. *Journal of Hepatology*, 71(4), 793–801.

Younossi, Z. M., Koenig, A. B., Abdelatif, D., Fazel, Y., Henry, L., & Wymer, M. (2016). Global epidemiology of nonalcoholic fatty liver disease—meta-analytic assessment of prevalence, incidence, and outcomes. *Hepatology*, 64(1), 73–84.

Younossi, Z. M., Loomba, R., Anstee, Q. M., Rinella, M. E., Bugianesi, E., Marchesini, G., Neuschwander-Tetri, B. A., Serfaty, L., Negro, F., Caldwell, S. H., Ratziu, V., Corey, K. E., Friedman, S. L., Abdelmalek, M. F., Harrison, S. A., Sanyal, A. J., Lavine, J. E., Mathurin, P., Charlton, M. R., ... Lindor, K. (2018). Diagnostic modalities for nonalcoholic fatty liver disease, nonalcoholic steatohepatitis, and associated fibrosis. *Hepatology*, 68(1), 349–360.

CHAPTER 63

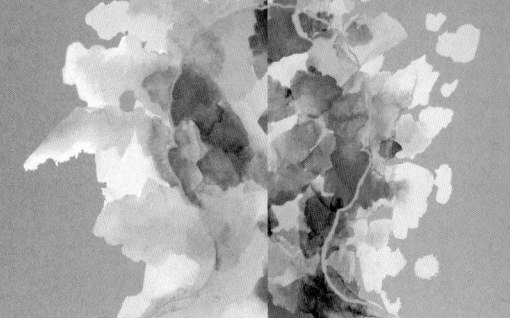

Weight

Morgan Weinert

I. Introduction and general background

Although obesity is strongly linked to diseases such as diabetes and heart disease, it is *health behaviors* that cause these diseases, not obesity itself. For example, data from the National Health and Nutrition Examination Survey (NHANES) of 1999–2004 showed that half of the patients labeled "overweight" and one-third of the patients labeled "obese" were found to be "metabolically fit" based on their measures of high-density lipoprotein (HDL) cholesterol, blood pressure, C-reactive protein (CRP), triglycerides, insulin resistance, and fasting plasma glucose. Notably, the same study showed that approximately one-quarter of patients considered "normal weight" had cardiometabolic risk factors based on the same measurements (Bombak, 2014). A more recent study looking at NHANES data used waist-to-hip ratio, lack of diabetes, and systolic blood pressure to determine "metabolic health." Using these parameters, 41% of people with classified as overweight or obese were considered "metabolically healthy" and had the same mortality risk as people of "normal weight" who were metabolically healthy (Zembic et al., 2021).

The Framingham Heart Study, key in guiding how healthcare providers approach cardiovascular disease (CVD), also demonstrates that behaviors, rather than weight alone, are responsible for poor cardiovascular health. Overweight patients who did not gain or lose weight during the study had comparable CVD risk to patients with stable "normal weight" (Pereira, 2018). This study and others underline that the behaviors that often lead to weight gain are the behaviors that should be targeted and modified for improved metabolic and cardiovascular health. In fact, many studies have shown that weight regain after intentional weight loss and weight "cycling" (the act of gaining and losing weight many times) are often more damaging than maintaining a higher weight (Montani et al., 2006). It is a disservice to our patients to reinforce the belief that increased weight is the only enemy.

Diet, exercise, mental health, and relationships all affect the health of patients, regardless of their weight. Micha et al. (2017) found that consumption of foods high in sodium, excessive intake of sugar-sweetened beverages, and low consumption of fruits and vegetables were dietary behaviors linked to cardiometabolic deaths. Cardiorespiratory fitness, as measured by peak rate of oxygen use during exercise, and postexercise heart rate recovery were better predictors of CVD risk than weight (Swainson et al., 2018). Common symptoms of anxiety and depression, such as anhedonia, social isolation, and overeating, can lead to weight gain, and the social stigma of obesity can cause or worsen these mood disorders (Simon et al., 2006). Relationships with healthcare providers as well as peers, partners, and parents affect the way our patients feel about their bodies and can lead to poor eating habits and dysphoric body image (Handford et al., 2018).

Reframing the approach to working with overweight patients is crucial in addressing the behaviors that cause ill health. As healthcare providers, it is critical that a healthy diet, regular exercise, mental health care, and healthy relationships are at the core of all the lifestyle interventions we prescribe, regardless of a patient's weight or perceived health.

A. Social determinants of health

Many factors affect a patient's ability to access healthy food and engage in physical activity. Where a person lives, their access to transportation, how close they live to an open space or a gym, job hours, and access to childcare all influence a person's ability to include regular physical activity in their life (Althoff et al., 2017). A person's access to healthy food is correlated with living near grocery stores, fewer fast-food restaurants in their neighborhood, having a higher income, and having a college education (Althoff et al., 2022). In addition to food and exercise, stress and poor sleep affect a person's weight (Lakerveld & Mackenbach, 2017). All these factors overlap to increase, or decrease, a person's ability to engage in healthy behaviors.

Poverty is a major social determinant of health that is often associated with poor access to grocery stores and reliance on fast food for ease of access and cost. In the United States, poverty disproportionately affects people of color. Additionally, people of color are more likely to receive poor health care as a result of provider ignorance or bias and have higher rates of post-traumatic stress disorder (PTSD) and depression than White people (American Psychological Association, 2017). Chronic stress, discrimination, and vigilance affect metabolism and can lead to the development of central obesity (Hicken et al., 2018). It is important to consider these complex environmental factors when discussing healthy behaviors and weight with patients. Asking about access to healthy foods, mental health, and other stressors ensures more appropriate, inclusive health education and support.

B. *Weight bias and mental health*

Advising a patient to lose weight is rarely a successful intervention and can negatively affect both the provider–patient relationship and the patient's self-esteem. Patients who are considered overweight or obese are more likely to experience healthcare-related stress and avoidance due to weight-based stigma (Mensinger et al., 2018). These same patients are also more likely to have their health concerns ignored because their provider assumes any health problems are due to their weight or because the provider carries bias against overweight and obese people. For instance, one study by Miller et al. (2018) showed that providers are more likely to judge the pain of overweight and obese patients as "less intense," "more exaggerated," and "less in need of treatment" compared with people of "normal" weight.

The internal and external stigma and bias experienced by overweight and obese people in health care, employment, education, and social relationships can lead to the development of eating disorders, depression, and poor self-image (Ciciurkaite & Perry, 2018). Studies have shown that experiencing this sort of stigma leads to increased mortality and chronic disease and often leads to increased weight gain (Tomiyama et al., 2018). Weight-based discrimination is also associated with increased suicidal ideation (Hunger et al., 2019). Societal expectations of thinness and social and familial pressures to conform to these expectations are also key factors in the development of disordered eating (Culbert et al., 2015). In fact, Giel et al. (2022) found that up to 30% of obese patients coming to their provider for help with weight loss met criteria for having binge-eating disorder. Removing blame and judgment about weight from our conversations with patients will decrease the risk of disordered eating, unhealthy weight loss, and poor self-image (Hoyt et al., 2019).

C. *Etiologies of obesity*

When looking for the etiology of a patient's weight gain, it is important to tease apart causation and association. Obesity and type 2 diabetes are often co-occurring, but the diabetes did not necessarily cause the weight gain, and vice versa. As discussed earlier, it is health behaviors that contribute to the development of diabetes, and those health behaviors often also cause weight gain.

1. Diseases that may have weight gain as a sign or symptom due to hormonal/metabolic imbalance:
   a. Hypothyroidism
   b. Cushing syndrome
   c. Hypogonadism
   d. Hypothalamic injuries
   e. Polycystic ovary syndrome (PCOS)
   f. Pseudo-hypoparathyroidism
   g. Insulinoma
2. Diseases that can co-occur with obesity:
   a. Diabetes mellitus type 2
   b. Cardiovascular disease
   c. Dyslipidemia
   d. Hypertension
   e. Sleep apnea
   f. Fertility issues
   g. Nonalcoholic fatty liver disease (NAFLD)
3. Medications that may have weight gain as a side effect (Bessesen & Perreault, 2022):
   a. Second-generation (atypical) antipsychotics (olanzapine, quetiapine, risperidone, clozapine)
   b. Antidepressants (amitriptyline, doxepin, mirtazapine, paroxetine)
   c. Antiseizure medications (gabapentin, valproate, carbamazepine)
   d. Oral contraceptives
   e. Protease inhibitors and integrase inhibitors
   f. Steroids

II. **Database**

A. *Subjective*

A thorough history is beneficial to understand why the patient may be gaining weight and also to understand what barriers may be keeping them from accessing a healthy diet, engaging in regular exercise, and establishing or maintaining emotional well-being. The history should consider the following factors.

1. Social history:
   a. Environment: Where does the patient live and work? Can they access safe spaces for recreation? Do they live near stores that sell fresh, diverse, healthy foods?
   b. Employment: Does the patient have a sedentary job or an active one? Do they have enough time in their day to exercise or cook healthy meals? Do they make enough money to afford healthy foods?
   c. Childhood and adolescence: Was the patient overweight as a child/adolescent? Did they have access to healthy food and exercise? Were they bullied/criticized due to their weight?
   d. Drugs, tobacco, and alcohol: Does the patient use any substances? Do they use these substances to suppress their appetite (stimulants, tobacco)? Do any of the drugs they use increase appetite or have excess calories (alcohol, marijuana)?
   e. Social supports: Who in the patient's life supports them in a healthy lifestyle? Who may be contributing to disordered eating or exercise habits?

2. Dietary habits: Ask the patient to recall an average day of eating. How often does the patient eat out? What do they drink most days? Do they have access to fresh fruits and vegetables? How frequently do they snack?
3. Exercise habits: How often is the patient able to get their heart rate elevated? Do they engage in sports or other recreational activities? Do they have access to outdoor space or a gym? Are there physical issues that are preventing them from regular exercise?
4. Mental health: Do they have a history of binge eating, anorexia, laxative use, and so forth? Do they have a mental illness that may be causing over- or undereating (e.g., anxiety, depression, bipolar disorder)? How is their self-esteem? What may trigger them to eat "unhealthy" foods or avoid exercise?
5. Family history: Are their family members overweight? Did anyone in the family have diabetes, hypertension, CVD, and so forth? Did their family members have disordered eating or exercise habits? What norms and values did their family have around food and weight?
6. Past medical history: History of bariatric surgeries? Gallbladder disease? Hypertension? Dyslipidemia? Diabetes or prediabetes? Infertility? NAFLD? Current medications, including those that may increase weight?
7. A review of systems can help identify signs and symptoms of underlying disease (e.g., endocrine issues) and open up conversation about how current behaviors may be affecting the patient's health. Some issues may be more common in people who are overweight, but it is critical that providers do not assume that a sign or symptom is due to a patient's weight. All patients deserve a thorough workup of their complaint, regardless of weight or health status. Issues and symptoms commonly seen in patients with higher weight that require thorough workup include:
    a. Head, eyes, ears, nose, and throat (HEENT): vision changes, dental health, snoring, difficulty swallowing
    b. Cardiac: chest pain, heart palpitations, edema
    c. Pulmonary: easily fatigued or short of breath with exertion, daytime somnolence
    d. Gastrointestinal (GI): abdominal pain, stooling frequency, stool consistency/color, reflux, flatulence, bloating
    e. Genitourinary (GU): menstrual cycle regularity and associated symptoms (dysmenorrhea, etc.); sexual health, function, and pleasure; fertility, contraception
    f. Skin: rashes (especially under the pannus, breasts), striae, dry skin, acne, easy bruising
    g. Musculoskeletal (MSK): joint pain, myalgias, decreased range of motion
    h. Neurological: dizziness, weakness, syncope or pre-syncope, sensation in extremities, seizures
    i. Endocrine: heat or cold intolerance, unwanted hair growth or hair loss
    j. Psychological: mood, suicidal ideation, self-esteem/self-image, emotional lability

B. Objective
1. A thorough, informed, and medically necessary exam should be given to all patients regardless of weight. It is inappropriate to forgo an exam for convenience or discomfort or skip a diagnostic test due to a patient's size. Similarly, do not give unnecessary exams and tests because of presumed health conditions due to someone's size. For example, the America Diabetes Association suggests testing A1c every 3 years starting at age 35 in asymptomatic adults. More frequent testing of asymptomatic people is only indicated in overweight people who also have risk factors such as a first-degree relative with diabetes, elevated HDL, or hypertension (American Diabetes Association, 2022).

    The following physical exam findings may necessitate further workup to rule out secondary causes of obesity:
    a. Hypothyroidism: cool, dry skin; hoarse voice; facial edema; thick tongue; delayed or absent deep tendon reflexes
    b. Cushing syndrome: "moon face"; dark/coarse hair on face, chest, back; central obesity; purple striae, ecchymosis
    c. Hypogonadism: short stature, lack of secondary sex characteristics, poor muscle development
    d. Pseudo-hypoparathyroidism: short stature, round face, developmental delays, joint deformity, cataracts, papilledema
2. Diagnostic testing that can give insight on health status and rule out secondary causes of obesity:
    a. Regular preventive care diagnostics: complete metabolic panel (CMP), fasting glucose, A1c, fasting lipids, sexually transmitted infection (STI) testing, Patient Health Questionnaire–9 (PHQ-9), Generalized Anxiety Disorder–7 (GAD-7)
    b. To rule out thyroid dysfunction: thyroid-stimulating hormone (TSH)
    c. To rule out asthma/chronic obstructive pulmonary disease (COPD) in someone who complains of shortness of breath: pulmonary function tests and arterial blood gases
    d. To rule out heart failure in someone who complains of edema, fatigue, or shortness of breath: echocardiogram, brain natriuretic peptide (BNP)
    e. To rule out Cushing syndrome: cortisol levels and dexamethasone suppression test
    f. To rule out hypogonadism: growth hormone, testosterone
    g. To rule out PCOS and evaluate fertility: testosterone, follicle-stimulating hormone (FSH), luteinizing hormone (LH), prolactin
    h. Metabolic syndrome (a.k.a. syndrome x or insulin resistance) is the presence of at least three of the following indicators: increased blood

pressure, increased waist circumference, elevated triglycerides, lowered HDL, and/or elevated fasting glucose (Meigs, 2021). This constellation of measurements is important to include in the physical examination of an overweight patient because studies have shown that people with metabolic syndrome are more likely to develop cardiovascular disease (International Diabetes Federation [IDF], 2006). It is important to note that obesity as measured by waist circumference (to determine if the patient has central obesity) is one of the five indicators—not weight measured with body mass index (BMI) (IDF, 2006). This again emphasizes that weight alone should not be used as evidence of increased risk for cardiovascular disease. Many social determinants of health increase a person's risk of developing metabolic syndrome, including poverty, a diet high in carbohydrates or sugar-sweetened beverages, poor cardiovascular health, and a family history of metabolic syndrome (Meigs, 2021). Health behaviors and medications that may increase the risk include cigarette smoking and second-generation antipsychotics (e.g., olanzapine, clozapine, quetiapine) (Meigs, 2021).

i. BMI and waist circumference are two common measures used to classify people as overweight or obese. Discussion of these categories of objective measurement have been intentionally omitted from this chapter due to their inaccuracies in determining health status and because data show that gender and race inequality are inherent in both measures.

BMI is a calculation of weight and height developed in 1832 by Adolphe Quetelet, the same man who developed the racist and ableist pseudoscience of anthropometry. Quetelet was a sociologist and mathematician who was committed to finding the mean of a population using measurements taken almost exclusively from White men as the "ideal." This, of course, means that the equation cannot be generalized to women or people of color. Unfortunately, BMI was adopted by the medical community in the 1970s and popularized as a way of measuring health. People of color and women are more likely to be categorized as "overweight" or "obese" when using BMI as a measure, which may lead to healthcare discrimination, stigma, and gatekeeping from procedures or treatments (Stern, 2021). Additionally, waist circumference charts are also based on studies done in predominantly White European populations (Lear et al., 2009) and may not be generalizable to other populations. Simply using a person's height and weight or waist circumference to determine their spot on the wellness bell curve does not consider other measures of health that are more relevant and based in modern science.

III. Assessment

The assessment of a patient's weight should always be firmly centered on the patient's goals, with nonjudgmental, compassionate conversation about potential health issues uncovered during the visit. If secondary causes of weight gain have been ruled out, the patient should be asked to guide the plan of care. If a patient does not bring up a desire to lose weight, it should not be assumed that it is their goal. Was the only "abnormality" uncovered during the visit that the patient is overweight, but all other health indicators are within normal limits? If so, there is no indication to lecture the patient on weight loss. The clinician's role is to ensure the patient's preventive care needs have been met and that they have the information they need to continue living a healthy life.

If a patient has a health condition that has a high risk for worsening or developing harmful consequences (e.g., prediabetes or dyslipidemia), it is important to have an honest, but nonshaming, conversation with the patient that does not center on weight loss as the only solution to achieving health. Eating more whole foods, more fiber, less saturated fat, and less sugar and getting more exercise should be health behaviors that we encourage all patients to strive for—not just those who are overweight. Does the patient have joint pain? It may be that excess weight is causing more stress on the patient's joints, but simply telling the patient to "exercise more" when they are in pain is only going to erode the patient–provider relationship. Ask the patient what their movement goals are and develop a plan of care that brings them to comfortable functionality in an achievable manner.

Utilize motivational interviewing to uncover the patient's goals and any barriers that may be preventing forward movement. If the patient is interested in eating more vegetables, for example, ask open-ended questions about why they want to eat more vegetables, how they plan on getting more vegetables into their diet, when they plan on starting to eat more vegetables, and what sorts of vegetables they think they'd be most excited about eating. This will help turn a vague goal ("eating more vegetables") into a robust goal that considers the patient's strengths. Help the patient to identify potential barriers to their goal, with the result of a specific, measurable, attainable, relevant, time-based (SMART) goal: "For the next 3 months, I will start adding frozen vegetables into at least two of the meals I cook at home each week since they're affordable and don't take a lot of prep."

Care based in the harm-reduction paradigm will honor the patient's choices while continuing to support them in making the healthiest choices possible. For example, a patient who is unwilling to start a medication for high blood pressure after education on the risks of untreated hypertension may be willing to change other behaviors. They may be open to discussing some other behaviors shown to reduce blood pressure, such as reducing or quitting smoking or caffeine consumption, managing stress, or increasing physical activity, and brainstorming ways that they can feel empowered to achieve these nonmedication interventions.

If the patient sees the clinician supporting their autonomy and actively meeting them where they're at, they will be more likely to continue to stay engaged in your care.

IV. Plan

A key piece of primary care for all patients is providing resources and tools for healthy eating, regular physical activity, healthy relationships, and improving mental health. Providers also play an important role in steering patients away from ineffective and potentially dangerous weight-loss and exercise fads, as well as identifying and addressing eating disorders, especially when patients inquire about weight loss.

Certain indications have evidence for focusing on weight loss for improved health outcomes. For instance, a reduction of 5%–10% of body weight has been shown to improve fatty liver disease (Chalasani et al., 2018), and an 11-pound weight loss has been shown to alleviate symptomatic knee osteoarthritis by 50% (Shahid et al., 2022). It is also necessary to inform patients when weight gain or loss can be indicative of an underlying health problem, such as thyroid disorders or other metabolic issues. When patients have requested help in losing weight, the provider should provide information about evidence-based, safe weight-loss interventions. Many advertised programs and diets have very little (if any) evidence to support long-term weight loss and maintenance over time. In fact, it is the norm for people in these programs to lose weight quickly and then gain much of that weight back (if not more) in the months and years that follow (Rothblum, 2018). Discussing the risks and benefits of interventions and performing a thorough informed consent for interventions that may have serious side effects are critical to ethical practice and protecting the health of patients.

V. Management

A. Healthy foods

Many patients benefit from basic nutrition education, such as how to read a nutrition panel, and the different ways that macronutrients affect the body. Connecting patients with a registered dietician (RD) can help patients learn about healthy food choices, appropriate portions, and how to identify high-calorie foods such as sugar-sweetened beverages. If access to an RD is limited, supplement basic education during the visit with resources such as ChooseMyPlate.gov. This U.S. Department of Agriculture–sponsored website offers basic nutritional education in different languages and provides patients with tools to make healthier dietary choices. When counseling patients on food, it is important to assess their access to fresh and healthy foods. If patients report food insecurity, it may be appropriate to provide a referral to social work to find food shelves nearby or facilitate enrollment in programs such as the Supplemental Nutrition Assistance Program (SNAP).

B. Diets

Helping patients find a diet that is healthy and fits with their lifestyle is one way to encourage sustainable healthy changes instead of "quick fixes." There are many diets advertised to patients, but these show little difference in outcomes (Johnston et al., 2014). Low-carbohydrate diets, low-fat diets, fasting diets, and more all lead to weight loss due to caloric restriction, or "calories in, calories out." Weight loss occurs when eating fewer calories than are needed to support that day's activities (Johnston et al., 2014).

Patients provided information about caloric restriction should be encouraged to target a daily caloric intake goal that is reasonable, healthy, and maintainable in the long term. The diet should be varied to ensure appropriate intake of macro- and micronutrients and should consist mainly of healthy, minimally processed ingredients. To calculate a patient's basal metabolic rate (BMR), use the Mifflin–St. Jeor or Harris–Benedict equations, which are easily available in many online calculators (e.g., http://www.bmrcalculator.org). These equations use age, sex, weight, and height to estimate how many calories are essential for basic bodily function. Patients who restrict their daily calories below this number risk fatigue, hair loss, infertility, and other metabolic complications. It is critical to counsel patients to eat enough to support their basic caloric needs, as well as to compensate for any physical activity they engage in throughout the day. For instance, if a patient's BMR is 1,800 calories and they are moderately active, they will need to eat about 2,700 calories to maintain their weight, and they would need to eat about 2,200 calories to lose approximately 1 pound per week of body weight. There are many online calculators available to estimate these numbers. Patients should be counseled that it is not recommended to lose more than 1–2 pounds per week on average (Centers for Disease Control and Prevention [CDC], 2022).

The Mediterranean diet and the Dietary Approaches to Stop Hypertension (DASH) diet are two evidence-based dietary interventions that show demonstrable reduction in CVD. The Mediterranean diet helps improve patients' triglycerides, whereas the DASH diet works to lower blood pressure. The DASH diet encourages patients to focus on foods that are low in fat and sodium and high in potassium, magnesium, calcium, fiber, and protein (National Heart, Lung, and Blood Institute [NHLBI], 2021). The Mediterranean diet encourages eating more plant-based foods and whole grains and limiting meats other than seafood, which is encouraged to be eaten weekly (Mayo Clinic, 2021). Both diets stress that highly processed foods and foods with added sugars or salt should be eaten rarely. These are both diets that highlight how foods can support overall health, rather than focusing on weight loss alone.

Fad diets are prolific and are rarely supported by any evidence that they are effective in substantial weight loss or maintenance. These sorts of diets advertise fast and significant weight loss through products or programs that often require membership or frequent purchases. It is important to remember that the weight-loss industry is worth billions of dollars—these fad diets can't be too successful, or they'd go out of business! More importantly, many of these diets encourage unhealthy behaviors like severe calorie restriction, "cleanses," and supplementing fresh foods with bars and shakes. Even popular diet concepts like "low carb" or "high protein" carry very little evidence for efficacy and long-term success (Perreault & Delahanty, 2021).

C. *Regular physical activity*

Ideally, patients should do an activity that increases their heart rate for about 30 minutes a day, 5 days a week for cardiovascular health (CDC, 2022). For bone health, it's also important to do muscle-strengthening activities 2 days a week (CDC, 2022). Talking to patients about what sort of activity they enjoy may increase the odds that they will participate. Patients may benefit from being reminded that physical activity doesn't have to take place in a gym. Walking around the neighborhood, cleaning the house, playing outside with kids, gardening, and engaging in recreational sports are all good options for meeting physical activity recommendations. Providers may also reassure patients that the recommended 30 minutes of exercise can be divided into shorter chunks throughout the day. Providers may also recommend local programs at community centers that may offer low-income memberships for gym access or aerobics classes. Many insurance plans also offer discounts to gyms for patients who want to get a membership.

D. *Mental health and therapeutic interventions*

Cognitive–behavioral therapy (CBT) is a widely accepted psychotherapeutic intervention to help people lose weight. CBT can be done in individual or group therapy and is considered the "gold standard" of therapeutic interventions for weight loss. Many studies show that it is helpful in reducing weight and improving quality of life overall for patients (dos Santos Moraes et al., 2021). Acceptance-based therapies, such as acceptance and commitment therapy (ACT), and dialectical behavior therapy (DBT) also show success in helping patients lose weight and successfully maintain their weight loss. These sorts of therapies seem to be more efficacious for people who struggle with emotional eating or have not had success with other interventions (Niemeier et al., 2012). Hypnosis and mindfulness are emerging as popular additions to more traditional therapies and may be useful when combined with other weight-loss interventions (Pellegrini et al., 2021).

Although there is no formal recommendation for routine screening for eating disorders, providers should be aware of signs and symptoms of these disorders, including rapid weight loss or weight gain, amenorrhea, and bradycardia (U.S. Preventive Services Task Force [USPSTF], 2022). Overweight people are consistently underdiagnosed and undertreated for eating disorders, so it is important to assess appropriately when red flags for disordered eating are seen (Ralph, 2022). Screening tools for eating disorders include the Eating Disorder Screen for Primary Care (EDS-PC) and Screen for Disordered Eating (USPSTF, 2022).

E. *Medication management*

Many medications have been marketed to help patients lose weight, and when combined with lifestyle interventions, these can result in weight loss of 4%–8% (Perreault, 2022). The following are medications that are commonly suggested when medication management is desired or indicated for weight loss. If a weight-loss medication is initiated, counsel the patient that outcomes are better with regular exercise and a healthy diet (Shi et al., 2022). It is important to note that all these medications are contraindicated for use in pregnant people.

1. The glucagon-like peptide-1 (GLP-1) agonists liraglutide and semaglutide are some of the newer medications that have shown some efficacy in weight loss and target CVD and diabetes and are now considered first line as a weight-loss drug (Perreault, 2022). Both medications are administered subcutaneously: liraglutide daily, semaglutide weekly. One systemic review and meta-analysis showed that semaglutide dosed at 2.4 mg/week has better outcomes and fewer side effects when compared with other weight-loss drugs (Shi et al., 2022). The most common side effects of GLP-1 agonists are nausea, diarrhea, and vomiting. They are contraindicated for use in people who have a personal history of pancreatitis and in people who have had certain cancers (Perreault, 2022).

2. Phentermine-topiramate is a pill dosed once daily and is one of the most efficacious medications for weight lowering (Shi et al., 2022). Side effects are anticholinergic in nature and can also include mood and cognitive issues (Perreault, 2022). A systemic review and meta-analysis showed that phentermine-topiramate results in more adverse effects than other weight-loss drugs (Shi et al., 2022). It is contraindicated in people with a history of kidney stones and those with glaucoma, cardiovascular disease, or hyperthyroidism (Perreault, 2022). Phentermine has also commonly been prescribed as a stand-alone agent for weight loss (Perreault, 2022).

3. Orlistat is a pill taken three times a day that increases the amount of fat excreted through stool. In addition to weight loss, it also improves low-density lipoprotein (LDL) cholesterol (Shi et al., 2022). Orlistat's side effects are not serious but may be very embarrassing for patients and lead to discontinuation. They include flatus and fecal incontinence (Perreault, 2022). Most of these side effects can be minimized by maintaining a low-fat diet. This pill can cause renal and liver issues in some people and should not be used in people who have preexisting absorption issues or in patients with gallbladder or kidney stones (Perreault, 2022). In one review,

Orlistat was no more efficacious than lifestyle change alone (Shi et al., 2022).
4. Bupropion is commonly used off-label to help reduce appetite and has been approved by the U.S. Food and Drug Administration (FDA) in combination with naltrexone as a weight-loss aid. Headache, insomnia, dizziness, and constipation are common side effects with bupropion-naltrexone (Perreault, 2022). This medication is contraindicated in people who use opioids or buprenorphine, have a seizure disorder, or have hepatic dysfunction (Perreault, 2022). This medication is also contraindicated in people with cardiac issues because it can increase heart rate and blood pressure (Perreault, 2022).
5. Phentermine, diethylpropion, benzphetamine, and phendimetrazine are scheduled medications approved for short-term (less than or equal to 12 weeks total) use as weight-loss aids, but they should be used with extreme caution because of the risk of abuse, anticholinergic side effects, and increase in heart rate and blood pressure (Perreault, 2022). They should not be used in people with existing heart disease or hyperthyroidism. Lorcaserin, sibutramine, ephedrine, and phenylpropanolamine have all been removed from the market due to significant adverse events (Perreault, 2022).
6. It is important to counsel patients that over-the-counter weight-loss supplements and pills are neither efficacious nor regulated and can be dangerous.

F. *Bariatric surgeries*

Bariatric surgeries gained popularity in the mid-1990s as a way to lose a significant amount of weight in a short period of time (Faria, 2017). Between 1993 and 2016, 2 million patients received bariatric surgery, and the number of surgeries performed continues to increase every year (Lim, 2022). Over a quarter of a million bariatric surgeries were performed in the United States in 2019 alone (American Society for Metabolic and Bariatric Surgery, 2018). Initially, the practice guidelines for recommendation of bariatric surgery were very strict: Patients with obesity were first directed to implement exercise and lifestyle management with professionals in these fields, robust informed consent was required, and lifelong follow-up was maintained. Patients were required to be evaluated by a multidisciplinary team to review appropriateness for the surgery, and the surgeries were reserved for people considered "morbidly obese" (BMI >40) or people with a BMI of >35 at high risk of complications from comorbid conditions (Hubbard & Hall, 1991). As the surgeries have gained popularity, the guidelines have relaxed, and now patients with a BMI of >30 are considered candidates regardless of comorbidities. Additionally, the guidelines now indicate that failure of unsupervised diets is sufficient instead of required formal intervention from nutritionists and so forth (Burguera et al., 2007). This has resulted in more patients being directed to bariatric surgery as a "first-line" intervention for weight loss before other nonsurgical methods. Although bariatric surgeries are invasive procedures that should only be undertaken after thorough informed consent and trial of other methods, it is important to note that weight-loss surgery does have more sustained weight loss and remission of type 2 diabetes than other interventions (Iqbal et al., 2021).

There are four types of bariatric surgeries: Roux-en-Y and sleeve gastrectomy are the most common types, but adjustable gastric banding and biliopancreatic diversion surgeries are also routinely performed (Courcoulas et al., 2020). Single-anastomosis duodeno-ileal bypass with sleeve gastrectomy and intragastric balloon surgeries are both newer options that will not be discussed here. All of the interventions reduce the amount of calories taken into the body by either reducing the size of the stomach (sleeve gastrectomy, gastric banding, intragastric balloon) and/or routing the stomach to bypass parts of the GI tract (Roux-en-Y, biliopancreatic diversion, single-anastomosis duodeno-ileal bypass). Roux-en-Y surgeries are associated with the largest amount of weight loss but are also more commonly associated with a greater need for revision, intervention, and hospitalization compared with sleeve gastrectomy (Courcoulas et al., 2020). Gastric banding is associated with a slower rate of weight loss and higher rate of weight regain (Courcoulas et al., 2020). Biliopancreatic diversion is associated with stomach ulceration, protein malnutrition, anemia, and surgical complications, so is not a recommended first-line surgery (Telem et al., 2022).

Primary care providers should be comfortable with the management of patients who have undergone a gastric bypass surgery. All bariatric surgeries cause long-term malabsorption that must be assessed with lab monitoring at 3, 6, and 12 months after surgery and annually thereafter (Kushner et al., 2021). Common deficiencies are calcium, iron, selenium, copper, zinc, vitamin A, vitamin B_{12}, thiamine, vitamin C, vitamin D, folate, vitamin E, and vitamin K (Kushner et al., 2021). Physical exam and review of systems should assess for hair loss, memory issues, vision changes, confusion, stomatitis, weakness, neuropathy, impaired wound healing, and more (Kushner et al., 2021).

Bariatric surgeries can also affect the absorption of some medications (Lim, 2022). Before prescribing new medications, make sure they are compatible with the patient's surgical intervention. Patients who did not receive adequate counseling before surgery or who are complaining of stomach pain, gastroesophageal reflux disease (GERD), weight gain, and so forth may need additional support in "re-learning" how to eat with the revisions to their GI tract to avoid issues (Lim, 2022). Complications from bariatric surgeries that may be identified in primary care include ulcers, hernias, infertility, GERD, stomach rupture/leakage, metabolic complications, dumping syndrome, bone loss, secondary hyperparathyroidism, and other side effects of nutritional deficiencies (Lim, 2022).

Although bariatric surgery is an appealing intervention for many patients and providers, it is incredibly important that patients and providers are intimately familiar with the risks of surgery and the many possible complications in the long term. Patients are frequently lost to follow-up after bariatric surgery, which can result in weight regain, malnutrition, and other complications. In addition to general risks inherent with surgical procedures, studies show that these surgeries have anywhere from a 5% to 60% rate of required revision or other invasive intervention in the years following the initial surgical procedure (Courcoulas et al., 2020).

VI. Resources

A. Association for Size Diversity and Health: https://asdah.org/
B. Radical Health Alliance: https://www.radicalhealthalliance.org/
C. Health at Every Size: https://haescurriculum.com/
D. MyFitness Pal: https://www.myfitnesspal.com/
E. American Heart Association (AHA): http://www.heart.org
F. AHA "Move More" page: https://www.heart.org/en/healthy-living/fitness
G. Choose My Plate: https://www.myplate.gov
H. Supplemental Nutrition Assistance Program (SNAP): https://www.fns.usda.gov/snap/supplemental-nutrition-assistance-program
I. Dietary Guidelines for Americans: https://www.dietaryguidelines.gov/
J. CDC Physical Activity Guidelines: https://www.cdc.gov/physicalactivity/index.html
K. National Institute on Aging exercise page: https://www.nia.nih.gov/health/exercise-physical-activity

References

Althoff, T., Nilforoshan, H., Hua, J., & Leskovec, J. (2022). Large-scale diet tracking data reveal disparate associations between food environment and diet. *Nature Communications*, 13(1), 267. doi:10.1038/s41467-021-27522-y

Althoff, T., Sosic, R., Hicks, J. L., King, A. C., Delp, S. L., & Leskovec, J. (2017). Large-scale physical activity data reveals worldwide activity inequality. *Nature*, 547(7663), 336–351. doi:10.1038/nature23018

American Diabetes Association. (2022). Standards of medical care in diabetes—2022 abridged for primary care providers. *Clinical Diabetes*, 40(1), 10–38.

American Psychological Association. (2017). *Ethnic and racial minorities and socioeconomic status*. https://www.apa.org/pi/ses/resources/publications/minorities

American Society for Metabolic and Bariatric Surgery. (2018). *Estimate of bariatric surgery numbers, 2011–2018*. https://asmbs.org/resources/estimate-of-bariatric-surgery-numbers

Bessesen, D., & Perreault, L. (2022). Obesity in adults: Etiologies and risk factors. *UpToDate*. https://www.uptodate.com/contents/obesity-in-adults-etiologies-and-risk-factors

Bombak, A. (2014). Obesity, health at every size, and public health policy. *American Journal of Public Health*, 104(2), e61–e67.

Burguera, B., Arner, A. P., Baltasar, B. F., Barcelo, I. B., Breton, T. C., Casanueva, F. F., Couce, M. E., Dieguez, C., Fiol, M., Fernandez Real, J. M., Formiguera, X., Fruhbeck, G., Garcia Romero, M., Garcia Sanz, M., Ghigo, E., Gomis, R., Higa, K., Ibarra, O., ... Vila, M. (2007). Critical assessment of the current guidelines for the management and treatment of morbidly obese patients. *Journal Endocrinological Investigation*, 30(10), 844–852.

Centers for Disease Control and Prevention. (2022). *How much physical activity do adults need?* https://www.cdc.gov/physicalactivity/basics/adults/index.htm

Chalasani, N., Younossi, Z., Lavine, J. E., Charlton, M., Cusi, K., Rinella, M., Harrison, S. A., Brunt, E. M., & Sanyal, A. J. (2018). The diagnosis and management of nonalcoholic fatty liver disease: Practice guidance from the American Association for the Study of Liver Diseases. *Hepatology*, 67(1), 328–357.

Ciciurkaite, G., & Perry, B. L. (2018). Body weight, perceived weight stigma and mental health among women at the intersection of race/ethnicity and socioeconomic status: Insights from the modified labelling approach. *Sociology of Health and Illness*, 40(1), 18–37.

Courcoulas, A., Coley, Y., Clark, J.M., McBride, C.L., Cirelli, E. McTigue, K., Arterburn, D., Coleman, K. J., Wellman, R., Anau, J., Toh, S., Janning, C. D., Cook, A. J., Williams, N., Sturtevant, J. L., Horgan, C., Tavakkoli, A., & PCORnet Bariatric Study Collaborative. (2020). Interventions and operations 5 years after bariatric surgery in a cohort from the US National Patient-Centered Clinical Research Network Bariatric Study. *JAMA Surgery*, 155(3), 194–204. doi:10.1001/jamasurg.2019.5470

Culbert, K. M., Racine, S. E., & Klump, K. L. (2015). Research review: What we have learned about the causes of eating disorders—a synthesis of sociocultural, psychological, and biological research. *Journal of Child Psychology and Psychiatry*, 56(11): 1141–1164. doi:10.1111/jcpp.12441

Davies, N. (2016). Mental illness and obesity. *Psychiatry Advisor*. https://www.psychiatryadvisor.com/home/conference-highlights/aaic-2015-coverage/mental-illness-and-obesity/

Dos Santos Moraes, A., da Costa Padovani, R., La Scala Teixeira, C. V., Soria Cuesta, M. G., dos Santos Gil, S., de Paula, B., dos Santos, G. M., Goncalves, R. T., Damaso, A. R., Oyama, L. M., Gomes, R. J., & Caranti, D. A. (2021). Cognitive behavioral approach to treat obesity: A randomized clinical trial. *Frontiers in Nutrition*, 8, 611217. doi:10.3389/fnut.2021.611217

Faria, G. R. (2017). A brief history of bariatric surgery. *Porto Biomedical Journal*, 2(3), 90–92.

Giel, K. E., Bulik, C. M., Fernandez-Aranda, F., Hay, P., Keski-Rahkonen, A., Schag, K., Schmidt, U., & Zipfel, S. (2022). Binge eating disorder. *Nature Reviews Disease Primers*, 8(1), 16. doi:10.1038/s41572-022-00344-y

Handford, C. M., Rapee, R. M., & Fardouly, J. (2018). The influence of maternal modeling on body image concerns and eating disturbances in preadolescent girls. *Behaviour Research and Therapy*, 100, 17–23. doi:10.1016/j.brat.2017.11.001

Hicken, M. T., Lee, H., & Hing, A. K. (2019). The weight of racism: Vigilance and racial inequalities in weight related measures. *Social Science & Medicine, 199*, 157–166. doi:10.1016/j.socscimed.2017.03.058

Hoyt, C. L., Burnette, J. L., Thomas, F. N., & Orvidas, K. (2019). Public health messages and weight-related beliefs: Implications for well-being and stigma. *Frontiers in Psychology, 10*, 2806. doi:10.3389/fpsyg.2019.02806

Hubbard, V. S., & Hall, W. H. (1991). National Institutes of Health consensus development conference draft statement on gastrointestinal surgery for severe obesity 25–27 March 1991. *Obesity Surgery, 1*, 257–265.

Hunger, J. M., Dodd, D. R., & Smith, A. R. Weight-based discrimination, interpersonal needs, and suicidal ideation. *Stigma and Health, 5*(2), 217–224. doi:10.1037/sah0000188

Iqbal, I., Khan, M. A. A., Tariq, S., & Slusser, J. (2021). Role of bariatric surgery in managing metabolic syndrome. *Journal of the Endocrine Society, 5*(1), A475.

Johnston, B. C., Kanters, S., & Bandayrel, K. (2014). Comparison of weight loss among named diet programs in overweight and obese adults: A meta-analysis. *JAMA, 312*(9), 923–933.

Kushner, R. F., Herron, D. M., & Herrington, H. (2021). Bariatric surgery: Postoperative nutritional management. *UpToDate.* https://www.uptodate.com/contents/bariatric-surgery-postoperative-nutritional-management

Lakerveld, J., & Mackenbach, J. (2017). The upstream determinants of adult obesity. *Obesity Facts, 10*(3), 216–222.

Lear, S. A., James, P. T., Ko, G. T., & Kumanyika, S. (2009). Appropriateness of waist circumference and waist-to-hip ratio cutoffs for different ethnic groups. *European Journal of Clinical Nutrition, 64*(1), 42–61.

Lim, R. B. (2022) Bariatric procedures for the management of severe obesity: Descriptions. *UpToDate.* https://www.uptodate.com/contents/bariatric-procedures-for-the-management-of-severe-obesity-descriptions

Mayo Clinic. (2021, July 23). *Mediterranean diet for heart health.* https://www.mayoclinic.org/healthy-lifestyle/nutrition-and-healthy-eating/in-depth/mediterranean-diet/art-20047801

Meigs, J. B. (2021). Metabolic syndrome (insulin resistance syndrome or syndrome X). *UpToDate.* https://www.uptodate.com/contents/metabolic-syndrome-insulin-resistance-syndrome-or-syndrome-x

Mensinger, J. L., Tylka, T. L., & Calamari, M. E. (2018). Mechanisms underlying weight status and healthcare avoidance in women: A study of weight stigma, body-related shame and guild, and healthcare stress. *Body Image, 25*, 139–147.

Micha, R., Penalov, J. L., Cudhea, F., Imamura, F., Rehm, C. D., & Mozaffariam, D. (2017). Association between dietary factors and mortality from heart disease, stroke, and type 2 diabetes in the United States. *JAMA, 317*(9), 912–924.

Miller, M. M., Allison, A., Trost, Z., de Ruddere, L., Whellis, T., Goubert, L., & Hirsh, A. T. (2018). Differential effect of patient weight on pain-related judgements about male and female chronic low back pain patients. *Journal of Pain, 19*(1), 57–66.

Montani, J. P., Viecelli, A., Prévot, A., & Dulloo, A. G. (2006). Weight cycling during growth and beyond as a risk factor for later cardiovascular diseases: The "repeated overshoot" theory. *International Journal of Obesity, 30*(Suppl. 4), S58–S66.

National Heart, Lung and Blood Institute. (2021, December 9). *DASH eating plan.* https://www.nhlbi.nih.gov/education/dash-eating-plan

Niemeier, H. M., Leahey, T., Reed, K. P., Brown, R. A., & Wing, R. R. (2012). An acceptance-based behavioral intervention for weight loss: A pilot study. *Behavior Therapy, 43*(2), 427–435.

Pellegrini, M., Carletto, S., Scumaci, E., Ponzo, V., Ostacoli, L., & Bo, S. (2021). The use of self-help strategies in obesity treatment. A narrative review focused on hypnosis and mindfulness. *Current Obesity Reports, 10*(3), 351–364.

Perreault, L. (2022). Obesity in adults: Drug therapy. *UpToDate.* https://www.uptodate.com/contents/obesity-in-adults-drug-therapy

Perreault, L., & Delahanty, L. M. (2021). Obesity in adults: Dietary therapy. *UpToDate.* https://www.uptodate.com/contents/obesity-in-adults-dietary-therapy

Ralph, A. F., Brennan, L., Byrne, S., Caldwell, B., Farmer, J., Hart, L. M., Heruc, G. A., Maguire, S., Piya, M. K., Quin, J., Trobe, S. K., Wallis, A., Williams-Tchen, A. J., & Hay, P. (2022). Management of eating disorders for people with higher weight: Clinical practice guideline. *Journal of Eating Disorders, 10*(1), 121.

Rothblum, E. D. (2018). Slim chance for permanent weight loss. *Archives of Scientific Psychology, 6*, 63–69.

Shahid, A., Inam-Ur-Raheem, M., Iahtisham-Ul-Haq, M., Yasir Nawaz, M., Hamdan Rashid, M., Oz, F., Proestos C., & Muhammad Aadil, R. (2022). Diet and lifestyle modifications: An update on non-pharmacological approach in the management of osteoarthritis. *Journal of Food Processing and Preservation, 46*(8). doi:10.1111/jfpp.16786

Shi, Q., Wang, Y., Hao, Q., Vandvik, O., Guyatt, G., Li, J., Chen, Z., Xu, S., Shen, Y., Ge, L., Sun, F., Li, L., Yu, J., Nong, K., Zou, X., Zhu, S., Wang, C., Zhang, S., Qiao, Z., … Li, S. (2022). Pharmacotherapy for adults with overweight and obesity: a systematic review and network meta-analysis of randomized controlled trials. *The Lancet, 399*(10321), 259–269.

Simon, G. E., Von Korff, M., Saunders, K., Miglioretti, D. L., Crane, P. K., van Belle, G., & Kessler, R. C. (2006). Association between obesity and psychiatric disorders in the U.S. adult population. *Archives of General Psychiatry, 63*(7), 824–830. doi:10.1001/archpsyc.63.7.824

Stern, C. (2021). Why BMI is a flawed health standard, especially for people of color. *Washington Post.* https://www.washingtonpost.com/lifestyle/wellness/healthy-bmi-obesity-race-/2021/05/04/655390f0-ad0d-11eb-acd3-24b44a57093a_story.html

Swainson, M. G., Ingle, L., & Carroll, S. (2018). Cardiorespiratory fitness as a predictor of short-term and lifetime estimated cardiovascular disease risk. *Scandinavian Journal of Medicine & Science in Sports, 29*, 1402–1413. doi:10.1111/sms.13468

Tomiyama, J. A., Carr, D., Granberg, E. M., Major, B., Robinson, E., Sutin, A. R., & Brewis, A. (2018). How and why weight stigma drives the obesity "epidemic" and harms health. *BMC Medicine, 16*(1), 123.

U.S. Preventive Services Task Force. (2022). Screening for eating disorders in adolescents and adults. *JAMA, 327*(11), 1061–1067.

Zembic, A., Eckel, N., Stefan, N., Baudry, J., & Schulze, M. (2021). An empirically derived definition of metabolically healthy obesity based on risk of cardiovascular and total mortality. *JAMA Network Open, 4*(5), e218505. doi:10.1001/jamanetworkopen.2021.8505

CHAPTER 64

Substance Use and Substance Use Disorders

Pierre-Cedric Crouch and Pauli Grey

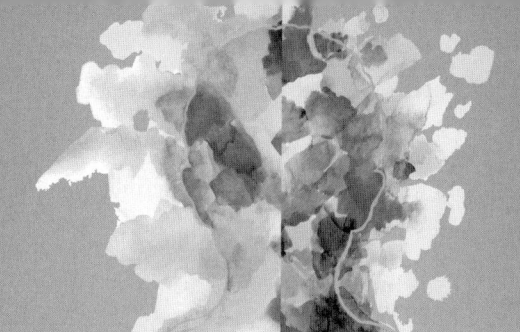

I. Introduction and general background

A. Prevalence and incidence
1. The Substance Abuse and Mental Health Services Administration (SAMHSA) conducts an annual household survey to track trends in substance use in the United States. The 2020 survey reported that 162.5 million (58.7%) people in the United States used a substance (including tobacco and alcohol) in the last 30 days, and an estimated 40.3 million people have an alcohol or drug use disorder (**Table 64-1**). While current trends cannot be established due to the COVID-19 pandemic, substance use has decreased over the years, except for cannabis (SAMHSA, 2021).
2. Overdose deaths have been increasing over the years and have been attributed to a rise in synthetic opioid use. Overdose deaths have quadrupled since 1999. Over 70% of the 70,630 overdose deaths in 2019 involved an opioid, and overdose deaths from synthetic opioids (e.g., fentanyl) increased by 15% in 2019 (National Center for Health Statistics, 2020).
3. The full repercussions of COVID-19 is not yet known, and it will take some time to fully understand the epidemic's impact on people who use substances. However, the early data suggest that overdose deaths continued to increase despite the COVID-19 pandemic. Alcohol-related deaths increased by 25% in 2020 (White et al., 2022). Opioid-related deaths increased by 38% in 2020, with a 55% increase in fentanyl-related deaths (National Institute on Drug Abuse, 2022). Racial disparities continued, with American Indian and Alaskan men and Black men having the highest rates of overdose deaths during the COVID-19 pandemic (Han et al., 2022).

B. Substance use treatment
1. There are no health specialties that are not affected by substance use disorders. Recognizing the symptoms of a substance use disorder is essential to everyone's practice. Despite some effective therapies, many people are not offered treatment and continue to suffer from a substance use disorder. In 2020, 41.1 million (14.9%) people needed treatment for substance use, yet only 4 million (1.4%) received some treatment for substance use (SAMHSA, 2021). Nurse practitioners are well placed to help identify people with substance use disorder and provide evidence-based treatment.
2. This chapter will cover opioids, stimulants, benzodiazepines, cannabis, tobacco, and alcohol. However, there are many other substances that people use.

II. Impact of stigmatizing language, language, and health disparities

A. Terminology
1. The terminology used to describe a group and the history of marginalization affects the provider's view of the patient and, most importantly, can affect the patient's view of the healthcare system. Conversations around substance use can make people feel uncomfortable. Using a substance does not mean a person has a substance use disorder. People can use substances for pleasure, with the use having no significant impact on their lives or ability to fulfill their daily responsibilities. Substance use disorders represent an treatable chronic illness. A person's decision to use substances is not a reflection of a moral failure, and it's not something one can easily stop. There is a complex path of trauma, shame, and reduced coping skills that can lead people to develop a substance use disorder. The role of the nurse practitioner is to support the patient where they are and support the patient in their goals, even if it is to continue using substances safely.

2. Words can create undue stigma, making it challenging to establish a therapeutic relationship with the patient. Stigmatizing language is disproportionately used in medical records to describe Black patients with a substance use disorder (Himmelstein et al., 2022). In another study, mental health clinicians were provided with two patient summaries. One patient was described as having a "substance use disorder," and the other patient was described as a "substance abuser." Mental health clinicians were more likely to recommend punitive measures and put the blame on the patient when "substance abuser" was used to describe a patient versus having a "substance use disorder" (Kelly & Westerhoff, 2010). This would indicate that the words used to describe a patient in a medical record can affect other providers' impressions of a patient. Overall, the general public's view of people who use substances often contains stigmatizing language and represents a negative view of people who use substances (Yang et al., 2017). These views can perpetuate stigma that can negatively influence providers and make accessing evidence-based treatments more difficult for patients (**Table 64-2**).

B. Health disparities and structural racism
   1. Health disparities and structural racism are present in substance use care and negatively affect a patient's ability to access care. Black patients are 70% less likely to receive a prescription for buprenorphine (Lagisetty et al., 2019). Women, Hispanic, and Black patients were less likely to obtain treatment after an overdose (Kilaru et al., 2020). Black patients are less likely to be enrolled in a substance use treatment center (Webb et al., 2021). Lesbian, gay, bisexual, transgender, and queer communities have higher rates of substance use disorders than the general population, attributed to discrimination and marginalization (Green & Feinstein, 2012).
   2. Substance use disorders should be treated as a public health issue and not a criminal matter to reduce stigma and improve access to care. Overdose prevention sites and safe consumption rooms decrease the use of substances in public, increase access to treatment, and prevent overdoses without increasing crime, drug use, or trafficking (Pauly et al., 2020; Potier et al., 2014). In addition, decriminalization of drugs does not affect the age of onset of drug use (Vicknasingam et al., 2018). Decriminalization in Portugal has led to a decrease in overdose deaths, a decrease in drug-related incarceration, a decrease in financial costs, and a decrease in high-risk opioid use, and it did not have an impact on

Table 64-1 Substance Use Estimates Among People in the United States Aged 12 and Over in 2020

Substance	Recent Use
Alcohol	138,500 (50%)
Tobacco	57,300 (20.7%)
Cannabis	49,600 (17.9%)
Prescription pain reliever misuse	9,300 (3.3%)
Hallucinogens	7,100 (2.6%)
Cocaine	5,200 (1.9%)
Prescription stimulant misuse	5,100 (1.8%)
Prescription benzodiazepine misuse	4,800 (1.7%)
Methamphetamine	2,500 (0.9%)
Inhalants	2,400 (0.9%)
Heroin	920 (0.3%)

Numbers listed in thousands.
Data trends not listed due to bias from COVID-19.
Data from Substance Abuse and Mental Health Services Administration. (2021). Key substance use and mental health indicators in the United States: Results from the 2020 National Survey on Drug Use and Health. https://www.samhsa.gov/data/

Table 64-2 Acceptable Terms to Use With Substance Use to Limit Stigma

Stigmatizing Term	Better Term	Rationale
Drug user, addict, alcoholic	A person who uses drugs or person who uses heroin	People are more than a diagnosis. Using person-first language keeps the focus on the person.
Drug habit	Disease or illness	A substance use disorder is a disease.
Relapsed	Return to use	A substance use disorder is a lifelong illness with periods of use and nonuse.
Clean	Nonuse	People are not dirty or clean. People are either using or not using substances.
Dirty or clean urine drug screen	Urine tested positive or negative for a substance	A urine drug screen is not dirty or clean. It's a lab test with a positive or negative result.
Drug abuse	Drug misuse	*Abuse* can have a negative connotation to it.

Table 64-3 Effects of Drugs

	Classification	Mechanism of Action	Effect
Heroin, fentanyl, oxycodone, hydromorphone	Opioid	Mu opioid receptor agonism	Euphoria, pain relief, sedation
Methamphetamine	Stimulant	Releases dopamine and prevents the reuptake of norepinephrine, serotonin, and dopamine	Euphoria, increased alertness, increased energy, tachycardia, and elevated blood pressure. Similar to cocaine but longer acting. Excess dopamine can cause psychosis.
Cocaine	Stimulant	Prevents reuptake dopamine, norepinephrine, and serotonin	Euphoria, increased alertness, increased energy, tachycardia, and elevated blood pressure. Similar to methamphetamine but shorter acting. Alcohol, when used with cocaine, creates an active metabolite, cocaethylene, which provides similar effects to cocaine but has a longer half-life than cocaine and can extend cocaine's euphoria (Jones, 2019).
Benzodiazepines	Sedative	Potentiates the gamma-aminobutyric acid (GABA) receptor, causing GABA to bind more tightly	Elevate mood, decrease anxiety, relaxation of social and personal inhibition
Tobacco	Stimulant	Nicotine receptor agonist	Mild stimulant, increased alertness, improved attention, and decreased appetite
Alcohol	Sedative	Stimulation of GABA and inhibition of glutamate	Euphoria, disinhibition, sedation, impaired memory, impaired coordination

Data from Miller, S., Fiellin, D., Rosenthal, R., & Saitz, R. (Eds.). (2019). The ASAM Principles of Addiction Medicine (6th ed.). Wolters Kluwer.

the price of drugs that would make them more accessible (European Monitoring Centre for Drugs and Drug Addiction, 2020a, 2020b; Félix & Portugal, 2017; Gonçalves et al., 2015).

III. Assessment

A. *How patients use drugs—some important considerations*
1. Substances are used in different ways, and people may use additional methods of using a substance that are not described in **Table 64-4**. It is important to ask how someone uses or may have used a substance in the past to assess risks for comorbid conditions like cellulitis, hepatitis C, or endocarditis. Some methods can be plausible ways to use but may not be routine. Fentanyl can be ingested, but this is not a common way to use fentanyl. Ingesting fentanyl may be related to a person trying to get rid of substances quickly to avoid arrest.
2. Substances may be purchased from a person illegally selling drugs, given by or stolen from friends or family, stolen from their place of work (e.g., health professionals), or even made at home with legally purchased chemicals. Drugs like heroin, fentanyl, methamphetamine, and cocaine tend to be bought by weight. The weight and potency of a substance are not standard, which makes it difficult to estimate how much a person uses or to attempt to convert their current use to a morphine equivalent for treatment. The patient's perceived dose is important to assess and helps estimate tolerance but is not used clinically otherwise.
3. Drugs may be prepacked in select volumes, or a person may purchase a specific dollar amount from someone selling as an "open bag," where the person scoops out the amount of the substance they feel is worth that dollar amount.
4. The weights are generally expressed as a fraction of a gram or ounce (Tweaker, 2020).
    a. A quarter is ¼ of a gram.
    b. A half is ½ of a gram.
    c. A sixteenth is 1/16 of an ounce (1.8 g) or may be known as a teenager.
    d. An eight is 1/8 of an ounce (3.5 g) or may be known as an 8-ball.
    e. An ounce is 28 grams.
5. Some drugs, like street-purchased benzodiazepines, are often "pressed pills" designed to look like pharmaceutically made benzodiazepines that

Table 64-4 How Drugs Are Used

Drug	Suppository or Pessary	Ingested	Snorted or Applied to Gums	Smoked	Intravenous, Intramuscular, or Subcutaneous
Heroin	■ Possible route but not common	■ Can be swallowed—less common because there is no rush feeling	■ White heroin can be crushed and snorted. ■ White heroin can be placed in a bottle with coins and shaken to pulverize. ■ It can be rubbed against the gums. ■ Tar heroin is not snorted.	■ Placed on foil and heated below. ■ Smoke is inhaled through a straw or cardboard from toilet paper to maximize smoke inhalation. ■ It can be smoked in a bulb pipe though there is a drug loss with smoke escaping from the bulb.	■ It is dissolved in water on an aluminum foil or a metal tealight candleholder. ■ Gentle heat is applied to help dissolve the drug into the water. ■ A small piece of cotton is placed in the liquid to filter insoluble particles. ■ A syringe is inserted into the cotton to pull the filtered liquid through. ■ The prepared syringe is injected into the vein, muscle, or under the skin. ■ Adding meth or cocaine to heroin will make it a "speedball" or "goofball" that helps enhance the heroin.
Fentanyl	■ Possible route but not common	■ Can be swallowed—less common because there is no rush feeling	■ It can be pulverized and snorted with a straw. ■ It can be rubbed against gums.	■ Placed on foil and heated below. ■ Smoke is inhaled through a straw or cardboard from toilet paper to maximize smoke inhalation. ■ It can be smoked in a bulb pipe, although there is a drug loss with smoke escaping from the bulb.	■ It is dissolved in water on an aluminum foil or a metal tealight candleholder. ■ Gentle heat is applied to help dissolve the drug into the water. ■ A small piece of cotton is placed in the liquid to filter insoluble particles. ■ A syringe is inserted into the cotton to pull the filtered liquid through. ■ The prepared syringe is injected into the vein, muscle, or under the skin. ■ Adding meth or cocaine to fentanyl will make it a "speedball" or "goofball" that helps enhance the fentanyl.
Oxycodone	■ Possible route but not common	■ Most often swallowed	■ It can be pulverized and snorted with a straw. ■ It can be rubbed against the gums.	■ Possible route but not common	■ It is dissolved in water on an aluminum foil or a metal tealight candleholder. ■ No heat is needed. ■ A small piece of cotton is placed in the liquid to filter insoluble particles. ■ A syringe is inserted into the cotton to pull the filtered liquid through. ■ The prepared syringe is injected into the vein, muscle, or under the skin. ■ Some tablets may have a coating, making them more difficult to dissolve.
Hydromorphone	■ Possible but not common	■ Most often swallowed	■ It can be pulverized and snorted with a straw. ■ It can be rubbed against the gums.	■ Not smoked	■ It is dissolved in water on an aluminum foil or a metal tealight candleholder. ■ No heat is needed. ■ A small piece of cotton is placed in the liquid to filter insoluble particles. ■ A syringe is inserted into the cotton to pull the filtered liquid through. ■ The prepared syringe is injected into the vein, muscle, or under the skin.

Methamphetamine	■ Dissolved in a liquid ■ Drawn up in a syringe without a needle ■ Inserted into rectum or vagina ■ More common method to enhance sexual pleasure	■ It can be swallowed or mixed into a beverage.	■ It can be pulverized and snorted with a straw. ■ It can be rubbed against gums.	■ It is smoked in a bulb or "bubble" pipe. ■ Hot railing involves heating the end of a glass straw, which is placed in a line of pulverized methamphetamine, and the resulting smoke is inhaled through the nose.	■ It is dissolved in water on aluminum foil or a metal tealight candleholder. ■ No heat is needed. ■ A small piece of cotton is placed in the liquid to filter insoluble particles. ■ A syringe is inserted into the cotton to pull the filtered liquid through. ■ The prepared syringe is injected into the vein. ■ Methamphetamine is not injected into the muscle or under the skin because it is not absorbed. ■ "Cold shake" preparation is where the drug is placed in a syringe filled with water and shaken to dissolve. This leaves some unfiltered drug particles, leading to "cotton fever" (not related to cotton), when people develop fevers, headaches, sweats, chills, muscle pain, and joint pain.
Cocaine—powder	■ Possible but not common	■ Possible but not common	■ It can be pulverized and snorted with a straw. ■ It can be rubbed against the gums.	■ It can be smoked or mixed in a tobacco cigarette.	■ It is dissolved in water on aluminum foil or a metal tealight candleholder. ■ No heat is needed. ■ A small piece of cotton is placed in the liquid to filter insoluble particles. ■ A syringe is inserted into the cotton to pull the filtered liquid through. ■ The prepared syringe is injected into the vein, muscle, or under the skin.
Cocaine—crack	■ Possible but not common	■ Possible but not common	■ It can be pulverized and snorted with a straw. ■ It can be rubbed against the gums.	■ It is smoked in glass straw pipe with metal filters. ■ Crack is cocaine mixed with baking soda to lower the melting point to allow for smoking.	■ It is mixed with citric acid or vitamin C in a 1:3 ratio with crack cocaine to dissolve in water on aluminum foil or a metal tealight candleholder. ■ No heat is needed. ■ A small piece of cotton is placed in the liquid to filter insoluble particles. ■ A syringe is inserted into the cotton to pull the filtered liquid through. ■ The prepared syringe is injected into the vein, muscle, or under the skin.
Benzodiazepines	■ Possible but not common	■ Can be swallowed—most common	■ It can be pulverized and snorted with a straw. ■ It can be rubbed against the gums.	■ It is not smoked.	■ It is not injected.

may not always contain benzodiazepines but include fentanyl or other substances that could lead to an overdose (O'Donnell et al., 2021). It is important to determine how the substances are acquired and counsel around the potential for a poisoned drug supply containing unknown substances.

IV. **Database (may include but is not limited to)**
A. *Subjective data*
   1. Evaluate substance use with the RIPTEAR framework (Yale University, n.d.).
      a. Risks of current use: Assessing risk of overdose and withdrawal. Was there a prior overdose?
      b. Initiation: At what age was each substance started?
         i. Early initiation may impact cognitive development.
      c. Patterns of use: How often, how much, which routes, who with, and where?
      d. Treatment attempts and outcome: history of residential treatment, medications, or therapy
      e. Effects of substance use: What are the good things about using substances? What purpose does it serve? What are the bad things? Has it affected your life goals and relationships?
      f. Abstinence: Describe periods of nonuse and what tools were in place that allowed them to succeed.
      g. Return to use prevention plan: Assess if the patient wants to continue using, cut down, or stop. Assess access to safer-use supplies, including naloxone, and never using alone.
   2. Medical and psychiatric history
      a. Current age
         i. Many states allow minors to access substance use treatment without parental notification. Verify current laws in your state.
      b. Current medications
         i. Assess for medications that risk misuse, sedation, or overstimulation (e.g., benzodiazepines with opioids, mixed amphetamine salts with methamphetamine).
      c. Allergies
      d. Surgeries and hospitalizations
         i. Note any upcoming surgeries, which may affect treatment options.
      e. Significant illnesses
         i. Renal disease and liver disease may affect treatment options.
         ii. Mental health diagnoses that need treatment
      f. Complications of substance use
         i. Heart failure
         ii. Endocarditis
         iii. Soft tissues infections
         iv. Osteomyelitis
         v. Abscesses
         vi. Emphysema
      g. Sexual health
         i. Type of sex the patient enjoys
         ii. Assess risk for sexually transmitted infections (STIs), including gonorrhea, chlamydia, syphilis, HIV, and trichomonas.
         iii. History of preexposure prophylaxis (PrEP) and postexposure prophylaxis for HIV
         iv. Use of substances when having sex
         v. Last menstrual period, if applicable, and the possibility of pregnancy
      h. Social history
         i. Current living situation
         ii. Food access
         iii. Source of financial support
         iv. Family and social support
         v. Family and social support views of substance use and recovery
         vi. History of violence or sexual abuse
         vii. Occupation
            a. This may restrict the ability to access methadone due to clinic opening times.
         viii. Access to safer-use supplies, including naloxone
         ix. Family history
         x. Substance use
B. *Objective data*
   1. Physical exam
      a. General: Poor hygiene may indicate a lack of resources or intoxication.
      b. Head, eyes, ears, nose, and throat (HEENT): Rhinorrhea may be indicative of opioid withdrawal.
      c. Eyes: Pupil size
         i. Dilated pupils indicative of withdrawal or stimulant intoxication
         ii. Pinpoint pupils indicative of opioid intoxication
         iii. Lateral gaze nystagmus and lateral rectus muscle paralysis may indicate Wernicke encephalopathy.
      d. Lungs: Decreased lung sounds may indicate emphysema.
      e. Skin: Goosebump flesh may indicate opioid withdrawal.
      f. Speech: May be pressured or slurred
      g. Thought process: Circumstantial or tangential when intoxicated
      h. Thought content: Auditory and visual hallucinations may indicate stimulant intoxication or alcohol withdrawal.
      i. Mood: Elevated mood may indicate intoxication with stimulants or anxious and irritable if in withdrawal.
      j. Neurological: Ataxia and encephalopathy may indicate Wernicke encephalopathy.
   2. Screening tools: Additional tools can be helpful to screen for alcohol use or assess withdrawal, but they are not required to make a diagnosis.
      a. The Alcohol Use Disorders Identification Test–Concise (Audit-C) is a brief three-question screener to assess hazardous alcohol use (Bush et al., 1998).

3. Tools to assess withdrawal
    a. Clinical Institute Withdrawal Assessment for Alcohol (CIWA): used to assess alcohol withdrawal (Sullivan et al., 1989) (**Table 64-5**)
    b. Clinical Opiate Withdrawal Scale (COWS): used to assess opioid withdrawal (Wesson & Ling, 2003) (**Table 64-6**)
    c. The Prediction of Alcohol Withdrawal Severity Scale (**Table 64-7**) can be used to help guide if a person with alcohol withdrawal can be treated as an outpatient or if the withdrawal is expected to be complicated and needs to be managed in the hospital. A score equal to or greater than 4 would indicate a need to manage withdrawal in the hospital (Maldonado et al., 2014).

4. Diagnostic tests
    a. Drug toxicology: Used to confirm the patient's history or inform them of substances they were unaware they used to prevent overdose. This is used to help guide treatment plans, not to punish or accuse patients. Verbal informed consent should be obtained when ordering a toxicology test. Be mindful of potential consequences for certain groups (e.g., pregnant individuals), which may trigger legal consequences. Each laboratory will have a different assay and capabilities to detect certain drugs. Drug detection depends on multiple factors, including the volume of substances consumed by the patient and when they last used (**Table 64-8**). Some benzodiazepines may not be

Table 64-5 Clinical Institute Withdrawal Assessment (CIWA) for Alcohol

Assessment and Questions	Scores	
NAUSEA AND VOMITING—Ask, "Do you feel sick to your stomach? Have you vomited?" Observation.	0 no nausea and no vomiting 1 mild nausea with no vomiting 2 3 4 intermittent nausea with dry heaves 5 6 7 constant nausea, frequent dry heaves, and vomiting	10-item scale with a maximum score of 67. Withdrawal treatment should be initiated with scores of 8 or more. Each item is individually assessed and scored during each assessment. Prior scores and information obtained in their history should not be used. CIWA can be observational or treatment based, where a score would trigger a specific dose of medication.
TREMOR—Arms extended and fingers spread apart. Observation.	0 no tremor 1 not visible, but can be felt fingertip to fingertip 2 3 4 moderate, with patient's arms extended 5 6 7 severe, even with arms not extended	
PAROXYSMAL SWEATS—Observation.	0 no sweat visible 1 barely perceptible sweating, palms moist 2 3 4 beads of sweat obvious on forehead 5 6 7 drenching sweats	
ANXIETY—Ask, "Do you feel nervous?" Observation.	0 no anxiety, at ease 1 mildly anxious 2 3 4 moderately anxious, or guarded, so anxiety is inferred 5 6 7 equivalent to acute panic states as seen in severe delirium or acute schizophrenic reactions	

(continues)

Table 64-5 Clinical Institute Withdrawal Assessment (CIWA) for Alcohol *(continued)*

Assessment and Questions	Scores
AGITATION—Observation.	0 normal activity 1 somewhat more than normal activity 2 3 4 moderately fidgety and restless 5 6 7 paces back and forth during most of the interview or constantly thrashes about
TACTILE DISTURBANCES—Ask, "Do you have any itching, pins-and-needles sensations, any burning, or any numbness, or do you feel bugs crawling on or under your skin?" Observation.	0 none 1 very mild itching, pins and needles, burning or numbness 2 mild itching, pins and needles, burning or numbness 3 moderate itching, pins and needles, burning or numbness 4 moderately severe hallucinations 5 severe hallucinations 6 extremely severe hallucinations 7 continuous hallucinations
AUDITORY DISTURBANCES—Ask, "Are you more aware of sounds around you? Are they harsh? Do they frighten you? Are you hearing anything that is disturbing to you? Are you hearing things you know are not there?" Observation.	0 not present 1 very mild harshness or ability to frighten 2 mild harshness or ability to frighten 3 moderate harshness or ability to frighten 4 moderately severe hallucinations 5 severe hallucinations 6 extremely severe hallucinations 7 continuous hallucinations
VISUAL DISTURBANCES—Ask, "Does the light appear to be too bright? Is its color different? Does it hurt your eyes? Are you seeing anything that is disturbing to you? Are you seeing things you know are not there?" Observation.	0 not present 1 very mild sensitivity 2 mild sensitivity 3 moderate sensitivity 4 moderately severe hallucinations 5 severe hallucinations 6 extremely severe hallucinations 7 continuous hallucinations
HEADACHE, FULLNESS IN HEAD—Ask, "Does your head feel different? Does it feel like there is a band around your head?" Do not rate for dizziness or lightheadedness. Otherwise, rate severity.	0 not present 1 very mild 2 mild 3 moderate 4 moderately severe 5 severe 6 very severe 7 extremely severe
ORIENTATION AND CLOUDING OF SENSORIUM—Ask, "What day is this? Where are you? Who am I?"	0 oriented and can do serial additions 1 cannot do serial additions or is uncertain about date 2 disoriented for date by no more than 2 calendar days 3 disoriented for date by more than 2 calendar days 4 disoriented for place/or person

Sullivan, J T et al. "Assessment of alcohol withdrawal: the revised clinical substitute withdrawal assessment for alcohol scale (CIWA-Ar)." British journal of addiction vol. 84,11 (1989): 1353–7. doi:10.1111/j.1360-0443.1989.tb00737.x

Table 64-6 Clinical Opiate Withdrawal Scale

Assessment and Observations	Scored Answers	Notes
Resting pulse rate (record beats per minute): measured after patient is sitting or lying for 1 minute	0 pulse rate 80 or below 1 pulse rate 81–100 2 pulse rate 101–120 4 pulse rate greater than 120	11-item assessment of withdrawal Scoring: 5–12 mild withdrawal 13–24 moderate withdrawal 25–36 moderately severe withdrawal Greater than 36 is severe withdrawal. It is used to assess withdrawal to initiate buprenorphine. The best practice is to ensure the inclusion of 2 or more objective assessments when starting buprenorphine to minimize subjective overrating.
Sweating: over past 1/2 hour not accounted for by room temperature or patient activity	0 no report of chills or flushing 1 subjective report of chills or flushing 2 flushed or observable moistness on face 3 beads of sweat on brow or face 4 sweat streaming off face	
Restlessness: observation during assessment	0 able to sit still 1 reports difficulty sitting still but is able to do so 3 frequent shifting or extraneous movements of legs/arms 5 Unable to sit still for more than a few seconds	
Pupil size	0 pupils pinned or normal size for room light 1 pupils possibly larger than normal for room light 2 pupils moderately dilated 5 pupils so dilated that only the rim of the iris is visible	
Bone or joint aches: If patient was having pain previously, only the additional component attributed to opiate withdrawal is scored.	0 not present 1 mild diffuse discomfort 2 patient reports severe diffuse aching of joints/muscles 4 patient is rubbing joints or muscles and is unable to sit still because of discomfort	
Runny nose or tearing: not accounted for by cold symptoms or allergies	0 not present 1 nasal stuffiness or unusually moist eyes 2 nose running or tearing 4 nose constantly running or tears streaming down cheeks	
Gastrointestinal (GI) upset over last 30 minutes	0 no GI symptoms 1 stomach cramps 2 nausea or loose stool 3 vomiting or diarrhea 5 multiple episodes of diarrhea or vomiting	
Tremor: observation of outstretched hands	0 no tremor 1 tremor can be felt, but not observed 2 slight tremor observable 4 gross tremor or muscle twitching	
Yawning: observation during assessment	0 no yawning 1 yawning once or twice during assessment 2 yawning three or more times during assessment 4 yawning several times a minute	

(continues)

Table 64-6 Clinical Opiate Withdrawal Scale (continued)

Assessment and Observations	Scored Answers	Notes
Anxiety or irritability	0 none 1 patient reports increasing irritability or anxiousness 2 patient is obviously irritable or anxious 4 patient is so irritable or anxious that participation in the assessment is difficult	
Gooseflesh skin	0 skin is smooth 3 piloerection of skin can be felt or hairs standing up on arms 5 prominent piloerection	

Reproduced from Wesson, D. R., & Ling, W. (2003). The Clinical Opiate Withdrawal Scale (COWS). Journal of Psychoactive Drugs, 35(2), 253–259. https://doi.org/10.1080/02791072.2003.10400007

Table 64-7 Prediction of Alcohol Withdrawal Severity Scale

Part A: Threshold criteria	
Have you consumed any amount of alcohol (i.e., been drinking) within the last 30 days? OR did the patient have a "+" blood alcohol level (BAL) on admission?	Y or N, no point If the answer to either is YES, proceed with test:
Part B: Based on patient interview	**1 point each**
Have you been recently intoxicated/drunk within the last 30 days?	
Have you ever undergone alcohol use disorder rehabilitation treatment or treatment for alcoholism (i.e., inpatient or outpatient treatment programs or AA attendance)?	
Have you ever experienced any previous episodes of alcohol withdrawal, regardless of severity?	
Have you ever experienced blackouts?	
Have you ever experienced alcohol withdrawal seizures?	
Have you ever experienced delirium tremens or DTs?	
Have you combined alcohol with other "downers," like benzodiazepines or barbiturates, during the last 90 days?	
Have you combined alcohol with any other substances of abuse during the last 90 days?	
Part C: Based on clinical evidence	**1 point each**
Was the patient's BAL on presentation >200?	
Is there evidence of increased autonomic activity (e.g., heart rate > 120 bpm, tremor, sweating, agitation, nausea)?	
Notes: Maximum score = 10. This instrument is intended as a SCREENING TOOL. The greater the number of positive findings, the higher the risk for the development of alcohol withdrawal syndrome (AWS). A score of ≥4 suggests HIGH RISK for moderate to severe (complicated) AWS; prophylaxis and/or treatment may be indicated.	Total Score:

Reproduced from Maldonado, J. R., Sher, Y., Ashouri, J. F., Hills-Evans, K., Swendsen, H., Lolak, S., & Miller, A. C. (2014). The "Prediction of Alcohol Withdrawal Severity Scale" (PAWSS): Systematic literature review and pilot study of a new scale for the prediction of complicated alcohol withdrawal syndrome. Alcohol (Fayetteville, N.Y.), 48(4), 375–390. https://doi.org/10.1016/J.ALCOHOL.2014.01.004

Table 64-8 Drug Detection Times

Drug	Detection Time
Amphetamine	3 days
Benzodiazepine	7 days
Barbiturates	4 days for short-acting and 14 days for long-acting
Cannabis	7 days for light use and 27 days for heavy use
Cocaine	3 days for light use and 22 days for heavy use
Opioids	3 days
LSD	5 days
Phencyclidine	7 days single dose and 21 days for chronic use

Data from Miller, S., Fiellin, D., Rosenthal, R., & Saitz, R. (Eds.). (2019). The ASAM Principles of Addiction Medicine (6th ed.). Wolters Kluwer.

Table 64-9 Causes of False-Positive Tests

Drug	False-Positive Trigger
Opiates	Poppy seeds, quinolones, rifampin
Methadone	Diphenhydramine, verapamil, quetiapine, promethazine, thioridazine
Buprenorphine	Tramadol
Cocaine	Coca-leaf tea, anesthetics containing cocaine
Amphetamines	Pseudoephedrine, bupropion, ranitidine, phenylpropanolamine, amantadine, desipramine, trazodone, chlorpromazine, selegiline, phentermine, benzphetamine, fluoxetine
Phencyclidine	Dextromethorphan, diphenhydramine, tramadol, venlafaxine
Cannabinoids	Dronabinol, efavirenz
Benzodiazepine	Sertraline

Reproduced from Moeller, K. E., Lee, K. C., & Kissack, J. C. (2008). Urine drug screening: Practical guide for clinicians. Mayo Clinic Proceedings, 83(1), 66–76. https://doi.org/10.4065/83.1.66

detected in a benzodiazepine test. Call the laboratory to confirm the detected medications. Urine is the most common substance tested, but blood, hair, saliva, and sweat can be used.
    i. Two methods of detection (Miller et al., 2019)
       a. Urine immunoassay
          i. Least expensive
          ii. It can be rapid and at the point of care.
          iii. Sensitivity and specificity may miss drugs or have false-positive results (**Table 64-9**).
       b. Mass spectrometry
          i. More costly
          ii. Done in a lab
          iii. Used to confirm an immunoassay if a valid result is needed
          iv. Medications may trigger false-positive results on a urine drug immunoassay.
       b. Blood alcohol level
          i. Indicator of recent intoxication
          ii. ≥200 increases the risk of severe withdrawal
       c. Liver enzymes
          i. Aspartate transaminase (AST) and alanine transaminase (ALT) may be elevated from substance use
          ii. An AST-to-ALT ratio of 2:1 may be indicative of alcohol use.

d. Renal function
   i. Used to assess the need for renal dosing of medications
e. Prothrombin time (PT)/international normalized ratio (INR)
   i. Used to evaluate liver health
f. Urine pregnancy test

V. Goals of clinical management
A. *Establish a trusting relationship so that the patient feels safe to return, no matter the outcomes.*
B. *Manage immediate withdrawal symptoms.*
   1. Benzodiazepine and ethyl alcohol or ethanol (ETOH) withdrawal can cause seizures and are most crucial to manage.
C. *Assess if the patient has a use disorder versus substance use.*
D. *Develop a multimodal patient-centered plan for treatment with a combination of medications and/or therapy.*

VI. Assessment
A. *The initial assessment determines whether the patient is experiencing withdrawal and the safest setting for the patient to be treated. Alcohol and benzodiazepine withdrawal can cause seizures and require special attention. Opioid, stimulant, tobacco, and cannabis withdrawal are not generally life-threatening and can be managed on an outpatient basis. Once the withdrawal is addressed, patients should be assessed for a substance use disorder and have an appropriate treatment plan.*
B. *Substance withdrawal is diagnosed using the criteria in the* **Diagnostic and Statistical Manual of Mental Disorders, 5th edition** *(American Psychiatric Association, 2013).*
   1. Alcohol withdrawal
      a. Cessation of alcohol use that has been heavy and prolonged
      b. Two or more of the following developing within several hours to a few days after the cessation of alcohol:
         i. Autonomic hyperactivity
         ii. Increased hand tremor
         iii. Insomnia
         iv. Nausea or vomiting
         v. Transient visual, tactile, or auditory hallucinations or illusions
         vi. Psychomotor agitation
         vii. Anxiety
         viii. Generalized tonic-clonic seizures
      c. Specifier: With perceptual disturbances
   2. Opioid withdrawal
      a. Cessation of opioid use that has been heavy and prolonged or administration of an opioid antagonist after a period of opioid use
      b. Three or more of the following developing in minutes to several days:
         i. Dysphoric mood
         ii. Nausea or vomiting
         iii. Muscle aches
         iv. Lacrimation or rhinorrhea
         v. Pupillary dilation, piloerection, or sweating
         vi. Diarrhea
         vii. Yawning
         viii. Fever
         ix. Insomnia
   3. Stimulant withdrawal
      a. Cessation of or reduction in prolonged amphetamine-type substance, cocaine, or other stimulant use
      b. Dysphoric mood and two or more of the following physiological changes, developing within a few hours to several days
         i. Fatigue
         ii. Vivid, unpleasant dreams
         iii. Insomnia or hypersomnia
         iv. Increased appetite
         v. Psychomotor retardation or agitation
   4. Tobacco withdrawal
      a. Daily use of tobacco for at least several weeks
      b. Abrupt cessation of tobacco use, or reduction in the amount of tobacco use, followed within 24 hours by four or more of the following:
         i. Irritability, frustration, or anger
         ii. Anxiety
         iii. Difficulty concentrating
         iv. Increased appetite
         v. Restlessness
         vi. Depressed mood
         vii. Insomnia
   5. Sedative, hypnotic, or anxiolytic withdrawal
      a. Cessation or reduction in sedative, hypnotic, or anxiolytic use that has been prolonged
      b. Two or more of the following, developing within several hours to a few days after the cessation of or reduction in sedative, hypnotic, or anxiolytic use:
         i. Autonomic hyperactivity
         ii. Hand tremor
         iii. Insomnia
         iv. Nausea or vomiting
         v. Transient visual, tactile, or auditory hallucinations or illusions
         vi. Psychomotor agitation
         vii. Anxiety
         viii. Grand mal seizures
      c. Specifier: With perceptual disturbances
   6. Cannabis withdrawal
      a. Cessation of cannabis use that has been heavy and prolonged
      b. Three or more of the following signs and symptoms developing within 1 week:
         i. Irritability, anger, or aggression
         ii. Nervousness or anxiety
         iii. Sleep difficulty
         iv. Decreased appetite or weight loss
         v. Restlessness
         vi. Depressed mood

vii. At least one of the following physical symptoms causing significant discomfort: abdominal pain, shakiness/tremors, sweating, fever, chills, or headache
C. *The diagnosis of a substance use disorder is based on criteria in the* **Diagnostic and Statistical Manual of Mental Disorders, 5th edition** *(American Psychiatric Association, 2013) and is based on the substance used. A person can have multiple substance use disorder diagnoses if different substances are used from different categories, such as methamphetamine and fentanyl, or a single diagnosis if all the substances used are in the same category, such as methamphetamine and cocaine. The specific substance can be listed in parentheses—for example, "Opioid use disorder (fentanyl)." Polysubstance use disorder is not a diagnosis and should not be used because it is not specific and can be stigmatizing.*
  1. Each use disorder corresponds to a specific substance.
     a. Opioid use disorder (fentanyl, heroin, oxycodone)
     b. Stimulant use disorder (methamphetamine, amphetamine, cocaine)
     c. Alcohol use disorder (alcohol)
     d. Cannabis use disorder (cannabis)
     e. Sedative, hypnotic, or anxiolytic use disorder (benzodiazepine)
     f. Tobacco use disorder (cigarettes, cigars, chewing tobacco, nicotine vaping)
  2. The criteria are based on the person's relationship to a substance.
  3. The quantity and frequency of substance use do not factor into a diagnosis.
  4. The criteria involve impaired control, social problems, risky use, or physical dependence.
     a. Impaired control
        i. The substance is often taken in larger amounts or over a longer period than was intended.
        ii. There is a persistent desire or unsuccessful efforts to cut down or control substance use.
     b. Social problems
        i. A great deal of time is spent in activities necessary to obtain the stimulant, use the stimulant, or recover from its effects.
        ii. Recurrent stimulant use resulting in a failure to fulfill major role obligations at work, school, or home
        iii. Continued stimulant use despite having persistent or recurrent social or interpersonal problems caused or exacerbated by the effects of the stimulant
        iv. Important social, occupational, or recreational activities are given up or reduced because of stimulant use.
     c. Risky use
        i. Recurrent stimulant use in situations in which it is physically hazardous
        ii. Stimulant use is continued despite knowledge of having a persistent or recurrent physical or psychological problem that is likely to have been caused or exacerbated by the stimulant.
     d. Physical dependence
        i. A strong desire or urge to use the stimulant (cravings)
        ii. Tolerance, as defined by either of the following:
           a. A need for markedly increased amounts of the stimulant to achieve intoxication or desired effect
           b. A markedly diminished effect with continued use of the same amount of the stimulant
           c. Tolerance does not count toward criteria if the substance is a prescribed part of the patient's treatment.
        iii. Withdrawal, as manifested by either of the following:
           a. The characteristic withdrawal syndrome for the substance
           b. The substance is taken to relieve or avoid withdrawal symptoms.
           c. Withdrawal does not count toward the criteria if the substance is prescribed as part of the patient's treatment.
     e. Severity specifier
        i. Mild: 2–3 criteria
        ii. Moderate: 4–5 criteria
        iii. Severe: 6 or more criteria
     f. Additional specifiers
        i. In early remission: nonuse with or without cravings for the last 3–12 months
        ii. In sustained remission: nonuse with or without cravings for over 12 months

VII. Plan
A. *Establishing a trusting relationship with the patient is essential to ensure the patient remains engaged in care.*
  1. Utilize motivational interviewing techniques to help patients develop their own goals and solutions.
  2. Do not force the patient to stop using substances or place other ideals to access services.
  3. Develop a plan based on the patient's goals to continue use, decrease use, or stop the use of substances.
     a. Do not shame or stigmatize a patient for wanting to continue to use substances.
     b. Returning to use with safer-use supplies is an appropriate plan.
  4. Provide initial treatment regardless of the patient's ability to follow up with a plan.
  5. Any positive healthcare interaction is helpful even if the patient does not engage in any care.
B. *Identify and support withdrawal management of their substances, keeping in mind that the patient can be in withdrawal from multiple substances at one time* (**Table 64-10**).

Table 64-10 Management of Withdrawal

Type of Withdrawal	Assessment Tool	Medications	Notes
ETOH withdrawal	PAWSS CIWA	Inpatient: CIWA: Symptom triggered with diazepam or lorazepam for people with cirrhosis or older than 70. Assess CIWA q4h. CIWA < 8 Day 1: Diazepam 5 mg PO q4h Day 2: Diazepam 5 mg PO q6h Day 3: Diazepam 5 mg q8h CIWA 8–16 Diazepam 10 mg q2h until CIWA is <8 CIWA 17–24 Diazepam 20 mg q1h until CIWA is <17 CIWA >24 Diazepam 20 mg Outpatient: Off-label, benzodiazepine-sparing mild withdrawal management with an eGFR >50 (Myrick et al., 2009) Day 1–3: Gabapentin 400 mg PO TID Day 4: Gabapentin 400 mg BID Day 5: Stop gabapentin Diazepam fixed taper (mild to moderate withdrawal) Day 1: Diazepam 10 mg q6h Day 2: Diazepam 10 mg q8 h Day 3: Diazepam 10 mg q12 h Day 4: Diazepam 10 mg at bedtime Day 5: Diazepam 10 mg at bedtime Thiamine replacement: All patients should receive thiamine. IV thiamine is preferred because of its bioavailability. Thiamine 100–200 mg PO or IV daily for 3–5 days can be used outpatient if withdrawal is mild. However, if signs of Wernicke encephalopathy are present (ataxia, lateral nystagmus, confusion), the patient must go to the hospital for thiamine 500 mg IV TID for 2–7 days, then 250 mg daily for 3–5 days, and then 100 mg daily until no longer at risk (Flannery et al., 2016).	The main goal is to prevent seizures, delirium tremens, and Wernicke encephalopathy. Patients with a history of seizures or severe withdrawal should be referred to an emergency room or a medical withdrawal program. The PAWSS can be used to determine if hospitalization is needed (Maldonado et al., 2014).
Opioid withdrawal	COWS	Medications Clonidine 0.1–0.3 mg q6h prn sweats and chills. Hold for SBP <100. Hydroxyzine 50 mg q6h prn anxiety and insomnia. Loperamide 2 mg PO prn loose stool. Max 16 mg a day. Ondansetron 4 mg q6h prn nausea and vomiting. Buprenorphine may be initiated, or the patient may be referred to a methadone clinic. Opioids may not be used in an outpatient setting to manage withdrawal but can be used in inpatient setting to treat symptoms.	Opioids may not be used to treat withdrawal in an outpatient setting. Although most opioid withdrawal is not fatal, it can be very uncomfortable, and the patient could benefit from inpatient treatment to access opioids and adjunctive therapy to feel well.

Type of Withdrawal	Assessment Tool	Medications	Notes
Stimulant withdrawal	No standard assessment	Supportive measures	There are no data to support treating stimulant withdrawal with stimulants. Withdrawal is generally not fatal; only supportive measures are needed to recover. Mirtazapine 15 mg at bedtime, increasing to 30 mg after 1 week, may help improve sleep and be part of an ongoing treatment plan.
Benzodiazepine withdrawal	CIWA	Inpatient: CIWA symptom triggered with lorazepam or diazepam as per alcohol withdrawal Outpatient: If on prescribed benzodiazepine, calculate the equivalent dose to a longer-acting benzodiazepine (e.g., diazepam). Reduce dose in weekly increments of 25%. The initial dose decrease is the easiest, with the last dose decrease being the most challenging. A taper may take a few weeks to several months. The patient needs to be agreeable to the time frame and dose changes. Provide frequent support and refer to mental health for support for anxiety, insomnia, PTSD, or other mental health condition that may have initiated the benzodiazepine use (National Center for PTSD, 2015).	Abrupt stopping of benzodiazepines can cause seizures. If available, a loading dose of phenobarbital may also be used in the inpatient setting.
Tobacco withdrawal	No standard assessment	May initiate nicotine replacement at equivalent doses of current nicotine use. ½ pack of cigarettes is a 21-mg nicotine patch. The patient may need two patches. 4-mg nicotine gum or lozenge is 1 cigarette.	
Cannabis withdrawal	No standard assessment	Cannabis withdrawal can be treated off-label with dronabinol 10 mg at bedtime and increased after 1 week to 20 mg BID for 8 weeks, then titrated down as tolerated over 2 weeks (Levin et al., 2011).	

BID, twice daily; *COWS*, Clinical Opiate Withdrawal Scale; *CIWA*, Clinical Institute Withdrawal Assessment for Alcohol; *eGFR*, estimated glomerular filtration rate; *ETOH*, ethyl alcohol or ethanol; *IV*, intravenous; *PAWSS*, Prediction of Alcohol Withdrawal Severity Scale; *PO*, per os (orally); *prn*, as needed; *PTSD*, posttraumatic stress disorder; *SBP*, systolic blood pressure; *TID*, three times daily.

C. Using medications to treat substance use disorders
 1. Clinicians can partner with patients to provide safe and effective medications for the management of many substance use disorders (**Table 64-11** and **Table 64-12**).
D. Using therapy to treat substance use disorders (**Table 64-13**)

VIII. Harm reduction

Safer use is an essential principle of harm reduction that can reduce the risk of overdose or complications from substance use for people who want to continue or reduce their use. The goal is to provide sterile equipment, safer-use strategies, and overdose prevention tools that can reduce HIV and hepatitis C transmission and increase the likelihood of a person accessing treatment (Fernandes et al., 2017; Platt et al., 2017).

A. All patients should be offered naloxone to reverse an overdose for use in the community.
 1. Naloxone is available as an injectable, auto-injector, and nasal spray.

Table 64-11 Medications for Treatment of Substance Use Disorders

Alcohol Use Disorder: The purpose of pharmacotherapy is to help decrease cravings and the amount of alcohol consumed. Extended-release naltrexone is a good first-step treatment with or without gabapentin if the patient can take pills.

Medication	Dosing	Advantages	Disadvantages	Common Side Effects	Pregnancy	FDA Approval	Notes
Acamprosate (Merck, 2012)	333 mg: take 2 pills by mouth 3 times a day.	Helps decrease alcohol cravings. Better for people who have already stopped drinking and want to continue to abstain from alcohol. Can be administered with methadone and buprenorphine if patient has an OUD.	Heavy pill burden. Not as effective as other medications.	Nausea, diarrhea	Not safe in pregnancy	FDA approved	Renal dosing 30-50 mL/min, 333 mg TID. Contraindicated in <30 mL/min.
Naltrexone PO or IM (Alkermes, 2013; Duramed Pharmaceuticals, 2013)	IM: Administer naltrexone 25 mg. Take 1 pill by mouth as a test dose, then naltrexone 380 mg IM q4 weeks. PO: Naltrexone 50 mg: take 1 pill by mouth daily. If daily dosing of naltrexone is difficult, as-needed dosing of taking naltrexone 50 mg on days with alcohol cravings or plans for drinking may be considered (Santos et al., 2022).	Helps decrease the amount of alcohol consumed. Better for people who are not on opioids. For people who want a monthly injection.	It can't be used in Child-Pugh C liver cirrhosis. Not studied with eGFR <30. It can't be used if the patient needs opioids. IM shouldn't be administered if the patient has an upcoming surgery.	Syncope, abdominal pain, nausea, vomiting, headache, anxiety IM: injection site pain	Not safe during pregnancy, although there is increasing data that it may be okay to do so with a risk-benefit discussion with the patient (Carits & Venkataramanan, 2020).	FDA approved	No long-acting opioids in the last 7 days and no short-acting opioids in the last 24 hours. Urine toxicology is helpful to ensure no opioids are present. Combining naltrexone with gabapentin may have improved outcomes (Anton et al., 2011). IM Naltrexone skips first-pass metabolism and may be easier on the liver. There are no guidelines for monitoring LFTs. PO version should not be used to co-treat AUD with OUD because poor adherence can lead to withdrawal, with the return to the use of opioids.

VIII. Harm reduction

Disulfiram (Physicians Total Care, 2012)	Disulfiram 250 mg: take 1 pill by mouth daily. May increase up to 500 mg daily.	For people who want a negative consequence to returning to use.	Negative reinforcement is less effective than other treatments.	Fatigue, headache, psychosis (rare) Disulfiram reaction from drinking alcohol: flushing, nausea, vomiting, respiratory difficulty, diaphoresis, thirst, chest pain, palpitation, dyspnea, hyperventilation, tachycardia, hypotension, syncope, confusion, vertigo, and blurred vision	Not safe in pregnancy	FDA approved	Must abstain from alcohol for 12 hours and avoid any alcohol for 2 weeks after stopping use.
Gabapentin (Pfizer, 2017)	Gabapentin 300 mg: take 1 pill by mouth 3 times a day. Increase to gabapentin 600 mg: take 1 pill by mouth 3 times a day.	Helps to reduce heavy drinking days and more days of nonuse Can manage mild withdrawal and support recovery	3-times-a-day dosing	Dizziness, somnolence, fatigue, weight gain, depression	May be safe in pregnancy	Not FDA approved	Risk of oversedation when combined with opioids or benzodiazepines
Topiramate (Janssen Pharmaceuticals, 2012)	Topiramate 25 mg: take 1 pill by mouth daily. Increase in 25- to 50-mg increments every week to a maximum of 300 mg per day. Doses over 50 mg should be split into twice-daily dosing.	Helps reduce heavy drinking days. It may help with a concurrent cocaine use disorder.	Slow titration to an effective dose. Drug interactions with oral contraceptive Twice-a-day dosing.	Paresthesia, change in taste, poor appetite, difficulty concentrating, or memory problems	Not safe in pregnancy	Not FDA approved	

(continues)

Table 64-11 Medications for Treatment of Substance Use Disorders

Medication	Dosing	Advantages	Disadvantages	Common Side Effects	Pregnancy	FDA Approval	Notes
Opioid Use Disorder	The goal of pharmacotherapy in OUD is to relieve cravings and withdrawal. Methadone has improved outcomes, and the frequent visits to a methadone clinic can provide some structure to the patient's day. Buprenorphine is easier to access and can provide faster relief. The patient can decide which is best and switch treatments if one does not work. Switching from methadone to buprenorphine is more challenging and should be done in conjunction with the methadone clinic. Naltrexone is abstinence therapy with lower success rates and should be reserved for patients who feel it is needed to succeed or if there are any legal issues for a licensed professional, who must not be on any opioids.						
Methadone (Roxane Laboratories, 2015)	Up-titrated over several weeks. Day 1 methadone: 40 mg Day 2 methadone: 50 mg Day 3 methadone: 60 mg Increased by 10 mg every 3–5 days as tolerated.	Provides relief of opioid cravings and withdrawal. Provides improved relief from withdrawal with full mu agonism.	It must be administered at a licensed methadone clinic. Methadone stacks on prior doses and gets to a steady state after 3–5 days, which increases the risk of oversedation. Slower than buprenorphine to get to a therapeutic dose.	Sedation, CNS depression, constipation, QTcF prolongation at doses >100 mg	Safe in pregnancy. May need increased doses after 2nd trimester and split twice-a-day dosing. There are no evidence-based guidelines, and dosing is patient centered and based on symptom control and sedation (Pace et al., 2014; Shiu & Ensom, 2012).	FDA approved	Patients may still need to use opioids while up-titrating their methadone dose. Methadone can be administered in inpatient setting without any special licenses. Methadone may not be prescribed in outpatient setting for OUD outside of a methadone clinic. However, up to 3 days of buprenorphine or methadone can be dispensed (not prescribed) after hospitalization or clinic visit with provider clearance by DEA (U.S. Drug Enforcement Administration, 2022).
Buprenorphine/naloxone, buprenorphine, extended-release buprenorphine (Indivior Inc., 2017; Reckitt Benckiser Pharmaceuticals Inc., 2010, 2011)	See the buprenorphine initiation table. Sublingual maintenance doses range from 8 to 24 mg daily.	Provides relief of opioid cravings and withdrawal. It can be accessed in any clinical setting with an X-waivered provider.	Must be accessed from an X-waivered provider.	Sublingual film: Nausea, vomiting, constipation, diarrhea, xerostomia, dizziness, fatigue, and headache. SQ: Injection site pain.	Safe in pregnancy. The naloxone in the sublingual film is safe to use during pregnancy (Link et al., 2020).	FDA approved	Patients may still use substances while on buprenorphine, but the euphoric effects will be blunted by the buprenorphine. Sublingual films may leave less residue and be preferred by patients.

(continued)

VIII. Harm reduction

	The effect on cravings and withdrawal lasts 24 hours, but the pain relief is around 8 hours. Splitting the dose to two or three times a day allows for better pain control. Extended-release buprenorphine: Must be on stable buprenorphine SL for seven days (may initiate after two days if needed). Extended-release buprenorphine 300 mg SQ every 4 weeks for the first two monthly doses. Then administer extended-release buprenorphine 100 mg SQ every 4 weeks. The dose may be kept at 300 mg if the patient responds better to the higher dose.	Can have monthly supplies. Less risk of sedation. Protective of overdose	It may not provide full relief to patients with a high opioid tolerance or who need the feeling of a full mu opioid agonist. It can cause precipitated withdrawal if initiated too quickly.		The naloxone in the sublingual films is not fully absorbed and should not affect care. The buprenorphine mono-product can be used if preferred. If the patient has chronic pain, may divide the dose into BID or TID dosing for additional pain relief.
Naltrexone (Alkermes, 2013)	Administer naltrexone 25 mg. Take 1 pill by mouth as a test dose, then naltrexone 380 mg IM q4 weeks.	Reduces the use of opioids. It is a monthly shot, reducing the pill burden.	It can't be used in Child-Pugh C liver cirrhosis. Not studied with eGFR < 30. It can't be used if the patient needs opioids.	Syncope, abdominal pain, nausea, vomiting, headache, anxiety, injection site pain.	Not safe during pregnancy, although there are increasing data that it may be okay to do	FDA approved	Do not use pill formulation for OUD. Incomplete adherence may cause withdrawal with any return to use. No long-acting opioids in the past 7 days and no short-acting opioids in the last 24 hours.

(continues)

Table 64-11 Medications for Treatment of Substance Use Disorders *(continued)*

Medication	Dosing	Advantages	Disadvantages	Common Side Effects	Pregnancy	FDA Approval	Notes
		Recommended for people who need to abstain for legal reasons or feel this is how they can achieve their goals.	IM shouldn't be administered if the patient has an upcoming surgery. IM Naltrexone skips first-pass metabolism and may be easier on the liver. There are no guidelines for monitoring LFTs.		so with a risk-benefit discussion with the patient (Caritis & Venkataramanan, 2020).		Urine toxicology is helpful to ensure no opioids are present.
Stimulant Use Disorder	There are no FDA-approved medications for stimulant use disorder. However, some have some potential to help, which can be trialed, especially if there is a co-occurring illness that could also benefit from the medication. The primary treatment is therapy and contingency management.						
Mirtazapine (Merck & Co., 2020)	Start mirtazapine 15 mg. Take 1 pill by mouth daily. Increase by 15 mg after 1 week to mirtazapine 30 mg. Take 1 pill by mouth daily.	It may reduce the frequency of stimulant use. It may be able to treat comorbid depression. It helps with sleep and weight gain, which may help people using stimulants.	Limited data. Weight gain may be an issue if the patient is overweight and has cardiac problems.	Weight gain and sedation	May be safe in pregnancy	Not FDA approved	The data are limited and primarily in MSM and transfemme communities. Do not start antidepressants in people with bipolar disorder who are not on a mood stabilizer or in a manic episode without a psychiatry consult to limit rapid mood cycling.
Bupropion and naltrexone (Alkermes, 2013; GlaxoSmithKline, 2017)	Start bupropion XL 150 mg daily. Increase in weekly intervals by 150 mg to a total of bupropion 450 mg. Take 1 pill by mouth daily.	It may reduce the frequency of stimulant use. It can be used to treat co-occurring tobacco use or alcohol use disorders.	Limited data. May not be able to obtain insurance coverage for q3 week administration.	Bupropion: tachycardia, diaphoresis, weight loss, constipation, nausea, vomiting, xerostomia, agitation,	Not safe during pregnancy, although there are increasing data that it may be okay to do so with a risk-benefit	Not FDA approved	Do not start antidepressants in people with bipolar disorder who are not on a mood stabilizer or in a manic episode without a psychiatry consult to limit rapid mood cycling.

VIII. Harm reduction

	Administer naltrexone 25 mg. Take 1 pill by mouth as a test dose, then naltrexone 380 mg IM q3 weeks.		dizziness, insomnia, and tremors. Naltrexone: syncope, abdominal pain, nausea, vomiting, headache, anxiety, injection site pain	discussion with the patient (Caritis & Venkataramanan, 2020).	No long-acting opioids in the past 7 days and no short-acting opioids in the last 24 hours. Urine toxicology is helpful to ensure no opioids are present.
Tobacco Use Disorder	The goal of pharmacotherapy for tobacco use disorder is to treat cravings and withdrawal to allow the patient to stop using tobacco. Varenicline may provide increased efficacy and is a good place to start if the patient wants to quit. Combinations may not improve outcomes, but they can be used based on patient preferences.				
Nicotine replacement: patches, gum, lozenges, inhaler, and nasal spray (GlaxoSmithKline, 2006, 2011, 2013; Pfizer, 2010b, 2019).	Replace current nicotine use and titrate down over time based on patient preferences for up to 24 weeks. Nicotine patches: available in 7 mg, 14 mg, 24 mg daily. Gum or lozenge also available. Inhaler: 10-mg cartridge. Inhale 6–16 cartridges/day for 3–6 weeks. Do not use it longer than 6 months. Nasal spray: 10-mL bottle. Use 2–4 sprays per hour up to 80 sprays per day. Do not use it for longer than 3 months. 1 cigarette = 2 mg (National Institute on Drug Abuse, 2021). 21-mg nicotine patch = 1/2 pack of cigarettes per day.	Allows for more immediate relief	Can be underdosed and seem ineffective	Spray or inhaler: headache, oral irritation, dyspepsia, nasal discomfort, throat irritation, rhinitis Patch: sleep disturbance when applied overnight. Gum, lozenge: increased blood pressure, palpitations, heartburn, dyspepsia, and oral irritation	May be safe in pregnancy	FDA approved	Combination therapy with varenicline may not improve outcomes (Baker et al., 2021). The efficacy of nicotine replacement decreases after 24 weeks (Schnoll et al., 2015). Nonuse in the first 2 weeks is the best predictor of long-term nonuse (Kenford et al., 1994). Nicotine patches deliver 24-hr nicotine and may affect sleep. However, the patient can remove the patch at bedtime.

(continues)

Table 64-11 Medications for Treatment of Substance Use Disorders *(continued)*

Medication	Dosing	Advantages	Disadvantages	Common Side Effects	Pregnancy	FDA Approval	Notes
Varenicline (Pfizer, 2010a)	Day 1-3: Varenicline 0.5 mg. Take 1 pill by mouth daily. Day 4-7: Varenicline 0.5 mg. Take 1 pill by mouth twice daily. Day 8: Varenicline 1 mg. Take 1 pill by mouth daily for 11 weeks.	May continue to smoke while on varenicline and stop or decrease when the patient chooses to.	Daily pill and will take time to get to a therapeutic dose.	Nausea, vomiting, abnormal dreams, depressed mood, headache, insomnia, and irritability	May be safe in pregnancy	FDA approved	Initial concerns about suicidal ideation had limited its initial use, but further research has proven varenicline is safe, and the black-box warning was removed. Mixed evidence on combining varenicline with nicotine patches or bupropion.
Bupropion SR (GlaxoSmithKline, 2019)	Bupropion SR 150 mg. Take 1 pill by mouth twice daily	May treat co-occurring depression	It cannot be used for patients with a seizure disorder or eating disorder history.	Tachycardia, diaphoresis, weight loss, constipation, nausea, vomiting, xerostomia, agitation, dizziness, insomnia, and tremors	May be safe in pregnancy	FDA approved	The sustained-release formulation is FDA approved for smoking cessation, although the XL formulation is also appropriate to use off-label. Do not start antidepressants in people with bipolar disorder who are not on a mood stabilizer or in a manic episode without a psychiatry consult to limit rapid mood cycling.
Benzodiazepine use disorder	There are no medications used for long-term treatment after withdrawal management. However, patients can be referred to therapy to help manage cravings.						
Cannabis use disorder	There are no medications used for long-term treatment after withdrawal management. However, patients can be referred to therapy to help manage cravings.						

AUD, alcohol use disorder; *BID*, twice daily; *CNS*, central nervous system; *DEA*, U.S. Drug Enforcement Administration; *eGFR*, estimated glomerular filtration rate; *FDA*, U.S. Food and Drug Administration; *IM*, intramuscular; *LFT*, liver function test; *MSM*, men who have sex with men; *OUD*, opioid use disorder; *PO*, per os (orally); *SQ*, subcutaneous; *SL*, sublingual; *SR*, sustained release; *TID*, three times daily; *XL*, extended release.

Table 64-12 Buprenorphine Initiation

Buprenorphine initiation	Buprenorphine is a partial agonist on the mu opioid receptor. Its inhibitory constant is lower than other opioids and even naloxone. This causes buprenorphine to remove existing opioids from the mu opioid receptor, resulting in precipitated withdrawal, which is extremely uncomfortable. There are multiple ways to initiate buprenorphine, including ones not outlined here, with the goal of getting to a therapeutic dose of buprenorphine without causing withdrawal. Slower initiations will limit withdrawal by allowing buprenorphine to replace an opioid as it leaves the opioid receptor naturally, but delays in getting to a therapeutic dose can limit a successful transition. Some patients may be comfortable going through the withdrawal for a traditional start, and others may have experienced precipitated withdrawal before and will only try a slow initiation. Assess the patient's comfort with withdrawal and any recent use of fentanyl or methadone in the last 24 hours to help guide which option is best (Ahmed et al., 2021; de Aquino et al., 2021; Ghosh et al., 2019).	
Buprenorphine/ naloxone	Stop all opioids. Assess COWS. Once COWS is >8 with 2 objective signs, administer buprenorphine 8 mg. Reassess after 2 hours. Administer an additional 8 mg for a total of 16 mg on the first day. Continue 16-mg daily dose or increase to 24 mg daily.	It can be done at home and does not need to be supervised. An app is available to guide patients (listed in the patient resources section).
Buprenorphine 3-day microinitiation	Day 1: Buprenorphine/naloxone film 0.5 mg QID (1/4 of a 2-mg film) Day 2: Buprenorphine/naloxone film 1 mg QID (1/2 of a 2-mg film) Day 3: Buprenorphine/naloxone film 2 mg QID Day 6: Buprenorphine/naloxone film 8–16 mg daily.	The patient may continue to use opioids during the titration. Administer buprenorphine 1 hour before any opioids. Buprenorphine film is preferred as it is easier to cut into quarters, but pills can be used if the pill is cut without much crumbling. If unable to cut films or pills into quarters for day 1, may use 2× buprenorphine 20 mcg transdermal to equal 0.5 mg buprenorphine/naloxone SL. Outpatient: The patient will need to use opioids to help minimize withdrawal. Inpatient: Patients can receive prn opioids to relieve withdrawal symptoms. Buprenorphine should be administered 1 hour before or after any other opioids to limit withdrawal.
Buprenorphine 5-day microinitiation	Day 1: Buprenorphine/naloxone film 0.5 mg once (1/4 of a 2-mg film) Day 2: Buprenorphine/naloxone 0.5 mg film BID (1/4 of a 2-mg film) Day 3: Buprenorphine/naloxone film 1 mg BID (1/4 of a 2-mg film) Day 4: Buprenorphine/naloxone film 2 mg BID Day 5: Buprenorphine/naloxone film 2 mg QID Day 6: Buprenorphine/naloxone film 8–16 mg daily.	The patient may continue to use opioids during the titration. Administer buprenorphine 1 hour before any opioids. Buprenorphine film is preferred as it is easier to cut into quarters, but pills can be used if the pill is cut without much crumbling. If unable to cut films or pills into quarters for day 1, may use 2× buprenorphine 20 mcg transdermal to equal 0.5 mg buprenorphine/naloxone SL. Outpatient: The patient will need to use opioids to help minimize withdrawal. Inpatient: Patients can receive prn opioids to relieve withdrawal symptoms. Buprenorphine should be administered 1 hour before or after any other opioids to limit withdrawal.

(continues)

Table 64-12 Buprenorphine Initiation *(continued)*

Extended-release buprenorphine	The patient must be on a stable dose of sublingual buprenorphine between 8 and 24 mg for at least 2–7 days. Extended-release buprenorphine is administered in 300-mg subcutaneous q 4 weeks. Standard dosing is to receive 300 mg for the first 2 months, then decrease to 100 mg monthly	Minimum 26 days between doses. Delays of 2 weeks are not expected to influence the treatment effect. May continue 300-mg follow-up doses after month 2 if needed for symptom control. The patient may need additional sublingual buprenorphine/naloxone 2 mg q6h prn withdrawal or cravings not relieved by extended-release buprenorphine. The injection is administered in the lower abdomen. The injection can be painful. For anesthesia, ice may be applied for 20 minutes to the area prior to injection, or 3 mL of 1% buffered lidocaine may be administered into the injection area.

BID, twice daily; *COWS*, Clinical Opiate Withdrawal Scale; *QID*, four times per day; *prn*, as needed; *SL*, sublingual.

Table 64-13 Therapy Options for Substance Use Disorders

	Opioid Use Disorder	Stimulant Use Disorder	Alcohol Use Disorder	Benzodiazepine Use Disorder	Tobacco Use Disorder	Cannabis Use Disorder
Brief Intervention (Bernstein et al., 2005; Beyer et al., 2019; Little et al., 2016; Roy-Byrne et al., 2014; Saitz et al., 2014)	May be effective	Minimal to no effect on use	Effective in less severe alcohol use disorder	No data. May be helpful.	May be effective	No data. May be helpful.
Contingency Management (Ainscough et al., 2017; Benishek et al., 2014; Bolívar et al., 2021; Hirchak et al., 2021; Secades-Villa et al., 2015; Volpp et al., 2009)	Reduce the frequency of use	Reduce the frequency of use	Limited data	No data. May be helpful.	Limited data. May be helpful.	Limited data. May be helpful.
Cognitive–Behavioral Therapy (Gates et al., 2016; Harada et al., 2018; Otto et al., 2010; Rawson et al., 2002; Ray et al., 2020; Secades-Villa et al., 2015)	Minimal to no effect	Minimal to no effect	Effective in reducing use	Limited data. May be helpful.	Limited data. May be helpful.	May be helpful
Psychotherapy (Carroll et al., 2004; Kang et al., 1991; Taylor et al., 2017; Woody et al., 1995)	Limited data. May be helpful.	Not effective	Not effective	No data	No data	No data

	Opioid Use Disorder	Stimulant Use Disorder	Alcohol Use Disorder	Benzodiazepine Use Disorder	Tobacco Use Disorder	Cannabis Use Disorder
Self-Help Group Therapy (12-step) (Christo & Franey, 1995; Darker et al., 2015; Gossop et al., 2008; Hoffmann et al., 1983; Kelly et al., 2020; Stead et al., 2017; Walsh et al., 1991; Witbrodt et al., 2012; Woodhead et al., 2020)	Minimal to no effect on use	Minimal to no effect on use	Effective with frequent participation	Not effective	Group and individual counseling are helpful.	Limited data. May be effective.
Residential Treatment (Bonn-Miller et al., 2011; Gossop et al., 2003; Guydish et al., 1999; Keen et al., 2001; Simpson et al., 1999; Walsh et al., 1991; Ware et al., 2021)	Programs 90 days or longer reduce the frequency of use.	Programs 90 days or longer reduce the frequency of use.	Programs 90 days or longer reduce the frequency of use.	No data	No data	Limited data. May be helpful.

2. It can be prescribed as naloxone 4 mg intranasal. Administer one full nasal spray into one nostril upon signs of opioid overdose. Call 911. May repeat in the other nostril once if there is no response within 3 minutes.
3. Newer 8-mg formulations are available, although there is no evidence to support the need for a higher dose. Administering too much naloxone can increase the patient's discomfort (Carpenter et al., 2020).
4. Community members and healthcare providers are encouraged to keep naloxone on them.
5. Naloxone should be used in the community on anyone who is unresponsive and in whom an opioid overdose is suspected, with the following steps:
    a. Assess the patient for response through verbal "Are you okay?" and tactile stimulus (arm touch, then sternal rub if no response).
    b. Provide a "verbal naloxone" to the patient by stating, "I'm going to give you Narcan if you don't respond," before administering naloxone to ensure the patient has overdosed and can't respond.
    c. If there is no response, initiate Basic Life Support and call 911.
    d. If opioid overdose is suspected, administer naloxone 4 mg intranasal.
    e. Repeat after 3 minutes in the other nostril. It is essential to ensure that 3 minutes have passed to avoid over-administering naloxone (Adapt Pharma, 2015).
    f. Stay with the patient until emergency services arrive. Naloxone wears off after 90 minutes, and the patient can become sedated again.
    g. The goal of naloxone is to restore breathing and not to remove all opioids from the body. Administering too much naloxone is uncomfortable for the patient and may create distrust or fear of coming to a healthcare provider.
    h. There has been a recent increase in the use of xylazine as an adulterant in opioids to enhance the sedative effects. Xylazine is an alpha2-adrenoceptor agonist that is not reversed by naloxone. If a patient does not respond after multiple doses of naloxone and xylazine use is suspected, the patient should receive oxygen and respiratory support, including up to intubation, until the xylazine is metabolized (Friedman et al., 2022).
B. *Safer-use strategies can be discussed with the patient to support any incremental changes to reduce their risk of complications or overdose.*
    1. Snorting and smoking have a decreased overdose risk compared to injecting.
    2. Injecting into the upper extremities is safer. Avoid neck and face.
    3. Clean skin with alcohol and use sterile equipment to limit infections.
    4. Never use alone. Use with someone who can monitor and administer naloxone if needed. Put the Never Use Alone phone number 1-877-696-1996 in the patient's phone.

5. Never share equipment, and use new equipment frequently.
6. Tolerance is lowered after a period of nonuse (e.g., after a hospitalization). If returning to use, start with lower doses.
7. Test substances with home fentanyl test strips or refer to substance testing centers.
8. If using with other people, color code or label the equipment to minimize the chance of sharing.

C. *Safer-use supplies provide sterile equipment to limit infections. The goal is that the equipment is used once and then tossed, with a new set used each time.*
 1. Syringe access laws vary by state and will determine the ease of availability of supplies and the chance the person has to reuse supplies.
 2. Refer patients to safer-use centers to access clean supplies.
 3. Some states allow for getting needles at a pharmacy without a prescription.
 4. Safer-use supplies can be mailed to a patient's home or picked up at a syringe access center in the community. See resources for patients section.

D. *Healthcare maintenance specific to substance use*
 1. HIV screening
    a. Test for HIV with an HIV fourth-generation antibody and antigen test every 3–6 months (DiNenno et al., 2019).
    b. HIV PrEP decreases the risk of HIV in people who inject drugs (Choopanya et al., 2013).
       i. PrEP may be offered to people who inject drugs to decrease their risk of HIV.
       ii. If the risk of HIV is only from needles, the patient may benefit from accessing clean needles versus trying to incorporate a daily pill.
 2. Hepatitis C screening
    a. People who share drug injection equipment or other preparation equipment should be screened for hepatitis C every 3–6 months with a hepatitis C virus (HCV) antibody for people who have never had hepatitis C or an HCV RNA for people who have cleared or cured hepatitis C (Schillie et al., 2020).
 3. Hepatitis B screening
    a. Screen for hepatitis B with hepatitis B virus (HBV) antibody, HBV antigen, and HBV total core antibody, and offer the hepatitis B vaccine (Schillie et al., 2019).
 4. Hepatitis A screening
    a. Screen for hepatitis A with a hepatitis A virus (HAV) total antibody and offer a hepatitis A vaccine (Nelson et al., 2021).
 5. Sexual health screening
    a. Order rapid plasma regain (RPR) for syphilis screening every 3–6 months
    b. Gonorrhea and chlamydia nucleic acid amplification test (NAAT) for body parts used for sex (oral, vaginal or frontal, penile, or anal) every 3–6 months (Workowski et al., 2021)
 6. Screen for abuse and intimate partner violence and refer to care (Curry et al., 2018).

IX. Follow-up
A. There is no evidence-based follow-up schedule, and it should be a shared decision with the patient and provider.
B. Patients may benefit from frequent contacts for additional support, which can be shared interdisciplinary (e.g., alternating weekly visits with a therapist and provider).
C. Returning to use is anticipated and should not be considered a failure.
D. Work with the patient to identify a new plan to manage the triggers that caused them to return to use and repeat the process.
E. Any positive change is celebrated.
F. When in doubt, always be present and welcome the patient back.

X. Resources for patients who use substances
A. *Never Use Alone:* Nonjudgmental, nonreportable phone support to help monitor a person when they use substances. They will ask for a name, location, and phone number. If the person becomes unresponsive, emergency services will be notified of an "unresponsive person" (1-877-696-1996).
B. *Next Distro:* Online Harm Reduction Service to mail safer-use supplies and naloxone. The patient can sign up at https://nextdistro.org.
C. *Syringe Access Centers:* Many but not all communities have access to Syringe Access Centers, which can provide safer-use supplies, fentanyl test strips, and naloxone. A directory of Syringe Access Centers can be found at https://www.nasen.org.
D. *Safer-Use Techniques:* https://injectingadvice.com provides guidance on how to use substances safely.
E. *Buprenorphine home initiation:* The Buprenorphine Home Induction App is available in the Apple App Store and Google Play Store. The app guides the patient through a traditional buprenorphine initiation.

XI. Resources for clinicians
A. *National Clinician Consultation Center Substance Use Warmline* Free clinician-to-clinician advice on managing substance use disorders (Table 64-13). Consultation is available Monday to Friday, 9 a.m. to 8 p.m. ET, at (855)300-3595. https://nccc.ucsf.edu/clinical-resources/substance-use-resources/
B. Before 2023, prescribing buprenorphine required a DEA license with an X-waiver which involved additional training and restricted the provider to a limited number of patients. The Consolidated Appropriations Act of 2023 eliminated the requirement for an X-waiver with the goal of facilitating broader access to buprenorphine by empowering more providers to prescribe it. Any provider with a valid DEA for schedule III medications may prescribe buprenorphine with no restrictions on the number

of patients, if permitted by applicable state law, with no additional registration (SAMSHA, 2023).

1. Buprenorphine training is still recommended though not required and available for free through the American Psychiatric Nurses Association: https://www.apna.org/continuing-education/mat-waiver-training/.

C. National Harm Reduction Coalition Resources and education for the provider to learn about safer drug use and how to best help your patients through harm reduction. https://Harmreduction.org

D. Drug prices. https://Streetrx.com provides crowd-sourced drug pricing information by the community. Although not scientific, it can help estimate the price of drugs in an area.

References

Adapt Pharma. (2015). *Narcan: Highlights of prescribing information.* https://www.accessdata.fda.gov/drugsatfda_docs/label/2015/208411lbl.pdf

Ahmed, S., Bhivandkar, S., Lonergan, B. B., & Suzuki, J. (2021). Microinduction of buprenorphine/naloxone: A review of the literature. *American Journal on Addictions, 30*(4), 305–315. doi:10.1111/AJAD.13135

Ainscough, T. S., McNeill, A., Strang, J., Calder, R., & Brose, L. S. (2017). Contingency Management interventions for non-prescribed drug use during treatment for opiate addiction: A systematic review and meta-analysis. *Drug and Alcohol Dependence, 178,* 318–339. doi:10.1016/j.drugalcdep.2017.05.028

Alkermes. (2013). *Vivitrol: Highlights of prescribing information.* https://www.accessdata.fda.gov/drugsatfda_docs/label/2013/021897s020s023lbl.pdf

American Psychiatric Association. (2013). *Diagnostic and Statistical Manual of Mental Disorders* (5th ed.). doi:10.1176/appi.books.9780890425596

Anton, R. F., Myrick, H., Wright, T. M., Latham, P. K., Baros, A. M., Waid, L. R., & Randall, P. K. (2011). Gabapentin combined with naltrexone for the treatment of alcohol dependence. *American Journal of Psychiatry, 168*(7), 709. doi:10.1176/APPI.AJP.2011.10101436

Baker, T. B., Piper, M. E., Smith, S. S., Bolt, D. M., Stein, J. H., & Fiore, M. C. (2021). Effects of combined varenicline with nicotine patch and of extended treatment duration on smoking cessation: A randomized clinical trial. *JAMA, 326*(15), 1485–1493. doi:10.1001/JAMA.2021.15333

Benishek, L. A., Dugosh, K. L., Kirby, K. C., Matejkowski, J., Clements, N. T., Seymour, B. L., & Festinger, D. S. (2014). Prize-based contingency management for the treatment of substance abusers: A meta-analysis. *Addiction, 109*(9), 1426–1436. doi:10.1111/ADD.12589

Bernstein, J., Bernstein, E., Tassiopoulos, K., Heeren, T., Levenson, S., & Hingson, R. (2005). Brief motivational intervention at a clinic visit reduces cocaine and heroin use. *Drug and Alcohol Dependence, 77*(1), 49–59. doi:10.1016/j.drugalcdep.2004.07.006

Beyer, F. R., Campbell, F., Bertholet, N., Daeppen, J. B., Saunders, J. B., Pienaar, E. D., Muirhead, C. R., & Kaner, E. F. S. (2019). The Cochrane 2018 review on brief interventions in primary care for hazardous and harmful alcohol consumption: A distillation for clinicians and policy makers. *Alcohol and Alcoholism, 54*(4), 417–427. doi:10.1093/alcalc/agz035

Bolívar, H. A., Klemperer, E. M., Coleman, S. R. M., DeSarno, M., Skelly, J. M., & Higgins, S. T. (2021). Contingency Management for patients receiving medication for opioid use disorder: A systematic review and meta-analysis. *JAMA Psychiatry, 78*(10), 1092–1102. doi:10.1001/JAMAPSYCHIATRY.2021.1969

Bonn-Miller, M. O., Vujanovic, A. A., & Drescher, K. D. (2011). Cannabis use among military veterans after residential treatment for posttraumatic stress disorder. *Psychology of Addictive Behaviors, 25*(3), 485–491. doi:10.1037/A0021945

Bush, K., Kivlahan, D. R., McDonell, M. B., Fihn, S. D., & Bradley, K. A. (1998). The AUDIT Alcohol Consumption Questions (AUDIT-C): An effective brief screening test for problem drinking. *Archives of Internal Medicine, 158*(16), 1789–1795. doi:10.1001/ARCHINTE.158.16.1789

Caritis, S. N., & Venkataramanan, R. (2020). Naltrexone use in pregnancy: A time for change. *American Journal of Obstetrics and Gynecology, 222*(1), 1–2. doi:10.1016/J.AJOG.2019.08.041

Carpenter, J., Murray, B. P., Atti, S., Moran, T. P., Yancey, A., & Morgan, B. (2020). Naloxone dosing after opioid overdose in the era of illicitly manufactured fentanyl. *Journal of Medical Toxicology, 16*(1), 41–48. doi:10.1007/S13181-019-00735-W

Carroll, K. M., Fenton, L. R., Ball, S. A., Nich, C., Frankforter, T. L., Shi, J., & Rounsaville, B. J. (2004). Efficacy of disulfiram and cognitive behavior therapy in cocaine-dependent outpatients: A randomized placebo-controlled trial. *Archives of General Psychiatry, 61*(3), 264–272. doi:10.1001/ARCHPSYC.61.3.264

Center for Behavioral Health Statistics and Quality. (2021). *Racial/ethnic differences in substance use, substance use disorders, and substance use treatment utilization among people aged 12 or older (2015–2019)* (Publication No. PEP21-07-01-001). Substance Abuse and Mental Health Services Administration. https://www.samhsa.gov/data/

Choopanya, K., Martin, M., Suntharasamai, P., Sangkum, U., Mock, P. A., Leethochawalit, M., Chiamwongpaet, S., Kitisin, P., Natrujirote, P., Kittimunkong, S., Chuachoowong, R., Gvetadze, R. J., McNicholl, J. M., Paxton, L. A., Curlin, M. E., Hendrix, C. W., & Vanichseni, S. (2013). Antiretroviral prophylaxis for HIV infection in injecting drug users in Bangkok, Thailand (the Bangkok Tenofovir Study): A randomised, double-blind, placebo-controlled phase 3 trial. *Lancet, 381*(9883), 2083–2090. doi:10.1016/S0140-6736(13)61127-7

Christo, G., & Franey, C. (1995). Drug users' spiritual beliefs, locus of control and the disease concept in relation to Narcotics Anonymous attendance and six-month outcomes. *Drug and Alcohol Dependence, 38*(1), 51–56. doi:10.1016/0376-8716(95)01103-6

Curry, S. J., Krist, A. H., Owens, D. K., Barry, M. J., Caughey, A. B., Davidson, K. W., Doubeni, C. A., Epling, J. W., Grossman, D. C., Kemper, A. R., Kubik, M., Kurth, A., Landefeld, C. S., Mangione, C. M., Silverstein, M., Simon, M. A., Tseng, C. W., & Wong, J. B. (2018). Screening for intimate partner violence, elder abuse, and abuse of vulnerable adults: US Preventive Services Task Force final recommendation statement. *JAMA, 320*(16), 1678–1687. doi:10.1001/JAMA.2018.14741

Darker, C. D., Sweeney, B. P., Barry, J. M., Farrell, M. F., & Donnelly-Swift, E. (2015). Psychosocial interventions for benzodiazepine harmful use, abuse or dependence. *Cochrane Database of*

Systematic Reviews, 2015(5), CD009652. doi:10.1002/14651858.CD009652.PUB2

de Aquino, J. P., Parida, S., & Sofuoglu, M. (2021). The pharmacology of buprenorphine microinduction for opioid use disorder. *Clinical Drug Investigation*, 41(5), 425–436. doi:10.1007/S40261-021-01032-7/TABLES/2

DiNenno, E. A., Prejean, J., Irwin, K., Delaney, K. P., Bowles, K., Martin, T., Tailor, A., Dumitru, G., Mullins, M. M., Hutchinson, A. B., & Lansky, A. (2019). Recommendations for HIV screening of gay, bisexual, and other men who have sex with men—United States, 2017. *Morbidity and Mortality Weekly Report*, 66(31), 830–832. doi:10.15585/MMWR.MM6631A3

Duramed Pharmaceuticals. (2013). *Revia: Highlights of prescribing information*.

European Monitoring Centre for Drugs and Drug Addiction. (2020a). *Statistical bulletin 2020—overdose deaths*. https://www.emcdda.europa.eu/data/stats2020/drd

European Monitoring Centre for Drugs and Drug Addiction. (2020b). *Statistical bulletin 2020—problem drug use*. https://www.emcdda.europa.eu/data/stats2020/pdu

Félix, S., & Portugal, P. (2017). Drug decriminalization and the price of illicit drugs. *International Journal on Drug Policy*, 39, 121–129. doi:10.1016/J.DRUGPO.2016.10.014

Fernandes, R. M., Cary, M., Duarte, G., Jesus, G., Alarcão, J., Torre, C., Costa, S., Costa, J., & Carneiro, A. V. (2017). Effectiveness of needle and syringe programmes in people who inject drugs—an overview of systematic reviews. *BMC Public Health*, 17(1). doi:10.1186/S12889-017-4210-2

Flannery, A. H., Adkins, D. A., & Cook, A. M. (2016). Unpeeling the evidence for the banana bag: Evidence-based recommendations for the management of alcohol-associated vitamin and electrolyte deficiencies in the ICU. *Critical Care Medicine*, 44(8), 1545–1552. doi:10.1097/CCM.0000000000001659

Friedman, J., Montero, F., Bourgois, P., Wahbi, R., Dye, D., Goodman-Meza, D., & Shover, C. (2022). Xylazine spreads across the US: A growing component of the increasingly synthetic and polysubstance overdose crisis. *Drug and Alcohol Dependence*, 233, 109380. doi:10.1016/J.DRUGALCDEP.2022.109380

Gates, P. J., Sabioni, P., Copeland, J., le Foll, B., & Gowing, L. (2016). Psychosocial interventions for cannabis use disorder. *Cochrane Database of Systematic Reviews*, 2016(5), CD005336. doi:10.1002/14651858.CD005336.PUB4

Ghosh, S. M., Klaire, S., Tanguay, R., Manek, M., & Azar, P. (2019). A review of novel methods to support the transition from methadone and other full agonist opioids to buprenorphine/naloxone sublingual in both community and acute care settings. *Canadian Journal of Addiction*, 10(4), 41–50. doi:10.1097/CXA.0000000000000072

GlaxoSmithKline. (2006). *NicoDerm: Drug facts*. https://www.accessdata.fda.gov/drugsatfda_docs/label/2006/020165s023lbl.pdf

GlaxoSmithKline. (2011). *Nicorette gum: Drug facts*. https://www.accessdata.fda.gov/drugsatfda_docs/label/2012/018612s061_020066s042lbl.pdf

GlaxoSmithKline. (2013). *Nicorette lozenge: Drug facts*. https://www.accessdata.fda.gov/drugsatfda_docs/label/2013/021330Orig1s016lbl.pdf

GlaxoSmithKline. (2017). *Wellbutrin XL: Highlights of prescribing information*. https://www.accessdata.fda.gov/drugsatfda_docs/label/2017/021515s036lbl.pdf

GlaxoSmithKline. (2019). *Wellbutrin SR: Highlights of prescribing information*. https://www.accessdata.fda.gov/drugsatfda_docs/label/2019/020358s061lbl.pdf

Gonçalves, R., Lourenço, A., & da Silva, S. N. (2015). A social cost perspective in the wake of the Portuguese strategy for the fight against drugs. *International Journal on Drug Policy*, 26(2), 199–209. doi:10.1016/J.DRUGPO.2014.08.017

Gossop, M., Marsden, J., Stewart, D., & Kidd, T. (2003). The National Treatment Outcome Research Study (NTORS): 4-5 year follow-up results. *Addiction*, 98(3), 291–303. doi:10.1046/J.1360-0443.2003.00296.X

Gossop, M., Stewart, D., & Marsden, J. (2008). Attendance at Narcotics Anonymous and Alcoholics Anonymous meetings, frequency of attendance and substance use outcomes after residential treatment for drug dependence: A 5-year follow-up study. *Addiction*, 103(1), 119–125. doi:10.1111/J.1360-0443.2007.02050.X

Green, K. E., & Feinstein, B. A. (2012). Substance use in lesbian, gay, and bisexual populations: An update on empirical research and implications for treatment. *Psychology of Addictive Behaviors*, 26(2), 265–278. doi:10.1037/A0025424

Guydish, J., Sorensen, J. L., Chan, M., Werdegar, D., Bostrom, A., & Acampora, A. (1999). A randomized trial comparing day and residential drug abuse treatment: 18-month outcomes. *Journal of Consulting and Clinical Psychology*, 67(3), 428–434. doi:10.1037//0022-006X.67.3.428

Han, B., Einstein, E. B., Jones, C. M., Cotto, J., Compton, W. M., & Volkow, N. D. (2022). Racial and ethnic disparities in drug overdose deaths in the US during the COVID-19 pandemic. *JAMA Network Open*, 5(9), e2232314–e2232314. doi:10.1001/JAMANETWORKOPEN.2022.32314

Harada, T., Tsutomi, H., Mori, R., & Wilson, D. B. (2018). Cognitive-behavioural treatment for amphetamine-type stimulants (ATS)-use disorders. *Cochrane Database of Systematic Reviews*, 12(12). doi:10.1002/14651858.CD011315.PUB2

Himmelstein, G., Bates, D., & Zhou, L. (2022). Examination of stigmatizing language in the electronic health record. *JAMA Network Open*, 5(1). doi:10.1001/JAMANETWORKOPEN.2021.44967

Hirchak, K. A., Lyons, A. J., Herron, J. L., Kordas, G., Shaw, J. L., Jansen, K., Avey, J. P., McPherson, S. M., Donovan, D., Roll, J., Buchwald, D., Ries, R., & McDonell, M. G. (2021). Contingency management for alcohol use disorder reduces cannabis use among American Indian and Alaska Native adults. *Journal of Substance Abuse Treatment*, 137, 108693. doi:10.1016/J.JSAT.2021.108693

Hoffmann, N. G., Harrison, P. A., & Belille, C. A. (1983). Alcoholics Anonymous after treatment: Attendance and abstinence. *International Journal of the Addictions*, 18(3), 311–318. doi:10.3109/10826088309039350

Indivior Inc. (2017). *Sublocade: Highlights of prescribing information*. https://www.accessdata.fda.gov/drugsatfda_docs/label/2017/209819s000lbl.pdf

Janssen Pharmaceuticals. (2012). *Topamax: Highlights of prescribing information*. https://www.accessdata.fda.gov/drugsatfda_docs/label/2012/020844s041lbl.pdf

Jones, A. W. (2019). Forensic drug profile: Cocaethylene. *Journal of Analytical Toxicology*, 43(3), 155–160. doi:10.1093/JAT/BKZ007

Kang, S. Y., Kleinman, P. H., Woody, G. E., Millman, R. B., Todd, T. C., Kemp, J., & Lipton, D. S. (1991). Outcomes for cocaine abusers after once-a-week psychosocial therapy. *American Journal of Psychiatry*, 148(5), 630–635. doi:10.1176/AJP.148.5.630

Keen, J., Oliver, P., Rowse, G., & Mathers, N. (2001). Residential rehabilitation for drug users: A review of 13 months' intake to a therapeutic community. *Family Practice*, 18(5), 545–548. doi:10.1093/FAMPRA/18.5.545

Kelly, J. F., Humphreys, K., & Ferri, M. (2020). Alcoholics Anonymous and other 12-step programs for alcohol use disorder.

Cochrane Database of Systematic Reviews, 3(3), CD012880. doi:10.1002/14651858.CD012880.PUB2

Kelly, J. F., & Westerhoff, C. M. (2010). Does it matter how we refer to individuals with substance-related conditions? A randomized study of two commonly used terms. *International Journal on Drug Policy*, 21(3), 202–207. doi:10.1016/J.DRUGPO.2009.10.010

Kenford, S. L., Fiore, M. C., Jorenby, D. E., Smith, S. S., Wetter, D., & Baker, T. B. (1994). Predicting smoking cessation. Who will quit with and without the nicotine patch. *JAMA*, 271(8), 589–594. doi:10.1001/jama.271.8.589

Kilaru, A. S., Kilaru, A. S., Xiong, A., Lowenstein, M., Meisel, Z. F., Perrone, J., Khatri, U., Mitra, N., & Delgado, M. K. (2020). Incidence of treatment for opioid use disorder following nonfatal overdose in commercially insured patients. *JAMA Network Open*, 3(5). doi:10.1001/JAMANETWORKOPEN.2020.5852

Lagisetty, P. A., Ross, R., Bohnert, A., Clay, M., & Maust, D. T. (2019). Buprenorphine treatment divide by race/ethnicity and payment. *JAMA Psychiatry*, 76(9), 979–981. doi:10.1001/JAMAPSYCHIATRY.2019.0876

Levin, F. R., Mariani, J. J., Brooks, D. J., Pavlicova, M., Cheng, W., & Nunes, E. V. (2011). Dronabinol for the treatment of cannabis dependence: A randomized, double-blind, placebo-controlled trial. *Drug and Alcohol Dependence*, 116(1–3), 142–150. doi:10.1016/J.DRUGALCDEP.2010.12.010

Link, H. M., Jones, H., Miller, L., Kaltenbach, K., & Seligman, N. (2020). Buprenorphine-naloxone use in pregnancy: A systematic review and meta-analysis. *American Journal of Obstetrics & Gynecology MFM*, 2(3), 100179. doi:10.1016/j.ajogmf.2020.100179

Little, M. A., Talcott, G. W., Linde, B. D., Pagano, L. A., Messler, E. C., Ebbert, J. O., & Klesges, R. C. (2016). Efficacy of a brief tobacco intervention for tobacco and nicotine containing product use in the US Air Force. *Nicotine & Tobacco Research*, 18(5), 1142–1149. doi:10.1093/NTR/NTV242

Maldonado, J. R., Sher, Y., Ashouri, J. F., Hills-Evans, K., Swendsen, H., Lolak, S., & Miller, A. C. (2014). The "Prediction of Alcohol Withdrawal Severity Scale" (PAWSS): Systematic literature review and pilot study of a new scale for the prediction of complicated alcohol withdrawal syndrome. *Alcohol*, 48(4), 375–390. doi:10.1016/J.ALCOHOL.2014.01.004

Merck. (2012). *Campral: Highlights of prescribing information*. https://www.accessdata.fda.gov/drugsatfda_docs/label/2012/021431s015lbl.pdf

Merck & Co. (2020). *Remeron: Highlights of prescribing information*. https://www.accessdata.fda.gov/drugsatfda_docs/label/2020/020415s029,%20021208s019lbl.pdf

Miller, S., Fiellin, D., Rosenthal, R., & Saitz, R. (Eds.). (2019). *The ASAM principles of addiction medicine* (6th ed.). Wolters Kluwer.

Moeller, K. E., Lee, K. C., & Kissack, J. C. (2008). Urine drug screening: Practical guide for clinicians. *Mayo Clinic Proceedings*, 83(1), 66–76. doi:10.4065/83.1.66

Myrick, H., Malcolm, R., Randall, P. K., Boyle, E., Anton, R. F., Becker, H. C., & Randall, C. L. (2009). A double-blind trial of gabapentin versus lorazepam in the treatment of alcohol withdrawal. *Alcoholism, Clinical and Experimental Research*, 33(9), 1582–1588. doi:10.1111/J.1530-0277.2009.00986.X

National Center for Health Statistics. (2020). *Wide-Ranging Online Data for Epidemiologic Research (WONDER)*. http://wonder.cdc.gov/

National Center for PTSD. (2015). *Effective treatments for PTSD: Helping patients taper from benzodiazepines*. https://www.pbm.va.gov/PBM/AcademicDetailingService/Documents/Academic_Detailing_Educational_Material_Catalog/59_PTSD_NCPTSD_Provider_Helping_Patients_Taper_BZD.pdf

National Institute on Drug Abuse. (2021). *Tobacco, nicotine, & vaping (e-cigarettes)*. https://teens.drugabuse.gov/drug-facts/tobacco-nicotine-vaping-e-cigarettes

National Institute on Drug Abuse. (2022). *Overdose death rates*. https://nida.nih.gov/drug-topics/trends-statistics/overdose-death-rates

Nelson, N. P., Weng, M. K., Hofmeister, M. G., Moore, K. L., Doshani, M., Kamili, S., Koneru, A., Haber, P., Hagan, L., Romero, J. R., Schillie, S., & Harris, A. M. (2021). Prevention of hepatitis A virus infection in the United States: Recommendations of the Advisory Committee on Immunization Practices, 2020. *MMWR Recommendations and Reports*, 69(5), 1–38. doi:10.15585/MMWR.RR6905A1

O'Donnell, J., Tanz, L. J., Gladden, R. M., Davis, N. L., & Bitting, J. (2021). Trends in and characteristics of drug overdose deaths involving illicitly manufactured fentanyls—United States, 2019–2020. *Morbidity and Mortality Weekly Report*, 70(50), 1740–1746. doi:10.15585/MMWR.MM7050E3

Otto, M. W., McHugh, R. K., Simon, N. M., Farach, F. J., Worthington, J. J., & Pollack, M. H. (2010). Efficacy of CBT for benzodiazepine discontinuation in patients with panic disorder: Further evaluation. *Behaviour Research and Therapy*, 48(8), 720–727. doi:10.1016/J.BRAT.2010.04.002

Pace, C. A., Kaminetzky, L. B., Winter, M., Cheng, D. M., Saia, K., Samet, J. H., & Walley, A. Y. (2014). Postpartum changes in methadone maintenance dose. *Journal of Substance Abuse Treatment*, 47(3), 229–232. doi:10.1016/J.JSAT.2014.04.004

Pauly, B., Wallace, B., Pagan, F., Phillips, J., Wilson, M., Hobbs, H., & Connolly, J. (2020). Impact of overdose prevention sites during a public health emergency in Victoria, Canada. *PloS One*, 15(5). doi:10.1371/JOURNAL.PONE.0229208

Pfizer. (2010a). *Chantix: Highlights of prescribing information*. https://www.accessdata.fda.gov/drugsatfda_docs/label/2010/021928s014s017lbl.pdf

Pfizer. (2010b). *Nicotrol NS*. https://www.accessdata.fda.gov/drugsatfda_docs/label/2010/020385s010lbl.pdf

Pfizer. (2017). *Neurontin: Highlights of prescribing information*. https://www.accessdata.fda.gov/drugsatfda_docs/label/2017/020235s064_020882s047_021129s046lbl.pdf

Pfizer. (2019). *Nicotrol inhaler*. https://www.accessdata.fda.gov/drugsatfda_docs/label/2019/020714s018lbl.pdf

Physicians Total Care. (2012). *Antabuse*. https://dailymed.nlm.nih.gov/dailymed/drugInfo.cfm?setid=12850de3-c97c-42c1-b8d3-55dc6fd05750

Platt, L., Minozzi, S., Reed, J., Vickerman, P., Hagan, H., French, C., Jordan, A., Degenhardt, L., Hope, V., Hutchinson, S., Maher, L., Palmateer, N., Taylor, A., Bruneau, J., & Hickman, M. (2017). Needle syringe programmes and opioid substitution therapy for preventing hepatitis C transmission in people who inject drugs. *Cochrane Database of Systematic Reviews*, 9(9), CD012021. doi:10.1002/14651858.CD012021.PUB2

Potier, C., Laprévote, V., Dubois-Arber, F., Cottencin, O., & Rolland, B. (2014). Supervised injection services: What has been demonstrated? A systematic literature review. *Drug and Alcohol Dependence*, 145, 48–68. doi:10.1016/J.DRUGALCDEP.2014.10.012

Rawson, R. A., Huber, A., McCann, M., Shoptaw, S., Farabee, D., Reiber, C., & Ling, W. (2002). A comparison of contingency management and cognitive-behavioral approaches during methadone maintenance treatment for cocaine dependence. *Archives of General Psychiatry*, 59(9), 817–824. doi:10.1001/ARCHPSYC.59.9.817

Ray, L. A., Meredith, L. R., Kiluk, B. D., Walthers, J., Carroll, K. M., & Magill, M. (2020). Combined pharmacotherapy and cognitive behavioral therapy for adults with alcohol or substance use disorders: A systematic review and meta-analysis. *JAMA Network Open, 3*(6). doi:10.1001/JAMANETWORKOPEN.2020.8279

Reckitt Benckiser Pharmaceuticals Inc. (2010). *Suboxone: Highlights of prescribing information.* https://www.accessdata.fda.gov/drugsatfda_docs/label/2010/022410s000lbl.pdf

Reckitt Benckiser Pharmaceuticals Inc. (2011). *Subutex: Highlights of prescribing information.*

Roxane Laboratories. (2015). *Dolophine: Highlights of prescribing information.* https://www.accessdata.fda.gov/drugsatfda_docs/label/2015/006134s038lbl.pdf

Roy-Byrne, P., Bumgardner, K., Krupski, A., Dunn, C., Ries, R., Donovan, D., West, I. I., Maynard, C., Atkins, D. C., Graves, M. C., Joesch, J. M., & Zarkin, G. A. (2014). Brief Intervention for problem drug use in safety-net primary care settings. *JAMA, 312*(5), 492. doi:10.1001/jama.2014.7860

Saitz, R., Palfai, T. P. A., Cheng, D. M., Alford, D. P., Bernstein, J. A., Lloyd-Travaglini, C. A., Meli, S. M., Chaisson, C. E., & Samet, J. H. (2014). Screening and brief intervention for drug use in primary care: The ASPIRE randomized clinical trial. *JAMA, 312*(5), 502–513. doi:10.1001/JAMA.2014.7862

SAMSHA. (2023, October 10). *Waiver Elimination (MAT Act).* https://www.samhsa.gov/medications-substance-use-disorders/waiver-elimination-mat-act

Santos, G.-M., Ikeda, J., Coffin, P., Walker, J. A., Matheson, T., Ali, A., Mclaughlin, M., Jain, J., Arenander, J., Vittinghoff, E., & Batki, S. (2022). Targeted oral naltrexone for mild to moderate alcohol use disorder among sexual and gender minority men: A randomized trial. *American Journal of Psychiatry, 179*(12), 915–926. doi:10.1176/APPI.AJP.20220335

Schillie, S., Vellozzi, C., Reingold, A., Harris, A., Haber, P., Ward, J. W., & Nelson, N. P. (2019). Prevention of hepatitis B virus infection in the United States: Recommendations of the Advisory Committee on Immunization Practices. *MMWR Recommendations and Reports, 67*(1), 1–31. doi:10.15585/MMWR.RR6701A1

Schillie, S., Wester, C., Osborne, M., Wesolowski, L., & Ryerson, A. B. (2020). CDC recommendations for hepatitis C screening among adults—United States, 2020. *MMWR Recommendations and Reports, 69*(2), 1–17. doi:10.15585/MMWR.RR6902A1

Schnoll, R. A., Goelz, P. M., Veluz-Wilkins, A., Blazekovic, S., Powers, L., Leone, F. T., Gariti, P., Wileyto, E. P., & Hitsman, B. (2015). Long-term nicotine replacement therapy: A randomized clinical trial. *JAMA Internal Medicine, 175*(4), 504–511. doi:10.1001/JAMAINTERNMED.2014.8313

Secades-Villa, R., Vallejo-Seco, G., García-Rodríguez, O., López-Núñez, C., Weidberg, S., & González-Roz, A. (2015). Contingency management for cigarette smokers with depressive symptoms. *Experimental and Clinical Psychopharmacology, 23*(5), 351–360. doi:10.1037/PHA0000044

Shiu, J. R., & Ensom, M. H. H. (2012). Dosing and monitoring of methadone in pregnancy: Literature review. *Canadian Journal of Hospital Pharmacy, 65*(5), 380–386. doi:10.4212/CJHP.V65I5.1176

Simpson, D. D., Joe, G. W., Fletcher, B. W., Hubbard, R. L., & Anglin, M. D. (1999). A national evaluation of treatment outcomes for cocaine dependence. *Archives of General Psychiatry, 56*(6), 507–514. doi:10.1001/ARCHPSYC.56.6.507

Stead, L. F., Carroll, A. J., & Lancaster, T. (2017). Group behaviour therapy programmes for smoking cessation. *Cochrane Database of Systematic Reviews, 3*(3), CD001007. doi:10.1002/14651858.CD001007.PUB3

Substance Abuse and Mental Health Services Administration. (2021). *Key substance use and mental health indicators in the United States: Results from the 2020 National Survey on Drug Use and Health.* https://www.samhsa.gov/data/

Sullivan, J. T., Sykora, K., Schneiderman, J., Naranjo, C. A., & Sellers, E. M. (1989). Assessment of alcohol withdrawal: The revised clinical institute withdrawal assessment for alcohol scale (CIWA-Ar). *British Journal of Addiction, 84*(11), 1353–1357. doi:10.1111/J.1360-0443.1989.TB00737.X

Taylor, M., Petrakis, I., & Ralevski, E. (2017). Treatment of alcohol use disorder and co-occurring PTSD. *American Journal of Drug and Alcohol Abuse, 43*(4), 391–401. doi:10.1080/00952990.2016.1263641

Tweaker. (2020). *Weights & measures.* https://tweaker.org/crystal-meth/weights-measures/

U.S. Drug Enforcement Administration. (2022). *DEA's commitment to expanding access to medication-assisted treatment.* https://www.dea.gov/press-releases/2022/03/23/deas-commitment-expanding-access-medication-assisted-treatment

Vicknasingam, B., Narayanan, S., Singh, D., & Chawarski, M. (2018). Decriminalization of drug use. *Current Opinion in Psychiatry, 31*(4), 300–305. doi:10.1097/YCO.0000000000000429

Volpp, K. G., Troxel, A. B., Pauly, M. V., Glick, H. A., Puig, A., Asch, D. A., Galvin, R., Zhu, J., Wan, F., DeGuzman, J., Corbett, E., Weiner, J., & Audrain-McGovern, J. (2009). A randomized, controlled trial of financial incentives for smoking cessation. *New England Journal of Medicine, 360*(7), 699–709. doi:10.1056/NEJMSA0806819

Walsh, D. C., Hingson, R. W., Merrigan, D. M., Levenson, S. M., Cupples, L. A., Heeren, T., Coffman, G. A., Becker, C. A., Barker, T. A., Hamilton, S. K., McGuire, T. G., & Kelly, C. A. (1991). A randomized trial of treatment options for alcohol-abusing workers. *New England Journal of Medicine, 325*(11), 775–782. doi:10.1056/NEJM199109123251105

Ware, O. D., Manuel, J. I., & Huhn, A. S. (2021). Adults with opioid and methamphetamine co-use have lower odds of completing short-term residential treatment than other opioid co-use groups: A retrospective health services study. *Frontiers in Psychiatry, 12.* doi:10.3389/FPSYT.2021.784229

Wesson, D. R., & Ling, W. (2003). The Clinical Opiate Withdrawal Scale (COWS). *Journal of Psychoactive Drugs, 35*(2), 253–259. doi:10.1080/02791072.2003.10400007

White, A. M., Castle, I.-J. P., Powell, P. A., Hingson, R. W., & Koob, G. F. (2022). Alcohol-related deaths during the COVID-19 pandemic. *JAMA.* doi:10.1001/JAMA.2022.4308

Witbrodt, J., Mertens, J., Kaskutas, L. A., Bond, J., Chi, F., & Weisner, C. (2012). Do 12-step meeting attendance trajectories over 9 years predict abstinence? *Journal of Substance Abuse Treatment, 43*(1), 30–43. doi:10.1016/J.JSAT.2011.10.004

Woodhead, E. L., Brief, D., Below, M., & Timko, C. (2020). Participation in 12-step programs and drug use among older adults with cannabis use disorder: Six-month outcomes. *Journal of Drug Issues, 51*(1), 38–49. doi:10.1177/0022042620957013

Woody, G. E., McLellan, A. T., Luborsky, L., & O'Brien, C. P. (1995). Psychotherapy in community methadone programs: A validation study. *American Journal of Psychiatry, 152*(9), 1302–1308. doi:10.1176/AJP.152.9.1302

Workowski, K. A., Bachmann, L. H., Chan, P. A., Johnston, C. M., Muzny, C. A., Park, I., Reno, H., Zenilman, J. M., & Bolan, G. A. (2021). Sexually transmitted infections treatment guidelines, 2021. *MMWR Recommendations and Reports, 70*(4), 1–187. doi:10.15585/MMWR.RR7004A1

Yale University. (n.d.). *Evaluate with RIPTEAR.*

Yang, L. H., Wong, L. Y., Grivel, M. M., & Hasin, D. S. (2017). Stigma and substance use disorders: An international phenomenon. *Current Opinion in Psychiatry, 30*(5), 378. doi:10.1097/YCO.0000000000000351

CHAPTER 65

Thyroid Disorders

JoAnne M. Saxe

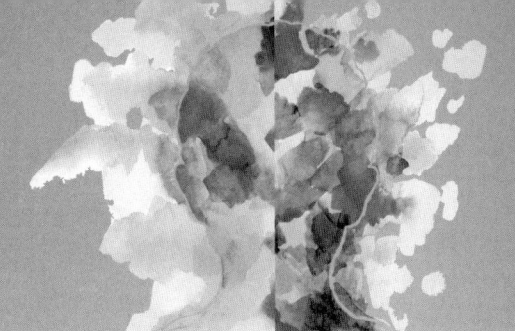

I. Introduction and general background

The adult thyroid gland is responsible for the production of hormones (L-thyroxine [T_4] and 3,5,3'-triiodothyronine [T_3]) that influence a variety of metabolic processes. Its structure and function are contingent on an intact axis between this gland and the hypothalamus and pituitary glands. Specifically, the hypothalamus secretes thyrotropin-releasing hormone (TRH), which stimulates the pituitary to produce and release thyroid-stimulating hormone (TSH). TSH triggers the production and secretion of T_3 and T_4 from the thyroid. Through a positive–negative feedback loop, these glands, when normally functioning, regulate T_3 and T_4 secretion so that metabolic homeostasis is ensured (**Figure 65-1**).

Thyroid gland integrity is dependent on adequate dietary intake of several micronutrients, most notably, iodine, iron, and selenium (Rayman, 2019). If iodine deficiency ensues, thyroid enlargement (goiter) and/or thyroid dysfunction (hypothyroidism or hyperthyroidism) are potential sequelae. Thyroid metabolism is also dependent on adequate stores of iron and selenium. It is recommended that persons with hypothyroidism in general and autoimmune-related thyroid diseases be assessed and treated for iron-deficiency anemia, in addition to the treatment of the thyroid disorder, because inadequate stores of iron can impair the production of thyroid hormones (Ihnatowicz et al., 2020; Rayman, 2019). Although there is insufficient evidence to support the use of selenium supplementation in the treatment of related thyroid disorders (i.e., hypothyroidism, subclinical hypothyroidism, autoimmune thyroid disease, thyroid cancer, and goiter), it is prudent to ensure an adequate dietary intake of selenium, particularly in regions with low levels of selenium intake (e.g., eastern European and Middle Eastern countries, China), given the substantiated role that this element plays in regard to thyroid health (Rayman, 2019; Stoffaneller & Morse, 2015).

Globally, iodine deficiency is the most common cause of thyroid dysfunction. In regions where there is ample iodine supply, most thyroid disorders are due to an underlying autoimmune disorder, which is related to a complex interface between genetic factors, host factors (e.g., intestinal microbiota), environmental factors (e.g., intake of endocrine-disruptive medications and products), additional nutritional factors (e.g., diets high in red and/or processed meat, wheat and refined grains, and fatty dairy products), pregnancy, and/or aging (American College of Obstetrics and Gynecology [ACOG], 2020; Ihnatowicz et al., 2020; Rayman, 2019; Tonstad et al., 2015; Vieira et al., 2014). Commonly presenting thyroid conditions are primary hypothyroidism (with or without goiter); hyperthyroidism (with or without goiter); and thyroid nodules, which may be benign or malignant (Esfandiari & McPhee, 2019).

A. *Primary hypothyroidism*
   1. Definition and overview
      This is a condition in which there is a loss of thyroid function as a result of the intrinsic thyroid pathology. Primary hypothyroidism accounts for over 99% of all cases of hypothyroidism (Chaker et al., 2017). (Note: Secondary and tertiary hypothyroidism, which are uncommon conditions, are due to pathology in the pituitary gland and hypothalamus, respectively.)

      The most common causes of primary hypothyroidism in iodine-sufficient countries are related to:
   a. Thyroid inflammatory diseases, with the majority being on the autoimmune spectrum (e.g., Hashimoto thyroiditis [chronic autoimmune thyroiditis], postpartum thyroiditis, and subacute thyroiditis). The initial presentation of thyroid inflammatory diseases, however, may be a transient presentation of thyrotoxicosis (a term referring to any condition that causes elevated levels of circulating thyroid hormones) followed by a euthyroid state (a period of normal thyroid hormone levels) prior to developing hypothyroidism, which may be permanent or transitory. For

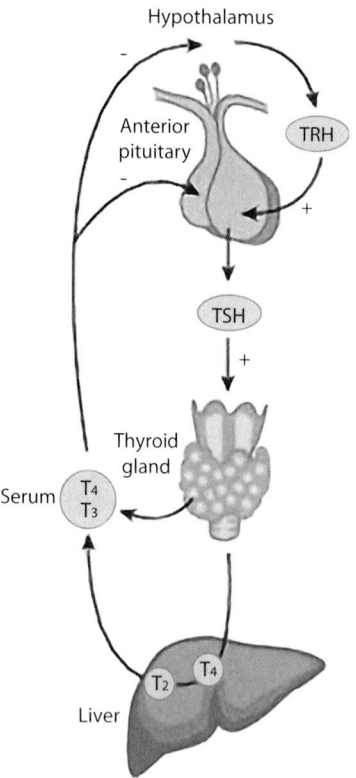

Figure 65-1 Hypothalamus, Anterior pituitary, Thyroid gland, Serum, Liver

example, in the case of the subacute, viral-related thyroiditis, there is an increase in circulating thyroid hormones as a result of thyroid tissue damage, not due to alterations in thyroid functionality. As such, most individuals return to a euthyroid state within a few months after the resolution of the infectious process.
   b. Radioiodine-induced or surgically induced interventions
   c. Various medications (e.g., amiodarone and lithium) (Jameson et al., 2018a; McDermott, 2020; Saxe, 2004).
   2. Epidemiology
   As noted by the ACOG (2020), several studies have noted that the prevalence of overt hypothyroidism ranges from 0.2% to 5.3% in Europe and from 0.3% to 3.7% in the United States. However, the prevalence of subclinical hypothyroidism (a person who has abnormalities in chemical markers, an elevated TSH, and normal free T_4 hormone, yet is clinically euthyroid) in similar populations is estimated to be between 3% and 10% (Schübel et al., 2017). Per several surveys, females are 10 times more likely to have primary hypothyroidism than males (note that gender was conveyed in binary terms), with the female population over the age of 40 having the greatest prevalence (ACOG, 2020; Hollowell et al., 2002; Madariaga et al., 2014; Wang & Crapo, 1997). (Note: This author did not appreciate any frequency data pertaining to hypothyroidism specifically related to transgender individuals.) Additionally, in the United States, hypothyroidism has been reported to be more common in White, non-Hispanic Americans and Mexican Americans than in Black, non-Hispanic Americans (Hollowell et al., 2002). There is a need for research to determine the interrelationships between the multiple health determinants that influence this variability.

B. **Hyperthyroidism**
   1. Definition and overview
   Hyperfunctioning of the thyroid gland can result from a variety of diseases. The most common causes of hyperthyroidism are:
      a. Diffuse toxic goiter (commonly known as *Graves disease*), which is an autoimmune disorder
      b. Toxic multinodular goiter
      c. Autonomously functioning thyroid adenoma (also known as *toxic uninodular goiter*) (ACOG, 2020; Vanderpump, 2011)

      As previously noted, thyroid inflammatory diseases (e.g., Hashimoto thyroiditis, postpartum thyroiditis) may cause a transient thyrotoxicosis. In these conditions, tissues throughout the body are subjected to elevated levels of circulating thyroid hormones as a result of thyroid tissue damage, not from excessive synthesis and secretion of thyroid hormones, as seen with Graves disease (Cooper & Ladenson, 2017).
   2. Epidemiology
   Data from the Whickham survey and other studies indicate that the prevalence and incidence of hyperthyroidism in males are low (Vanderpump, 2011; Wang & Crapo, 1997). In females, the prevalence of overt hyperthyroidism is between 0.5% and 2% (note that gender was conveyed in binary terms) (Vanderpump, 2011). As with primary hypothyroidism, hyperthyroidism, all causes combined, is most commonly seen in females during and after the fourth decade of life (Cooper & Ladenson, 2017; Wang & Crapo, 1997), yet with significant variability in prevalence noted in different regions of the world (Vanderpump, 2011). (Note: This author did not appreciate any frequency data pertaining to hyperthyroidism specifically related to transgender persons.)

C. *Thyroid nodules*
   1. Definition and overview
   Thyroid nodules may be functional (secrete thyroid hormones) or nonfunctional and are usually benign. However, a malignancy should be suspected, particularly if an individual has the following risk profile: <45 years of age; history of external head or neck ionizing radiation; predominant nodule or recent growth of a nodule, particularly if it does not alter thyroid function; associated hoarseness and dysphagia; higher body weight; alcohol and/or tobacco use; flame-retardant exposure; and a family history of medullary cancer of the thyroid and/or hereditary thyroid cancer syndromes (e.g., Cowden disease and familial adenomatous polyposis)

(Cooper & Ladenson, 2017; Metzger, 2016; Seib & Sosa, 2019).

2. Epidemiology

Thyroid nodules are common entities. The prevalence rates of nodules vary by detection method (e.g., palpation, ultrasound, or other imaging), with rates of up to 50% of individuals who have had a thyroid ultrasound (Cooper & Ladenson, 2017). Most of the detected nodules are benign, and they are more commonly noted in females than in males (Cooper & Ladenson, 2017). (Note: This author did not appreciate any frequency data pertaining to thyroid nodules specifically related to transgender individuals.) Except for malignant nodules, thyroid nodules are more prevalent with increasing age, as noted by incidence rates (Cooper & Ladenson et al., 2017; Howlader et al., 2014). There has been, however, a rising incidence of thyroid malignancies in the United States since 1975. The age-adjusted incidence rate for thyroid cancer was 4.85/100,000 in 1975 (National Cancer Institute, 2021). The age-adjusted rate of new cases of thyroid cancer was 15.5 per 100,000 per year based on 2014–2018 reported cases (National Cancer Institute, 2021). This increase in case rates is largely due to the incidental finding of thyroid nodules and malignancies via imaging that has been completed for unrelated reasons (Cooper & Ladenson, 2017; Seib & Sosa, 2019).

II. Database (may include but is not limited to)

A. *Subjective*

1. Primary hypothyroidism
   a. Past health history
      i. Medical history: autoimmune thyroid disorders that can be associated with other autoimmune diseases, such as celiac disease, type 1 diabetes mellitus, pernicious anemia, rheumatoid arthritis, and systemic lupus erythematosus, and secondary or tertiary hypothyroidism caused by pituitary or hypothalamic diseases (low TSH and low free FT_4), respectively.
      ii. Surgical history: thyroid or pituitary surgery
      iii. Obstetric and gynecological history: recent pregnancy or parturition
      iv. Trauma history: brain trauma
      v. Exposure history: radiation (e.g., radioiodine therapy or external head and neck irradiation) and other toxins (e.g., flame retardants)
      vi. Medication history: medications or supplements that influence the synthesis of thyroid hormones (e.g., amiodarone, lithium, and iodine)
   b. Family history
      i. Thyroid diseases
      ii. Other endocrinopathies
      iii. Autoimmune disorders
   c. Occupational and environmental history: work-related exposures to radiation or radioactive iodine and other toxins, such as flame retardants and mercury
   d. Personal and social history: iodine-deficient diet (uncommon in regions that have iodination programs), dietary intake of iron and selenium, and country of origin to note if iodine deficiency or excess and/or selenium deficiency is/are common.
   e. Review of systems: Signs and symptoms vary depending on the degree of thyroid dysfunction. The individual with subclinical hypothyroidism or mild hypothyroidism is frequently asymptomatic. Persons with moderate dysfunction often notice constitutional, and skin signs and symptoms. The individual with advanced disease often has multisystem signs and symptoms. The person with long-standing, undiagnosed, and severe thyroid hormone deficiency may present with myxedema coma. The diagnosis of this condition is usually determined by objective data because the individual is obtunded.
      i. Constitutional signs and symptoms: fatigue, weight gain, or cold intolerance
      ii. Skin, hair, and nails: dry skin, puffy and doughy skin, and coarse hair or hair loss
      iii. Ear, nose, and throat: decreased hearing, hoarseness, dysphagia, or dysarthria
      iv. Cardiac: chest pain
      v. Abdomen: constipation
      vi. Genitourinary: oligomenorrhea and menorrhagia
      vii. Musculoskeletal: joint stiffness or pain and myalgias
      viii. Neurologic: paresthesias, lethargy, less expressive at rest, depressed mood, and/or rarely ataxic gait

2. Hyperthyroidism
   a. Past health history
      i. Medical illnesses: Graves disease, toxic uninodular or multinodular goiter, or rarely pituitary TSH-secreting tumor
      ii. Surgical history: thyroid surgery
      iii. Obstetric and gynecological history: recent pregnancy or parturition
      iv. Exposure history: toxins (e.g., flame retardants)
      v. Medication history: medications or supplements that influence the production of thyroid hormones (e.g., antithyroid drug use [propylthiouracil (PTU) or methimazole], amiodarone, lithium, exogenous thyroid hormone supplements, and iodine)
   b. Family history
      i. Thyroid diseases
      ii. Other endocrinopathies
      iii. Autoimmune diseases

c. Personal and social history: a recent intake of an iodine-rich diet in an individual who previously had an iodine-deficient diet (geographic regions that may not have iodination programs and that have limited access to iodine-containing foods are certain regions in South America, Africa, and Asia), long-term exposure to excessive iodine intake, and country of origin to note if iodine deficiency or excess and/or selenium deficiency is/are common
d. Occupational and environmental history: work-related exposures to toxins, such as flame retardants and mercury
e. Review of systems: signs and symptoms vary depending on the degree of thyroid dysfunction. The individual with subclinical and mild hyperthyroidism may be relatively asymptomatic. Persons with moderate dysfunction often notice constitutional signs and symptoms, palpitations, increased bowel motility, and neurologic signs and symptoms, as described next. The individual with advanced disease often has multisystem symptomatology.
  i. Constitutional signs and symptoms: weakness, fatigue in the elderly, increased appetite, weight loss, insomnia, or heat intolerance
  ii. Skin: increased perspiration; pretibial myxedema in Graves disease
  iii. Eyes: proptosis in Graves disease
  iv. Ear, nose, and throat: hoarseness or dysphagia
  v. Pulmonary: dyspnea
  vi. Cardiac: chest pain or palpitations
  vii. Abdomen: increased bowel motility that often results in frequent bowel movements
  viii. Genitourinary: irregular menses or amenorrhea
  ix. Neurologic: tremors, or nervousness and anxiety
3. Thyroid nodules
  a. Past health history
    i. Medical history: thyroid disorders, including thyroid cancer, and autoimmune disorders that may cause a nodular gland (e.g., Graves disease)
    ii. Surgical history: thyroid surgery
    iii. Exposure history: radiation (e.g., radioiodine therapy or external head and neck irradiation)
    iv. Medication history: medications or supplements that influence hormone production (e.g., lithium and iodine)
  b. Family history: thyroid diseases, including goitrous thyroid conditions and thyroid cancer
  c. Occupational and environmental history: work-related exposures to radiation or radioactive iodine and other toxins, such as mercury
  d. Personal and social history
    i. Iodine-deficient diet or iodine-excessive diet (see primary hypothyroidism and hyperthyroidism for discussion)
    ii. Regular ingestion of dietary goitrogens (e.g., certain cruciferous vegetables, such as turnips, and beans, such as lima beans) (Eastman & Zimmermann, 2018)
    iii. Tobacco use
    iv. Alcohol intake
  e. Review of systems
    The nodules may be nonfunctional, in which case the individual is clinically euthyroid. However, the nodules or nodular gland may be hypofunctioning (resulting in signs and symptoms consistent with hypothyroidism) or autonomously functioning (resulting in signs and symptoms of hyperthyroidism). See the previous discussion on primary hypothyroidism or hyperthyroidism, respectively, if an altered thyroid hormone status is suspected.
    It is important to inquire about symptoms, such as dysphagia, caused by an enlarged gland or hoarseness suggestive of malignant vocal cord infiltration (Cooper & Ladenson, 2017).
B. *Objective*
  1. Physical examination findings (**Table 65-1**)
  2. Supporting data from relevant diagnostic tests (**Tables 65-2** and **65-3**)

III. Assessment
A. *Determine the diagnosis.*
  1. Primary hypothyroidism
  2. Hyperthyroidism
  3. Thyroid neoplasms (benign or malignant)
  4. Other conditions that may explain the patient's presentation
    a. Pituitary disease
    b. Hypothalamic disease
    c. Cardiovascular disease
    d. Extrathyroidal malignancy
    e. Psychiatric disorder
B. *Severity*
  Assess the severity of the disease: distinguish early and mild disease with few or no signs and symptoms from advanced and/or life-threatening disease with multisystem symptomatology and findings.
C. *Significance and motivation*
  1. Assess the significance of the problem to the patient and significant others.
  2. Determine the patient's willingness and ability to follow the treatment plan.

IV. Goals of clinical management
A. *Screening or diagnosing thyroid disease*
  Choose a cost-effective approach for screening or diagnosing thyroid disease.

Table 65-1 Physical Examination Findings

Condition	Associated Findings (May or May Not Include)
Primary hypothyroidism	Assess: 1. Vital signs: hypothermia, bradypnea (advanced manifestation), bradycardia, and/or increase in weight 2. General appearance: flat affect and/or dull facial expressions 3. Skin/hair: dry skin (early manifestation) to pasty, rough, and spongy skin (advanced manifestation); coarse hair (early manifestation) to hair loss (advanced manifestation) 4. Eyes: periorbital edema (advanced manifestation) 5. Ears, nose, and throat: enlarged tongue (advanced manifestation) 6. Thyroid: nonpalpable gland to a symmetrically enlarged and smooth gland to a multinodular enlarged gland 7. Lungs: crackles (advanced manifestation) 8. Cardiovascular: (+) S_4, (+) S_3, and jugular venous distention (advanced manifestations) 9. Abdomen: diminished bowel sounds 10. Neurologic: decreased tendon reflexes or enhanced relaxation phase, depressed mood, inattentiveness, and/or somnolence; or obtunded (advanced manifestation)
Hyperthyroidism	Assess: 1. Vital signs: tachycardia and/or decrease in weight 2. General appearance: restless 3. Skin/hair: moist and warm skin, pretibial myxedema (most suggestive of Graves disease), and/or fine and very smooth hair 4. Eyes: exophthalmos/proptosis due to Graves disease and/or eye signs related to sympathetic hyperstimulation (lid lag, lid retraction, diminished blinking, inability to crease the eyebrows on upward stare) 5. Thyroid: single nodule (toxic uninodular goiter); tender or painless, symmetrically enlarged gland (thyroiditis) or diffusely enlarged (Graves disease); and/or thyroid bruit (Graves disease) 6. Lungs: crackles 7. Cardiovascular: systolic murmur and/or (+) S_4, (+) S_3; jugular venous distention 8. Abdomen: enhanced bowel sounds 9. Neurologic: increased tendon reflexes and/or fine tremor of the hands and tongue
Thyroid nodules	The associated findings are contingent on the functional status of the thyroid: 1. Nonfunctional nodule(s): Exam will be relevant only for a thyroid gland with palpable nodule(s) or asymmetry of the gland. 2. Hypofunctioning multinodular gland: See the Primary Hypothyroidism Associated Findings section. 3. Autonomously functioning nodule(s): See the Hyperthyroidism Associated Findings section. 4. Lymph nodes: Assess lymph nodes of the head and neck (may suggest a malignancy).

Table 65-2 Common Thyroid Tests*

Test	Definition	Clinical Implications	Comments
Serum-free T_4 (FT_4)	Measurement of the metabolically active T_4 (unbound to thyroid-binding globulin)	Decreased in primary hypothyroidism Increased in thyrotoxicosis	May be increased by various drugs or conditions in individuals who are clinically euthyroid
Serum T_3	Measurement of bound and free serum levels of T_3	Increased in T_3 thyrotoxicosis	May be increased by various drugs or conditions in individuals who are clinically euthyroid

(continues)

Table 65-2 Common Thyroid Tests* *(continued)*

Test	Definition	Clinical Implications	Comments
Highly sensitive thyroid-stimulating hormone (TSH)	Measurement of TSH, an anterior pituitary hormone that stimulates growth and function of thyroid cells	Sensitive and specific test for the initial assessment of thyroid dysfunction Increased in primary hypothyroidism Decreased in most forms of thyrotoxicosis	Acceptable or optimal TSH ranges may vary for persons who are pregnant or elderly and/or have a history of pituitary gland disease or thyroid cancer. Values may be altered by certain drugs (e.g., aspirin and lithium).
Serum antithyroid antibodies (e.g., antithyroid peroxidase antibodies [also known as *antithyroid microsomal antibody*], antithyroglobulin antibodies, and TSH receptor–stimulating, TSH receptor–binding, and TSH receptor–blocking antibodies)	Measurement of immunologic markers for autoimmune thyroid diseases	Increased antithyroid peroxidase antibodies and/or thyroglobulin antibodies are seen in Hashimoto thyroiditis and Graves disease. TSH receptor–stimulating antibodies (also known as *thyroid-stimulating immunoglobulin*) are commonly seen in persons with Graves disease.	May be increased in clinically euthyroid individuals
Radioactive iodine uptake	Measurement of thyroid function via uptake of radioactive iodine (^{123}I) or technetium ^{99m}Tc pertechnetate (^{99m}TcO4)	Used to evaluate defects in thyroid hormone production Low uptake of radioactive iodine noted with non–iodine-deficient hypothyroidism, thyroiditis, and factitious thyrotoxicosis Increased uptake is often seen with Graves disease and toxic multinodular and uninodular goiter.	Variety of medications may interfere with uptake of the radioisotope. This test is usually not necessary for the basic evaluation of most thyroid disorders. Contraindications are iodine allergy, pregnancy, and lactation.
Thyroid scintiscan	Visualization of the thyroid gland via a scintillation camera after the administration of a radioactive isotope (e.g., ^{123}I or ^{99m}TcO4)	This test provides information about the structure and function of the thyroid gland. Increased uptake of the radioactive isotope is noted in a (hot) hyperfunctioning gland or nodule (e.g., Graves disease and toxic uninodular goiter, respectively). Decreased uptake is seen in hypothyroidism or nonfunctioning (cold) nodule (e.g., thyroid cancer).	Variety of medications may interfere with uptake of the radioisotope. This test is usually not indicated for the evaluation of primary hypothyroidism. Contraindications are iodine allergy, pregnancy, or lactation.

* Normal ranges may vary from one clinical laboratory to another. Please refer to the respective clinical lab for reference ranges.

Data from Saxe, J. M. (2004). Thyroid diseases. In W. L. Star, L. L. Lommel, & M. T. Shannon (Eds.), *Women's primary health care: Protocols for practice* (2nd ed., pp. 10-33–10-39). San Francisco, CA: UCSF Nursing Press; reassessed and adapted Fischbach, F.T., & Fischbach, M.A. (2018). A manual of laboratory and diagnostic tests (10th ed.). Philadelphia, PA: Wolters Kluwer and Jameson, Jameson J, & Mandel S.J., & Weetman A.P. (2018b). Thyroid gland physiology and testing. Jameson J, & Fauci A.S., & Kasper D.L., & Hauser S.L., & Longo D.L., & Loscalzo J(Eds.), Harrison's Principles of Internal Medicine, (20th ed., Chapter 375) McGraw Hill. Retrieved July 24, 2021, from https://accessmedicine-mhmedical-com.ucsf.idm.oclc.org/content.aspx?bookid=2129&sectionid=179924504; Used with permission from the UCSF Nursing Press.

Table 65-3 Supporting Data From Other Relevant Diagnostics Studies*

Condition	Diagnostic Test	Results
Primary hypothyroidism	■ Serum sodium ■ Serum cholesterol ■ Complete blood count ■ Electrocardiogram and/or echocardiogram	■ Decreased (advanced disease) ■ Increased ■ Mild normocytic, normochromic anemia, commonly referred to as an *anemia of chronic disease* (Note: A low hematocrit, hemoglobin, and mean corpuscular volume may be present that could be consistent with iron-deficiency anemia, which may influence successful treatment of a thyroid disorder. A follow-up serum ferritin and additional iron studies would help to differentiate between the anemia of chronic disease/inflammation and iron-deficiency anemia.) ■ Changes secondary to a hypometabolic state and/or congestive heart failure
Thyrotoxicosis and hyperthyroidism	■ Complete blood count ■ Erythrocyte sedimentation rate (ESR) ■ Electrocardiogram and/or echocardiogram	■ Mild normocytic, normochromic anemia may occur with autoimmune-related hyperthyroidism ■ Elevated white blood count (WBC) with some of the thyroid inflammatory conditions (e.g., subacute thyroiditis) ■ Elevated ESR with some of the thyroid inflammatory conditions (e.g., subacute thyroiditis) ■ Changes secondary to a hypermetabolic state and/or congestive heart failure
Thyroid nodules	■ Hypofunctioning gland (see Primary Hypothyroidism) ■ Hyperfunctioning gland (see Thyrotoxicosis) ■ Thyroid ultrasonography ■ Fine-needle aspiration (FNA) biopsy	■ Differentiates a solid from a cystic (a fluid-filled nodule that is usually benign) nodule ■ Benign, malignant, or suspicious/indeterminate

* Not usually indicated for confirming the diagnosis of thyroid dysfunction but rather for assessing target organ damage or thyroid cancer.

B. *Treatment*
Select a treatment plan that returns the patient to a euthyroid state in a safe, effective and economical manner.

C. *Patient adherence*
Select an approach that maximizes patient adherence.

V. Plan

A. *Screening*
Per the U.S. Preventive Services Task Force (2015), there is insufficient evidence to support routine screening for thyroid disorders in nonpregnant, asymptomatic (average-risk) adults. Additionally, the American College of Obstetricians (2020), the American Association of Clinical Endocrinologists, and the American Thyroid Association (Garber et al., 2012) do not support general screening for thyroid disease in pregnancy because the detection and management of subclinical hypothyroidism and hyperthyroidism in pregnancy have not been correlated with improved pregnancy, fetal, or infant outcomes. Some authorities (Garber et al., 2012; Slovik, 2021b) recommend a "case-finding" approach for asymptomatic, at-risk populations (e.g., adults >60 years of age, individuals with autoimmune diseases and/or a history of infertility, persons taking medications that may affect thyroid function, and/or those with a strong family history of thyroid diseases). If the clinician and patient determine that the benefits of screening or case finding for thyroid disease outweigh the disadvantages of this process, the initial screening test should be the highly sensitive TSH because it is more sensitive and specific than the FT_4 and the FT_4I (Jameson et al., 2018b). If the highly sensitive TSH is high or low, the clinician should use the suggested diagnostic approach in **Table 65-4**.

B. *Diagnostic tests*
See Tables 65-2 and 65-3 for the description of relevant diagnostic studies and Table 65-4 for the suggested approach to the assessment of thyroid dysfunction.

1. Common thyroid studies may include but are not limited to highly sensitive TSH, free T_4 (FT_4), T_3, serum antithyroid antibodies, radioactive iodine uptake, and thyroid scintigraphy.
2. Thyroid ultrasonography with a survey of cervical lymph nodes is indicated for an individual with

Table 65-4 The Assessment of Thyroid Dysfunction

Order the highly sensitive thyroid-stimulating hormone (TSH) test		
↓	↓	↓
Normal TSH→ Are secondary causes of hypothyroidism suspected?	**Increased TSH→** Order a serum FT_4	**Decreased TSH→** Order a serum FT_4
No→ No further testing is indicated. The patient is clinically euthyroid.	Decreased FT_4—primary hypothyroidism	Increased FT_4—primary hyperthyroidism→ Order TSH receptor–stimulating antibodies ■ If the antibodies are elevated, the person has an autoimmune thyroid disease (e.g., Graves disease). ■ If the antibodies are normal, the patient probably has a non–immune-mediated form of thyrotoxicosis (e.g., toxic uninodular goiter). ■ Consult with a physician to determine the need for a thyroid scintiscan.
Yes→ Order a serum FT_4	Increased FT_4—pituitary (TSH-induced) thyrotoxicosis	Normal FT_4—subclinical hyperthyroidism or a rare form of primary hyperthyroidism called T_3 toxicosis Does the patient have signs and symptoms consistent with thyrotoxicosis?
Decreased FT_4→ Consult with a physician to determine the necessity for a thyrotropin-releasing hormone (TRH) stimulation test (a test for assessing the hypothalamic–pituitary function).	Normal FT_4—subclinical hypothyroidism→ Order thyroid peroxidase antibodies. ■ If the antibodies are elevated, the person has compensated chronic Hashimoto thyroiditis (subclinical hypothyroidism). ■ If the antibodies are normal, consult with a physician to determine the necessity for a TRH stimulation test.	Yes→ Order T_3 Increased T_3—T_3 toxicosis ■ Consult with a physician to determine the need for a thyroid scintiscan. ■ Normal→ Consult with a physician for other diagnostic considerations

Reproduced from Saxe, J. M. (2004). Thyroid diseases. In W. L. Star, L. L. Lommel, & M. T. Shannon (Eds.), *Women's primary health care: Protocols for practice* (2nd ed., pp. 10-33–10-39). San Francisco, CA: UCSF Nursing Press; reassessed and adapted Fischbach, F.T., & Fischbach, M.A. (2018). A manual of laboratory and diagnostic tests (10th ed.). Philadelphia, PA: Wolters Kluwer and Jameson, Jameson J, & Mandel S.J., & Weetman A.P. (2018b). Thyroid gland physiology and testing. Jameson J, & Fauci A.S., & Kasper D.L., & Hauser S.L., & Longo D.L., & Loscalzo J(Eds.), Harrison's Principles of Internal Medicine, (20th ed., Chapter 375) McGraw Hill. Retrieved July 24, 2021, from https://accessmedicine-mhmedical-com.ucsf.idm.oclc.org/content.aspx?bookid=2129&sectionid=179924504; Used with permission from the UCSF Nursing Press.

thyroid nodules noted on physical examination so as to differentiate between solid and cystic lesions or those who have a neck mass of questionable thyroid origin (Haugen et al., 2016).

3. Fine-needle aspiration is necessary to rule out a cancerous nodule, not purely cystic nodules (Haugen et al., 2016).
4. Extrathyroidal diagnostic studies are warranted for assessing the status of other systems that may be affected by altered thyroid functions (Table 65-3).

C. *Management (includes treatment, consultation, referral, and follow-up care)*
   1. Primary hypothyroidism
      a. Emphasize avoidance of specific exposures (e.g., bisphenol A in plastic water bottles and work-related radiation) and, if possible, medications (e.g., lithium) that may negatively affect the thyroid gland.
      b. Ensure adequate dietary iodine intake in populations in which iodine deficiency is common. All U.S. women who are planning pregnancy, pregnant, or breastfeeding should take a multivitamin containing 150 micrograms of iodine per day because mild iodine deficiency is common (American Thyroid Association, 2013).
      c. Recommend a diet that is rich in a variety of plant-based foods and with fish, seafood, lean red meats, and poultry included in moderation, which will support healthy gut microbiota and immune function, and assure adequate intake of selenium and other micronutrients

(Myers, 2015; National Institutes of Health, 2021; Tonstad et al., 2015; Vieira et al., 2014).
   d. Arrange a hospital admission for patients with severe cardiopulmonary compromise.
   e. Begin oral replacement with L-thyroxine (a synthetic T_4 hormone). Note: To date, there is no evidence that one type of L-thyroxine medication has greater efficacy than another. Yet, as noted by Katz (2023) via his review of the literature, there are data that these products do have differences in bioavailability. As such, patients should be maintained on the same L-thyroxine formulation.
      i. Suggested initial dosing for a young adult without cardiac disorders: 50–100 mcg/day
      ii. Suggested initial dosing for an elder or an individual with heart conditions: 25 mcg/day
   f. Increase dosage by 25–50 mcg every 4–6 weeks until the person's highly sensitive TSH is within normal parameters. The usual replacement dose is 1.6–1.7 mcg/kg/day for adults (Cooper & Ladenson, 2017).
   g. Sustain a full replacement of L-thyroxine, which is usually 100–150 mcg daily.
   h. Check the person's highly sensitive TSH every 6–12 months or as needed to assess the response to chronic therapy and to determine the need for any adjustment in daily doses (Slovik, 2021b).
2. Hyperthyroidism
   a. Reduce the intake of iodine if thought to be a contributing factor.
   b. Emphasize avoidance of specific exposures (e.g., mercury) and, if possible, medications (e.g., amiodarone) that may negatively affect the thyroid gland.
   c. Recommend a diet that is rich in a variety of plant-based foods, with fish, seafood, lean red meats, and poultry included in moderation. See the primary hypothyroidism management section for details.
   d. Start the use of β-blocking agents (e.g., propranolol, 20 mg every 6 hours) to blunt the symptoms and signs of hyperthyroidism (e.g., palpitations, heat intolerance, nervousness, and tremor), if not contraindicated (Slovik, 2021a).
   e. Consult with a physician for the use and dosing of antithyroid agents (e.g., thionamide drugs, such as methimazole [usual starting dose 10–15 mg/day, yet higher doses may be required for persons with large goiters or more severe hyperthyroidism], propylthiouracil [PTU; average starting dose of PTU is 300 mg/day (100 mg every 8 hours)], or iodide [dosing varies according to the specific condition]) (Slovik, 2021a). PTU should be given to pregnant women during the first trimester of pregnancy because methimazole can cause teratogenic effects (Hackmon et al., 2012). Although the thionamide drugs have an overall low rate of serious adverse effects, hepatotoxicity, vasculitis, and agranulocytosis are the most serious adverse sequelae. PTU is more likely to cause fulminant hepatic failure and vasculitis than methimazole. Cholestatic jaundice is more likely to occur with methimazole than PTU. An autoimmune agranulocytosis can occur with both agents but may be less likely to occur in low doses of methimazole (less than or equal to 30 mg/day) than with PTU. Iodide is usually reserved for individuals in thyroid storm and for those being prepared for thyroid surgery (Katz, 2023).
   f. Refer the patient to a physician specialist for ablative therapy with radioactive agents (e.g., radioactive iodine) or subtotal thyroidectomy.
   g. Refer the patient to an ophthalmologist for the assessment and management of Graves ophthalmopathy disease, also known as thyroid eye disease.
   h. Facilitate a hospital admission for the person with severe cardiopulmonary and/or neurologic compromise.
   i. Assess TSH levels annually or as needed after the individual is in remission to determine the adequacy of treatment and the earliest evidence of overtreatment (evidence of hypothyroidism). If the values are abnormal, assess the FT_4 or serum T_3 levels. TSH receptor antibodies should also be obtained if the individual has Graves disease. Consult with or refer to a physician for additional treatment if these tests are abnormal (Slovik, 2021a).
   j. Screen and treat for osteoporosis in cisgender and transgender females with hyperthyroidism (Radix & Deutsch, 2016).
3. Thyroid nodules
   a. Refer the patient with a solitary nodule or a dominant nodule within a multinodular gland to an endocrinologist for further diagnostic evaluation (fine-needle aspiration and possible thyroid scintigraphy) and for therapeutic interventions (e.g., L-thyroxine suppressive or replacement therapy or surgical therapy).
   b. Emphasize the importance of avoiding exposures that can increase the risk for thyroid cancer (e.g., work-related mercury and radiation exposure).
   c. Stop goiter-producing medications, if possible (e.g., lithium). Consultation with the prescribing provider should be considered.
   d. Use the hypothyroidism treatment guidelines (see the management section) for the person with a hypofunctioning multinodular goiter (e.g., chronic thyroiditis).
   e. Use the hyperthyroidism treatment guidelines (see the management section) for the individual with a toxic multinodular goiter.

D. Patient education
1. Information
   Provide verbal and, preferably, written information regarding:
   a. Risk reduction and screening (e.g., dietary recommendations, stress management and relapse prevention in autoimmune-mediated thyroid disease, and osteoporosis screening for cisgender and transgender females with hyperthyroidism)
   b. The disease process, including signs and symptoms and underlying etiologies
   c. Diagnostic tests, including a discussion about preparation, cost, the actual procedure(s), and aftercare
   d. Management (rationale, action, use, drug interactions, side effects, associated risks, and cost of therapeutic interventions; need for adhering to long-term treatment plans) (Saxe, 2004).
2. Counseling: preconception counseling as indicated for childbearing persons.

VI. Self-management resources and tools
A. Patient education
   1. American Thyroid Association (ATA)
      The ATA's (2024) website has patient education brochures and frequently-asked-question documents in English and Spanish. The documents, albeit useful and accurate, have an average grade 9–10 reading level via the Flesch–Kincaid assessment tool. Additionally, there are few photographs, figures, or graphs to facilitate further understanding of challenging concepts.
   2. Geisinger's Health Library (powered by Krames online)
      The Geisinger's Health Library (2009–2024) includes consumer-friendly resources on common thyroid problems. The Flesch–Kincaid reading level is approximately grade 7. This educational resource includes colorful illustrations and culturally appropriate images.
B. Community support groups and resources
   1. ATA
      The ATA (2024) has support group postings (e.g., thyroid patient education health forum).
   2. U.S. Department of Agriculture (USDA), Food and Nutrition Service
      Some individuals may need nutritional support resources to ensure a balanced diet that includes an adequate intake of macronutrients and micronutrients needed for thyroid and immune function. For details about specific programs, go to the USDA (2024) website.

References

American College of Obstetrics and Gynecology. (2020). Thyroid disease in pregnancy: ACOG practice bulletin, Number 223. *Obstetrics and Gynecology*, 135(6), e261–e274. doi:10.1097/AOG.0000000000003893

American Thyroid Association. (2013). *ATA statement on the potential risks of excess iodine ingestion and exposure.* https://www.thyroid.org/ata-statement-on-the-potential-risks-of-excess-iodine-ingestion-and-exposure/

American Thyroid Association. (2024). *ATA patient information.* http://www.thyroid.org/thyroid-information/

Chaker, L., Bianco, A. C., Jonklaas, J., & Peeters, R. P. (2017). Hypothyroidism. *Lancet*, 23, 390(10101), 1550–1562. doi:10.1016/S0140-6736(17)30703-1

Cooper, D. S., & Ladenson, P. W. (2017). The thyroid gland. In D. G. Gardner D. Shoback (Eds.), *Greenspan's basic & clinical endocrinology* (10th ed., Chapter 7). McGraw-Hill.

Eastman, C. J., & Zimmermann, M. B. (2018). The iodine deficiency disorders. In K. R. Feingold, B. Anawalt, & A. Boyce, et al. (Eds.), *Endotext*. MDText.com. https://www.ncbi.nlm.nih.gov/books/NBK285556/

Esfandiari, N. H., & McPhee, S. J. (2019). Thyroid disease. In G. D. Hammer & S. J. McPhee (Eds.), *Pathophysiology of disease: An introduction to clinical medicine* (8th ed., Chapter 20). McGraw-Hill. https://accessmedicine.mhmedical.com/content.aspx?bookid=2468&sectionid=198224090

Fischbach, F. T., & Fischbach, M. A. (2018). *A manual of laboratory and diagnostic tests* (10th ed.). Wolters Kluwer.

Garber, J. R., Cobin, R. H., Gharib, H., Hennessey, J. V., Klein, I., Mechanick, J. I., Pessah-Pollack, R., Singer, P. A., Woeber, K. A., & American Association of Clinical Endocrinologists and American Thyroid Association Taskforce on Hypothyroidism in Adults. (2012). Clinical practice guidelines for hypothyroidism in adults: Cosponsored by the American Association of Clinical Endocrinologists and the American Thyroid Association. *Endocrine Practice*, 18(6), 988–1028. doi:10.4158/EP12280.GL

Hackmon, R., Blichowski, M., & Koren, G. (2012). The safety of methimazole and propylthiouracil in pregnancy: a systematic review. *Journal of Obstetrics and Gynaecology Canada*, 34(11), 1077–1086. doi:10.1016/S1701-2163(16)35438-X

Haugen, B. R., Alexander, E. K., Bible, K. C., Doherty, G. M., Mandel, S. J., Nikiforgov, Y. E., Pacini, F., Randolph, G. W., Sawka, A. M., Schlumberger, M., Schuff, K. G., Sherman, S. I., Sosa, J. A., Steward, D. L., Tuttle, R. M., & Wartofsky, L. (2016). American Thyroid Association management guidelines for adult patients with thyroid nodules and differentiated thyroid cancer. *Thyroid*, 26(1), 1–133. doi:10.1089/thy.2015.0020

Hollowell, J. G., Staehling, N. W., Flanders, W. D., Hannon, W. H., Gunter, E. W., Spencer, C. A., & Braverman, L. E. (2002). Serum TSH, T(4), and thyroid antibodies in the U.S. population (1988 to 1994). National Health and Nutrition Examination Survey (NHANES III). *Journal of Clinical Endocrinology and Metabolism*, 87(2), 489–499. doi:10.1210/jcem.87.2.8182

Howlader, N., Noone, A. M., Krapcho, M., Garshell, J., Miller, D., Altekruse, S. F., Kosary, C. L., Yu, M., Ruhl, J., Tatalovich, Z.,

Mariotto, A., Lewis, D. R., Chen, H. S., Feuer, E. J., & Cronin, K. A. (Eds.). (2014). *SEER cancer statistics review, 1975–2011*. National Cancer Institute. http://seer.cancer.gov/archive/csr/1975_2011/

Ihnatowicz, P., Drywień, M., Wątor, P., & Wojsiat, J. (2020). The importance of nutritional factors and dietary management of Hashimoto's thyroiditis. *Annals of Agricultural and Environmental Medicine, 27*(2), 184–193. doi:10.26444/aaem/112331

Jameson, J., Mandel, S. J., & Weetman, A. P. (2018a). Hypothyroidism. In J. Jameson, A. S. Fauci, D. L. Kasper, S. L. Hauser, D. L. Longo, & J. Loscalzo (Eds.), *Harrison's principles of internal medicine* (20th ed., Chapter 376). McGraw-Hill. https://accessmedicine-mhmedical-com.ucsf.idm.oclc.org/content.aspx?bookid=2129&sectionid=179924583

Jameson, J., Mandel, S. J., & Weetman, A. P. (2018b). Thyroid gland physiology and testing. J. Jameson, A. S. Fauci, D. L. Kasper, S. L. Hauser, D. L. Longo, & J. Loscalzo (Eds.), *Harrison's principles of internal medicine* (20th ed., Chapter 375). McGraw-Hill. https://accessmedicine-mhmedical-com.ucsf.idm.oclc.org/content.aspx?bookid=2129&sectionid=179924504

Katz M. D. (2023, in press). Thyroid disorders. Chisholm-Burns, M. A., Schwinghammer, T. L., Malone, P. M., Kolesar, J. M., Bookstaver, P., & Lee, K. C. (Eds.), *Pharmacotherapy Principles & Practice, 7e*. McGraw Hill.

Krames Patient Education- A Product of Staywell. (2009-2024). Common thyroid problems. https://myhealthlibrary.kramesonline.com/HealthSheets/3,S,82164

Madariaga, A. G., Palacios, S. S., Guillén-Grima, F., & Galofré, J. C. (2014). The incidence and prevalence of thyroid dysfunction in Europe: A meta-analysis. *Journal of Clinical Endocrinology & Metabolism, 99*(3), 923–931. doi:10.1210/jc.2013-2409

McDermott, M. T. (2020). Hypothyroidism. *Annals of Internal Medicine, 173*(1), ITC1–ITC16, doi:10.7326/AITC202007070

Metzger, R. (2016). *Prevalence of thyroid cancer in Cowden syndrome and FAP drives new screening recommendations*. https://consultqd.clevelandclinic.org/prevalence-thyroid-cancer-cowden-syndrome-fap-drives-new-screening-recommendations/

Myers, A. (2015). *The autoimmune solution: Prevent and reverse the full spectrum of inflammatory symptoms and diseases*. HarperOne.

National Cancer Institute. (2021). *SEER cancer stat facts: Thyroid cancer*. https://seer.cancer.gov/statfacts/html/thyro.html

National Institutes of Health. (2021). *Selenium: Fact sheet for health professionals*. https://ods.od.nih.gov/factsheets/Selenium-Health Professional/

Radix, A., & Deutsch, M. B. (2016). *Bone health and osteoporosis*. https://transcare.ucsf.edu/guidelines/bone-health-and-osteoporosis

Rayman, M. P. (2019). Multiple nutritional factors and thyroid disease, with particular reference to autoimmune thyroid disease. *Proceedings of the Nutrition Society, 78*(1), 34–44. doi:10.1017/S0029665118001192

Saxe, J. M. (2004). Thyroid diseases. In W. L. Star, L. L. Lommel, & M. T. Shannon (Eds.), *Women's primary health care: Protocols for practice* (2nd ed., pp. 10-33–10-39). UCSF Nursing Press.

Schübel, J., Feldkamp, J., Bergmann, A., Drossard, W., & Voigt, K. (2017). Latent hypothyroidism in adults. *Deutsches Arzteblatt international, 114*(25), 430–438. doi:10.3238/arztebl.2017.430

Seib, C. D., & Sosa, J. A. (2019). Evolving understanding of the epidemiology of thyroid cancer. *Endocrinology and Metabolism Clinics of North America, 48*(1), 23–35. doi:10.1016/j.ecl.2018.10.002

Slovik, D. M. (2021a). Approach to the patient with hyperthyroidism. In A. H. Goroll & A. G. Mulley (Eds.), *Primary care medicine: Office evaluation and management of the adult patient* (8th ed., Chapter 103). Wolters Kluwer Health.

Slovik, D. M. (2021b). Approach to the patient with hypothyroidism Mulley (Eds.), *Primary care medicine: Office evaluation and management of the adult patient* (8th ed., Chapter 104). Wolters Kluwer Health.

Stoffaneller, R., & Morse, N. L. (2015). A review of dietary selenium intake and selenium status in Europe and the Middle East. *Nutrients, 7*(3), 1494–1537. doi:10.3390/nu7031494

Tonstad, S., Nathan, E., Oda, K., & Fraser, G. E. (2015). Prevalence of hyperthyroidism according to type of vegetarian diet. *Public Health Nutrition, 18*(8), 1482–1487. doi:10.1017/S1368980014002183

U.S. Department of Agriculture. (2021). *Food and Nutrition Service*. https://www.fns.usda.gov/.

U.S. Preventive Services Task Force. (2014). *Evidence summary: Thyroid dysfunction screening*. https://www.uspreventiveservicestaskforce.org/uspstf/recommendation/thyroid-dysfunction-screening

Vanderpump, M. P. J. (2011). The epidemiology of thyroid disease. *British Medical Bulletin, 99*, 39–51. doi:10.1093/bmb/ldr030

Vieira, S. M., Pagovich, O. E., & Kriegel, M. A. (2014). Diet, microbiota and autoimmune diseases. *Lupus, 23*(6), 518–526. doi:10.1177/0961203313501401

Wang, C., & Crapo, L. M. (1997). The epidemiology of thyroid disease and implications for screening. *Endocrinology and Metabolism Clinics of North America, 26*(1), 189–218. doi:10.1016/s0889-8529(05)70240-1

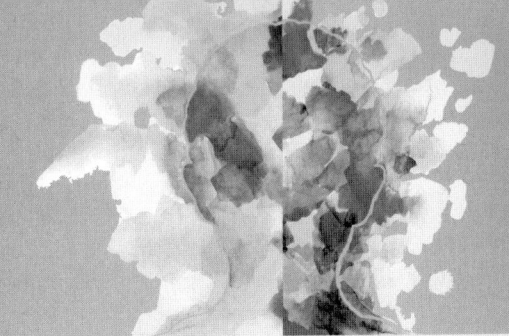

CHAPTER 66

Upper Back and Neck Pain Syndromes

Sandra Jo Domeracki and Rossana Segovia

I. Introduction and general background

The cervical and thoracic spine can be the source of many pain syndromes that affect the neck, thorax, and upper extremities. Given their anatomical proximity and the frequency of misattribution of the symptom origin, the purpose of this chapter is to focus on the most common cervical and thoracic pain syndromes. Of note, the upper extremities (e.g., forearm and hands) and associated conditions are covered elsewhere in this textbook and therefore are not covered in this chapter. Further, although the shoulder is not covered here in detail, it is important to recognize that neck pain can be a manifestation of shoulder conditions, such as rotator cuff derangement (VanBaak & Aerni, 2020), acute and chronic muscular injuries (Monica et al., 2016), osteoarthritis of the shoulder joint (Mehl et al., 2018), and even vaccination complications of deltoid intramuscular injection (i.e., shoulder injury related to vaccine administration [SIRVA]) (Shahbaz et al., 2019).

The cervical (C) spine is a complex anatomic structure composed of vertebrae, intervertebral discs, joints, the spinal cord, nerve roots, blood vessels, muscles, and ligaments. The atlanto-occipital joints (C0–C1) are the two uppermost joints, which are responsible for flexion, extension, and side flexion. The atlantoaxial joint (C1–C2) is the most mobile joint of the spine, axial rotation being its principal movement. The facet joints, also known as *apophyseal* or *zygapophyseal* joints, allow flexion, extension, and twisting motions. This mobility can be a source of degeneration, most often seen at the C4–C7 levels.

Approximately 25% of the height of the cervical spine is from the intervertebral discs, which are responsible for the spine's lordotic shape. The nucleus pulposus of the disc acts as a cushion to axial compression; the disc's annulus fibrosus withstands tension within the disc. The cervical vertebrae support the weight of the head and neck (approximately 15 lb). The vertebral arch protects the spinal cord. Cervical nerve roots are named for the vertebra below each root (e.g., the C5 nerve root is between the C4 and C5 vertebrae). For the rest of the spine, in contrast, the nerve root is named for the vertebra above (Magee & Manske, 2021). This change in the nerve root location is due to the presence of eight cranial nerve roots and seven cervical vertebral levels.

Given the cervical spine's complex structure, it is vulnerable to injuries and disorders that can produce pain and restrict mobility. Neck pain is generally perceived "as arising in a region bounded superiorly by the superior nuchal line, laterally by the lateral margins of the neck, and inferiorly by an imaginary transverse line through the T1 spinous process" (Bogduk, 2011, p. 369). This helps to define where the patient is feeling the pain. The causes of neck pain are various and can be classified as acute (duration of ≤3 months) or chronic (duration of >3 months).

The most common cause of neck pain is mechanical injury, often caused by repetitive everyday activities such as poor posture, repetitive movements, or nonergonomic workstations. More serious injuries, typically acute trauma, can occur as a result of sports, motor vehicle accidents (MVAs), or work-related events.

Nonmechanical causes of pain are less common and are often of an inflammatory or infectious nature, presenting with "red flags" that should be considered in any differential of neck pain (e.g., nuchal rigidity is a classic such finding). Other causes of neck pain that should not be overlooked include referred pain and other visceral conditions that can present acutely. By gender, women seem to have an increased incidence of spinal conditions, such as scoliosis in adolescence, osteoporosis with vertebral body fractures, and increased kyphosis after menopause. Men, however, have an increased incidence of kyphosis in adolescence, ankylosing spondylitis in mid-adulthood, and diffuse idiopathic skeletal hyperostosis in later adulthood (Armstrong & Hubbard, 2016).

The anatomical arrangement of the upper spine and thorax provides for structural protection for the vital organs of the heart, lungs, and liver. It also forms a cavity for the lungs to expand and contract safely (Magee & Manske, 2021). The thoracic spine has very limited motion because the ribs are firmly attached to both the spine posteriorly and the sternum anteriorly.

The lower three ribs do not join together anteriorly but do function to protect the vital organs while still allowing for slightly more motion. The joints between the thoracic vertebra (T12) and the lumbar vertebra (L1) allow for twisting movements from side to side. Although the thoracic spine is relatively stable because of its solid construction, this does not prevent it from being a source of radicular symptoms and pain.

The cervical rib is also a bone anomaly to consider. This is often described as an additional rib, which typically arises from the seventh cervical vertebra but can also originate from the fifth or sixth cervical vertebrae. It commonly occurs bilaterally and is more frequent in women. (Spadliński et al., 2016). The cervical rib can cause vascular or neurologic symptoms in the upper extremity (Povlsen et al., 2014) as a result of compression of nerves or blood vessels. The extra rib can be one of the various causes of thoracic outlet syndrome because of the differences in the shape of the bones of the spinal column, abnormal bands of tissue beneath the skin, and abnormalities of how muscles in the side of the neck attach to these bones.

Muscular thoracic pain is commonly caused by irritation or tension of the muscles and can be categorized as myofascial pain. The cause of such pain may be poor posture, mechanical injury, or referred pain from the neck. Joint dysfunction where the ribs attach to the spine can also be a source of symptoms in the thoracic spine. Genetic or injury-related conditions such as vertebral fractures, kyphosis, and scoliosis can also greatly affect an individual's well-being. Compression fractures of the vertebra at the thoracic level can be a result of osteoporosis, especially in the elderly, or cancer that has spread to the bones. Kyphosis and scoliosis in the thoracic area can be due to poor posture or deformity and can cause a great deal of chronic pain. Some common spinal disorders, such as a herniated disc, spinal stenosis, degenerative disc disease, or spinal instability, are not as common in the thoracic spine because of the great stability of this section of the spine.

Regarding cultural aspects, sources of pain disparities can be complex within and across racial and ethnic groups (Manchikanti et al., 2009). Contributors to such disparities can include differential risk (e.g., due to vulnerable occupations); lack of access to care, culturally appropriate or otherwise; and fiscal instability, leading to continued exposure to cumulative trauma.

A. *Mechanical spine disease (acute)*
  1. Definition and overview
     a. Cervical spine pain: Cervical spine problems that provoke subacute or chronic pain account for thousands of primary care evaluations each year. The majority of patients suffer from acute cervical strains or osteoarthritis (OA). Neck pain can be caused by muscle strains, ligament sprains, arthritis, or nerve or artery impingement. Most strains and sprains recover in 2–4 weeks with conservative treatment. Arthritic neck pain also often responds to medication and physical therapy in the acute phase. In contrast to chronic pain, acute musculoskeletal neck pain is a common problem in the general population that frequently leads to emergency department evaluation.
     b. Thoracic spine pain: The thoracic spine has not been studied as much as the cervical or lumbar spine from an epidemiologic perspective in both vocational and avocational settings. Pain arising from the thoracic spine, however, can be just as disabling, causing major physical burdens on the individual and their participation in the workforce. Conditions such as osteoporosis, hyperkyphosis, and ankylosing spondylitis have been linked to thoracic spinal pain and dysfunction (Briggs, Smith, et al., 2009). Other conditions, such as thoracic nerve impingement, often correlate with the size and location of the disc herniation. Occupational and vocational activities that require prolonged sitting may predispose individuals to thoracic spinal pain, as is similar for lumbar spine pain. Roquelaure et al. (2014) found that thoracic spine pain, for men in particular, was increased with prolonged driving of cars or buses but not with driving of industrial vehicles (i.e., tractors or forklift trucks). This is similar to the findings from a large survey of bus drivers in San Francisco (Krause et al., 1997). Thoracic spine pain in this setting is most likely related to postural constraints of the upper back rather than to mechanical vibration because newer cars and buses do not generate sufficient vibration energy to be the source of such thoracic pain. But there can be sources of high vibration that do cause pain, such as with agricultural equipment drivers, who may experience whole-body vibration (WBV), which has been associated with lifetime, transient, and chronic spine pain and symptoms (Mayton et al., n.d.).
  2. Prevalence and incidence
     a. Cervical spine pain: Neck pain is a common condition, and the prevalence rises with age. The lifetime prevalence of neck pain is quite high. Neck pain is especially common in the middle-aged population (e.g., 45–60 years of age) (Corwell & Davis, 2020). The prevalence of cervical facet joint pain in patients with chronic pain after whiplash injury is a common scenario. The prevalence of cervical pain and stiffness in epidemiologic studies varies greatly. A study by Gordon et al. (2002) pointed out that one in every five patients who went to an orthopedist

suffered from a cervical syndrome. In both the United States and Japan, cervical pain syndrome is the second-most-common cause for consultations and visits in pain clinics. Notably, neck and shoulder pain are a frequent health problem for employees.

Globally, the annual prevalence of work-related neck and shoulder pain has been estimated to range from 27.1% to 47.8%. Therefore, the identification and recognition of risk factors for neck/shoulder pain in the workplace is important in the prevention of recurrent and chronic pain (Sterud et al., 2014).

b. Thoracic spine pain: The thoracic spine has long been considered the "Cinderella" region of the spine because there is a paucity of literature regarding it, along with the etiology and epidemiology of thoracic spine pain (Heneghan & Rushton, 2016). There is also limited research on the prevalence of and risk factors for thoracic spine disorders, which may lead to an unfounded belief that the clinical and public health significance of thoracic spine disorders is less compared to disorders at other spinal levels. Despite this misconception, evidence suggests that pain or dysfunction in the thoracic spine is not uncommon in the adult population (Briggs, Smith, et al., 2009).

Indeed, 3% to 23% of patients evaluated in interventional pain management settings have acute thoracic pain syndromes. The prevalence of thoracic pain was estimated at 13% of the population compared to 43% in the lumbar spine and 44% in the cervical spine during a 1-year period when a study was done in 2009 (Manchikanti et al., 2009).

Moreover, a survey of factory workers found a 5% prevalence of thoracic pain, which did not show any association with age. This evaluation also showed the prevalence of cervical and lumbar pain to be 24% and 34%, respectively, with increasing prevalence with age in both cases (Manchikanti et al., 2009).

B. *Cervicothoracic myofascial pain syndrome*
  1. Definition and overview
  Myofascial pain syndrome, which is also known as *regional pain syndrome*, is characterized by hyperirritability areas in the body referred to as *trigger points*. These trigger points are conceptualized to arise from taut bands in the skeletal muscle. The syndrome usually accompanies a pain pattern that is specific to the muscle area involved. Eventually, according to models of this condition, the muscle becomes weak and stiff as a result of the chronicity of the symptoms, which leads to decreased range of motion. This pain may go undertreated because of a lack of awareness among clinicians (Jalil et al., 2009). This is also a musculoskeletal syndrome that has evoked debate and controversy (Marovino & Quinton, 2008). Not all of the motor and sensory symptoms of myofascial pain syndrome have to be present in order for this to be clinically diagnosed. The presence of the taut band with its zone of tenderness in the muscle involved is one important feature of myofascial pain that distinguishes it from other types of muscle pain. The ability to reproduce pain in the individual while examining the tender zone and its taut band is very important (Gerwin, 2014).

  a. Primary and secondary cervicothoracic myofascial pain syndrome has been reported in individuals with chronic tension-type headaches. Migraine symptoms of nausea and photosensitivity can be associated with active myofascial trigger-point pain (Gerwin, 2014). Neck and shoulder muscles such as the sternocleidomastoid, scalene, levator scapulae, trapezius, suboccipital, and posterior cervical muscles can directly cause neck pain. Postural stress, such as a forward head position (FHP) and anteriorly rotated shoulders, is a factor causing trigger-point–related neck pain. Mahmoud et al. (2019) found in their systemic review that age played an important role as a confounding factor in relation to this. Their results also demonstrated that adults with neck pain had increased FHP compared to asymptomatic adults.

  Both shoulder pain and decreased or restricted range of motion can be directly related to primary trigger-point myofascial pain resulting from overuse of certain muscles. For example, the subscapularis muscle can be triggered by poor body posture, biomechanics, and injury.
  b. Cervical whiplash: Cervical whiplash injuries can become chronic pain in 20%–40% of cases, and 50% of these cases are related to injury to one or more cervical facet joints (Gerwin, 2001).
  c. Chronic myofascial cervical and/or thoracic pain syndrome: Chronic myofascial pain syndrome can involve other muscle groups and regions because of stresses that may develop along the skeletal chain.

  When a muscle in this functional unit does not work effectively because of tender trigger points, it is theorized to become weak and lose its ability to lengthen, which prevents a normal range of motion. This in turn can create a "chain reaction" as other muscles try to compensate for this loss and become overused and chronically shortened (Fricton, 2016; Giamberardino et al., 2011).

  2. Prevalence and incidence
  The prevalence of myofascial pain syndrome in the United States is approximately 9 million persons. In Canada, population prevalence rate estimates are similar. It affects men and women equally but is more prevalent in people greater than 60 years

of age. No data are available to suggest a relationship between myofascial pain and ethnicity, socioeconomic status, or geographical location (Bordoni et al., 2022).
C. *Scalene muscle pain and thoracic outlet syndrome*
  1. Definition and overview
  Both scalene muscle pain and thoracic outlet syndrome can be overlooked by providers because the symptoms mimic those of cervical radiculopathy arising from disc herniation. Scalene muscle pain and thoracic outlet syndrome have also been associated with other neuropathic diseases, such as carpal tunnel syndrome and peripheral polyneuropathy, because of their presentation with referred pain to the distal extremities.
     a. Scalene myofascial pain syndrome: Scalene myofascial pain syndrome is a regional pain that originates over the neck area and radiates down to the arm. It may present as primary or secondary to underlying cervical pathology.
     b. Thoracic outlet syndrome (TOS): TOS is caused by compression of nerves or blood vessels in the thoracic outlet, which refers to the area between the neck and the axilla, including the anterior shoulders and anterior chest. An important distinction that has been identified in studies is the categorization of vascular versus neurogenic presentations (Hooper et al., 2010). Overall, TOS has been the subject of considerable debate in terms of its frequency, etiology, and treatment (Doneddu et al., 2017).
  2. Prevalence and incidence
     a. Scalene myofascial pain syndrome: In one study, it was found that 31% of patients complaining of scalene muscle pain had acute trigger points, which have also been described in all age groups and in both sexes (Fomby & Mellion, 1997). The syndrome most often occurs between the ages of 30 and 60 years; prevalence declines with advancing age. A study done in the 1950s studied asymptomatic U.S. Air Force recruits and found tender spots indicative of latent trigger points in 54% of the women and 45% of the men. The study also noted referred pain with palpation in 5% of the recruits (Fomby & Mellion, 1997).
     b. TOS: A survey done in 2009 (Manchikanti et al.) on factory workers and their prevalence of thoracic pain demonstrated a 5% prevalence of thoracic pain that was not associated with age. TOS is generally diagnosed between 20 and 50 years of age; however, it can be found in teenagers and rarely in children. Neurogenic TOS is found three to four times more commonly in women compared to the vascular type but is more equal between nonathletic women and men. For competitive athletic individuals, the vascular forms of TOS is more common in men than women (Hooper et al., 2010).
D. *Osteoarthritis*
  1. Definition and overview
     a. OA (also called *degenerative joint disease* or *osteoarthrosis*): OA is the most common form of arthritis and occurs when cartilage in the joints wears down over time. Treatment can relieve pain and help patients maintain their activities of daily living.
     b. Spondylosis is degeneration of the discs and vertebrae, causing compression of the spinal cord in the neck. OA is the most common cause, most often affecting middle-aged and older people. This is the most common cause of spinal cord dysfunction in the older-than-55 population (Steinberg et al., 1999).
  2. Prevalence and incidence
     a. In a study by Hirpara et al. (2012), it was noted that the prevalence of cervical spondylosis is similar for both sexes, although the degree of severity is greater for males. Moreover, spondylotic changes in the cervical spine occurred at solitary disc space levels in about 15%–40% of patients, whereas in the majority, this occurred at multiple levels. The discs between the third and seventh cervical vertebrae are most commonly affected. Repeated occupational trauma may also contribute to the development of cervical spondylosis. For example, there was an increased incidence in patients who carried heavy loads on their heads or shoulders, as well as in dancers, gymnasts, and patients with spasmodic torticollis (Hirpara et al., 2012).

     Of note, osteoarthritis and associated conditions not mentioned in this chapter will be discussed in more detail elsewhere in this textbook.
E. *Strains and sprains*
  1. Definition and overview
     a. Musculoskeletal strains and sprains (arising from work or sports and other avocations) occur when there is an injury to the muscles of the neck caused by prolonged or repetitive neck extension or flexion. This is often related to poor posture at work, such as repetitive leaning or bending of the neck and nonergonomic workstations, or during hobbies, such as knitting or crocheting. Repetition of the motion causes constant insult to the affected area and prevents healing (Steinberg et al., 1999). Poor remote home office work ergonomic factors are likely to contribute to this problem in the future.
  2. Prevalence and incidence
     a. According to a study published by Cohen (2015, p. 284), "neck pain is the fourth leading cause of disability, with an annual prevalence rate exceeding 30%." This rate includes all types of causes of neck pain; however, most episodes of acute neck pain will resolve with or without treatment, as in the case of strains. Half of these "individuals

will continue to experience some degree of pain or frequent occurrences" (Cohen, 2015, p. 284).
   b. A review article by Briggs, Bragge, et al. (2009) reported that the range of prevalence estimates of thoracic back pain in the general population is very broad because of many factors, including the different types and causes, as well as duration. There was a higher estimated prevalence for thoracic back pain in children and adolescents, especially for females. In children and adolescents, thoracic back pain was associated with female gender, postural changes associated with backpack use, backpack weight, other musculoskeletal symptoms, participation in specific sports, chair height at school, and difficulty with homework (Briggs, Bragge, et al., 2009). In adults, thoracic back pain was associated with other concurrent musculoskeletal symptoms and difficulty in performing activities of daily living.

F. *Spinal deformities*
   1. Definition and overview
      a. *Spinal deformities* refers to conditions in which the spine has an abnormal curvature or alignment. The two most common cervical/thoracic spinal deformities are scoliosis and hyperkyphosis.
      b. Scoliosis: Scoliosis is defined as a lateral curvature of the spine that may occur in children or adults. Scoliosis can cause back pain, abnormal gait, uneven hips, and different leg lengths for adolescents and even more severe symptoms when found in adults. Most cases of scoliosis are mild, but some children develop spine deformities that continue to get more severe as they grow. Severe scoliosis can be disabling. An especially severe spinal curve can reduce the amount of space within the chest, making it difficult for the lungs to function properly. There are two types of scoliosis. One is postural (Grade I), which is without any bony changes or muscular weakness; the second type is structural (Grade II and III), which is a defect in bone (Shakil, 2014).
      c. Scoliosis can also be classified according to etiology:
         i. Congenital scoliosis, caused by a bone abnormality present at birth
         ii. Paralytic scoliosis is the result of abnormal muscles or nerves. This most frequently is seen in people with spina bifida or cerebral palsy or in people with various conditions that are accompanied by or result in paralysis. Historically, poliomyelitis was an important cause of this disorder (Tassadaq & Osama, 2021).
         iii. Idiopathic scoliosis is the most common type of scoliosis and has no specific identifiable cause. It can affect persons of any age range, with adolescent idiopathic scoliosis (AIS) and adult degenerative scoliosis being some of the common presentations. There are many theories, but none of them have been found to be conclusive. Genetic and hereditary causes are widely accepted as the etiology for this classification of scoliosis (Shakil, 2014).
      d. Hyperkyphosis: The forward bend to the spine is called *kyphosis* and is marked by a small anterior concavity resulting from the shape of vertebral bodies and intervertebral discs. The "normal" range for adults is between 20° and 40° of curvature kyphosis (Roghani et al., 2017). There are three types of kyphosis: congenital, developmental, and traumatic.
      e. There are two types of congenital kyphosis. Type I deformity is the failure of formation and failure of segmentation of a portion of one or more vertebral bodies that usually worsens with growth. The deformity is usually visible at birth as a lump or bump on the infant's spine. Type II deformity is the failure of segmentation that occurs as two or more vertebrae fail to separate and form normal discs and rectangular bones. This type of kyphosis is often more likely to be diagnosed later, after the child is walking (Scoliosis Research Society, 2022).
      f. Postural kyphosis is postural in origin, especially with young patients. In older patients, it may be related to weakened bones (i.e., osteoporosis) or spinal fractures. Postural kyphosis is corrected when the patient stands up straight. Patients with postural kyphosis have no abnormalities in the shape of the vertebrae.
      g. Scheuermann kyphosis (juvenile kyphosis) is defined as rigid (structural) kyphosis because the front sections of the vertebrae grow slower than the back sections. This occurs during a period of rapid bone growth, usually between the ages of 12 and 15 years of age in males or a few years earlier in females.
      h. Posttraumatic kyphosis occurs most commonly in the thoracolumbar and lumbar regions. This type of kyphosis is most common in patients with severe neurologic deficits, such as quadriplegia or paraplegia.
      i. Congenital kyphosis occurs in girls more commonly than in boys. It occurs in any part of the spinal column, but the apex is often located between T10 and L1.
      j. Neuromuscular kyphosis is characterized by injury of the upper motor neurons (e.g., cerebral palsy, syringomyelia), spinal cord injury, or diseases of the lower motor neurons (e.g., poliomyelitis, spinal muscular atrophy) (Yaman & Dalbayrak, 2014).
   2. Prevalence and incidence
      a. The prevalence of spinal deformity and scoliosis in the adult population is not well established

but has been reported to be up to 32% of the population. A study targeting elderly volunteers showed a prevalence of more than 60%. The prevalence of degenerative scoliosis ranges from 6% to 68%. Many cases of degenerative scoliosis are undiagnosed, but elderly patients often seek care because of back and leg pain that may be caused by scoliosis and associated spinal stenosis (Kotwal et al., 2011).
   b. The prevalence of adult scoliosis cited in the literature ranges variably depending on severity (Correa & Watkins-Castillo, n.d., para. 2). Moreover, a conservative estimate of 2.5% of the prevalence of adult scoliosis reported yields an incidence of a minimum of 5.88 million adults in the United States with adult scoliosis. In 2010–2011 alone, there were an estimated 1.61 million of these adults who received treatment as either an inpatient or outpatient. Estimates for the prevalence of kyphosis were approximated to 17% as the primary diagnosis in hospital and emergency departments (Correa & Watkins-Castillo, n.d.).

II. Database (may include but is not limited to)
Because cervical, thoracic, and/or cervicothoracic pain is usually multifactorial, it is important to determine if the pain is caused by spinal or extra spinal (soft tissue) injury or a serious infectious or inflammatory disorder.

A. *Subjective*
   1. History of presenting illness: Description of the pain, including onset, location, duration, radiation, character and quality, and aggravating and alleviating factors. Determine modifying factors, such as rest, activity, and changes in position; course of symptoms; and accompanying symptoms, such as numbness, tingling, weakness, paresthesias, and incontinence. If a traumatic injury, delineate the mechanism of the injury.
      Additional important questions: Is there any pain with inspiration or expiration or both? Is the pain affected by coughing or sneezing or straining? Is there any particular posture that intensifies or eases the pain? Is the skin in the thoracic area intact? Has there been any recent spinal manipulation of the neck (e.g., physical therapy, chiropractic) as a source of trauma? Any issues with sleep or upon arising (e.g., to consider torticollis)? Any dizziness/lightheadedness, headaches, or feelings of coldness in the upper extremities (TOS)?
   2. Past medical, surgical, and other health history
      a. Medical illnesses: cardiovascular, diabetes mellitus, carpal tunnel syndrome, cancer, osteoporosis, rheumatoid or other inflammatory arthritis, scoliosis, OA, fibromyalgia, herpes zoster, prior neck or low back disorders (work related or not), MVA, risk factors for aneurysm, infection, immuno-suppressive disorder
      b. Surgical or trauma history (prior surgery to cervical spine, shoulder, chest, or lumbar spine; recent surgery)
      c. Medication history: medications for the symptoms or any other disorders
   3. Family history: history of any musculoskeletal disorders (e.g., scoliosis, kyphosis, spondylosis, stenosis) or connective tissue disorders (e.g., Marfan syndrome)
   4. Occupational and environmental history: If currently working, type of work; specific tasks, frequency of tasks, length of time performing same task, and length of time doing the same jobs; ergonomic factors; and chemical exposures. For past work history, assess change in duties, job, or ability to work altogether because of pain or injury. Inquire as to current or prior workers' compensation claims and outcome (e.g., if discharged from care or considered "permanent and stationary"). It is also good to know if there are any associated restrictions or accommodations that have been prescribed. Investigate environmental history (e.g., recent bystander exposure to neurotoxins if paresthesias present).
   5. Personal and social history and health-related behaviors: housing situation (alone or accompanied), hobbies, exercise, support system, smoking cigarettes, ethanol consumption, and substance use
   6. Review of systems
      a. Constitutional signs and symptoms: fever, chills, weight loss, and poor appetite (suggesting infectious or malignancy etiology)
      b. Ear, nose, and throat: worsening of neck pain when swallowing (esophageal disorders), headache, visual changes, nuchal rigidity (infectious or malignancy)
      c. Skin: rash, pain, numbness, or tingling, itching in area
      d. Cardiac and pulmonary: cough, dyspnea, worsening with inspiration, chest pressure, pain, arm pain, anxiety, or diaphoresis (myocardial infarction, angina, or lung cancer)
      e. Abdomen: anorexia, nausea, vomiting, heartburn, gas/flatulence, and change in bowel function or stool function (gastrointestinal disorders)
      f. Musculoskeletal: active range of motion, activities of daily living (ADLs), instrumental activities of daily living (IADLs), pain with or without movement, swelling, redness, warmth, clicking, or locking
      g. Neurologic: depressive symptoms, fatigue, headaches (multifactorial mechanical pain), numbness, tingling, weakness, vertigo, or balance disturbances

B. *Objective*
   1. Physical examination findings (**Tables 66-1** through **66-3**)

Table 66-1 Physical Examination Findings

Joint clearing reduces or eliminates scar tissue within the joints, which can limit surrounding joint mobility and cause pain. Manually move scar tissue from joint area. This will enable one to perform a more reliable examination.

Inspection	Overall spinal and total body posture to determine if asymmetry contributes to problems (e.g., head tilt that can occur with torticollis). Check for hyperkyphosis (round back, humpback, flat back, or dowager's hump) and scoliosis and the level of the deformity. Observe for breathing patterns. Observe for chest deformities such as pigeon chest, funnel chest, or barrel chest. Observe for scapular and clavicular symmetry and muscle atrophy. Loss of cervical lordosis is present with painful acute sprains, fractures, and infectious or neoplastic processes.
Palpation	Palpate the spinous process to define the alignment of the spine. Determine tenderness level, muscle tightness, and spasms. Palpation pressure may provoke paresthesias or numbness and tingling. Palpate anterior and posterior thoracic area, including neck and shoulders. Palpate the spinous process to define the alignment of the spine. C7 is the most prominent spinous process. The top of the thyroid cartilage is parallel to C4, and the cricoid cartilage is parallel to C6. Paraspinous muscles, trapezii, the medial border of the scapula, and sternocleidomastoid muscle palpation may provoke tenderness.
Range of motion (ROM) *Stabilize the trunk so that motion does not occur in the thoracic spine but in the neck only.*	Flexion and extension are estimated visually in degrees. Flexion limitation can also be measured as the distance the chin lacks in touching the sternum. Rotation and lateral bending of neck: the degree of motion is the angle between the vertical axis and midaxis of the face. Rotation is estimated in degrees. Limited range of motion of the neck is usually common and may present in all planes. Forward flexion (normal ROM 20°–45°) and extension (normal ROM 25°–45°). Flexion limitation can also be measured with a tape measure. Measure the spine while the patient is in a normal standing position from C7 to T12; then ask the patient to bend forward and measure again. A 2.7-cm (1.1-inch) difference in length is considered normal. Lateral flexion is about 20°–40° to each side. A tape measure can be used to measure the distance from the floor. The distance should be equal bilaterally. Rotation is about 35°–50°. Ask the patient either to cross the arms in front or place the hands on opposite shoulders and then rotate to both sides. To avoid lumbar and hip rotation, the patient can be asked to perform this part of the exam while sitting. Costovertebral expansion is measured by chest expansion using a measuring tape at the level of the fourth intercostal space. The patient is asked to exhale as much as possible to take the measurement. Then the patient is asked to inhale as much as possible and hold the breath while measuring again. The normal difference between the two is 3–7.5 cm (~1–2.75 inches).
Neurologic and motor	**Assess:** **C5 Level** Deltoid—C5 axillary nerve (Abduct the shoulder to 90°. Push down on the arm to resist activity of the deltoid. True weakness of this muscle should be a uniform giving-way motion.) Biceps—C5–C6 musculocutaneous nerve (Ask patient to flex the elbow in the supinated position against resistance.) Biceps reflex Sensation—lateral arm: axillary nerve **C6 Level** Wrist extensor group—C6 radial nerve Biceps—C6 musculocutaneous nerve Brachioradialis reflex Sensation—lateral forearm: musculocutaneous nerve **C7 Level** Triceps—C7 radial nerve (With the patient supine and the shoulder flexed about 90 degrees, ask the patient to extend the elbow against resistance.) Wrist flexor group—C7 median and ulnar nerves Finger extensor—C7 radial nerve Triceps reflex Sensation—middle finger

(continues)

Table 66-1 Physical Examination Findings (continued)

	C8 Level
	No reflex. Examination is limited to muscle strength and sensation tests.
	Finger flexors (Stabilize the long, index, and little fingers in extension and ask the patient to flex the fingers as you apply resistance.)
	Sensation—ring and little fingers of the hands and distal half of the forearm ulnar side (Neurologic examination is usually normal in cervical strain.)
	Resisted isometric movements are a gross test, and subtle alterations in strength are hard to determine. If the muscles tested have been injured, contracting them will provoke pain.
	This exam is done while the patient is in a sitting position. The examiner must be standing with one leg behind the patient's buttocks and with the arms around the patient's chest and back (hugging). Tell the patient, "Don't let me move you," and proceed with forward flexion, extension, side flexion (right/left), and rotation (right/left).
	Nerve root tested, flexion: T6–T12
	Nerve root tested, extension: T1–T12
	Nerve root tested, rotation and side bending: T1–T12 and L1
	Nerve root tested, elevation of the ribs: C3–C8, T1–T12, and intercostals 2–5
	Nerve root tested, depression of the ribs: T6–T12, L1–L3

Data from Magee, D. (2008). *Orthopedic physical assessment* (5th ed.). Musculoskeletal Rehabilitation Series. St. Louis, MO: Saunders Elsevier.

Table 66-2 Special Tests

Spurling test	Have the patient extend the neck while tilting the head to the side. With one hand and doing the same for each side, lightly compress downward on the head in order to axially load the cervical spine. This narrows the neural foramen and increases or reproduces radicular arm pain that is associated with disc herniation or cervical spondylosis (Armstrong & Hubbard, 2016).
Axial loading test (compression test)	Push down on the patient's head. This provokes neck pain in some patients with disc problems; however, increased low back pain indicates a nonorganic finding. Avoid this test if you are highly suspicious of vertebral damage or facture (Armstrong & Hubbard, 2016).
Hoffmann test	With the patient relaxed in a seated position and the hand cradled in the clinician's hand, flick the third fingernail and look for index finger and thumb flexion. If present, it is a sign of long-tract spinal cord involvement in the neck (Armstrong & Hubbard, 2016).
Distraction test	Place one hand with palm open under the patient's chin, the other hand on the occiput, then gradually lift the head to remove its weight from the neck. If the patient experiences a relief in symptoms, it demonstrates the effect of neck traction by widening the neural foramen (Hoppenfeld, 1976).
Adson test	Take the patient's radial pulse; abduct, extend, and externally rotate the patient's arm. Ask the patient to take a deep breath and to turn their head toward the arm being tested. If there is compression of the subclavian artery, you will feel a marked diminution or absence of the radial pulse (Hoppenfeld, 1976).
Upper limb neural tension test 1a (ULTT1a)	Depress the shoulder, abduct the arm to 110°, and flex the elbow 90°. Then externally rotate the shoulder to 90°, extend your patient's wrist and fingers, and slowly extend the elbow.
Slump test (sitting dural stretch test)	The patient should be sitting on the exam table. The patient is asked to slump (the spine flexes forward, and the shoulders sag forward) while the examiner holds the chin and head of the patient erect. If no symptoms are produced, flex the neck of the patient and hold the head down; if no symptoms are produced, passively extend one of the patient's knees; if no symptoms are produced, passively dorsiflex the foot of the same leg. The test is considered positive when the symptoms diminish with a sensitizing maneuver of cervical extension. This is repeated on the other side of the leg. Rationale: This maneuver increases the stress on the intercostal nerves. The pain is usually produced at the site of the injured area.

Data from Magee, D. (2008). *Orthopedic physical assessment* (5th ed.). Musculoskeletal Rehabilitation Series. St. Louis, MO: Saunders Elsevier.

Table 66-3 Referred Pain Patterns

Referred Pain Pattern	Muscle Involved
Spine to the line along the medial border aspect of the scapula	Iliocostalis muscle
Adjacent to the spine	Multifidus muscle
Scapular area to posterior-anterior arm down to the fifth finger	Serratus superior muscle
Medial border of the arm to medial fourth and fifth fingers	Serratus posterior muscle
Lateral chest wall to lower medial border of the scapula	Serratus anterior muscle
Medial border of the scapula	Rhomboids muscle
Upper thoracic spine to medial border of the scapula	Trapezius muscle
Inferior angle of the scapula to posterior shoulder and iliac crest	Latissimus dorsi muscle
Neck/shoulder angle to posterior shoulder and along medial edge of the scapula	Levator scapula muscle

Data from Magee, D. (2008). *Orthopedic physical assessment* (5th ed.). Musculoskeletal Rehabilitation Series. St. Louis, MO: Saunders Elsevier.

Table 66-4 Red-Flag Conditions

Presentation	Etiologies	Comments
Possible cauda equina syndrome	Possible tumor, fracture, or infection	
Saddle anesthesia	Major trauma, such as motor vehicle accident or fall from height	Age >50 or <20
Recent onset of bladder dysfunction, such as urinary retention, increased frequency, or overflow incontinence	Tumor or minor trauma (even strenuous lifting in older or potentially osteoporotic patient)	
Severe or progressive neurologic deficit in the lower extremity Pain that worsens when supine; severe nighttime pain	Spinal infection: recent bacterial infection (e.g., urinary tract infection), intravenous drug abuse, or immune suppression (from steroids, transplant, HIV, tumor/cancer)	Assess for constitutional symptoms, such as recent fever or chills or unexplained weight loss.
■ Unexpected laxity of the anal sphincter or perianal or perineal sensory loss ■ Major motor weakness: quadriceps (knee extension weakness), ankle plantar flexors, evertors, and dorsiflexors (foot drop)	Nerve root impingement	

Other red-flag or "don't miss" conditions to consider include carotid artery dissection, meningitis, nonspinal causes of pain (e.g., angina pectoris, esophageal obstruction, apical lung tumor, biliary disease), compression of cervical cord, and myelopathy.

Data from U.S. Agency for Health Care Policy and Research. (1994). *Acute low back problems in adults: Assessment and treatment. Quick reference guide for clinicians: Clinical practice guideline #14.* Rockville, MD: Author

III. Assessment
A. Determine the cause of the neck pain, if acute or chronic.
B. Determine if the patient needs immediate referral for consultation (e.g., progressive neurologic symptoms or fracture). See **Table 66-4** for red-flag conditions.
C. Determine if the condition is work related.
D. Assess the patient's ability to perform their usual activities (i.e., ADLs, IADLs).
E. Assess the patient's pain control and coping abilities.

IV. Goals of clinical management
A. Evidence-based management of the patient's cervical and/or thoracic pain presentation

B. Cost-effective plan of treatment
C. Appropriate management of the patient's condition if work related
D. Selection of management approach that maximizes the patient's adherence to the plan of care

V. Plan
A. Diagnostic criteria for non–red-flag conditions (**Table 66-5**)
B. Other diagnostic tests that may be included
  1. Blood tests: erythrocyte sedimentation rate, rheumatoid factor, antinuclear antibody if suspecting systemic, infectious, and inflammatory conditions; cardiac enzymes, if indicated
  2. Tuberculosis screening (tuberculin skin test or QuantiFERON® test, if indicated.
  3. Imaging: cervical/thoracic spine radiograph series, shoulder radiograph series, chest radiograph if indicated based on clinical pulmonary presentation, computerized axial tomography, or magnetic resonance imaging if patient presents with soft tissues and disc signs and symptoms, and is not responding to standard treatment within expected time period
  4. Electromyelogram or nerve conduction study to rule out other structures causing the neurologic symptoms when the diagnosis is unclear
C. Treatment (**Table 66-6**)
D. Patient education
  1. Discuss nature of condition and expected time of recovery.
    a. Discuss proper posture and body mechanics.
    b. Discuss frequent breaks and how ergonomic setup of a workstation can be modified to improve symptoms.
    c. Explain proper use of supportive devices such as neck pillows.
    d. Discuss need for a lifelong stretching and conditioning exercise program for maintenance and prevention of further disability.
    e. Discuss stress reduction techniques.
    f. Discuss medication use and compliance and other symptom-relief modalities.
    g. If determined to be work related, discuss process of reporting the injury to the employer and assuming care with the employer's occupational health system.
E. Follow-up (acute and chronic)
  The follow-up time frame is based on the plan of care and the acuity and severity of the patient's presentation. If imaging has been ordered, follow-up should be prompted to communicate the results to the patient. If the patient is taken off work, appropriate follow-up is necessary to determine whether the patient is ready to return to work and at what capacity.

VI. Self-management resources and tools
A. Patient education internet-based materials
  1. OrthoInfo, http://www.orthoinfo.org, for spine conditioning program exercises
  2. Dynamic Chiropractic, http://www.dynamicchiropractic.com, for corrective exercises for thoracic kyphosis
  3. National Institute of Arthritis and Musculoskeletal and Skin Diseases (NIAMS), http://www.niams.nih.gov/, for back pain management and exercises
  4. Neck Injuries and Disorders (U.S. National Library of Medicine, 2017), http://www.nlm.nih.gov/medlineplus/neckinjuriesanddisorders.html

Table 66-5 Diagnostic Criteria Non–Red-Flag Conditions

Probable Diagnosis	Mechanism	Common Symptoms	Common Signs	Tests and Results
Regional neck pain	Unknown	Diffuse pain	None	None indicated
Cervical strain	Flexion–extension or rotation force, blow to the head or neck	Neck pain, difficult or decreased motion	Limited range of motion because of pain	None indicated
Cervical nerve root compression with radiculopathy	Degenerative condition, trauma	Dermatomal sensory changes, motor weakness	Specific motor, sensory, and reflex changes	None indicated for 4–6 weeks, unless progressive motor weakness
Spinal stenosis	Older patients: degenerative disc disease Younger patients: congenital stenosis	Neck, shoulder, and posterior arm pain; paresthesias in the same distribution as the pain	Weakness of the shoulder girdle and upper arms Signs worse with extension, improved with flexion of the neck	Computed tomography or magnetic resonance imaging shows spinal stenosis.

Data from Glass, L. S., & Harris, J. S. (2004). *Occupational medicine practice guidelines: Evaluation and management of common health problems and functional recovery in workers* (2nd ed.). Beverly Farms, MA: OEM Press

Table 66-6 Clinical Characteristics and Management of Cervicothoracic Spine Pain

Condition	Clinical Characteristics	Management
Cervical strain and sprain	Most patients can report specific mechanism of injury. May not notice pain immediately, but after several hours, may have tightness in the neck. Some may report nausea. Physical examination may only show mild abnormalities. May have tenderness, edema, spasms, headaches, and dizziness. With moderate injuries, may present with radicular symptoms.	Diagnostic workup: Cervical radiograph to rule out fracture or dislocation if suspected. Treatment: Rest in comfortable position; soft cervical collar is appropriate for 1 or 2 days if in the acute phase. Cold packs applied for 15 minutes four to six times a day, then heat. May also alternate cold and heat if combination promotes better relief. Gentle stretches of the neck and shoulders (early movements of the stable spine promote recovery). Analgesics according to symptoms, especially for nighttime pain. Muscle relaxants are appropriate in the acute phase to relieve spasms and aid with nighttime sleep. Physical therapy can be helpful, especially in the first 4 weeks. Encourage early return to normal activities, including work, if appropriate.
Acute disc herniation	Pain is usually aggravated by cough, sneeze, strain, and other activities that prolong static position of the neck, especially in flexion–extension and rotation. Lifting, pushing, and pulling may also aggravate the pain. Usually, there is tenderness to palpation of the spinous process. Distraction test relieves the pain; compression test increases the pain. Usually, there are associated muscle spasms and trigger-point tenderness.	Diagnostic workup: radiograph may be normal or show degenerative disc disease. May need magnetic resonance imaging (MRI), computed tomography (CT), or electromyogram/nerve conduction studies (EMG/NCS) if indicated based on presenting symptoms. Treatment: Conservative treatment in the acute phase, absent major progressing symptoms. Rest by limiting activities; encourage soft pillows, elevation of the head of the bed, and soft collar. Physical therapy can be helpful and may possibly include traction as well as exercises for functional range of motion and strength. Heat or cold compress to the neck for 15 minutes as tolerated can also be recommended. Nonsteroidal anti-inflammatory drugs (NSAIDs) and muscle relaxants used in the acute phase. Patients should be reassured that most disc herniations resolve without residual problems. If symptoms do not resolve within 3–6 weeks, epidural injection may be appropriate, depending on presentation of symptoms and degree of limitation in activities of daily living.
Chronic disc degeneration (spondylosis or osteoarthritis)	Most common presentations are stiffness and chronic pain that worsen with upright activity. Some patients may report grinding or popping in the neck region. Referred pain to shoulder and arm, paraspinous process spasms, headaches, fatigue, and sleep disturbances. Difficulty with basic activities of daily living.	Diagnostic tests: Anteroposterior and lateral radiograph shows sclerosis in the intervertebral disc area with osteophytes (bone spurs) projecting anteriorly. Osteophytes may also project posteriorly, causing stenosis of the cervical canal. Anterior subluxation of one vertebra over the other may also be appreciated. Degenerative findings, usually at the C5–C6 and C6–C7 levels. Treatment: Usually responsive to traction. NSAIDs and muscle relaxants are helpful, especially at nighttime. Cervical pillow, cervical roll, and physical therapy may be appropriate. Epidural injection may also be appropriate. In chronic cases without resolution of major symptoms and with radicular involvement, decompression and fusion surgery may be appropriate.

(continues)

Table 66-6 Clinical Characteristics and Management of Cervicothoracic Spine Pain *(continued)*

Condition	Clinical Characteristics	Management
Cervical radiculopathy	Patients present with neck pain along with radicular pain associated with numbness and paresthesias in the upper extremity along the distribution of the nerve root involved. Muscle spasms or fasciculations may also be present in the myotomes involved. Other symptoms may be weakness, lack of coordination, difficulty with handwriting and performing fine manipulative tasks, dropping objects, and decreased strength. If stenosis of the cervical canal, patient may present with lower extremity symptoms and bowel or bladder dysfunction.	Diagnostic tests: Plain radiographs may identify spondylosis or degeneration of the disc and the facet. MRI or CT with intrathecal contrast confirms the diagnosis. However, this is not routine care unless symptoms are progressive. EMG/NCS helps determine the location of the neurologic dysfunction and is commonly used presurgically. Treatment: In most cases, it resolves spontaneously within 6–12 weeks. Nonnarcotic analgesic is usually helpful. May also use short course of oral steroids if appropriate. Physical therapy, which may include traction, is useful in the first 2–4 weeks.
Cervical fracture	Patient may present with severe neck pain, paraspinous muscle spasms, and point tenderness to the area of fracture. Pain radiates to the shoulder or arm and may be associated with radicular symptoms if nerve root involvement is present.	Diagnostic tests: Anteroposterior, lateral, and odontoid views are the standard. Lateral radiograph should include the occiput superiorly and the top of T1 inferiorly. Swimmer's view may also be indicated to visualize the cervicothoracic junction. If no fracture is seen, it should be evaluated for instability. Treatment: Immobilization of cervical spine during transportation to emergency department. Patients whose initial radiograph was negative for fracture but continue to have pain may use cervical collar. Repeat radiograph if symptoms persist past 7–10 days. NSAIDs and analgesics are also appropriate.
Cervicothoracic myofascial syndrome	Deep aching pain in a muscle, pain that persists or worsens. Cervical spine range of motion is often limited and painful. May be described as lumpiness or painful bump in the trapezius or cervical paraspinal muscles. Massage is often helpful, as is superficial heat. Patient's sleep may be interrupted because of pain The cervical rotation required for driving is difficult to achieve Patient may describe pain radiating into the upper extremities, accompanied by numbness and tingling, making discrimination from radiculopathy or peripheral nerve impingement difficult Dizziness or nausea may be a part of the symptomatology The patient experiences typical patterns of radiating pain referred from trigger points	Diagnostic workup: Diagnosis is typically made after diagnosis of cervical disc prolapse has been ruled out. Positive Spurling's test will indicate cervical disc prolapse. Cervical radiograph and MRI can be done to assist with ruling out cervical presentation. Treatment: Manual therapy techniques targeting the myofascial system (Edmondston & Singer, 1997). Trigger-point injections. Acupuncture. Physical therapy or physical therapy interventions to address postural impairments. NSAIDs, muscle relaxants, foam roller, and heat therapy.

Condition	Clinical Characteristics	Management
Scalene muscle pain	Pain in cervical region radiating to occiput, nuchal muscles, shoulders, and upper extremities. Stiffness. Tenderness to the trapezius, levator scapulae, rhomboids, supraspinatus, and infraspinatus. Unilateral neck/shoulder pain.	Diagnostic workup: Same as previously. Treatment: Same as previously.
Thoracic outlet syndrome (TOS)	Symptoms are often vague and variable. Paresthesias from the neck to the shoulder, arm, medial forearm, and fingers. If vascular, intermittent swelling and discoloration of the arm. Aching, fatigue, and weakness. Symptoms can worsen if arm is in overhead position. Tenderness.	Diagnostic workup: Venous ultrasound studies, Doppler ultrasound, and angiography in the seated position for arterial TOS, EMG/NCS. Treatment: Physical therapy, Edgelow Program, NSAIDs, lifestyle changes, ergonomic changes. Surgical recommendation: Depending on nature of disease.
Scoliosis	Pain localized to area of deformity. Radicular pain, if associated with compression.	Diagnostic workup: Weight-bearing full-length posterior-anterior and lateral x-rays. EMG/NCS is rare but can be done if suspecting neuropathy. NSAIDs, exercise programs, swimming, bracing in children only. Physical therapy can be helpful as well if the condition is painful.
Hyperkyphosis	Pain related to activity if poor posture	Diagnostic workup: Weight-bearing anterior-posterior and lateral x-rays. Treatment: Observation or exercise program and physical therapy. Bracing only in noncongenital situations. Surgery depending on severity of deformity.

Other conditions to consider include cervical discogenic pain, diffuse skeletal hyperostosis, ossifications of the posterior longitudinal ligament, and posterior chest wall pain syndrome.

Data from Green, W. B. (2001). *Essentials of musculoskeletal care* (2nd ed.). Rosemont, IL: American Academy of Orthopaedic Surgeons; Griffin, L. Y. (2005). *Essentials of musculoskeletal care* (3rd ed.). Rosemont, IL: American Academy of Orthopaedic Surgeons and American Academy of Pediatrics; Steinberg, G., Akins, C., & Baran, D. (1999). *Orthopaedics in primary care* (3rd ed.). Hagerstown, MD: Lippincott Williams & Williams.

5. Congenital kyphosis (Scoliosis Research Society, 2022): http://www.srs.org/patients-and-families/conditions-and-treatments/parents/kyphosis/congenital-kyphosis
6. Neck and back: http://orthoinfo.aaos.org/menus/spine.cfm
7. Community support groups:
   a. WebMD® Health Community: http://exchanges.webmd.com
   b. Back Pain Support Group: http://back-pain.supportgroups.com/
   c. Health Boards: https://www.healthboards.com/

VII. Clinical evaluation of patients in medically underserved areas and low- and middle-income communities with spine-related complaints includes:
A. History to identify signs or symptoms suggesting serious pathology and psychological factors
B. Physical examination to identify neurological deficits and range of motion
C. Diagnostic imaging only when severe or progressive neurologic deficits are present or when serious underlying conditions are suspected on the basis of history and physical examination
D. No routine ordering of diagnostic imaging in the initial assessment or routine performance of electromyography and nerve conduction studies for diagnosis of radiculopathy
E. No discography for the assessment of spinal disorders (Nordin et al., 2018)

References

Armstrong, A. D., & Hubbard, M.C. (2016). *Essentials of musculoskeletal care* (5th ed.). American Academy of Orthopaedic Surgeons.

Bogduk, N. (2011). The anatomy and pathophysiology of neck pain. *Physical Medicine and Rehabilitation Clinics of North America, 22*(3), 367–382, vii. doi:10.1016/j.pmr.2011.03.008

Bordoni, B., Sugumar, K., & Varacallo, M. (2022, February 12). Myofascial pain. *StatPearls*. https://www.ncbi.nlm.nih.gov/books/NBK535344/

Briggs, A. M., Bragge, P., Smith, A. J., Govil, D., & Straker, L. M. (2009). Prevalence and associated factors for thoracic spine pain in the adult working population: A literature review. *Journal of Occupational Health, 51*(3), 177–192. doi:10.1539/joh.k8007

Briggs, A. M., Smith, A. J., Straker, L. M., & Bragge, P. (2009). Thoracic spine pain in the general population: Prevalence, incidence and associated factors in children, adolescents, and adults. A systematic review. *BMC Musculoskeletal Disorders, 10*, 77). doi:10.1186/1471-2474-10-77

Cohen, S. P. (2015). Epidemiology, diagnosis, and treatment of neck pain. *Mayo Clinic Proceedings, 90*(2), 284–299. doi:10.1016/j.mayocp.2014.09.008

Correa, A., & Watkins Castillo, S. I. (n.d.). Prevalence of adult scoliosis: Spinal curvature. *Bone and Joint Initiative USA*. https://www.boneandjointburden.org/2014-report/iiid21/prevalence-adult-scoliosis

Corwell, B. N., & Davis, N. L. (2020). The emergent evaluation and treatment of neck and back pain. *Emergency Medicine Clinics of North America, 38*(1), 167–191. doi:10.1016/j.emc.2019.09.007

Doneddu, P. E., Coraci, D., De Franco, P., Paolasso, I., Caliandro, P., & Padua, L. (2017). Thoracic outlet syndrome: Wide literature for few cases. Status of the art. *Neurological Sciences, 38*, 383–388. doi:10.1007/s10072-016-2794-4

Edmondston, S. J., & Singer, K. P. (1997). Thoracic spine: Anatomical and bio-mechanical considerations for manual therapy. *Manual Therapy, 2*(3), 132–143. doi:10.1054/math.1997.0293

Fomby, E. W., & Mellion, M. B. (1997). Identifying and treating myofascial pain syndrome. *Physician and Sports Medicine, 25*(2), 67–75. doi:10.3810/psm.1997.02.1674

Fricton, J. (2016). Myofascial pain: Mechanisms to management. *Oral and Maxillofacial Surgery Clinics of North America, 28*(3), 289–311. doi:10.1016/j.coms.2016.03.010

Gerwin, R. D. (2001). Classification, epidemiology, and natural history of myofascial pain syndrome. *Current Pain Headache Reports, 5*(5), 412–420. doi:10.1007/s11916-001-0052-8

Gerwin, R. D. (2014). Diagnosis of myofascial pain syndrome. *Physical Medicine and Rehabilitation Clinics of North America, 25*(2), 341–355. doi:10.1016/j.pmr.2014.01.011

Giamberardino, M. A., Affaitati, G., Fabrizio, A., & Costantini, R. (2011). Myofascial pain syndromes and their evaluation. *Best Practice & Research Clinical Rheumatology, 25*(2), 185–198. doi:10.1016/j.berh.2011.01.002

Gordon, S. J., Trott, P., & Grimmer, K. A. (2002). Waking cervical pain and stiffness, headache, scapular, or arm pain: Gender and age effects. *Australian Journal of Physiotherapy, 48*(1), 9–15. doi:10.1016/s0004-9514(14)60277-4

Heneghan, N. R., & Rushton, A. (2016). Understanding why the thoracic region is the "Cinderella" region of the spine. *Manual Therapy, 21*, 274–276. doi:10.1016/j.math.2015.06.010

Hirpara, K. M., Butler, J. S., Dolan, R. T., O'Byrne, J. M., & Poynton, A. R. (2012). Nonoperative modalities to treat symptomatic cervical spondylosis. *Advances in Orthopedics*, 294857. doi:10.1155/2012/294857

Hooper, T. L., Denton, J., McGalliard, M. K., Brismee, J-M., & Sizer, P. S. Jr. (2010). Thoracic outlet syndrome: A controversial clinical condition. Part 1: Anatomy, and clinical examination/diagnosis. *Journal of Manual & Manipulative Therapy, 18*(2), 74–83. doi:10.1179/106698110X12640740712734

Hoppenfeld, S. (1976). *Physical examination of the spine and extremities*. Appleton-Century-Crofts.

Jalil, N. A., Sulaiman, Z., Awang, M. S., & Omar, M. (2009). Retrospective review of outcomes of a multimodal chronic pain service in a major teaching hospital: A preliminary experience in Universiti Sains Malaysia. *Malaysian Journal of Medical Sciences, 16*, 55–65.

Kotwal, S., Pumberger, M., Hughes, A., & Girardi, F. (2011). Degenerative scoliosis: A review. *HSS Journal, 7*(3), 257–264. doi:10.1007/s11420-011-9204-5

Krause, N., Ragland, N., Greiner, B. A., Fisher, J. M., Holman, B. L., & Selvin, S. (1997). Physical workload and ergonomic factors associated with prevalence of back and neck pain in urban transit operators. *Spine, 22*(18), 2117–2126. doi:10.1097/00007632-199709150-00010

Magee, D. J., & Manske, R. C. (2021). *Orthopedic physical assessment* (7th ed.). Saunders Elsevier.

Mahmoud, N. F., Hassan, K. A., Abdelmajeed, S. F., Moustafa, I. M., & Silva, A. G. (2019). The relationship between forward head posture and neck pain: A systematic review and meta-analysis. *Current Reviews in Musculoskeletal Medicine, 12*(4), 562–577. doi:10.1007/s12178-019-09594-y

Manchikanti, L., Singh, V., Datta, S., Cohen, S., & Hirsch, J. (2009). Comprehensive review of epidemiology, scope, and impact of spinal pain. *Pain Physician, 12*(4), E35–E70.

Marovino, T., & Quinton, J. (2008). Unraveling the mysteries of myofascial pain syndromes. *Practical Pain Management, 8*(6). https://www.practicalpainmanagement.com/pain/myofascial/unraveling-mysteries-myofascial-pain-syndromes

Mayton, A. G., Kittusamy, N. K., Ambrose, D. H., Jobes, C. C., & Legalt, M. L. (n.d.). *Jarring/jolting and musculoskeletal symptoms among farm equipment operators*. https://www.cdc.gov/niosh/mining/userfiles/works/pdfs/jjeam.pdf

Mehl, J., Imhoff, A. B., & Beitzel, K. (2018). Omarthrose: Pathogenese, Diagnostik und konservative Therapieoptionen [Osteoarthritis of the shoulder: pathogenesis, diagnostics and conservative treatment options]. *Orthopade, 47*(5), 368–376. doi:10.1007/s00132-018-3542-7

Monica, J., Vredenburgh, Z., Korsh, J., & Gatt, C. (2016). Acute shoulder injuries in adults. *American Family Physician, 94*(2), 119–127.

Nordin, M., Randhawa, K., Torres, P., Yu, H., Haldeman, S., Brady, O., Côté, P., Torres, C., Modic, M., Mullerpatan, R., Cedraschi, C., Chou, R., Acaroğlu, E., Hurwitz, E. L., Lemeunier, N., Dudler, J., Taylor-Vaisey, A., & Sönmez, E. (2018). The Global Spine Care Initiative: A systematic review for the assessment of spine-related complaints in populations with limited resources and in low- and middle-income communities. *European Spine Journal, 27*(Suppl. 6), 816–827. doi:10.1007/s00586-017-5446-3

Povlsen, B., Hansson, T., & Pilsen, S. D. (2014). Treatment for thoracic outlet syndrome. *Cochrane Database of Systematic Reviews, 2014*(26), CD007218. doi:10.1002/14651858.CD007218.pub3

Roghani, T., Zavieh, M. K., Manshadi, F. D., King, N., & Katzman, W. (2017). Age-related hyperkyphosis: Update of its potential causes and clinical impacts-narrative review. *Aging Clinical and Experimental Research, 29*(4), 567–577. doi:10.1007/s40520-016-0617-3

Roquelaure, Y., Bodin, J., Ha, C., Le Marec, F., Fouquet, N., Ramond-Roquin, A., Goldberg, M., Descatha, A., Petit, A., & Imbernon, E. (2014). Incidence and risk factors for thoracic spine pain in the working population: The French Pays de la Loire study. *Arthritis Care & Research*, *66*(11), 1695–1702. doi:10.1002/acr.22323

Scoliosis Research Society. (2022). *Congenital kyphosis*. http://www.srs.org/patients-and-families/conditions-and-treatments/parents/kyphosis/congenital-kyphosis

Shahbaz, M., Blanc, P. D., Domeracki, S. J., & Guntur, S. (2019). Shoulder injury related to vaccine administration (SIRVA): An occupational case report. *Workplace Health & Safety*, *67*(10), 501–505. doi:10.1177/2165079919875161

Shakil, H. (2014). Scoliosis: Review of types of curves, etiological theories and conservative treatment. *Journal of Back and Musculoskeletal Rehabilitation*, *27*(2), 111–115. doi:10.3233/BMR-130438

Spadliński, Ł., Cecot, T., Majos, A., Stefańczyk, L., Pietruszewska, W., Wysiadecki, G., Topol, M., & Polguj, M. (2016). The epidemiological, morphological, and clinical aspects of the cervical ribs in humans. *BioMed Research International*, 8034613. doi:10.1155/2016/8034613

Steinberg, G., Akins, C., & Baran, D. (1999). *Orthopaedics in primary care* (3rd ed.). Lippincott Williams & Williams.

Sterud, T., Johannessen, H. A., & Tynes, T. (2014). Work-related psychosocial and mechanical risk factors for neck/shoulder pain: A 3-year follow-up study of the general working population in Norway. *International Archives of Occupational and Environmental Health*, *87*(5), 471–481. doi:10.1007/s00420-013-0886-5

Tassadaq, N., & Osama, M. (2021). Occurrence of paralytic scoliosis in patients with poliomyelitis reporting at Fauji Foundation Hospital, Rawalpindi. *Journal of Pakistan Medical Association*, *71*(2[B]), 737–739. doi:10.47391/JPMA.986

U.S. National Library of Medicine. (2017). *Neck injuries and disorders*. https://medlineplus.gov/neckinjuriesanddisorders.html

VanBaak, K., & Aerni, G. (2020). Shoulder conditions: Rotator cuff injuries and bursitis. FP Essentials, *491*, 11–16.

Yaman, O., & Dalbayrak, S. (2014). Kyphosis: Diagnosis, classification, and treatment methods. *Turkish Neurosurgery*, *24*(1).

CHAPTER 67

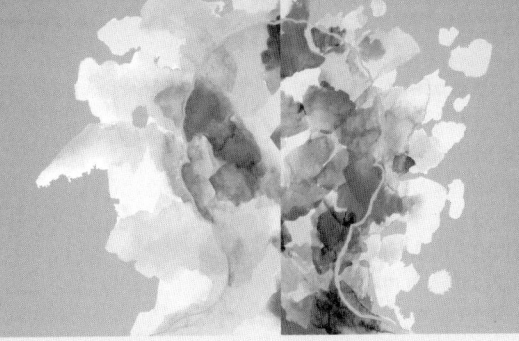

Upper Extremity Tendinopathy: Shoulder (Bicipital and Rotator Cuff), Elbow, and De Quervain Tendinopathy

Nicole L. Collman

I. Introduction and general background

Upper extremity musculoskeletal complaints are common conditions advanced practice nurses will encounter in the clinical setting. Tendon pain has historically been referred to as *tendinitis*, which implies an acute inflammatory condition. *Tendinosis* and *tendinopathy* are both terms that have been used to describe chronic tendon complaints (Scott et al., 2015). All three clinical terms have been used for the diagnosis of pain/swelling of injured tendons without distinguishing between the presence or absence of inflammation. *Tendinopathy* has become the accepted clinical terminology to describe persistent tendon pain related to repeated mechanical loading or overuse (Scott et al., 2015, 2020). Tendon injuries of the upper extremity can present acutely (<4 weeks), subacutely (5–12 weeks), chronically (>12 weeks), or in an acute-on-chronic manner (Scott et al., 2020). Common upper extremity tendinopathy is typically localized to the shoulder (rotator cuff and biceps tendinopathy), elbow (medial and lateral elbow tendinopathy), and wrist (de Quervain tendinopathy).

Tendons connect muscles to bones and facilitate joint movement. Individuals are predisposed to overuse tendinopathy as a result of various intrinsic factors: age over 35, obesity, prior tendon injury, anatomic and biomechanical abnormalities, gender, medications, and comorbidities. Extrinsic factors also contribute to this condition: improper training, poor movement patterns, including repetition and overuse, environmental conditions, poor ergonomics and awkward postures, and poor equipment (Harris-Adamson et al., 2014; Jozsa & Kannus, 1997; Kirchgesner et al., 2014; Lui, 2017; Raynor & Kuhn, 2016; van der Molen et al., 2017; Werner et al., 2005).

Although rare, drug-induced tendinopathy or tendon rupture is also a factor that clinicians need to consider when evaluating tendon injuries. To date, four main drug classes have been associated with tendinopathies: quinolones, long-term glucocorticoids, statins, and aromatase inhibitors (Kirchgesner et al., 2014; Marie et al., 2008). The specific pathophysiological mechanisms responsible for tendon damage remain unknown. Risk factors for the development of drug-induced tendinopathies include age over 60; preexisting tendinopathy; and concurrent use of drugs associated with tendinopathies, especially high-dose corticosteroids (Khaliq & Zhanel, 2003; Kirchgesner et al., 2014). Timing of symptom onset varies depending on the drug class, from a median time of 9 days for quinolones to 8–10 months for statins, 4 months to several years for systemic glucocorticoids, and 2 weeks to 19 months for aromatase inhibitors (Kirchgesner et al., 2014).

Metabolic disorders such as diabetes mellitus (DM), obesity, high cholesterol, gout, and hypothyroidism have also been associated with tendinopathy (Abate et al., 2013, Olivia et al., 2013). DM induces structural, inflammatory, and vascular changes in tendons that may predispose these patients to a greater risk of tendinopathy (Lui, 2017). Obesity affects tendons in a number of ways: excess weight can affect the load-bearing capacity of tendons, and bioactive peptides released by adipocytes can negatively affect tendons at the cellular level, causing chronic, low-grade inflammation (Abate et al., 2016).

A. Diagnosis: biceps tendinopathy
   1. Definition and overview
      The biceps muscle is made up of a long and short head, each with a unique tendon origin on the scapula. The primary biomechanical roles of the biceps brachii muscle are to flex and supinate the elbow. The long head of the biceps brachii is more susceptible to injury compared to the short head. The long head of the biceps tendon helps stabilize the anterior shoulder and assists with shoulder range of motion. Patients with biceps tendinopathy present with progressive anterior shoulder pain and complain of point tenderness located within the bicipital groove and may report clicking or popping sensations experienced in the anterior shoulder. Biceps tendinopathy is a common cause of anterior shoulder pain. Isolated biceps tendinopathy is uncommon, and the condition often coexists with other rotator cuff pathology and impingement (Linaker & Walker-Bone, 2015). Risk factors for biceps tendinopathy include:
      a. Repetitive overhead activities, especially throwing sports
      b. Degenerative changes of soft tissue and bone associated with the aging process
      c. Secondary tendinopathy with associated shoulder pathology (e.g., impingement syndrome, rotator cuff disease)
      d. Occupational risk factors, particularly jobs involving exposure to combinations of overhead work, arm/hand elevation, heavy loads, vibration, forceful work, and repetition (van der Molen et al., 2017)
   2. Prevalence and incidence
      The overall prevalence of primary, isolated biceps tendinopathy is difficult to determine. A systematic review of the prevalence of shoulder pain in the general population (age over 18 and under 70) found the frequency to be between 7% and 27% (Luime et al., 2004). A large population-based study in the United Kingdom found that the point prevalence in adults of "shoulder pain" was between 18% and 25% (Walker-Bone et al., 2004). Patients with primary isolated biceps tendinitis tend to be younger and participate in overhead sports such as baseball, softball, and volleyball (Patton & McCluskey, 2001).

B. Diagnosis: rotator cuff tendinopathy
   1. Definition and overview
      The shoulder is a ball-and-socket joint with a shallow socket, which allows the shoulder joint to have the most motion of any joint. The surrounding ligaments and muscles stabilize the joint. The rotator cuff comprises four muscles: the subscapularis, the supraspinatus, the infraspinatus, and the teres minor. Shoulder pain is frequently caused by acute or chronic injury to the rotator cuff, most often the supraspinatus tendon or muscle. Patients with rotator cuff tendinopathy present with shoulder pain when reaching overhead and during activities of daily living (e.g., dressing, grooming hair). Overhead reaching may mechanically compress or irritate the subacromial tendon structures between the humeral head and the acromion, a condition known as *shoulder impingement syndrome*. Pain is often localized to the lateral deltoid area, and patients report difficulty sleeping on the affected shoulder. Biceps tendinopathy and shoulder bursitis can also present concurrently with rotator cuff tendinopathy. A 2019 systematic review and meta-analysis by Leong et al. revealed that risk factors for rotator cuff tendinopathy include:
      a. Repetitive overhead activities, either occupationally or sports related, specifically elevating the shoulder above 90°
      b. Age over 50
      c. DM
      d. Occupational risk factors such as heavy manual work, repetitive work, high frequency of work, and vibration work
      Other risk factors include anatomic variants (down-sloped or hooked acromion types), scapular instability, weakness of the rotator cuff muscles, and poor postural alignment (Dela Rosa et al., 2001)
   2. Prevalence and incidence
      The prevalence of shoulder pain in the general population (age over 18 and under 70) can range between 7% and 27%. The incidence of nontraumatic rotator cuff tendinopathy and shoulder symptoms (shoulder pain or burning) in the working population can be as high as 14% to 18% in occupations with high force and low, medium, or high repetitive job demands involving the upper extremities (Silverstein et al., 2006).

C. Diagnosis: elbow tendinopathy: medial (golf) and lateral (tennis)
   1. Definition and overview
      The lateral and medial epicondyles are bony prominences that can be easily palpated on their respective sides of the distal humerus proximal to the elbow joint. The lateral epicondyle is the origin for the wrist extensor muscles of the forearm, and the medial epicondyle is the origin for the wrist flexors of the forearm. Chronic pain in the region of the lateral epicondyle is termed *lateral elbow tendinopathy* (LET), commonly referred to as *tennis elbow* or *lateral epicondylitis*. Patients with LET report pain at the lateral elbow, which can radiate down the forearm when the arm and wrist are extended. Symptoms include pain when lifting objects, using a computer mouse, twisting towels, shaking hands, or performing a back-handed tennis stroke. Chronic

pain in the region of the medial epicondyle is termed *medial elbow tendinopathy* (MET) or *golfer's elbow* or *medial epicondylitis*. Patients with MET report pain at the medial elbow when the wrist is flexed and the forearm is pronated. Symptoms include pain with gripping or squeezing objects, opening jars or doors, or swinging a golf club. Despite the reference to sports-related activities, athletes are not the only individuals to develop these conditions. Risk factors for LET and MET:

   a. There is an association between physically forceful occupational activities (especially high force combined with high repetition or awkward posture of wrists and hands) and the incidence of LET and MET (Descatha et al., 2016; van Rijn et al., 2009). Work involving exposure to hand/arm vibration is associated with MET (van Rijn et al., 2009). A 2021 systematic review by Curti et al. found that there was limited evidence of a *causal* relationship between occupational exposure to biomechanical risk factors and LET and insufficient evidence to support a *causal* relationship for MET.
   b. Age >40 (Fan et al., 2014)
   c. Former or current smoker (Shiri et al., 2006)
   d. Athletes, particularly those who play tennis or golf (Fedorczyk et al., 2021)
2. Prevalence and incidence
   The incidence of LET is higher than that of MET (da Costa et al., 2015). A large population-based study of adults in the United States found an annual incidence of LET at 15.1 cases/10,000 (Degen et al., 2018). In the general Finnish population, the prevalence of LET was estimated at 1.3% and MET at 0.4% based on self-reported symptoms and clinical signs in a standardized health examination performed by a physician (Shiri et al., 2006). A large longitudinal cohort study of newly hired workers from a variety of industries in the United States found that after a 3-year follow-up, 6.9% had symptoms and physical exam findings of LET and/or MET (Descatha et al., 2013). In a systematic literature review, van Rijn et al. (2009) found that the prevalence of LET and MET in workers whose jobs required repetitive work varied from 1.3% to 12.2% and from 0.2% to 3.8%, respectively. A study of meat-processing workers in Finland found the rate of epicondylitis in strenuous jobs (meat cutters, packers, and sausage makers) to be between 5.2 and 8.9 cases per 100 workers per year, and the rate in non-strenuous jobs was found to be 1 case per 100 workers per year (Kurppa et al., 1991).

D. Diagnosis: de Quervain tendinopathy
   1. Definition and overview
      Two of the main tendons of the thumb (abductor pollicis longus and extensor pollicis brevis) pass through the first dorsal compartment (extensor retinaculum) located on the radial side of the wrist. De Quervain disease is precipitated by thickening of the tendons and the surrounding retinaculum (Ilyas et al., 2007). It is characterized by pain and tenderness at the level of the first dorsal compartment over the radial styloid (Ilyas et al., 2007). Patients may report pain when opening jars, wringing towels, cutting with scissors, or playing piano (Lee et al., 2021). Resisted thumb extension is usually painful, and either a Finkelstein or Eichhoff test is typically positive. More recently, the wrist hyperflexion and abduction of the thumb (WHAT) test has shown better sensitivity and specificity compared to the Eichhoff maneuver (Goubau et al. 2014). The WHAT test involves having the patient fully flex their affected wrist and keep their thumb extended and abducted while the examiner applies abducted resistance to the thumb (Goubau et al., 2014). Risk factors for de Quervain tendinopathy include:
      a. Age over 40 (Wolf et al., 2009)
      b. Female gender (Wolf et al., 2009)
      c. Pregnancy and lactation (Afshar & Tabrizi, 2021)
      d. High-frequency smartphone use (Morgan et al., 2020)
      e. Occupational biomechanical risk factors that have been *associated* with the incidence of de Quervain disease include repeated or sustained wrist bending for >2 hours per day and repeated movements associated with the twisting or driving of screws >2 hours per day (Petit Le Manac'h et al., 2011). In contrast, a 2013 systematic review and meta-analysis conducted by Stahl et al. found no *causal* relationship between de Quervain disease and occupational risk factors.
      f. Increasing hours of computer work has been associated with de Quervain disease as a result of contact stress or sustained wrist postures (American College of Occupational and Environmental Medicine [ACOEM], 2021a).
      g. Athletes who participate in racquet sports, rowing, golf, volleyball (thought to be caused by repetitive microtrauma from impact of the ball on the dorsal radial wrist), and bowling (Patrick & Hammert, 2020)
   2. Prevalence and incidence
      A large U.S. population–based study found the overall incidence rate of de Quervain tendinopathy to be 2.54 per 100,000 person-years for females and 1 per 100,000 person-years for males (Hassan et al., 2022).

II. Database (including but not limited to)
A. *Subjective*
   For all soft tissue complaints:
   1. History of presenting illness: description of the pain, including onset, location, duration, radiation, character, quality, and timing, as well as aggravating and alleviating factors. Determine modifying factors, such as rest, activity, and changes in posture or position.

Inquire about the course of symptoms, including any recent change in activities, job duties, or new equipment (desk, computer, mouse, tablet, racquet, etc.). If acute onset of pain or trauma, determine exact mechanism of the injury. Ask the patient about their theory as to the causation of the problem.
2. Concurrent medical problems: liver or kidney disease, cardiovascular, pulmonary, gastrointestinal, autoimmune disorders (including psoriasis, inflammatory and arthritis), degenerative arthritis, diabetes, hyperlipidemia, gout, or thyroid disorder
3. Past conditions: prior soft tissue complaints or injuries, neck pain or trauma, fractures, workers' compensation claims, history of cancer, infectious diseases, gastrointestinal (GI) bleeds (helpful for determining drug therapy choices)
4. Past surgical history: any history of surgery to the affected area
5. Accidental trauma: including motor vehicle accidents
6. Obstetric and gynecological history: current pregnancy or lactation
7. Medications: nonsteroidal anti-inflammatory drugs (NSAIDs), oral or topical; any current over-the-counter topical or oral medications for pain; history of cortisone injections; medications associated with tendinopathy, such as recent quinolone use (within past 1–2 weeks), long-term glucocorticoids (months to years), statins (8–10 months), and aromatase inhibitors (2 weeks to 19 months)
8. Allergies: including sensitivity to aspirin or NSAIDs
9. Family history: arthritis, psoriasis, autoimmune and inflammatory conditions, diabetes, gout, skeletal deformities
10. Occupational illnesses/injuries; disability, compensation
    a. Hours, tasks, responsibilities
    b. Exposures: psychological, social, physical (e.g., any work activity that involves repetitive or awkward postures; lifting, pushing, or pulling; contact stress; vibration; and/or cold temperature)
    c. Computer, phone, and tablet work: ergonomic equipment and adjustment of workstation, percentage of time spent at computer workstation, and ratio of keyboard versus mouse versus 10-key use
    d. Protective equipment used: splints, elbow pads or braces, ergonomic equipment (sit–stand desk, ergonomic keyboard or mouse or dictation equipment)
    e. Coworkers with similar symptoms
    f. Symptoms relieved on days away from work or made worse by certain work activities
    g. Relationships with coworkers and supervisors, job satisfaction
    h. Past or current workers' compensation claims
11. Hobbies, sports, leisure activities
    a. Any hobby and/or sport involving repetitive or awkward postures; lifting, pushing, or pulling; contact stress; vibration; and/or cold temperature (past and current)
    b. High-risk sports (tennis or racquet sports, golf, volleyball, bowling, throwing sports, or rowing); musical instruments; needlework (e.g., crocheting, knitting, needlepoint); home computer, smartphone, tablet, or gaming console usage (including amount of screen time per day); motorcycle or four-wheeler; vibrating tools
12. Personal and social history
    a. Functional impact of symptoms on activities of daily living (e.g., dressing, bathing, grooming, etc.) or instrumental activities of daily living (e.g., shopping, housekeeping, food preparation, and caregiving); trouble turning a doorknob or using a screwdriver (pronation or supination of elbow)
    b. Substances: smoking and alcohol use (abuse screening may be indicated for possible osteonecrosis); intravenous drug use (if suspicion for infection is present)
    c. Sleep quality and quantity; impact of symptoms on sleep (e.g., unable to sleep on affected side or wakes with numbness in hand or fingers)
    d. Frequency and type of exercise (stretching and flexibility, strength, endurance conditioning, overtraining, and postural awareness)
    e. Exposure to intimate partner violence
13. Review of systems
    a. Constitutional signs and symptoms: fatigue, fever, weight loss or gain, and night sweats
    b. Skin, hair, and nails: erythema or warmth to affected area
    c. Musculoskeletal: hand dominance; pain level on a 0–10 numerical or visual analogue scale; quality of pain (e.g., burning, aching, or electric-shock pain); radiation of pain; pain at rest or with activity; stiffness; limitations in motion (acute or chronic); presence of swelling; crepitus or popping, clicking, catching of joints; locking of digits; giving way of joints; nighttime wakening with symptoms; and presence of pain in distal or proximal joints
    d. Neurologic: paresthesias or motor weakness
    e. Respiratory: shortness of breath, wheeze, cough, sputum, hemoptysis, pneumonia, tuberculosis (referred pain to shoulder from the lungs)
    f. Abdominal: any abdominal pain, changes in appetite, bowel patterns, nausea or vomiting (referred pain to shoulder from the abdomen)

B. Objective
   1. Physical examination findings
      a. Vital signs: temperature, height and weight, and pain level
      b. General appearance, posture, overall conditioning
      c. Skin: pallor, surgical scars, erythema, warmth, swelling, crepitus, and tenderness

d. Musculoskeletal
   i. Inspection: It is important to inspect both extremities and have adequate exposure (ask patient to remove clothing and don a gown) so that subtle differences in muscle atrophy and deformities can be appreciated. Assess any bony deformities and muscle atrophy or asymmetry (e.g., long-standing rotator cuff tendinopathy may reveal atrophy of the supraspinatus or infraspinatus muscles).
   ii. Palpation: Assess for localized tenderness over specific muscles or tendons. Palpation over the proximal long head of the biceps tendon often elicits tenderness in patients with *biceps tendinopathy*. Palpation over the subacromial area of the shoulder may elicit tenderness with *rotator cuff tendinopathy* or bursitis. Palpation over the lateral epicondyle and wrist extensor muscle mass or medial epicondyle and wrist flexor muscle mass will elicit tenderness in patients with *elbow tendinopathy* (LET or MET, respectively). Palpation over the first dorsal compartment over the radial styloid will elicit tenderness in patients with *de Quervain tendinopathy*.
   iii. Assess anatomic distribution of pain and paresthesias.
   iv. Perform joint range of motion (ROM), including examination of the joint above and below the presenting area to rule out referred pain. Examiners may choose to perform simultaneous, bilateral shoulder joint ROM to detect subtle differences between extremities.
   v. Perform special maneuvers (**Table 67-1**). A combination of special maneuvers may provide better accuracy (Hedegus et al., 2012).
e. Neurologic: sensory loss mapping, motor strength, deep tendon reflexes

Table 67-1 Provocative Physical Examination Maneuvers for Selected Tendinopathy Diagnosis

Special Test	Diagnosis	How to Perform
Palpation of bicipital groove: https://meded.ucsd.edu/clinicalmed/joints2.htm	Bicipital tendinopathy	The bicipital groove can be palpated by locating the greater tuberosity of the humerus and then moving the fingers slightly medially to locate the groove. It can be helpful to keep the affected arm flexed at 90° and then internally and externally rotate the arm while palpating; examiner will feel the tendon roll under their fingers. A positive test is tenderness with palpation in this region.
Yergason test: https://meded.ucsd.edu/clinicalmed/joints2.htm	Bicipital tendinopathy	Place the patient's arm at their side at 70° with the forearm fully pronated. Ask the patient to supinate their arm against the examiner's resistance. Pain reproduced in the region of the long head of the biceps tendon is considered a positive test.
Neers test: https://meded.ucsd.edu/clinicalmed/joints2.htm	Shoulder impingement	Stabilize the patient's scapula with one hand and grasp elbow with other hand. The patient is asked to internally rotate their arm so that the thumb is pointing down. The examiner elevates the patient's arm overhead. Pain with this maneuver suggests impingement.
Hawkins-Kennedy test: https://meded.ucsd.edu/clinicalmed/joints2.htm	Shoulder impingement	Stabilize the patient's shoulder with one hand, with the patient's elbow flexed at 90° and shoulder elevated to 90°. The examiner internally rotates the shoulder (thumb down). Pain with this maneuver suggests impingement. This maneuver can detect more subtle impingement than the Neers test.
Painful arc	Rotator cuff tendinopathy	Patient actively abducts shoulder beyond 90°. Pain with active abduction suggests rotator cuff tendinopathy and is most useful when combined with the Neer and Hawkins-Kennedy tests.
Resisted wrist extension: https://meded.ucsd.edu/clinicalmed/joints4.htm	Lateral elbow tendinopathy	Resisted extension of the wrist reproduces pain in the lateral epicondyle region for a positive test.

(continues)

Table 67-1 Provocative Physical Examination Maneuvers for Selected Tendinopathy Diagnosis *(continued)*

Special Test	Diagnosis	How to Perform
Book test	Lateral elbow tendinopathy	Patient holds a reasonably heavy book in the hand of the affected arm, which is raised, the elbow fully extended, palm facing down. Discomfort at the lateral epicondyle while holding the book is a positive test.
Resisted wrist flexion: https://meded.ucsd.edu/clinicalmed/joints4.htm	Medial elbow tendinopathy	Resisted flexion of the wrist reproduces pain in the medial epicondyle region for a positive test.
Modified book test	Medial elbow tendinopathy	Patient grips a 3- to 5-pound weight in the hand of the affected arm, which is raised, the elbow fully extended, palm facing upward. Discomfort at the medial epicondyle while gripping the weight is a positive test.
Finkelstein test:	de Quervain tendinopathy	Examiner grasps patient's thumb firmly with one hand while supporting the forearm. The patient's wrist and forearm are in a neutral position. Examiner applies a firm traction to the patient's thumb, pulling it in a longitudinally and ulnar direction. Pain reported over the first extensor compartment (i.e., distal to the lateral aspect of radial styloid and proximal to the anatomic snuff box) indicates a positive test. This test can stress and produce discomfort in other unrelated joints, reducing the sensitivity and specificity of maneuver.
Eichhoff test (commonly mistaken for Finkelstein test): https://meded.ucsd.edu/clinicalmed/joints3.htm	de Quervain tendinopathy	Patient makes a fist around flexed thumb and gently ulnar deviates the wrist. Pain reported over the first extensor compartment is a positive test.
Wrist hyperflexion and abduction of the thumb (WHAT) test	de Quervain tendinopathy	Patient fully flexes their affected wrist and keeps their thumb extended and abducted while the examiner applies abducted resistance to the thumb.

i. There are four major muscles of the rotator cuff; each of the four muscles can be tested individually for strength (and discomfort). Weakness in the muscle may indicate a partial or complete tear of a muscle or tendon, and pain while testing may indicate specific rotator cuff tendinopathy (**Table 67-2**).
2. Supporting data from relevant diagnostic tests
   a. Laboratory data to determine presence of metabolic disorders: fasting blood sugar, hemoglobin A1c, serum uric acid level, lipid panel
   b. Rheumatoid factor, anti-cyclic citrullinated peptide (anti-CCP) antibody, antinuclear antibody, erythrocyte sedimentation rate (if suspect an inflammatory rheumatologic condition)
   c. Thyroid-stimulating hormone (if suspect hypothyroidism)
   d. Radiograph (e.g., for acute trauma to rule out fracture, to assess acromion type, or if suspicion of arthritis)
   e. Nerve conduction studies (if suspect a peripheral nerve entrapment syndrome or cervical radiculopathy)
   f. Electromyogram (if suspect cervical radiculopathy)
   g. Ultrasound (e.g., for imaging of the biceps tendon if rupture is suspected or for staging of elbow tendinopathy)
   h. Magnetic resonance imaging (MRI) is used to rule out a rotator cuff tear when conservative treatment fails or for clinical suspicion of tear. MRI may be helpful for evaluating injuries to the labrum, glenohumeral joint, and other adjacent structures.

III. Assessment
   A. Determine the likely diagnosis based on patient's history, subjective and objective supporting data (**Table 67-3**).
      1. The O'VINDICATES mnemonic is helpful in developing a broad and thorough differential:
         O—Occupational
         V—Vascular

Table 67-2 Isometric Rotator Cuff Muscle Testing

Muscle of the Rotator Cuff	Function	Isometric Strength Testing
Supraspinatus: https://meded.ucsd.edu/clinicalmed/joints2.html	Connects top of scapula to humerus. Major role in shoulder abduction and stabilization.	Perform "empty can" or Jobe test: The examiner places patient's straight arm at 90° of abduction and 30° of forward flexion, then internally rotates the patient's arm (thumb pointing down or "emptying cans"). Ask patient to resist examiner's attempt to depress arm. Weakness suggests partial- or full-thickness tear of the supraspinatus muscle/tendon. Pain with this maneuver suggests tendinopathy.
Infraspinatus: https://meded.ucsd.edu/clinicalmed/joints2.html	Connects the scapula to the humerus. Primarily responsible for external rotation of the shoulder, along with the teres minor to a minor degree.	Start with the patient's arm adducted and elbow flexed to 90° with forearm in neutral position (thumbs up). Patient is asked to attempt to externally rotate their arm against examiner's resistance. Weakness suggests partial- or full-thickness tear of the infraspinatus or teres minor muscle/tendon. Pain with this maneuver suggests tendinopathy.
Teres minor: https://meded.ucsd.edu/clinicalmed/joints2.html	Connects the scapula to the humerus. Responsible for external rotation to a minor degree (same function as the infraspinatus).	Same as infraspinatus
Subscapularis: https://meded.ucsd.edu/clinicalmed/joints2.html	Connects the scapula to the humerus with the muscle origin on the anterior surface of the scapula	Perform the Gerber Lift-Off test: Ask patient to place one hand behind their back with palm facing out and lift off against the examiner's resistance. Weakness suggests partial- or full-thickness tear of the subscapularis muscle/tendon. Pain with this maneuver suggests tendinopathy.

Table 67-3 Differential Diagnoses of Upper Extremity Complaints

Probable Diagnosis	History and Epidemiology	Examination Findings	Differential Diagnoses
Biceps tendinopathy	Isolated tendinitis in young or middle-aged patients Degenerative tendinopathy in older patients Repetitive overhead activities, especially throwing sports Secondary to other associated shoulder pathology Occupational factors—overhead work, repetitive activities, heavy loads, vibration Progressive anterior shoulder pain	Anterior shoulder pain Point tenderness over bicipital groove Positive Yergason test	Rotator cuff pathology Glenohumeral arthritis Adhesive capsulitis (frozen shoulder) Acromioclavicular (AC) joint injury or arthritis Referred pain from chest or abdomen Humeral head osteonecrosis Subacromial bursitis Labral tears
Rotator cuff tendinopathy	Age > 50 Repetitive overhead activities Pain increases with overhead reaching Diabetes mellitus Obesity	Subacromial tenderness Pain with impingement testing (Neer and Hawkins tests) Normal strength but may be painful Normal passive range of motion	Rotator cuff tear Adhesive capsulitis Arthritis (glenohumeral or AC joint) Subscapular bursitis Biceps tendinopathy

(continues)

Table 67-3 Differential Diagnoses of Upper Extremity Complaints (continued)

Probable Diagnosis	History and Epidemiology	Examination Findings	Differential Diagnoses
Lateral elbow tendinopathy	Lateral extra-articular elbow and proximal extensor muscle pain Age > 40 Obesity Former or current smoker Athletes—tennis players Repetitive movements of the wrist and elbow Pain with shaking hands, twisting towels, lifting objects, and backhand tennis stroke	Lateral epicondyle pain Positive book test and pain with resisted wrist extension Normal range of motion (ROM) of joint	Arthritis Fracture or other acute trauma, usually with history of trauma Neurologic—radial tunnel syndrome or cervical radiculopathy Intraarticular pathology
Medial elbow tendinopathy	Medial extra-articular elbow and proximal flexor muscle pain Age > 40 Obesity Former or current smoker Athletes—golf and tennis players, baseball pitchers, and weight lifters Repetitive movements of the forearm and wrist and forceful gripping during heavy labor	Medial epicondyle pain Pain with resisted wrist flexion and positive modified book test Normal ROM of joint	Arthritis Fracture or other acute trauma, usually with history of trauma Neurologic—cubital tunnel syndrome or cervical radiculopathy Ulnar collateral ligament injury (particularly with throwing injuries) Intraarticular pathology
de Quervain tendinopathy	Pain and tenderness at the first dorsal compartment of the radial wrist, usually in the dominant hand Age > 40 Women Pregnancy and lactation Smartphone use and increased hours at the computer Athletes—racquet sport players, rowers, golfers, and bowlers Occupations with repeated wrist bending or twisting	Pain and enlargement over the first dorsal compartment of the radial wrist Positive WHAT, Finkelstein, and/or Eichhoff tests	Arthritis of the trapeziometacarpal joint Ganglion cyst Neurologic—radial nerve entrapment Gout or pseudogout Fracture or other acute trauma, usually with history of trauma

I—Infectious
N—Neoplastic
D—Degenerative
I—Inflammatory
C—Congenital
A—Autoimmune
T—Trauma
E—Endocrine/Metabolic
S—Social/Psychological

B. Determine if the condition is acute, subacute, or chronic.
C. Determine if the condition is work related.
D. Assess the patient's ability to perform their usual actives, including occupational job duties.

IV. Goals of clinical management
A. Cost-effective and evidence-based assessment of the patient's upper extremity tendinopathy

In the absence of red-flag conditions (trauma, infection or systemic symptoms, history of cancer [especially lung], deformity, pain at rest, focal motor weakness or sensory loss), most upper extremity tendinopathies can be diagnosed with a thorough history and physical examination. Additional diagnostic procedures (MRI) or referrals to specialists can be made if there is no improvement in 4–6 weeks of conservative treatment.

B. Evidence-based management of the patient's upper extremity tendinopathy and strong patient adherence

It is important to select a treatment plan that engages the patient in a self-care, sports-medicine approach. Tendinopathies are chronic injuries that are usually slow to resolve and can require months of adherence in an active rehabilitation program. Careful supervision by a physiotherapist is important to ensure a controlled and progressive rehabilitation program.

C. *Selection of appropriate activity modifications for both work-related and non–work-related activities*
Development of a plan of care that limits the volume and intensity of work, reduces the aggravating activities, corrects biomechanical factors, and gradually increases the tendon-loading activities.

V. Plan

A. *Diagnostic tests*
   1. Initial laboratory and diagnostic studies
      a. In the absence of red-flag conditions or trauma, most initial tendinopathy workups do not include diagnostic studies. Imaging may be ordered at the initial visit if there is a presence of red-flag conditions:
         i. Trauma, either acute or prior history of fracture or dislocation, or presence of a deformity
         ii. Clinical suspicion for infection or systemic symptoms
         iii. History of cancer (especially lung) or with long-term smoking history (especially with shoulder complaints)
         iv. Pain at rest, focal motor weakness, or sensory loss
         v. Progressive neurologic or vascular compromise
      b. Plain radiographs do not reveal tendinopathy unless chronic calcification is present. According to the American College of Radiology (2021) Appropriateness Criteria, plain radiographs are usually appropriate as a best initial study (vs. MRI) for chronic wrist pain, chronic elbow pain, or chronic shoulder pain to identify coexisting or predisposing factors (arthritis, bony anatomic variations, or bone or soft tissue tumors). In general, plain radiographs are not indicated in patients with suspected tendinopathy.
      c. Failure of conservative therapy
         If, after 4–6 weeks of conservative therapy, the patient is showing no signs of improvement in symptoms, additional diagnostic studies may be ordered and/or specialty consultation can be considered.

B. *Management*
   1. Initial care
      Initial care for chronic upper extremity tendinopathy includes activity modification, relative rest, pain control, rehabilitative exercise, and protection. It may take more than 6 months for complete symptom resolution (Kane et al., 2019).
      a. Activity modification: reduction in or abstinence from inciting activities
         A period of modified duty for work-related tasks may be indicated for occupationally related symptoms—for example, a 5-minute break for every hour of repetitive activities to allow for stretching and rest. Explicit limitations of overhead work or lifting of heavy objects are often needed in shoulder tendinopathies (ACOEM, 2021c). Primary care providers need to be cautious when writing work restrictions and provide specific guidance, focusing on what the employee is able to do (e.g., "able to lift up to 10 pounds" or "able to use computer workstation for 30 minutes every hour over 8-hour shift") and not recommending general, nonspecific work restrictions (e.g., "light duty"). Removal from a specific job task may be needed. The goal should be to keep the employee at work, doing either alternative work or modified work (ACOEM, 2021a, 2021b, 2021c).
      b. Bracing and splints
         Bracing, splints, and other compressive supports can reduce strain on surrounding muscle groups and can also be a form of rest; however, prolonged immobilization can lead to stiffness and atrophy and should be used in combination with physical therapy. Slings and shoulder supports are not recommended for subacute or chronic shoulder pain (ACOEM, 2021c). Counterforce bracing or compression sleeves may be helpful for patients with elbow tendinopathy. A thumb-spica forearm splint is recommended to be worn during waking hours for de Quervain tendinopathy (ACOEM, 2021a).
      c. Pain control
         i. Cryotherapy: Although histopathological evidence of inflammation is not present in chronic tendinopathies, cryotherapies can be effective for temporary relief of pain (ACOEM, 2021c).
         ii. NSAIDs: Traditionally, heavy emphasis has been placed on anti-inflammatory treatments; however, with advancements in the understanding of tendinopathies, it is clear that it is a degenerative process and not an inflammatory process. When not contraindicated due to allergy, renal or hepatic function, or bleeding risk, NSAIDs are only recommended for purposes of pain relief. A short course of 7–10 days of scheduled NSAID therapy can alleviate pain in acute injuries. Topical NSAIDs can be a good option for short-term pain control and have fewer systemic side effects than oral medications, but systematic reviews have found no difference in treatment outcomes (Bisset et al., 2005).
         iii. Acetaminophen is recommended for shoulder pain, particularly for those with a contraindication to NSAIDs (ACOEM, 2021c).
         iv. Glucocorticoid injections: For patients with rotator cuff tendinopathy, glucocorticoid steroid injections are generally reserved for patients with pain that has not responded to NSAIDs or acetaminophen,

where ongoing pain has prevented the patient from participating in physical therapy, or in patients whose symptoms did not improve after 6–8 weeks of initial conservative therapy (Hopewell et al., 2021). A similar approach is taken for biceps tendinopathy, with glucocorticoid injections reserved for patients who do not respond to initial conservative treatment (Nho et al., 2010). For LET, glucocorticoid injections may improve short-term outcomes but have been associated with worse long-term outcomes (Olaussen et al., 2015). For patients experiencing severe symptoms, a single injection can provide short-term relief so that the patient can participate in a physical therapy program. Glucocorticoid injections for MET have the same indication as for LET. An initial glucocorticoid injection for de Quervain tendinopathy is recommended for patients with severe symptoms or for those who do not respond to NSAIDs and splinting (ACOEM, 2021a). In these patients, a second injection may be given for those who have an unsuccessful response to the first injection (ACOEM, 2021a).
     v. Topical nitroglycerin: This may be a useful adjunct to physical therapy for patients with persistent discomfort from rotator cuff tendinopathy or elbow tendinopathy (Challoumas et al., 2019). Although the exact mechanism is unknown, it is thought to enhance collagen synthesis in damaged tendons.
    vi. Platelet-rich plasma (PRP) and other biologic injections: Systematic reviews have found that PRP is not effective therapy for elbow tendinopathy (Sirico et al., 2017), but it may provide benefit in the long-term for rotator cuff tendinopathy (Lin et al., 2020).
  d. Rehabilitative exercise: Physical therapy is the primary treatment for rotator cuff tendinopathy and the often-associated biceps tendinopathy. Physical therapy for rotator cuff and biceps tendinopathy generally involves shoulder mobilization, strengthening exercises and correction of any asymmetry or muscle imbalances, correction of posture, and post-recovery ongoing exercises. For elbow tendinopathies, moderately to severely affected patients benefit from a supervised physical or occupational therapy program (ACOEM, 2021b).
  e. Equipment check: If the patient participates in sporting activities (tennis, golf), the patient should be encouraged to consult with a pro to ensure proper fit of equipment to the patient. A racquet with a smaller head and lighter weight and looser-strung racquets will reduce the strain and stress on the muscles of the forearm. Additionally, golf clubs that reduce the transmission of shock to the elbow may be helpful.
  f. Ergonomic interventions: Ergonomics is an expansive discipline that addresses design and intervention. It encompasses a wide variety of topics related to the human interface with the work environment, including physical, cognitive, and organizational ergonomics (Emerson & Finch, 2021). Ergonomic interventions that reduce the force, repetition, vibration, contact stress, or exposure to cold temperatures are theoretically helpful (ACOEM, 2021a). A referral to a certified ergonomist or human factors engineer can be useful for modifying the work activity, redesigning the workstation, or recommending organizational or management relief (ACOEM, 2021a). If the condition is work related, the provider can issue a prescription requesting an ergonomic evaluation of the employee's workstation. If not work related, the provider can assist the patient in requesting an ergonomic modification of the workplace as a reasonable accommodation request under the Americans With Disabilities Act (ADA).
2. Referral and consultation
  a. Acupuncture: Studies of acupuncture for the treatment of tendinopathy are limited but have found that it can provide short-term benefit for the reduction of acute pain while the patient participates in an exercise rehabilitation program (ACEOM, 2021a, 2021b, 2021c).
  b. Myofascial release and soft tissue friction massage. Massage is purported to improve tendon function by increasing circulation and tendon nutrition; however, there are no controlled studies demonstrating the efficacy (Lee et al., 2021).
  c. Rehabilitation specialist or orthopedic surgeon: Consultation with a rehabilitation specialist for complex cases or cases that do not respond to conventional therapy may be beneficial for a more tailored rehabilitation plan. Refer to a surgical specialist if a surgical intervention is needed (e.g., shoulder arthroscopy or surgical release of the first dorsal compartment).
  d. If condition is work related, the case needs to be reported to the patient's employer and the employer's workers' compensation program.
3. Follow-up care
  After initial assessment of the injury, the patient should return to the clinic within 2–3 weeks for reevaluation of symptoms and function. This follow-up visit is helpful to determine if the patient is beginning to respond to treatment or whether there is a need for further diagnostic workup or referrals. Once an appropriate management plan has been established, periodic visits can be made to assess work abilities and return to sporting activities.

C. Patient education: review
1. Self-care activities are important for improving overall physical conditioning: stretching, postural awareness, and core strengthening. Educate the patient on the need to take rest breaks and stretch, especially during any repetitive work at home and on the job. Reinforce that tendinopathies are chronic injuries. The mainstay of treatment requires active and regular participation in an exercise program performed by the patient, and recovery may require an extended period of time.
2. Review the management plan, including any medications and potential side effects, and follow-up care.
3. If symptoms are caused by work activities, review any state-specific reporting requirements and advise the patient to have an interactive discussion with management on work abilities, job duties, and equipment needs. Encourage the patient to remain in the workplace and utilize the workplace as part of the therapeutic treatment plan to avoid prolonged disability and lost wages.
4. Encourage primary prevention of injuries and utilize ergonomic interventions at work and home to prevent reinjury and injury to others.

VI. Self-management resources and tools
A. **Occupational Safety and Health Administration Ergonomics eTools:** consumer-oriented web-based training tools on occupational safety and health topics, including evaluating computer workstations and a purchase guide for computer workstations: http://www.osha.gov/etools
B. **The National Institute for Occupational Safety and Health (NIOSH):** A resource for workplace health and safety topics, including ergonomics and musculoskeletal disorders. Ergonomic interventions by industry are available for consumers: http://www.cdc.gov/niosh/topics/ergonomics
C. **MedlinePlus:** http://www.medlineplus.gov
D. **OrthoInfo (from the American Academy of Orthopedic Surgeons):** patient education for common orthopedic conditions and high-quality patient handouts available for download or printing: http://www.orthoinfo.aaos.org

Acknowledgments

The author wishes to thank Barbara J. Burgel, a *fabulous* colleague and mentor, for her previous edition of this chapter, for the constructive feedback, and for exceptional support of the process. Thank you to Dr. Michael Fischman for your thoughtful and meticulous editorial review.

References

Abate, M., Salini, V., & Andia, I. (2016). How obesity affects tendons? In P. Ackermann & D. Hart (Eds.), *Advances in Experimental Medicine and Biology* (pp. 167–177). Springer. doi:10.1007/978-3-319-33943-6_15

Abate, M., Schiavone, C., Salini, V., & Andia, I. (2013). Occurrence of tendon pathologies in metabolic disorders. *Rheumatology, 52*(4), 599–608. doi:10.1093/rheumatology/kes395

Afshar, A., & Tabrizi, A. (2021). Pregnancy-related hand and wrist problems. *Archives of Bone and Joint Surgery, 9*(3), 345–349. doi:10.22038/abjs.2020.50995.2531

American College of Occupational and Environmental Medicine. (2021a). *Hand, wrist, and forearm disorders*. https://www.mdguidelines.com/acoem/disorders/hand-wrist-and-forearm-disorders

American College of Occupational and Environmental Medicine. (2021b). *Elbow disorders*. https://app.mdguidelines.com/state-guidelines/ca-mtus/elbow-disorders

American College of Occupational and Environmental Medicine. (2021c). *Rotator cuff tendinopathies*. https://app.mdguidelines.com/state-guidelines/ca-mtus/shoulder-disorders/treatment-recommendations/rotator-cuff/

American College of Radiology. (2021). *Appropriateness criteria*. https://www.acr.org/Clinical-Resources/ACR-Appropriateness-Criteria

Bisset, L., Paungmali, A., Vicenzino, B., & Beller, E. (2005). A systematic review and meta-analysis of clinical trials on physical interventions for lateral epicondylalgia. *British Journal of Sports Medicine, 39*(7), 411–422. doi:10.1136/bjsm.2004.016170

Challoumas, D., Kirwan, P. D., Borysov, D., Clifford, C., McLean, M., & Millar, N. L. (2019). Topical glyceryl trinitrate for the treatment of tendinopathies: A systematic review. *British Journal of Sports Medicine, 53*(4), 251–262. doi:10.1136/bjsports-2018-099552

Curti, S., Mattioli, S., Bonfiglioli, R., Farioli, A., & Violante, F. S. (2021). Elbow tendinopathy and occupational biomechanical overload: A systematic review with best-evidence synthesis. *Journal of Occupational Health, 63*(1), e12186. doi:10.1002/1348-9585.12186

da Costa, J. T., Baptista, J. S., & Vaz, M. (2015). Incidence and prevalence of upper-limb work related musculoskeletal disorders: A systematic review. *Work, 51*(4), 635–644. doi:10.3233/WOR-152032

Degen, R. M., Conti, M. S., Camp, C. L., Altchek, D. W., Dines, J. S., & Werner, B. C. (2018). Epidemiology and disease burden of lateral epicondylitis in the USA: Analysis of 85,318 patients. *HSS Journal, 14*(1), 9–14. doi:10.1007/s11420-017-9559-3

Dela Rosa, T. L., Wang, A. W., & Zheng, M. H. (2001). Tendinosis of the rotator cuff: A review. *Journal of Musculoskeletal Research, 5*(3), 143.

Descatha, A., Albo, F., Leclerc, A., Carton, M., Godeau, D., Roquelaure, Y., Petit, A., & Aublet-Cuvelier, A. (2016). Lateral epicondylitis and physical exposure at work? A review of prospective studies and meta-analysis. *Arthritis Care & Research, 68*(11), 1681–1687. doi:10.1002/acr.22874

Descatha, A., Dale, A. M., Jaegers, L., Herquelot, E., & Evanoff, B. (2013). Self-reported physical exposure association with medial and lateral epicondylitis incidence in a large longitudinal study. *Occupational and Environmental Medicine*, 70(9), 670–673. doi:10.1136/oemed-2012-101341

Emerson, S. A., & Finch, D. (2021). The injured worker: Onsite evaluation and services. In T. M. Skirven, A. L. Osterman, J. M. Fedorczyk, P. C. Amadio, S. B. Feldscher, & E. K. Shin (Eds.), *Rehabilitation of the hand and upper extremity* (7th ed., Vol. 2, pp. 1704–1752). Elsevier.

Fan, Z. J., Bao, S., Silverstein, B. A., Howard, N. L., Smith, C. K., & Bonauto, D. K. (2014). Predicting work-related incidence of lateral and medial epicondylitis using the strain index. *American Journal of Industrial Medicine*, 57(12), 1319–1330. doi:10.1002/ajim.22383

Fedorczyk, J. M., Day, J. M., Lucado, A. M., & Vincent, J. (2021). Therapy management of lateral elbow tendinopathy. In T. M. Skirven, A. L. Osterman, J. M. Fedorczyk, P. C. Amadio, S. B. Feldscher, & E. K. Shin (Eds.), *Rehabilitation of the hand and upper extremity* (7th ed., Vol. 1, pp. 518–531). Elsevier.

Goubau, J. F., Goubau, L., Van Tongel, A., Van Hoonacker, P., Kerckhove, D., & Berghs, B. (2014). The wrist hyperflexion and abduction of the thumb (WHAT) test: A more specific and sensitive test to diagnose de Quervain tenosynovitis than the Eichhoff's test. *Journal of Hand Surgery*, 39(3), 286–292. doi:10.1177/1753193412475043

Harris-Adamson, C., You, D., Eisen, E. A., Goldberg, R., Rempel, D. (2014). The impact of posture on wrist tendinosis among blue-collar workers: The San Francisco study. *Human Factors*, 56(1), 143–150. doi:10.1177/0018720813502807

Hassan, K., Sohn, A., Shi, L., Lee, M., & Wolf, J. M. (2022). De Quervain tenosynovitis: An evaluation of the epidemiology and utility of multiple injections using a national database. *Journal of Hand Surgery*, 47(3), 284.e1–284.e6. doi:10.1016/j.jhsa.2021.04.018

Hegedus, E. J., Goode, A. P., Cook, C. E., Michener, L., Myer, C. A., Myer, D. M., & Wright, A. A. (2012). Which physical examination tests provide clinicians with the most value when examining the shoulder? Update of a systematic review with meta-analysis of individual tests. *British Journal of Sports Medicine*, 46(14), 964–978. doi:10.1136/bjsports-2012-091066

Hopewell, S., Keene, D. J., Marian, I. R., Dritsaki, M., Heine, P., Cureton, L., Dutton, S. J., Dakin, H., Carr, A., Hamilton, W., Hansen, Z., Jaggi, A., Littlewood, C., Barker, K. L., Gray, A., Lamb, S. E., & GRASP Trial Group. (2021). Progressive exercise compared with best practice advice, with or without corticosteroid injection, for the treatment of patients with rotator cuff disorders (GRASP): A multicentre, pragmatic, 2 × 2 factorial, randomised controlled trial. *Lancet*, 398(10298), 416–428. doi:10.1016/S0140-6736(21)00846-1

Ilyas, A. M., Ast, M., Schaffer, A. A., & Thoder, J. (2007). De Quervain tenosynovitis of the wrist. *Journal of the American Academy of Orthopaedic Surgeons*, 15(12), 757–764. doi:10.5435/00124635-200712000-00009

Jozsa, L. G., & Kannus, P. (1997). *Human tendons: Anatomy, physiology, and pathology*. Human Kinetics.

Kane, S. F., Olewinski, L. H., & Tamminga, K. S. (2019). Management of chronic tendon injuries. *American Family Physician*, 100(3), 147–157.

Khaliq, Y., & Zhanel, G. G. (2003). Fluoroquinolone-associated tendinopathy: A critical review of the literature. *Clinical Infectious Diseases*, 36(11), 1404–1410. doi:10.1086/375078

Kirchgesner, T., Larbi, A., Omoumi, P., Malghem, J., Zamali, N., Manelfe, J., Lecouvet, F., Vande Berg, B., Djebbar, S., & Dallaudière, B. (2014). Drug-induced tendinopathy: From physiology to clinical applications. *Joint Bone Spine*, 81(6), 485–492. doi:10.1016/j.jbspin.2014.03.022

Kurppa, K., Viikari-Juntura, E., Kuosma, E., Huuskonen, M., & Kivi, P. (1991). Incidence of tenosynovitis or peritendinitis and epicondylitis in a meat-processing factory. *Scandinavian Journal of Work, Environment & Health*, 17(1), 32–37. doi:10.5271/sjweh.1737

Lee, M. P., Biafora, S. J., & Zelouf, D. S. (2021). Management of hand and wrist tendinopathies. In T. M. Skirven, A. L. Osterman, J. M. Fedorczyk, P. C. Amadio, S. B. Feldscher, & E. K. Shin (Eds.), *Rehabilitation of the hand and upper extremity* (7th ed., Vol. 1, pp. 498–517). Elsevier.

Leong, H. T., Fu, S. C., He, X., Oh, J. H., Yamamoto, N., & Hang, S. (2019). Risk factors for rotator cuff tendinopathy: A systematic review and meta-analysis. *Journal of Rehabilitation Medicine*, 51(9), 627–637. doi:10.2340/16501977-2598

Lin, M. T., Wei, K. C., & Wu, C. H. (2020). Effectiveness of platelet-rich plasma injection in rotator cuff tendinopathy: A systematic review and meta-analysis of randomized controlled trials. *Diagnostics*, 10(4), 189. doi:10.3390/diagnostics10040189

Linaker, C. H., & Walker-Bone, K. (2015). Shoulder disorders and occupation. *Best Practice & Research. Clinical Rheumatology*, 29(3), 405–423. doi:10.1016/j.berh.2015.04.001

Lui, P. (2017). Tendinopathy in diabetes mellitus patients—epidemiology, pathogenesis, and management. *Scandinavian Journal of Medicine & Science in Sports*, 27(8), 776–787. doi:10.1111/sms.12824

Luime, J. J., Koes, B. W., Hendriksen, I. J., Burdorf, A., Verhagen, A. P., Miedema, H. S., & Verhaar, J. A. (2004). Prevalence and incidence of shoulder pain in the general population; a systematic review. *Scandinavian Journal of Rheumatology*, 33(2), 73–81. doi:10.1080/03009740310004667

Marie, I., Delafenêtre, H., Massy, N., Thuillez, C., Noblet, C., & Network of the French Pharmacovigilance Centers. (2008). Tendinous disorders attributed to statins: A study on ninety-six spontaneous reports in the period 1990–2005 and review of the literature. *Arthritis and Rheumatism*, 59(3), 367–372. doi:10.1002/art.23309

Morgan, S. D., Sivakumar, B. S., An, V. G., Sevao, J., & Graham, D. J. (2020). A review of de Quervain's stenosing tenovaginitis in the context of smartphone use. *Journal of Hand Surgery Asian-Pacific Volume*, 25(2), 133–136. doi:10.1142/S2424835520300029

Nho, S. J., Strauss, E. J., Lenart, B. A., Provencher, M. T., Mazzocca, A. D., Verma, N. N., & Romeo, A. A. (2010). Long head of the biceps tendinopathy: Diagnosis and management. *Journal of the American Academy of Orthopaedic Surgeons*, 18(11), 645–656. doi:10.5435/00124635-201011000-00002

Olaussen, M., Holmedal, Ø., Mdala, I., Brage, S., & Lindbœk, M. (2015). Corticosteroid or placebo injection combined with deep transverse friction massage, Mills manipulation, stretching and eccentric exercise for acute lateral epicondylitis: A randomised, controlled trial. *BMC Musculoskeletal Disorders*, 16, 122. doi:10.1186/s12891-015-0582-6

Oliva, F., Berardi, A. C., Misiti, S., & Maffulli, N. (2013). Thyroid hormones and tendon: current views and future perspectives. Concise review. *Muscles, Ligaments and Tendons Journal*, 3(3), 201–203.

Patrick, N. C., & Hammert, W. C. (2020). Hand and wrist tendinopathies. *Clinics in Sports Medicine*, 39(2), 247–258. doi:10.1016/j.csm.2019.10.004

Patton, W. C., & McCluskey, G. M., 3rd. (2001). Biceps tendinitis and subluxation. *Clinics in Sports Medicine*, 20(3), 505–529. doi:10.1016/s0278-5919(05)70266-0

Petit Le Manac'h, A., Roquelaure, Y., Ha, C., Bodin, J., Meyer, G., Bigot, F., Veaudor, M., Descatha, A., Goldberg, M., & Imbernon, E. (2011). Risk factors for de Quervain's disease in a French working population. *Scandinavian Journal of Work, Environment & Health*, 37(5), 394–401. doi:10.5271/sjweh.3160

Raynor, M., & Kuhn, J. E. (2016). Utility of features of the patient's history in the diagnosis of atraumatic shoulder pain: A systematic review. *Journal of Shoulder and Elbow Surgery, 25*(4), 688–694.

Scott, A., Backman, L. J., & Speed, C. (2015). Tendinopathy: Update on pathophysiology. *Journal of Orthopaedic and Sports Physical Therapy, 45*(11), 833–841. doi:10.2519/jospt.2015.5884

Scott, A., Squier, K., Alfredson, H., Bahr, R., Cook, J. L., Coombes, B., de Vos, R. J., Fu, S. N., Grimaldi, A., Lewis, J. S., Maffulli, N., Magnusson, S. P., Malliaras, P., Mc Auliffe, S., Oei, E., Purdam, C. R., Rees, J. D., Rio, E. K., Gravare Silbernagel, K., ... Zwerver, J. (2020). ICON 2019: International Scientific Tendinopathy Symposium consensus: Clinical terminology. *British Journal of Sports Medicine, 54*(5), 260–262. doi:10.1136/bjsports-2019-100885

Shiri, R., Viikari-Juntura, E., Varonen, H., & Heliövaara, M. (2006). Prevalence and determinants of lateral and medial epicondylitis: A population study. *American Journal of Epidemiology, 164*(11), 1065–1074. doi:10.1093/aje/kwj325

Silverstein, B. A., Viikari-Juntura, E., Fan, Z. J., Bonauto, D. K., Bao, S., & Smith, C. (2006). Natural course of nontraumatic rotator cuff tendinitis and shoulder symptoms in a working population. *Scandinavian Journal of Work, Environment & Health, 32*(2), 99–108. doi:10.5271/sjweh.985

Sirico, F., Ricca, F., DI Meglio, F., Nurzynska, D., Castaldo, C., Spera, R., & Montagnani, S. (2017). Local corticosteroid versus autologous blood injections in lateral epicondylitis: Meta-analysis of randomized controlled trials. *European Journal of Physical and Rehabilitation Medicine, 53*(3), 483–491. doi:10.23736/S1973-9087.16.04252-0

Stahl, S., Vida, D., Meisner, C., Lotter, O., Rothenberger, J., Schaller, H. E., & Stahl, A. S. (2013). Systematic review and meta-analysis on the work-related cause of de Quervain tenosynovitis: A critical appraisal of its recognition as an occupational disease. *Plastic and RECONSTRUCTIVE surgery, 132*(6), 1479–1491. doi:10.1097/01.prs.0000434409.32594.1b

van der Molen, H. F., Foresti, C., Daams, J. G., Frings-Dresen, M., & Kuijer, P. (2017). Work-related risk factors for specific shoulder disorders: A systematic review and meta-analysis. *Occupational and Environmental Medicine, 74*(10), 745–755. doi:10.1136/oemed-2017-104339

van Rijn, R. M., Huisstede, B. M., Koes, B. W., & Burdorf, A. (2009). Associations between work-related factors and specific disorders at the elbow: A systematic literature review. *Rheumatology, 48*(5), 528–536. doi:10.1093/rheumatology/kep013

Walker-Bone, K., Reading, I., Coggon, D., Cooper, C., & Palmer, K. T. (2004). The anatomical pattern and determinants of pain in the neck and upper limbs: An epidemiologic study. *Pain, 109*(1–2), 45–51. doi:10.1016/j.pain.2004.01.008

Werner, R. A., Franzblau, A., Gell, N., Ulin, S. S., & Armstrong, T. J. (2005). A longitudinal study of industrial and clerical workers: Predictors of upper extremity tendonitis. *Journal of Occupational Rehabilitation, 15*(1), 37–46. doi:10.1007/s10926-005-0872-1

Wolf, J. M., Sturdivant, R. X., & Owens, B. D. (2009). Incidence of de Quervain's tenosynovitis in a young, active population. *Journal of Hand Surgery, 34*(1), 112–115. doi:10.1016/j.jhsa.2008.08.020

Index

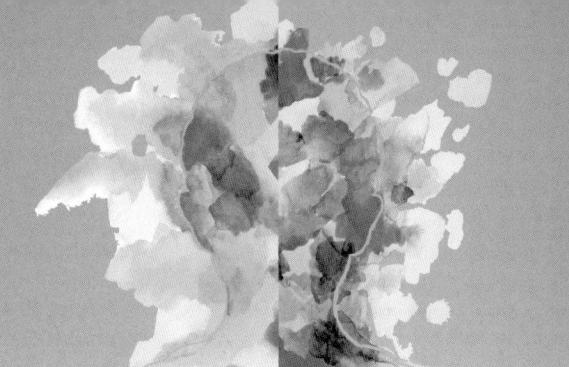

Note: Page numbers followed by *b*, *f*, or *t* represent boxes, figures, or tables, respectively.

A

AACAP (American Academy of Child and Adolescent Psychiatry), 120, 125–126
AADE. *See* American Association of Diabetes Educators (AADE)
AAHIVM (American Academy of HIV Medicine), 697
AAP. *See* American Academy of Pediatrics (AAP)
abdominal bloating, 726
abdominal pain, 726
ABI (Ankle-Brachial Index), 583*t*
abnormal uterine bleeding (AUB), 173–183
   assessment of, 177–178
   clinical management goals, 178
   clinical presentations of, 173, 174*t*
   COEIN etiologies, 175–176
   databases used for, 176–177
   diagnostic testing for, 178, 178–180*t*, 180
   etiologies of, 173, 174*t*
   overview of, 173–176
   PALM (structural) etiologies, 174–175
   physical examination, 177
   treatment and management of, 180–183
abortion care
   assessment of, 199–200
   barriers to, 188–189
   clinical management, goals of, 200
   databases used for, 193–194, 196–199
   diagnostic tests for, 200–202
   healthcare providers and, 189
   medication abortion, 190–192, 192*t*, 195*t*
   options counseling, 193, 193–194*t*
   overview of, 187
   physical examinations of, 199
   procedural abortion, 192–193, 195*t*
   resources and tools, 205–206
   in sociopolitical context, 188
   treatment and management of, 200–205
   unintended pregnancy rates and, 187–188
abrupt medication discontinuation syndromes, 576

abuse. *See* Maltreatment of children; Physical abuse; Substance use and abuse
abusive head trauma (AHT), in children, 135
ACA (Affordable Care Act), 53
acetaminophen, 572
Achenbach Child Behavior Checklist, 104
ACHES mnemonic, 267*t*
ACOG. *See* American Congress of Obstetricians and Gynecologists (ACOG)
Acquired Immune Deficiency Syndrome. *See* HIV (human immunodeficiency virus); postexposure prophylaxis (PEP), for HIV infection
activities of daily living (ADLs), 592, 650
acupressure wrist bands, 378
acute bleeding, 181
acute heart failure, 658
acute retroviral syndrome (ARS), 689
acute wounds, 579
AD. *See* atopic dermatitis (AD)
AD (Alzheimer disease), 587–588, 589–590, 590*t*
ADA. *See* American Diabetes Association (ADA)
addiction. *See* Substance use and abuse
addiction specialist, 575
adenomyosis, 175
ADHD. *See* attention-deficit/hyperactivity disorder (ADHD)
adjunctive therapies, on chronic wound care, 585–586
adolescence, defined, 35
Adolescent Health Working Group, 39
adult health maintenance and promotion
   developmental disabilities and, 479–493
   transgender and gender expansive adults and, 495–501
adult health maintenance and promotion. *See also specific issues*
adult presentations. *See also specific disorders*
   anemia, 505–517
   anxiety, 521–528

   asthma, 529–543
   cancer survivorship, 545–551
   chronic nonmalignant pain, 569–576
   chronic obstructive pulmonary disease, 553–566
   chronic wound care, 579–586
   dementia, 587–596
   depression, 599–612
   diabetes mellitus, 615–626
   epilepsy, 627–635, 629*t*
   gastroesophageal reflux disease, 637–643
   heart failure, 655–664
   herpes simplex infections, 665–672
   HIV-infected adults, primary care of, 675–697
   hypertension, 701–708
   intimate partner violence, 711–716
   irritable bowel syndrome, 721–726
   lipid disorders, 729–740
   nonalcoholic fatty liver disease, 757–762
   substance use and abuse, 775–801
   thyroid disorders, 805–814
   upper back and neck pain syndromes, 817–829
   upper extremity tendinopathy, 833–843
   weight, 765–772
advanced practice nurses (APNs), 129, 134
AEDs (antiepileptic drugs), 628, 629, 630–633*t*
Affordable Care Act (ACA), 53, 188, 545
Ages and Stages Questionnaire (Squires et al.), 70
agoraphobia, 524
AHA (American Heart Association), 656, 663, 740, 772
AHT (abusive head trauma), 135
AIDS. *See* HIV (human immunodeficiency virus); postexposure prophylaxis (PEP), for HIV infection
airway inflammation, 529
alcohol consumption. *See also* Substance use and abuse
   drug use screening and, 38
   hypertension and, 705
alcohol withdrawal, 786, 788*t*

847

Index

allergens
  12–26 years, 36
  asthma and, 82, 530, 535
  atopic dermatitis and, 90, 95
  fatigue and, 104
  skin testing for, 82, 91
allergic rhinitis, 89
Allergy & Asthma Network Mothers of Asthmatics, 87
allergy immunotherapy, 85
α_2-adrenergic agonists, 109
5α-reductase inhibitors, 228
Alzheimer disease (AD), 587–588, 589–590, 590t
Alzheimer's Association, 596, 654
Alzheimer's Disease Education and Referral Center, 596
amenorrhea
  assessment of, 215–216
  associated with pituitary dysfunction, 211–212
  clinical management goals, 216
  databased used for, 213–214
  diagnostic testing for, 215, 216–217, 216–217t
  etiologies of, 213–214, 213–214t
  hypothalamic, 211
  outflow tract/uterus disorders and, 212
  overview of, 211–213
  PCOS and, 211–221
  physical examination findings, 215, 215t
  primary ovarian insufficiency and, 212
  self-management resources and tools, 221
  treatment and management of, 217–221
American Academy of Allergy, Asthma and Immunology, 87, 541
American Academy of Child and Adolescent Psychiatry (AACAP), 120, 125–126
American Academy of Family Physicians, 6, 363, 668
American Academy of HIV Medicine (AAHIVM), 697
American Academy of Pediatrics (AAP)
  on developmental and behavioral problems, 53
  on healthy babies, 4
  on parenting, 6
  on post-NICU patients, 9, 14
American Association of Diabetes Educators (AADE), 395
  lifestyle behaviors, 393
American Cancer Society, 551
American College of Cardiology Foundation, 655, 656
American College of Nurse-Midwives, 327, 363
American Congress of Obstetricians and Gynecologists (ACOG), 327
  on AUB, 183
  on carrier screening, 332
  on gestational diabetes mellitus, 391

on postpartum care, 345
on preeclampsia, 401–402
on VBAC, 363
American Diabetes Association (ADA), 391, 395, 626
American Geriatrics Society, 654
American Geriatrics Society Beer, 654
American Heart Association (AHA), 656, 663, 740, 772
American Lung Association, 87, 541
American Pain Society, 576
American Society for Clinical Oncology (ASCO), 545, 549
American Society of Hematology, 517
American Thyroid Association, 814
American Urological Association symptom score, 225–226f
amniocentesis, 334–335
amphetamine salts, 107
androgen insensitivity, 212
anemia, 505–517
  assessment of, 512–515, 514t
  classification of, 505–506, 507t
  clinical management goals for, 515, 516t
  databases used for, 510–511
  defined, 505
  differentiation of, 507t
  hemolytic, 509, 511, 514, 517
  macrocytic, 509–510, 511–512, 514–515, 517
  megaloblastic, 509, 511–512, 514–515, 517
  microcytic, 506–508, 510–511, 515, 517
  nonmegaloblastic, 509
  normocytic, 508–509, 511, 514, 517
  overview of, 505–506
  patient education and, 517
  physical examinations for, 512, 513t
  screening, 19, 27
  self-management resources and tools, 517
  sideroblastic, 508, 510–511, 513–514, 515, 517
  treatment of, 515–517
anemia of chronic disease (ACD), 508–509, 511, 514, 517
aneuploidy, fetal, 329
anhedonia, 115
Ankle-Brachial Index (ABI), 583t
ankyloglossia. See tongue-tie
anorectal trauma, in children, 137
anterior shoulder pain, 834
anti-IgE therapy, 537
anticipated early death, infants with, 12
anticonvulsants, 572
antidepressants, 122–123, 525, 572, 605–610f, 611t
antiepileptic drugs (AEDs), 628, 629, 630–633t
antihistamines, 84, 97, 379
antiretroviral therapy (ART), 675, 678–679, 680t

anxiety, 521–528
  ADHD and, 102
  assessment of, 522–524
  children/adolescents and, 527
  database used for, 522
  menopause transition and, 278
  overview of, 521–522
  patient education and, 527–528
  postpartum, 417
  during pregnancy, 372
  psychosocial treatment, 526–527
  self-management resources and tools, 527–528
  special populations and, 527
  treatment of, 524–527, 526t
Anxiety and Depression Association of America, 528
Apgar scores, 4, 12
aphasia syndromes, 588
apnea
  fatigue and, 104
  in infants, 10
APNs (advanced practice nurses), 129, 134
ARS (acute retroviral syndrome), 689
arterial ulcers, 579–580
arthritis. See osteoarthritis (OA)
ASD (autism spectrum disorders), 481–482
Asherman syndrome, 212
Ask Suicide-Screening Questions (ASQ), 121
Association of Asthma Educators, 541
Association of Nurses in AIDS Care (ANAC), 697
asthma, in adolescents/adults, 529–543
  action plan for, 541, 542–543f
  assessment of, 531–533
  biologics, 537
  clinical management goals to control, 534
  database used for, 530–531
  diagnostic screening and testing of, 531, 534
  etiology of, 529
  management of, 534–538, 536–537t
  overview of, 529–530
  patient education and training in, 538–541, 538–540b
  severity/control/response to treatment, 531, 532t, 533t
asthma, in children, 77–87
  assessment of, 78–81
  atopic dermatitis and, 89
  classifying severity/control of, 78–81, 79–80t
  clinical management goals in, 81
  databases used for, 77–78
  defined, 77
  medication for, 81t, 83–84
  overview of, 77
  prevalence and incidence, 77
  treatment and management of, 82
atomoxetine, 109

atopic dermatitis (AD), 89–98
  assessment of, 91
  clinical management goals in, 91–92
  conditions and features associated with, 91, 93f
  databases used for, 90–91
  defined, 89
  diagnostic tests for, 91, 94t
  differential diagnoses, 91, 94f
  etiology, 89–90
  overview of, 89
  phases of, 91, 92f
  prevalence and incidence, 89
  psychosocial and emotional support and, 98
  self-management of, 98
  signs/symptoms of, 91
  treatment and management of, 92, 94–97
  triggering factors for, 90, 90f
atopic eczema. See atopic dermatitis (AD)
attention-deficit/hyperactivity disorder (ADHD), 101–111
  assessment of, 106–107
  database used for, 104–106
  incidence and prevalence, 102–103
  long-term issues, 111
  medications for, 107, 108t, 109–110
  overview of, 101–104
  physical examination for, 106
  screening tools for, 104, 105t
  transition to adulthood, 111
  treatment and management of, 107, 109–111
atypical ulcers, 581
AUB. See abnormal uterine bleeding (AUB)
Autism. See also Developmental delay and autism, screening for
  screening for, 53–72
autism spectrum disorders (ASD), 481–482
azithromycin, 562

B

babies, healthy, 3–6
back pain. See low back pain (LBP)
bariatric surgery, 151, 771–772
Barrett esophagus, 637
battering. See intimate partner violence (IPV)
bazedoxifene, 282
BBD (bladder and bowel dysfunction), 155, 156
Beck Depression Inventory–Primary Care Version (U.S. Preventive Services Task Force), 38
Bedwetting Store, 169
behavior changes in adults. See lifestyle changes
behavioral-variant frontotemporal dementia (bvFTD), 588
benign prostatic hyperplasia (BPH), 223–229
  assessment of, 227
  clinical management goals for, 227
  database used for, 224–227, 225–226f
  defined, 223
  diagnostic screening and tests for, 227
  family and social histories of, 224
  management and treatment for, 227–228
  overview of, 223–224
  patient education and, 228
  physical examination of, 226–227
  prevalence and incidence of, 223–224
  self-management resources and tools, 228–229
benzodiazepines, 525, 789t
β^2-agonists, 529
beta blockers, 662t
bicipital tendinopathy, 834
bioidentical hormone therapy, 283
biomarkers, 592–593
BIPOC (Black, Indigenous, and People of Color), 321–322
bipolar disorder, perinatal, 417
bipolar spectrum disorder, 120
birth control. See contraception
Birth to 5: Watch Me Thrive! (U.S. Departments of Health and Human Services and Education), 53
birth weight, 13, 13t
"black box" labeling, 122–123
Black, Indigenous, and People of Color (BIPOC), 321–322
Black Mamas Matter Alliance, 327
bladder and bowel dysfunction (BBD), 155, 156
bladder disorders. See urinary incontinence (UI)
bladder training, 312, 312t
bladder wall muscle, 155
bleeding
  acute, 181
  chronic, 181
blindness, 645
blood pressure (BP), 401t, 701, 702, 702t. See also hypertension (HTN)
  accurate measurements, steps for
blood pressure screening
  0–3 years, 18
  3–6 years, 27
BMI (body mass index), 149, 768
BODE index, 558, 559t
body mass index (BMI), 149, 768
BPH. See benign prostatic hyperplasia (BPH)
BPH. See Benign prostatic hyperplasia (BPH)
brain imaging, 592–593
breastfeeding, bottle feeding vs., 4, 10
Brief Early Childhood Screening Assessment (Fallucco et al.), 70
Bright Futures: Guidelines for Health Supervision of Adolescents (American Academy of Pediatrics and the Maternal Child Health Bureau), 39
bronchial thermoplasty (BT), 537
bronchitis, chronic. See chronic obstructive pulmonary disease (COPD)
bronchodilators, 561

bruises on children, 135
BT (bronchial thermoplasty), 537
buprenorphine, 576, 797–798t, 800
bupropion, 110
burns on children, 135
bvFTD (behavioral-variant frontotemporal dementia), 588

C

cabergoline, 219–220
calcineurin inhibitors, topical, 96
California Diabetes and Pregnancy Program, 395
cancer screening for cervical, vaginal, and vulvar cancers, 38
cancer survivorship, 545–551
  assessment of, 549
  clinical management goals, 549–550
  consultations and referrals, 550–551
  database used for, 547
  defined, 545
  diagnostic testing and, 547–549
  epidemiology, 546
  healthcare disparities and financial toxicity, 546–547
  late effects for cancer treatment, 548–549t
  overview of, 545
  patient education on, 550
  physical examination findings, 547, 548–549t
  self-management resources, 551
Cancer.Net, 551
cannabis withdrawal, 786–787, 789t
cardiovascular disease (CVD), 729. See also Heart failure
  HIV and, 680
Caregiver Strain Index (CSI), 596
caregivers, 593, 596, 654
carrier screening for recessive conditions, 331–332
catch-up growth. See also growth trends
CBT (cognitive-behavioral therapy), 123–125, 526
CDC. See Centers for Disease Control and Prevention (CDC)
cell-free fetal DNA testing, 329–331
CenteringPregnancy (prenatal care model), 337, 338t
Centers for Disease Control and Prevention (CDC), 551, 663
  on asthma in children, 87
  Division of Diabetes, 395
  on HIV/AIDS, 676–677
  on immunization schedules, 443, 460–467f
  sex-specific BMI-for-age growth charts, 145
  sexually transmitted infection treatment guidelines and original sources, 471–473t
  on weight, 769

central sensitization, 291–292, 296
cephalosporins, 97
cerebral palsy (CP), 480–481
cervical spine pain, 818. See also upper back/neck pain
cervicothoracic myofascial pain syndrome, 819–820
cesarean deliveries, 3, 363. See also vaginal birth after cesarean (VBAC)
chamomile, 373
CHC (combined hormonal contraception), 181, 252–254, 264, 265, 266–267, 267t
CHCs. See combined hormonal contraceptives (CHCs)
chest radiographs, 82
child abuse and neglect. See maltreatment of children
Child Abuse Prevention and Treatment Act, 129
Child Protective Services (CPS), 132
child sex trafficking (CPS), 132
Child Welfare and Information Gateway, 141
Childbirth Connection, 327
children. See pediatric health maintenance and promotion
chlamydia screening, 38
chorionic villus sampling (CVS), 334
chronic bleeding, 181
chronic kidney disease (CKD), HIV and, 681
chronic lung disease (CLD), in infants, 9–10
chronic neuropsychiatric conditions, 101
chronic nonmalignant pain (CNP), 569–576
 assessment of, 571
 clinical management goals, 571
 databases used for, 570–571
 defined, 569–570
 diagnostic screening and tests, 571
 management and treatment of, 571–576
 overview of, 569–570
 patient education, 576
 physical examination findings, 570–571
 prevalence of, 569–570
 support resources and tools, 576
chronic obstructive pulmonary disease (COPD), 553–566
 action at national level, 566
 combined assessment of, 558
 defined, 553
 epidemiology, 554
 lung development, age, and sex, 565
 management and treatment of, 558–564, 560f
 National Action Plan, 566
 nonpharmacologic therapies, 562–563
 overview of, 553
 pathophysiology, 553
 physical examination findings, 555
 risk factors, 554
 socioeconomic status, 566
 specific population, 564–566

 spirometric testing for, 555
 taxonomy, 554
chronic pelvic pain (CPP)
 assessment of, 293
 causes of, 289–290
 clinical management goals for, 293
 conditions with, 290t
 database used for, 292–293, 292f
 defined, 289
 diagnostic screening and tests for, 293
 family and social histories of, 292
 management and treatment for, 293–297, 294–296t
 overview of, 289–292, 290t
 patient and provider education resources, 296, 297
 physical examination of, 292
chronic wound care, 579–586
 assessment of, 583
 database used for, 581–583
 debridement, 584–585
 diagnostic screening and tests for, 584
 management and treatment of, 584–586
 overview of, 579
 wound dressing categories, 584, 585t
 wound healing, phases of, 580
Citizens United for Research in Epilepsy (CURE), 635
client education. See patient and family education and resources
clinical depression, 120
Clinical Institute Withdrawal Assessment (CIWA), 781–782t
Clinical Opiate Withdrawal Scale, 784t
clonidine, 283
CNP. See chronic nonmalignant pain (CNP)
coagulopathy, 175
COC (combined oral contraceptives) pills, 181, 252–255, 258, 267–268
COEIN etiologies (coagulopathy, ovulatory, endometrial, iatrogenic, not yet classified), 175–176
cognitive-behavioral therapy (CBT), 123–125, 526
coitus interruptus. See withdrawal method
cold sores. See herpes simplex virus (HSV) infections
combined hormonal contraception (CHC), 181, 252–254, 264, 265, 266–267, 267t
combined oral contraceptives (COC) pills, 181, 252–255, 258, 267–268
commercial sexual exploitation of children (CSEC), 132
common adult presentations. See adult presentations
common obstetric presentation. See obstetric presentations
common pediatric presentations. See pediatric presentations
Communication and Symbolic Behavior Scales Developmental Profile (Wetherby&Prizant), 70

communication with developmentally disabled adults, 481–482
complementary and alternative medicine (CAM), 284
complete abortion, 232t
condoms, 259–260, 265, 268
conduct disorder, 102
Confusion Assessment Method (CAM), 648
congenital hypothyroid screening of infants, 5
congenital scoliosis, 821
consent, patient, adolescents and, 35–36
constipation, 725–726
 during pregnancy, 381, 383
contraception, 243–269. See also specific methods
 assessment of, 265
 clinical management goals for, 265
 database used for, 264–265
 diagnostic screening and tests for, 265
 family and social histories of, 264
 general guidelines for, 266t
 management and treatment for, 265–269, 266t, 267t
 overview of, 243–264, 244–252t
 patient and provider education resources, 265–269
contraceptive ring, 252, 253, 262, 267
contraindications, for stimulants, 110
controlled substances. See opioid(s)
controller medications, 84, 535
COPD. See chronic obstructive pulmonary disease (COPD)
COPD Assessment Test (CAT), 554, 556f
copper T 380A Intrauterine Contraception (IUC) (ParaGard), 257–258, 265, 268
cortical inhibitory pathway, 155
corticosteroids, 96, 561, 561f
counseling. See patient and family education and resources
CP (cerebral palsy), 480–481
CPP. See chronic pelvic pain (CPP)
CPS (Child Protective Services), 132
CRAFFT (mnemonic), 38
Crisaborole, 98
CSEC (commercial sexual exploitation of children), 132
CURE (Citizens United for Research in Epilepsy), 635
Current Procedural Terminology (CPT), 53
Cushing disease, 212
CVD. See cardiovascular disease (CVD)
CVS (chorionic villus sampling), 334
cyclothymia, 120

D

dating violence. See intimate partner violence (IPV)
daytime urinary incontinence, 156–157
DCM (dilated cardiomyopathy), 655
De Quervain's tenosynovitis, 833

degenerative joint disease.
See osteoarthritis (OA)
degenerative scoliosis, 821–822
delirium, 646–647, 648, 650, 651, 651t
dementia, 587–596
    assessment of, 593
    caregiver status, 596
    causes of, 587, 588t
    clinical management goals for, 593
    database used for, 589–593, 590t
    diagnostic tests for, 592t, 593
    frontotemporal, 588–589, 591
    management and treatment of, 593–595, 594t
    mixed, 589
    overview of, 587–588, 588t
    physical examination, 592
    vascular, 588, 591
Dementia with Lewy bodies (DLB), 588, 591, 593
Department of Health and Human Services (DHHS), 675
Depot medroxyprogesterone acetate (DMPA), 181
depression, adults, 599–612
    assessment of, 602–603
    databases used for, 601–602, 601t
    definition of, 599
    diagnostic screening and tests, 600f, 602, 604
    management and treatment of, 603–604, 604f, 605–610f, 611t
    medications causing, 603
    menopause transition and, 278
    overview of, 599–601, 600f
    patient and family education on, 610–612
    physical examination findings, 602
    postpartum, 414–417
    in pregnancy, 372
    primary care treatment algorithm for, 604f
    self-management resources and tools, 611–612
    symptoms, 418t
Depression and Bipolar Support Alliance, 612
depression, childhood, 38
depression, pediatric, 115–126
    ADHD and, 104
    assessment of, 119–121
    databases used for, 116–119
    medication for, 122–125, 124–125t
    overview of, 115–116
    physical examination, 118–119
    self-management resources in, 125–126
    treatment and management of, 122–125
dermatitis. See atopic dermatitis (AD)
detrusor muscle, 155
development and behavior appraisal.
See also developmental delay and autism, screening for
    0–3 years, 20
    3–6 years, 26
    6–11 years, 30
    infants and, 11
    screening tests and tools, 54–56
developmental delay and autism, screening for, 53–72. See also development and behavior appraisal
    clinician resources for, 70–71
    overview of, 53–54
    psychometrics, 70–71
    surveillance and screening algorithm for, 55–70, 55–56f, 58–69t
    tools for, 58–69t
developmental disabilities (DDs), adults with, health maintenance for, 479–493
    assessment of, 485–486
    databases used for, 483–485
    defined, 480
    diagnostic tests, 486, 488–491t
    healthcare maintenance guidelines for, 488–491t
    interdisciplinary healthcare teams and, 485, 486f
    overview of, 479–483
    patient education, 492
    physical examination considerations and, 485, 487f
    self-management resources and tools, 493
    treatment of, 491–492
Developmental Disabilities Assistance and Civil Rights Act of 2000, 480
developmental kyphosis, 821
developmental screening tools, 58–69t
developmental surveillance and screening algorithm, 55–70, 55–56f, 58–69t
dextroamphetamine, 109
DHHS (Department of Health and Human Services), 675
diabetes mellitus, 615–626. See also gestational diabetes mellitus (GDM)
    assessment of, 617, 617t
    clinical management goals for, 617–618, 617t
    database used for, 615–616
    diagnosis screening and tests for, 616, 617t
    foot ulcers and, 580
    HIV and, 680
    language and, 625–626
    management and treatment of, 618–626, 618t, 619t, 621–624t, 621f
    overview of, 615
    patient and family education on, 626
    physical examinations for, 616
    self-management resources and tools, 626
diabetic foot ulcers, 580
Diagnostic and Statistical Manual for Mental Disorders (DSM)
    on anxiety, 521
    on autism spectrum disorders, 481
    on depression, 599, 602–603
    on transgender and gender expansive adults, 496
Diagnostic and Statistical Manual of Mental Disorders, 5th edition (DSM-5), 119
diagnostic screening and tests
    for 0–3 years, 21
    for 3–6 years, 27
    for 6–11 years, 31
    for 12–26 years, 38
    for abortion care, 200–202
    for ADHD, 104–106
    for amenorrhea and PCOS, 216–217, 216–217t
    for anemia in adults, 505t, 512–515, 516t
    for asthma, 78, 82, 531
    for atopic dermatitis, 91, 94t
    for AUB, 178, 178–180t, 180
    for benign prostatic hyperplasia, 227
    for cancer survivorship, 550
    for chronic nonmalignant pain, 571
    for chronic obstructive pulmonary disease, 554–558
    for chronic pelvic pain, 293
    for contraception, 265
    for dementia, 592t, 593
    for depression in adults, 600f, 602–603
    for diabetes in pregnancy, 391, 392t
    for diabetes mellitus, 616, 617t
    for early pregnancy loss, 236
    for epilepsy, 628, 629
    for GERD, 640
    for heart failure, 657–658
    for HIV, 681, 689
    for HSV infections, 669
    for human lactation, 426, 428–429, 431, 434
    for hypertension, 703, 705t
    for IBS, 723, 724–725t
    for infants, 5
    for intimate partner violence, 716
    for lipid disorders, 731–732
    for low back pain, 748–749
    maltreatment of children and, 139–140
    for menopause transition, 279
    for nonalcoholic fatty liver disease, 758
    for obesity, 148–149
    for perinatal mood and anxiety disorders, 413–414
    for post-NICU patients, 13
    postpartum, 349
    for preeclampsia-eclampsia, 401–402
    pregnancy and, 323–327, 324b, 339
    prenatal genetic, 329–335
    for sexual dysfunction, 303–304
    substance use and abuse, 780–781, 787, 800
    for thyroid disorders, 808, 809–811t, 811
    transgender and gender diverse, 43
    for transgender and gender expansive adults, 498, 498t

diagnostic screening and tests (*Continued*)
  for upper back/neck pain, 824*t*, 826, 826*t*
  for upper extremity tendinopathy, 837, 838, 841
  for urinary incontinence in children, 162–163, 163–164*f*
  for urinary incontinence in women, 310–311
  for weight, 767–768
diaphragm, 260–261, 265, 268
diarrhea, 725
diastolic heart failure, 655
diastolic HTN, 701
diet
  history and obesity, 766
  interventions and patient motivation, 769
differential diagnoses
  for anemia in adults, 505*t*, 512–515
  for asthma, 78, 531
  for atopic dermatitis, 91, 94*f*
  for heart failure, 657
  for preeclampsia-eclampsia, 401
  during pregnancy, 375, 378
  for urinary incontinence in women, 309, 309*t*
dilated cardiomyopathy (DCM), 655
discomforts, of pregnancy, 371–383
  musculoskeletal pain, 373–376
  overview of, 371–372
  poor quality of sleep, 372–373
diuretic therapy, 663*t*
DLB (dementia with Lewy bodies), 588, 591, 593
DMPA (depot medroxyprogesterone acetate), 181
domestic violence. *See* intimate partner violence (IPV)
dopamine agonists, 219–220
dopamine antagonists, 380
Down syndrome, 482
drugs and alcohol use. *See* substance use and abuse
Dupilumab (injection), 98
dysfunctional uterine bleeding (DUB). *See* abnormal uterine bleeding (AUB)
dyslipidemia screening, 31, 38
  0–3 years, 19
  3–6 years, 27
dysmenorrhea, 291, 293–294
dyspnea, 655
dysthymia, 119, 599

E

Early and Periodic Screening, Diagnostic, and Treatment (EPSDT), 53
early pregnancy failure, 231
early pregnancy loss (EPL), 231–240
  assessment of, 235–236
  clinical management goals for, 236
  database used for, 233–235
  defined, 231
  diagnostic screening and tests for, 236
  family and social histories of, 233–234
  management and treatment for, 236–240
  overview of, 231–233, 232*t*
  patient education and, 239–240
  physical examination of, 234–235
  review of systems, 236
  terminology, 232*t*
Early Screening for Autism and Communication Disorders (Wetherby et al.), 70
economic abuse, 711
ectopic pregnancy (EP), 200, 232*t*
eczema. *See* atopic dermatitis (AD)
Edinburgh Postnatal Depression Screening (EPDS), 414, 419
education. *See* patient and family education and resources
elbow tendinopathy, 833–834, 838
elderly. *See* older adults
emergency contraception (EC), 258–259, 264, 265, 268
emotional abuse, 711
emotional or psychologic abuse. *See* maltreatment of children
emotional/psychologic abuse, 131
emphysema. *See* chronic obstructive pulmonary disease (COPD)
end-of-life and palliative care, 596, 661
endometrial etiologies, 176
endometriosis and adenomyosis, 291, 294–295
enuresis risoria, 157
environmental history. *See* family and social histories
EP (ectopic pregnancy), 200, 232*t*
EPDS (Edinburgh Postnatal Depression Screening), 414, 419
epilepsy, 483, 627–635, 629*t*
  assessment of, 628
  clinical management goals for, 628–629
  database used for, 627–628
  defined, 627
  diagnostic screening and tests for, 628, 629
  overview of, 627
  physical examination for, 628
  referral guidelines, 634
  self-management resources, 634–635
  treatment and management of, 629, 634*t*
Epilepsy Therapy Project, 634
EPL. *See* early pregnancy loss (EPL)
EPSDT (Early and Periodic Screening, Diagnostic, and Treatment), 53
erythropoiesis, 505
escitalopram, 123
esophageal carcinoma, 637
estrogen therapy, 279–280, 280*t*, 283*t*
estrogen use, 499*t*
estrogens, 279

ethnicity-based health issues
  HIV and, 677
  hypertension and, 705
exacerbations of COPD, 563–564, 565*f*
Executive Function Performance Test, 592
exercise. *See* physical activity
external condom, 259–260, 265, 268
external sphincter muscle, 155

F

falls, as geriatric syndromes, 646, 647, 648, 650–651
FAM (fertility awareness method), 262–263, 262*t*, 265, 268
familial transmission of depression, 116
family and social histories
  0–3 years, 19
  3–6 years, 25
  6–11 years, 30
  12–26 years, 36
  abortion care, 198–199
  amenorrhea and, 214
  of anemia in adults, 510–513
  asthma and, 77, 531
  atopic dermatitis and, 90–91
  AUB and, 177
  benign prostatic hyperplasia and, 224
  cancer survivorship and, 547
  chronic nonmalignant pain and, 570
  of chronic pelvic pain, 292
  chronic wound care and, 581
  of contraception, 264
  COPD and, 554
  depression and, 116–117, 601–602
  of developmentally disabled adults, 485
  diabetes mellitus and, 615–616
  of early pregnancy loss, 233–234
  epilepsy and, 627
  GERD and, 638
  heart failure and, 656
  HSV and, 667–668
  hypertension and, 702–703
  IBS and, 723
  infants, 4
  lipid disorders and, 731
  low back pain and, 746
  maltreatment of children and, 133
  obesity and, 147
  PCOS and, 214
  of post-NICU patients, 12
  postpartum care and, 347
  preeclampsia-eclampsia and, 400
  pregnancy and, 323
  of preterm birth, 406–407
  substance use and abuse, 780
  thyroid disorders and, 807–808
  transgender and gender diverse, 42
  transgender and gender expansive adults and, 497
  upper back/neck pain and, 822

upper extremity tendinopathy and, 837
weight and, 766–767
Family Caregiver Alliance, 596, 654
family education. *See* patient and family education and resources
fatigue. *See* sleep
FDA. *See* U.S. Food and Drug Administration (FDA)
FemCap cervical cap, 260, 265, 268
feminizing therapy, 499t
fertility awareness method (FAM), 262–263, 262t, 265, 268
fetal fibronectin (fFN), 407
fever blisters. *See* herpes simplex virus (HSV) infections
fFN (fetal fibronectin), 407
FHA (functional hypothalamic amenorrhea), 211
first well-baby visits, 3–6
First Year Inventory (Rowberry), 70
fluoxetine, 123
fluvoxamine, 123
folate (folic acid) deficiency, 510, 511–512, 514, 517
Food and Drug Administration. *See* U.S. Food and Drug Administration (FDA)
forced expiratory volume (FEV), 531, 534, 555
forced vital capacity (FVC), 534, 555
formal developmental assessments, infant, 11
fractures, in children, 135
frailty, 645, 647, 648, 650
frontotemporal dementia (FTD), 588–589, 591
Functional Activities Questionnaire, 592
functional bowel disorder. *See* irritable bowel syndrome (IBS)
functional hypothalamic amenorrhea (FHA), 211

G

gabapentin, 283
galactagogues, 429b
galactopoiesis (lactogenesis III), 424
gastroesophageal reflux disease (GERD), 637–643
  assessment of, 639
  clinical management goals, 640
  databases used for, 638–639
  defined, 637
  diagnostic screening and tests for, 640
  in infants, 10
  management and treatment of, 640–641, 642t, 643
  overview of, 637–638, 638t
  patient education and resources on, 643
  pregnancy and, 381, 382t
gastrointestinal tract during pregnancy, 376–380, 377t, 379t

GDM (gestational diabetes mellitus) in pregnancy, 389–395
Geisinger's Health Library, 814
gender dysphoria, 43
gender identity disorder. *See* prenatal genetic diagnosis; prenatal genetic screening
generalized anxiety disorder, 424, 521
Generalized Anxiety Disorder 7-item (GAD-7), 521, 522, 523f
Genetic Information Nondiscrimination Act (GINA), 332
genetic testing, 332, 333f
genetics
  disorders, 482–483
  transmission of depression, 116
genital HSV, 665, 667f
genitourinary syndrome of menopause (GSM), 277, 284
GERD. *See* gastroesophageal reflux disease (GERD)
Geriatric Depression Scale, 592, 596, 601
geriatric syndromes, 645–654
  assessment of, 650–651
  clinical management goals, 651
  database used for, 647–648, 650
  defined, 645
  delirium, 646–647
  diagnostic tests for, 651, 652t, 653–654
  falls, 646, 648
  frailty, 645, 647, 648
  online resources for clinicians/patients/caregivers, 654
  physical examinations for, 648, 649f, 650t
  sensory impairment, 645–646, 648
  treatment and management of, 651–654
  urinary incontinence, 646, 648
geriatrics. *See* older adults
Gerontological Advanced Practice Nurses Association, 654
Gestational diabetes mellitus (GDM), in pregnancy, 389–395, 615. *See also* Diabetes mellitus
  clinical management goals for, 391–392
  defined, 389–390
  GDM A1/A2, postpartum management of, 394–395
  lifestyle behaviors, 393–394
  methods to diagnose, 391, 392t
  overview of, 389–390
  people with, resources for, 395
  prevalence and incidence, 390
giggle incontinence (enuresis risoria), 157
Global Initiative for Chronic Obstructive Lung Disease (GOLD), 553, 554, 555, 557f, 558, 558f, 559t, 565
goiter. *See* thyroid disorders
gonadal dysgenesis, 212
gonadotropin-releasing hormone agonists, 182
gonorrhea screening, 38

growth trends
  infants and, 5
  post-NICU patients and, 13
GSM (genitourinary syndrome of menopause), 277, 284
gynecology. *See also specific issues*
  abnormal uterine bleeding. *See* abnormal uterine bleeding (AUB)
  amenorrhea and PCOS, 211–221
  menopause transition, 275–285
  urinary incontinence, 309–316

H

H2RA (histamine-2 receptor antagonists), 380–381, 382t
Hartford Institute for Geriatric Nursing, 654
HDL. *See* high-density lipoprotein (HDL)
health assessment form, 483
health boards, 829
health education. *See* patient and family education and resources
health histories
  0–3 years, 19
  3–6 years, 25
  6–11 years, 29–30
  12–26 years, 36
  abortion care, 194, 196–197
  ADHD in children and, 106–107
  of adults with developmental disabilities, 484–485
  amenorrhea and, 213–214
  anemia and, 510–513
  asthma and, 77, 531
  atopic dermatitis and, 90
  AUB and, 176–177
  cancer survivorship and, 547
  chronic nonmalignant pain and, 570
  COPD and, 554
  depression and, 601–602
  diabetes mellitus and, 615–616
  epilepsy and, 627–628
  heart failure and, 656
  HSV and, 667–668
  hypertension and, 702–703
  IBS and, 723
  of infants, 4
  lipid disorders and, 731
  low back pain and, 746
  nonalcoholic fatty liver disease, 758
  obesity and, 147
  PCOS and, 214
  of post-NICU patients, 12
  preeclampsia-eclampsia and, 400
  of preterm birth, 406–407
  PTB risk and, 406–407
  substance use and abuse, 780
  thyroid disorders and, 807–808
  transgender and gender diverse, 42
  of transgender and gender expansive adults, 497

health histories (*Continued*)
  upper back/neck pain and, 822
  upper extremity tendinopathy and, 835–836
  urinary incontinence in children, 159–160
  weight and, 766–767
  wound care and, 581
health maintenance and promotion, adult, 443–476
  assessment of, 470, 474*b*
  clinical management goals for, 470, 474
  database used for, 470, 471–473*t*, 474, 475–476*t*
  overview of, 443
healthcare disparity, 479
Healthy People 2030 (U.S. Department of Health & Human Services), 36
hearing impairment, 645–646, 647, 650
hearing screening
  0–3 years, 5, 11, 18
  3–6 years, 27
  6–11 years, 31
heart failure, 655–664
  assessment of, 657
  clinical management goals, 657
  database used for, 656–657
  defined, 655
  diagnostic tests for, 657–658
  overview of, 655–656
  physical examinations for, 657
  treatment and management for, 658, 659*f*, 660, 660*b*, 663–664
heartburn. *See also* gastroesophageal reflux disease (GERD)
  during pregnancy, 380–381, 382*t*
HEEADSSS (mnemonic), 37
HELLP (hemolysis, elevated liver enzymes, and low platelets) syndrome, 378, 381, 397
hemiplegic cerebral palsy, 481
hemoglobin, and hematocrit screening, 38
hemolytic anemia, 509, 511, 514, 517
hepatitis A screening, 800
hepatitis B screening, 800
hepatitis C screening, 800
hepcidin, 508
Herpes Resource Center, 672
herpes simplex virus (HSV) infections, 97, 665–672
  assessment of, 668
  clinical management goals, 668
  database used for, 667–668
  diagnostic screening and tests for, 669
  overview of, 665
  treatment and management of, 669–670, 671*t*
  types of, 665–666
HG (hyperemesis gravidarum), 377
high-density lipoprotein (HDL), 729, 757
histamine-2 receptor antagonists (H2RA), 380–381, 382*t*

HIV (human immunodeficiency virus), 675–697. *See also* postexposure prophylaxis (PEP), for HIV infection
  antiretroviral therapy, 679
  assessment of, 691
  Black Americans, 677
  cardiovascular disease, 681
  care continuum, 680, 680*f*
  cisgender women, 677
  clinical management goals, 691
  database used for, 689–691
  diagnostic screening and tests, 681, 689
  epidemiology, 675–678, 676*t*
  global epidemic, 678
  immunizations for, 682, 686–688*t*
  linkage to care and partner services, 689
  malignancies, 681–682
  national screening recommendations, 688–689
  pathogenesis, 678–679, 680*f*
  patient education on, 697
  postmenopausal cisgender women of, 691
  prevention of, 696
  renal disease, 682
  screening for, 38, 800
  screening tests, 689
  stigma, 675
  T2DM, 681
  transgender people, 677–678, 695–696
  treatment and management of, 691, 693, 694–695*t*, 695–696
  U.S. geography, 677
  viral hepatitis, 682
hormone therapy (HT), 279–283
Hospital Elder Life Program, 654
HSV infections. *See* herpes simplex virus (HSV) infections
HT (hormone therapy), 279–283
HTN. *See* hypertension (HTN)
human lactation, 423–437
  clinical management goals for, 434
  contraindications, 435–436
  database used for, 434
  galactopoiesis (lactogenesis III), 424
  involution, 424
  low supply, 425–426, 426–428*t*
  mastitis, 431, 434–435, 435*t*
  nursing session, tools for evaluation of, 430*b*
  overview of, 423
  pain with nursing, 430–431, 431–434*t*
  prescribing medications, 436
  resources, 437
  secretory activation (lactogenesis II), 424
  secretory differentiation (lactogenesis I), 423–424
  stages of, 423–424
  tongue-tie, 426, 428–430
human sexual response, 301
hydatidiform mole, 232*t*
hydration, during pregnancy, 378
5-hydroxytryptamine 3-receptor antagonists, 380

hyperemesis gravidarum (HG), 377
Hyperglycemia and Adverse Pregnancy Outcomes (HAPO), 390–391
hyperkyphosis, 821
hyperprolactinemia, 212, 220
hypertension (HTN), 701–708
  assessment of, 703–705
  classification of, 701
  clinical management goals, 705
  database used for, 702–703
  defined, 701
  diagnostic screening and tests for, 703, 705*t*
  follow-up, 708
  management and treatment of, 705–708, 706–707*t*
  patient education on, 708
  in pregnancy. *See* preeclampsia-eclampsia
  prevalence of, 701
  screening, 27
  substances associated with, 704*t*
hyperthyroidism, 805–806, 813
hypertriglyceridemia, 730
hypoglycemia, 616. *See also* diabetes mellitus
hypothalamic amenorrhea, 211, 217–219. *See also* amenorrhea; polycystic ovarian syndrome (PCOS)
hypothalamic-pituitary-adrenal axis (HPA), 116
hypothalamic-pituitary-ovarian (HPO) axis, 173, 211
hypothyroidism, 211
hysterectomy, 183, 365–366

I

IADLs (instrumental activities of daily living), 650
IADPSG (International Association of Diabetes and Pregnancy Study Groups), 390–391
IASP (International Association for Study of Pain), 576
iatrogenic etiologies, 176
IBS. *See* irritable bowel syndrome (IBS)
ibuprofen, 182
ICA (Interstitial Cystitis Association), 292
ID (intellectual disability), 480
idiopathic scoliosis, 821
IgE sensitization, 82, 529
ILAE (International League Against Epilepsy), 627
immunizations
  0–3 years, 19
  3–6 years, 27
  6–11 years, 31
  12–26 years, 36, 38
  infants, 5
implant (Nexplanon), 256, 268
incomplete abortion, 232*t*

independent reports on maltreatment of children, 138, 138t
Individuals with Disabilities Education Improvement Act (IDEA), 53
inevitable abortion, 232t
Infant and Toddler Checklist (Wetherby et al.), 70
infants, healthy, 3–6
Infectious Disease Society of America (IDSA), 675
inhaled corticosteroid-formoterol (ICS-formoterol), 84
inhalers, 538, 538–540b
inherited disorders, 729–730
INJECTABLE progestins, 255–256, 268
injuries, 130
Innovative Education in Reproductive Health (IERH), 239
insomnia, during pregnancy, 372–373
Institute of Medicine (IOM), 545
instrumental activities of daily living (IADLs), 650
Instrumental Activities of Daily Living Scale, 592
insulins, 620, 623–624t
intellectual disability (ID), 480
interdisciplinary healthcare teams, 485, 486f
internal condom, 259–260, 265, 268
International Association for Study of Pain (IASP), 576
International Association of Diabetes and Pregnancy Study Groups (IADPSG), 390–391
International Children's Continence Society, 169
International Classification of Diseases–10 codes, 571
International League Against Epilepsy (ILAE), 627
International Pelvic Pain Society (IPPS), 292
Interstitial Cystitis Association (ICA), 292
intimate partner violence (IPV), 188, 711–716
　assessment of, 715t
　clinical management goals for, 715
　consequences of, 712
　database used for, 715
　diagnostic testing for, 716
　physical examination for, 715, 715t
　population considerations, 713
　prevalence and incidence, 712
　risk factors, 712–713
　screening, 713–715
　self-management resources and tools, 716
　treatment and management of, 715
　types of, 711
intrauterine pregnancy (IUP), 232t
intravenous fluid therapy, 379
involution, 424
iodine deficiency, and thyroid disorder, 805
IOM (Institute of Medicine), 545

IPPS (International Pelvic Pain Society), 292
IPV. *See* intimate partner violence (IPV)
iron deficiency anemia, 506–508, 510, 512, 515
irritable bowel syndrome (IBS), 291, 296, 721–726
　assessment of, 723
　clinical management goals, 723
　database used for, 723
　defined, 721
　diagnostic testing for, 723, 724–725t
　epidemiology, 721–722
　FODMAP diet, 725t
　overview of, 721–722
　pathophysiology of, 722
　patient and family education on, 726
　physical examination for, 723
　symptoms of, 721
　treatment and management of, 723, 725–726
Irritable Bowel Syndrome Association, 726
irritants, asthma and, 83, 530

J

John A. Hartford Foundation, 654
Johns Hopkins Medicine, 228–229
Joint National Committee on Prevention, Detection, Evaluation, and Treatment of High Blood Pressure (JNC 7), 701–702
Joslin Diabetes Center, 626
Journey Forward, 551
Juvenile Diabetes Research Foundation International, 626

K

kyphosis, 821–822

L

labor management, preterm, 405–410
lactation. *See* human lactation
lactational amenorrhea method (LAM), 262–263, 262t, 265, 268
lateral epicondylitis, 834, 837
LBP. *See* low back pain (LBP)
lead screening
　0–3 years, 19
　3–6 years, 27
　6–11 years, 31
learning disabilities, screening for, 105–106
left ventricular heart failure, 655
legal issues
　implications of reporting child maltreatment, 138t
leiomyomas, 175, 182
LES (lower esophageal sphincter), 637

lesbian, gay, bisexual, transgender, and queer (LGBTQ), 188
Levine Quantitative Swab Technique, 582b
levonorgestrel intrauterine device (LNG IUD), 256–257, 265, 268
life expectancy, adults with developmental disabilities, 479
lifestyle changes
　for hypertension, 705
　and menopause transition, 284
　for obesity and weight loss, 149–150, 151f, 770, 771
lipid disorders, 729–740
　assessment of, 732
　classifications of, 729–730
　clinical management goals, 732
　database used for, 731–732
　defined, 729
　diagnostics tests for, 732–734
　hypertriglyceridemia, 735–736
　interprofessional team use and referral, 739
　overview of, 729
　patient education, 740
　prevalence of, 729
　primary prevention strategies, 736–737
　treatment and management of, 732, 734
　treatment of hypercholesterolemia, 737–739
Livestrong, 551
low back pain (LBP)
　assessment of, 749
　causes of, 743, 744t
　database used for, 743–744, 745t, 746–749
　diagnostic screening and tests for, 748–749
　management and treatment of, 749–752, 754–755
　overview of, 743
　patient education on, 751
　physical examinations for, 745t, 746–748
　pregnancy and, 373–376
low-density lipoprotein (LDL), 695
low supply, human lactation, 425–426, 426–428t
low transverse cesarean sections (LTCS), 363
lower esophageal sphincter (LES), 637
LTCS (low transverse cesarean sections), 363
lung disease. *See* asthma; chronic obstructive pulmonary disease (COPD)
lymphadenopathy, 91

M

macrocytic anemia, 509–510, 511–512, 514–515, 517
magnetic resonance imaging (MRI), 375

major depressive disorders (MDD), 116, 119
malignancy, 175
maltreatment of children, 129–141. *See also specific types* of abuse
    assessment of, 138–139
    databases used for, 133–138
    independent report triggers for, 138, 138t
    overview of, 129–130
    physical examination findings in, 135, 136t, 137–138
    safety, 139
    treatment and management of, 139–140
mandatory reporting, on maltreatment of children, 138–139, 138t
mania, 418t
March of Dimes, 14, 327
masculinizing therapy, 499t
mastitis, 431, 434–435
    causes, treatment, and prevention, 435t
Mayo Clinic, 221, 643
MCV (mean cell volume), 505–506, 512
MDD (major depressive disorder), 116, 119
mean cell volume (MCV), 505–506, 512
medical child abuse, 131–132
medical history. *See* health histories
medical nutrition therapy (MNT), 619
medication abortion (MAB), 190–192, 192t, 195t
medications. *See also* pharmacotherapy/ psychotherapy; *specific medications*
    12–26 years, 36
    asthma and, 78
    causing depression, 603
    monitoring, 123
    weight gain and, 766
medroxyprogesterone acetate (MPA), 181–182
megaloblastic anemias, 509, 511–512, 514–515, 517
Memorial Sloan Kettering Cancer Center Integrative Medicine, 551
Mended Hearts, 664
menopause transition, 275–285
    assessment of, 278–279
    clinical management goals in, 279
    overview of, 275
    treatment and management of, 279–285
    types of, 275
menorrhagia, 173, 276
menstrual cycle. *See also* amenorrhea; polycystic ovarian syndrome (PCOS)
    changes in, 276, 278
    phases of, 173
mental status examination (MSE), 118
Merck Manual Consumer Version, 229
methotrexate, 193
methylxanthines, 559, 561
microcytic anemias, 506–508, 510–511, 512, 515, 517

Mifepristone (Mifeprex), 191, 192t
miscarriage, 231
Misoprostol (Cytotec), 191–192, 192t
missed abortion, 232t
mixed dementia, 589
MNT (medical nutrition therapy), 619
mobile apps, depression and, 612
Modified Checklist for Autism in Toddlers (Robins et al.), 70
Modified Medical Research Council (MMRC) dyspnea scale, 554, 555f, 558
monophasic COC, 182
monosymptomatic enuresis, 157
Montreal Cognitive Assessment (MOCA), 648, 649f
mood and cognition, menopause transition and, 278
mortality/morbidity
    maternal, 366
    neonatal, 366
    from preeclampsia, 397
Motherisk, 378
MPA (medroxyprogesterone acetate), 181–182
MSE (mental status examination), 118
mucolytics, 562
Müllerian abnormalities, 212
multi-infarct dementia, 588
multidisciplinary treatment teams. *See* interdisciplinary healthcare teams
musculoskeletal neck pain, acute, 818
musculoskeletal pain, in pregnancy, 373–376
    differential diagnosis and management of, 373, 374t
    "red flag" symptoms, 375, 375t
    types of, 373
musculoskeletal strains/sprains, 820–821
myofascial pain syndrome, 819–820
myofascial pelvic pain syndrome, 291, 295

N

NAFC (National Association for Continence), 316
NAMS (North American Menopause Society), 285
National Alliance on Mental Illness (NAMI), 528, 612
National Association for Continence (NAFC), 316
National Association of Pediatric Nurse Practitioners, 28
National Cancer Institute (NCI), 545, 551
National Center for Health Care Technology, 363
National Center for PTSD, 528
National Center for Transgender Equality (NCTE), 501
National Center for Victims of Crime's Stalking Resource Center, 715

National Child Abuse and Neglect Data System (NCANDS), 130
National Coalition for Cancer Survivorship (NCCS), 545, 551
National Coalition of Anti-Violence Programs, 715
National Comprehensive Cancer Network (NCCN), 549
National Diabetes Education Program, 626
National Health and Nutrition Examination Survey (NHANES), 701, 765
National Heart, Lung, and Blood Institute, 87, 534
National Institute for Diabetes, Digestive and Kidney Diseases (NIDDK), 316
National Institute for Mental Health (NIMH), 528
National Institute of Allergy and Infectious Disease, 672
National Institute of Arthritis and Musculoskeletal and Skin Diseases (NIAMS), 826
National Institute of Child and Human Development, 363
National Institute of Mental Health (NIMH), 611
National Institute on Aging, 654
National Institutes of Health (NIH), 6, 228, 517
    on BMI, 768
    on GDM, 391
    on GERD, 643
    on IBS, 726
    on VBAC, 363
National Intimate Partner and Sexual Violence Survey (NISVS), 712
National Jewish Medical and Research Center, 87, 97
National Library of Medicine (Medline Plus), 228
National Online Resource Center on Violence Against Women, 715
National Sexual Violence Resource Center, 715
National Women's Health Information Center, 327
natural family planning (NFP), 262–263, 262t, 265, 268
nausea and vomiting of pregnancy (NVP), 377–380
    pharmacotherapy for, 379
NCANDS (National Child Abuse and Neglect Data System), 130
neck pain. *See* upper back/neck pain
negative predictive value (NPV), of screening tests, 71
neglect, child, 131. *See also* maltreatment of children
    physical examination for, 138
neonatal intensive care unit (NICU), 9–14
nerve root, 746
neural tube defects (NTD), 329
neurobehavioral and sensory deficits, 11

neurologic examinations, 747
neuromuscular scoliosis, 821
neuropsychiatric conditions, and ADHD, 106
New York Heart Association (NYHA), 656
newborns, 3–6
NICE, 239
NICU patients, 9–14
NIDDK (National Institute for Diabetes, Digestive and Kidney Diseases), 316
nighttime intermittent incontinence, 157–158
NIPT (noninvasive prenatal testing), 329–331
nocturnal enuresis, 157–158
nonalcoholic fatty liver disease (NAFLD), 757–762
   assessment, 759–761
   clinical management goals of, 761–762
   database used for, 758–759
   definition of, 757
   history for, 758
   liver test, 759t
   motivation and ability, 761
   patient education, 762
   physical examination, 759t
   Prevalence and high-risk of, 757
   screening of, 758
   severity, 760–761
   significance, 761
   treatment and management of, 762
nonalcoholic steatohepatitis (NASH), 757
nonhormonal drugs, and menopause transition, 283–284
noninvasive prenatal testing (NIPT), 329–331
nonmalignant pain, chronic (CNP). *See* chronic nonmalignant pain (CNP)
nonmonosymptomatic enuresis, 157
nonoccupational postexposure prophylaxis (nPEP). *See also* postexposure prophylaxis (PEP), for HIV infection
nonsteroidal anti-inflammatory drugs (NSAIDs), 182, 572
nonstimulant medications, and ADHD, 109–110
nonviable pregnancy, 232t
norepinephrine reuptake inhibitors, 109
normocytic anemia, 508–509, 511, 514, 517
North American Menopause Society (NAMS), 285
not yet classified etiologies, 176
NSAIDs (nonsteroidal anti-inflammatory drugs), 182, 572
nuchal line, 817
nuchal translucency (NT), 329
nursing session, tools for evaluation of, 430b
nutrition
   0–3 years, 20
   3–6 years, 25–26
   6–11 years, 30
   on chronic wound care, 585
   infants and, 4, 11
   post NICU infants and, 12
   postpartum care, 348
   pregnancy and, 323, 341, 341t, 378
   and preterm labor risk, 408
NVP. *See* nausea and vomiting of pregnancy (NVP)

O

OAB (overactive bladder), 310, 313, 314t
obesity
   in adolescents, 146
   assessment of, 149
   databases used for, 147–149, 148f
   diagnostic testing for, 148–149
   in early childhood, 146
   etiology of, 766
   in infancy, 145
   in school-age children, 146
   in special populations, 146–147
   treatment and management of, 149–151, 150f, 151f
obsessive–compulsive disorder (OCD)
   postpartum, 417
obstetric health maintenance and promotion. *See also specific issues*
   medical consultation/interprofessional collaboration/transfer of care during, 355–359
   postpartum visits, 345–353
   prenatal genetic screening and diagnosis, 329–335
   prenatal visits, initial, 321–327
   prenatal visits, return, 337–343
obstetric presentations. *See also specific issues*
   discomforts of pregnancy, 371–383
   gestational diabetes mellitus in pregnancy, 389–395
   preterm labor management, 405–410
   trial of labor vs. vaginal birth after cesarean, 365–367
obstructive pulmonary disease, chronic. *See* chronic obstructive pulmonary disease (COPD)
occupational and environmental history, asthma and, 78
occupational exposures (PEP). *See* postexposure prophylaxis (PEP), for HIV infection
occupational safety and health administration Ergonomics eTool, 843
Office of Developmental Primary Care, University of California, 493
OGTT (oral glucose tolerance test), 391
older adults. *See also* dementia
   anxiety disorders and, 527
   individualizing screening decisions, 443, 468–470, 469f
   life expectancy, 469f

Omalizumab (Xolair), 84
opiates
   risk assessment, 571
opioid(s)
   long-term, 569
   medication strategies, 573–576
   overdose, 573f
   risk assessment, 571
   safety, 569
   withdrawal, 786, 788t
oppositional defiant disorder, 102
oral glucose tolerance test (OGTT), 391
oral health
   0–3 years, 19
   6–11 years, 31
   12–26 years, 36
oral systemic corticosteroids, 84
order serum testing, 402
osteoarthritis (OA), 820
osteoporosis, 284–285
outflow tract/uterus disorders, and amenorrhea, 212, 220
ovarian disorders, 220. *See also* amenorrhea; polycystic ovarian syndrome (PCOS)
overactive bladder (OAB), 156, 313, 314t
overweight. *See* obesity
ovulatory disorders, 175–176

P

pain
   nipple or breast/chest, causes of, 431–434t
   with nursing, 430–431, 431–434t
painful bladder syndrome/interstitial cystitis, 291, 295–296, 295t
palliative care, 596, 661
PALM (polyps, adenomyosis, leiomyomas, malignancy), 174–175
Panel on Antiretroviral Guidelines for Adults and Adolescents (PAGAA), 675
panic attack, 523
panic disorder, 521, 522, 523–524
parent-child interactions
   0–3 years, 17, 20
   3–6 years, 25
   6–11 years, 29, 31
   12–26 years, 35, 39
   infants, 5
   post-NICU patients and, 13
parent education. *See* patient and family education and resources
Parents' Evaluation of Developmental Status (Glascoe), 70
passive vs. active immunizations. *See also* immunizations
patch, 252, 253, 254, 267
pathologic reflux, 10
pathophysiology, theories for ADHD, 103–104

patient and family education and resources
    0–3 years, 22
    3–6 years, 27–28
    6–11 years, 31, 32b
    12–26 years, 39
    abortion care, 202–204
    on ADHD, 107, 111, 111b
    on adults with developmental
        disabilities, 492, 492f
    on amenorrhea and PCOS, 221
    on anemia, 517
    on anxiety disorders, 527–528
    on asthma, 85–86
    on atopic dermatitis in children, 98
    on AUB, 183
    on cancer survivorship, 550
    on chronic nonmalignant pain, 576
    on chronic wound care, 586
    on COPD, 558–559
    on depression, 610–612
    on diabetes mellitus, 626
    on epilepsy, 634
    on GDM, 391–392
    on GERD, 643
    on geriatric syndromes, 654
    on heart failure, 663–664
    on HIV, 697
    on HSV infections, 670
    on hypertension, 708
    on IBS, 726
    on infants, 6
    for intimate partner violence, 715
    on lipid disorders, 740
    on maltreatment in children, 141
    on menopause transition, 285
    on NAFLD, 762
    on post-NICU patients, 14
    on postpartum care, 351–352
    on preeclampsia-eclampsia, 402–403
    on pregnancy, 325–326f, 327, 340–341f, 342, 376, 378
    on prenatal genetic diagnosis, 335
    sexual dysfunction, 307
    on tendinopathy, 842
    on thyroid disorders, 814
    transgender and gender diverse, 49
    on transgender and gender expansive
        adults, 501
    on upper back/neck pain, 826, 829
    urinary incontinence in children, 169
    on urinary incontinence in women, 316
    on weight, 769
patient consent. See consent, patient
Patient Health Questionnaire (PHQ), 592, 596
Patient Health Questionnaire (PHQ-9), 121, 600f
Patient Health Questionnaire (PHQ-2), 414, 419, 601
Patient Health Questionnaire for
    Adolescents, 38
PCOS. See polycystic ovarian
    syndrome (PCOS)

PDE4 inhibitor, 562
Peak Expiratory Flow Rate Monitoring, 538, 540b
pediatric health maintenance and
    promotion
    0–3 years, 17–22
    3–6 years, 25–28
    6–11 years, 29–32
    12–26 years, 35–39
    developmental delay and autism,
        screening for, 53–72
    first well-baby visits, 3–6
    post-neonatal intensive care unit (NICU)
        patients, 9–14
pediatric presentations
    asthma, 77–87
    attention-deficit/hyperactivity disorder
        (ADHD), 101–111
    depression, 115–126
    maltreatment, 129–141
    urinary incontinence, 155–169
Pediatric Symptom Checklist (Gardner
    et al.), 70
pelvic girdle pain (PGP), 373–376
Pelvic Pain Education Program (PPEP), 292
penile trauma, in children, 137
people living with HIV (PLWH), 675
PEP. *See* postexposure prophylaxis (PEP),
    for HIV infection
percutaneous tibial nerve stimulation
    (PTNS), 315
perinatal bipolar disorder, 417
perinatal mood and anxiety disorders
    (PMADs), 413–419
    diagnosis of, 414
    health disparities and special
        populations, 418–419
    overview of, 413
    prevalence of, 413
    screening recommendations for, 413–414
    types of, 414–418
permanent contraception, 263–264, 265, 268–269
persistent depressive disorder
    (dysthymia), 116
personal habits
    0–3 years, 20
    3–6 years, 27
    6–11 years, 30
    12–26 years, 37
    adults with developmental
        disabilities, 485
persons assigned male at birth (AMAB), 223
pessaries, 315
PGP (pelvic girdle pain), 373–376
pharmacotherapy/psychotherapy
    for anxiety disorders, 525, 526t
    for dementia, 593, 594t
    for heart failure, 660, 661, 661b
    for hypertension, 705, 706–707t
phenothiazines, 380
phenylketonuria (PKU) screening, 5
phototherapy, 97

PHQ (Patient Health Questionnaires), 592
physical abuse, 130–131. *See also*
    intimate partner violence (IPV);
    maltreatment of children
    defined, 711
    physical examination for, 135, 136t, 137
physical activity
    12–26 years, 39
    3–6 years, 27
    6–11 years, 30
    asthma and, 85
    diabetes and, 619, 619t
    diabetes in pregnancy and, 393
    hypertension and, 705
    pregnancy and, 376
    weight and, 768–770
physical examinations
    0–3 years, 18–21
    3–6 years, 26
    6–11 years, 31
    12–26 years, 37–38
    abortion care, 199
    for ADHD, 106
    of adults with developmental disabilities, 485, 487f
    amenorrhea and PCOS, 215, 215t
    for anemia, 512, 513t
    for anxiety, 522
    for asthma, 78, 531
    for atopic dermatitis, 91
    for AUB, 177
    of benign prostatic hyperplasia, 226–227
    for bicipital tendinopathy, 836–837, 837t
    cancer survivorship and, 547, 548–549t
    for chronic nonmalignant pain, 570–571
    of chronic pelvic pain, 292
    for chronic wound care, 583
    for COPD, 555
    for dementia, 592
    for depression, 602
    for diabetes mellitus, 616
    of early pregnancy loss, 234–235
    for epilepsy, 628
    for GERD, 639
    for geriatric syndromes, 648, 649f, 650t
    for heart failure, 657
    for herpes simplex infections, 668
    for hypertension, 703
    infants and, 4–5
    for intimate partner violence, 715, 715t
    for irritable bowel syndrome, 723
    for lipid disorders, 731
    for low back pain, 745t, 746–748
    for maltreatment in children, 135, 136t, 137–139
    nonalcoholic fatty liver disease, 758
    for obesity, 148
    for post-NICU patients, 13
    for preeclampsia-eclampsia, 400–401
    for pregnancy discomforts, 375
    for prenatal visits, 323
    substance use and abuse, 780
    for thyroid disorders, 808, 809t

transgender and gender diverse, 42–43
for transgender and gender expansive adults, 497
for upper back/neck pain, 823–824t
urinary incontinence in children, 160, 160–162t
physiologic reflux, 10
pituitary amenorrhea, 211–212, 219–220. *See also* amenorrhea; polycystic ovarian syndrome (PCOS)
placenta accreta, 365–366
placenta previa, 366
placental growth, 377
placental hormones, 389, 390t
Planned Parenthood Federation of America, 269
plasma glucose concentrations, clinical interpretations of, 617t
PNFA (progressive nonfluent aphasia), 588
POI (primary ovarian insufficiency), 212
polycystic ovarian syndrome (PCOS), 175, 211, 757. *See also* amenorrhea
assessment of, 215–216
databased used for, 214–215
defined, 212
diagnostic testing for, 216–217, 216–217t
overview, 212–213
physical examination findings, 215, 215t
self-management resources and tools, 221
polyps, 174–175, 182
positive predictive value (PPV), of screening tests, 71
post-neonatal intensive care unit (NICU) patients, 9–14
posterior pelvic pain provocation test, 375
postexposure prophylaxis (PEP), for HIV infection. *See also* HIV (human immunodeficiency virus)
discomforts. *See* discomforts, of pregnancy
hypertension in. *See* preeclampsia-eclampsia
postnatal growth restriction, 10
postnatal infection, 11
postpartum care, 345–353
assessment of, 349
clinical management goals for, 349
database used for, 346–349
medications and therapeutics, 350–351
overview, 345–346
treatment and follow-up, 349–350
postpartum depression (PPD), 414–417
posttraumatic stress disorder (PTSD), 418, 521, 522, 524, 526, 526t
postural kyphosis, 821
PPIs (proton pump inhibitors), 380–381, 382t, 640
Prediction of Alcohol Withdrawal Severity Scale, 784t
preeclampsia-eclampsia, 397–403
assessment of, 401–402
clinical management goals for, 401
clinical risk assessment for, 399, 399t

consultation and referral, 403
database used for, 400–401
diagnostic tests, 401–402
etiology of, 399
overview of, 397–400, 398t
physical examination for, 400–401
treatment/follow-up of, 402
pregnancy
abuse during, 339
anxiety disorders and, 527
complications, 356
constipation during, 381, 383
consultation and referral during, 334
dating of, 322, 322b
depression during, 372
diagnostic testing during, 339
fetal evaluation, 342, 342t
gestational diabetes mellitus in, 389–395
healthcare visits, 321–327
heartburn during, 380–381, 382t
medical consultation and referral during, 356–359, 356f, 358t
medical consultation/interprofessional collaboration/transfer of care during, 355–356
nutrition and, 341, 341t
patient education and counseling, 340–341f, 342
postterm, 342, 343t
signs of complications, 339t
pregnancy of unknown location (PUL), 232t
preimplantation genetic diagnosis, 335
premature and late premature infants, 3, 405–410
prenatal genetic diagnosis, 334–335
assessment of, 335
clinical management goals for, 335
database used for, 335
overview, 334
prenatal genetic screening, 329–335
assessment for, 333
clinical management goals for, 333
database used for, 332–333
overview of, 329
for trisomies/NTD/SLOS, 329–331, 330t
prenatal health care visits, 321–327, 337–343
preschoolers. *See* pediatric health maintenance and promotion
pressure injuries, 580–581
preterm birth (PTB), 405–410
assessment of, 406, 407
burden, 405–406
clinical management goals for, 408
database used for, 406–407
defined, 405
digital examinations of, 407
economic impact, 406
etiology, 405
health histories, 406–407
management and treatment of, 408–410
overview of, 405–406

pregnant people with diagnosis, 409–410
pregnant people with signs and symptoms, 409
prevalence/incidence, 405
racial disparities, 406
threatened, 407
preterm labor management, 405–410
primary care providers (PCPs), 189
primary care setting, anxiety disorders and, 521
primary hypothyroidism, 805, 813
primary ovarian insufficiency (POI), 212
procedural abortion, 192–193, 195t
prodromal psychosis, 120
progestin-only contraception. *See* progestin
progestin-only pills (POPs), 254–255, 267–268
progestogen therapy, 280–282
progressive nonfluent aphasia (PNFA), 588
Project Health, 501
prolactin-secreting tumors, 211
proton pump inhibitors (PPIs), 380–381, 382t, 640
pruritus, 91, 97
psychoeducation, and ADHD, 107
psychological abuse, 711
psychologic/emotional abuse, 131, 711
psychometrics, 70–71
psychosis
postpartum, 418
psychosocial and emotional support, atopic dermatitis and, 98
psychosocial assessment and support 12–26 years, 36–38
atopic dermatitis in children and, 98
interventions, 526–527
psychotherapy. *See* pharmacotherapy/psychotherapy
PTB (premature births). *See* preterm birth (PTB)
PTNS (percutaneous tibial nerve stimulation), 315
PTSD (posttraumatic stress disorder), 521, 522, 524, 526, 526t
puberty, 29, 530
pulmonary edema, 655
PUQE (pregnancy-unique quantification of emesis/nausea) index, 377, 377t
pyelonephritis, 375

Q

quadruple (quad) marker serum examination, 331

R

race. *See* ethnicity-based health issues
Rape, Abuse, and Incest National Network, 715

red blood cell (RBC)
   morphology, 506t
referrals
   for anxiety disorders, 527
   for cancer survivorship, 550–551
   chronic nonmalignant pain, 575
   for diabetes, 625
   for epilepsy, 634
   human lactation, 426, 429–430, 431, 434–435
   for postpartum care, 352–353
   for preeclampsia-eclampsia, 403
   for pregnancy, 327, 327b, 334
   during pregnancy, 356–359, 356f, 358t
   for tendinopathy, 842
referred neck pain, 817–818
regional pain syndrome, 819
relaxation training, 526–527
reliability, of screening tests, 70
reporting, mandatory
   on maltreatment of children, 138–139, 138t
reproductive coercion (RC), 188
Reproductive Health Access, 239
rescue medications, 83–84, 535
respiratory diseases. *See* asthma; chronic obstructive pulmonary disease (COPD)
respiratory syncytial virus (RSV), 11
RIPTEAR framework, 780
Risk Evaluation and Mitigation Strategy (REMS), 191
roflumilast, 562
Rome III criteria, for IBS diagnosis, 721
Roux-en-Y gastric bypass, 771
RSV (respiratory syncytial virus), 11

S

safety
   0–3 years, 22
   3–6 years, 27
   6–11 years, 30–32, 31–32, 32b
   12–26 years, 37, 39
   infants, 6
   maltreatment of children and, 139
scalene-myofascial pain syndrome, 820
Scheuermann's kyphosis, 821
schools
   12–26 years, 37
   3–6 years, 27
   6–11 years, 30
   asthma medications and, 86–87
sciatica, 747
scoliosis, 821–822
SCORAD (clinical tool), 91
screening tests. *See also specific type*
   accurate, characteristics of, 70–71
   standardized, 54
Screening Tool for Autism in Toddlers and Young Children (Stone et al.), 70

secondary disorders, 730
secretory activation (lactogenesis II), 424
secretory differentiation (lactogenesis I), 423–424
Seizure Tracker, 635
seizures. *See* epilepsy
selective serotonin reuptake inhibitors (SSRIs), 123, 124–125t, 283, 525
self-injurious behavior, 117
self-management resources, 39
senior citizens. *See* older adults
sensitivity, of screening tests, 71
sensory impairments, 645–646, 647, 648, 650
sequential integrated screening, 331
serotonin-norepinephrine reuptake inhibitors (SNRIs), 525, 572
sertraline, 123
serum integrated screening, 331
sexual abuse, 131, 711. *See also* maltreatment of children
   physical examination for, 137
sexual acting out, 133
sexual debut, 117
sexual dysfunction (SD)
   assessment of, 303
   clinical management goals for, 303
   database used for, 303
   defined, 301
   diagnostic screening and tests for, 303–304
   management and treatment for, 303–307, 304–305t
   medical conditions and medications affecting, 302t
   overview of, 301–302, 302t
   patient and provider education resources, 307
   prevalence of, 301–302
   risk factors for, 302
   self-help education, 307
   self-management resources and tools, 307
   types of, 301
sexual orientation/gender identity (SOGI), 42
sexually transmitted infections (STIs), 137, 716
short-acting β-agonists (SABA), 83–84
sickle cell screening, 5
side effects, of stimulant medications, 107
sideroblastic anemia, 508, 510–511, 513–514, 515, 517
Simon Foundation for Continence, 316
SisterSong, 327
skin disorders. *See* atopic dermatitis (AD)
sleep
   0–3 years, 20
   6–11 years, 30
   fatigue and, 104
   medications and, 107
   menopause transition and, 277
   poor quality, during pregnancy, 372–373

Smith-Lemli-Opitz syndrome (SLOS), 329–331
smoking. *See also* tobacco
   and asthma, 531
   and COPD, 555, 562, 564
   and hypertension, 705
SNRIs (serotonin-norepinephrine reuptake inhibitors), 525, 572
social and environmental risks
   12–26 years, 36, 37
   6–11 years, 30
   for asthma in children, 85
   for childhood maltreatment, 133–134
   for post-NICU patients, 11–12
   for urinary incontinence in children, 155–156
social anxiety disorder, 424, 521
Social Communication Questionnaire (Rutter et al.), 70
social history. *See* family and social histories
Society for Adolescent Health and Medicine (SAHM), 39
spastic diplegia, 481
specific IgE immunoassay (in vitro), 82
specificity, of screening tests, 71
spermicides, 261, 265, 268
spinal deformities, 821–822
spirometry, 82, 534, 534f, 555
spondylosis, 820
spontaneous abortion (SAB), 231, 232t
SSHADESS (mnemonic), 37
SSRIs (selective serotonin reuptake inhibitors), 123, 124–125t, 283, 525
Stages of Reproductive Aging Workshop (STRAW), 275
standardized screening tests, 54
statin therapy, 732
Stemmer's sign, 582b
stimulant medications, and ADHD, 107, 108t, 109
stimulant withdrawal, 786, 789t
STIs (sexually transmitted infections), 137
stomach acid, 380–381
strains/sprains, 820–821
STRAW (Stages of Reproductive Aging Workshop), 275
Strengths and Difficulties Questionnaire (Stone et al.), 70
stress incontinence, 157
stress UI (SUI), 309
Substance Abuse Mental Health Services Administration (SAMHSA), 115
substance use, 117–118
substance use and abuse, 37, 569, 571, 775–801
   assessment of, 777–780, 778–779t, 786–787
   clinical management goals, 786
   complications of, 780
   database used for, 780–781, 781–785t, 785

diagnostic screening and tests of, 780–781, 787, 800
drug detection times, 785t
drugs, effects of, 777t
false-positive tests, causes of, 785t
follow-up for, 800
harm reduction for, 789, 799–800
health disparities and structural racism, 776–777
management and treatment of, 787–789, 789–799t
overview, 775–777
patient and family education and resources, 800
physical examinations of, 780
prevalence and incidence, 775, 776t
terminology, 775–776, 776t
treatment, 775
sudden changes in behavior, 133
sudden death, and stimulants, 106
suicide
  12–26 years, 37
  depression and, 121
Suicide Assessment Five-Step Evaluation and Triage (SAFE-T), 121
suicide risk factors, 601t
supine active straight leg raise (SLR) test, 375
supplementary feeding, 430b
Surveillance, Epidemiology, and End Results (SEER) database, 546
Survey of Well-Being of Young Children (Sheldrick & Perrin), 70
syphilis screening, 38
Syringe Access Centers, 800
systolic heart failure, 655
systolic HTN, 701

T

TADS (Treatment for Adolescents with Depression Study), 123
teenagers. *See* pediatric health maintenance and promotion
tendinopathy. *See* upper extremity tendinopathy
Texas Functional Living Scale, 592
Th1 and Th2 cytokines, 529
thalassemia, 508, 510, 512–513, 514t, 515
thoracic outlet syndrome, 820
thoracoabdominal trauma, in children, 135–136
threatened abortion, 232t
thyroid disorders, 805–814
  assessment of, 808, 811, 812t
  clinical management goals for, 808
  databases used for, 807–808
  diagnostic screening and tests for, 808, 809–811t, 811–812
  management and treatment of, 812–813
  overview of, 805–806
  patient and family education and resources on, 814

thyroid nodules, 806–807, 813
thyroid-stimulating hormone (TSH), 805
tic disorders, 106
tissue biopsy, 583, 584
Title V, Social Security Act, 53
tobacco. *See also* smoking
  0–3 years, 18
  and asthma, 78
  and hypertension, 705
  withdrawal, 786, 789t
toddlers. *See* pediatric health maintenance and promotion
tongue-tie, 426, 428–430
topical analgesic creams and patches, 572
tracheal shaving, 500t
tracking medication effects, 110
trafficking and exploitation, of children, 132–133
tranexamic acid, 182
transfeminine, 499
transgender and gender diverse (TGD)
  assessment of, 43
  databases used for, 41–43
  definition, 41
  diagnostic tests for, 43
  overview of, 41
  physical examinations, 42–43
  self-management of resources and tools, 50
  treatment and management of, 44–49, 45–48t
transgender and gender expansive (TGE) adults, health maintenance for, 495–501
  assessment for, 498
  database used for, 497
  healthcare maintenance guidelines, 498t
  identity, 496–497
  overview of, 495–496
  physical examinations, 497
  resources and tools, 501
  surgical options for, 500, 500t
  treatment for, 498–500, 499t, 500t
Transgender Law Center, 501
transmasculine, 499–500
transvaginal ultrasound (TVUS), 183
traumatic kyphosis, 821
traumatic wounds, 579–580
Treatment for Adolescents with Depression Study (TADS), 123
trial of labor (TOL)
  contraindications for, 368, 368t
  VBAC vs., 365–367
tricyclic antidepressants, 572
trisomies, 329–331
tubal sterilization, 263–264, 265, 268–269
tuberculosis screening
  0–3 years, 18
  3–6 years, 27
  6–11 years, 31
  12–26 years, 38
TVUS (transvaginal ultrasound), 183

type 1 diabetes (T1D), 615, 620. *See also* diabetes mellitus
type 2 diabetes (T2D), 615, 620. *See also* diabetes mellitus

U

UI. *See* urinary incontinence (UI), in children; urinary incontinence (UI), in women
ulcers. *See* wound care
underactive bladder, 156–157
University of Michigan Chronic Pain Guide, 292
upper back/neck pain, 817–829
  assessment of, 825, 825t
  causes of, 817
  clinical management goals for, 825–826
  databases used for, 822, 826
  diagnostic screening and tests for, 824t, 826, 826t
  mechanical spine disease, acute, 818–819
  musculoskeletal strains and sprains, 820–821
  myofascial pain syndrome, 819–820
  osteoarthritis, 820
  overview of, 817–818
  patient education and resources on, 826, 829
  physical examination findings, 823–824t
  scalene muscle pain/thoracic outlet syndrome, 820
  treatment and management of, 827–829t
upper extremity tendinopathy, 833–843
  assessment of, 838, 840
  clinical management goals for, 840–841
  databased used for, 835–838, 837t
  diagnostic tests for, 837, 838, 841
  overview of, 833
  treatment and management of, 841–843
upper GI (UGI) tract, 638
urge incontinence (UUI), 310, 313, 314t
urinary diary, 310, 311t
urinary incontinence (UI), in children, 155–169
  assessment of, 160
  clinical management goals, 160, 162
  databases used in, 158–160
  daytime, 156–157
  defined, 155
  diagnostic tests for, 162–163, 163–164f
  night, 157–158
  overview of, 155–158
  physical examination findings and, 160, 160–162t
  treatment and management of, 162–163, 163–164f, 164–168t, 169
  voiding and elimination history and, 158–159, 158t, 159f

urinary incontinence (UI), in women, 309–316
  assessment of, 311–312
  clinical management goals for, 312
  initial evaluation of, 310–311
  nonpharmacologic treatment for, 312–313, 313t, 314t
  overview of, 309
  pharmacologic treatment for, 313–315, 313t, 314t
  prevalence of, 310
  self-management resources and tools, 316
  treatment and management of, 312–316
  types of, 309–310, 309t
  urinary diary, 310, 311t
urinary tract infections (UTIs), 155
Urology Care Foundation, 229
U.S. Department of Health and Human Services (USDHHS), 675
U.S. Environmental Protection Agency, 541
U.S. Food and Drug Administration (FDA), 122, 123, 191, 510
U.S. Preventive Services Task Force (USPSTF), 443, 601, 603, 654, 668–669
  age-based recommendations for screening and interventions, 444–448t
  characteristic-based recommendations for screening and interventions, 449–457t
  recommendations for preventive medications, 458–459t
  on screening for lipid disorders, 732
  screening/counseling recommendations, 471–473t
U.S. Preventive Task Force, 116
USMEC, 269
uterine bleeding. *See* abnormal uterine bleeding (AUB)
uterine ruptures, 365
UTIs (urinary tract infections), 155
UUI (urge incontinence), 310, 313, 314t

V

vaccinations. *See* immunizations
vaginal birth after cesarean (VBAC), 365–367
  overview, 365
  person-centered decision-making model, 364f
  success factors, 367–368, 367t
  success rates, 367–368, 367t
  trial of labor vs., 365–367
  values clarification tool, 365f
vaginal deliveries, 3
vaginal pH regulator gel, 261–262, 265
vaginal reflux and postvoid dribbling, 156
vaginal/rectal electrical stimulation, 315
validity, of screening tests, 70–71
Vancouver Coastal Health Clinic, 501
vascular dementia, 588f, 591
vasculitic ulcers, 581
vasomotor symptoms, 276–277, 278
VBAC. *See* vaginal birth after cesarean (VBAC)
venous ulcers, 579
vision screening
  0–3 years, 18–19
  3–6 years, 27
  6–11 years, 31
  infants and, 11
visual impairment, 645–646, 647, 651
vitamin B$_{12}$ deficiency, 509–510, 511, 514–515, 517
voiding
  dysfunctional, 156
  and elimination history, 158–159, 158t, 159f

  postponement, 156
  process of, 155
von Willebrand disease (VWD), 175
vulnerable child syndrome, 12
vulvar/vaginal trauma, in children, 137
VWD (von Willebrand disease), 175

W

weight, 765–772
  assessment of, 768–769
  in children, 765
  consequences of, 768
  databases used for, 766–768
  diagnostic testing for, 767–768
  diet interventions and, 769
  medication management, 770–771
  mental health and therapeutic interventions, 770
  mental illness and, 766
  overview of, 765
  patient and family education and resources on, 646–647
  treatment and management of, 769–772
weight loss
  hypertension and, 705
  urinary incontinence in women and, 313
well babies visits, 3–6
wet-wrap dressings, 96–97
whiplash, 819
withdrawal method, 264, 265
Women's Health Initiative (WHI), 282
workplace modification during pregnancy, 376
World Health Organization (WHO), 391, 505, 701
World Professional Association for Transgender Health (WPATH), 500, 501